# Patient
# Drug Facts

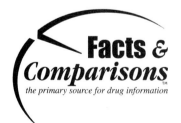

**Facts &**
*Comparisons*™
*the primary source for drug information*

# Patient Drug Facts, Second Edition

Adapted from *Professional's Guide to Patient Drug Facts* loose-leaf drug information service through the July 2003 update.

ISBN 1-57439-166-6

Printed in the United States of America

The information contained in this publication is intended to supplement the knowledge of health care professionals regarding patient drug information. This information is advisory only and is not intended to replace sound clinical judgment or individualized patient care in the delivery of health care services. The information is derived from literature research and is subject to review by the Editors and the Editorial Panel. However, Wolters Kluwer Health, Inc. disclaims all warranties, whether expressed or implied, including any warranty as to the quality, accuracy, or suitability of this information for any particular purpose.

Indexing by Coughlin Indexing Services, Inc., Annapolis, Maryland.

The information contained in *Patient Drug Facts* is available for licensing as source data. For more information on data licensing, please call 1-800-223-0554.

**Facts and Comparisons®**
part of **Wolters Kluwer Health**
**111 West Port Plaza Dr., Suite 300**
**St. Louis, Missouri 63146-3098**
**www.drugfacts.com**
**314-216-2100/800-223-0554**

# Patient
# Drug Facts

| | |
|---|---|
| **Executive Vice President** | Kenneth H. Killion |
| **Publisher** | Cathy H. Reilly |
| **Senior Managing Editor** | Renée M. Wickersham |
| **Managing Editor** | Angela J. Schwalm |
| **Senior Editor** | Kimberly A. Faulhaber |
| **Assistant Editors** | Jennifer A. Guimaraes |
| | Nicholas R. Weber |
| **Quality Control Editor** | Susan H. Sunderman |
| **SGML Specialist** | Linda M. Jones |
| **Composition Specialist** | Jennifer M. Reed |
| **General Manager, Disease & Drug Information** | Renée Rivard, PharmD |
| **National Sales Manager** | Donald M. McQuade |
| **Director of Marketing** | Mark A. Sohasky |

**Consulting Editors**

**Associate Editor**
Timothy R. Covington, PharmD, MS
Anthony and Marianne Bruno
 Professor of Pharmacy
Director, Managed Care Institute
School of Pharmacy, Samford University
Birmingham, Alabama

**Assistant Editors**
Lawrence R. Borgsdorf, PharmD, FCSHP
Pharmacist Specialist-
 Ambulatory Care
Kaiser Permanente
Bakersfield, California

Richard M. Oksas, PharmD, MPH
Family Practice Pharmacist
Natividad Medical Center
Salinas, California

Karen J. Tietze, PharmD
Professor of Clinical Pharmacy
Philadelphia College of Pharmacy
University of the Sciences in
 Philadelphia
Philadelphia, Pennsylvania

# Table of Contents

**Preface** . . . . . . . . . . . . . . . . . . . . . . . . . . . . . . . . . . . . . . . . . . . . . .  vii

**Introduction** . . . . . . . . . . . . . . . . . . . . . . . . . . . . . . . . . . . . . . . .  ix

**Guidelines For Use** . . . . . . . . . . . . . . . . . . . . . . . . . . . . . . .  xi

**Chapters** (A detailed table of contents appears at the beginning of each chapter.)

| | | |
|---|---|---|
| 1. | Nutritionals . . . . . . . . . . . . . . . . . . . . . . . . . . . . . . . . . . . | 1 |
| 2. | Blood Modifiers . . . . . . . . . . . . . . . . . . . . . . . . . . . . | 67 |
| 3. | Hormones . . . . . . . . . . . . . . . . . . . . . . . . . . . . . . . . . | 125 |
| 4. | Cardiovasculars . . . . . . . . . . . . . . . . . . . . . . . . . . . | 303 |
| 5. | Respiratories . . . . . . . . . . . . . . . . . . . . . . . . . . . . | 453 |
| 6. | Central Nervous System Agents . . . . . . . . . . . . . . . . . | 577 |
| 7. | Gastrointestinals . . . . . . . . . . . . . . . . . . . . . . . . . | 901 |
| 8. | Anti-Infectives . . . . . . . . . . . . . . . . . . . . . . . . . . | 1011 |
| 9. | Vaccines . . . . . . . . . . . . . . . . . . . . . . . . . . . . . . . . | 1233 |
| 10. | Ophthalmics and Otics . . . . . . . . . . . . . . . . . . . . . | 1291 |
| 11. | Topicals . . . . . . . . . . . . . . . . . . . . . . . . . . . . . . . | 1385 |
| 12. | Antineoplastics . . . . . . . . . . . . . . . . . . . . . . . . . . | 1527 |
| 13. | Miscellaneous Agents . . . . . . . . . . . . . . . . . . . . . . | 1623 |
| 14. | Home Testing Kits . . . . . . . . . . . . . . . . . . . . . . . . . | 1749 |

**Appendices**

The Home Medicine Cabinet . . . . . . . . . . . . . . . . . . . .  A-3

Oral Dosage Forms that Should Not Be Crushed or Chewed . . . . . . . . . . . . . . . . . . . . . . . . . . . . . . . . .  A-7

International System of Units . . . . . . . . . . . . . . . . . . . .  A-21

Normal Laboratory Values . . . . . . . . . . . . . . . . . . . . .  A-23

FDA Pregnancy Categories . . . . . . . . . . . . . . . . . . . .  A-31

Poison Center Hotline . . . . . . . . . . . . . . . . . . . . . . . .  A-33

Drug Names that Look Alike and Sound Alike  . . . . . .  A-35

**Index** . . . . . . . . . . . . . . . . . . . . . . . . . . . . . . . . . . . . . . . . . . . . .  I-1

# Preface

The contemporary health care landscape is changing rapidly. The focus on quality of care and improved health outcomes is growing in intensity. Payers of health care goods and services are experiencing sticker shock, and they expect more value for each dollar spent on health care. Thus, managed care and managed cost are increasingly pervasive elements on one's professional life.

Drugs are the "best buy" in American health care. The total annual expenditure for drug therapy represents 7% to 10% of the total health care expenditure; however, 85% to 90% of patients with acute or chronic diseases get well or better because of drug therapy. The return-on-investment with regard to drug therapy is profound and irrefutable.

Drugs are truly two-edged swords. They have the potential to not only do great good but also great harm if used inappropriately. Providers of health care are being increasingly challenged to do the following:

- Promote safe, appropriate, effective, and economical drug use.

- Assist in producing optimal therapeutic outcomes by fostering precision in drug therapy management.

- Foster the evolution and delivery of highly cognitive, interactive, problem-based, outcome-oriented pharmaceutical care that maximizes the benefit of drug therapy while operating to prevent, identify, and resolve drug-related problems and therapeutic misadventures.

Optimal pharmacotherapy is central to the quest for disease management quality. System failures in drug therapy management are abundant, and there is much room for improvement.

Selected evidence of system failures in drug therapy management is included below:

- Approximately 30% to 50% of the 1.8 to 2 billion prescriptions dispensed annually are not taken properly by the patient.

- Approximately 7% to 8% of diagnosed patients never get their prescription(s) filled – the ultimate noncompliance error.

- The annual *direct* cost of therapeutic noncompliance and drug-induced morbidity and mortality is estimated to be $50 to $80 billion. The *indirect* cost (eg, lost productivity, lost wages) is estimated to be an additional $50 billion per year.[1,2]

- The economic consequences of managing the complications of inappropriate or mismanaged drug therapy exceeds the annual cost of all diabetes care ($45.2 billion in 1994) and approaches the cost of managing all cardiovascular disease ($117 to $154 billion in 1994).

- As many as 28% of hospital admissions (more than 8 million per year) at a cost in excess of $47 billion annually appear to be due to drug-related morbidity and mortality.[2]

- It is estimated that 115 million physician visits per year (17.3% of all physician office visits), at an annual cost of approximately $7.5 billion, are due to drug-induced problems and therapeutic misadventures.[2,3]

- Approximately 140,000 Americans die annually from failure to consume drugs properly.

- Approximately 23% of nursing home admissions result from the inability of patients to manage medication use in the home.

- The compliance rate to prescribed antihypertensive therapy in patients diagnosed for at least 3 years is approximately 32%.

- The compliance rate to immunosuppressant therapy in outpatient organ transplant recipients is only 82%.

- Approximately 24% to 66% of antibiotic use in hospitals is either inappropriate or unnecessary as judged by expert panels of infectious disease physicians.

- Noncompliance of prescribed drug therapy produces a loss of more than 20,000,000 workdays per year.

These facts dramatically reveal, and place into perspective, the need for application of information included in *Patient Drug Facts.* This publication is designed to serve as a clear, concise, and current reference source and information tool for health care providers in optimizing pharmacotherapy, improving health outcomes, and minimizing drug-induced adverse events. The format and language of *Patient Drug Facts* is designed to present drug information in a user-friendly format.

*Patient Drug Facts* contains vital information on the most frequently prescribed and consumed prescription and nonprescription drugs. The hundreds of monographs provide product information on over 6500 generic and brand name drugs. Proper use of this reference has contributed – and will continue to contribute – to improved drug therapy management and health outcomes.

Timothy R. Covington, PharmD, MS<br>
Associate Editor

---

[1] Noncompliance with Medications: An Economic Tragedy With Important Implications for Health Care Reform. Baltimore, MD: The Task Force for Compliance, 1993.

[2] Johnson JA, Bootman JL. Drug-Related Morbidity and Mortality – A Cost-of-Illness Model. *Arch Intern Med* 1995;155(Oct 9):1949-1956.

[3] Schappert SM. National Ambulatory Medical Care Survey: 1991 Summary. Hyattsville, MD: National Center for Health Statistics, 1993 (No. 230).

# Introduction

Patient drug information provides a dilemma. The health care community wishes to inform – not scare – and wants to spend quality time with patients. Whether the learning process takes place in a classroom, counseling session, or at the prescription counter, *Patient Drug Facts* can be instrumental.

Communication courses and teaching courses tell us we must set the stage for learning and remembering with our audience. The same is true for patient counseling. First, we must tell the patient what it is we plan to talk about (state our objectives). Second, we must tell them what they need to know (provide instructions) and allow time for their questions and feedback. Lastly, we must repeat what we told them (restate the objectives). Ideally, the next time we see the patient we can ask them questions and reinforce the learning process.

**Our Objectives for *Patient Drug Facts* are:**

1. To provide information for health care providers to tell patients what they need to know about their medications.

2. To provide a standardized, concise format for patient instruction and learning in a classroom or patient counsulting session or at the prescription counter.

The National Council on Patient Information and Education (NCPIE) has set guidelines to help patients "get the answers." These guidelines provide us with the groundwork for our first objective. *Patient Drug Facts* provides the answers for the NCPIE questions and much more.

| NCPIE Questions |
| --- |
| 1. What is the name of the drug and what is it supposed to do? Is this the brand or generic name? Is a generic version available? **Type of Drug, How the Drug Works, Uses** |
| 2. How and when do I take it – and for how long? **Guidelines for Use** (and prescription on product label) |
| 3. What foods, drinks, other medicines, dietary supplements, or activities should I avoid while taking this drug? **Precautions, Drug Interactions, Guidelines for Use** |
| 4. Are there any side effects, and what do I do if they occur? **Precautions, Side Effects, Guidelines for Use** |
| 5. When should I expect this drug to begin to work, and how will I know if it's working? **Guidelines for Use** |
| 6. Will this drug work safely with other drugs I am taking? **Precautions, Drug Interactions, Guidelines for Use** |
| 7. Is there any written information available about this drug? **PDF monographs** can be copied and highlighted for an individual patient in the course of specific patient-related consultation. |

In addition to answering the NCPIE questions, *Patient Drug Facts* contains an appendix for quick reference on necessary household medicines, oral dosage forms that should not be crushed or chewed, an international system of units, normal laboratory values, FDA pregnancy categories, the poison center hotline, and drug names that look alike and sound alike.

Our second objective is to provide a standard, concise format for patient education and learning in a classroom or patient counseling session or at the prescription counter. The monographs are grouped together by therapeutic class. The product listings are located at the beginning of the monographs, which allows the reader to immediately make an association between the trade name and the generic name of the drug. Common dosage forms and dosage strengths available to consumers are listed. Generic availability is also indicated. After the product list, the standardized presentation of information includes: Type of Drug, How the Drug Works, Uses, Drug Interactions, Side Effects, and Guidelines for Use.

The format is important in providing a guide for patient counseling. The *Patient Drug Facts* format outlines information for a brief patient encounter in a clear, concise manner. It provides the name of the drug, how it works, what it is used for, when it cannot be used, and guidelines for proper use. The information provided in the monographs reminds the patient counselor of important and unique characteristics of a particular drug or drug group (eg, the drug causes the urine to turn yellow or the undissolved capsule may appear in the stool).

We feel we have met our goal to develop a tool for health care providers to use during patient drug information counseling. *Patient Drug Facts* is adaptable for use in the classroom or at the prescription counter. As always, we are interested in your comments and suggestions for future updates and additions.

# Guidelines For Use

*Patient Drug Facts* is a comprehensive drug information compendium organized by therapeutic class. A general table of contents, detailed chapter table of contents, a comprehensive alphabetical index, and cross references enable the reader to quickly locate needed information. The following pages explain in detail the organization and contents of *Patient Drug Facts*. All readers are urged to review this information to ensure efficient and effective use of *Patient Drug Facts.*

## Editorial Overview

The core of information for monographs in *Patient Drug Facts* is based on the Facts and Comparisons database. We have included information on prescription and over-the-counter medications that are predominantly used in an outpatient environment (ie, drugs used specifically in a hospital environment are not included).

General prescribing information is presented in a standardized format and the technical language has been translated to assist the health care provider in effective communication with, and counseling of, patients.

Because the material has been written with the patient in mind, a monograph can be photocopied, highlighted, and used as a tool with an individual patient in the course of a specific patient-related consultation.

## Editorial Panel

The Editorial Panel for *Patient Drug Facts* is an interdisciplinary group of established and respected clinicians and educators. The panel includes recognized experts in the fields of pharmacology, pharmacy practice, and drug information. These experts provide direction for *Patient Drug Facts,* as well as write and review monograph material.

The *Drug Facts and Comparisons* Editorial Advisory Panel consists of physicians, pharmacologists, and pharmacists. This panel reviews monographs and provides editorial direction for the entire Facts and Comparisons database.

## Organization

*Patient Drug Facts* is divided into chapters. The first page of each chapter has a detailed Table of Contents of the information presented in that chapter. Each chapter is divided into therapeutic groups and subgroups according to the use of the drug. Products similar in content or use are listed together.

## Index

The alphabetical index lists drugs by their generic name, brand name, and therapeutic group names. Additionally, many synonyms and therapeutic uses for agents are included.

## Appendix

The appendix provides supplementary listing for quick reference on the following topics:

*The Home Medicine Cabinet* – A suggested listing of the basic medicines and equipment patients should keep in their medicine chests.

*Oral Dosage Forms That Should Not be Crushed or Chewed* – A listing of drugs that must be swallowed whole to be effective.

*International System of Units* – *SI* is a modernized version of the metric system designed to revise the present confused measurement system and to improve test-result communications.

*Normal Laboratory Values* – Guidelines for normal laboratory values.

*FDA Pregnancy Categories*– Five categories that indicate the potential of a systemically absorbed drug for causing birth defects.

*Poison Center Hotline* – National toll-free poison center hotline information.

*Drug Names That Look Alike and Sound Alike* – A listing of drug names that can easily be confused because of similar spellings or pronunciations.

## Product Listings

Tables of individual products are found at the beginning of each monograph. Most of the products listed are protected by patent and their names are trademarked and registered. Listing of specific products is only an indication of availability on the market and does not constitute an endorsement or recommendation. Prescription products that contain identical amounts of active ingredients are listed together for comparison. **Listing of products together does not imply that they are therapeutically equivalent or legally interchangeable.** Drug product interchange is regulated by state law. Caution is particularly advised when comparing sustained-release, timed-release, or repeat-action dosage forms.

The format and components of the product listings are discussed below and illustrated on the opposite page.

① The therapeutic class and/or the generic titles appear at the beginning of the monograph. All drugs in a therapeutic class are listed in alphabetical order.

② Generic product availability is indicated in the last column.

③ Generic names of the products are indicated by bold-face print.

④ Brand name examples of the products are indicated in italics. The listing of brand name products has been included to provide examples of common names of products to help the patient identify the drug he/she is taking. While we have made a sincere attempt to include as many brand names as possible, we do not purport this listing as comprehensive. Brand name products that are identical in formulation are listed together in alphabetical order. Products most similar in formulation are listed next to each other. This format makes it easy to compare identical, similar, or related products.

⑤ Products are grouped by dosage form. Available strengths of the product are included.

⑥ Distribution status of products is indicated as *Rx* (prescription or legend), controlled substance status (*c-II, c-III,* etc.) or *otc* (nonprescription or over-the-counter).

*Cough* is a normal protective reflex. It helps clear mucus, irritants and other foreign matter from the throat, trachea and lungs. Caution is advised in attempting to suppress a productive cough (mucus is coughed up). The productive cough is essential to the removal of foreign debris. If mucus is not removed from the lungs, it may support growth of bacteria and make breathing more difficult. Moderate cough suppression may be used to reduce discomfort and allow sleep, but do not attempt to completely suppress a productive cough.

The dry, nonproductive cough is a good candidate for theapeutic cough suppression. If such coughs are persistent, bothersome or sleep disrupting, they may respond well to treatment with antitussives. ②

| Generic Name ——③<br>*Brand Name Examples* | Supplied As | Generic<br>Available |
|---|---|---|
| *Rx* **Benzonatate** | | |
| *Tessalon Perles* | **Capsules:** 100 mg | No |
| *otc* **Dextromethorphan HBr** | | |
| ④———*Mediquell* | **Chewy squares:** 15 mg | No |
| *Hold, Sucrets Cough Control* | **Lozenges:** 5mg | No |
| *Benylin DM[1], Congespirin for* ⑤ *Children, Cremacoat 1[1], DM Cough[1], Pedia Care 1, Pertussin[1], St. Joseph Cough* | **Syrup:** 5 mg/tsp, 7.5 mg/tsp, 10 mg/tsp, 15 mg/tsp | No |
| *Delsym[1]* | **Liquid, sustained action:** Equivalent to 30 mg dextromethorphan HBr/tsp | No |
| **Diphenhydramine HCl** | | |
| *otc Beldin[1], Benylin Cough[1], Bydramine Cough[1], Diphen Cough, Gen-D-phen[1], Hydramine Cough[1], Nordryl Cough[1]* | **Syrup:** 12.5 mg/tsp, 13.3 mg/tsp | Yes |
| *Rx Hydramyn[1], Tusstat[1], Valdrene[1]* | **Syrup:** 12.5 mg/tsp, 13.3 mg/tsp | Yes |
| **Nonnarcotic Antitussive Combinations** | | |
| *otc Spec-T[2]* | **Lozenges:** 10 mg dextromethorphan HBr and 10 mg benzocaine | No |
| *otc Formula 44 Cough Control Disks* | **Lozenges:** 5 mg dextromethorphan HBr and 1.25 mg benzocaine | No |
| *otc Vick's Cough Silencers[2]* | **Lozenges:** 2.5 mg dextromethorphan HBr and 1 mg benzocaine | No |

⑥ (bracket grouping the two Diphenhydramine HCl rows)

[1] Contains alcohol.
[2] Contains the dye tartrazine.

**Type of Drug:**
Cough medicine; cough suppressants.

# Drug Monographs

Patient counseling information is presented in the text of the drug monographs. General information on a group of closely related drugs may be presented in a group monograph (eg, Antibiotics — Cephalosporins). Information relating to a particular drug is presented in an individual monograph under the generic name of the drug (eg, Antianxiety — Meprobamate). All monographs are divided into sections identified with bold titles for ease in locating the desired information.

## Drug Class

A brief statement describing the class of the drug or drugs represented in the monographs can be found in the **Drug Class** section. When appropriate, slang terms often used by patients may be included (eg, diuretics, "water pills").

## How the Drug Works

This section briefly describes, in simplified language, the mechanism of action of the drug(s) represented in the monograph. This section tells the patient how the drug works in the body. For detailed information on mechanisms of action, pharmacology, and pharmacokinetics, refer to *Drug Facts and Comparisons.*

## Uses

The Food and Drug Administration's (FDA) approved indications for the drug or drugs represented in the monograph are listed.

Occasionally, a drug may be prescribed by the doctor for a use not officially recognized by the FDA. These unofficial uses are listed under *Unlabeled Uses.*

## Precautions

This section contains brief statements in simplified language derived from the Contraindications, Warnings, and Precautions sections of appropriate drug literature.

Two important statements found in this section list conditions in which the drug or drugs in the monograph should be used with caution or not at all.

*Do not use in the following situations:*

This list specifies those disease states and conditions in which the drug should NOT be used. If the patient has one of the conditions listed, contact his or her doctor.

*Use with caution in the following situations:*

This list specifies conditions in which the use of the drug may be hazardous to the patient. Consider contacting the patient's doctor if the patient has one of the conditions listed.

Examples of other items covered in the Precautions section include:

| | |
|---|---|
| breastfeeding | photosensitivity |
| children | pregnancy |
| diabetic patients | sulfite sensitivity |
| elderly patients | superinfection |
| lab tests | tartrazine |

## Drug Interactions

A list of potential drug-drug and drug-food interactions is provided. Drugs are listed by drug class or generic name. An example drug product is provided.

clarithromycin *(Biaxin)*. . . . . . . . generic name (only brand name available)

phenytoin (eg, *Dilantin*). . . . . . . generic name (one example of the brand name products available)

tricyclic antidepressants
(eg, amitriptyline). . . . . . . . . drug class (one example of a generic drug in this drug class)

## Side Effects

Side effects that have been reported are listed by organ system (eg, Digestive Tract, Nervous System). Occasionally, side effects specific to a drug or drug class are listed.

## Guidelines for Use

This boxed section includes Patient Information available in drug literature. The statements included in this list should reflect standard "Caution Label" ("sticker") language. The guidelines section also highlights other significant information that is important to verbally communicate to the patient.

## Vitamins

Recommended Dietary Allowances of Vitamins and Minerals, 3

Recommended Dietary Allowances of Vitamins and Minerals Table, 5

Vitamin A, 7

Vitamin $B_1$ (Thiamine), 10

Vitamin $B_2$ (Riboflavin), 12

Vitamin $B_3$ (Nicotinic Acid/Niacin), 13

Vitamin $B_5$ (Pantothenic Acid), 16

Vitamin $B_6$ (Pyridoxine), 17

Vitamin C (Ascorbic Acid), 19

Vitamin D, 22

Vitamin E, 26

## Minerals and Electrolytes

Calcium, 28

Electrolyte Mixtures, Oral, 32

Fluoride, 34

Magnesium, 38

Potassium, 40

Zinc, 43

## Vitamin Combinations

Vitamins A and D, 45

Vitamin B, 46

Vitamin B with C, 47

Vitamin B with Folic Acid, 49

Calcium and Vitamin D, 51

## Nutritional Supplements

Amino Acids, 53

Amino Acid Combinations, 54

Bioflavonoids, 56

Fish Oils, 58

Levocarnitine, 60

Lipotropic Products, 62

Para-Aminobenzoic Acid (PABA), 64

Recommended Dietary Allowances (RDA) are published by the Food and Nutrition Board, National Research Council-National Academy of Sciences, as a guide for nutritional problems and to provide standards of good nutrition for different age groups. They are revised periodically.

The RDA values are *not requirements*; they are *recommended* daily intakes of certain essential nutrients. Based on available scientific knowledge, they are believed to be adequate for known nutritional needs for most *healthy* people under usual environmental stresses. The recommended allowances vary for age and sex, with extra allowances for women during pregnancy and breastfeeding. The most commonly used RDA values (the "reference male" and the "reference female") are those of adults 23 to 50 years of age. With the exception of energy (kilocalories [kcal]), the RDA provide for individual requirement variations and prevent symptoms of clinical deficiency of 97% of the population.

RDAs have been established for many essential nutrients; however, present knowledge of human nutritional needs of pantothenic acid and biotin is incomplete. Therefore, to ensure adequate nutrient intake, obtain the recommended allowances from as varied a selection of foods as possible.

Nutritionists suggest that dietary planning include regular intake of each of the four basic food groups:
Milk, cheese, dairy products — Minimum 2 servings/day.
Meat, poultry, fish, beans — Minimum 2 servings/day.
Vegetables, fruit — Minimum 4 servings/day.
Bread, cereal (whole-grain and enriched or fortified) — Minimum 4 servings/day.

Such a balance, in sufficient quantities, will provide approximately 1200 kcal, enough protein, and most of the vitamins and minerals required daily. A person may increase nutrient and energy intake by consuming larger quantities (or more servings/day) of the four basic food groups. Nutrient and energy intake may also be increased by selecting food from a fifth group, fats-sweets-alcohol, which provides mainly energy.

RDA quantities apply only to healthy people and are not intended to cover therapeutic nutritional requirements in disease or other abnormal states (eg, metabolic disorders, weight reduction, chronic disease, drug therapy). Although certain single nutrients in larger quantities may have pharmacologic actions, these are unrelated to nutritional functions. There is no convincing evidence that consuming excessive quantities of single nutrients will cure or prevent nonnutritional diseases.

The "official" listings of United States Recommended Daily Allowances (US-RDAs) should not be confused with the RDA values. US-RDAs are derived from the 1968 RDA and serve as legal standards for nutritional labeling of food and dietary food and dietary supplement products controlled by the US Food and Drug Administration. Generally, they represent the higher value of the male or female RDA and are grouped into only three age brackets plus one category for pregnant or breastfeeding women. Prior to 1972, these allowances were erroneously listed as minimum daily requirements (MDR). A second fallacy perpetuated by the US-RDA labeling of foods is the implication that a food is defective if it does not contain all of the officially established nutrients in their full US-RDA quantities. No individual food is nutritionally complete, but several foods together should complement each other to provide maximal nutrient balance and to minimize naturally occurring toxic principles consumed from any individual foodstuff.

The RDAs for adult males and adult females are included in each individual vitamin monograph. The table on the following page presents the listing of vitamin and mineral RDA values for all age groups as published in *Recommended Dietary Allowances,* 10th Edition, National Academy of Sciences, Washington, D.C., 1989.

*If you have any questions, consult your doctor, pharmacist, or health care provider.*

Reproduced from: *Recommended Dietary Allowances*, 10th edition, 1989, National Academy of Sciences, National Academy Press, Washington, DC.

| RECOMMENDED DIETARY ALLOWANCES[1] | | | | | | | | | | | | |
|---|---|---|---|---|---|---|---|---|---|---|---|---|
| Patient Parameters | | | | | | Minerals | | | | | | |
| Age (years) or Condition | Weight[2] (kg) | Weight[2] (lb) | Height[2] (cm) | Height[2] (in) | Protein g | Calcium mg | Phosphorus mg | Magnesium mg | Iron mg | Zinc mg | Iodine μg | Selenium μg |
| **Infants** | | | | | | | | | | | | |
| 0.0-0.5 | 6 | 13 | 60 | 24 | 13 | 400 | 300 | 40 | 6 | 5 | 40 | 10 |
| 0.5-1 | 9 | 20 | 71 | 28 | 14 | 600 | 500 | 60 | 10 | 5 | 50 | 15 |
| **Children** | | | | | | | | | | | | |
| 1-3 | 13 | 29 | 90 | 35 | 16 | 800 | 800 | 80 | 10 | 10 | 70 | 20 |
| 4-6 | 20 | 44 | 112 | 44 | 24 | 800 | 800 | 120 | 10 | 10 | 90 | 20 |
| 7-10 | 28 | 62 | 132 | 52 | 28 | 800 | 800 | 170 | 10 | 10 | 120 | 30 |
| **Males** | | | | | | | | | | | | |
| 11-14 | 45 | 99 | 157 | 62 | 45 | 1200 | 1200 | 270 | 12 | 15 | 150 | 40 |
| 15-18 | 66 | 145 | 176 | 69 | 59 | 1200 | 1200 | 400 | 12 | 15 | 150 | 50 |
| 19-24 | 72 | 160 | 177 | 70 | 58 | 1200 | 1200 | 350 | 10 | 15 | 150 | 70 |
| 25-50 | 79 | 174 | 176 | 70 | 63 | 800 | 800 | 350 | 10 | 15 | 150 | 70 |
| 51 + | 77 | 170 | 173 | 68 | 63 | 800 | 800 | 350 | 10 | 15 | 150 | 70 |
| **Females** | | | | | | | | | | | | |
| 11-14 | 46 | 101 | 157 | 62 | 46 | 1200 | 1200 | 280 | 15 | 12 | 150 | 45 |
| 15-18 | 55 | 120 | 163 | 64 | 44 | 1200 | 1200 | 300 | 15 | 12 | 150 | 50 |
| 19-24 | 58 | 128 | 164 | 65 | 46 | 1200 | 1200 | 280 | 15 | 12 | 150 | 55 |
| 25-50 | 63 | 138 | 163 | 64 | 50 | 800 | 800 | 280 | 15 | 12 | 150 | 55 |
| 51 + | 65 | 143 | 160 | 63 | 50 | 800 | 800 | 280 | 10 | 12 | 150 | 55 |
| Pregnant | | | | | 60 | 1200 | 1200 | 320 | 30 | 15 | 175 | 65 |
| Lactating – 1st 6 mo. | | | | | 65 | 1200 | 1200 | 355 | 15 | 19 | 200 | 75 |
| 2nd 6 mo. | | | | | 62 | 1200 | 1200 | 340 | 15 | 16 | 200 | 75 |

[1] The allowances, expressed as average daily intakes over time, are intended to provide for individual variations among most normal persons as they live in the US under usual environmental stresses. Diets should be based on a variety of common foods in order to provide other nutrients for which human requirements have been less well defined.

[2] Weights and heights of Reference Adults are actual medians for the US population of the designated age, as reported by NHANES II. The median weights and heights of those under 19 years of age were taken from Hamill PV et al. *Am J Clin Nutr* 1979;32:607-29. The use of these figures does not imply that the height-to-weight ratios are ideal.

# RECOMMENDED DIETARY ALLOWANCES OF VITAMINS AND MINERALS

## RECOMMENDED DIETARY ALLOWANCES[1]

| Patient Parameters | | | | | Fat-Soluble Vitamins | | | | Water-Soluble Vitamins | | | | | | |
|---|---|---|---|---|---|---|---|---|---|---|---|---|---|---|---|
| Age (years) or Condition | Weight[2] (kg) | Weight[2] (lb) | Height[2] (cm) | Height[2] (in) | Vitamin A (μg RE[3]) | Vitamin D (IU[4]) | Vitamin E (IU[5]) | Vitamin K (μg) | Ascorbic Acid (C) (mg) | Thiamine (B₁) (mg) | Riboflavin (B₂) (mg) | Niacin (B₃) (mg) | Pyridoxine (B₆) (mg) | Folate (μg) | Cyanocobalamin (B₁₂) (μg) |
| **Infants** | | | | | | | | | | | | | | | |
| 0.0-0.5 | 6 | 13 | 60 | 24 | 375 | 300 | 4 | 5 | 30 | 0.3 | 0.4 | 5 | 0.3 | 25 | 0.3 |
| 0.5-1 | 9 | 20 | 71 | 28 | 375 | 400 | 6 | 10 | 35 | 0.4 | 0.5 | 6 | 0.6 | 35 | 0.5 |
| **Children** | | | | | | | | | | | | | | | |
| 1-3 | 13 | 29 | 90 | 35 | 400 | 400 | 9 | 15 | 40 | 0.7 | 0.8 | 9 | 1 | 50 | 0.7 |
| 4-6 | 20 | 44 | 112 | 44 | 500 | 400 | 10 | 20 | 45 | 0.9 | 1.1 | 12 | 1.1 | 75 | 1 |
| 7-10 | 28 | 62 | 132 | 52 | 700 | 400 | 10 | 30 | 45 | 1 | 1.2 | 13 | 1.4 | 100 | 1.4 |
| **Males** | | | | | | | | | | | | | | | |
| 11-14 | 45 | 99 | 157 | 62 | 1000 | 400 | 15 | 45 | 50 | 1.3 | 1.5 | 17 | 1.7 | 150 | 2 |
| 15-18 | 66 | 145 | 176 | 69 | 1000 | 400 | 15 | 65 | 60 | 1.5 | 1.8 | 20 | 2 | 200 | 2 |
| 19-24 | 72 | 160 | 177 | 70 | 1000 | 400 | 15 | 70 | 60 | 1.5 | 1.7 | 19 | 2 | 200 | 2 |
| 25-50 | 79 | 174 | 176 | 70 | 1000 | 200 | 15 | 80 | 60 | 1.5 | 1.7 | 19 | 2 | 200 | 2 |
| 51 + | 77 | 170 | 173 | 68 | 1000 | 200 | 15 | 80 | 60 | 1.2 | 1.4 | 15 | 2 | 200 | 2 |
| **Females** | | | | | | | | | | | | | | | |
| 11-14 | 46 | 101 | 157 | 62 | 800 | 400 | 12 | 45 | 50 | 1.1 | 1.3 | 15 | 1.4 | 150 | 2 |
| 15-18 | 55 | 120 | 163 | 64 | 800 | 400 | 12 | 55 | 60 | 1.1 | 1.3 | 15 | 1.5 | 180 | 2 |
| 19-24 | 58 | 128 | 164 | 65 | 800 | 400 | 12 | 60 | 60 | 1.1 | 1.3 | 15 | 1.6 | 180 | 2 |
| 25-50 | 63 | 138 | 163 | 64 | 800 | 200 | 12 | 65 | 60 | 1.1 | 1.3 | 15 | 1.6 | 180 | 2 |
| 51 + | 65 | 143 | 160 | 63 | 800 | 200 | 12 | 65 | 60 | 1 | 1.2 | 13 | 1.6 | 180 | 2 |
| **Pregnant** | | | | | 800 | 400 | 15 | 65 | 70 | 1.5 | 1.6 | 17 | 2.2 | 400 | 2.2 |
| Lactating – 1st 6 mo. | | | | | 1300 | 400 | 18 | 65 | 95 | 1.6 | 1.8 | 20 | 2.1 | 280 | 2.6 |
| 2nd 6 mo. | | | | | 1200 | 400 | 16 | 65 | 90 | 1.6 | 1.7 | 20 | 2.1 | 260 | 2.6 |

1 The allowances, expressed as average daily intakes over time, are intended to provide for individual variations among most normal persons as they live in the US under usual environmental stresses. Diets should be based on a variety of common foods in order to provide other nutrients for which human requirements have been less well defined.

2 Weights and heights of Reference Adults are actual medians for the US population of the designated age, as reported by NHANES II. The median weights and heights of those under 19 years of age were taken from Hamill PV et al. *Am J Clin Nutr* 1979;32:607-29. The use of these figures does not imply that the height-to-weight ratios are ideal.

3 Retinol equivalents. 1 retinol equivalent = 1 μg retinol or 6 μg β-carotene.

4 As cholecalciferol. 10 μg cholecalciferol = 400 IU of vitamin D.

5 α-Tocopherol equivalents. 1 mg d-α-tocopherol = α-TE = 1.49 IU.

| Generic Name<br>*Brand Name Examples* | Supplied As | Generic<br>Available |
|---|---|---|
| **Vitamin A** | | |
| *otc* *Palmitate-A 5000, Vitamin A and Beta Carotene, Vitamin A Palmitate* | **Tablets:** 5000 IU, 10,000 IU, 15,000 IU, 25,000 IU | Yes |
| *Vitamin A* | **Capsules:** 10,000 IU, 25,000 IU | Yes |
| *Rx* *Vitamin A* | **Capsules:** 25,000 IU | Yes |

For a complete listing of Recommended Dietary Allowances, see the RDA table.

## Type of Drug:

Fat-soluble vitamin. Vitamin that can be stored by the body.

## How the Drug Works:

Vitamin A is essential for vision (prevents night blindness), dental development, growth, hydrocortisone synthesis, reproduction, and normal skin.

## Uses:

To treat or prevent vitamin A deficiency.

## Precautions:

*Do not use in the following situations:*
> allergy to vitamin A
> hypervitaminosis A (overuse of vitamin A)
> oral use in malabsorption syndrome

*Kidney disease:* Patients with chronic kidney failure may develop vitamin A toxicity.

*Multiple vitamin deficiency:* It is unusual for vitamin A deficiency to occur alone. Other vitamin supplements may be needed. Consult your pharmacist or doctor.

*Acne:* Taking large doses of vitamin A (100,000 to 300,000 IU/day) by mouth has not been shown to be effective in the treatment of acne. Topical vitamin A derivatives (retinoic acid [tretinoin] and isotretinoin) have been found to be effective.

*Pregnancy:* Adequate studies have not been done in pregnant women. Use only if clearly needed and potential benefits outweigh the possible hazards to the fetus. Safety of amounts greater than 5000 IU daily during pregnancy has not been established.

*Breastfeeding:* The US-RDA of vitamin A is 1300 mcg retinol equivalents in the first 6 months for nursing mothers and 1200 mg retinol equivalents in the second 6 months. Human milk supplies sufficient vitamin A for infants unless the mother's diet is inadequate.

## Drug Interactions:

Tell your doctor or pharmacist if you are taking or if you are planning to take any over-the-counter or prescription medications or dietary supplements with vitamin A. Doses of one or both drugs may need to be modified or a different drug may need to be prescribed. The following drugs and drug classes interact with vitamin A:

> aminoglycosides (eg, neomycin)
> mineral oil

## Side Effects:

Every drug is capable of producing side effects. Many vitamin A users experience no, or minor, side effects. The frequency and severity of side effects depend on many factors including dose, duration of therapy, and individual susceptibility. Possible side effects include:

*Acute Toxicity (occurs 8 to 12 hours after a large dose):* Headache; nausea; vomiting; blurred or double vision; drowsiness; feeling of whirling motion; bulging fontanelle (soft spot) in infants.

*The following are symptoms of hypervitaminosis A (toxicity after long-term use):*

*Digestive Tract:* Stomach discomfort; vomiting; appetite loss; nausea.

*Nervous System:* Unusual tiredness; dizziness; irritability; headache; bulging eyes; drowsiness.

*Skin:* Cracking of lips or skin; hair loss; scaling; itching; redness; inflammation of tongue, lips, and gums; yellowing of skin and eyes; face inflammation; sticky skin.

*Other:* Slow growth; night sweats; bone and joint pain; swelling of legs and ankles; decreased menstrual periods; dry mucous membranes; eye inflammation; blurred vision.

## Guidelines for Use:

- Dosage will be individualized.
- Most people on balanced diets do not need vitamin supplements. People with hepatic cirrhosis, biliary tract or pancreatic disease, sprue, cystic fibrosis, or digestive tract diseases who are unable to digest fats are at risk for vitamin A deficiency.
- *Recommended Dietary Allowances (RDAs)* —
  Adult males: 1000 mcg retinol equivalents
  Adult females: 800 mcg retinol equivalents
- Do not take more than the recommended doses.
- Notify your doctor if signs of overdosage occur: Nausea, vomiting, headache, bulging fontanelle (soft spot) in infants, dizziness, feeling of whirling motion, drowsiness, blurred vision.
- *Common sources of vitamin A* — Liver, sweet potatoes, carrots, dark green leafy vegetables, whole milk, butter, cheese, egg yolk, meat, fish, squash, cantalopes.
- *Other vitamin A sources* — Fortified foods, multivitamins, and cod liver oil. Vitamin A is stored in the liver. Consider all possible sources of vitamin A before taking a supplement. Doses of vitamin A over 25,000 IU daily should be taken only with a doctor's order.
- Store as directed on container or package.

*If you have any questions, consult your doctor, pharmacist, or health care provider.*

| Generic Name<br>*Brand Name Examples* | Supplied As | Generic<br>Available |
|---|---|---|
| **Thiamine HCl/Vitamin B₁** | | |
| *Rx Thiamine HCl* | **Injection:** 100 mg/mL | Yes |
| *otc Betalin S* | **Tablets:** 50 mg, 100 mg,<br>250 mg, 500 mg | Yes |
| *otc Thiamilate* | **Tablets, enteric coated:** 20 mg | No |

For a complete listing of Recommended Dietary Allowances, see the RDA table.

## Type of Drug:
Water-soluble vitamin. Vitamin not stored by the body.

## How the Drug Works:
Thiamine (vitamin B₁) is important in carbohydrate (sugar and starch) metabolism, maintenance of normal growth, and transmission of nerve impulses.

## Uses:
To treat or prevent thiamine deficiency (a severe form is called beriberi). Beriberi may cause vomiting, rapid heart rate, abnormal skin sensations in the hands and feet, loss of muscle strength, appetite loss, difficulty breathing, pounding in the chest, fluid retention, greenish stools, voice loss, and muscle wasting or rigidity.

*Unlabeled Use(s):* Oral thiamine has been used as a mosquito repellant; however, effectiveness has not been proven.

## Precautions:
*Do not use in the following situations:* Allergy to thiamine.

*Use with caution in the following situations:* Wernicke-Korsakoff syndrome.

*Multiple vitamin deficiencies:* It is unusual for thiamine deficiency to occur alone. Other vitamin supplements may be needed. Consult your pharmacist or doctor.

*Pregnancy:* This drug appears to be safe for use during pregnancy. However, no drug should be used during pregnancy unless clearly needed. Use only in amounts recommended by your doctor.

*Breastfeeding:* It is not known whether thiamine appears in breast milk. Consult your doctor before you begin breastfeeding.

## Side Effects:
Every drug is capable of producing side effects. Many thiamine users experience no, or minor, side effects. The frequency and severity of side effects depend on many factors including dose, duration of therapy, and individual susceptibility. Possible side effects include:

*Nervous System:* Weakness; restlessness.

*Skin:* Itching; rash; hives; sweating; bluish skin discoloration; tenderness or hardening of the skin at injection site (injection only).

*Other:* Feeling of warmth; nausea; fluid retention; tightness of throat; low blood pressure; fluid accumulation in the lungs; dizziness.

---

## Guidelines for Use:

- Most people on balanced diets do not need vitamin supplements. People with excessive alcohol intake, long-term dialysis, malapsorption, excessive carbohydrate intake, excessive coffee or tea intake, appetite loss, chronic diarrhea, bilary disease, liver dysfunction, or hyperthyroidism are at risk for thiamine deficiency.
- Do not take enteric-coated tabets with dairy products.
- *Recommended Dietary Allowances (RDAs) —*
  Adult males: 1.2 to 1.5 mg
  Adult females: 1 to 1.1 mg
- *Common sources of thiamine* — Pork, liver, brewer's yeast, legumes, beef, milk, nuts, whole grains, enriched flour.
- Store at controlled room temperature (59° to 86°F). Protect from moisture.

---

*If you have any questions, consult your doctor, pharmacist, or health care provider.*

| Generic Name | Supplied As | Generic Available |
|---|---|---|
| *otc* **Riboflavin/Vitamin B$_2$** | **Tablets:** 50 mg, 100 mg, 400 mg | Yes |

For a complete listing of Recommended Dietary Allowances, see the RDA table.

## Type of Drug:
Water-soluble vitamin. Vitamin not stored by the body.

## How the Drug Works:
Riboflavin (vitamin B$_2$) acts in a variety of important metabolic processes in the body and promotes healthy skin and vision.

## Uses:
To treat and prevent riboflavin deficiency. Symptoms of riboflavin deficiency include itching and burning eyes, lips, mouth, or tongue; sensitivity to light; sore throat; mouth or tongue inflammation; scrotal or vulval skin changes; skin inflammation; red eyes; cataract formation; dry lips and corners of the mouth; or scaly skin inflammation on the face and scalp.

## Precautions:
*Multiple vitamin deficiencies:* It is unusual for riboflavin deficiency to occur alone. Other vitamins and protein may also be needed. Consult your pharmacist or doctor.

*Pregnancy:* Adequate, well-controlled studies have failed to demonstrate risk to the fetus. In doses that exceed RDA, risk cannot be ruled out. However, potential benefits to the mother may justify the potential risks to the fetus. Consult your doctor.

*Breastfeeding:* Riboflavin is excreted in breast milk. Consult your doctor before you begin breastfeeding.

---

### Guidelines for Use:
- Most people on balanced diets do not need vitamin supplements. People with excessive alcohol intake, malabsorption, or poor diets are at risk for riboflavin deficiency.
- Dosage for treatment of deficiency states is 5 to 10 mg/day
- May cause a yellow discoloration of the urine when taken in large doses.
- *Recommended Dietary Allowances (RDAs)* —
  Males: 1.4 to 1.8 mg
  Females: 1.2 to 1.3 mg
- *Common sources of riboflavin* – Meats, poultry, fish, dairy products, broccoli, turnips, asparagus, spinach, enriched and fortified grains, cereals, and bakery products.
- Store at controlled room temperature (59° to 86°F). Protect from moisture.

---

*If you have any questions, consult your doctor, pharmacist, or health care provider.*

| Generic Name<br>*Brand Name Examples* | Supplied As | Generic<br>Available |
|---|---|---|
| *Rx* **Nicotinic Acid/Niacin**[1] | **Capsules, sustained-release**: 500 mg | Yes |
| | **Capsules, timed-release**: 500 mg | Yes |
| *Niacor* | **Tablets**: 500 mg | Yes |
| *otc* **Nicotinic Acid/Niacin**[1] | **Tablets**: 50 mg, 100 mg, 250 mg, 500 mg | Yes |
| | **Tablets, sustained-release**: 500 mg | Yes |
| | **Tablets, timed-release**: 250 mg, 500 mg | Yes |
| | **Capsules, extended-release**: 250 mg, 400 mg | Yes |
| | **Capsules, sustained-release**: 125 mg, 500 mg | Yes |
| | **Capsules, timed-release**: 250 mg, 500 mg | Yes |
| *Slo-Niacin* | **Tablets, controlled-release**: 250 mg, 500 mg, 750 mg | Yes |
| *Nicotinex* | **Elixir**: 50 mg/5 mg | No |
| *otc* **Nicotinamide/ Niacinamide** | **Tablets**: 100 mg, 500 mg | Yes |

[1] Some products may be available *Rx* according to distributor discretion.

For a complete listing of Recommended Dietary Allowances, see the RDA table.

## Type of Drug:

Water-soluble vitamin. Vitamin not stored by the body. Nicotinamide (niacinamide) is chemically related to niacin.

## How the Drug Works:

Niacin (nicotinic acid) is a biochemical entity involved in fat metabolism, tissue respiration, and energy production. Vitamins do not give people energy, even though they are involved in the energy production process in the body.

Niacin and nicotinamide both act as vitamins in the body. However, only niacin dilates blood vessels in the face, neck, and chest and lowers cholesterol and triglyceride levels in the blood.

## Uses:

The following information pertains primarily to uses of niacin in doses greater than the Recommended Dietary Allowance (RDA).

To prevent or to treat niacin deficiency. Niacin requirements may be increased during periods of increased calorie use (recovery from illness or injury).

To prevent and to treat pellagra. Pellagra is rare. It occurs most frequently in alcoholics, the poorly-nourished elderly, and people on unusual diets. It also occurs in areas where much corn is eaten, because the niacin in corn is bound to indigestible constituents, making it unavailable for use by the body.

## Precautions:

*Do not use in the following situations:*

| | |
|---|---|
| allergy to niacin or any of its ingredients | liver disease |
| bleeding, arterial | peptic ulcer, active |

*Use with caution in the following situations:*

| | |
|---|---|
| alcoholics | heart disease |
| angina, unstable | jaundice, history of |
| bleeding, arterial, history of | liver disease, history of |
| diabetes | MI, acute phase |
| gallbladder disease | peptic ulcer, history |
| gout | |

*Diabetes mellitus:* Niacin may decrease glucose tolerance. Diet or blood sugar lowering drugs may have to be adjusted. Consult your doctor before taking niacin supplements.

*Gout:* Niacin may cause an increase in uric acid levels, possibly causing a gout attack.

*Pregnancy:* Adequate studies have not been done in pregnant women. Use doses in excess of the RDA only if clearly needed and potential benefits to the mother outweigh the possible hazards to the fetus.

*Breastfeeding:* Niacin appears in breast milk. Consult your doctor before you begin breastfeeding.

*Children:* Safety and efficacy in children have not been established in doses that exceed the RDA.

*Lab tests* may be required to monitor therapy. Tests may include lipids (cholesterol and triglycerides), blood glucose, and liver function tests.

## Drug Interactions:

Tell your doctor or pharmacist if you are taking or if you are planning to take any over-the-counter or prescription medications or dietary supplements with niacin. Doses of one or both drugs may need to be modified or a different drug may need to be prescribed. The following drugs and drug classes interact with niacin:

beta blockers (eg, propranolol)
HMG-CoA reductase inhibitors (eg, lovastatin)
sulfinpyrazone (eg, *Anturane*)

## Side Effects:

Every drug is capable of producing side effects. Many niacin users experience no, or minor, side effects. The frequency and severity of side effects depend on many factors including dose, duration of therapy, and individual susceptibility. Possible side effects include:

*Digestive Tract:* Stomach distress or pain; nausea; vomiting; diarrhea; indigestion; activation of peptic ulcer.

*Skin:* Rash; hives; itching; dry skin; flushing; tingling of skin; sensation of warmth; thickening and brownish discoloration of the skin in bony folds.

*Other:* Headache; low blood pressure; dimming of vision; abnormal heart rhythms; liver dysfunction; lab test abnormalities; elevated blood sugar; yellowing of the skin or eyes; gout; vision changes.

---

### Guidelines for Use:

- Most people on balanced diets do no need vitamin supplements.
- *Recommended Dietary Allowances (RDAs) —*
  Adult males: 15 to 20 mg
  Adult females: 13 to 15 mg
- *For hyperlipidemia —* Usual target dosage is 1 to 2 g 2 or 3 times daily. Do not exceed 6 g/day.
  *For pellagra —* Take up to 500 mg/day.
- *Niacinamide —* Usual dosage is 100 to 500 mg/day.
- *Sustained-, extended-, or timed-release products —* Take whole. Do not break, crush, or chew before swallowing.
- Do not substitute sustained-, extended-, or timed-release preparations for immediate-release (crystalline) nicotinic acid.
- May cause stomach upset. Take with meals.
- If dizziness occurs, avoid sudden changes in posture.
- Flushing appears frequently with oral therapy and generally begins 20 minutes after ingestion and lasts 30 to 60 minutes. Flushing is transient and will usually subside after 3 to 6 weeks of continued therapy. The flush response can be reduced by slowly increasing the dose (100 mg 3 times daily each week), administering with food or milk, or by administering either a nonsteroidal anti-inflammatory drug (eg, ibuprofen) or aspirin 60 minutes prior to niacin administration.
- Discontinue use and contact a doctor if any of the following symptoms occur: Persistent flu-like symptoms (nausea, vomiting, general unwell feeling); hives; loss of appetite; decreased urine output associated with dark-colored urine; muscle discomfort such as tender, swollen muscles or muscle weakness; irregular heartbeat; or dimming of vision.
- *Common sources of niacin —* Liver, meat, fish, chicken, nuts, legumes, green vegetables, yeast, potatoes, and whole-grain enriched cereals and breads.
- Lab tests may be required to monitor therapy. Be sure to keep appointments.
- Store at controlled room temperature (59° to 86°F).

---

*If you have any questions, consult your doctor, pharmacist, or health care provider.*

| Generic Name | Supplied As | Generic Available |
|---|---|---|
| *otc* **Calcium Pantothenate/ Vitamin B₅** | **Tablets:** 100 mg (= to 92 mg pantothenic acid), 218 mg (= to 200 mg pantothenic acid), 545 mg (= to 500 mg pantothenic acid) | Yes |

For a complete listing of Recommended Dietary allowances, see the RDA table.

## Type of Drug:
Water-soluble vitamin. Pantothenic acid. Vitamin not stored by the body.

## How the Drug Works:
Calcium pantothenate (vitamin B₅) in the formation and metabolism of carbohydrates (sugars), fatty acids, and hormones in the body.

## Uses:
To treat pantothenic acid deficiency. Most people on regular diets do not need pantothenic acid supplements. Symptoms of deficiency are very rare and may include fatigue, headache, sleep disturbances, stomach cramps, vomiting, gas, muscle cramps, abnormal skin sensations in the arms and legs, and impaired coordination.

## Precautions:
*Multiple vitamin deficiencies:* It is unusual for pantothenic acid deficiency to occur alone. Other vitamins may be needed; consult your pharmacist or doctor.

*Pregnancy:* This drug appears to be safe for use during pregnancy. However, no drug should be used during pregnancy unless clearly needed. Adequate studies have not been done in pregnant women taking doses that exceed the recommended daily allowance (RDA); therefore, use only if clearly needed and potential benefits to the mother outweight possible hazards to the fetus.

*Breastfeeding:* Pantothenic acid appears in breast milk. Consult your doctor before you begin breastfeeding.

### Guidelines for Use:
- Most people on balanced diets do not need vitamin supplements.
- *Recommendation for adults* — An approximate dietary intake of 4 to 7 mg/day has been recommended.
- *Common sources of pantothenic acid* — Meat, poultry, fish, cereals, fruits, vegetables, milk, and egg yolks.
- Store at controlled room temperature (59° to 86°F). Protect from moisture.

*If you have any questions, consult your doctor, pharmacist, or health care provider.*

| Generic Name<br>*Brand Name Examples* | Supplied As | Generic<br>Available |
|---|---|---|
| **Pyridoxine/Vitamin B$_6$** | | |
| *otc Nestrex* | **Tablets**: 25 mg | Yes |
| *otc Vitamin B$_6$* | **Tablets**: 25 mg, 50 mg,<br>100 mg, 200 mg, 250 mg,<br>500 mg | Yes |
| *otc Aminoxin* | **Tablets, enteric-coated**: 20 mg | No |
| *Rx Pyridoxine HCl* | **Injection**: 100 mg/mL | Yes |

For a complete listing of Recommended Dietary Allowances, see the RDA table.

## Type of Drug:
Water-soluble vitamin. Vitamin not stored by the body.

## How the Drug Works:
Pyridoxine acts in protein, carbohydrate, and fat metabolism in the body.

## Uses:
To treat or prevent pyridoxine deficiency. Symptoms of a severe deficiency include dry, oily, or flaky skin around the eyes, nose, and mouth; mouth inflammation; abnormal blood counts; convulsions; irritability; or numbness or tingling in the hands or feet.

## Precautions:
*Do not use in the following situations:* Allergy to pyridoxine.

*Multiple vitamin deficiency:* It is unusual for pyridoxine deficiency to occur alone. Other vitamin supplements may be needed; consult your pharmacist or doctor.

*Abuse and dependence:* Withdrawal symptoms (eg, loss of coordination, numbness of the hands or feet) may occur after suddenly stopping 200 mg/day doses taken for longer than 2 months.

*Pregnancy:* This drug appears to be safe for use during pregnancy. However, drugs should not be used during pregnancy unless clearly needed. Adequate studies have not been done in pregnant women taking doses that exceed the RDA; therefore, use only if clearly needed and potential benefits to the mother outweigh possible hazards to the fetus.

*Breastfeeding:* Pyridoxine appears in breast milk. Seizures in nursing infants have been reported. Consult your doctor before you begin breastfeeding.

*Children:* Safety and efficacy have not been established for use in children in doses that exceed the RDA.

## Drug Interactions:

Tell your doctor or pharmacist if you are taking or if you are planning to take any over-the-counter or prescription medications or dietary supplements with pyridoxine. Doses of one or both drugs may need to be modified or a different drug may need to be prescribed. The following drugs and drug classes interact with pyridoxine:

hydantoins (eg, phenytoin)
levodopa (eg, *Larodopa*)

phenobarbital (eg, *Solfoton*)
primidone (eg, *Mysoline*)

## Side Effects:

Every drug is capable of producing side effects. Many pyridoxine users experience no, or minor, side effects. The frequency and severity of side effects depend on many factors including dose, duration of therapy, and individual susceptibility. Possible side effects include:

*Skin:* Numbness or tingling on skin or in fingers and toes; numbness around mouth; abnormal skin sensations.

*Other:* Unstable walk; awkwardness of hands; decreased sensation to touch, temperature, and vibration perception; drowsiness; clumsiness; sensitivity to light.

---

### Guidelines for Use:

- Most people on balanced diets do not need vitamin supplements. Those on certain prescription drugs (eg, isoniazid, oral contraceptives, hydralazine); who are pregnant; who have kidney failure, liver disease, or malignancies; and chronic alcoholics are at risk for pyridoxine deficiency.
- *Recommended Dietary Allowances (RDAs)* —
  Adult males: 1.7 to 2 mg
  Adult females: 1.4 to 1.6 mg
- *Enteric-coated tablets* — Do not cut, crush, or chew. Swallow whole with a glass of water.
- *Common sources of pyridoxine* — Liver, eggs, meat, whole-grain breads and cereals, soybeans, vegetables, peanuts, walnuts, and corn.
- Store at controlled room temperature (59° to 86°F). Protect from moisture.

---

*If you have any questions, consult your doctor, pharmacist, or health care provider.*

| Generic Name<br>*Brand Name Examples* | Supplied As | Generic<br>Available |
|---|---|---|
| **Ascorbic Acid/Vitamin C** | | |
| otc *Vitamin C* | **Tablets**: 250 mg, 500 mg, 1000 mg | Yes |
| otc *Vitamin C* | **Capsules:** 750 mg | Yes |
| otc *Cevi-Bid* | **Tablets, timed-release:** 500 mg, 1000 mg | Yes |
| otc *N'ice Vitamin C Drops* | **Lozenges:** 60 mg | Yes |
| otc *Cecon* | **Oral solution:** 100 mg/mL | Yes |
| otc *Dull-C* | **Powder:** 1060 mg/g | Yes |
| otc *Vita-C* | **Crystals:** 1000 mg/g | Yes |
| Rx *Cenolate* | **Injection:** 500 mg/mL | Yes |
| otc **Calcium Ascorbate** | **Tablets:** 500 mg | Yes |
| | **Powder:** 814 mg/g | Yes |

For a complete listing of Recommended Dietary Allowances, see the RDA table.

## Type of Drug:

Water-soluble vitamin with antioxidant properties. Vitamin not stored by the body.

## How the Drug Works:

Vitamin C is involved with several functions in the body, including the following: Utilization of carbohydrates; formation of fats and proteins; maintenance of blood vessels; cell respiration; formation of connective tissues (eg, collagen); promotion of growth, tissue repair, and wound healing; aiding tooth and bone formation; increasing iron absorption; resistance to infections.

## Uses:

To prevent and treat scurvy (vitamin C deficiency), characterized by slow wound healing, defects in tooth formation (children), faulty bone development (children), bleeding gums and loose teeth, irritability, easy bruising, joint pain, fatigue, and muscle weakness.

Scurvy is a rare condition in the US. It develops only when psychiatric illness, alcoholism, age, disease of the digestive system, food fads, poverty, or ignorance result in inadequate nutrition. It may also develop in infants whose formulas lack adequate vitamin C.

*Unlabeled Use(s):* Vitamin C may occasionally be used as a supplement in patients with chronic illnesses, infections, conditions with fever, burns, and certain types of blood disorders, and in infants or smokers. It may be used to improve the general health and well-being of institutionalized elderly patients; to promote healing after surgery, trauma, and fractures; to prevent the common cold; to treat asthma; and to decrease recovery time from cold sores, pressure sores, rectal polyps, and other lesions. It is also used as a urinary acidifier at high doses.

## Precautions:

*Use with caution in the following situations:* Kidney stones or a history of kidney stones

*Lab test interference:* Vitamin C doses over 500 mg may cause false-negative urine sugar results in some tests. Also, vitamin C use 48 to 72 hours before certain types of tests for blood in the stool may cause false-negative results. Use with caution.

*Drug interactions:* Large doses (more than 2 g/day) may affect the pH of urine, making it more acidic. Changes in urine pH may cause the effects of other medications to be exaggerated (increased) or may decrease their effectiveness.

*Kidney stone formation:* Kidney stone formation with vitamin C is more likely if large doses are taken over long periods of time. Symptoms include severe flank pain associated with nausea and vomiting, difficult or painful urination, and blood in the urine.

*Pregnancy:* Adequate studies have not been done in pregnant women. Use only if clearly needed and potential benefits outweigh the possible hazards to the fetus.

*Breastfeeding:* Vitamin C appears in breast milk. Consult your doctor before you begin breastfeeding.

*Tartrazine:* Some of these products may contain the dye tartrazine (FD&C Yellow No. 5), which can cause allergic reactions in certain individuals. Check the package label when available or consult your pharmacist or doctor.

## Drug Interactions:

Tell your doctor or pharmacist if you are taking or planning to take any over-the-counter or prescription medications or dietary supplements with vitamin C. Doses of one or both drugs may need to be modified or a different drug may need to be prescribed. The following drugs and drug classes interact with vitamin C:

> contraceptives, oral (eg,*Ortho-Novum*)
> sulfonamides (eg,*Gantrisin*)
> warfarin (eg, *Coumadin*)

## Side Effects:

Every drug is capable of producing side effects. Many vitamin C users experience no, or minor, side effects. The frequency and severity of side effects depend on many factors, including dose, duration of therapy, and individual susceptibility. Possible side effects include:

*Digestive Tract:* Diarrhea; mouth sores; nausea; vomiting; stomach upset; heartburn.

*Other:* Kidney stones; fatigue; flushing; headache; sleeplessness; sleepiness.

## Guidelines for Use:

- Most people on a balanced diet do not need vitamin supplements.
- *Recommended Dietary Allowances (RDAs) —* Adults: 60 mg
- *Tablets —* May discolor slightly. This does not affect potency.
- *Powder/Crystals —* Dissolve the recommended dose in a glass of water or juice.
- *Solution —* Add recommended dose to any desired liquid (eg, milk, juice).
- Total vitamin C intake includes the amounts taken in the diet, plus supplements. This total should not substantially exceed the RDA.
- *Common sources of vitamin C –* Strawberries, citrus fruit, tomatoes, potatoes, leafy vegetables, cabbage greens, and melons.
- Store at controlled room temperature (59° to 86°F). Keep containers tightly closed.

*If you have any questions, consult your doctor, pharmacist, or health care provider.*

| Generic Name<br>*Brand Name Examples* | Supplied As | Generic<br>Available |
|---|---|---|
| *Rx* **Calcifediol**[1] | | |
| *Calderol* | **Capsules:** 20 mcg, 50 mcg | No |
| *Rx* **Calcitriol**[1] | | |
| *Rocaltrol* | **Capsules:** 0.25 mcg, 0.5 mcg | No |
| *Rocaltrol* | **Oral solution:** 1 mcg/mL | No |
| *Calcijex* | **Injection:** 1 mcg/mL, 2 mcg/mL | No |
| *otc* **Cholecalciferol ($D_3$)**[1] | | |
| *Delta D3, Vitamin D3* | **Tablets:** 400 IU, 1000 IU | Yes |
| *Rx* **Dihydrotachysterol (DHT)**[2] | | |
| *Hytakerol* | **Capsules:** 0.125 mg | No |
| *DHT* | **Tablets:** 0.125 mg, 0.2 mg, 0.4 mg | No |
| *DHT Intensol* | **Solution:** 0.2 mg/mL | No |
| **Ergocalciferol ($D_2$)**[1] | | |
| *otc Calciferol Drops* | **Solution:** 200 IU/drop | No |
| *otc Drisdol* | **Solution:** 200 IU/drop | No |
| *otc Delta-D2* | **Tablets:** 400 IU | Yes |
| *Rx Drisdol*[3] | **Capsules:** 50,000 IU | No |
| *Rx Calciferol* | **Injection, in oil:** 500,000 IU/mL | No |
| *Rx* **Paricalcitol**[4] | | |
| *Zemplar* | **Injection:** 5 mcg/mL | No |

[1] 1 mg = 40,000 IU.
[2] 1 mg DHT is approximately equal to 3 mg vitamin $D_2$, which is equal to 120,000 IU.
[3] Contains tartrazine.
[4] Synthetic vitamin D analog.

For a complete listing of Recommended Dietary Allowances, see the RDA table.

## Type of Drug:

Fat-soluble vitamin. Essential vitamin that can be stored by the body. Natural supply of vitamin D depends largely upon exposure to the ultraviolet (UV) light of the sun.

## How the Drug Works:

Vitamin D promotes proper absorption and use of calcium and phosphate by the body and normal bone development and maintenance. It also helps regulate parathyroid hormone levels and is involved in magnesium metabolism.

## Uses:

As a dietary supplement (cholecalciferol).

To prevent and treat rickets, a vitamin D deficiency disease characterized by weak bones, deformed skeleton, bowed legs, deformed spine, "potbelly" appearance, sometimes flat feet, stunted growth, soft bones, and deformed joints (ergocalciferol, cholecalciferol).

To help regulate levels of parathyroid hormone (DHT, calcitriol, calcifediol, ergocalciferol, paricalcitol).

To prevent and treat postsurgical and other types of tetany (severe muscle spasms due to low calcium levels) (DHT).

To treat low calcium levels and bone disease in patients on chronic kidney dialysis (calcitriol, calcifediol, ergocalciferol).

## Precautions:

*Do not use in the following situations:*

abnormal sensitivity to effects of vitamin D (eg, become toxic at lower doses)
allergy to vitamin D or any of its ingredients
high calcium levels
kidney function, decreased (ergocalciferol)
malabsorption syndrome (oral forms)
vitamin D toxicity

*Use with caution in the following situations:*

bone lesions
coronary artery disease (in elderly patients)
hypoparathyroidism
kidney disease
kidney stones

*Hypercalcemia:* Instruct patients to discontinue therapy immediately and contact their physician if signs or symptoms of high blood calcium develop. Symptoms may include the following: Weakness; headache; tiredness; vomiting; nausea; dry mouth; constipation; muscle pain; bone pain; metallic taste; increased urinary frequency; increased thirst; loss of appetite; weight loss; increased urinary frequency at night; eye inflammation; any other unusual symptoms.

*Pregnancy:* Adequate studies have not been done in pregnant women. Use only if clearly needed and potential benefits outweigh the possible hazards to the fetus.

*Breastfeeding:* Vitamin D is excreted in breast milk. Do not breastfeed while using calcitriol. Consult your doctor before using other vitamin D supplements during breastfeeding.

*Children:* Safety and effectiveness in children of doses exceeding the RDA and in children undergoing dialysis have not been established.

*Lab tests* will be required to monitor therapy. Tests may include blood calcium, magnesium, and phosphorus; kidney function; and urine tests.

*Tartrazine:* Some of these products may contain the dye tartrazine (FD&C Yellow No. 5), which can cause allergic reactions in certain individuals. Check the package label when available or consult your doctor or pharmacist.

## Drug Interactions:

Tell your doctor or pharmacist if you are taking or planning to take any over-the-counter or prescription medications or dietary supplements with vitamin D. Doses of one or both drugs may need to be modified or a different drug may need to be prescribed. The following drugs and drug classes interact with vitamin D.

cholestyramine (eg, *Questran*)
digitalis glycosides (eg, digoxin)
magnesium-containing
 antacids (eg, *Maalox*)
mineral oil

phosphate or vitamin D-related
 compounds
thiazide diuretics (eg, hydrochlorothiazide)
verapamil (eg, *Calan*)

## Side Effects:

Every drug is capable of producing side effects. Many vitamin D users experience no, or minor, side effects. The frequency and severity of side effects depend on many factors, including dose, duration of therapy, and individual susceptibility. Possible side effects include:

*Digestive Tract:* Loss of appetite; stomach pain or cramps; constipation; digestive tract bleeding; excessive thirst; nausea; vomiting; dry mouth; metallic taste.

*Nervous System:* Weakness; irritability; headache; drowsiness.

*Renal:* Increased urinary frequency; increased urination at night.

*Other:* Muscle or bone pain; increased blood pressure; itching; runny nose; sensitivity to light; weight loss; decreased sex drive; pneumonia; chills; fever; flu-like symptoms; irregular heartbeat; fluid retention; increased body temperature; pounding in the chest.

## Guidelines for Use:

- Dosage will be individualized. Do not change the dose or stop taking unless advised to do so by your doctor.
- *Recommended Dietary Allowances (RDAs) —* Adults (24 years of age or older): 200 IU
- *Calciferol in oil injection* - For intramuscular administration only. Do not administer intravenously or subcutaneously.
- *Common sources of vitamin D –* Fortified milk and milk products, eggs, fish liver oils (eg, cod oil), livers of animals that eat fish.
- The total amount of vitamin D taken each day includes both dietary intake and supplements. Do not take more than the RDA unless advised to do so by your doctor.
- Carefully measure liquid doses of vitamin D-containing products because some doseforms are very concentrated. Do not exceed recommended volume.
- Eating a balanced diet and periodic exposure to sunlight usually satisfies normal vitamin D requirements. Never use vitamin supplements as a substitute for a balanced diet.
- Compliance with dosage instructions, diet, and calcium supplementation are essential, especially in patients undergoing dialysis.
- Swallow tablets and capsules whole. Do not crush or chew.
- Drink plenty of fluids while taking vitamin D.
- Overdosage of any form of vitamin D is dangerous. Discontinue therapy and notify your doctor if any of the following occurs: Weakness, drowsiness, headache, metallic taste, loss of appetite, weight loss, nausea, vomiting, stomach pain or cramps, diarrhea, constipation, excessive thirst, excessive urine output, dry mouth, muscle or bone pain. These may be caused by high blood calcium levels.
- Avoid use of nonprescription drugs, including magnesium-containing antacids, multivitamins containing vitamin D, and natural products unless such use has been discussed with your doctor.
- Patients with digestive tract, liver, or biliary disease associated with vitamin D malabsorption require intramuscular administration of vitamin D.
- The effects of dihydrotachysterol can last for up to 1 month after stopping treatment. The effects of ergocalciferol can last for 2 or more months after stopping treatment.
- Avoid simultaneous use of mineral oil while taking vitamin D products.
- Lab tests may be required to monitor treatment. Be sure to keep appointments.
- Store at controlled room temperature (59° to 86°F). Protect from heat and light.

*If you have any questions, consult your doctor, pharmacist, or health care provider.*

| Generic Name<br>*Brand Name Examples* | Supplied As | Generic<br>Available |
|---|---|---|
| *otc* **Vitamin E**[1] | | |
| *Dry E 400, E-Pherol* | **Tablets:** 100 IU, 200 IU,<br>400 IU, 500 IU, 800 IU | Yes |
| *Vitamin E 400 I.U.,*<br>*Vitamin E 1000 I.U., Vita-*<br>*Plus E* | **Capsules:** 200 IU, 400 IU,<br>1000 IU | Yes |
| *d'ALPHA E 400 ,*<br>*d'ALPHA E 1000, E-400*[2]*,*<br>*Formula E-400, Mixed E*<br>*400, Mixed E 1000* | **Softgels:** 100 IU, 200 IU,<br>400 IU, 600 IU, 1000 IU | Yes |
| *Aquavit-E* | **Drops:** 15 IU/0.3 mL | No |
| *Vitamin E* | **Liquid:** 1150 IU/1.25 mL | Yes |

[1] The exact number of IU per mg of vitamin E varies depending on the vitamin E source. One mg of vitamin E equals 0.9 to 1.5 IU of vitamin E.
[2] Also available with 50 mcg of selenium.

For a complete listing of Recommended Dietary Allowances, see the RDA table.

## Type of Drug:
Fat-soluble vitamin; essential vitamin with antioxidant properties.

## How the Drug Works:
Vitamin E prevents destructive "oxidation" reactions in the body. It helps red blood cells maintain their integrity, decreases platelet clumping, and may be an important biochemical component of certain human enzyme systems.

## Uses:
A dietary supplement used to treat or prevent vitamin E deficiency.

*Unlabeled Use(s):* Occasionally doctors may prescribe vitamin E for premature infants to prevent bleeding in the brain and for those on oxygen therapy to reduce the possibility of lung and eye problems. It has also been used in cancer, skin problems, night leg cramps, sexual problems, heart disease, aging, premenstrual problems, and to increase athletic performance.

## Precautions:
*Do not use in the following situations:* Intravenously.

*Multiple vitamin deficiencies:* It is unusual for vitamin E deficiency to occur alone. Other vitamins may be needed; consult your pharmacist or doctor.

*Breastfeeding:* Vitamin E appears in breast milk. Consult your doctor before you begin breastfeeding.

## Drug Interactions:

Tell your doctor or pharmacist if you are taking or if you are planning to take any over-the-counter or prescription medications or dietary supplements with vitamin E. Doses of one or both drugs may need to be modified or a different drug may need to be prescribed. Oral anticoagulants (eg, *Coumadin*) interact with vitamin E.

## Side Effects:

Every drug is capable of producing side effects. Many vitamin E users experience no, or minor, side effects. The frequency and severity of side effects depend on many factors including dose, duration of therapy, and individual susceptibility. Possible symptoms of toxicity include: Nausea; gas; diarrhea; unusual tiredness or weakness; stomach cramps; headache; blurred vision; breast enlargement.

## Guidelines for Use:

- Most people on balanced diets do not need vitamin supplements. People with cystic fibrosis or gastrointestinal diseases who are unable to digest or absorb fats, premature or underfed infants, and people with specific blood disorders may be at risk for vitamin E deficiency.
- *Recommended Dietary Allowances (RDAs) —*
  Adult males: 15 IU
  Adult females: 12 IU
- *Vitamin E drops —* Use included marked dropper to measure dose. Drops may be administered directly on the tongue or mixed with liquid (eg, milk, formula, juice) or semi-liquid food (eg, applesauce, cereal).
- Swallow capsules whole. Do not crush or chew.
- *Common sources of vitamin E –* Vegetable oils, seeds, corn, soy, margarine, leafy vegetables, milk, eggs, meat, whole wheat flour, and nuts. Consider all possible dietary sources of vitamin E before using a supplement.
- Store in a dry, air-tight container.

*If you have any questions, consult your doctor, pharmacist, or health care provider.*

| Generic Name<br>*Brand Name Examples* | Supplied As (mg of<br>elemental calcium/dose unit) | Generic<br>Available |
|---|---|---|
| *otc* **Calcium Glubionate**<br>(6.5% Ca) | | |
| *Calcionate, Calciquid* | **Syrup:** 115 mg Ca/5 mL | No |
| *otc* **Calcium Gluconate**<br>(9.3% Ca) | **Tablets:** 50 mg Ca, 60 mg Ca,<br>90 mg Ca | Yes |
| | **Powder:** 89 mg Ca/g | Yes |
| *otc* **Calcium Lactate**<br>(13% Ca) | **Tablets:** 84 mg Ca | Yes |
| | **Capsules:** 96 mg Ca | Yes |
| *otc* **Calcium Citrate** (21% Ca) | | |
| *Cal-Citrate, Citracal,*<br>*Citracal Caplets + D* | **Tablets:** 200 mg Ca, 250 mg<br>Ca, 315 mg Ca | Yes |
| *Citracal Liquitab[1]* | **Tablets, effervescent:**<br>500 mg Ca | No |
| *otc* **Dibasic Calcium Phos-<br>phate Dihydrate**<br>(23% Ca) | **Tablets:** 112 mg Ca | Yes |
| *otc* **Tribasic Calcium Phos-<br>phate** (39% Ca) | | |
| *Posture, Posture-D* | **Tablets:** 600 mg Ca | No |
| *Posture-D* | **Tablets, chewable:** 600 mg Ca | No |
| *otc* **Calcium Carbonate**<br>(40% Ca) | **Powder:** 800 mg Ca/g | Yes |
| *Cal-Carb Forte, Caltrate*<br>*600, Caltrate 600+D, Cal-*<br>*trate 600 Plus, Caltrate*<br>*600+Soy, Nephro-Calci,*<br>*Os-Cal 250+D[2], Os-Cal*<br>*500[2], Os-Cal 500+D[2],*<br>*Oysco 500[2], Oyst-Cal*<br>*500[2], Oyst-Cal-D[2], Oyst-*<br>*Cal-D 500[2], Oystercal*<br>*500, Oystercal-D 250* | **Tablets:** 250 mg Ca, 500 mg<br>Ca, 600 mg Ca | Yes |
| *Florical* | **Tablets:** 145 mg Ca with<br>8.3 mg sodium fluoride | No |

| Generic Name<br>*Brand Name Examples* | Supplied As (mg of<br>elemental calcium/dose unit) | Generic<br>Available |
|---|---|---|
| *Alka-Mints, Amitone, Cal-*<br>*Carb Forte, Cal-Mint, Cal-*<br>*cichew, Caltrate 600 Plus,*<br>*Chooz[1], Dicarbosil, Malla-*<br>*mint, Os-Cal, Rolaids[2],*<br>*Tums, Tums 500, Tums*<br>*E-X[2], Tums E-X Sugar*<br>*Free, Tums Ultra[2]* | **Tablets, chewable:** 168 mg<br>Ca, 200 mg Ca, 220 mg Ca,<br>260 mg Ca, 300 mg Ca,<br>340 mg Ca, 350 mg Ca,<br>400 mg Ca, 500 mg Ca,<br>600 mg Ca | Yes |
| *Super Calcium 1200* | **Capsules:** 600 mg Ca | No |
| *Florical* | **Capsules:** 145 mg Ca with<br>8.3 mg sodium fluoride | No |

[1] Contains phenylalanine.
[2] Contains tartrazine.

The amount of calcium provided by a product varies with the calcium salt (formulation) contained in the product. For example, the salt calcium glubionate contains 6.5% calcium (Ca), while the calcium carbonate formulations are 40% Ca. The percentage of calcium represents elemental, or active calcium. Therefore, 1500 mg of calcium glubionate only contains 98 mg of elemental calcium, while 1500 mg of calcium carbonate contains 600 mg of elemental calcium.

For a complete listing of Recommended Dietary Allowances, see the RDA table.

## Type of Drug:

Mineral; calcium supplement.

## How the Drug Works:

Calcium is the fifth most abundant element in the body. The majority is in the bones. It is essential for normal development and maintenance of bones; normal functioning of nerves and muscles; normal heart functioning; normal blood clotting; and normal functioning of a variety of cells, glands, and enzyme systems.

## Uses:

As a dietary supplement, especially at times when dietary intake may be inadequate (eg, children and teens, the elderly, during pregnancy and breastfeeding, after menopause, patients with kidney failure).

To treat and prevent calcium deficiency (eg, osteoporosis, rickets, osteomalacia, hypoparathyroidism).

To treat muscle cramps caused by low calcium levels.

*Unlabeled Use(s):* Doctors may occasionally prescribe calcium for high blood pressure in patients with calcium deficiency.

## Precautions:

*Do not use in the following situations:*
    high blood calcium levels
    kidney stones
    low blood phosphate levels

*Use with caution in the following situations:*
    constipation
    kidney disease (calcium citrate only)
    low stomach acid levels (all except calcium lactate)

*Pregnancy and breastfeeding:* Do not take more than the RDA without first contacting your doctor.

*Adequate calcium intake:* Adequate calcium intake is particularly important during periods of bone growth in childhood and adolescence, and during pregnancy and breastfeeding. An adequate intake of calcium is also necessary in adults, especially those over 40 years of age, to help prevent the development of osteoporosis.

*Vitamin D:* Vitamin D facilitates the absorption of calcium from the digestive tract. A vitamin D deficiency can interfere with calcium balance in the body. This is a concern for the elderly because of limited exposure to the sun, reduced intake of dairy products, and decreased absorption because of the natural aging process. Consult your doctor before increasing vitamin D intake above the RDA.

*Phenylketonuria:* Some of these products contain phenylalanine. Check package label when available or consult your doctor or pharmacist.

*Lab tests* may be required to monitor therapy. Tests may include kidney function and calcium and phosphate blood levels.

*Tartrazine:* Some of these products contain tartrazine (FD&C Yellow No. 5), which may cause allergic reactions in certain individuals. Check package label when available or consult your doctor or pharmacist.

## Drug Interactions:

Tell your doctor or pharmacist if you are taking or if you are planning to take any over-the-counter or prescription medications or dietary supplements with calcium. Doses of one or both drugs may need to be modified or a different drug may need to be prescribed. The following drugs and drug classes interact with calcium:

atenolol (eg, *Tenormin*)
fiber (eg, bran)
iron salts (eg, *Feosol*)
hydantoins (eg, phenytoin)
quinolone antibiotics (eg, ciprofloxacin)
sodium polystyrene sulfonate
  (eg, *Kayexalate*)

tetracycline (eg, *Achromycin V*)
thiazide diuretics
  (eg, hydrochlorothiazide)
valproic acid (eg, *Depakote*)
verapamil (eg, *Calan*)

## Side Effects:

Every drug is capable of producing side effects. Many calcium users experience no, or minor, side effects. The frequency and severity of side effects depend on many factors including dose, duration of therapy, and individual susceptibility. Possible side effects of high calcium levels include: Loss of appetite; nausea; vomiting; dry mouth; increased urination; constipation; stomach pain; thirst; confusion; delirium.

## Guidelines for Use:

- Calcium products are confusing. Calcium salts and elemental, or active, calcium vary from product to product. Read the "Supplemental Facts" on the package to determine the serving size and amount of elemental calcium per serving.
- Divide total daily dose into 2 or 3 separate doses.
- Take with a glass of water with or after meals to increase absorption by the body.
- Make sure you are taking your RDA of vitamin D every day. If you are taking a multivitamin containing vitamin D you may not need a calcium product that also contains vitamin D. Do not exceed the RDA of vitamin D without consulting your doctor.
- Some tablets and capsules are larger than others. Ease of swallowing may be a consideration in product selection.
- *Chewable tablets* — Chew well before swallowing. May be followed with a glass of water.
- *Effervescent tablets* — Allow the tablet to stop fizzing before taking.
- Notify your doctor if loss of appetite, nausea, vomiting, constipation, stomach pain, dry mouth, thirst, or increased urination occurs.
- Do not take more than 2000 mg of elemental calcium daily (including calcium in diet, vitamins, and supplements), unless advised to do so by your doctor.
- *Recommended Dietary Allowances (RDA)* —
  Adult males: 1200 mg
  Adult females: 1200 mg
- *Common sources of calcium* — Dairy products, calcium fortified foods, and some leafy green vegetables (eg, broccoli, kale, collards).
- Products derived from bonemeal or dolomite have been reported to contain toxic metals (eg, lead, arsenic, mercury). These products have been associated with problems involving the nervous system, digestive system, skin, and blood. Some health authorities suggest avoiding these products.

*If you have any questions, consult your doctor, pharmacist, or health care provider.*

| | Brand Name Examples | Electrolyte content (mEq/L) | | | | Calories/ fl. oz. |
|---|---|---|---|---|---|---|
| | | Sodium | Potassium | Chloride | Citrate | |
| otc | Rehydralyte Solution | 75 | 20 | 65 | 30 | 3 |
| otc | Infalyte Oral Solution | 50 | 25 | 45 | 34 | 4.2 |
| otc | Pediatric Electrolyte Solution | 45 | 20 | 35 | 48 | 3 |
| otc | Gerber Pediatric Electrolyte Solution, Pedialyte Freezer Pops, Pedialyte Solution | 45 | 20 | 35 | 30 | 3 |

## Type of Drug:

Electrolyte solutions and oral rehydration solutions.

## How the Drug Works:

Used properly, mixtures with electrolytes, water, and sugar prevent dehydration (fluid loss) or achieve rehydration and maintain strength and a feeling of well-being. They contain sodium, chloride, potassium, and bicarbonate to replace depleted electrolytes and restore acid-base balance and sugar, which aids in sodium and water absorption by the body.

## Uses:

For maintenance of water and electrolytes following corrective intravenous therapy for severe diarrhea, for maintenance to replace mild-to-moderate fluid loss when food and liquid intake are discontinued, and for the restoration of fluid and electrolytes lost in diarrhea and vomiting in infants and children.

## Precautions:

*Do not use in the following situations:*

diarrhea, severe and continuing
kidney disease, severe
obstructed bowel

shock, prolonged
vomiting, severe and
unremitting

*Pregnancy and breastfeeding:* A pregnant or breastfeeding woman should consult a doctor before using these products.

## Guidelines for Use:

- Dosage will be individualized. Follow the package directions or your doctor's instructions when using these products.
- Use only the recommended volumes to avoid excessive electrolyte ingestion.
- Do not mix with other electrolyte-containing liquids (eg, milk, fruit juices, sports drinks).
- Store opened solutions in the refrigerator. Discard any remaining solution after 48 hours.

*If you have any questions, consult your doctor, pharmacist, or health care provider.*

| Generic Name<br>*Brand Name Examples* | Supplied As | Generic<br>Available |
|---|---|---|
| Rx **Fluoride, Oral** | **Drops**: 0.125 mg/drop (from ≈ 0.275 mg sodium fluoride) | Yes |
| *Fluoritab, Luride Lozi-Tabs* | **Tablets, chewable**: 0.25 mg (from 0.55 mg sodium fluoride) | No |
| *Fluoritab, Luride Lozi-Tabs, Pharmaflur 1.1* | **Tablets, chewable**: 0.5 mg (from 1.1 mg sodium fluoride) | Yes |
| *Fluoritab, Flura-Loz, Luride Lozi-Tabs, Pharmaflur* | **Tablets, chewable** 1 mg (from 2.2 mg sodium fluoride) | Yes |
| *Fluoritab* | **Drops**: 0.25 mg/drop (from 0.55 mg sodium fluoride) | No |
| *Luride, Pediaflor* | **Drops**: 0.5 mg /mL (from 1.1 mg sodium fluoride) | Yes |
| **Fluoride, Topical** | | |
| otc *ACT[1], ACT for Kids, Fluorigard[1]* | **Rinse**: 0.02% (from 0.05% sodium fluoride) | No |
| otc *Phos-Flur* | **Rinse**: 0.044% sodium fluoride, acidulated phosphate fluoride | No |
| Rx *Fluorinse* | **Rinse**: 0.09% (from 0.2% sodium fluoride) | No |
| Rx *Gel-Kam, PerioMed* | **Rinse**: 0.1% when diluted (from 0.63% stannous fluoride) | No |
| Rx *PreviDent[2]* | **Rinse**: 0.2% neutral sodium fluoride | No |
| Rx *Gel-Tin, Just for Kids, OMNI* | **Gel**: 0.1% (from 0.4% stannous fluoride) | No |
| otc *Stop* | **Gel**: 0.1% (from 0.4% stannous fluoride) | No |
| Rx *Karigel, Karigel Maintenance Neutral, PreviDent, SF 1.1%* | **Gel**: 0.5% (from 1.1% sodium fluoride) | No |
| Rx *NeutraCare, Phos-Flur* | **Gel**: 0.5% (from 1.1% sodium fluoride and acidulated phosphate fluoride) | No |
| Rx *Thera-Flur-N* | **Gel drops**: 0.5% (from 1.1% sodium fluoride) | No |
| Rx *PreviDent 5000 Plus, SF 5000 Plus* | **Cream**: 1.1% sodium fluoride | No |

[1] Contains tartrazine.
[2] Contains alcohol.

The amount of fluoride provided by a product varies with the fluoride salt (formulation) contained in the product. The table above lists the fluoride salts by the amount of fluoride contained in the formulation.

## Type of Drug:

Mineral.

## How the Drug Works:

Fluoride acts on teeth before (tablets, drops) and after (rinses, gels, creams) they erupt to make them more resistant to cavities by increasing tooth resistance to acid and bacteria decay.

## Uses:

To help prevent cavities when water supplies are low in fluoride (0.7 parts per million [ppm] or less), to prevent decalcification under and around orthodontic brackets, and to control rampant dental decay after xerostomia (dry mouth)-producing radiotherapy of head and neck tumors.

*Unlabeled Use(s):* Occasionally doctors may prescribe sodium fluoride for osteoporosis.

## Precautions:

*Do not use in the following situations:*
allergy to the drug or any of its ingredients
drinking water with a fluoride content greater than 0.7 ppm
low-sodium diet

*Concurrent use with fluoridated drinking water:* Fluoride tablets and drops provide systemic fluoride to the body. Fluoridated drinking water also provides systemic fluoride. Excessive fluoride ingestion can damage the teeth (dental fluorosis). Depending on the amount of fluoride in your drinking water (eg, 0.7 ppm), some of these products should not be used or the dose should be reduced. If you move from one community to another, fluoridation levels may change and dosage adjustments will need to be made. Check with your doctor or dentist. This is not a concern with topical fluoride products.

*Gum tissues:* Gum tissues may be sensitive to some flavors or to the alcohol contained in some of the topical products.

*Pregnancy:* There are no adequate and well-controlled studies in pregnant women. Use only if clearly needed and the potential benefits to the mother outweigh the possible risks to the fetus.

*Breastfeeding:* It is not known if fluoride appears in breast milk. Consult your doctor before you begin breastfeeding.

*Children:* Do not use drops or chewable tablets in children under 6 months of age. Consult your doctor before using a rinse in a child under 6 years of age. Use of a cream, rinse, or gel in pediatric patients should be supervised by an adult to prevent swallowing of the product. Do not use topical products in children under 6 years of age, unless advised to do so by your doctor.

*Tartrazine:* Some of these products may contain the dye tartrazine (FD&C Yellow No. 5), which can cause allergic reactions in certain individuals. Check package label when available or consult your doctor or pharmacist.

## Drug Interactions:

Tell your doctor or pharmacist if you are taking or if you are planning to take any over-the-counter or prescription medications or dietary supplements with fluoride. Doses of one or both drugs may need to be modified or a different drug may need to be prescribed. Dairy products and calcium supplements may interact with fluoride drops and tablets.

## Side Effects:

Every drug is capable of producing side effects. Many fluoride users experience no, or minor, side effects. The frequency and severity of side effects depend on many factors including dose, duration of therapy, and individual susceptibility. Possible side effects include:

*Other:* Rash; gum irritation (topical products only).

## Guidelines for Use:

- Use exactly as directed by your doctor or dental professional.
- Do not stop using or change the dose, unless advised to do so by your doctor.
- For best results, do not eat, drink, or rinse mouth for 30 minutes after topical application.
- Do not swallow topical doseforms.
- *Tablets and drops* — Do not eat or drink dairy products within 1 hour of administration. Take with meals if stomach upset occurs.
- *Tablets* — Dissolve in the mouth, chew, swallow whole, add to drinking water or fruit juice, or add to water for use in infant formulas or other nondairy food.
- *Drops* — Take orally, undiluted, or mix with fluids or nondairy food.
- *Cream* — Use once a day in place of your regular toothpaste, unless advised otherwise by your dentist. Brush thoroughly for 2 minutes, then spit out. Pediatric patients 6 to 16 years of age should rinse out their mouth thoroughly after use.
- *Gel* — Once daily, following brushing and flossing, apply with a toothbrush or mouth tray and allow to remain on teeth for 1 minute and then spit out. Pediatric patients 6 to 16 years of age should rinse out their mouth thoroughly after use.
- *Gel drops* — Apply once daily with applicators supplied by your dentist. Apply 4 to 8 drops as required to cover the inner surface of each applicator. Spread gel drops with tip of bottle. Place applicator over upper and lower teeth at the same time. Bite down lightly for 6 minutes. Remove applicators and rinse mouth. Clean applicators with cold water.
- *Rinse* — Use once daily or as directed by your dental professional. Most effective immediately after brushing and flossing just prior to bedtime. Vigorously swish between teeth for 1 minute. Spit out remaining solution. Do not swallow rinse. Do not dilute acidulated gels or rinses in a porcelain or glass container; use plastic.
- Notify your dentist if your teeth become spotted or stained.
- Fluoride helps to reduce cavity formation but does not replace good oral hygiene practices (eg, brushing, flossing). See your dental professional regularly.
- Store at controlled room temperature (59° to 86°F).

*If you have any questions, consult your doctor, pharmacist, or health care provider.*

# MINERALS AND ELECTROLYTES — MAGNESIUM

| Generic Name<br>*Brand Name Examples* | Supplied As | Generic<br>Available |
|---|---|---|
| *otc* **Magnesium Amino Acid Chelate** | | |
| *Chelated Magnesium, Magnesium AA* | **Tablets:** 100 mg | No |
| *otc* **Magnesium Carbonate** | | |
| *Mag-Carb* | **Capsules:** 72 mg | No |
| *otc* **Magnesium Chloride Hexahydrate** | | |
| *Mag-SR, Slow-Mag* | **Tablets, sustained release:** 64 mg | No |
| *otc* **Magnesium Citrate** | **Tablets:** 100 mg | Yes |
| *otc* **Magnesium Gluconate Dihydrate** | | |
| *Almora, Magonate* | **Tablets:** 27 mg | Yes |
| *Magtrate* | **Tablets**: 29 mg | No |
| *Magonate* | **Liquid**: 54 mg/5 mL | No |
| *Magonate Natal* | **Liquid**: 3.52 mg/mL | No |
| *otc* **Magnesium Lactate** | | |
| *Mag-Tab SR* | **Tablets, sustained release**: 84 mg | No |
| *otc* **Magnesium Oxide** | | |
| *Mag-Ox 400* | **Tablets**: 241.3 mg | Yes |
| *Uro-Mag* | **Capsules**: 84.5 mg | No |

The amount of magnesium provided by a product varies with the magnesium salt (formulation) contained in the product. The table above lists the magnesium salts by the amount of magnesium contained in the formulation.

For a complete listing of Recommended Dietary Allowances, see the RDA table at the beginning of this chapter.

## Type of Drug:
Electrolyte. Dietary supplement.

## How the Drug Works:
Magnesium is needed for normal enzyme activity, muscle contraction, and nerve conduction.

## Uses:
To reverse or prevent magnesium deficiency. Magnesium deficiency may occur due to prolonged diarrhea, vomiting, chronic alcoholism, malabsorption syndromes, hemodialysis, kidney disease, electrolyte abnormalities, or diuretic use.

*Unlabeled Use(s):* Occasionally doctors may prescribe pyridoxine/magnesium oxide combinations to prevent recurrence of calcium oxalate kidney stones.

## Precautions:

*Use with caution in the following situations:* Kidney disease.

## Drug Interactions:

Tell your doctor or pharmacist if you are taking or planning to take any over-the-counter or prescription medications or dietary supplements with magnesium. Doses of one or both drugs may need to be modified or a different drug may need to be prescribed. The following drugs and drug classes interact with magnesium:

aminoquinolones (eg, chloroquine)
fluoroquinolones (eg, ciprofloxacin)

nitrofurantoin (eg, *Macrodantin*)
penicillamine (eg, *Cuprimine*)
tetracyclines (eg, oxytetracycline)

## Side Effects:

Every drug is capable of producing side effects. Many magnesium users experience no, or minor, side effects. The frequency and severity of side effects depend on many factors including dose, duration of therapy and individual susceptibility. Possible side effects at high doses include diarrhea.

---

## Guidelines for Use:

- Dosage will be individualized.
- Excessive doses may cause diarrhea and gastrointestinal irritation.
- *Recommended Dietary Allowances (RDAs)* —
  Adult males: 350 to 400 mg
  Adult females: 280 to 300 mg
- Swallow sustained-release tablets whole. Do not crush or chew.
- *Common sources of magnesium* — Bananas, avocados, roasted peanuts, legumes, unmilled grains, green vegetables.
- Magnesium-containing antacids may also be used as dietary supplements. See the Antacids monograph in the Gastrointestinal Drugs chapter.
- Store at controlled room temperature (59° to 86°F) in a dry place. Keep out of the reach of children.

---

*If you have any questions, consult your doctor, pharmacist, or health care provider.*

| Generic Name<br>*Brand Name Examples* | Supplied As | Generic<br>Available |
|---|---|---|
| *Rx* **Potassium Chloride** | | |
| *K⁺8, K⁺10, K-Dur 10, K-Dur 20, K-Tab, Kaon-Cl 10, Klor-Con 8, Klor-Con 10, Klotrix, Slow-K* | **Tablets, controlled release:** 8 mEq, 10 mEq, 20 mEq | Yes |
| *K-Lyte/Cl, K-Lyte/Cl 50* | **Effervescent tablets:** 25 mEq, 50 mEq | No |
| *Micro-K Extencaps, Micro-K 10 Extencaps* | **Capsules, controlled release:** 8 mEq, 10 mEq | Yes |
| *Kaochlor¹, Kaochlor-SF, Kaon-Cl, Kay Ciel, Rum-K* | **Liquid:** 15 mEq/5 mL, 20 mEq/5 mL, 30 mEq/5 mL | Yes |
| *K-Lor, Kay Ciel, Klor-Con, Klor-Con/25* | **Powder:** 20 mEq/packet, 25 mEq/packet | Yes |
| *otc* **Potassium Gluconate** | **Tablets:** 2.1 mEq | Yes |
| *otc Potassium 99* | **Tablets:** 2.5 mEq | Yes |
| *otc K-99* | **Capsules:** 2.5 mEq | No |
| *Rx Kaon Elixir* | **Liquid:** 20 mEq/15 mL | Yes |
| **Potassium Combina-<br>tions²** | | |
| *Rx Effer-K, K-Lyte DS, Klor-Con/EF* | **Effervescent tablets:** 25 mEq, 50 mEq | Yes |
| *Rx Tri-K* | **Liquid:** 45 mEq/15 mL | No |

¹ Contains tartrazine.
² As potassium gluconate, potassium acetate, potassium bicarbonate, or potassium citrate.

The amount of potassium provided by a product varies with the potassium salt (formulation) contained in the product. For example, the salt potassium chloride contains 13.4 mEq potassium per gram of salt, while potassium gluconate contains only 4.5 mEq potassium per gram of salt.

## Type of Drug:
Essential electrolyte. Dietary supplement.

## How the Drug Works:
Potassium is involved in many biochemical processes in the body. It is required for normal functioning of cells, nerve conduction, muscle contractions, kidney function, and acid-base balance.

## Uses:
To treat or prevent hypokalemia (low potassium blood levels) when dietary intake is inadequate. Low potassium levels may also be caused by some diseases, severe or prolonged episodes of vomiting or diarrhea, or by certain medicines (eg, potassium-losing diuretics). Symptoms of low potassium levels include weakness, constipation, fatigue, or weakening of reflexes.

## Precautions:

*Do not use in the following situations:*

allergy to potassium supplements or any of their ingredients

Addison's disease, untreated

anticholinergic drugs, concurrent use

conditions predisposing to high potassium levels (eg, dehydration, heat cramps)

delay in passage through gastrointestinal tract (tablets only)

high blood potassium levels

kidney disease, severe

*Use with caution in the following situations:*

digestive tract diseases

kidney disease

potassium-sparing diuretics, concurrent use (solid doseforms only)

*Digestive tract disease:* Solid doseforms, especially enteric-coated products, of potassium supplements should not be used by any patient who may have difficulty passing the tablet through the digestive tract. Some preparations may cause ulcers on the esophagus (food pipe), stomach, and intestines. Potassium supplementation should be taken as a liquid preparation by these individuals.

*Heart patients:* Too much or too little potassium can adversely affect the heart. Be sure that your doctor and pharmacist are aware of any heart medications you are taking.

*Pregnancy:* There are no adequate and well-controlled studies in pregnant women. Use only if clearly needed and potential benefits to the mother outweigh the possible hazards to the fetus.

*Breastfeeding:* Safety for use during breastfeeding has not been established. Consult your doctor before you begin breastfeeding.

*Children:* Safety and effectiveness in children have not been established.

*Lab tests* may be required to monitor therapy. Tests may include serum potassium levels, electrolytes, and electrocardiograms.

*Tartrazine:* Some of these products may contain the dye tartrazine (FD&C Yellow No. 5), which can cause allergic reactions in certain individuals. Check package label when available or consult your doctor or pharmacist.

## Drug Interactions:

Tell your doctor or pharmacist if you are taking or planning to take any over-the-counter or prescription medications or dietary supplements with potassium supplements. Doses of one or both drugs may need to be modified or a different drug may need to be prescribed. The following drugs and drug classes interact with potassium supplements:

ACE inhibitors (eg, captopril, enalapril)

anticholinergics (eg, *Banthine*) (solid doseforms only)

potassium-sparing diuretics (eg, amiloride)

salt substitutes

## Side Effects:

Every drug is capable of producing side effects. Many potassium users experience no, or minor, side effects. The frequency and severity of side effects depend on many factors including dose, duration of therapy, and individual susceptibility. Possible side effects include:

*Digestive Tract:* Stomach pain or discomfort; nausea; vomiting; black, tarry stools; throat pain when swallowing; diarrhea; gas.

*Nervous System:* Confusion; unusual tiredness or weakness; anxiety.

*Respiratory System:* Shortness of breath; breathing difficulties.

*Other:* Tingling or numbness of hands, feet, or lips; feeling of heaviness or weakness of the arms or legs; high blood potassium levels; irregular heart rhythm.

## Guidelines for Use:

- Dosage will be individualized.
- Do not stop taking or change the dose, unless advised to do so by your doctor.
- May cause stomach upset. Take after meals or with food and with a full glass of water or other liquid.
- Do not crush or chew tablets or capsules. Swallow whole.
- *Liquids, powders, and effervescent tablets* — Must be dissolved or diluted before using. The package label will recommend the amount (eg, 4 ounces) of cold water, juice, or other beverage in which the medicine should be dissolved or mixed. After thoroughly dissolving or mixing, drink slowly over a 5- to 10-minute period.
- *Wax matrix products* — Following the release of potassium chloride, the wax matrix of the tablets, which is not absorbable, is excreted in the stool. This is normal and no cause for concern.
- Do not use salt substitutes, which contain additional potassium, except on the advice of your doctor.
- Notify your doctor immediately if you experience tingling of the hands and feet; abnormal heartbeat; unusual tiredness or weakness; a feeling of heaviness in the arms or legs; severe vomiting; stomach pain or swelling; black, tarry stools; indigestion; or if you have trouble swallowing the tablets or capsules or they seem to stick in your throat.
- Over-the-counter (OTC) potassium products contain very little potassium and cannot be substituted for prescription-strength potassium products.
- Too much or too little potassium can adversely affect the heart. Be sure your doctor and pharmacist are aware of any heart medications you are taking.
- *Common sources of potassium* — Beef, veal, ham, chicken, turkey, fish, milk, bananas, dates, prunes, raisins, avocado, watermelon, cantaloupes, apricots, molasses, beans, yams, broccoli, brussel sprouts, lentils, potatoes, spinach.
- Lab tests may be required to monitor therapy. Be sure to keep appointments.
- Keep out of the reach of children.

*If you have any questions, consult your doctor, pharmacist, or health care provider.*

| Generic Name<br>*Brand Name Examples* | Supplied As | Generic<br>Available |
|---|---|---|
| *otc* **Zinc Gluconate**<br>(14.3% zinc) | **Tablets:** 10 mg, 15 mg, 30 mg,<br>50 mg, 100 mg | Yes |
| | **Lozenges:** 10.5 mg, 23 mg,<br>30 mg | Yes |
| **Zinc Sulfate** (23% zinc) | | |
| *otc* *Orazinc 110, Zinc 15* | **Tablets:** 15 mg, 25 mg | No |
| *otc* *Orazinc 220, Zinc-220* | **Capsules:** 50 mg | Yes |
| *Rx* *Zincate* | **Capsules:** 50 mg | Yes |

The amount of zinc provided by a product varies with the zinc salt (formulation) contained in the product. For example, the salt zinc sulfate contains 23% zinc and zinc gluconate contains 14.3% zinc. The table above lists the zinc products by the amount of zinc contained in the product.

For a complete listing of Recommended Dietary Allowances, see the RDA table at the beginning of this chapter.

## Type of Drug:
Mineral; trace element.

## How the Drug Works:
Zinc is needed for normal tissue growth and repair and for protein and carbohydrate metabolism.

## Uses:
To treat or prevent zinc deficiency. Symptoms of zinc deficiency include appetite loss; growth retardation; impaired taste or smell; hair loss; dwarfism; rashes; skin lesions; swelling or inflammation of the mouth, tongue, or eyelids; hangnails; and impaired wound healing.

*Unlabeled Use(s):* Occasionally doctors may prescribe zinc for the common cold, acrodermatitis enteropathica (a severe digestive tract and skin disorder of early childhood), delayed wound healing, acne, rheumatoid arthritis, and senile dementia.

## Precautions:
*Do not use in the following situations:* Allergy to zinc supplements or any of their ingredients.

*Pregnancy:* Because zinc deficiency is very rare, routine use of zinc supplementation during pregnancy is not recommended.

*Breastfeeding:* Breast milk concentrations of zinc decrease over time following delivery; extra dietary intake of zinc 7 mg/day for the first 6 months of breastfeeding and 4 mg/day during the second 6 months is recommended.

*Children:* Consult your doctor regarding use in children under 12 years of age.

## Drug Interactions:

Tell your doctor or pharmacist if you are taking or planning to take any over-the-counter or prescription medications or dietary supplements with oral zinc supplements. Doses of one or both drugs may need to be modified or a different drug may need to be prescribed. The following products interact with oral zinc supplements:

fluoroquinolones (eg, ciprofloxacin)
tetracyclines (eg, oxytetracycline)

## Side Effects:

Every drug is capable of producing side effects. Many zinc users experience no, or minor, side effects. The frequency and severity of side effects depend on many factors including dose, duration of therapy, and individual susceptibility. Possible side effects include:

*Digestive Tract:* Nausea; vomiting.

---

### Guidelines for Use:

- Dosage will be individualized.
- If stomach upset or nausea occurs, take with food or liquid.
- Avoid taking with foods high in bran, calcium, phosphorus, or phytate.
- Do not exceed the prescribed or recommended dose. Vomiting is likely to occur with doses greater than 2 g.
- *Recommended Dietary Allowance (RDA) —*
  Adults: 12 to 15 mg
- *Common sources of zinc —* Cooked dry beans, meat, eggs, liver, seafoods, wheat germ, whole grain products.
- Store at controlled room temperature (59° to 86°F). Protect from moisture. Keep out of the reach of children.

---

*If you have any questions, consult your doctor, pharmacist, or health care provider.*

| Vitamins A and D Combinations *Brand Name Examples* | Vitamin A (IU) | Vitamin D (IU) | Vitamin C (mg) |
|---|---|---|---|
| *otc* *Vitamin A & D Tablets* | 10,000/tablet | 400/tablet | |
| *otc* *Tri-Vi-Sol Drops, Vi-Daylin ADC Oral Solution* | 1500/mL | 400/mL | 35/mL |
| *otc* *Norwegian Cod Liver Oil Capsules* | 1250/capsule | ≈ 130/capsule | |
| *otc* *Scott's Emulsion* | 1250/5 mL | 100/5 mL | |
| *otc* *Cod Liver Oil USP, Norwegian Cod Liver Oil* | 5000/5 mL 5000/5 mL 4600/5 mL | 500/5 mL 400/5 mL 460/5 mL | |

For a complete listing of Recommended Dietary Allowances, see the RDA table at the beginning of this chapter. For more information, see the Vitamin A and Vitamin D monographs in this chapter.

## Type of Drug:
Vitamin combinations.

## Uses:
Dietary supplement.

---

**Guidelines for Use:**
- Dosage will be individualized.
- Do not exceed the recommended dose, unless advised to do so by your doctor.
- Most people on regular diets do not need vitamin supplements.
- *Capsules* — Take with meals. Store in a cool, dry place.
- *Drops* — Administer directly into mouth using dropper, or mix with formula, fruit juice, cereal, or other food. Store at room temperature. Protect from light.
- *Emulsion* — Shake well before using. Store at room temperature.
- Keep out of the reach of children.

---

*If you have any questions, consult your doctor, pharmacist, or health care provider.*

| | Vitamin B Combinations<br>*Brand Name Examples* | B$_1$<br>(mg) | B$_2$<br>(mg) | B$_3$<br>(mg) | B$_5$<br>(mg) | B$_6$<br>(mg) | B$_{12}$<br>(mcg) |
|---|---|---|---|---|---|---|---|
| *otc* | Neurodep-Caps Capsules | 125 | | | | 125 | 1000 |
| *otc* | B Complex Tablets | 25 | 25 | 100 | 25 | 25 | 25 |
| *otc* | Apatate Liquid, Apatate Tablets | 15 | | | | 0.5 | 25 |
| *otc* | Orexin Chewable Tablets | 8.1 | | | | 4.1 | 25 |
| *otc* | B-Complex and B-12 Tablets | 7 | 14 | 4.5 | | | 25 |
| *otc* | Super B Complex Capsules | 3 | 6 | 1 | | | 3 |
| *otc* | Gevrabon Liquid | 0.83 | 0.42 | 8.3 | 1.67 | 0.17 | 0.17 |
| *otc* | Brewers Yeast 500 Tablets | 0.4 | 0.1 | 1.2 | | | |
| *otc* | Natural Brewers Yeast 7½ grs Tablets | 0.12 | 0.04 | 0.4 | | | |

Content in the table above is given per serving of capsule, tablet, or teaspoon (5 milliliters). Products containing the greatest amount of Vitamin B$_1$ are listed first.

For a complete listing of Recommended Dietary Allowances, see the RDA table at the beginning of this chapter. For more information, see the Vitamin B monographs in this chapter.

## Type of Drug:
Vitamin combinations.

## Uses:
Dietary supplement.

## Guidelines for Use:
- Dosage will be individualized.
- Do not exceed the recommended dose, unless advised to do so by your doctor.
- Most people on regular diets do not need vitamin supplements.
- Store at controlled room temperature (59° to 86°F). Protect from moisture.

*If you have any questions, consult your doctor, pharmacist, or health care provider.*

| Vitamin B with C Combinations Brand Name Examples | $B_1$ (mg) | $B_2$ (mg) | $B_3$ (mg) | $B_5$ (mg) | $B_6$ (mg) | $B_{12}$ (mcg) | C (mg) |
|---|---|---|---|---|---|---|---|
| otc Optimum Stress Formula Capsules[1,2] | 75 | 37 | 150 | 75 | 45 | 25 | 600 |
| otc Enviro-Stress Tablets[1] | 50 | 50 | 100 | 50 | 50 | 25 | 600 |
| otc T-Vites Tablets | 25 | 25 | 150 | 25 | 25 | | 100 |
| otc ThexForte Caplets | 25 | 15 | 100 | 10 | 5 | | 500 |
| Rx B C w/Folic Acid Plus Tablets[2] | 20 | 20 | 100 | 25 | 25 | 50 | 500 |
| otc Vicon-C Capsules, Viogen-C Capsules | 18 | 10 | 95 | 22 | 4 | | 300 |
| Rx Berocca Tablets[1], B-Plex Tablets[1], Strovite Tablets[1,3] | 15 | 15 | 100 | 18 | 4 | 5 | 500 |
| otc Surbex-T Filmtabs | 15 | 10 | 100 | 20 | 5 | 10 | 500 |
| otc Glutofac Caplets[1] | 15 | 10 | 50 | 20 | 50 | 12 | 300 |
| otc Arcobee with C Caplets, Therapeutic B Complex with C Capsules[3], Vita-Bee w/C Captabs | 15 | 10 | 50 | 10 | 5 | | 300 |
| otc B-Complex plus C High Potency Timed-Release Tablets | 10 | 10 | 50 | 10 | 5 | 10 | 200 |
| otc Surbex with C Filmtabs | 6 | 6 | 30 | 10 | 2.5 | 5 | 250 |
| otc Nephro-Vite OTC Tablets[1] | 1.5 | 1.7 | 20 | 10 | 10 | 6 | 60 |
| Rx Nephro-Vite Rx Tablets[1] | 1.5 | 1.7 | 20 | 10 | 10 | 6 | 60 |
| Rx Nephrocaps Capsules[1] | 1.5 | 1.7 | 20 | 5 | 10 | 6 | 100 |

[1] Contains folic acid
[2] Contains iron (ferrous fumarate).
[3] Contains tartrazine.

Content in the table above is given per capsule or tablet. Products containing the greatest amount of Vitamin $B_1$ are listed first.

For a complete listing of Recommended Dietary Allowances, see the RDA table at the beginning of this chapter. For more information, see the Vitamin B and Vitamin C monographs in this chapter.

## Precautions:

*Tartrazine:* Some of these products contain the dye tartrazine (FD&C Yellow No. 5), which can cause allergic reactions in some individuals. Check package label when available or consult your doctor or pharmacist.

---

### Guidelines for Use:

- Most people on regular diets do not need vitamin supplements.
- Do not exceed the recommended dose, unless advised to do so by your doctor.
- Store at controlled room temperature (59° to 86°F) in a dry place.

---

*If you have any questions, consult your doctor, pharmacist, or health care provider.*

## Vitamin B with Folic Acid Combinations

| | Brand Name Examples | B₁ (mg) | B₂ (mg) | B₃ (mg) | B₅ (mg) | B₆ (mg) | B₁₂ (mcg) | FA (mg) | Other content |
|---|---|---|---|---|---|---|---|---|---|
| otc | Balanced B-100 Capsules, Super DEC B-100 Tablets, Vitamin B-100 Complex Tablets | 100 | 100 | 100 | 100 | 100 | 100 | 0.4 | Biotin, choline, inositol, PABA |
| otc | B-100 Ultra B Complex Timed-Release Tablets, Mega-B Tablets | 100 | 100 | 100 | 100 | 100 | 100 | 0.1 | Biotin, choline, inositol, lecithin, PABA, |
| otc | Balanced B-50 Capsules, Super Quints B-50 Tablets | 50 | 50 | 50 | 50 | 50 | 50 | 0.4 | Biotin, choline, inositol, PABA |
| otc | B-50 Caps Capsules, B-50 Super B Complex Tablets | 50 | 50 | 50 | 50 | 50 | 50 | 0.1 | Biotin, choline, inositol, lecithin,PABA |
| otc | Quin B Strong B-25 Tablets | 25 | 25 | 100 | 25 | 25 | 25 | 0.4 | Biotin, choline, inositol, PABA |
| otc | Parvlex Tablets | 20 | 20 | 20 | 10 | 10 | 50 | 0.4 | Copper, iron, manganese |
| otc | Kobee Tablets | 10 | 10 | 50 | 10 | 10 | 10 | 0.4 | Biotin, choline, inositol, PABA |
| otc | B-Complex with Vitamin B-12 Tablets | 1.5 | 1.7 | 20 | 10 | 2 | 6 | 0.4 | |
| otc | Vitamin B12 with Folic Acid Tablets | | | | | | 500 | 0.4 | |

Content in the table above given per tablet or 15 mL. Products containing the greatest amount of Vitamin B₁ are listed first.

For a complete listing of Recommended Dietary Allowances, see the RDA table. For more information, see the Vitamin B monographs in this chapter and the Folic Acid monograph in the Blood Modifiers chapter.

# VITAMIN COMBINATIONS — VITAMIN B WITH FOLIC ACID

## Type of Drug:
Vitamin and mineral combinations.

## Uses:
Dietary supplement.

---

### Guidelines for Use:
- Dosage will be individualized.
- Do not exceed the recommended dose, unless advised to do so by your doctor.
- Most people on regular diets do not need vitamin supplements.

---

*If you have any questions, consult your doctor, pharmacist, or health care provider.*

| Calcium and Vitamin D Combinations<br>*Brand Name Examples* | Elemental<br>Calcium (mg) | Vitamin<br>D<br>(IU) |
|---|---|---|
| otc *Calcium 600 mg with D Tablets, Calcium 600 with Vitamin D Tablets, Caltrate 600+D Tablets* | 600 | 200 |
| otc *Calcarb 600 with Vitamin D Tablets, Calcium 600-D Tablets, Posture D-Chewable Tablets, Posture D-Tablets* | 600 | 125 |
| otc *Os-Cal 500+D Tablets[1], Parva-Cal 500 Tablets* | 500 | 200 |
| otc *Calcium 500 mg with D Tablets[1], Oysco 500+D Tablets, Oyst-Cal-D 500 Tablets[1], Oystercal-D 500 Tablets* | 500 | 125 |
| otc *Citrus Calcium+D Tablets* | 315 | 200 |
| otc *Calcet Tablets[1]* | 300 | 200 |
| otc *Os-Cal 250+D Tablets, Oyst-Cal-D Tablets[1], Oystercal-D 250 Tablets, Oysco D Tablets* | 250 | 125 |
| otc *Parva-Cal 250 Tablets* | 250 | 100 |
| otc *Dical-D Tablets* | 117 | 133 |

[1] Contains tartrazine.

Content in the table above given per capsule or tablet. Products containing the greatest amount of elemental calcium are listed first.

A variety of calcium salts are available. Some are derived from natural products such as bone or oyster shell. Calcium carbonate and calcium phosphate products contain the highest amount of calcium per serving (approximately 40%). Calcium lactate and calcium gluconate contain the least amount of calcium per serving.

For a complete listing of Recommended Dietary Allowances, see the RDA table at the beginning of this chapter. For more information, see the Vitamin D monograph and the Calcium monograph in this chapter.

## Type of Drug:
Vitamin and mineral combinations.

## Uses:
Dietary supplement.

## Precautions:
*Tartrazine:* Some of these products contain the dye tartrazine (FD&C Yellow No. 5), which can cause allergic reactions in certain individuals. Check package label when available or consult your doctor or pharmacist.

## Guidelines for Use:

- Dosage will be individualized.
- Take in divided doses with meals to enhance absorption.
- Do not exceed the recommended dose, unless advised to do so by your doctor.
- Most people on regular diets do not need vitamin supplements.
- Store at room temperature (59° to 86°F). Keep out of the reach of children.

*If you have any questions, consult your doctor, pharmacist, or health care provider.*

| Generic Name | Supplied As | Generic Available |
|---|---|---|
| *otc* **L-Lysine** | **Tablets:** 500 mg, 1000 mg | Yes |
| | **Capsules:** 500 mg | Yes |

## Type of Drug:

Essential amino acid (an amino acid required by the body). Nutritional supplement.

## Uses:

To improve use of vegetable protein in the body.

*Unlabeled Use(s):* Occasionally doctors may recommend L-lysine for herpes simplex infections (eg, fever blisters).

---

### Guidelines for Use:

- Dosage will be individualized.
- Do not exceed the recommended dose, unless advised to do so by your doctor.
- Most people on regular diets do not need nutritional supplements.
- Store at controlled room temperature (59° to 86°F). Protect from moisture. Keep out of the reach of children.

---

*If you have any questions, consult your doctor, pharmacist, or health care provider.*

| | Brand Name Examples | Amino Acids | Vitamins/Minerals |
|---|---|---|---|
| otc | A/G-Pro | **Tablets:** 542 mg protein hydrolysate (45% amino acids), 50 mg L-lysine, 12.5 mg L-methionine | 10.33 mg $B_6$, 6.7 mg vitamin C, with copper, iodine, iron, potassium, zinc, magnesium, manganese |
| otc | Dequasine | **Tablets:** 20 mg L-lysine, 50 mg L-cysteine, 150 mg dl-methionine, 50 mg N-acetylcysteine | 200 mg vitamin C, with calcium, copper, iodine, iron, magnesium, molybendum, manganese, potassium, zinc |
| otc | Jets | **Tablets, chewable:** 300 mg L-lysine | 25 mg vitamin C, 25 mcg $B_{12}$, 5 mg $B_6$, 10 mg $B_1$ |
| otc | NeuRecover-DA | **Capsules:** 460 mg L-phenylalanine, 25 mg L-glutamine | 333.3 IU vitamin A, 2.4 mg $B_1$, 0.85 mg $B_2$, 33 mg $B_3$, 15 mg $B_5$, 3 mg $B_6$, 5 mcg, $B_{12}$, 100 mg C, 5 IU E, with folic acid, biotin, calcium, chromiun, iron, magnesium, zinc |
| otc | NeuRecover-SA | **Capsules:** 250 mg L-phenylalanine, 150 mg L-tyrosine, 50 mg L-glutamine | 167 mg vitamin $B_1$, 2.5 mg $B_2$, 16.6 mg $B_3$, 15 mg $B_5$, 3.3 mg $B_6$, 5 mcg $B_{12}$, 100 mg C, with folic acid, calcium, chromium, iron, magnesium, zinc |
| otc | NeuroSlim | **Capsules:** 500 mg D/L-phenylalanine, 15 mg L-glutamine, 25 mg L-tyrosine, 10 mg L-carnitine, 10 mg L-arginine pyroglutamate, 10 mg ornithine aspartate | 0.33 mg vitamin $B_1$, 0.5 mg $B_2$, 3.3 mg $B_3$, 0.12 mg $B_5$, 0.33 mg $B_6$, 1 mcg $B_{12}$, 5 IU E, with biotin, folic acid, iron, zinc, chromium, selenium, calcium, iodine, copper, magnesium |
| otc | PDP Liquid Protein | **Liquid:** 15 g protein (from protein hydrolysate)/30 mL | |

For a complete listing of Recommended Dietary Allowances, see the RDA table at the beginning of this chapter. For more information, see the Amino Acids monograph and the individual vitamin and mineral monographs in this chapter.

## Type of Drug:

Dietary supplement.

## Uses:

To prevent or treat a variety of rare deficiency disorders. Science-based clinical evaluations of safety and efficacy for inferred therapeutic value are lacking. Use with caution.

---

### Guidelines for Use:

- Dosage will be individualized.
- Do not exceed the recommended dose, unless advised to do so by your doctor.
- Most people on regular diets do not need dietary supplements.

---

*If you have any questions, consult your doctor, pharmacist, or health care provider.*

|  | Brand Name Examples | Supplied As |
|---|---|---|
| otc | C Factors "1000" Plus | **Tablets:** 1000 mg vitamin C, 250 mg citrus bioflavonoids complex, 50 mg rutin, 20 mg hesperidin complex |
| otc | Extra Potency Ester-C Plus | **Tablets:** 1000 mg vitamin C, 200 mg citrus bioflavonoids complex, 25 mg acerola, 25 mg rutin, 25 mg rose hips, 125 mg calcium |
| otc | Flavons | **Tablets:** 500 mg citrus bioflavonoids |
| otc | Pan-C 500 | **Tablets:** 100 mg hesperidin, 100 mg citrus bioflavonoids, and 500 mg vitamin C |
| otc | Peridin-C | **Tablets:** 150 mg hesperidin complex, 50 mg hesperidin methyl chalcone (bioflavonoids), and 200 mg vitamin C |
| otc | Quercetin | **Tablets:** 50 mg, 250 mg quercetin (from eucalyptus) |
| otc | Rutin | **Tablets:** 50 mg rutin |
| otc | Span C | **Tablets:** 300 mg citrus bioflavonoids, 200 mg vitamin C |
| otc | Tri Super Flavons | **Tablets:** 100 mg hesperidin, 900 mg citrus bioflavonoids |
| otc | Ester-C Plus 500 mg Vegicaps | **Capsules:** 500 mg vitamin C, 62 mg calcium, 25 mg citrus bioflavonoid complex, 10 mg acerola, 10 mg rose hips, 5 mg rutin |
| otc | Ester-C Plus Multi-Mineral Formula Vegicaps | **Capsules:** 425 mg vitamin C, 50 mg citrus bioflavonoid complex, 12.5 mg acerola, 12.5 mg rose hips, 5 mg rutin, 25 mg calcium, 13 mg magnesium, 12.5 mg potassium, 2.5 mg zinc |
| otc | P-1000 | **Capsules:** 1000 mg lemon bioflavonoids complex |

## Type of Drug:

Water-soluble vitamins not stored by the body. Vitamin P. Citrus bioflavonoids.

## Uses:

There is no established need for bioflavonoids in human nutrition, nor is there a recommended dietary allowance. There is little evidence that bioflavonoids are effective for any medical condition.

## Guidelines for Use:

- Dosage will be individualized.
- Do not exceed the recommended dose, unless advised to do so by your doctor.
- Most people on regular diets do not need dietary supplements.
- *Common dietary sources of bioflavonoids* — Fruits, vegetables, nuts, seeds, grains, tea, wine.

*If you have any questions, consult your doctor, pharmacist, or health care provider.*

| | Brand Name Examples | Fish oil (mg/capsule) | Omega-3 Fatty Acid Content | | Other Content |
|---|---|---|---|---|---|
| | | | EPA | DHA | |
| otc | Mega-MaxEPA Capsules | 1275 | 225 | 150 | 2.5 IU vitamin C |
| otc | Marine Lipid Concentrate Capsules | 1200 | 360 | 240 | 5 IU vitamin E |
| otc | Sea-Omega 30 Capsules | 1200 | 180 | 140 | 2 IU vitamin E |
| otc | Sea-Omega 50 Capsules | 1000 | 300 | 200 | 1 IU vitamin E |
| otc | EPA Capsules | 1000 | 180 | 120 | 5 IU vitamin E |
| otc | Max EPA Capsules | 1000 | 180 | 120 | 2 IU vitamin E |
| otc | EPA Capsules, Optimal Omega Capsules | 1000 | 180 | 120 | 1 IU vitamin E |
| otc | Omega-3 700 Capsules | 700 | 400 | 300 | 2 mg vitamin C, 2 IU vitamin E |
| otc | Sam-EPA Capsules | 500 | 300 | 200 | 1 IU vitamin E |

Cold-water fish oils contain large amounts of omega-3 polyunsaturated fatty acids (eg, eicosapentaenoic acid [EPA] and docosahexaenoic acid [DHA]).

## Type of Drug:

Fish oils, omega-3 (N-3) polyunsaturated fatty acids; nutritional supplement.

## How the Drug Works:

Omega-3 fatty acids appear to act on several factors which may contribute to the development of certain types of heart disorders (especially the development of fatty deposits in the heart blood vessels).

They possibly decrease the levels of fats in the blood by reducing the amount of fats produced by the liver, or by increasing the excretion of fats from the body.

Studies have indicated that diets high in omega-3 fatty acids may lower total cholesterol levels and very low-density lipoproteins (VLDL). However, some studies indicate that fish oils may actually raise LDL cholesterol levels. HDL cholesterol levels appear not to be affected as much as LDL levels.

Some studies indicate that fish oils may produce some anti-inflammatory effects by interfering with the normal inflammatory processes in the body.

It has been observed that fish oils may promote the development of beneficial prostaglandins. Prostaglandins are hormones made locally by tissues throughout the body. The fish oils seem to favor the development of protective types of prostaglandins, thereby helping to reduce chemical reactions in the body, which can contribute to blood clot and plaque formation, which, in turn, can clog blood vessels.

## Uses:
To supplement the diet of people at early risk for heart diseases affecting the blood vessels of the heart (coronary artery disease). The American Heart Association recommends eating fish; however, it does not find justification for fish oil capsule supplements.

*Unlabeled Use(s):* Occasionally doctors may prescribe omega-3 fatty acids as adjunctive treatment for rheumatoid arthritis, psoriasis, and other inflammatory diseases.

## Precautions:
*Use with caution in the following situations:*

anticoagulant (eg, warfarin) therapy, concurrent

aspirin use, concurrent

surgery, recent

type 2 diabetes mellitus

*Pregnancy and breastfeeding:* Do not use fish oil products until further information is available.

*Children:* Dot use fish oil products until further information is available.

## Side Effects:
Every drug is capable of producing side effects. Many fish oil users experience no, or minor, side effects. The frequency and severity of side effects depend on many factors including dose, duration of therapy, and individual susceptibility. Diarrhea has been reported in patients taking 4 to 6 capsules daily.

---

### Guidelines for Use:
- Dosage will be individualized.
- Do not exceed the recommended dose, unless advised to do so by your doctor.
- Consult your doctor if you plan to take large amounts of fish oils or you plan to take them for a long period of time.
- It is not known whether fish oils can reduce the incidence of heart disease. At this time, health authorities do not know whether or not fish oil supplements can be recommended as a measure for preventing heart disease or other diseases.
- People who consider taking fish oils to reduce their risks for heart disease should also make appropriate lifestyle changes. These include reduced intake of fats, cholesterol, salt, and alcohol in the diet; elimination of smoking; appropriate exercise; and control of blood pressure.
- Fish oil supplements do not replace prescription medicines that lower cholesterol (eg, lovastatin). Do not stop prescription cholesterol medicines when starting fish oil supplements, unless advised to do so by your doctor.

---

*If you have any questions, consult your doctor, pharmacist, or health care provider.*

| Generic Name<br>*Brand Name Examples* | Supplied As | Generic<br>Available |
|---|---|---|
| **Levocarnitine<br>(L-Carnitine)** | | |
| *otc* L-Carnitine | **Tablets**: 500 mg | Yes |
| *otc* L-Carnitine | **Capsules:** 250 mg, 500 mg | Yes |
| *Rx* Carnitor | **Tablets:** 330 mg | No |
| *Rx* Carnitor | **Oral solution:** 100 mg/mL | No |
| *Rx* Carnitor | **Injection:** 500 mg/2.5 mL,<br>1 g/5 mL | No |

## Type of Drug:
Amino acid derivative.

## How the Drug Works:
Occurring naturally in the body, L-carnitine is needed by the body for energy metabolism and to properly use fats.

## Uses:
To supplement the diet of people born with primary carnitine deficiency. Symptoms of primary carnitine deficiency include low blood sugar, lethargy, liver problems, heart problems, muscle weakness, neurologic disturbances, and impaired growth and development in infants.

*Carnitor* is used for the acute and chronic treatment of patients with internal metabolism errors that cause a secondary carnitine deficiency. It is also used for the prevention and treatment of carnitine deficiency in patients with end-stage kidney disease who are also undergoing dialysis.

*Unlabeled Use(s):* Occasionally doctors may prescribe L-carnitine for modifying abnormal plasma lipoprotein patterns.

## Precautions:
*Do not use in the following situations:* Allergy to L-carnitine or any of its ingredients.

*Kidney disease:* Patients with kidney disease taking D, L-carnitine (not L-carnitine) have, on rare occasions, noted mild muscle weakness.

*Pregnancy:* There are no adequate and well-controlled studies in pregnant women. Use only if clearly needed and the potential benefits to the mother outweigh the possible risks to the fetus.

*Breastfeeding:* It is not known if L-carnitine appears in breast milk. Consult your doctor before you begin breastfeeding.

*Lab tests* may be required to monitor therapy. Tests include blood chemistries, vital signs, plasma L-carnitine concentrations, and overall clinical condition.

## Side Effects:

Every drug is capable of producing side effects. Many L-carnitine users experience no, or minor, side effects. The frequency and severity of side effects depend on many factors including dose, duration of therapy, and individual susceptibility. Possible side effects include:

*Digestive Tract:* Nausea; vomiting; stomach cramps; diarrhea.

*Other:* Body odor.

---

### Guidelines for Use:

- Dosage will be individualized.
- *Capsules and tablets* — Take on an empty stomach.
- *Oral solution* — Take alone or dissolve in drinks or liquid food. Consume slowly. Space doses evenly (eg, every 3 or 4 hours), preferably with or after meals.
- D, L-carnitine, sold in health food stores as vitamin $B_T$, inhibits L-carnitine and can cause a deficiency.
- Lab tests may be required to monitor therapy. Be sure to keep appointments.
- Store at controlled room temperature (59° to 86°F).

---

*If you have any questions, consult your doctor, pharmacist, or health care provider.*

| Generic Name<br>*Brand Name Examples* | Supplied As | Generic<br>Available |
|---|---|---|
| *otc* **Choline** | **Tablets:** 250 mg, 300 mg, 500 mg, 650 mg | Yes |
| *otc* **Choline Bitartrate** | **Capsules:** 350 mg | Yes |
| | **Powder** | Yes |
| *otc* **Inositol** | **Tablets:** 250 mg, 650 mg | Yes |
| | **Capsules:** 500 mg | Yes |
| | **Powder** | Yes |
| *otc* **Lipotropic Combinations** | | |
| *Lecithin* | **Capsules:** 400 mg, 500 mg, 1200 mg, 1360 mg | Yes |
| *PhosChol* | **Capsules:** 900 mg | No |
| *Lecithin* | **Granules** | Yes |
| *PhosChol* | **Liquid:** 3000 mg/5 mL | No |

The need for lipotropics in human nutrition has not been established. The lipotropic factors choline, inositol, and betaine have not been proven therapeutically valuable, although they have been used for treatment of liver disorders and disturbed fat metabolism.

## Type of Drug:
Lipotropic.

## How the Drug Works:
Lipotropic products increase the removal of, or decrease, fat deposits in the liver.

## Uses:
To treat liver disorders and fat metabolism diseases.

*Unlabeled Use(s):* Occasionally doctors may prescribe choline for tardive dyskinesia, Huntington chorea, Tourette syndrome, Friedreich ataxia, presenile dementia, fatty liver, cirrhosis, Alzheimer disease, and eyelid spasms.

## Side Effects:
Every drug is capable of producing side effects. Many lipotropic product users experience no, or minor, side effects. The frequency and severity of side effects depend on many factors including dose, duration of therapy, and individual susceptibility. Possible side effects for choline include: Depression; uncontrollable urination; fishy odor; nausea; vomiting; diarrhea; stomach discomfort.

**Guidelines for Use:**
- Dosage will be individualized.
- Do not exceed the recommended dose, unless advised to do so by your doctor.
- Take with plenty of liquids.

*If you have any questions, consult your doctor, pharmacist, or health care provider.*

| Generic Name<br>*Brand Name Examples* | Supplied As | Generic<br>Available |
|---|---|---|
| *otc* **Para-Aminobenzoic Acid (PABA)** | **Tablets:** 100 mg | Yes |
| *Rx* **Potassium Para-Amino-benzoate (KPAB)** | | |
| *Potaba* | **Tablets:** 500 mg | No |
| | **Capsules:** 500 mg | No |
| | **Powder (Envules):** 2 g | No |

## Type of Drug:

Accessory food factor naturally associated with B-complex vitamins.

## How the Drug Works:

A component of several important biochemical processes, PABA and KPAB, working by undefined mechanisms, may prevent or reduce inappropriate fibrosis (making of fibrous tissue). It has no nutrient value. It is not a true vitamin.

## Uses:

*KPAB only* — To treat scleroderma, dermatomyositis, morphea, linear scleroderma, pemphigus, and Peyronie disease.

## Precautions:

*Do not use in the following situations:*

allergy to PABA or KPAB
sulfonamide anti-infective therapy, concurrent

*Use with caution in the following situations:*

appetite loss
nausea
kidney disease or impairment

*Pregnancy:* Adequate studies have not been done in pregnant women. Use only if clearly needed and potential benefits outweigh the possible hazards to the fetus.

*Breastfeeding:* It is not known if PABA appears in breast milk. Consult your doctor before you begin breastfeeding.

## Drug Interactions:

Tell your doctor or pharmacist if you are taking or if you are planning to take any over-the-counter or prescription medications or dietary supplements with PABA or KPAB. Doses of one or both drugs may need to be modified or a different drug may need to be prescribed. The following drugs and drug classes interact with PABA or KPAB.

dapsone
sulfonamides (eg, sulfisoxazole)

## Side Effects:

Every drug is capable of producing side effects. Many PABA or KPAB users experience no, or minor, side effects. The frequency and severity of side effects depend on many factors including dose, duration of therapy, and individual susceptibility. Possible side effects include:

*Digestive Tract:* Loss of appetite; nausea; vomiting; stomach upset.

*Other:* Fever; itching; rash; decreased white blood cell count; liver toxicity.

---

### Guidelines for Use:

- Average adult daily dosage is 12 g, given in 4 to 6 separate doses. Six (6) tablets or capsules can be given 4 times daily, usually with meals and at bedtime with a snack. Tablets, capsules, and powder (envules) must be taken with an adequate amount of liquid or food to prevent stomach upset. Envules contain 2 g of potassium para-aminobenzoate powder each. Six (6) envules are given for a total of 12 g daily.
- Take with food to minimize stomach upset.
- If a dose is missed, take it as soon as possible. If several hours have passed or if it is nearing time for the next dose, do not double the dose in order to catch up, unless advised to do so by your doctor. If more than one dose is missed, or it is necessary to establish a new dosage schedule, contact your doctor or pharmacist.
- If loss of appetite or nausea occurs, stop therapy until you are eating normally again.
- Although not a vitamin, this food factor is found naturally associated with B-complex vitamins. Small amounts are found in cereal, eggs, milk, and meats.

---

*If you have any questions, consult your doctor, pharmacist, or health care provider.*

**Iron-Containing Products,** 69

**Iron Combinations**
Iron with Vitamin C, 73
Iron with Vitamins, 74
Iron with Vitamin $B_{12}$ and Intrinsic
Factor, 75

**Folic Acid,** 77

**Leucovorin,** 79

**Vitamin $B_{12}$,** 81

**Antiplatelet Agents**
Aggregation Inhibitors, 84
Aggregation Inhibitors/
Vasodilators, 88
Anagrelide, 90
Dipyridamole, 92
Dipyridamole/Aspirin, 94

**Anticoagulants**
Heparin, 97
Low Molecular Weight Heparins, 100
Coumarin Derivatives, 104

**Thrombolytic Agents,** 109

**Pentoxifylline,** 112

**Phytonadione (Vitamin K),** 114

**Sodium Phenylbutyrate,** 116

**Recombinant Human
Erythropoietin,** 118

**Colony Stimulating Factors,** 121

| Generic Name *Brand Name Examples* | Supplied As | Generic Available |
|---|---|---|
| *otc* **Ferrous Sulfate** | | |
| *Feratab, Mol-Iron* | **Tablets:** 195 mg, 300 mg, 324 mg | Yes |
| *Fero-Gradumet Filmtab* | **Tablets, timed release:** 525 mg | No |
| *Ferospace* | **Capsules:** 250 mg | Yes |
| *Fer-In-Sol[1]* | **Syrup:** 90 mg/tsp | No |
| *Feosol[1]* | **Elixir:** 220 mg/tsp | Yes |
| *Fen-gen-sol[1], Fer-In-Sol[1], Fer-Iron[1]* | **Drops:** 75 mg/0.6 mL | Yes |
| *otc* **Ferrous Sulfate Exsiccated** | | |
| *Feosol* | **Tablets:** 200 mg | No |
| *Slow FE* | **Tablets, slow release:** 160 mg | No |
| *Fer-In-Sol* | **Capsules:** 190 mg | No |
| *Feosol, Ferralyn Lanacaps, Ferra-TD* | **Capsules, timed release:** 159 mg, 250 mg | Yes |
| *otc* **Ferrous Gluconate** | | |
| *Fergon, Ferralet* | **Tablets:** 300 mg, 320 mg, 325 mg | Yes |
| *Ferralet Slow Release* | **Tablets, sustained release:** 320 mg | No |
| *Simron* | **Capsules:** 86 mg | No |
| *Fergon[1]* | **Elixir:** 300 mg/tsp | No |
| *otc* **Ferrous Fumarate** | | |
| *Femiron, Ferretts, Fumasorb, Fumerin, Hemocyte, Ircon, Nephro-Fer* | **Tablets:** 63 mg, 106 mg, 195 mg, 200 mg, 324 mg, 325 mg, 350 mg | Yes |
| *Feostat* | **Tablets, chewable:** 100 mg | No |
| *Span-FF* | **Capsules, controlled release:** 325 mg | No |
| *Feostat* | **Suspension:** 100 mg/tsp | No |
| *Feostat* | **Drops:** 45 mg/0.6 mL | No |

| Generic Name<br>_Brand Name Examples_ | Supplied As | Generic<br>Available |
|---|---|---|
| _otc_ **Polysaccharide-Iron Complex** | | |
| _Niferex_ | **Tablets:** 50 mg iron | No |
| _Hytinic, Niferex-150, Nu-Iron 150_ | **Capsules:** 150 mg iron | No |
| _Niferex[1,2,3], Nu-Iron[1,2]_ | **Elixir:** 100 mg iron/tsp | No |
| _otc_ **Modified Iron Products** | | |
| _Fermalox_ | **Tablets:** 200 ferrous sulfate, 100 mg magnesium hydroxide, 100 mg aluminum hydroxide | No |
| _Ferocyl, Ferro-Sequels_ | **Tablets, sustained release:** 150 mg ferrous fumarate, 100 mg docusate sodium | No |
| _Ferro-Docusate T.R., Ferro-Dok TR, Ferro-DSS S.R._ | **Capsules, timed released:** 150 mg ferrous fumarate, 100 mg docusate sodium | No |

[1] Contains alcohol.
[2] Sugar free.
[3] Dye free.

The amount of elemental iron provided by a product varies with the iron salt (formulation) contained in the product. For example, ferrous sulfate contains 20% elemental iron and ferrous gluconate contains 11.6% elemental iron. The above table lists the amount of iron salts (not elemental iron). Iron is also available in combination with other vitamins and minerals and by injection (eg, iron dextran). For a complete listing of Recommended Dietary Allowances, see the RDA table in the Nutritionals chapter.

## Type of Drug:
Iron supplements.

## How the Drug Works:
Iron, a mineral found in some foods, is needed to make hemoglobin, a component of red blood cells. Hemoglobin allows red blood cells to carry oxygen throughout the body.

## Uses:
To prevent or treat iron deficiency anemia.

_Unlabeled Use(s):_ Occasionally doctors may prescribe iron supplementation for patients receiving epoetin therapy.

## Precautions:
_Do not use in the following situations:_
allergy to any ingredients in these products
iron overload (eg, hemachromatosis)
non-iron deficiency anemias or blood disorders (eg, hemolytic anemia)
normal iron balance

*Use with caution in the following situations:*

| | |
|---|---|
| chronic fatigue of unknown cause | peptic ulcer |
| | ulcerative colitis |
| enteritis (inflammation of small intestine) | |

*Occult blood tests:* Iron products may skew results of occult blood tests.

*Children:* Children are particularly sensitive to accidental overdoses of iron-containing products. Immediately report any suspected overdoses to your local Poison Control Center.

*Tartrazine:* Some of these products may contain the dye tartrazine (FD&C Yellow No. 5) which can cause allergic reactions in certain individuals. Check package label when available or consult your doctor or pharmacist.

*Sulfites:* Some of these products may contain sulfite preservatives which can cause allergic reactions in certain individuals (eg, asthmatics). Check package label when available or consult your doctor or pharmacist.

## Drug Interactions:
Tell your doctor or pharmacist if you are taking or if you are planning to take any over-the-counter or prescription medications or dietary supplements while taking this medicine. Doses of one or both drugs may need to be modified or a different drug may need to be prescribed. The following drugs and drug classes interact with this medicine.

| | |
|---|---|
| antacids (eg, *Maalox*) | levodopa (eg, *Dopar*) |
| chloramphenicol *(Chlor-omycetin)* | methyldopa (eg, *Aldomet*) |
| | penicillamine (eg, *Cuprimine*) |
| cimetidine *(Tagamet)* | tetracyclines (eg, *Achromycin V*) |
| fluorquinolones (eg, *Cipro*) | vitamin C |

## Side Effects:
Every drug is capable of producing side effects. Many patients experience no, or minor, side effects. The frequency and severity of side effects depend on many factors including dose, duration of therapy and individual susceptibility. Possible side effects include:

*Iron Overdose –* Unexplained tiredness; nausea; vomiting; abdominal pain; black, tarry stools; weak, rapid pulse; decreased blood pressure; dehydration; coma; fast breathing.

*Digestive Tract:* Stomach upset; appetite loss; nausea; vomiting; constipation; diarrhea; dark stools; staining of teeth (liquids only).

## Guidelines for Use:

- Certain foods (eg, eggs, milk, coffee, tea) may decrease iron absorption. Take on an empty stomach with water. However, if stomach upset occurs, take after meals or with food.
- Do not chew or crush sustained-release preparations.
- Avoid taking antacids, fluoroquinolones or tetracycline at the same time. Allow 1 to 2 hours between iron and the antacid or antibiotics.
- Drink liquid iron preparations mixed in water or juice and through a straw to prevent staining of teeth.
- Medication may cause black stools, constipation or diarrhea.
- Discontinue medication and contact your doctor immediately if you experience unexplained tiredness, nausea, vomiting, abdominal pain, black tarry stools, weak rapid pulse, decreased blood pressure or dehydration.
- If a dose is missed, take it as soon as possible. If several hours have passed or if it is nearing time for the next dose, do not double the dose in order to "catch up" (unless advised to do so by your doctor). If more than one dose is missed or it is necessary to establish a new dosage schedule, contact your doctor or pharmacist.
- *Recommended Dietary Allowances (RDA)* — Adults: males and females over 50 years of age, 10 mg; females 11 to 50 years of age, 15 mg; pregnancy, 30 mg (if this increased requirement cannot be met by ordinary diets, the use of supplemental iron may be recommended); breastfeeding, 15 mg.
- *Common sources of iron:* Meat, eggs, vegetables, fortified or enriched cereals.
- In a true iron deficiency state, iron doses are higher than the RDA. Discuss the desired dose and duration of therapy with your doctor if you are iron deficient.

*If you have any questions, consult your doctor, pharmacist, or health care provider.*

Content given per capsule or tablet.

| Iron with Vitamin C<br>*Brand Name Examples* | Iron<br>(mg) | Vitamin C | |
|---|---|---|---|
| | | Ascorbic Acid<br>(mg) | Sodium Ascorbate<br>(mg) |
| otc  *Vitron-C-Plus Tablets* | 132 | 250 | |
| otc  *Ferancee-HP Tablets* | 110 | 600 | |
| otc  *Hemaspan Tablets[2]* | 110 | 200 | |
| otc  *Fero-Grad-500 Filmtabs[2]* | 105 | | 500 |
| otc  *Fe-O.D. Tablets[2]* | 100 | 500 | |
| otc  *Ferancee Tablets[1,3]* | 67 | 150 | |
| otc  *Vitron-C Tablets[3]* | 66 | 125 | |
| otc  *Ferromar Caplets [2]* | 65 | 200 | |
| otc  *Irospan Capsules[2],<br>Irospan Tablets[2]* | 60 | 150 | |
| otc  *Niferex w/Vitamin C<br>Tablets[3]* | 50 | 100 | 169 |
| otc  *Mol-Iron w/Vitamin C<br>Tablets* | 39 | 75 | |

[1] Contains the dye tartrazine.
[2] Timed release.
[3] Chewable.

For more information, see Iron-Containing Products monograph and individual drug monographs. Products containing the greatest amount of iron are listed first.

*If you have any questions, consult your doctor, pharmacist, or health care provider.*

Content given per capsule or tablet. Products containing the greatest amount of elemental iron are listed first.

| Iron with Vitamins<br>*Brand Name Examples* | Elemental<br>Iron<br>(mg) | Vitamin<br>B$_{12}$<br>(mcg) | Vitamin<br>C<br>(mg) | Folic Acid<br>(mg) |
|---|---|---|---|---|
| *otc* *Tolfrinic Tablets* | 200 | 25 | 100 | |
| *Rx* *Fe-Tinic 150 Forte Capsules, Niferex-150 Forte Capsules* | 150 | 25 | | 1 |
| *otc* *Iberet Filmtabs*[1] | 150 | 25 | 150 | |
| *Rx* *Hemocyte-F Tablets* | 106 | | | 1 |
| *Rx* *Hemocyte Plus Tablets* | 106 | 15 | 200 | 1 |
| *Rx* *Iberet-Folic-500 Filmtabs*[1] | 105 | 25 | 500 | 0.8 |
| *Rx* *Fero-Folic-500 Filmtabs*[1] | 105 | | 500 | 0.8 |
| *otc* *Generet-500 Tablets*[1]*, Iberet-500 Filmtabs*[1] | 105 | 25 | 500 | |
| *otc* *Iron-Folic 500 Tablets*[1] | 105 | 25 | 500 | 0.8 |
| *otc* *Ircon-FA Tablets* | 82 | | | 0.8 |
| *Rx* *Fumatinic Capsules*[2] | 66 | 5 | 60 | |
| *Rx* *Nephron FA Tablets*[3] | 66 | 6 | 40 | 1 |
| *otc* *Parvlex Tablets* | 29 | 50 | 50 | 0.4 |

[1] Controlled release.
[2] Extended release with a trace amount of intrinsic factor.
[3] Contains 75 mg docusate sodium.

*If you have any questions, consult your doctor, pharmacist, or health care provider.*

## Iron with Vitamin $B_{12}$ and Intrinsic Factor

| Brand Name Examples | Elemental Iron (mg) | $B_{12}$ (mcg) | IFC (mg) | $B_1$ (mg) | $B_2$ (mg) | $B_3$ (mg) | C (mg) | Folic Acid (mg) |
|---|---|---|---|---|---|---|---|---|
| Rx TriHemic 600 Tablets[1] | 115 | 25 | 75 | | | | 600 | 1 |
| Rx Contrin Capsules, Foltrin Capsules, Trinsicon Capsules | 110 | 15 | 240 | | | | 75 | 0.5 |

[1] Contains 50 mg docusate sodium and 30 IU vitamin E.

These products contain Intrinsic Factor derived from stomach extract to promote the absorption of vitamin $B_{12}$. Although previously used to treat anemias responding to oral therapy, injectable cobalamin is preferred for $B_{12}$ deficiencies, including pernicious anemia. Content given per capsule or tablet. Products containing the greatest amount of iron are listed first.

## Type of Drug:
Dietary and therapeutic supplement.

## Uses:
To prevent and treat iron deficiency or iron deficiency anemia associated with certain nutritional deficiencies (eg, vitamin $B_{12}$).

Ascorbic acid (vitamin C) may enhance the absorption of some forms of iron.

## Precautions:
*Do not use in the following situations:*

allergy to any ingredients in these products
iron overload (eg, hemochromatosis)

non-iron deficiency anemias or blood disorders (eg, hemolytic anemia)
normal iron balance

*Use with caution in the following situations:*

chronic fatigue of unknown cause
enteritis (inflammation of intestine)

peptic ulcer
ulcerative colitis

*Occult blood tests:* Iron products may skew results of occult blood tests.

*Children:* Children are particularly sensitive to accidental overdoses of iron-containing products. Immediately report any suspected overdoses to your local Poison Control Center.

## Drug Interactions:
Tell your doctor or pharmacist if you are taking or if you are planning to take any over-the-counter or prescription medications or dietary supplements while taking this medicine. Doses of one or both drugs may

need to be modified or a different drug may need to be prescribed. The following drugs and drug classes interact with this medicine.

antacids (eg, *Maalox*)
chloramphenicol (*Chlor-
omycetin*)
cimetidine (eg, *Tagamet*)
fluoroquinolones (eg, ciprofloxacin)

levodopa (eg, *Dopar*)
methyldopa (eg, *Aldomet*)
penicillamine (eg, *Cuprimine*)
tetracyclines (eg, doxycycline)
vitamin C

## Side Effects:

Every drug is capable of producing side effects. Many patients experience no, or minor, side effects. The frequency and severity of side effects depend on many factors including dose, duration of therapy, and individual susceptibility. Possible side effects include:

*Iron Overdose:* Unexplained tiredness; nausea; vomiting; abdominal pain; black, tarry stools; weak, rapid pulse; decreased blood pressure; dehydration; coma; fast breathing.

*Digestive Tract:* Stomach upset; appetite loss; nausea; vomiting; constipation; diarrhea; dark stools.

---

### Guidelines for Use:

- Take on an empty stomach with water. If stomach upset occurs, take after meals or with food. Do not chew or crush sustained release preparations. Sustained release products may be better tolerated.
- Avoid taking antacids, cholestyramine, or tetracycline at the same time. Take 1 hour before or 2 hours after the antacid, cholestyramine, or tetracycline.
- Medication may cause black stools, constipation, nausea, vomiting, pain, or diarrhea. Inform your doctor if any of these occur and are intolerable.
- *Recommended Dietary Allowances (RDA) for Iron —*
  Adult males: 10 mg.
  Adult females: 15 mg if menstruating, 10 mg if not menstruating.
  During pregnancy: 30 mg. If this increased requirement cannot be met by ordinary diets, the use of supplemental iron may be recommended.
  During breastfeeding: 15 mg.
- In a true iron deficiency state, iron doses are higher than the RDA. Discuss the desired dose and duration of therapy with your doctor if you are iron-deficient.
- Accidental overdose of iron-containing products is a leading cause of fatal poisoning in children. Keep these products out of reach of children. In case of accidental overdose, call a poison control center immediately.
- Sustained release iron products may not be as effective as regular release products due to delayed absorption of iron.
- Lab tests may be required to monitor therapy. Be sure to keep appointments.
- Store at room temperature (59° to 86°F) in a tightly closed container.

---

*If you have any questions, consult your doctor, pharmacist, or health care provider.*

| Generic Name<br>*Brand Name Examples* | Supplied As | Generic<br>Available |
|---|---|---|
| **Folic Acid**[1] | | |
| *otc* Folic Acid | **Tablets:** 0.4 mg, 0.8 mg | Yes |
| *Rx* Folic Acid | **Tablets:** 1 mg | Yes |
| *Rx* Folvite | **Injection:** 5 mg/mL | Yes |

## Type of Drug:

Folate; folacin; pteroylglutamic acid.

## How the Drug Works:

Folic acid stimulates the production of red and white blood cells and platelets (used in clotting). Folic acid acts on megaloblastic bone marrow to produce a normoblastic marrow.

## Uses:

To treat anemia (low red blood cell count) caused by folic acid deficiency due to digestive disorders (eg, sprue), poor diet, pregnancy, infancy, or childhood. Folic acid is rarely taken alone.

## Precautions:

*Do not use in the following situations:* Allergy to folic acid or any of its ingredients.

*Use with caution in the following situations:*
alcoholism
anemia due to vitamin $B_{12}$ deficiency
epilepsy controlled with phenytoin, primidone, or phenobarbital
non-folic acid deficiency anemias (eg, pernicious anemia)

*Pregnancy:* Folic acid is often prescribed during pregnancy and is safe when used as directed. Folic acid requirements are markedly increased during pregnancy, and deficiency will likely result in fetal damage.

*Breastfeeding:* Folic acid appears in breast milk. Usually, amounts present in breast milk are adequate to fulfill infant requirements, but the lactating mother may require folic acid supplementation. Consult your doctor before you begin breastfeeding.

## Drug Interactions:

Tell your doctor or pharmacist if you are taking or if you are planning to take any over-the-counter or prescription medications or dietary supplements with folic acid. Doses of one or both drugs may need to be modified or a different drug may need to be prescribed.

alcohol
antimetabolites (eg, methotrexate)
barbiturates (eg, phenobarbital)
hydantoins (eg, phenytoin)
nitrofurantoin (eg, *Furadantin*)
primidone (eg, *Mysoline*)
pyrimethamine (eg, *Daraprim*)

## Side Effects:

Every drug is capable of producing side effects. Many folic acid users experience no, or minor, side effects. The frequency and severity of side effects depend on many factors including dose, duration of therapy, and individual susceptibility. Possible side effects include: Difficulty breathing; itching; skin redness or rash; general body discomfort; flushing.

In higher doses (15 mg/day), additional possible side effects include: Loss of appetite; nausea; stomach bloating or swelling; gas; bitter or bad taste; altered sleep patterns; difficulty in concentrating; irritability; overactivity; excitement; depression; confusion; impaired judgment; decreased vitamin $B_{12}$ levels (in patients receiving prolonged therapy).

---

### Guidelines for Use:

- Take only when recommended by your doctor.
- *Treatment of Anemia –*
  Usual therapeutic (treatment) dose for anemia: Up to 1 mg daily.
  Usual maintenance dose once amenia has been corrected:
    Infants: 0.1 mg/day.
    Children under 4 years of age: Up to 0.3 mg/day.
    Adults and children over 4 years of age: 0.4 mg/day.
    Pregnant and breastfeeding women: 0.8 mg/day.
- In the presence of alcoholism, hemolytic anemia, anticonvulsant therapy, or chronic infection, the maintenance dose may need to be increased.
- Except during pregnancy and lactation, folic acid should not be given in doses greater than 0.4 mg/day until pernicious anemia has been ruled out.
- Oral administration is preferred. Intramuscular, intravenous, and subcutaneous routes may be used if the disease is severe, or if oral absorption is impaired.
- Store at room temperature (59 to 86°F). Protect from light and moisture.

---

*If you have any questions, consult your doctor, pharmacist, or health care provider.*

| Generic Name Brand Name Examples | Supplied As | Generic Available |
|---|---|---|
| **Leucovorin Calcium**[1] | | |
| *Rx Wellcovorin* | **Tablets:** 5 mg, 10 mg, 15 mg, 25 mg | Yes |

[1] This product is also available as an injection.

## Type of Drug:

Folic acid derivative; folinic acid, citrovorum factor.

## How the Drug Works:

Leucovorin is a faster acting and more potent form of folic acid. It interferes with the harmful action of folic acid-inhibiting drugs such as methotrexate.

## Uses:

*Tablets and injection:* To lessen the toxicity and counteract the adverse effects of large doses of some drugs that are folic acid antagonists (eg, methotrexate).

*Injection:* To treat anemias due to folic acid deficiency when oral folic acid therapy is not possible.

## Precautions:

*Do not use in the following situations:*
   pernicious anemia and other anemias due to a vitamin $B_{12}$ deficiency

*Pregnancy:* Adequate studies have not been done in pregnant women. Use only if clearly needed and potential benefits outweigh the possible hazards to the fetus.

*Breastfeeding:* It is not known if leucovorin appears in breast milk. Consult your doctor before you begin breastfeeding.

*Lab tests* may be required during treatment with leucovorin. Tests may include complete blood counts, electrolyte and liver function tests.

## Drug Interactions:

Tell your doctor or pharmacist if you are taking or if you are planning to take any over-the-counter or prescription medications or dietary supplements with leucovorin. Doses of one or both drugs may need to be modified or a different drug may need to be prescribed. The following drugs and drug classes interact with leucovorin.

   anticonvulsants (eg, phenytoin)
   fluorouracil (*Adrucil*)
   methotrexate (*Mexate*)

## Side Effects:

Every drug is capable of producing side effects. Many leucovorin users experience no, or minor, side effects. The frequency and severity of side effects depend on many factors including dose, duration of therapy and individual susceptibility. Possible side effects include: Allergic reactions (eg, difficulty breathing, itching, skin redness/rash).

---

### Guidelines for Use:

- Take only under medical supervision.
- Itching, rash, difficult breathing or other signs of hypersensitivity should be reported immediately.

---

*If you have any questions, consult your doctor, pharmacist, or health care provider.*

| Generic Name | Supplied As | Generic Available |
|---|---|---|
| *otc* **Vitamin B$_{12}$**[1,2] | **Tablets:** 25 mcg, 50 mcg, 100 mcg, 250 mcg, 500 mcg, 1000 mcg | Yes |
| | **Nasal gel:** 400 mcg/unit | No |

[1] This product is also available as an injection (*Rx*).
[2] Some products may be available sugar free.

For a complete listing of Recommended Dietary Allowances, see the RDA table in the Nutritionals chapter.

## Type of Drug:

Water-soluble vitamin. Vitamin that can be stored by the body. Vitamin B$_{12}$ includes cyanocobalamin and hydroxocobalamin.

## How the Drug Works:

Vitamin B$_{12}$ is needed for normal growth and reproduction of red blood cells, muscle and nerve tissue. It is usually adequately provided by the diet.

## Uses:

To treat diagnosed vitamin B$_{12}$ deficiency that may be due to pernicious anemia, inadequate diet, digestion disorders (sprue), trauma, surgery, cancer or infections.

Vitamin B$_{12}$ requirements may increase during pregnancy, in vegetarians, after blood loss, during illnesses involving the liver and kidneys, in hemolytic anemia and in thyrotoxicosis.

*Unlabeled Use(s):* Occasionally doctors may prescribe hydroxocobalamin for cyanide poisoning associated with sodium nitroprusside.

## Precautions:

*Do not use in the following situations:*
    allergy to cobalt
    allergy to vitamin B$_{12}$ or any component of the formulation

*Use with caution in the following situations:*

| | |
|---|---|
| bone marrow suppressant drugs (eg, chloramphenicol) | iron deficiency Leber disease |
| folic acid deficiency | polycythemia vera |
| infection | uremia |

*Eye problems:* Use of vitamin B$_{12}$ may worsen Leber disease, a rare hereditary eye condition.

*Single deficiency* (vitamin B$_{12}$ alone) is rare. Expect multiple vitamin deficiency in any dietary deficiency.

*Pregnancy:* Adequate studies have not been done in pregnant women. However, B$_{12}$ is an essential vitamin and needs are increased during pregnancy.

*Breastfeeding:* Vitamin B$_{12}$ appears in breast milk. Consult your doctor before you begin breastfeeding.

*Lab tests* may be necessary to determine progress of therapy.

## Drug Interactions:

Tell your doctor or pharmacist if you are taking or planning to take any over-the-counter or prescription medications or dietary supplements while taking this drug. Doses of one or both drugs may need to be modified or a different drug may need to be prescribed. The following drugs and drug classes interact with this drug:

alcohol (excessive intake)
aminosalicylic acid (*Paser*)
chloramphenicol (eg, *Chloromy-cetin*)

colchicine
folic acid
omeprazole (eg, *Prilosec*)

## Side Effects:

Every drug is capable of producing side effects. Many patients experience no, or minor, side effects. The frequency and severity of side effects depend on many factors including dose, duration of therapy, and individual susceptibility. Possible side effects include:

*Injectable vitamin B$_{12}$:* Discomfort following injection; pain at injection site; blood clots in arms or legs; breathing difficulties; congestive heart failure; anaphylactic shock; death.

*Skin:* Rash; itching; hives; bruising.

*Other:* Fever; vision difficulties; feeling of swelling of the entire body; mild diarrhea; abnormal blood counts.

## Guidelines for Use:

- *Recommended Dietary Allowance (RDA) —*
  Adult males: 2 mcg
  Adult females: 2 mcg
  Pregnant women: 2.2 mcg
  Breastfeeding women: 2.6 mcg
  Infants and children: 0.3 to 2 mcg
  Doses larger than the RDA are used to treat vitamin B$_{12}$ deficiency.
- A well-balanced diet is necessary. Correct poor eating habits. Strict vegetarian diets containing no animal products (including milk products and eggs) do not supply vitamin B$_{12}$. Vegetarians should take vitamin B$_{12}$ supplements regularly.
- *Common sources of vitamin B$_{12}$ —* Meat, liver.
- Initially, vitamin B$_{12}$ may be given daily.
- In some cases, vitamin B$_{12}$ must be continued indefinitely to prevent the return of anemia and to prevent damage to the central nervous system.
- Although oral dosing of vitamin B$_{12}$ is convenient, injections may be required.
- Folic acid is sometimes taken with vitamin B$_{12}$ but is not a substitute for it. In pernicious anemia, folic acid may effectively return the blood profile to normal while nerve damage due to vitamin B$_{12}$ deficiency progresses.

*If you have any questions, consult your doctor, pharmacist, or health care provider.*

| Generic Name<br>*Brand Name Example* | Supplied As | Generic<br>Available |
|---|---|---|
| *Rx* **Cilostazol** | | |
| *Pletal* | **Tablets**: 50 mg, 100 mg | No |
| *Rx* **Clopidogrel Bisulfate** | | |
| *Plavix* | **Tablets**: 75 mg (as base) | No |
| *Rx* **Ticlopidine HCl** | | |
| *Ticlid* | **Tablets**: 250 mg | Yes |

## Type of Drug:

Antiplatelet agents.

## How the Drug Works:

Platelets are components of the blood that aid in clot formation. Blood clots often form on platelets that have clumped together. These medicines help prevent blood clots from forming by preventing platelets from clumping together. In addition, cilostazol may dilate (widen) arteries in the legs to improve circulation.

## Uses:

*Cilostazol:* To reduce the symptoms of intermittent claudication (ie, leg weakness, muscle pain, limping after walking) resulting in an increased walking distance before symptoms start.

*Clopidogrel:* To reduce the chances of stroke, heart attack, or death caused by blood clots in patients who have had a recent heart attack or stroke or who have peripheral arterial disease (hardening of the arteries or poor circulation).

To reduce the chances of heart attack, stroke, or death in patients with acute coronary syndrome (incomplete heart attack or rapidly worsening angina-type chest pain) who are going to be treated with medicines or heart surgery.

*Ticlopidine:* To reduce the risk of stroke caused by blood clots in patients who have experienced stroke precursors (eg, transient ischemic attacks, transient blindness, minor stroke), and in patients who have had a completed stroke caused by a blood clot. It is used in patients who are intolerant or allergic to aspirin therapy or have failed aspirin therapy for stroke prevention.

Used in combination with aspirin for 30 days to reduce the risk of blood clots forming in stents in patients who have had stents placed in their arteries.

*Unlabeled Use(s):* Occasionally doctors may prescribe ticlopidine to improve blood flow in the lower extremities, reduce neurological deficit in patients with subarachnoid hemorrhage, as an aid in open heart surgery, or as treatment of sickle cell disease or primary glomerulonephritis. Further studies are needed to establish usefulness in these situations.

## Precautions:

*Do not use in the following situations:*

allergy to the drug or any of its ingredients
aplastic anemia, history of (ticlopidine only)
blood clotting disorders or active bleeding (eg, bleeding peptic ulcer, bleeding in the brain)
congestive heart failure (cilostazol only)
liver disease, severe (ticlopidine only)
low blood platelet count (ticlopidine only)
low white blood cell count (ticlopidine only)
thrombotic thrombocytopenia (TTP), history of (ticlopidine only)

*Use with caution in the following situations:*

gastrointestinal bleeding, history of
kidney disease (ticlopidine only)
liver disease
trauma, surgery, or diseases that increase risk of bleeding
ulcers, stomach or intestinal

*Pregnancy:* There are no adequate and well-controlled studies in pregnant women. Use only if clearly needed and the potential benefits outweigh the possible hazards to the fetus.

*Breastfeeding:* It is not known if these drugs appear in breast milk. Because of the potential for adverse effects in a nursing infant, a decision should be made whether to discontinue nursing or the drug, taking into account the importance of the drug to the mother. Consult your doctor before you being breastfeeding.

*Children:* Safety and effectiveness have not been established.

*Lab tests* are required during treatment with ticlopidine. Tests may include complete blood counts, platelet counts, and liver function tests.

## Drug Interactions:

Tell your doctor or pharmacist if you are taking or planning to take any over-the-counter or prescription medications or dietary supplements with these drugs. Drug doses may need to be modified or a different drug prescribed. The following drugs and drug classes interact with these drugs:

aspirin
azole antifungals (eg, ketoconazole) (cilostazol only)
cimetidine (eg, *Tagamet*) (ticlopidine only)
digoxin (eg, *Lanoxin*) (ticlopidine only)
diltiazem (eg, *Cardizem*) (cilostazol, clopidrogel only)
grapefruit juice (cilostazol, clopidrogel only)
hydantoins (eg, phenytoin)
(ticlopidine only)

macrolide antibiotics (eg,
erythromycin) (cilostazol only)
NSAIDs (eg, ibuprofen) (clopidrogel only)
omeprazole (eg, *Prilosec*) (cilostazol, clopidrogel only)
theophyllines (eg, amino-
phylline) (ticlopidine only)
warfarin (eg, *Coumadin*) (clopidrogel only)

## Side Effects:

Every drug is capable of producing side effects. Many patients experience no, or minor, side effects. The frequency and severity of side effects depend on many factors including dose, duration of therapy, and individual susceptibility. Possible side effects include:

*Circulatory System:* Pounding in the chest (palpitations); fast heartbeat; chest pain; high blood pressure.

*Nervous System:* Headache; depression; dizziness; fatigue; feeling of whirling motion (vertigo).

*Skin:* Rash; bruising; itching; bleeding under the skin; skin disorder.

*Digestive Tract:* Diarrhea; nausea; indigestion; stomach pain; vomiting; gas; appetite loss; light-colored stool; constipation; bleeding ulcer.

*Urinary and Reproductive Tract:* Dark urine; blood in urine; urinary tract infection.

*Respiratory System:* Upper respiratory infection; difficulty breathing; bronchitis; increased cough; runny nose; nosebleed; sore throat.

*Other:* Abnormal blood counts; yellow skin or eyes; sore throat; back, joint, muscle, or body pain; infection; swelling of the arms or legs; bleeding in the brain; swelling; weakness; accidental injury; flu-like symptoms; abnormal lab tests (eg, liver function).

## Guidelines for Use:

- Dosage is individualized. Take exactly as prescribed.
- Do not stop taking or change the dose, unless instructed by your doctor.
- Take cilostazol at least 30 minutes before or 2 hours after meals.
- Take clopidrogel without regard to food. Take with food if stomach upset occurs.
- Take ticlopidine with food or just after eating to minimize stomach discomfort and increase absorption of the drug.
- If a dose is missed, take it as soon as possible. If several hours have passed or it is nearing time for the next dose, do not double the dose to catch up, unless instructed by your doctor. If more than one dose is missed or it is necessary to establish a new dosage schedule, contact your doctor or pharmacist.
- It may take a few weeks for cilostazol to start working. Treatment for up to 12 weeks may be required before walking-distance benefits are experienced.
- Contact your doctor immediately if you experience any signs of infection such as fever, chills, or sore throat.
- It may take longer than usual to stop bleeding when taking these drugs. Report any unusual bleeding, bruising, or dark-colored stool to your doctor.
- Tell your dentist or doctor that you are taking one of these drugs before any surgery is scheduled (including tooth extraction) and before any new drug is prescribed.
- Notify your doctor immediately if you are taking ticlopidine and experience severe or persistent diarrhea, seizures, rashes, pinpoint bleeding beneath the skin, bleeding from the nose or gums, pale color, weakness on a side of the body, difficulty speaking, or any signs of liver damage such as yellow skin or eyes, dark urine, or light-colored stool.
- Lab tests will be required to monitor therapy with ticlopidine. Be sure to keep appointments.
- Store at controlled room temperature (59° to 86°F).

*If you have any questions, consult your doctor, pharmacist, or health care provider.*

| Generic Name<br>*Brand Name Example* | Supplied As | Generic<br>Available |
|---|---|---|
| *Rx* **Treprostinil Sodium** | | |
| *Remodulin* | **Injection**: 1 mg/mL, 2.5 mg/mL,<br>5 mg/mL, 10 mg/mL | No |

## Type of Drug:
Antiplatelet agent; pulmonary artery vasodilator.

## How the Drug Works:
Pulmonary artery hypertension is excessive blood pressure in the pulmonary arteries (arteries in the lung). Treprostinil dilates (widens) pulmonary arteries and reduces elevated blood pressure in the pulmonary arteries. It also keeps platelets (blood cells that aid in blood clot formation) from clumping together.

## Uses:
For the treatment of pulmonary arterial hypertension (PAH) in patients with New York Heart Association (NYHA) Class II through IV symptoms to reduce symptoms (eg, difficulty breathing, chest pain, fatigue) associated with exercise.

## Precautions:
*Do not use in the following situations:* Allergy to the drug or any of its ingredients.

*Use with caution in the following situations:*
  kidney disease
  liver disease

*Pregnancy:* There are no adequate and well-controlled studies in pregnant women. Use only if clearly needed and the potential benefits outweigh the possible risks to the fetus.

*Breastfeeding:* It is not known if treprostinil appears in breast milk. Consult your doctor before you begin breastfeeding.

*Children:* Safety and effectiveness in children younger than 16 years of age have not been established.

## Drug Interactions:
Tell your doctor or pharmacist if you are taking or planning to take any over-the-counter or prescription medications or dietary supplements with this drug. Drug doses may need to be modified or a different drug prescribed. The following drugs and drug classes interact with this drug:

  anticoagulants (eg, warfarin)
  blood pressure-reducing agents (eg, diuretics, antihypertensive agents, vasodilators)

## Side Effects:

Every drug is capable of producing side effects. Many patients experience no, or minor, side effects. The frequency and severity of side effects depend on many factors including dose, duration of therapy, and individual susceptibility. Possible side effects include:

*Circulatory System:* Low blood pressure; widening of the blood vessels (vasodilation).

*Other:* Infusion site reaction (eg, redness, hardness, induration, rash); infusion site pain, bleeding, or bruising; headache; rash; jaw pain; itching; dizziness; diarrhea; nausea.

---

### Guidelines for Use:

- This medicine will usually be prepared and administered by your health care provider in a medical setting, but may be administered at home if your doctor feels it is safe to do so.
- Dosage is individualized. Take exactly as prescribed.
- Do not stop taking or change the dose, unless instructed by your doctor.
- If medicine needs to be stopped, the dose will usually be slowly reduced before being stopped completely.
- Notify your doctor if your symptoms worsen or if you experience persistent headache, persistent nausea, or bothersome infusion site reactions.
- *For home infusion* — This drug is administered by continuous subcutaneous (SC; beneath the skin) catheter, through an infusion pump. Carefully follow the storage, preparation, administration, and disposal techniques taught to you by your health care provider. Ensure that a backup infusion pump and subcutaneous infusion sets are readily available should a problem develop with the pump or infusion set you are using. Check infusion pump function and catheter frequently. Implement corrective actions as taught by your health care provider if a pump malfunction is noted or if the catheter becomes kinked or dislodged. Store at controlled room temperature (59° to 86°F).

---

*If you have any questions, consult your doctor, pharmacist, or health care provider.*

| Generic Name<br>*Brand Name Example* | Supplied As | Generic<br>Available |
|---|---|---|
| *Rx* **Anagrelide HCl** | | |
| *Agrylin* | **Capsules**: 0.5 mg, 1 mg | No |

## Type of Drug:
Antiplatelet agent.

## How the Drug Works:
It is not known exactly how anagrelide reduces blood platelet levels. It is thought that it may slow down how fast platelets are produced and released by the bone marrow.

## Uses:
For the treatment of patients with essential thrombocytothemia (too many blood platelets) to reduce the elevated platelet count and the risk of clotting and associated symptoms.

## Precautions:
*Do not use in the following situations:* Allergy to the drug or any of its ingredients.

*Use with caution in the following situations:*
heart disease, known or suspected
kidney disease
liver disease

*Pregnancy:* There are no adequate and well-controlled studies in pregnant women. Use only if clearly needed and the potential benefits outweigh the possible risks to the fetus.

*Breastfeeding:* It is not known if this drug is excreted in breast milk. Consult your doctor before you being breastfeeding.

*Children:* Safety and effectiveness in patients younger than 16 years of age have not been established.

*Lab tests* will be required to monitor therapy. Tests include cardiovascular exams, blood counts, and kidney and liver function monitoring.

## Drug Interactions:
Tell your doctor or pharmacist if you are taking or planning to take any over-the-counter or prescription medications or dietary supplements while taking this drug. Drug doses may need to be modified or a different drug prescribed. Sucralfate (*Carafate*) may interact with anagrelide.

## Side Effects:

Every drug is capable of producing side effects. Many patients experience no, or minor, side effects. The frequency and severity of side effects depend on many factors including dose, duration of therapy, and individual susceptibility. Possible side effects include:

*Circulatory System:* Fast heartbeat; pounding in the chest (palpitations); heart failure; chest pain.

*Digestive Tract:* Diarrhea; stomach pain; nausea; gas; vomiting; indigestion; appetite loss.

*Other:* Headache; weakness; swelling; pain; dizziness; difficulty breathing; rash; hives; abnormal skin sensations; back pain; general body discomfort.

---

### Guidelines for Use:

- Dosage is individualized. Take exactly as prescribed.
- Do not stop taking or change the dose, unless instructed by your doctor.
- Dosage will usually be slowly increased to achieve maximum benefit.
- Take without regard to meals. Take with food if stomach upset occurs.
- If a dose is missed, take it as soon as possible. If several hours have passed or it is nearing time for the next dose, do not double the dose to catch up, unless instructed by your doctor. If more than one dose is missed or it is necessary to establish a new dosage schedule, contact your doctor or pharmacist.
- Women of childbearing potential must use adequate contraception while taking this drug. It may cause fetal harm when administered to a pregnant woman.
- Lab tests will be required to monitor therapy. Be sure to keep appointments.
- Store at controlled room temperature (59° to 77°F) in a light-resistant container.

*If you have any questions, consult your doctor, pharmacist, or health care provider.*

| Generic Name<br>*Brand Name Example* | Supplied As | Generic<br>Available |
|---|---|---|
| *Rx* **Dipyridamole**[1] | | |
| *Persantine* | **Tablets:** 25 mg, 50 mg, 75 mg | Yes |

[1] Also available as an intravenous injection.

## Type of Drug:
Antiplatelet agent.

## How the Drug Works:
Platelets are components of the blood that aid in clot formation. Blood clots often form on platelets that have clumped together. Dipyridamole helps prevent blood clots from forming by preventing platelets from clumping together.

## Uses:
Given in combination with oral anticoagulants (eg, warfarin) to prevent blood clot formation after heart valve surgery.

*Unlabeled Use(s):* Occasionally doctors may prescribe dipyridamole with aspirin to prevent heart attacks and reduce heart attack damage.

## Precautions:
*Do not use in the following situations:* Allergy to the drug or any of its ingredients.

*Use with caution in the following situations:*
coronary artery disease, severe
liver disease
low blood pressure

*Hypotension (low blood pressure):* Dipyridamole may aggravate light-headedness in people with low blood pressure. Use caution when rising from a sitting or lying position.

*Pregnancy:* There are no adequate and well-controlled studies in pregnant women. Use only if clearly needed and the potential benefits outweigh the possible risks to the fetus.

*Breastfeeding:* Dipyridamole appears in breast milk. Consult your doctor before you begin breastfeeding.

*Children:* Safety and effectiveness have not been established in children younger than 12 years of age.

*Lab tests* may be required to monitor therapy. Tests include liver function monitoring.

## Drug Interactions:

Tell your doctor or pharmacist if you are taking or planning to take any over-the-counter or prescription medications or dietary supplements while taking this drug. Drug doses may need to be modified or a different drug prescribed. The following drugs or drug classes interact with this drug:

adenosine (*Adenocard*)
cholinesterase inhibitors (eg, tacrine)

## Side Effects:

Every drug is capable of producing side effects. Many patients experience no, or minor, side effects. The frequency and severity of side effects depend on many factors including dose, duration of therapy, and individual susceptibility. Possible side effects include:

*Digestive Tract:* Stomach ache; diarrhea; vomiting.

*Other:* Dizziness; light-headedness; fainting; headache; rash; flushing; itching; abnormal liver tests.

---

### Guidelines for Use:

- Dosage is individualized. Take exactly as prescribed.
- Do not stop taking or change the dose, unless instructed by your doctor.
- Take without regard to food, but take with food is stomach upset occurs.
- If a dose is missed, take it as soon as possible. If several hours have passed or it is nearing time for the next dose, do not double the dose to catch up, unless instructed by your doctor. If more than one dose is missed or it is necessary to establish a new dosage schedule, contact your doctor or pharmacist.
- If using this medicine in combination with oral anticoagulants (eg, warfarin), do not take aspirin, unless instructed by your doctor.
- Lab tests may be required to monitor therapy. Be sure to keep appointments.
- Store at room temperature (59° to 86°F).

---

*If you have any questions, consult your doctor, pharmacist, or health care provider.*

| Generic Name<br>*Brand Name Example* | Supplied As | Generic<br>Available |
|---|---|---|
| Rx **Dipyridamole<br>and Aspirin** | | |
| *Aggrenox* | **Capsules**: 200 mg extended-release dipyridamole/25 mg aspirin | No |

## Type of Drug:
Combination antiplatelet agent.

## How the Drug Works:
Aspirin and dipyridamole work together to prevent blood clots from forming by preventing platelets from clumping together. Platelets are parts of the blood that aid in clot formation.

## Uses:
To reduce the risk of stroke in patients who have had transient ischemia of the brain (TIAs) or complete ischemic stroke because of blood clots.

## Precautions:
*Do not use in the following situations:*

      allergy to dipyridamole, aspirin, NSAIDs, or any of their ingredients
      asthma, nasal polyps, and rhinitis syndrome
      viral infections with or without fever, in children or teenagers

*Use with caution in the following situations:*

| | |
|---|---|
| alcohol use | kidney disease |
| bleeding abnormalities | liver disease |
| coronary artery disease | low blood pressure |
| gastrointestinal bleeding or ulcers | peptic ulcer disease |

*Reye syndrome:* There is a risk of Reye syndrome in children and teenagers when using aspirin in certain viral illnesses. Do not use in children or teenagers with viral infections with or without fever.

*Pregnancy:* There are no adequate and well-controlled studies in pregnant women. Use only when clearly needed and potential benefits outweigh the possible risks to the fetus. Avoid the combination in the third trimester of pregnancy because of the aspirin component.

*Breastfeeding:* Dipyridamole and aspirin are excreted in breast milk. Consult your doctor before you begin breastfeeding.

*Children:* Safety and effectiveness have not been established. This product is not recommended in children and teenagers because of the aspirin component.

*Lab tests* may be required during treatment. Tests include liver and kidney function, blood counts, urine tests, and bleeding tests.

## Drug Interactions:

Tell your doctor or pharmacist if you are taking or planning to take any over-the-counter or prescription medications or dietary supplements with this drug. Drug doses may need to be modified or a different drug prescribed. The following drugs and drug classes interact with this drug:

ACE inhibitors (eg, captopril)
acetazolamide (eg, *Diamox*)
adenosine (*Adenocard*)
anticoagulants (eg, warfarin)
beta blockers (eg, propranolol)
cholinesterase inhibitors
 (eg, tacrine)
diuretics (eg, furosemide)
heparin

hypoglycemics, oral
 (eg, sulfonylureas)
methotrexate (eg, *Rheumatrex*)
NSAIDs (eg, ibuprofen)
phenytoin (eg, *Dilantin*)
uricosuric agents
 (eg, probenecid)
valproic acid (eg, *Depakene*)

## Side Effects:

Every drug is capable of producing side effects. Many patients experience no, or minor, side effects. The frequency and severity of side effects depend on many factors including dose, duration of therapy, and individual susceptibility. Possible side effects include:

*Nervous System:* Headache; forgetfulness; convulsions; confusion; drowsiness; dizziness; fainting; weakness.

*Digestive Tract:* Stomach pain; indigestion; heartburn; nausea; vomiting; diarrhea; coffee-ground or bloody vomit; appetite loss; dark or bloody stools; rectal bleeding; stomach bleeding; hemorrhoids.

*Other:* Unusual bleeding or bruising; nosebleed; anemia; joint, chest, muscle, or back pain; arthritis; rash; itching; hives; general body discomfort; coughing; upper respiratory tract infection; accidental injury; heart failure; abnormal tissue growth; fatigue.

## Guidelines for Use:

- Dosage is individualized. Take exactly as prescribed.
- Do not stop taking or change the dose, unless instructed by your doctor.
- Swallow capsules whole. Do not crush or chew.
- Take with food if stomach upset occurs.
- Do not interchange with individual components of aspirin and dipyridamole.
- If a dose is missed, take it as soon as possible. If several hours have passed or it is nearing time for the next dose, do not double the dose to catch up, unless instructed by your doctor. If more than one dose is missed or it is necessary to establish a new dosage schedule, consult your doctor or pharmacist.
- Patients who consume 3 or more alcoholic drinks every day are at a higher risk of gastrointestinal bleeding while taking aspirin.
- Do not use in children or teenagers with viral infections with or without fever because of the risk of Reye syndrome associated with use of aspirin in certain viral illnesses.
- Do not use other aspirin-containing products, unless instructed by your doctor.
- Notify your doctor if you are pregnant, become pregnant, plan to become pregnant, or are breastfeeding.
- Contact your doctor immediately if you experience signs and symptoms of unusual bleeding, gastrointestinal bleeding (eg, bloody vomit, dark tarry stools), or recurrent signs of stroke or TIA.
- Notify your doctor if you experience bothersome side effects such as headache, indigestion, stomach pain, nausea, dizziness, or excessive bruising.
- Do not take aspirin if you have a known allergy to NSAIDs, asthma, rhinitis, or nasal polyps.
- Lab tests may be required to monitor treatment. Be sure to keep appointments.
- Store at room temperature (59° to 86°F) in a dry place.

*If you have any questions, consult your doctor, pharmacist, or health care provider.*

| Generic Name<br>*Brand Name Examples* | Supplied As | Generic<br>Available |
|---|---|---|
| Rx **Heparin Sodium** | | |
| *Heparin Sodium, Unit-<br>Dose* | **Injection**: 1000 units/dose,<br>2500 units/dose, 5000 units/<br>dose, 7500 units/dose,<br>10,000 units/dose, 20,000 units/<br>dose | Yes |
| *Heparin Sodium, Multiple<br>Dose Vials* | **Injection**: 1000 units/mL,<br>2000 units/mL, 2500 units/mL,<br>5,000 units/mL, 10,000 units/<br>mL, 20,000 units/mL,<br>40,000 units/mL | Yes |
| *Heparin Sodium, Single<br>Dose Ampules and Vials* | **Injection**: 1000 units/mL,<br>5000 units/mL, 10,000 units/mL,<br>20,000 units/mL, 40,000 units/<br>mL | Yes |

## Type of Drug:
Injectable anticoagulant; "blood thinner."

## How the Drug Works:
Heparin blocks the formation of fibrin (the framework for blood clots), preventing blood clots from forming. It will not dissolve already-formed blood clots, but will prevent them from becoming larger.

## Uses:
To prevent blood clots from forming.

To treat the extension of existing blood clots in veins, arteries, lungs, or heart.

To prevent blood-clotting complications of arterial and heart surgery, blood transfusions, artificial circulation (eg, heart-lung device), dialysis procedures, and blood samples for laboratory purposes.

*Unlabeled Use(s):* To reduce the risk of heart attack or stroke; to decrease angina attacks.

## Precautions:
*Do not use in the following situations:*
>absence of blood coagulation tests (full-dose heparin only)
>allergy to the drug or any of its ingredients
>bleeding, uncontrolled
>intramuscular (IM; into a muscle) injection
>low platelet count, severe

*Use with caution in the following situations:*

bleeding disorders (eg, hemophilia)
brain, spinal, or eye surgery
during or immediately following
spinal tap, spinal anesthesia,
or major surgery (especially of
the brain, spinal cord, or eye)
heart problems (eg, aneurysm)

high blood pressure, severe
increased lipoproteins (type III
hyperlipidemia)
kidney disease, severe
liver disease, severe
menstruation
ulcers

*Allergy:* Heparin is derived from animal (pork) tissue. Use with caution if there is a history of allergies.

*Pregnancy:* There are no adequate and well-controlled studies in pregnant women. Use only if clearly needed and potential benefits outweigh the possible risks to the fetus. Heparin does not cross the placenta, but bleeding problems can occur.

*Breastfeeding:* Heparin does not appear in breast milk. Consult your doctor before you begin breastfeeding.

*Children:* Safety and effectiveness have not been established in newborns.

*Elderly:* Patients older than 60 years of age require lower doses. Frequent monitoring is required.

*Lab tests* are required to monitor treatment. Tests include Partial Thromboplastin Time (PTT), Activated Coagulation Time (ACT), Activated Partial Thromboplastin Time (APTT), platelet count, hematocrit, potassium, and occult blood tests for the stool and urine.

## Drug Interactions:

Tell your doctor or pharmacist if you are taking or planning to take any over-the-counter or prescription medications or dietary supplements while taking this drug. Drug doses may need to be modified or a different drug prescribed. The following drugs and drug classes interact with this drug:

anticoagulants, oral (eg, warfarin)
antihistamines (eg, diphenhydramine)
cephalosporins (eg, cephalexin)
dextran (eg, *Macrodex*)
digitalis (eg, digoxin)
dipyridamole (eg, *Persantine*)

hydroxychloroquine (*Plaquenil*)
nicotine (cigarette smokers)
NSAIDs (eg, ibuprofen)
penicillins (eg, amoxicillin)
salicylates (eg, aspirin)
streptokinase (*Streptase*)
tetracyclines (eg, doxycycline)
ticlopidine (eg, *Ticlid*)

## Side Effects:

Every drug is capable of producing side effects. Many patients experience no, or minor, side effects. The frequency and severity of side effects depend on many factors including dose, duration of therapy, and individual susceptibility. Possible side effects include:

*Digestive Tract:* Nausea; vomiting; stomach pain; tarry stools.

*Circulatory System:* Bleeding; chest pain; increased blood pressure.

*Respiratory System:* Asthma; difficulty breathing or swallowing.

*Skin:* Hives; itching; burning; irritation; mild pain, redness, or bruising at injection site; hair loss; unusual bleeding or bruising; discoloration.

*Other:* Chills; fever; tearing; joint pain; painful sustained erection; headache; abnormal blood counts; shock; swelling; osteoporosis (long-term use); decreased blood platelets.

---

### Guidelines for Use:

- This medicine may be administered by your health care provider in a medical setting.
- Given continuously or intermittently intravenously (IV; into a vein) or subcutaneously (SC; beneath the skin) several times daily. IM use is to be avoided.
- Notify your doctor if you experience unusual bleeding or bruising, itching, chills, fever, or difficulty breathing.
- Lab tests are required to monitor therapy. Be sure to keep appointments.
- Store at controlled room temperature (59° to 86°F).

---

*If you have any questions, consult your doctor, pharmacist, or health care provider.*

| Generic Name<br>*Brand Name Example* | Supplied As | Generic<br>Available |
|---|---|---|
| Rx **Dalteparin Sodium** | | |
| *Fragmin*[1] | **Injection**: 2500 IU/0.2 mL,<br>5000 IU/mL, 7500 IU/0.3 mL,<br>10,000 IU/mL, 25,000 IU/mL | No |
| Rx **Enoxaparin Sodium** | | |
| *Lovenox* | **Injection**: 30 mg/0.3 mL,<br>40 mg/0.4 mL, 60 mg/0.6 mL,<br>80 mg/0.8 mL, 100 mg/mL,<br>120 mg/0.8 mL, 150 mg/mL | No |
| Rx **Tinzaparin Sodium** | | |
| *Innohep*[1,2] | **Injection**: 20,000 IU/mL | No |

[1] Multiple-dose vials contain benzyl alcohol.
[2] Contains sulfite preservative.

## Type of Drug:

Low molecular weight heparins (LMWHs); injectable anticoagulants; "blood thinners."

## How the Drug Works:

Low molecular weight heparins prevent blood clots from forming. They will not dissolve already-formed blood clots but may keep them from getting bigger and breaking loose (embolus).

## Uses:

*Dalteparin, enoxaparin:* For the prevention of deep vein thrombosis (DVT), which may lead to pulmonary embolism (PE) (blood clots in the lung) in patients undergoing hip replacement surgery (during and following hospitalization), knee replacement surgery (enoxaparin only), abdominal surgery in patients who are at risk for blood clotting complications, or in patients at risk for blood clotting complications due to severely restricted mobility during acute illness (enoxaparin only). Abdominal surgery patients at risk for blood clotting complications include those who are older than 40 years of age, obese, undergoing surgery under general anesthesia lasting longer than 30 minutes, or who have additional risk factors such as cancer or a history of DVT or PE.

For the prevention of ischemic complications of unstable angina and non-Q-wave myocardial infarction when coadministered with aspirin.

*Enoxaparin:* In conjunction with warfarin sodium (eg, *Coumadin*) for inpatient treatment of acute DVT with or without PE or for outpatient treatment of acute DVT without PE.

*Tinzaparin:* In conjunction with warfarin sodium for inpatient treatment of acute DVT with or without PE.

## Precautions:

*Do not use in the following situations:*
> allergy to the drug or any of its ingredients
> allergy to heparin
> allergy to pork products
> allergy to sulfites (tinzaparin only)
> bleeding, active major
> regional anesthesia for unstable angina or non-Q-wave MI
> > (dalteparin only)
> thrombocytopenia (low platelet count) with positive test for
> > antiplatelet antibody

*Use with caution in the following situations:*
> antiplatelet agent therapy, current
> bleeding disorders
> diabetic retinopathy
> elderly
> endocarditis, bacterial
> gastrointestinal disease (eg, ulcers or bleeding)
> heparin-induced thrombo-cytopenia (low platelet levels), history of
> high blood pressure, severe and uncontrolled
> hypertensive retinopathy
> kidney disease, severe
> liver disease, severe
> prosthetic heart valves (enoxaparin only)
> stroke, hemorrhagic (bleeding)
> surgery, recent (brain, spine, or eye)

*Benzyl alcohol:* Some of these products contain benzyl alcohol, which has been linked to fatal "gasping syndrome" in premature infants. Use with caution.

*Sulfites:* Some of these products contain sulfite preservatives that can cause allergic reactions in certain individuals (eg, patients with asthma). Consult your doctor or pharmacist.

*Pregnancy:* There are no adequate and well-controlled studies in pregnant women. A few spontaneous fetal deaths have been reported in enoxaparin-treated pregnant women with prosthetic heart valves. Use only if clearly needed and the potential benefits outweigh the possible risks to the fetus.

*Breastfeeding:* It is not known if these drugs appear in breast milk. Consult your doctor before you begin breastfeeding.

*Children:* Safety and effectiveness have not been established.

*Elderly:* The risk of enoxaparin-associated bleeding and other serious side effects increases with age. Elimination of enoxaparin is delayed in elderly patients. Use with caution.

*Lab tests* may be required to monitor therapy. Tests may include complete blood counts, urinalysis, neurological tests, and stool occult blood tests.

## Drug Interactions:

Tell your doctor or pharmacist if you are taking or planning to take any over-the-counter or prescription medications or dietary supplements while taking these drugs. Drug doses may need to be modified or a different drug prescribed. The following drugs and drug classes interact with these drugs:

anticoagulants, oral (eg, warfarin)
platelet inhibitors (eg, aspirin and other salicylates, dipyridamole, NSAIDs, sulfinpyrazone, dextran, ticlopidine)

## Side Effects:

Every drug is capable of producing side effects. Many patients experience no, or minor, side effects. The frequency and severity of side effects depend upon many factors including dose, duration of therapy, and individual susceptibility. Possible side effects include:

*Digestive Tract:* Constipation; nausea; vomiting; stomach pain; diarrhea; gas; indigestion.

*Circulatory System:* Changes in blood pressure; chest pain; abnormal heart rhythm; anemia; fast heartbeat.

*Nervous System:* Dizziness; sleeplessness; confusion; headache.

*Urinary and Reproductive Tract:* Blood in the urine; urinary tract infection; difficult or painful urination.

*Other:* Pain, redness, hardness, or bruising at the injection site; heavy or unusual bleeding or bruising; black stools; fever; swelling of the arms or legs; abnormal blood counts; lab test abnormalities; fever; difficulty breathing; pneumonia; nosebleed; back pain; impaired hearing; pain; infection; rash.

## Guidelines for Use:

- Dosage is individualized. Use exactly as prescribed.
- Do not stop taking or change the dose, unless instructed by your doctor.
- Follow the storage, preparation, administration, and disposal techniques taught to you by your health care provider.
- This medicine is administered once or twice daily. When it is started and how long therapy lasts depends on many factors, including the condition being treated. Your health care provider will advise you on how often to administer and for how long.
- Administer subcutaneously (SC; beneath the skin) only; do not administer intramuscularly (IM; into a muscle) or intravenously (IV; into a vein). Injections are given around the navel, upper thigh, or buttocks; change the injection site with each dose.
- If a dose is missed, inject as soon as possible. If more than 6 hours have passed or it is nearing time for the next dose, do not double the dose to catch up, unless instructed by your doctor. If more than one dose is missed or it is necessary to establish a new dosing schedule, contact your doctor or pharmacist.
- Do not rub or massage the injection site after completing the injection. Excessive bruising may occur. If bruising does occur, it may be lessened by an ice cube massage of the site prior to injection.
- Contact your doctor if you experience bleeding, unusual bruising, dizziness, light-headedness, itching, rash, fever, swelling of the arms or legs, or difficulty breathing.
- Low molecular weight heparins are not interchangeable with each other or with heparin. Each of these medicines has its own instructions for use.
- Lab tests may be required to monitor therapy. Be sure to keep appointments.
- Do not use if solution is discolored or contains particles.
- Store at controlled room temperature (59° to 77°F for enoxaparin, dalteparin; 59° to 86°F for tinzaparin).

*If you have any questions, consult your doctor, pharmacist, or health care provider.*

# ANTICOAGULANTS –
## COUMARIN DERIVATIVES

| Generic Name<br>*Brand Name Examples* | Supplied As | Generic<br>Available |
|---|---|---|
| **Anisindione** | | |
| *Rx* *Miradon* | **Tablets:** 50 mg | No |
| *Rx* **Dicumarol** | **Tablets:** 25 mg | Yes |
| **Warfarin Sodium** | | |
| *Rx* *Coumadin* | **Tablets:** 1 mg, 2 mg, 2.5 mg,<br>4 mg, 5 mg, 7.5 mg, 10 mg | No |
| *Rx* *Coumadin* | **Injection:** 2 mg/mL | No |

All of the products listed on this table are coumarin derivatives; however, they or their brand names are not interchangeable. For example, dicumarol cannot be used for anisindione, or *Coumadin* cannot be used for generic warfarin. Daily dose may vary depending on individual needs. Do not adjust the dose without consulting your pharmacist or doctor.

## Type of Drug:
Coumarin; anticoagulants, anti-clotting drugs; warfarin, blood thinners.

## How the Drug Works:
Coumarin prevents the liver from making substances needed to form blood clots. Anticoagulants are often given after stopping injectable heparin. Anticoagulants will not dissolve already-formed blood clots or repair tissue damage caused by blood clots.

## Uses:
To prevent or treat blood clots in veins.

To prevent or treat blood clots in the lungs.

To prevent blood clots associated with atrial fibrillation.

*Warfarin* — To reduce the risk of recurrence of a heart attack or a stroke after a heart attack, and to prevent blood clots after heart valve replacement or in patients with damaged heart valves.

*Anisindione, dicumarol* — To treat coronary blockage.

*Unlabeled Use(s):* Occasionally doctors may prescribe anticoagulants to prevent heart attack or symptoms which precede stroke. Warfarin has also been prescribed with cancer drugs and radiation for treatment of small cell lung cancer.

## Precautions:
*Do not use in the following situations:*

abnormal bleeding, history
abortion, threatened
alcoholism
allergy to this medicine
anesthesia, spinal
aneurysm

arthritis (anisindione only)
bleeding (eg, hemophilia, ulcers,
 genital or respiratory bleeding)
blood disease (anisindione only)
bruising

cancer, abdominal (dicumarol, anisindione)
colitis, ulcerative (anisindione only)
diverticulitis (anisindione only)
drainage (anisindione only)
emaciation (excessive leanness)
endocarditis, bacterial
high blood pressure, severe
inflammation or fluid around the heart
intrauterine device (IUD) insertion
kidney disease, serious (dicumarol, anisindione)
leukemia (anisindione only)
liver disease, serious (dicumarol, anisindione)
malnutrition (anisindione only)
polycythemia vera (eg, increase in blood volume) (anisindione only)
preeclampsia or eclampsia
pregnancy
prostate surgery
psychotic mental disorder
senility, unsupervised
spinal tap (puncture)
stroke, recent
surgery of eye, brain or central nervous system or resulting in large open surfaces
surgery, major
uncooperative patients
vitamin C deficiency (anisindione only)
vitamin K deficiency (dicumarol, anisindione)
wounds, open

*Use with caution in the following situations:*
absorption problems
allergic or anaphylactic disorders, severe
anemia, severe
antibiotic therapy
biliary tract abnormalities (anisindione only)
blood clots, recent
catheter use
congestive heart failure
dental procedures
diabetes, severe
diarrhea
drainage tubes, use (dicumarol only)
elderly
fever (anisindione, dicoumerol)
gastrointestinal bleeding, history
heart attack, recent
heart rhythm problems
high blood pressure
high cholesterol (anisindione only)
high triglycerides (anisindione only)
hyperthyroidism (anisindione only)
infections
injections, intramuscular
intestinal flora disturbances
jaundice (anisindione only)
kidney disease
liver disease
menstruation
polycythemia vera (increase in blood volume) (warfarin, dicumarol)
postpartum (after childbirth) (dicumarol only)
preparatory bowel sterilization (anisindione only)
protein C deficiency
protein C resistance
stomach bleeding, history of
stroke, history of
surgery with large exposed raw surfaces
surgery, recent
surgery/trauma, with potential internal bleeding
tuberculosis, active (dicumarol only)
vascular damage (anisindione only)
vasculitis (warfarin, dicumarol)
X-ray therapy (anisindione only)

*Lab tests:* Treatment with anticoagulants may be different with each patient. Dosage is controlled by lab tests. Tests may include kidney or liver function tests, prothrombin time (protime, PT) or INR (Interactional Normalized Ratio). Testing may be daily in the beginning of treatment. Once the dosage is stabilized, testing is every 4 to 6 weeks. Be sure to keep appointments.

*Pregnancy:* Do not use during pregnancy. The risk of use in a pregnant woman clearly outweighs any possible benefit.

*Breastfeeding:* Anticoagulants appear in breast milk. Nursing is not recommended while using anticoagulants.

*Children:* Safety and effectiveness have not been established.

*Elderly:* Elderly patients may be more sensitive to these agents.

## Drug Interactions:

Tell your doctor or pharmacist if you are taking or if you are planning to take any over-the-counter or prescription medications or dietary supplements while taking this medicine. Doses of one or both drugs may need to be modified or a different drug may need to be prescribed. The following drugs and drug classes interact with this medicine.

acetaminophen (eg, *Tylenol*)
adrenocortical steroids
 (eg, corticotropin)
alcohol
allopurinol (eg, *Zyloprim*)
aminoglutethimide (*Cytadren*)
aminoglycosides, oral
 (eg, neomycin)
aminosalicylic acid (*Pasar*)
amiodarone (*Cordarone*)
anabolic steroids
 (eg, oxandrolone)
androgens (eg, testosterone)
anesthetics, inhalation
antacids
antihistamines (eg, terfenadine)
azole antifungal agents
 (eg, metronidazole)
barbiturates (eg, phenobarbital)
beta blockers
 (eg, propranolol)
carbamazepine (eg, *Tegretol*)
cephalosporins (eg, cefaclor)
chloral hydrate
chloramphenicol (*Chloro-
mycetin*)
chlordiazepoxide (eg, *Librium*)
chlorpropamide (eg, *Diabinese*)
cholestyramine (eg, *Questran*)
chymotrypsin (*Catarase*)
cimetidine (eg, *Tagamet*)
clofibrate (eg, *Atromid-S*)

contraceptives, oral (eg, *Ortho-
Novum*)
corticosteroids (eg, prednisone)
cyclophosphamide
 (eg, *Cytoxan*)
dextran (eg, *Gentran*)
dextrothyroxine (*Choloxin*)
diazoxide (*Proglycam*)
dicloxacillin (eg, *Dynapen*)
diflunisal (*Dolobid*)
dipyridamole (*Persantine*)
disopyramide (eg, *Norpace*)
disulfiram (eg, *Antabuse*)
diuretics (eg, thiazides)
erythromycin (eg, *E-Mycin*)
estrogens (eg, estradiol)
ethacrynic acid (*Edecrin*)
ethchlorvynol (*Placidyl*)
etretinate (*Tegison*)
fenoprofen (eg, *Nalfon*)
fluorouracil (eg, *Adrucil*)
gemfibrozil (*Lopid*)
glucagon
glutethimide
griseofulvin (eg, *Grisactin*)
haloperidol (eg, *Haldol*)
hydantoins (eg, phenytoin)
hydrochloroquine (*Plaquenil*)
influenza vaccine
ifosfamide (*Ifex*)
isoniazid (eg, *Nydrazid*)
lovastatin (*Mevacor*)

magnesium salts (eg, *Milk of Magnesia)*
MAO inhibitor antidepressants (eg, phenelzine)
mefenamic acid (*Ponstel*)
meprobamate (eg, *Meprospan*)
methyldopa (eg, *Aldomet*)
methylphenidate (eg, *Ritalin*)
mineral oil
mitotane (*Lysodren*)
moricizine (*Ethmozine*)
nalidixic acid (*NegGram*)
nonsteroidal anti-inflammatory agents (eg, ibuprofen)
omeprazole (*Prilosec*)
paraldehyde (*Paral*)
penicillins (eg, amoxicillin)
pentoxifylline (*Trental*)
primadone (*Mysoline*)
propafenone (*Rythmol*)
propoxyphene (eg, *Darvon*)
quinidine (eg, *Quinora*)
quinine
quinolones (eg, ciprofloxacin)
rifamycins (eg, rifampin)
ranitidine (eg, *Zantac*)

salicylates (eg, aspirin)
serotonin reputake inhibitor antidepressants (eg, fluoxetine)
spironolactone (eg, *Aldactone*)
sucralfate (*Carafate*)
sulfonamides, (eg, sulfamethoxazole/trimethoprim)
sulfinpyrazone (eg, *Anturane*)
tamoxifen (*Nolvadex*)
tetracyclines (eg, doxycycline)
thioamines (eg, propylthiouracil)
thiopurines (eg, azathioprine)
thrombolytic agents (eg, alteplase)
thyroid hormones (eg, levothyroxine)
ticlopidine (*Ticlid*)
tolbutamide (eg, *Orinase*)
trazodone (eg, *Desyrel*)
tricyclic antidepressants (eg, amitriptyline)
valproic acid (eg, *Depakene*)
vitamin C
vitamin E
vitamin K

## Side Effects:

Every drug is capable of producing side effects. Many patients experience no, or minor, side effects. The frequency and severity of side effects depend on many factors including dose, duration of therapy and individual susceptibility. Possible side effects include:

*Hemorrhage* – Bloody or tarry stools; blood in urine; red or dark urine; excessive menstrual bleeding; unusual bleeding or bruising.

*Digestive Tract:* Diarrhea; nausea; vomiting; stomach pain; mouth sores; appetite loss.

*Skin:* Dermatitis; hives; purple toes; gangrene.

*Other:* Hair loss; yellowing of skin or eyes; fever; chills; chest, abdomen or joint pain; shortness of breath; difficulty breathing or swallowing; swelling; shock; paralysis; headache; drowsiness; sore throat; blurred vision; orange-red discoloration of urine; inability to urinate (anisindione only); sustained and painful erection.

## Guidelines for Use:

- Use exactly as prescribed. Strict adherence to prescribed dosage schedule is necessary.
- Dosing is individualized and may have to be frequently adjusted based on lab test results.
- *Injection* — Follow the injection procedure taught to you by your health care provider.
- If a dose is missed, take it as soon as possible. If several hours have passed or if it is nearing time for the next dose, do not double the dose to catch up, unless advised by your doctor. If more than one dose is missed, contact your doctor or pharmacist.
- Do not take or discontinue any other medication except on advice of your pharmacist or doctor.
- Avoid alcohol, aspirin, topical pain killers, large amounts of green leafy vegetables, or drastic changes in dietary habits.
- Inform your doctor if you are pregnant, become pregnant, are planning to become pregnant, or if you are breastfeeding.
- Contact your doctor if you experience diarrhea, infection, fever, pain, swelling, discomfort, prolonged bleeding from cuts, increased menstrual flow or vaginal bleeding, blood in urine, nosebleeds, bleeding from gums when brushing, other unusual bleeding or bruising, red or dark brown urine, red or tar black stools, purple toes, toe pain or tenderness, rash, ulcers, or hair loss.
- *Anisindione* — Contact your doctor if you experience excessive fatigue, chills, fever, or sore throat.
- Contact your doctor before undergoing dental work or elective surgery.
- Warfarin may cause a red-orange discoloration of urine.
- All of the products listed on this table are coumarin derivatives; however, they are not interchangeable.
- Lab tests will be required to monitor therapy. Be sure to keep appointments.
- *Injection* — Visually inspect solution for particles or discoloration.
- Store reconstituted injection solution at room temperature (59° to 86°F). Do not refrigerate. Use within 4 hours. Discard any unused solution.
- Store tablets at room temperature (59° to 77°F) in a tight, light-resistant container.

*If you have any questions, consult your doctor, pharmacist, or health care provider.*

| Generic Name<br>*Brand Name Examples* | Supplied As | Generic<br>Available |
|---|---|---|
| *Rx* **Alteplase, Recombinant** | | |
| *Activase* | **Powder for injection,<br>lyophilized**: 50 mg/vial,[1]<br>100 mg/vial[1] | No |
| *Rx* **Anistreplase** | | |
| *Eminase* | **Powder for injection,<br>lyophilized**: 30 units | No |
| *Rx* **Reteplase, Recombinant** | | |
| *Retavase* | **Powder for injection,<br>lyophilized**: 18.1 mg reteplase[2] | No |
| *Rx* **Streptokinase** | | |
| *Streptase* | **Powder for injection,<br>lyophilized**: 250,000 IU,<br>750,000 IU, 1,500,000 IU | No |
| *Rx* **Tenecteplase** | | |
| *TNKase* | **Powder for injection,<br>lyophilized**: 50 mg[1] | No |

[1] Contains L-arginine, phosphoric acid, polysorbate 80.
[2] Contains L-arginine.

## Type of Drug:

Blood clot dissolvers.

## How the Drug Works:

Thrombolytic agents dissolve blood clots and restore blood circulation to affected body tissue.

## Uses:

To dissolve blood clots, including those blocking coronary arteries in acute heart attacks.

*Alteplase:* To help manage acute ischemic strokes in adults to reduce the chances of disability, or to reduce the incidence of congestive heart failure (CHF) and death due to heart attack.

*Streptokinase:* To dissolve large blood clots in legs.

*Unlabeled Use(s):* Occasionally doctors may prescribe alteplase for the treatment of unstable angina pectoris (chest pain).

## Precautions:

*Do not use in the following situations:*

abnormal bleeding conditions
allergy to the thrombolytic agent
  or any of its ingredients
bleeding into or around the brain
brain aneurysm

brain cancer
cardiopulmonary resuscitation
  (CPR), recent
cerebrovascular accident
  (stroke), history of

high blood pressure, severe, uncontrolled
internal bleeding
low platelet count
seizures at onset of stroke
stroke, previous (within 2 to 3 months)
surgery or trauma to head or spine (within 2 to 3 months)

*Use with caution in the following situations:*
bacterial endocarditis
black or tarry stools
bleeding
blood clot in heart chamber
brain blood vessel disease
childbirth
diabetic bleeding retinopathy
gastrointestinal bleeding, recent
genitourinary bleeding, recent
high blood pressure
infections involving the heart
kidney disease
liver disease
major surgery or trauma, recent
older than 75 years of age
pregnancy
readministration (alteplase, anistrepalse, streptokinase, tenecteplase only)
stroke, history of

*Abnormal heartbeats:* Use of thrombolytic agents to dissolve clots in coronary arteries (acute heart attack) may result in abnormal heartbeat. Heart rate will need to be monitored during and following therapy.

*Pregnancy:* Safety for use during pregnancy has not been established. Use only if clearly needed and the potential benefits to the mother outweigh the possible hazards to the fetus.

*Breastfeeding:* It is not known if thrombolytic agents appear in breast milk. Consult your doctor before you begin breastfeeding.

*Children:* Safety and effectiveness have not been established.

*Lab tests* will be required to monitor therapy. Tests may include platelet counts, thrombin time (TT), activated partial thromboplastin time (APTT), prothrombin time (PT), fibrinogen levels, hematocrit counts, as well as the monitoring of blood pressure, heart rate and rhythm, and other vital signs (eg, respirations, temperature).

## Drug Interactions:
Tell your doctor or pharmacist if you are taking or will be taking any over-the-counter or prescription medications or dietary supplements while taking a thrombolytic agent. Doses of one or both drugs may need to be modified or a different drug may need to be prescribed. The following drugs and drug classes interact with thrombolytic agents:

anticoagulants (eg, warfarin)
antiplatelet agents (eg, *Persantin*)
aspirin
heparin (eg, *Hep-Lock*)
indomethacin (eg, *Indocin*)

## Side Effects:

Every drug is capable of producing side effects. Many thrombolytic agent users experience no, or minor, side effects. The frequency and severity of side effects depend on many factors including dose, duration of therapy, and individual susceptibility. Possible side effects include:

*Bleeding:* Bleeding at puncture and incision sites; bleeding from rectum, stomach, lungs, gums, mouth, nose, or urinary tract.

*Digestive Tract:* Nausea; vomiting.

*Circulatory System:* Internal bleeding; irregular heartbeat; changes in blood pressure.

*Skin:* Rash; unusual bruising.

*Other:* Fever; chills; difficult or fast breathing; back pain.

---

### Guidelines for Use:

- This medicine will be prepared and administered intravenously (into a vein) by your health care provider in a medical setting.
- Dosage is individualized.
- Effectiveness depends on how quickly the drug is given.
- Bleeding is a common side effect of thrombolytic agent therapy.
- Notify your doctor immediately if you experience fever, shivering, chills, rash, hives, swelling, or difficult or rapid breathing.

---

*If you have any questions, consult your doctor, pharmacist, or health care provider.*

| Generic Name<br>*Brand Name Examples* | Supplied As | Generic<br>Available |
|---|---|---|
| **Pentoxifylline** | | |
| *Rx  Trental* | **Tablets, controlled release:**<br>400 mg | No |

## Type of Drug:
Hemorrheologic agent; a drug that improves blood flow.

## How the Drug Works:
Pentoxifylline improves blood flow by reducing the thickness of the blood and improving red blood cell flexibility.

## Uses:
To treat circulatory conditions in the arms and legs (eg, intermittent claudication) that cause discomfort. It does not, however, cure these conditions.

*Unlabeled Use(s):* Occasionally doctors may prescribe pentoxifylline for cerebrovascular problems, circulatory and problems caused by diabetes, leg ulcers, sickle cell anemia, strokes, high altitude sickness, hearing problems, eye circulation disorders and Reynaud syndrome.

## Precautions:
*Do not use in the following situations:*
allergy to pentoxifylline, caffeine, theophylline or theobromine
cerebral and/or retinal bleeding

*Use with caution in the following situations:*
arteriosclerosis (hardening of the arteries)
kidney disease
peptic ulcers
surgery, recent

*Pregnancy:* Adequate studies have not been done in pregnant women, or animal studies may have shown a risk to the fetus. Use only if clearly needed and potential benefits outweigh the possible hazards to the fetus.

*Breastfeeding:* Pentoxifylline appears in breast milk. Consult your doctor before you begin breastfeeding.

*Children:* Safety and effectiveness in children have not been established.

*Lab tests* or exams may be required to monitor therapy. Be sure to keep appointments. Tests may include prothrombin time and exams for bleeding (eg, hematocrit/hemoglobin).

## Drug Interactions:

Tell your doctor or pharmacist if you are taking or planning to take any over-the-counter or prescription medications or dietary supplements while taking this medicine. Doses of one or both drugs may need to be modified or another drug may need to be prescribed. The following drugs and drug classes interact with this medicine:

anticoagulants, oral (eg, warfarin)
theophylline (eg, *Slo-Phyllin*)

## Side Effects:

Every drug is capable of producing side effects. Many patients experience no, or minor, side effects. The frequency and severity of side effects depend on many factors including dose, duration of therapy and individual susceptibility. Possible side effects may include:

*Digestive Tract:* Stomach ache; nausea; vomiting; indigestion.

*Nervous System:* Dizziness; headache.

### Guidelines for Use:

- Use exactly as prescribed.
- Take 1 tablet, three times daily with meals. A lower dose may be necessary if side effects occur. Consult your doctor.
- Do not crush, chew or break tablet.
- If a dose is missed, take it as soon as possible. If several hours have passed or if it is nearing time for the next dose, do not double the dose in order to "catch up" (unless advised to do so by your doctor). If more than one dose is missed or it is necessary to establish a new dosage schedule, contact your doctor or pharmacist.
- Improvement may take 2 to 4 weeks to notice and up to 8 weeks for maximum relief.
- If severe indigestion, nausea, vomiting, nervousness, dizziness or headache occur, contact your doctor immediately.
- May cause dizziness. Use caution while driving or performing other tasks requiring alertness, coordination or physical dexterity.
- Store at room temperature (59° to 86°F). Protect from light.

*If you have any questions, consult your doctor, pharmacist, or health care provider.*

| Generic Name<br>*Brand Name Examples* | Supplied As | Generic<br>Available |
|---|---|---|
| *Rx* **Phytonadione** | | |
| *Mephyton* | **Tablets:** 5 mg | No |
| *AquaMEPHYTON* | **Injection:** 2 mg/mL, 10 mg/mL | Yes |

## Type of Drug:
Antihemorrheologic; antibleeding agent.

## How the Drug Works:
Phytonadione stimulates the production of certain factors needed for blood to clot.

## Uses:
To treat certain bleeding disorders caused by a lack of vitamin K or interference with the way vitamin K works.

## Precautions:
*Do not use in the following situations:* Allergy to this medicine.

*Use with caution in the following situations:* Anticoagulant use, liver disease.

*Injection:* Phytonadione should be given under the skin or in the muscle. Injection into the vein (IV) may lead to shock, heart attack, stopped breathing and death. IV injection should only be used when the other methods are not possible and the serious risk involved is considered justified.

*Pregnancy:* Adequate studies have not been done in pregnant women, or animal studies may have shown a risk to the fetus. Use only if clearly needed and potential benefits outweigh the possible risk to the fetus.

*Breastfeeding:* Phytonadione appears in breast milk. Consult your doctor.

*Children:* Safety and effectiveness have not been established. Certain blood and liver problems in infants may be related to phytonadione use. Do not exceed recommended dosage.

*Lab tests* will be required. Tests may include prothrombin time monitoring.

## Drug Interactions:
Tell your doctor or pharmacist if you are taking or planning to take any over-the-counter or prescription medications or dietary supplements. Doses of one or both drugs may need to be adjusted or a different drug may need to be prescribed. Anticoagulants (eg, warfarin) and mineral oil interact with this medicine.

## Side Effects:

Every drug is capable of producing side effects. Many patients experience no, or minor, side effects. The frequency and severity of side effects depend on many factors including dose, duration of therapy and individual susceptibility. Possible side effects include: Temporary flushing and taste changes; pain, swelling and tenderness at the injection site; allergic reactions.

---

### Guidelines for Use:

- Results are not immediate.
- Store at room temperature. Protect from light.

---

*If you have any questions, consult your doctor, pharmacist, or health care provider.*

| Generic Name<br>*Brand Name Example* | Supplied As | Generic<br>Available |
|---|---|---|
| *Rx* **Sodium Phenylbutyrate** | | |
| *Buphenyl* | **Tablets:** 500 mg | No |
| *Buphenyl* | **Powder:** 3.2 g/tsp, 9.1 g/tbsp | No |

## Type of Drug:
Urea cycle disorder treatment.

## How the Drug Works:
Sodium phenylbutyrate forms a substance needed for the elimination of nitrogen waste (ammonia) from the body.

## Uses:
Adjunctive therapy for chronic management of patients with urea cycle disorder and in infants with enzymatic deficiencies that result in elevated levels of ammonia in the blood.

## Precautions:
*Do not use in the following situations:*
> to manage acute elevated ammonia blood levels

*Use with caution in the following situations:*
congestive heart failure (CHF)
kidney disease
liver disease
nerve impairment
sodium retention causing fluid retention (edema, swelling, water retention)

*Pregnancy:* Adequate studies have not been done in pregnant women, or animal studies may have shown a risk to the fetus. Use only if clearly needed and the potential benefits outweigh the possible hazards to the fetus.

*Breastfeeding:* It is not known if sodium phenylbutyrate appears in breast milk. Consult your doctor before you begin breastfeeding.

*Children:* Use of the tablets in newborns, infants and children under 44 lbs is not recommended.

*Lab tests* will be required to monitor therapy. Tests may include: Blood counts and ammonia and amino acid blood levels.

## Drug Interactions:
Tell your doctor or pharmacist if you are taking or planning to take any over-the-counter or prescription medication or dietary supplements while taking this medicine. Doses of one or both drugs may need to be modified or a different drug may need to be prescribed. The following drugs and drug classes interact with this medicine:

corticosteroids (eg, prednisone)
haloperidol (eg, *Haldol*)
probenecid (eg, *Benemid*)
valproate (eg, *Depakote*)

## Side Effects:

Every drug is capable of producing side effects. Many patients experience no, or minor, side effects. The frequency and severity of side effects depend upon many factors including dose, duration of therapy and individual susceptibility. Possible side effects include:

*Digestive Tract:* Stomach pain; nausea; vomiting; constipation; rectal bleeding; appetite loss; peptic ulcers.

*Nervous System:* Depression; drowsiness; fatigue; light-headedness; headache.

*Circulatory System:* Anemia; abnormal heartbeat.

*Other:* Menstrual problems; body odor; unpleasant taste sensation; fainting; weight gain; rash; swelling; kidney problems; abnormal lab tests.

---

### Guidelines for Use:

- Dosage is individualized. Take exactly as prescribed.
- *Tablets* — Take in equally divided amounts 3 times daily with meals.
- *Powder* — Take in equally divided amounts with each meal or feeding, 4 to 6 times daily. Mix with food (solid or liquid). Avoid acidic drinks. Shake lightly before use.
- If a dose is missed, take it as soon as possible. If several hours have passed or it is nearing time for the next dose, do not double the dose to catch up, unless instructed by your doctor. If more than one dose is missed or it is necessary to establish a new dosage schedule, contact your doctor or pharmacist.
- A special diet will be needed to derive the most benefit in using this drug.
- Sodium phenylbutyrate may have to be taken for life unless you receive a liver transplant.
- May cause drowsiness, fatigue, fainting, or light-headedness. Use caution while driving or performing other tasks that require alertness, coordination, or physical dexterity until tolerance is determined.
- Contact your doctor immediately if you experience decreased mental awareness, vomiting, combativeness, slurred speech, unstable gait, unconsciousness, or fever.
- Store at room temperature (59° to 86°F). Keep bottle tightly closed.

---

*If you have any questions, consult your doctor, pharmacist, or health care provider.*

| Generic Name<br>*Brand Name Examples* | Supplied As | Generic<br>Available |
|---|---|---|
| *Rx* **Darbepoetin Alfa** | | |
| *Aranesp* | **Injection**: 25 mcg/mL, 40 mcg/mL, 60 mcg/mL, 100 mcg/mL, 200 mcg/mL | No |
| *Rx* **Epoetin Alfa** | | |
| *Epogen, Procrit* | **Injection:** 2000 units/mL, 3000 units/mL, 4000 units/mL, 10,000 units/mL, 20,000 units/mL, 40,000 units/mL | No |

## Type of Drug:
Blood modifier; antianemia.

## How the Drug Works:
Epoetin alfa and darbepoetin alfa are synthetic copies of the natural hormone produced by the kidney, which stimulate production of oxygen-carrying red blood cells by the bone marrow.

## Uses:
*Darbepoetin:* To treat anemia associated with chronic kidney failure, including patients on and not on dialysis.

To treat anemia in patients with nonmyeloid malignancies where anemia is caused by coadministered chemotherapy.

*Epoetin:* To treat anemia and decrease the need for blood transfusions in patients with anemia associated with chronic kidney failure, including patients on and not on dialysis.

To treat anemia and decrease the need for blood transfusions in patients with anemia due to zidovudine (AZT) therapy for HIV infection.

To treat anemia and decrease the need for blood transfusions in patients with nonmyeloid (non-bone marrow) cancer who develop anemia because of chemotherapy. It is intended for patients who will be receiving chemotherapy for at least 2 months.

To increase a patient's red blood cell production before certain elective surgeries to reduce the need for blood transfusions.

*Unlabeled Use(s):* Doctors nay occasionally prescribe epoetin for pruritus associated with kidney failure.

## Precautions:
*Do not use in the following situations:*
allergy to human albumin (epoetin, darbepoetin with albumin only)
allergy to mammalian (animal) cell-derived products (epoetin only)
allergy to the drug or any of its ingredients
high blood pressure, uncontrolled

*Use with caution in the following situations:*

anemia due to iron or folate deficiencies, hemolysis or gastrointestinal bleeding
anemia, severe (chronic kidney
failure) (epoetin only)
blood disease

cardiac disease, preexisting
(epoetin only)
high blood pressure, preexisting
porphyria (epoetin only)
seizures

*Pregnancy:* There are no adequate and well-controlled studies in pregnant women. Use only if clearly needed and the potential benefits to
the mother outweigh the possible hazards to the fetus.

*Breastfeeding:* It is not known if these drugs appear in breast milk.
Consult your doctor before you begin breastfeeding.

*Children:* Safety and effectiveness of epoetin in children less than one
month of age on dialysis have not been established. Safety and effectiveness of epoetin in children for other uses have not been established.
Safety and effectiveness of darbepoetin in children have not been
established.

*Lab tests* and exams will be required to monitor therapy. Tests may include
blood pressure, blood cell and platelet counts, bleeding time, kidney
function tests, fluid and electrolyte tests, serum chemistry, and iron evaluation tests.

## Drug Interactions:

Tell your doctor or pharmacist if you are taking or planning to take any over-
the-counter or prescription medications or dietary supplements while
taking a recombinant human erythropoietin. Drug doses may need to be
modified or a different drug prescribed.

## Side Effects:

Every drug is capable of producing side effects. Many patients experience
no, or minor, side effects. The frequency and severity of side effects
depend upon many factors including dose, duration of therapy, and individual susceptibility. Possible side effects include:

*Digestive Tract:* Nausea; vomiting; diarrhea; stomach pain; constipation.

*Nervous System:* Headache; fatigue; weakness; dizziness; seizures;
abnormal skin sensations; sleeplessness.

*Circulatory System:* Changes in blood pressure; chest pain; irregular heart
beat; congestive heart failure; blood clots (eg, pain and swelling of the
lower legs).

*Respiratory System:* Congestion; shortness of breath; cough; upper respiratory infection.

*Other:* Joint, muscle, limb, back, or body pain; fluid retention; bleeding,
pain, or tenderness at injection site; rash; itching; fever; infection;
swelling of the arms or legs (edema); flu-like symptoms.

# RECOMBINANT HUMAN ERYTHROPOIETIN

## Guidelines for Use:

- Follow the storage, preparation, injection, and disposal procedures taught to you by your health care provider.
- Dosage is individualized. Take exactly as prescribed.
- *Epoetin* — Use this medicine three times weekly.
- *Darbepoetin* — Use this medicine once weekly.
- The dose may be changed by your doctor, depending on how you respond to the injections. Do not change the dose or stop taking, unless instructed by your doctor.
- Talk to your doctor about what to do if you miss a dose.
- Do not use a vial if there are any particles or discoloration.
- Do not mix with other injectable medications.
- Continue to follow the diet or dialysis prescribed by your doctor, even when you start to feel better.
- *High blood pressure* — It is important to follow the blood pressure monitoring and therapy recommendations and diet restrictions established by your doctor while taking this medicine.
- Discontinue use and contact your doctor immediately at the first appearance of rash or other signs of allergic reactions (eg, hives).
- Do not reuse needles or syringes. Dispose of used needles and syringes in the puncture-resistant container provided with your medication as directed by your doctor.
- Take supplemental iron and vitamins as directed by your doctor.
- Contraceptive measures (ie, birth control) are recommended to prevent pregnancy during treatment.
- May cause dizziness or seizures. Use caution when driving or performing other tasks requiring alertness, coordination, or physical dexterity until tolerance is determined.
- Lab tests and exams will be required to monitor therapy. Be sure to keep appointments.
- *Single-dose vials (1 mL)* — Contains no preservatives. Use only one dose per vial. Discard any unused portions.
- *Multi-dose vials (2 mL)* — Contains preservatives. Discard 21 days after first use.
- Refrigerate at 36° to 46°F. Do not freeze or shake. Protect from light.

*If you have any questions, consult your doctor, pharmacist, or health care provider.*

| Generic Name<br>*Brand Name Example* | Supplied As | Generic<br>Available |
|---|---|---|
| *Rx* **Filgrastim** | | |
| *Neupogen* | **Injection**: 300 mcg/mL,<br>480 mcg/1.6 mL vials; 300 mcg/<br>0.5 mL, 480 mcg/0.8 mL<br>syringes | No |
| *Rx* **Pegfilgrastim** | | |
| *Neulasta* | **Injection**: 6 mg/0.6 mL<br>syringes | No |
| *Rx* **Sargramostim** | | |
| *Leukine* | **Injection**: 250 mcg/vial (powder<br>for injection), 500 mcg/mL[1] | No |

[1] Contains benzyl alcohol.

## Type of Drug:

Granulocyte colony- or white blood cell-stimulating factor.

## How the Drug Works:

Colony stimulating factors are synthetic copies of the natural product that stimulates production of infection—fighting white blood cells (granulocytes) by the bone marrow.

## Uses:

*Filgrastim:* To decrease the incidence of infections due to neutropenia (low white blood cell counts) in cancer patients who are receiving white blood cell-suppressing anticancer drugs.

To reduce the duration of neutropenia and its symptoms (eg, fever, infections) in cancer patients undergoing chemotherapy followed by bone marrow transplantation.

For chronic use to reduce the incidence and duration of the symptoms of neutropenia (eg, fever, infections, mouth or throat ulcers) in patients with severe chronic neutropenia (SCN).

*Pegfilgrastim:* To decrease the incidence of infections due to neutropenia (low white blood cell counts) in cancer patients who are receiving white blood cell-suppressing anticancer drugs.

*Sargramostim:* For use after induction of chemotherapy in patients 55 years of age or older with acute myelogenous leukemia (AML) to shorten time to neutrophil (white blood cell) recovery to lower the risks of severe and life-threatening infections.

To speed up bone marrow recovery in patients with non-Hodgkin lymphoma (NHL), acute lymphoblastic leukemia (ALL), and Hodgkin disease undergoing bone marrow transplantation (BMT).

For bone marrow transplant patients in whom engraftment of bone marrow is delayed or has failed.

*Unlabeled Use(s):* Occasionally doctors may prescribe filgrastim for AIDS, aplastic anemia, hairy cell leukemia, drug-induced or congenital agranulocytosis, or developmental defects of the spinal cord.

## Precautions:

*Do not use in the following situations:*
>allergy to *E. coli*-derived proteins (filgrastim, pegfilgrastim only)
>allergy to the drug or any of its ingredients
>chemotherapy, current
>immature white blood cells in the bone marrow or peripheral blood (sargramostim only)
>radiation therapy, concurrent

*Use with caution in the following situations:*
chemotherapy, previous
congestive heart failure (CHF) (sargramostim only)
fluid retention (sargramostim only)
heart disease, preexisting
hypothyroid (underactive thyroid) (filgrastim only)
hypoxia (low oxygen level in the blood) (sargramostim only)
kidney disease (sargramostim only)
liver disease (sargramostim only)
lung disease (sargramostim only)
lung infiltrates (sargramostim only)
myeloid (bone marrow) cancer (filgrastim, pegfilgrastim only)
radiation therapy, previous
sickle cell disease (filgrastim, pegfilgrastim only)

*Adult respiratory distress syndrome (ARDS):* ARDS has been reported in neutropenic patients receiving colony stimulating factors. Notify your doctor if you experience fever or difficulty breathing.

*Benzyl alcohol:* Sargramostim injection contains benzyl alcohol, which has been associated with a fatal "gasping syndrome" in premature infants. Do not administer to neonates.

*First dose effects:* A syndrome with respiratory distress, hypoxia, flushing, low blood pressure, fainting, or fast heartbeat has occurred following the first administration of sargramostim in a particular cycle. These signs have resolved with treatment and usually do not recur with subsequent doses in the same cycle of treatment.

*Pregnancy:* There are no adequate and well-controlled studies in pregnant women. Use only if clearly needed and potential benefits outweigh the possible risk to the fetus.

*Breastfeeding:* It is not known if colony stimulating factors appear in breast milk. Consult your doctor before you begin breastfeeding.

*Children:*

*Filgrastim* – Serious long-term risks associated with daily filgrastim have not been identified in children 1 month to 16 years of age with severe chronic neutropenia. Safety and effectiveness in neonates and patients with autoimmune neutropenia of infancy have not been established.

*Pegfilgrastim* – Safety and effectiveness have not been established. Do not use the 6 mg fixed-dose single-use syringe formulation in infants, children, and smaller adolescents weighing less than 45 kg.

*Sargramostim* – Safety and effectiveness have not been established.

*Lab tests* and exams will be required to monitor therapy. Tests include white blood cell and platelet counts and liver and kidney tests.

## Drug Interactions:

Tell your doctor or pharmacist if your are taking or planning to take any over-the-counter or prescription medication or dietary supplements while taking these drugs. Drug doses may need to be modified or a different drug prescribed. Drugs that may stimulate release of white blood cells from the bone marrow, such as corticosteroids (eg, hydrocortisone) or lithium (eg, *Eskalith*) may interact with these drugs.

## Side Effects:

Every drug is capable of producing side effects. Many patients experience no, or minor, side effects. The frequency and severity of side effects depend on many factors including dose, duration of therapy, and individual susceptibility. Possible side effects include:

*Digestive Tract:* Nausea; vomiting; diarrhea; appetite loss; gastrointestinal upset or bleeding; inflammation of the mouth; stomach pain or bloating; indigestion; bloody vomit or stools; difficulty swallowing; constipation; taste sensation changes; sore throat.

*Nervous System:* Weakness; dizziness; general body discomfort; nervous system disorder; headache; abnormal skin sensations; sleeplessness; anxiety.

*Circulatory System:* Blood disorder; chest pain; changes in blood pressure; unusual bleeding or bruising; heart problems; fast heartbeat.

*Respiratory System:* Difficulty breathing; lung disorder; runny nose; cough.

*Skin:* Hair loss; rash; itching; skin disorders; injection site reaction.

*Other:* Fever; fatigue; chills; infection; weight changes; allergic reactions; sweating; mucous membrane disorder; fluid retention; swelling of the arms and legs; urinary tract disorder; abnormal kidney function; joint, bone, back, or muscle pain; nosebleed; abnormal lab tests; abnormal blood counts; blood in urine; enlargement of the spleen; general pain.

**Guidelines for Use:**

- Follow the storage, preparation, injection, and disposal procedures taught to you by your health care provider.
- Dosage is individualized. Take exactly as prescribed.
- Do not stop taking or change the dose, unless instructed by your doctor.
- Talk to your doctor about what to do if you miss a dose.
- Do not use if there are particles or discoloration in the injection solution.
- Contact your doctor immediately if you experience rash, difficulty breathing, flushing, dizziness, light-headedness, fainting, fast heart-beat, or upper abdominal or shoulder pain.
- Lab tests and exams will be required to monitor therapy. Be sure to keep appointments.
- Do not mix with any other injectable medications.
- Syringes and vials of filgrastim and pegfilgrastim contain no preserva-tives.
- Store in refrigerator (36° to 46°F). Do not freeze or shake. Filgrastim may be allowed to reach room temperature for up to 24 hours before injection. Discard vial or syringe if left at room temperature for longer than 24 hours. Pegfilgrastim may be allowed to reach room tempera-ture for up to 48 hours before injection. Discard syringe if left at room temperature for longer than 48 hours. If accidentally frozen, allow to thaw in the refrigerator before injecting. Discard if frozen a second time.

*If you have any questions, consult your doctor, pharmacist, or health care provider.*

**Octreotide Acetate,** 127

**Sex Hormones**
Anabolic Steroids, 130
Mifepristone, 134
Androgens, 137
Androgen Hormone Inhibitors, 141
Estrogens, 144
Estrogen Combinations, 150
Selective Estrogen Receptor Modulator, 153
Progestins, 156
Contraceptive Methods, 160
Medroxyprogesterone Acetate, 161
Medroxyprogesterone Acetate/Estradiol Cypionate, 163
Etonogestrel/Ethinyl Estradiol, 166
Oral Contraceptives, 170
Emergency Contraceptives, 179
Contraceptive Systems
Intrauterine Progesterone, 182
Levonorgestrel Implant, 185
Levonorgestrel-Releasing Intrauterine, 188
Contraceptive Transdermal Systems
Norelgestromin/Ethinyl Estradiol, 192

**Fertility Agents**
Choriogonadotropin Alfa, 195
Chorionic Gonadotropin, 197
Urofollitropin, 200
Follitropin Alfa, 202
Follitropin Beta, 204
Clomiphene, 206
Menotropins, 209

**Gonadotropin-Releasing Hormones**
Nafarelin, 212

**Danazol,** 215

**Posterior Pituitary Hormones**
Desmopressin Acetate, 218

**Growth Hormones**
Somatrem, 221
Somatropin, 223

**Adrenal Cortical Steroids**
Corticotropin, 226
Glucocorticoids, 230
Corticosteroids, Topical, 238
Corticosteroid Combinations, Topical, 245
Mineralocorticoid, 249

**Adrenal Steroid Inhibitors**
Aminoglutethimide, 253

**Antidiabetic Agents**
Insulin, 255
Alpha-Glucosidase Inhibitors, 264
Thiazolidinediones, 267
Sulfonylureas, 270
Meglitinides, 275
Metformin, 278
Glyburide/Metformin, 281

**Glucose Elevating Agents**
Glucagon, 284

**Thyroid Drugs**
Antithyroid Agents, 286
Iodine Products, 289
Thyroid Hormones, 291

**Calcitonin,** 294

**Bisphosphonates,** 297

**Imiglucerase,** 301

| Generic Name<br>*Brand Name Example* | Supplied As | Generic<br>Available |
|---|---|---|
| *Rx* **Octreotide Acetate**<br>*Sandostatin* | **Injection:** 0.05 mg/mL, 0.1 mg/mL, 0.2 mg/mL, 0.5 mg/mL, 1 mg/mL | No |

## Type of Drug:

Synthetic hormone closely related to the natural hormone somatostatin (growth hormone inhibitor).

## How the Drug Works:

Octreotide reduces blood levels of a variety of hormones (eg, growth hormone) and chemical messengers (eg, gastrin).

## Uses:

To reduce the blood levels of growth hormone and IGF-I in patients with acromegaly who have had inadequate response to or cannot be treated with surgical resection, pituitary irradiation and bromocriptine mesylate at maximally tolerated doses. The goal is to achieve normalization of growth hormone and IGF-I levels.

To treat symptoms of patients with metastatic carcinoid tumors where it suppresses or inhibits severe diarrhea and flushing episodes.

Treatment of the profuse watery diarrhea associated with vasoactive intestinal peptide (VIP) tumors.

*Unlabeled Use(s):* Occasionally doctors may prescribe this medicine to reduce output from gastrointestinal or pancreatic sores; treat variceal bleeding, diarrheal states associated with a variety of conditions, irritable bowel syndrome, dumping syndrome, enteric fistula, pancreatitis, pancreatic surgery, glucagonoma, insulinoma, gastrinoma (Zollinger-Ellison syndrome), intestinal obstruction, local radiotherapy, thyrotropin- and TSH-secreting tumors; for chronic pain management, antineoplastic (anti-cancer) therapy or to decrease insulin requirements in diabetes mellitus.

## Precautions:

*Do not use in the following situations:* Sensitivity to any component of this medicine.

*Use with caution in the following situations:*
diabetes
kidney disease

*Pregnancy:* Studies in pregnant women or in animals have been judged not to show a risk to the fetus. However, no drug should be used during pregnancy unless clearly needed.

*Breastfeeding:* It is not known if octreotide appears in breast milk. Consult your doctor before you begin breastfeeding.

*Elderly:* Lower doses may be necessary.

*Lab tests* may be required to monitor therapy. Lab tests may include blood tests and thyroid function tests.

## Drug Interactions:

Tell your doctor or pharmacist if you are taking or if you are planning to take any over-the-counter or prescription medications or dietary supplements while taking this medicine. Doses of one or both drugs may need to be modified or a different drug may need to be prescribed. The following drugs and drug classes may interact with this medicine.

beta blockers (eg, propranolol)
calcium channel blockers
 (eg, nifedipine)
cyclosporine (eg, *Sandimmune*)

drugs to control fluid and electrolyte balance
hypoglycemic agents, oral
 (eg, sulfonylureas)
insulin

## Side Effects:

Every drug is capable of producing side effects. Many patients experience no, or minor, side effects. The frequency and severity of side effects depend on many factors including dose, duration of therapy and individual susceptibility. Possible side effects include:

*Digestive Tract:* Diarrhea; loose stools; nausea; stomach pain; vomiting; gas; bloating; constipation.

*Nervous System:* Headache; dizziness; tiredness; weakness; depression.

*Circulatory System:* Slow or irregular heart rate.

*Skin:* Injection site pain or bruising; swelling; itching; hair loss; bruising; flushing.

*Other:* Gallbladder problems, especially stones or biliary sludge; back or joint pain; cold or flu symptoms; visual problems; blurred vision; frequent urination; urinary tract infection; changes in blood sugar levels; underactive thyroid; goiter.

## Guidelines for Use:

- Use exactly as prescribed.
- Follow the injection procedures taught to you by your health care provider. Use proper technique; inject deep under the skin, not into muscle. Rotate injection sites.
- If a dose is missed, inject it as soon as possible. If several hours have passed or if it is nearing time for the next dose, do not double the dose in order to "catch up" (unless advised to do so by your doctor). If more than one dose is missed or it is necessary to establish a new dosage schedule, contact your doctor or pharmacist.
- *Diabetics* — Insulin requirements may increase or decrease. Be prepared to monitor blood sugar more often.
- May cause dizziness. Use caution when driving or performing other tasks requiring alertness, coordination or physical dexterity.
- Lab tests may be required to monitor therapy. Be sure to keep appointments.
- Visually inspect solution for particles or discoloration before use.
- *Ampules* — Open just prior to administration. Discard any unused portion.
- *Vials* — Discard any unused portion within 14 days of first use.
- Store at room temperature (70° to 86°F) away from light, for up to 14 days. For prolonged storage, store in the refrigerator (36° to 46°F) away from light. Solution may be warmed to room temperature naturally. Do not warm artificially.

*If you have any questions, consult your doctor, pharmacist, or health care provider.*

| | Generic Name<br>*Brand Name Examples* | Supplied As | Generic<br>Available |
|---|---|---|---|
| *C-III* | **Nandrolone Decanoate** | | |
| | *Deca-Durabolin*[1] | **Injection (in oil)**: 50 mg/mL,<br>100 mg/mL, 200 mg/mL | No |
| *C-III* | **Oxandrolone** | | |
| | *Oxandrin* | **Tablets:** 2.5 mg | No |
| *C-III* | **Oxymetholone** | | |
| | *Anadrol-50* | **Tablets:** 50 mg | No |
| *C-III* | **Stanozolol** | | |
| | *Winstrol* | **Tablets:** 2 mg | No |

[1] Contains benzyl alcohol.

All of the products listed in the preceding table are anabolic steroids; however, they are not interchangeable. For example, oxandrolone cannot be used for oxymetholone. Daily dose may vary depending on individual needs. Do not change the dose without consulting your pharmacist or doctor.

## Type of Drug:

Synthetic hormones (anabolic steroids) closely related to the androgen testosterone (male sex hormone).

## How the Drug Works:

Anabolic steroids promote body tissue-building processes and reverse destructive tissue-depleting processes. They also decrease normal testosterone production by the testicles.

## Uses:

*Nandrolone and oxymetholone* — To treat certain types of anemia.

*Oxandrolone* — To treat weight loss due to severe illness, following extensive surgery, and in some patients who, without definite reasons, fail to gain or maintain normal weight.

To relieve bone pain caused by osteoporosis (brittle bones).

To prevent the breakdown of protein associated with prolonged corticosteroid (eg, prednisone) use.

*Stanozolol* — To decrease the frequency and severity of hereditary angioedema attacks.

*Unlabeled Use(s):* Occasionally doctors may prescribe oxandrolone for alcoholic hepatitis, short stature associated with Turner syndrome, HIV wasting syndrome, and HIV-associated muscle weakness.

## Precautions:

*Do not use in the following situations:*

allergy to the anabolic steroid or any of its ingredients

breast cancer, females with excess calcium in blood or males

for enhancement of physical appearance or athletic performance

hypercalcemia (excess calcium in blood) (oxandrolone only)

liver disease, severe (oxymetholone only)

nephrosis

pregnancy

prostate gland cancer

*Use with caution in the following situations:*

diabetes

elderly males

heart disease

hyperlipidemia

kidney disease

liver disease

migraine

seizure disorder (eg, epilepsy)

*Athletic performance:* Anabolic steroids have not been shown to enhance athletic ability. An athlete's motivation to use steroids includes: Increased muscle mass and strength; decreased muscle recovery time, allowing more frequent weight training; decreased healing time after muscle injury; increased aggressiveness. The increase in muscle size and weight gain is partially attributed to increased sodium and water retention. The serious health hazards associated with anabolic steroids minimize any real or perceived gain in performance. Effects of these agents may persist for up to 6 months after the last dose. Adverse effects may be serious and irreversible.

*Benzyl alcohol:* Some of these products contain benzyl alcohol, which has been associated with fatal "gasping syndrome" in premature infants. Consult your doctor or pharmacist.

*Edema:* Edema (swelling), with or without congestive heart failure, may occur. Use with caution in patients with heart, kidney, or liver disease; epilepsy; migraine; or other conditions that may be aggravated by fluid retention. In addition to discontinuation of the drug, diuretic therapy may be required.

*High serum cholesterol:* Anabolic steroids may lower high-density lipoprotein (HDL) ("good" cholesterol) and raise low-density lipoprotein (LDL) ("bad" cholesterol). This effect may increase the risk of atherosclerosis (hardening of the arteries) and coronary artery disease.

*Leukemia:* Leukemia has been observed in patients with aplastic anemia treated with oxymetholone, but the role of oxymetholone is unclear.

*Liver disease:* Liver cysts and tumors have occurred during treatment with anabolic steroids. They are often not recognized until a life-threatening condition develops. Stopping the medicine usually results in shrinking or complete disappearance of the lesions.

*Males after puberty:* Anabolic steroids may inhibit function of the testes, aggravate acne, decrease sperm count, promote development of breast tissue, cause the testes to shrink, and lead to impotence.

*Women:* Anabolic steroids may produce irreversible virilization (eg, deepening of voice, unusual hair growth, enlargement of the clitoris) in females. Women should be carefully monitored and drug therapy stopped at the first sign of virilization (eg, menstrual irregularities).

*Pregnancy:* Do not use during pregnancy. The risk of use in a pregnant woman clearly outweighs any possible benefit. Anabolic steroids may cause masculinization of the female fetus.

*Breastfeeding:* It is not known if anabolic steroids appear in breast milk. Because of the potential for serious adverse effects, decide whether to discontinue nursing or the drug. Consult your doctor before you begin breastfeeding.

*Children:* The adverse effects of use in young children are not fully understood. Anabolic steroids may interfere with growth to normal adult height. Use with caution.

*Elderly:* Anabolic steroids may increase risk of prostate enlargement or prostate cancer. Use with caution.

*Lab tests* may be required to monitor therapy. Tests may include liver function, blood calcium levels, cholesterol levels, and hemoglobin tests.

## Drug Interactions:

Tell your doctor or pharmacist if you are taking or if you are planning to take any over-the-counter or prescription medications or dietary supplements while taking an anabolic steroid. Doses of one or both drugs may need to be modified or a different drug may need to be prescribed. Anticoagulants (eg, warfarin) interact with anabolic steroids.

## Side Effects:

Every drug is capable of producing side effects. Many anabolic steroid users experience no, or minor, side effects. The frequency and severity of side effects depend on many factors including dose, duration of therapy, and individual susceptibility. Possible side effects include:

*Males (before puberty):* Increased size of penis; increased frequency of erections.

*Males (after puberty):* Breast enlargement; changes in sex drive; impotence; persistent, painful erections; shrinking of testes; decreased semen volume; bladder irritation; inhibition of testicular function.

*Females:* Excessive growth of body hair; hoarseness or deepening of the voice; enlargement of the clitoris; changes in sex drive; changes in menstruation; male pattern baldness.

*Digestive Tract:* Nausea; vomiting; diarrhea.

*Nervous System:* Sleeplessness; dependency; depression; excitability.

*Skin:* Yellowing of the skin or eyes; acne.

*Other:* Fluid retention; ankle swelling; electrolyte imbalance; abnormal cholesterol levels; abnormal lab tests; liver disease; elevated blood sugar.

## Guidelines for Use:

- Dosage is individualized. Take exactly as prescribed.
- Do not change the dose or stop taking, unless advised by your doctor.
- The injectable form of nandrolone will usually be prepared and administered by your health care provider in a medical setting.
- May cause nausea or gastrointestinal upset.
- *Diabetic patients* — Glucose tolerance may be altered. Monitor blood sugar closely and report any changes to your doctor.
- *Seizure disorders* — Epileptic patients may note an increase in seizure frequency; notify your doctor if this occurs.
- Notify your doctor if you experience nausea, vomiting, yellowing of skin color, or ankle swelling.
- Female patients should notify their doctor if they experience hoarseness, deepening of the voice, changes in body hair growth, menstrual changes, male-pattern baldness, or acne.
- Male patients should notify their doctor if they experience too frequent or persistent erections of the penis or development or worsening of acne.
- Tell your doctor if you are pregnant, planning to become pregnant, or breastfeeding.
- Do not use to enhance physical appearance or athletic performance.
- Effects of anabolic steroids may persist for up to 6 months after the last dose; some adverse effects are irreversible.
- Maximum benefit may not be reached for several months.
- Lab tests may be required to monitor therapy. Be sure to keep appointments.
- Store tablets at controlled room temperature (59° to 86°F).

*If you have any questions, consult your doctor, pharmacist, or health care provider.*

| Generic Name <br> *Brand Name Example* | Supplied As | Generic Available |
|---|---|---|
| *Rx[1]* **Mifepristone** | | |
| *Mifeprex* | **Tablets**: 200 mg | No |

[1] Mifepristone will be supplied only to licensed physicians who sign and return a Prescriber's Agreement.

## Type of Drug:
Uterine-active agent; abortifacient.

## How the Drug Works:
The hormone progesterone acts on the uterus in a pregnant woman to help maintain the pregnancy. Mifepristone blocks the action of progesterone on the uterus, resulting in termination of pregnancy.

## Uses:
For the medical termination of intrauterine pregnancy through 49 days of pregnancy. For purposes of this treatment, pregnancy is dated from the first day of the last menstrual period in a presumed 28-day cycle with ovulation occurring at mid-cycle. The duration of pregnancy may be determined from menstrual history and by clinical examination.

*Unlabeled Use(s):* Occasionally, doctors may prescribe mifepristone for postcoital contraception, intrauterine fetal death, unresectable meningioma, endometriosis, and Cushing syndrome.

## Precautions:
*Do not use in the following situations:*

adnexal mass, undiagnosed
adrenal failure, chronic
allergy to mifepristone or any of its ingredients
allergy to misoprostol or any other prostaglandin
anticoagulant therapy, concurrent
bleeding disorder
corticosteroid therapy, concurrent long-term
ectopic pregnancy, confirmed or suspected
inadequate access to medical facilities equipped to provide emergency treatment
intrauterine device (IUD) in place
porphyrias, inherited

*Use with caution in the following situations:* Patient is over 35 years of age and smokes 10 or more cigarettes/day.

*Incomplete abortion:* If mifepristone results in incomplete abortion, surgical intervention may be necessary.

*Pregnancy:* Mifepristone is indicated for use in the termination of pregnancy (through 49 days of pregnancy) and has no other approved indication for use during pregnancy. Birth defects may occur if treatment fails and pregnancy is allowed to go to term.

*Breastfeeding:* It is not known if mifepristone appears in breast milk. Consult your doctor before you begin breastfeeding.

*Children:* Safety and effectiveness in children have not been established.

## Drug Interactions:

Tell your doctor or pharmacist if you are taking or planning to take any over-the-counter or prescription medications or dietary supplements while taking mifepristone. Doses of one or both drugs may need to be modified or a different drug may need to be prescribed. The following drugs or drug classes interact with mifepristone:

carbamazepine (eg, *Tegretol*)
dexamethasone (eg, *Decadron*)
erythromycin (eg, *E.E.S.*)
grapefruit juice
itraconazole (*Sporanox*)
ketoconazole (eg, *Nizoral*)
phenobarbital
phenytoin (eg, *Dilantin*)
rifampin (eg, *Rifadin*)
St. John's Wort

## Side Effects:

Every drug is capable of producing side effects. Many mifepristone users experience no, or minor, side effects. The frequency and severity of side effects depend on many factors including dose, duration of therapy, and individual susceptibility. Possible side effects include:

*Nervous System:* Headache; dizziness; sleeplessness; anxiety; fainting; fatigue; weakness.

*Digestive Tract:* Stomach pain or cramping; indigestion; nausea; vomiting; diarrhea.

*Urinary and Reproductive Tract:* Uterine cramping and bleeding; vaginitis; pelvic pain.

*Other:* Abnormal blood counts; back pain; fever; leg pain; sinus congestion; viral infection; rigors (eg, chills, shaking).

## Guidelines for Use:

- Treatment with mifepristone and misoprostol for the termination of pregnancy requires 3 office visits. Mifepristone may be administered only in a clinic, medical office, or hospital, by or under the supervision of a physician able to assess how far the pregnancy has progressed and to diagnose ectopic pregnancies.
- Mifepristone should not be used by any patient who may be unable to understand the effects of the treatment procedure or follow the regimen. Each patient must understand the following:
  The necessity of completing the treatment schedule, including a follow-up visit about 14 days after taking mifepristone;
  that vaginal bleeding and uterine cramping probably will occur;
  that prolonged or heavy vaginal bleeding is not proof of a complete abortion;
  that if the treatment fails, there is a risk of fetal abnormalities;
  that incomplete abortions are managed by surgical procedures;
  the steps to take in an emergency situation, including precise instructions and a telephone number that can be called if she has any problems or concerns.
- *Day 1* — Patients must read the medication guide and read and sign the patient agreement before mifepristone is taken. Three 200 mg tablets (600 mg) of mifepristone are taken in a single oral dose.
- *Day 3* — The patient returns to the health care provider 2 days after taking mifepristone. Unless abortion has occurred and has been confirmed by clinical examination or ultrasonographic scan, the patient takes two 200 mcg tablets (400 mcg) of misoprostol orally. During the period immediately following the administration of misoprostol, the patient may need medication for cramps or gastrointestinal symptoms. The patient instructions should be given on what to do if significant discomfort, excessive bleeding, or other adverse reactions occur and a phone number to call if she has questions following the administration of misoprostol. In addition, the patient should have the name and phone number of the physician who will be handling emergencies.
- *Day-14, post-treatment examination* — Patients will return for a follow-up visit about 14 days after taking the mifepristone. The visit is very important to confirm by clinical examination or ultrasonographic scan that a complete termination of pregnancy has occurred. Patients who have an ongoing pregnancy at this visit have a risk of fetal malformation resulting from the treatment. Surgical termination is recommended to manage mifepristone treatment failures.
- Another pregnancy can occur following termination of pregnancy and before resumption of normal menses. Contraception can be initiated as soon as the termination of the pregnancy has been confirmed, or before resuming sexual intercourse.

*If you have any questions, consult your doctor, pharmacist, or health care provider.*

| Generic Name<br>*Brand Name Examples* | Supplied As | Generic<br>Available |
|---|---|---|
| *c-III* **Fluoxymesterone** | | |
| *Halotestin* | **Tablets:** 2 mg, 5 mg, 10 mg | Yes |
| *c-III* **Methyltestosterone** | **Tablets, buccal:** 10 mg | Yes |
| *Android* | **Tablets:** 10 mg, 25 mg | Yes |
| *Android, Testred, Virilon* | **Capsules:** 10 mg | No |
| *c-III* **Testosterone (in Aqueous Suspension)** | **Injection:** 25 mg/mL, 50 mg/mL, 100 mg/mL | Yes |
| *c-III* **Testosterone Cypionate (in Oil)** | | |
| *Depo-Testosterone, Depotest 100, Depotest 200* | **Injection:** 100 mg/mL, 200 mg/mL | Yes |
| *c-III* **Testosterone Enanthate (in Oil)** | | |
| *Delatestryl, Everone 200* | **Injection:** 100 mg/mL, 200 mg/mL | Yes |
| *c-III* **Testosterone Propionate (in Oil)** | **Injection:** 100 mg/mL | Yes |
| *c-III* **Testosterone Pellets** | | |
| *Testopel* | **Pellets:** 75 mg | No |
| *c-III* **Testosterone Transdermal** | | |
| *Androderm, Testoderm, Testoderm TTS* | **Transdermal System:** 2.5 mg, 4 mg, 5 mg, 6 mg/24 hours | No |

All of the products listed on this table are androgens; however, they are not interchangeable. For example, methyltestosterone cannot be used for fluoxymesterone. Daily dose may vary depending on individual needs.

## Type of Drug:
Male hormones.

## How the Drug Works:
Testosterone is the primary natural androgen (male sex hormone) produced by the testes. Androgens promote normal growth and development of male sex organs (eg, prostate, seminal vesicles, penis, scrotum) and affect fertility. They also produce the distinctive male characteristics of hair distribution, voice depth, fat distribution, and muscle development. Androgens contribute to growth during adolescence.

## Uses:

To treat testosterone deficiency. Prolonged treatment is required to maintain male sex characteristics.

For hormone deficiency due to developmental defects of the testes.

To treat delayed male puberty (brief treatment with low doses) in carefully selected patients.

To treat male impotence caused by androgen deficiency (methyltestosterone only).

Used for breast pain and swelling in women immediately after childbirth. Also used as secondary therapy in postmenopausal women for advanced, inoperable breast cancer that has spread to other areas, including bone.

*Unlabeled Use(s):* Testosterone enanthate has been studied for male contraception.

## Precautions:

*Do not use in the following situations:*

allergy to androgens, mercury compounds, or patch materials
cancer of the prostate gland or breast tissue (men)
females (*Androderm* and *Testoderm* only)

heart disease, serious
kidney disease, serious
liver disease, serious
pregnancy

*Use with caution in the following situations:*

breast cancer (women)
breast development, abnormal (men)
calcium blood level, increased (children)
delayed puberty, healthy males

elderly males
epilepsy
heart, liver or kidney disease
high cholesterol
migraine

*Males* frequently experience breast swelling or development. Reduced sperm counts may occur after prolonged use.

*Women* may show signs of masculinization: Deepening of voice, hair growth, acne, increased size of clitoris, menstrual changes. These symptoms usually follow high doses of androgens and should be tolerated during treatment for advanced breast cancer. Treatment may have to be discontinued. Consult your doctor. (The transdermal systems have not been tested in women and should not be used by women.)

*Product interchange:* Do not try to substitute short-acting and long-acting testosterone products. These products are not considered to be interchangeable.

*Athletic performance/physical appearance:* Androgens are not safe and effective for enhancement of athletic performance or physical appearance; use could produce serious adverse effects.

*Fluid retention:* Since androgens may cause fluid retention, use with caution in epilepsy, migraine, and heart, liver or kidney disease.

*Pregnancy:* Do not use during pregnancy. The risk of use in a pregnant woman clearly outweighs any possible benefit. Androgens may masculinize a female fetus.

*Breastfeeding:* It is not known if androgens appear in breast milk. Consult your doctor before you begin breastfeeding.

*Children: Androderm* has not been tested in males under 15 years of age. *Testoderm* has not been tested in males under 18 years of age. Use other androgens very cautiously in children under 18 years of age. Androgens may stop or stunt the growth process.

*Elderly:* Use with caution in elderly males. Androgens may increase risk of prostate enlargement or prostate cancer. An increase in sex drive may occur.

*Lab tests* may be required to monitor therapy. Be sure to keep appointments.

*Tartrazine:* Some of these products may contain the dye tartrazine (FD&C Yellow No. 5) which can cause allergic reactions in certain individuals. Check package label when available or consult your doctor or pharmacist.

## Drug Interactions:
Tell your doctor or pharmacist if you are taking or if you are planning to take any over-the-counter or prescription medications or dietary supplements while taking this medicine. Doses of one or both drugs may need to be modified or a different drug may need to be prescribed.The following drugs and drug classes interact with this medicine.

anticoagulants, oral
 (eg, *Coumadin*)
blood-sugar-lowering agents
 (eg, *Diabinese*)

imipramine (eg, *Tofranil*)
insulin

## Side Effects:
Every drug is capable of producing side effects. Many patients experience no, or minor, side effects. The frequency an severity of side effects depend on many factors including dose, duration of therapy and individual susceptibility. Possible side effects include:

*Female* – Irregular menstruation; absence of menstruation; deepening voice; enlargement of clitoris; changes in sex drive.

*Male* – Breast tenderness, swelling or development; decreased sperm count; erection problems (pain, frequency, increased duration); changes in sex drive; itching, blisters, bruising, hardening, redness, discomfort or irritation (patch only); enlargement of the prostate.

*Nervous System:* Headache; anxiety; depression; sleep disorders; memory loss; abnormal skin sensations.

*Skin:* Excessive growth of body hair; loss of scalp hair; acne; oily skin; changes in skin color (yellowing); rash; irritation (patch only).

*Other:* Fluid retention (edema); ankle swelling; nausea; pain at injection or implantation site; increased cholesterol; liver problems; vomiting; dilated pupils; abnormal bleeding or bruising; inflammation of the mouth (tablets only); stroke; black or tarry stools; urinary tract infection.

## Guidelines for Use:

- *Oral tablets* — May cause stomach upset.
- *Buccal tablets* — Do not swallow. Allow to dissolve between the gum and cheek. Avoid eating, drinking or smoking while tablet is in place.
- Notify your doctor if nausea, vomiting, swelling of the extremities (edema), prolonged or painful erections, or yellowing of the skin or eyes occurs.
- *Female patients* — Notify your doctor if hoarseness, deepening of the voice, hair growth changes, acne, menstrual irregularities or suspected pregnancy occur.
- Androgens are not effective and may be dangerous if used for fractures, surgery, convalescence, bleeding of the uterus or enhancement of athletic performance or physical appearance.
- *Brand interchange* — Do not change from one brand of these drugs to another without consulting your pharmacist or doctor.
- *Testosterone injections* — Shake well before using. Administer into buttock muscle only. Effects of *enanthate* and *cypionate* injections last about 4 weeks.
- *Transdermal systems* — Read patient instructions. Store at room temperature (59°-86° F) in provided pouch until ready to use. Carefully discard used patches to prevent accidental application or ingestion by others (eg, children, pets).
  *Androderm:* Place on clean dry non-scrotal skin (eg, back, abdomen, upper arm, thigh) every night. Rotate application sites, allowing 7 days between applications to the same site. Site should not be oily, damaged or irritated. Patch does not need to be removed during sexual intercourse or while bathing.
  *Testoderm:* Place on clean, dry scrotal skin. Scrotal hair should be dry-shaved for best contact. Do not use depilatories (chemical hair removers). System should be worn 22-24 hours, but can be removed for swimming or bathing and then reapplied. Lab tests should be made after 3 to 4 weeks of use.
- *Pellet implantation* — Report any unusual irritation or infection at the implant site. If treatment is discontinued, the pellets will have to be removed.
- Female sexual partners of male testosterone patients should contact a doctor if the following occur: changes in body hair distribution or increased acne.
- Do not alter the dose unless directed by your doctor.
- Diabetics may require insulin dose adjustments. Consult your doctor.
- Lab tests or exams may be necessary. Be sure to keep appointments.
- Store tablets in a closed container at room temperature.
- Avoid freezing injectable products.

*If you have any questions, consult your doctor, pharmacist, or health care provider.*

| Generic Name Brand Name Examples | Supplied As | Generic Available |
|---|---|---|
| Rx **Dutasteride** | | |
| *Avodart* | **Capsules**: 0.5 mg | No |
| Rx **Finasteride** | | |
| *Propecia* | **Tablets**: 1 mg | No |
| *Proscar* | **Tablets**: 5 mg | No |

## Type of Drug:

Enzyme inhibitors; androgen hormone inhibitors.

## How the Drug Works:

Dutasteride and finasteride inhibit the production of androgen, a hormone that is a major cause of prostate growth. By reducing the amount of androgen, dutasteride and finasteride help relieve urinary symptoms often associated with overdevelopment or enlargement of the prostate (benign prostatic hyperplasia [BPH]).

By inhibiting the production of androgen, finasteride interrupts processes that lead to male pattern baldness (hair loss on the crown of the head or the front scalp area).

## Uses:

*Dutasteride, Proscar:* To treat symptomatic benign prostatic hyperplasia (BPH) in men with an enlarged prostate to improve symptoms, reduce the risk of acute urinary retention, and reduce the risk of the need for prostate surgery. Not indicated for use in women or children.

*Propecia:* To treat male pattern hair loss (vertex and anterior mid-scalp). Effectiveness with other types of hair loss has not been determined. Not indicated for use in women or children.

*Unlabeled Use(s):* Finasteride is being investigated in combination with flutamide as therapy following radical prostatectomy. Other potential uses include prevention of the progression of first-stage prostate cancer, treatment of acne in women, abnormal hair growth.

## Precautions:

*Do not use in the following situations:*

allergy to the drug or any of its ingredients
breastfeeding
children (younger than 18 years of age)
pregnancy
women

*Use with caution in the following situations:*

liver disease
obstructive uropathy
urinary difficulty or blockage, major

*Pregnancy:* Do not use during pregnancy. The risk of use in a pregnant woman clearly outweighs any possible benefit. Not indicated for use in women. Women who are pregnant or may become pregnant should not handle broken or crushed tablets or capsules because of the potential for absorption and potential risk to a male fetus. Similarly, when a male patient's sexual partner is or may become pregnant, the patient should either avoid exposing his partner to his semen or discontinue therapy.

*Breastfeeding:* It is not known if these drugs appear in breast milk; they are not indicated for use in women. Consult your doctor before you begin breastfeeding.

*Children:* Safety and effectiveness have not been established; not indicated for use in patients younger than 18 years of age.

*Lab tests* may be required during and following treatment. Tests include prostate cancer screenings and urinary flow and volume monitoring.

## Drug Interactions:

Tell your doctor or pharmacist if you are taking or planning to take any over-the-counter or prescription medications or dietary supplements with these drugs. Drug doses may need to be modified or a different drug prescribed. Ritonavir (*Norvir*) interacts with dutasteride.

## Side Effects:

Every drug is capable of producing side effects. Many patients experience no, or minor, side effects. The frequency and severity of side effects depend on many factors including dose, duration of therapy, and individual susceptibility. Possible side effects include impotence, decreased sex drive, decreased amount of ejaculate, testicular pain, and breast tenderness and enlargement.

## Guidelines for Use:

- Read the patient information insert before beginning therapy.
- Dosage is individualized. Take exactly as prescribed.
- Do not stop taking or change the dose, unless instructed by your doctor.
- *Male pattern baldness* — In general, three months of daily treatment is necessary before benefit is observed. Continued use is recommended to sustain benefit. Stopping treatment can reverse results within 12 months.
- *Benign prostatic hyperplasia (BPH)* — Six to twelve months of treatment may be necessary to determine response.
- Take without regard to meals.
- Swallow dutasteride capsules whole.
- *Dutasteride long-term treatment* — The incidence of most drug-related adverse events (eg, impotence, decreased sex drive, ejaculation disorder) will decrease with duration of treatment. The incidence of drug-related breast tenderness and enlargement may remain constant during therapy.
- Women who are pregnant or may become pregnant should not handle broken or crushed tablets or capsules because of the potential for absorption and potential risk to male fetus. Similarly, when a male patient's sexual partner is or may become pregnant, the patient should either avoid exposing his partner to his semen or discontinue therapy.
- The amount of ejaculate may be decreased. This should not interfere with normal sexual function. However, impotence (erectile dysfunction) and decreased sex drive may occur.
- Men treated with dutasteride should not donate blood until at least 6 months have passed following their last dose to prevent pregnant women from receiving dutasteride through blood transfusion.
- Lab tests may be required during and following treatment. Be sure to keep appointments.
- Store at room temperature (59° to 86°F). Protect from light and moisture. Keep container tightly closed.

*If you have any questions, consult your doctor, pharmacist, or health care provider.*

| Generic Name<br>*Brand Name Examples* | Supplied As | Generic<br>Available |
|---|---|---|
| *Rx* **Conjugated Estrogens** | | |
| *Premarin* | **Tablets:** 0.3 mg, 0.625 mg,<br>0.9 mg, 1.25 mg, 2.5 mg | No |
| *Premarin* | **Vaginal cream:** 0.625 mg/g | No |
| *Premarin Intravenous* | **Injection:** 25 mg/vial | No |
| *Rx* **Dienestrol** | | |
| *Ortho Dienestrol* | **Vaginal cream:** 0.01% | No |
| *Rx* **Esterified Estrogens** | | |
| *Estratab, Menest* | **Tablets:** 0.3 mg, 0.625 mg,<br>1.25 mg, 2.5 mg | No |
| *Rx* **Estradiol** | | |
| *Estrace, Gynodiol* | **Tablets:** 0.5 mg, 1 mg, 1.5 mg,<br>2 mg[1] | Yes |
| *Estrace* | **Vaginal cream:** 0.01% | No |
| *Alora, Climara, Esclim,<br>Estraderm, FemPatch,<br>Vivelle, Vivelle-Dot* | **Transdermal system (patch):**<br>0.025 mg/day, 0.0375 mg/day,<br>0.05 mg/day, 0.075 mg/day,<br>0.1 mg/day | Yes |
| *Estring* | **Ring:** 2 mg | No |
| *Rx* **Estradiol Cypionate in<br>Oil** | | |
| *Depo-Estradiol, Depogen* | **Injection:** 5 mg/mL | Yes |
| *Rx* **Estradiol Hemihydrate** | | |
| *Vagifem* | **Vaginal tablets:** 25 mcg | No |
| *Rx* **Estradiol Valerate in Oil** | | |
| *Delestrogen, Valergen 20,<br>Valergen 40* | **Injection:** l0 mg/mL, 20 mg/mL,<br>40 mg/mL | Yes |
| *Rx* **Estrone Aqueous** | | |
| *Kestrone 5* | **Injection:** 5 mg/mL | Yes |
| *Rx* **Estropipate (Piperazine<br>Estrone Sulfate)** | | |
| *Ogen, Ortho-Est* | **Tablets:** 0.625 mg, 1.25 mg,<br>2.5 mg | Yes |
| *Ogen* | **Vaginal cream:** 1.5 mg/g | No |
| *Rx* **Ethinyl Estradiol** | | |
| *Estinyl* | **Tablets:** 0.02 mg[1], 0.05 mg | No |
| *Rx* **Synthetic Conjugated<br>Estrogens, A** | | |
| *Cenestin* | **Tablets:** 0.625 mg, 0.9 mg | No |

[1] *Estrace* 2 mg and *Estinyl* 0.02 mg contain the dye tartrazine.

All of the products listed in the previous table are estrogens; however, they are not interchangeable without dosage adjustments. For example, estradiol cannot be substituted for conjugated estrogens without changing the dose. Daily dose may vary depending on individual needs. Do not adjust the dose without consulting your pharmacist or doctor.

## Type of Drug:

Female hormones; estrogens.

## How the Drug Works:

Estrogens represent a group of several female hormones. The ovary produces and releases several natural estrogens until menopause occurs. All estrogens produce similar effects. They play a key role in the development and normal function of the reproductive system (including the vagina, uterus, fallopian tubes, and breasts) and secondary sex characteristics (eg, pubic hair) of women. Estrogens also assist in development and maintenance of strong bones.

## Uses:

To treat hot flashes associated with menopause.

To treat vulval, vaginal, and lower urinary tract tissue breakdown, drying, and thinning following menopause. Estrogen supplements may prevent or decrease complications.

To treat *kraurosis vulvae*, a condition involving the breakdown and drying of the external female genitalia (vulval area).

For estrogen replacement therapy after a failure of the ovaries due to menopause, disease, or surgical removal.

To treat advanced androgen-dependent cancer of the prostate gland in men.

To relieve the symptoms of breast cancer in selected men and women with metastatic disease.

*Conjugated estrogens, injection:* To treat abnormal uterine bleeding caused by hormone imbalance.

*Estradiol tablets and transdermal system (patch):* To prevent osteoporosis (brittle bones) related to a lack of estrogen after menopause. Therapy should be accompanied by a balanced diet, adequate daily calcium either through the diet or calcium supplements, adequate vitamin D, and weight-bearing exercises.

*Unlabeled Use(s):* Ethinyl estradiol has been used for treating Turner syndrome.

## Precautions:

*Do not use in the following situations:*

allergy to estrogens or any of their ingredients
blood clots, active
blood clots, history of with previous estrogen use
breast cancer, known or suspected

estrogen-dependent cancer, known or suspected
genital bleeding, abnormal undiagnosed
pregnancy, known or suspected

*Use with caution in the following situations:*

asthma
blood clots, risk factors or a history of
bone disease, metabolic
breast cancer, family history of, history of, or active
breast nodules
depression, history of
diabetes
endometrial cancer
endometriosis
epilepsy
fibrocystic breast disease
gallbladder disease
heart disease
high blood pressure

high blood calcium levels
immobilization, prolonged
jaundice, history of with pregnancy
kidney disease
liver disease
mammogram, abnormal
migraine headaches
narrow, short, or constricted vagina (estradiol ring only)
porphyria
stroke, history of
surgery
uterine cancer, history of
uterine fibroids, preexisting

*Blood Clots:* There is an increased risk of blood clots in men receiving estrogens for prostate cancer, in women using estrogens for postpartum breast engorgement, and in those taking oral contraceptives in general.

*Cancer Risk:* Estrogens may increase the risk of endometrial (lining of the uterus) cancer in postmenopausal women. Have regular physical examinations and contact your doctor if you experience persistent or recurrent abnormal vaginal bleeding.

*Concurrent progestin therapy:* A progestin agent is frequently added to long-term estrogen regimens in women who have a uterus. The addition of a progestin reduces the risk of estrogen-induced cancer of the uterus.

*History/physical exam:* Before beginning estrogen therapy, a complete medical and family history should be performed. Examinations every 12 months should include blood pressure tests, abdomen and pelvic organ examinations, and a Pap test (once a year). Patients should examine their breasts for lumps on a monthly basis. Women older than 40 years of age who take estrogens should have regular mammograms.

*Pregnancy:* Do not use during pregnancy. The risk of use in a pregnant woman clearly outweighs any possible benefit. Urinary system problems and testicular cancer have occurred in sons of women given diethylstilbestrol (DES) (not available in the US) during pregnancy. Daughters of women given DES during their pregnancy have shown an increased risk of developing vaginal or cervical cancer.

*Breastfeeding:* It is not known if estrogens appear in breast milk. Consult your doctor before you begin breastfeeding.

*Children:* Safety and effectiveness in children have not been established. Use with extreme caution in young patients who are still growing. Estrogens may interfere with normal bone development.

*Tartrazine:* Some of these products may contain the dye tartrazine (FD&C Yellow No. 5), which can cause allergic reactions in certain individuals. Check package label when available or consult your doctor or pharmacist.

## Drug Interactions:

Tell your doctor or pharmacist if you are taking or if you are planning to take any over-the-counter or prescription medications or dietary supplements while taking this medicine. Doses of one or both drugs may need to be modified or a different drug may need to be prescribed. The following drugs and drug classes interact with this medicine:

barbiturates (eg, phenobarbital)
corticosteroids
  (eg, prednisone)

hydantoins (eg, phenytoin)
rifampin (eg, *Rifadin*)
topiramate (*Topamax*)

## Side Effects:

Every drug is capable of producing side effects. Many patients experience no, or minor, side effects. The frequency and severity of side effects depend on many factors including dose, duration of therapy, and individual susceptibility. Possible side effects include:

*Urinary and Reproductive Tract:* Change in menstrual flow; abnormal vaginal bleeding; vaginal discomfort or pain; vaginal infection; unusual vaginal secretions; painful menstruation; absence of menstruation during or after treatment; premenstrual-like syndrome; increased size of uterine fibroids; urinary tract infection symptoms.

*Digestive Tract:* Nausea; vomiting; stomach pain or cramps; bloating; pancreatitis; diarrhea; gas; enlarged stomach; constipation; indigestion.

*Nervous System:* Headache; migraine; dizziness; depression; weakness; unusual, jerky body movements; sleeplessness; emotional instability; anxiety; nervousness.

*Skin:* Rash; hives; itching; skin discoloration, particularly on the face; scalp hair loss; excessive growth of body or facial hair.

*Local:* Pain at the injection site; redness; irritation or itching at patch application site.

*Other:* Intolerance to contact lenses; weight changes; breast tenderness or enlargement; breast milk secretion; sudden vision problems; abnormal blood glucose levels; swelling; high blood pressure; changes in sex drive; yellowing of skin or eyes; swelling of the arms or legs; vertigo (feeling of whirling motion); cough; abnormal lab tests; gallbladder disease; blood clots; steepening of corneal curvature; reduced carbohydrate tolerance; liver tumor development; runny nose; back, joint, muscle, or bone pain; sore throat; flu-like symptoms; hot flushes; palpitations (pounding in the chest); leg cramps; abnormal skin sensations.

## Guidelines for Use:

- Dosage is individualized.
- Carefully read the patient package insert available with your medicines.
- The lowest dose that will control symptoms should be chosen and medication should be discontinued as soon as possible.
- Notify your doctor immediately if you experience pain in the groin, calves, or chest; sudden shortness of breath; abnormal vaginal bleeding; missed menstrual period or suspected pregnancy; lumps in the breast; severe headache; dizziness; fainting; changes in vision or speech; weakness or numbness in an arm or leg; stomach pain, swelling, or tenderness; yellowing of the skin or eyes; severe depression; severe vomiting; or coughing up blood.
- Fluid retention caused by estrogens may aggravate asthma, epilepsy, migraine, heart disease, or kidney disease. Use with caution if you have any of these conditions.
- If a dose is missed, take it as soon as possible. If several hours have passed or if it is nearing time for the next dose, do not double the dose in order to catch up, unless advised to do so by your doctor. If several doses are missed, or it is necessary to establish a new dosage schedule, contact your doctor or pharmacist.
- While taking estrogens, it is important to visit your doctor at least once a year for a check-up. If members of your family have had breast cancer or if you have ever had breast lumps, you may need to have more frequent breast exams.
- Approximately every 6 months, you and your doctor should reevaluate whether or not you need to continue estrogen therapy.
- *Diabetic patients* — Glucose tolerance may be decreased. Monitor blood sugar closely and report changes to your doctor.
- When using estrogens to treat hot flashes and other symptoms of menopause, the dose may need to be changed occasionally. Discuss your symptoms with your doctor.
- Inform your doctor if you are pregnant, become pregnant, or are planning to become pregnant or if you are breastfeeding.
- Do not share your medicine with anyone else.
- *Brand interchange* — Do not change from one brand of these drugs to another without consulting your pharmacist or doctor. Products manufactured by different companies may not be equally effective and will require different doses.
- *Injections* — Visually inspect solutions for particles or discoloration. If you are self-administering, carefully follow the storage, preparation, and administration instructions provided by your health care provider.
- *Transdermal system (patch)* — Apply immediately after opening the pouch and removing the protective liner. Press firmly in place with the palm of the hand for approximately 10 seconds. Make sure there is good contact, especially around the edges. Avoid touching the sticky side of the patch with your fingers.
  Place adhesive side of the system on a clean, dry area of the skin on the trunk of the body that is not exposed to sunlight, preferably the buttocks or the abdomen. Do not apply to the breasts.

## Guidelines for Use: (cont.)

- *Transdermal system (patch)* (cont.)
  When it is time to change the patch, remove the old patch and discard. Apply a new patch on a different skin site.
  Rotate the application site with an interval of at least 1 week between applications to a particular site. The area selected should not be oily, damaged, or irritated. Avoid the waistline since tight clothing may rub the system off. Application to areas where sitting would dislodge the system should also be avoided.
  In the unlikely event that a system should fall off, the same system may be reapplied. If necessary, apply a new system. In either case, continue the original treatment schedule. If a rash or irritation develops at an application site, remove the patch and reapply at a different site. Contact your doctor if rash or irritation continues with each patch application.
  Contact with water while bathing, swimming, or showering will not affect the patch.
- *Vaginal creams* — Fill the applicator provided with the prescribed amount of cream. Insert the applicator high into the vagina. After use, clean applicator by removing the plunger from the barrel. Wash with mild soap and warm water. Do not boil or use hot water.
  Cream exposure has been reported to weaken latex condoms. The potential for creams to weaken and contribute to the failure of condoms, diaphragms, or cervical caps made of latex or rubber should be considered.
- *Vaginal ring* — Press the ring into an oval shape and insert as deeply as possible into the upper one-third of the vaginal vault. The ring will remain in place continuously for 3 months, after which it is removed and, if appropriate, replaced by a new ring.
  The exact position of the ring is not critical, although if you feel discomfort, it is probably not far enough inside the vagina. You should not feel the ring when it is in place and it should not interfere with sexual intercourse.
  Some women have experienced moving or gliding of the ring in the vagina. Instances of the ring being expelled from the vagina in connection with moving the bowels, strain, or constipation have been reported. If this occurs, the ring can be rinsed in lukewarm water and reinserted into the vagina.
  The ring should be removed if another intravaginally administered medication is being used.
  The ring may be removed by hooking a finger through the ring and pulling it out.
  Contact your doctor if signs of vaginal irritation develop.
- *Calcium* — If you are taking calcium supplements as part of the treatment to prevent osteoporosis, check with your doctor about the amounts recommended.
- *Storage* — Before reconstitution, store the conjugated estrogens injection in the refrigerator (36° to 46°F). Use the reconstituted solution within a few hours. Reconstituted solution is stable for 60 days in the refrigerator. All other doseforms can be stored at controlled room temperature (59° to 86°F).

*If you have any questions, consult your doctor, pharmacist, or health care provider.*

|  | Brand Name Examples | Estrogen | Progestin | Androgen |
|---|---|---|---|---|
| Rx | Depo-Testadiol injection, Depotestogen injection | 2 mg estradiol cypionate/mL |  | 50 mg testosterone cypionate/mL |
| Rx | Estratest tablets | 1.25 mg esterified estrogens |  | 2.5 mg methyl-testosterone |
| Rx | Estratest H.S. tablets | 0.625 mg esterified estrogens |  | 1.25 mg methyl-testosterone |
| Rx | Prempro tablets | 0.625 mg conjugated estrogens | 2.5 mg medroxy-progesterone acetate |  |
| Rx | Prempro tablets | 0.625 mg conjugated estrogens | 5 mg medroxy-progesterone acetate |  |
| Rx | Premphase tablets | 0.625 mg conjugated estrogens (days 1-14) |  |  |
|  |  | 0.625 mg conjugated estrogens (days 15-28) | 5 mg medroxy-progesterone acetate (days 15-28) |  |
| Rx | femhrt tablets | 5 mcg ethinyl estradiol | 1 mg norethindrone acetate |  |
| Rx | Activella tablets | 1 mg estradiol | 0.5 mg norethindrone acetate |  |
| Rx | Ortho-Prefest tablets | 1 mg estradiol (days 1-3) |  |  |
|  |  | 1 mg estradiol (days 4-6) | 0.09 mg norgestimate (days 4-6) |  |

| | Brand Name Examples | Estrogen | Progestin | Androgen |
|---|---|---|---|---|
| Rx | CombiPatch 9 cm² transdermal patch | 0.05 mg estradiol/ day | 0.14 mg norethindrone acetate/day | |
| | CombiPatch 16 cm² transdermal patch | 0.05 mg estradiol/ day | 0.25 mg norethindrone acetate/day | |

For complete information, see the Estrogens, Progestins, and Androgens monographs in this chapter.

## Type of Drug:

Combination hormone products.

## Uses:

*Estrogen and androgen combinations:* To treat moderate to severe vasomotor symptoms associated with menopause (feeling of warmth in the face, neck, or chest or sudden intense episodes of heat and sweating throughout the body) in patients who have not improved with treatment of estrogens alone.

To treat vulvar and vaginal atrophy associated with menopause.

*Estrogen and progestin combinations:* To treat moderate to severe vasomotor symptoms associated with menopause (feeling of warmth in the face, neck, or chest or sudden intense episodes of heat and sweating throughout the body) in patients who have not improved with treatment of estrogens alone.

To treat vulvar and vaginal atrophy associated with menopause (*femhrt* excluded).

To prevent osteoporosis (*Combi-Patch* excluded).

To treat low estrogen conditions caused by diseases such as hypogonadism or primary ovarian failure.

*Unlabeled Use(s):* There is no adequate evidence that estrogens are effective for nervous symptoms or depression that might occur during menopause; they should not be used to treat these conditions.

## Guidelines for Use:

- Dosage is individualized. Take exactly as prescribed.
- Do not change the dose or stop taking, unless directed by your doctor.
- Carefully read the patient package insert available with your medicine.
- Fluid retention may aggravate asthma, epilepsy, migraine, heart disease or kidney disease. Use with caution in these conditions.
- *Brand interchange* — Do not change from one brand of these drugs to another without consulting your pharmacist or doctor. Products manufactured by different companies may not be equally effective.
- If a dose is missed, take it as soon as possible. If several hours have passed or it is nearing time for the next dose, do not double the dose to catch up, unless advised by your doctor. If more than one dose is missed, or it is necessary to establish a new dosage schedule, contact your doctor or pharmacist.
- Store as directed by package labeling.

*If you have any questions, consult your doctor, pharmacist, or health care provider.*

| Generic Name<br>*Brand Name Example* | Supplied As | Generic<br>Available |
|---|---|---|
| *Rx* **Raloxifene HCl** | | |
| *Evista* | **Tablets:** 60 mg | No |

## Type of Drug:

Selective estrogen receptor modulator (SERM).

## How the Drug Works:

Raloxifene binds to estrogen receptors producing estrogen-like effects on some tissues and organs. Raloxifene reduces bone loss (prevents brittle bones) and elevated LDL ("bad") cholesterol values associated with menopause or hysterectomy (ovarian removal). However, unlike estrogen, raloxifene lacks estrogen-like effects on the uterus and breasts and does not reduce or eliminate hot flushes.

## Uses:

For the treatment and prevention of osteoporosis (brittle bones) in post-menopausal women.

## Precautions:

*Do not use in the following situations:*

allergy to raloxifene or any of its ingredients
blood clotting in legs, lungs, or eyes, history of
estrogen therapy, concurrent
immobilization, prolonged (post-surgical recovery, prolonged bed rest)
pregnancy
premenopausal women

*Use with caution in the following situations:*

breast abnormality, unexplained
breast cancer, history of
cholesterol-lowering agent therapy, concurrent
liver disease
uterine bleeding, unexplained

*Pregnancy:* Do not use during pregnancy. The risk of use in a pregnant woman clearly outweighs any possible benefit.

*Breastfeeding:* It is not known if raloxifene appears in breast milk. Do not use this drug while nursing.

*Children:* Raloxifene should not be used in pediatric patients.

## Drug Interactions:

Tell your doctor or pharmacist if you are taking or planning to take any over-the-counter or prescription medications or dietary supplements while taking raloxifene. Doses of one or both drugs may need to be modified or a different drug may need to be prescribed. The following drugs and drug classes interact with raloxifene:

cholestyramine (eg, *Questran*)
diazepam (eg, *Valium*)
diazoxide (*Proglycem*)
warfarin (eg, *Coumadin*)

## Side Effects:

Every drug is capable of producing side effects. Many raloxifene users experience no, or minor, side effects. The frequency and severity of side effects depend on many factors including dose, duration of therapy, and individual susceptibility. Possible side effects include:

*Digestive Tract:* Nausea; indigestion; vomiting; gas; stomach disorder; diarrhea.

*Nervous System:* Migraine; depression; sleeplessness; fainting; nerve pain; headache; loss of sensitivity to touch; vertigo (feeling of whirling motion).

*Respiratory System:* Nasal congestion; sore throat; sinusitis; increased cough; pneumonia; voice loss; bronchitis.

*Urinary and Reproductive Tract:* Vaginal inflammation; urinary tract infection; bladder inflammation; white vaginal discharge; uterine wall abnormality; breast pain; vaginal bleeding; urinary tract disorder.

*Skin:* Rash; sweating.

*Other:* Leg cramps; infection; hot flushes; flu-like syndrome; chest pain; fever; fluid retention; swelling of arms or legs; joint and muscle pain; joint swelling; weight gain; varicose vein; tendon disorder; eye inflammation.

## Guidelines for Use:

- Read patient package insert before beginning raloxifene therapy and re-read upon prescription renewal.
- Dosage is individualized. Take exactly as prescribed.
- Do not stop taking or change the dose unless directed by your doctor.
- Take this medicine once a day without regard to meals.
- If you miss a dose, start taking the medicine again as soon as possible on your normal schedule. You do not have to make up for the missed dose.
- Take raloxifene as long as your doctor prescribes it.
- Contact your doctor if you experience swelling of hands, feet, or legs, abnormal vaginal bleeding, or breast pain or enlargement.
- Inform your doctor if you are pregnant, become pregnant, plan to become pregnant, or are breastfeeding.
- Notify your doctor immediately if you experience pain in calves or leg swelling, sudden chest pain, shortness of breath, coughing blood, or changes in vision.
- Discontinue therapy 72 hours before and during prolonged immobilization such as postsurgical recovery and prolonged bed rest. Avoid prolonged restriction of movement during travel because of increased blood clotting risks.
- Raloxifene does not reduce hot flashes or flushes associated with menopause or estrogen deficiency. Hot flashes may occur upon beginning therapy.
- Take additional calcium and vitamin D if daily dietary intake is inadequate. Consider weight-bearing exercise and reduction of cigarette smoking and alcohol consumption.
- Store at room temperature (59° to 86°F).

*If you have any questions, consult your doctor, pharmacist, or health care provider.*

| Generic Name<br>*Brand Name Examples* | Supplied As | Generic<br>Available |
|---|---|---|
| *Rx* **Medroxyprogesterone Acetate** | | |
| *Provera* | **Tablets**: 2.5 mg, 5 mg, 10 mg | Yes |
| *Rx* **Megestrol Acetate** | | |
| *Megace* | **Tablets**: 20 mg, 40 mg | Yes |
| *Megace* | **Suspension**: 40 mg/mL | No |
| *Rx* **Norethindrone Acetate** | | |
| *Aygestin* | **Tablets**: 5 mg | Yes |
| *Rx* **Progesterone** | | |
| *Prometrium* | **Capsules**: 100 mg, 200 mg | No |
| *Crinone* | **Gel, vaginal**: 45 mg (4%),<br>90 mg (8%)/applicator | No |
| *Progesterone in oil* | **Injection**: 50 mg/mL | Yes |

## Type of Drug:
Female sex hormone.

## How the Drug Works:
Progesterone is the primary progestin produced by the female ovaries. Progestins prepare the uterus (womb) for implantation of a fertilized egg. They are also needed for the maintenance of pregnancy. However, when given as prescription medicine, they can inhibit the secretion of pituitary hormones, thus preventing ovulation, and may also inhibit spontaneous uterine contractions.

## Uses:
*Medroxyprogesterone acetate, norethindrone acetate, progesterone:* To treat secondary amenorrhea (absence of menstrual flow), abnormal bleeding from the uterus due to hormone imbalance, and to prevent abnormal uterine tissue growth in postmenopausal women taking estrogen.

*Megestrol acetate suspension:* For appetite enhancement in HIV-infected patients.

*Megestrol acetate tablets:* For treatment of advanced breast or endometrial cancer.

*Norethindrone:* To treat endometriosis.

*Progesterone gel:* To treat infertility as part of Assisted Reproductive Technology.

*Unlabeled Use(s):* Occasionally doctors may prescribe progesterone suppositories to treat premenstrual syndrome (PMS), to decrease spontaneous abortions, and to improve fertility. Other forms of progesterone have been used to treat premature labor and with estrogen replacement therapy for menopause. Medroxyprogesterone acetate may be prescribed to treat menopausal symptoms.

## Precautions:

*Do not use in the following situations:*

allergy to peanuts (progesterone capsules only)
allergy to the drug or any of its ingredients
blood clots, current or history of
breast cancer, known or suspected
genital cancer, known or suspected

liver disease, severe
miscarriage with some tissue still suspected in uterus
missed abortion
pregnancy, known or suspected
pregnancy test
stroke, current or history of
vaginal bleeding, undiagnosed

*Use with caution in the following situations:*

asthma
depression, current or history of
diabetes
epilepsy

heart disease
kidney disease
liver disease, mild to moderate
migraine headaches

*Blood clot disorders:* Blood clot disorders occasionally occur. Notify your doctor immediately if you experience pain in the calves or chest, sudden shortness of breath, coughing blood, sudden severe headache or vomiting, dizziness, fainting, visual or speech disturbances, or weakness or numbness in an arm or leg.

*Eyes:* Discontinue medication pending an eye exam if there is a loss or change in your vision, protrusion of the eyes, double vision, or migraines.

*Physical exams:* Physical exams should include self-examination of breasts (monthly), pelvic examination, and Pap smear test (yearly). Consult your doctor in all cases of unusual vaginal bleeding.

*Pregnancy:* Use during pregnancy is contraindicated. Progestin used during the first 4 months of pregnancy may cause masculinization of the female fetus as well as congenital heart and liver defects. Progesterone gel may be used during the first 12 weeks of pregnancy associated with Assisted Reproductive Technology to maintain the pregnancy.

*Breastfeeding:* Progestins appear in breast milk. Consult your doctor before you begin breastfeeding. Medroxyprogesterone may increase milk production and duration of production when taken after delivery.

*Children:* Safety and effectiveness have not been established.

*Lab tests* and exams will be required to monitor therapy. Tests include a pretreatment physical exam (including breast and pelvic organ exams and Pap smear).

## Drug Interactions:

Tell your doctor or pharmacist if you are taking or if you are planning to take any over-the-counter or prescription medications or dietary supplements while taking these drugs . Doses of one or both drugs may need to be modified or a different drug may need to be prescribed. The following drugs or drug classes interact with these drugs:

aminoglutethimide (*Cytadren*) (medroxyprogesterone acetate only)
ketoconazole (eg, *Nizoral*) (progesterone only)
rifampin (eg, *Rifadin*) (norethindrone only)

## Side Effects:

Every drug is capable of producing side effects. Many patients experience no, or minor, side effects. The frequency and severity of side effects depend on many factors including dose, duration of therapy, and individual susceptibility. Possible side effects include:

*Urinary and Reproductive Tract:* Change in menstrual flow; spotting; vaginal bleeding at abnormal times; unusual vaginal secretions; cervical eversion (turning outward); absence of menstrual flow; bladder problems; genital infection; impotence; decreased sex drive; pain during intercourse; breast pain or tenderness; breast enlargement (males or females); urinary tract infection; nipple discharge; genital pain; frequent or nighttime urination; cramps.

*Digestive Tract:* Nausea; constipation; vomiting; bloating; stomach pain or cramping; diarrhea; gas; mouth infection; indigestion; dry mouth; increased salivation.

*Nervous System:* Depression; sleeplessness; drowsiness; headache; dizziness; numbness in an arm or leg; confusion; convulsions; abnormal thinking; nervousness; irritability.

*Skin:* Discoloration of the skin; itching; rash; hives; acne; excessive hair growth; hair loss; herpes; sweating; pain, irritation, or discomfort at the injection site; abnormal skin sensations.

*Other:* Fluid retention (edema); weight changes; high blood pressure; changes in blood sugar; fever; vision changes; shortness of breath; pneumonia; infection; chest, joint, or back pain; yellowing of skin or eyes (jaundice); body pain; cough; sore throat; anemia; liver enlargement; abnormal heart rhythm; abnormal lab tests; weakness; pounding in the chest (palpitations); difficulty breathing; hot flashes; fatigue.

**Guidelines for Use:**

- Dosage is individualized. Use exactly as prescribed.
- Do not stop taking or change the dose, unless instructed by your doctor.
- Patient package inserts are available with most of these products. However, they are not required to be dispensed to cancer patients.
- *Oral dosage forms* — Take with food if stomach upset occurs. Take progesterone capsules with food to increase effectiveness.
- *Progesterone vaginal gel* — Do not use concurrently with any other intravaginal therapy. If other intravaginal therapy is to be used concurrently, administer 6 hours or more before or after progesterone vaginal gel.
- If a dose is missed, take it as soon as possible. If several hours have passed or it is nearing time for the next dose, do not double the dose to catch up, unless instructed by your doctor. If more than one dose is missed, or it is necessary to establish a new dosage schedule, contact your doctor or pharmacist.
- *Diabetic patients* — Glucose tolerance may be decreased. Monitor blood sugar closely and report any abnormal results to your doctor.
- Notify your doctor if you experience abnormal uterine bleeding, yellowing of the skin or eyes, breast lumps, or a feeling of depression.
- Notify your doctor immediately if you experience pain in the calves or chest, sudden shortness of breath, coughing blood, sudden severe headache or vomiting, dizziness, fainting, visual or speech disturbances, or weakness or numbness in an arm or leg.
- Dizziness or drowsiness may occur in some patients. Use caution when driving or performing other tasks requiring alertness, coordination, or physical dexterity.
- Inform your doctor if you are pregnant, become pregnant, are planning to become pregnant, or if you are breastfeeding.
- Fluid retention caused by progestins may aggravate asthma, epilepsy, migraine, heart disease, or kidney disease. Use with caution in these conditions.
- *Brand interchange* — Do not change from one brand of these drugs to another without consulting your doctor or pharmacist. Products manufactured by different companies may not be equally effective.
- Physical exams should include self-examination of breasts (monthly), pelvic examination, and Pap smear test (yearly). Consult your doctor in all cases of unusual vaginal bleeding.
- Lab tests will be required to monitor therapy. Be sure to keep appointments.
- Store at room temperature (59° to 86°F).

*If you have any questions, consult your doctor, pharmacist, or health care provider.*

For more information on individual methods, see the contraceptive mono-graphs in this chapter.

The following table gives ranges of pregnancy rates reported for various means of contraception. *The effectiveness of these means of contraception (except IUD, medroxyprogesterone injection, levonorgestrel implants, vasectomy, and tubal ligation) depends upon the degree of adherence to the method.*

| Pregnancy Rates for Various Means of Contraception (%)[1] | | |
|---|---|---|
| **Method of Contraception** | Typical[2] | Lowest[3] |
| **Oral Contraceptives** | | |
| **Combination (estrogen/progestin)** | 0.1 to 3.4 | 0.1 |
| **Progestin-only** | 0.5 to 1.5 | 0.5 |
| Mechanical/Chemical | | |
| **Cervical cap**[4] | | |
| **Multiparous** | 40 | 26 |
| **Nulliparous** | 20 | 9 |
| **Male condom without spermicide** | 12 to 14 | 3 |
| **Male condom with spermicide** | 4 to 6 | 1.8 |
| **Diaphragm**[4] | 20 | 6 |
| **Female condom** | 21 | 5 |
| **IUD** | $\leq$ 1 to 2 | $\leq$ 1 to 1.5 |
| **Levonorgestrel implants** | $\leq$ 1 | $\leq$ 1 |
| **Medroxyprogesterone injection** | $\leq$ 1 | $\leq$ 1 |
| **Spermicide alone** | 20 to 22 | 6 |
| **Rhythm (all types)** | 25 | 1 to 9 |
| **Vasectomy/Tubal Ligation** | $\leq$ 1 | $\leq$ 1 |
| **Withdrawal** | 40 to 50 | 30 |
| **No contraception** | 85 | 85 |

[1] During first year of continuous use.
[2] A typical couple who initiated a method that was either not always used correctly or was not used with every act of sexual intercourse, and who experienced an accidental pregnancy.
[3] The method of birth control was always used correctly with every act of sexual intercourse but the couple still experienced an accidental pregnancy.
[4] Used with spermicide.

*If you have any questions, consult your doctor, pharmacist, or health care provider.*

| Generic Name Brand Name Example | Supplied As | Generic Available |
|---|---|---|
| Rx **Medroxyprogesterone Acetate** | | |
| *Depo-Provera* | **Injection:** 150 mg/mL | No |

## Type of Drug:
Female hormone; birth control injection; contraceptive injection.

## How the Drug Works:
This hormone, when administered at the recommended dose, prevents ovulation by suppressing the follicle stimulating hormone (FSH) and the luteinizing hormone (LH). These changes result in endometrial thinning.

## Uses:
To prevent pregnancy. It is a long-term injectable contraceptive in women when administered at 3-month intervals.

## Precautions:
*Do not use in the following situations:*

allergy to any component of the formulation
breast cancer, known or suspected
clotting disorder, current or history of
liver disease
pregnancy, known or suspected
stroke, current or history of
vaginal bleeding, undiagnosed abnormal

*Use with caution in the following situations:*

asthma
depression
diabetes
epilepsy
heart disease
jaundice (yellowing of skin or eyes)
kidney disease
migraine

*Use of injectable medroxyprogesterone* may be associated with an increased risk of the following:

blood clots
ectopic pregnancy
osteoporosis
visual disorders

*Eye problems:* Do not readminister pending examination if there is a sudden partial or complete loss of vision or if there is a sudden onset of eyeball protrusion, double vision or migraine. Consult your doctor if you experience any of these.

*Pregnancy:* Do not use during pregnancy. The risk of use in a pregnant woman clearly outweighs any possible benefit.

*Breastfeeding:* Medroxyprogesterone appears in breast milk. Consult your doctor before you begin breastfeeding.

## Drug Interactions:

Tell your doctor or pharmacist if you are taking or if you are planning to take any over-the-counter or prescription medications or dietary supplements with medroxyprogesterone. Doses of one or both drugs may need to be modified or a different drug may need to be prescribed. Aminoglutethimide (*Cytadren*) interacts with medroxyprogesterone.

## Side Effects:

Every drug is capable of producing side effects. Many medroxyprogesterone users experience no, or minor, side effects. The frequency and severity of side effects depend on many factors including dose, duration of therapy and individual susceptibility. Possible side effects include:

*Urinary and Reproductive Tract:* Menstrual irregularities; decreased sex drive; failure to experience orgasm; vaginal infection; pelvic pain; breast pain; vaginal discharge.

*Digestive Tract:* Stomach pain/discomfort; nausea; bloating.

*Nervous System:* Headache; nervousness; dizziness; weakness; depression; sleeplessness.

*Other:* Weight changes; backache; leg cramps; acne; no hair growth or hair loss; rash; edema (fluid retention); hot flashes.

---

### Guidelines for Use:

- Patient labeling available with product.
- Menstrual cycle may be disrupted and irregular when beginning treatment. This should decrease to the point of an absence of menstruation as treatment continues.
- Notify your doctor if there is a sudden partial or complete loss of vision, double vision or if migraine occurs.

---

*If you have any questions, consult your doctor, pharmacist, or health care provider.*

| Generic Name<br>*Brand Name Example* | Supplied As | Generic<br>Available |
|---|---|---|
| Rx **Medroxyprogesterone Acetate/Estradiol Cypionate** | | |
| *Lunelle* | **Injection**: 25 mg/5 mg per 0.5 mL | No |

## Type of Drug:

Female hormone; monthly birth control injection; monthly contraceptive injection.

## How the Drug Works:

This drug prevents ovulation by inhibiting the release of certain hormones. Other effects that enhance contraceptive effectiveness include a thickening of cervical mucus (decreases sperm penetration) and thinning of the endometrium (retards implantation of a fertilized egg).

## Uses:

To prevent pregnancy.

## Precautions:

*Do not use in the following situations:*

allergy to any component of the formulation
breast, endometrial, or other estrogen-dependent cancer, known or suspected
cerebral vascular disease
clotting disorder, current or history of
coronary artery disease
diabetes with vascular involvement
heart disease, valvular
high blood pressure, severe
jaundice associated with pregnancy or hormonal contraceptive use, history of
liver disease
migraine headaches with neurological symptoms
pregnancy, known or suspected
smoking, heavy (15 or more cigarettes/day) and older than 35 years of age
stroke or history of stroke
vaginal bleeding, undiagnosed abnormal

*Use with caution in the following situations:*

depression, history of
diabetes
gallbladder disease
high cholesterol levels

*Use may be associated with an increased risk of the following:*

blood clots
gallbladder disease
heart disease
hypertriglyceridemia
liver disease
osteoporosis
stroke
visual disorders

*Pregnancy:* Do not use during pregnancy. The risk of use in a pregnant woman clearly outweighs any possible benefit.

*Breastfeeding:* It is not known if medroxyprogesterone/estradiol cypionate appears in breast milk. Consult your doctor before you begin breastfeeding.

*Children:* Safety and effectiveness have been established in women of reproductive age. Safety and effectiveness are expected to be the same for postpubertal adolescents 16 years of age or older. Use before the first menstruation is not indicated.

## Drug Interactions:

Tell your doctor or pharmacist if you are taking or planning to take any over-the-counter or prescription medications or dietary supplements with this medicine. Doses of one or both drugs may need to be modified or a different drug may need to be prescribed. The following drugs or drug classes interact with this medicine:

acetaminophen (eg, *Tylenol*)
aminoglutethimide (*Cytadren*)
antibiotics (eg, tetracycline)
anticonvulsants (eg, phenytoin)
ascorbic acid (vitamin C)
clofibrate (*Atromid-S*)
cyclosporine (eg, *Neoral*)
morphine (eg, *MS Contin*)
phenylbutazone
prednisolone (eg, *Prelone*)
rifampin (eg, *Rifadin*)
salicylic acid (eg, *Panscol*)
St. John's wort (hypericum perforatum)
temazepam (eg, *Restoril*)
theophylline (eg, *Slo-Phyllin*)

## Side Effects:

Every drug is capable of producing side effects. Many patients experience no, or minor, side effects. The frequency and severity of side effects depend on many factors including dose, duration of therapy, and individual susceptibility. Possible side effects include:

*Nervous System:* Headache; depression; emotional lability; dizziness; nervousness.

*Urinary and Reproductive Tract:* Changes in menstrual bleeding (eg, frequent, irregular, prolonged, infrequent, or absence of bleeding); vaginal yeast infection.

*Other:* Increased blood pressure; weight gain; fluid retention; visual changes or changes in contact lens tolerance; breast tenderness or pain; stomach pain; acne; hair loss; decreased sex drive; nausea.

## Guidelines for Use:

- Carefully read the patient labeling available with the product.
- The first intramuscular (IM; into the muscle) injection is given within the first 5 days of the onset of a normal menstrual period, within 5 days of a complete first trimester abortion, or at least 4 weeks postpartum if you are not breastfeeding. If you are breastfeeding, the first injection is administered at least 6 weeks postpartum.
- The second and subsequent injections are administered monthly (28 to 30 days) after the previous injection, not to exceed 33 days. If the patient has not adhered to the prescribed schedule, pregnancy should be considered and she should not receive another injection until pregnancy is ruled out. Shortening the injection interval could lead to a change in menstrual pattern. Do not use bleeding episodes to guide the injection schedule.
- If a patient misses 2 consecutive periods, pregnancy should be considered before initiating or continuing injections.
- Menstrual cycle may be disrupted and irregular when beginning treatment. Notify your doctor if abnormal bleeding persists or is severe.
- Notify your doctor if you experience a sudden partial or complete loss of vision, double vision, yellowing of the skin or eyes, chest pain, pain in the legs, dizziness, or migraines.
- Medroxyprogesterone/estradiol cypionate injection does not protect against HIV (the virus that causes AIDS) or any other sexually transmitted diseases.
- When switching from other contraceptive methods, the injection should be given in a manner that ensures continuous contraceptive coverage based on the mechanism of action of both methods (eg, patients switching from oral contraceptives should have their first injection within 7 days after taking their last active pill).

*If you have any questions, consult your doctor, pharmacist, or health care provider.*

| Generic Name<br>*Brand Name Example* | Supplied As | Generic<br>Available |
|---|---|---|
| Rx **Etonogestrel/Ethinyl Estradiol** | | |
| *NuvaRing* | **Vaginal ring**: 0.12 mg etono-gestrel, 0.015 mg ethinyl estra-diol/day | No |

## Type of Drug:

Combination contraceptive drug.

## How the Drug Works:

The primary effect is the inhibition of ovulation. Other effects include changing the cervical mucus and endometrium, which makes it more difficult for sperm to enter the uterus and for the egg to implant.

## Uses:

For the prevention of pregnancy.

## Precautions:

*Do not use in the following situations:*

abnormal genital bleeding
allergy to the device or any of
 its components
breast cancer, active or
 history of
cigarette smoking, heavy (15 or
 more cigarettes/day) and older
 than 35 years of age
coronary artery disease, active
 or history of
deep vein thrombosis, history of
diabetes with kidney, eye, nerve,
 or blood vessel complications
estrogen-dependent neoplasia
eye clots
headaches with neurological
 symptoms
heart disease, active or
 history of
high blood pressure, severe
jaundice
liver disease
pregnancy, known or suspected
prolonged bed rest following
 major surgery
stroke (cerebrovascular disease)
thromboembolic disorders,
 active or history of
thrombophlebitis (blood clots in
 legs, lungs, or eyes)

*Use with caution in the following situations:*

abnormal mammogram
breast cancer, family history of
breast nodules
conditions made worse by fluid
 retention (edema)
depression, history of
diabetes
dropped bladder
dropped uterus
fibrocystic disease
gallbladder disease
hyperlipidemia
kidney disease

*Combination hormonal contraceptive risks:* Women who use combination hormonal contraceptives have an increased risk of several serious conditions including myocardial infarction, thromboembolism, stroke, liver tumors, cancer, and gallbladder disease.

*Pregnancy:* Do not use during pregnancy. The risk of use in a pregnant woman clearly outweighs any possible benefit.

*Breastfeeding:* Etonogestrel/ethinyl estradiol appears in breast milk. Do not breastfeed while using this device.

*Children:* Safety and effectiveness in children younger than 16 years of age have not been established.

## Drug Interactions:

Tell your doctor or pharmacist if you are taking or planning to take any over-the-counter or prescription medications or dietary supplements while using this device. Doses of one or both drugs may need to be modified or a different drug may need to be prescribed. The following drugs and drug classes interact with this device:

acetaminophen (eg, *Tylenol*)
antibiotics (eg, ampicillin, tetracycline)
anticonvulsants (eg, phenytoin)
antifungals (eg, griseofulvin)
ascorbic acid (vitamin C)
atorvastatin (eg, *Lipitor*)
barbiturates (eg, phenobarbital)
benzodiazepines (eg, diazepam)
beta blockers (eg, propranolol)
carbamazepine (eg, *Tegretol*)
cyclosporine (eg, *Sandimmune*)
felbamate (eg, *Felbatol*)
itraconazole (*Sporanox*)

ketoconazole (eg, *Nizoral*)
morphine (eg, *MSIR*)
oxcarbazepine (eg, *Trileptal*)
prednisolone (eg, *Prelone*)
protease inhibitors (eg, saquinavir)
rifampin (eg, *Rifadin*)
salicylic acid
St. John's wort
temazepam (eg, *Restoril*)
theophylline (eg, *Theo-Dur*)
topiramate (eg, *Topamax*)
tricyclic antidepressants (eg, amitriptyline)

## Side Effects:

Every drug is capable of producing side effects. Many patients experience no, or minor, side effects. The frequency and severity of side effects depend on many factors including dose, duration of therapy, and individual susceptibility. Possible side effects include:

*Circulatory System:* Thrombophlebitis (leg clots); stroke; venous thrombosis; arterial thromboembolism; myocardial infarction (heart attack); increased blood pressure.

*Nervous System:* Depression; emotional instability; headache.

*Digestive Tract:* Nausea; vomiting; cramps; bloating.

*Urinary and Reproductive Tract:* Breakthrough bleeding or spotting; vaginal inflammation or discomfort; change in menstrual flow; temporary infertility after discontinuation of treatment; vaginal fungal infections; menstrual cramps.

*Other:* Decreased glucose tolerance in diabetic patients; fluid retention; upper respiratory tract infection; runny nose; device-related events (eg, foreign body sensation, coital problems, device explusion); gallbladder disease; lung clots (pulmonary embolism); liver tumors; retinal thrombosis; mesenteric thrombosis; swelling of legs; patchy pigmentation of skin; breast tenderness or enlargement; nipple discharge; weight changes; yellowing of the skin or eyes (jaundice); migraine; rash; intolerance to contact lenses.

## Guidelines for Use:

- Use exactly as prescribed.
- *Starting the contraceptive vaginal ring:*
  *If you have not used a hormonal contraceptive in the past month:* Counting the first day of menstruation as day 1, insert the contraceptive vaginal ring on or prior to day 5 of the cycle, even if you have not finished bleeding. During the first cycle, an additional method of contraception (eg, male condoms, spermicide) is recommended until after the first 7 days of continuous use.
  *If you are switching from a combination oral contraceptive:* Insert the vaginal ring any time within 7 days after the last tablet and no later than the day that a new cycle of pills would have started. No backup method is needed.
  *If you are switching from a progestin-only method:* Insert the vaginal ring any day of the month (do not skip any days between the last pill and the first day of vaginal ring use); or on the same day as contraceptive implant removal; or on the same day as removal of a progestin-containing IUD; or on the day when the next contraceptive injection would be due. Use an additional method of contraception (eg, male condoms, spermicide) for the first 7 days after insertion of the ring.
  *Following complete first-trimester abortion:* Start using the vaginal ring within the first 5 days following a complete first-trimester abortion. You do not need to use an additional method of contraception. If use of the vaginal ring is not started within 5 days following a first-trimester abortion, follow the instructions as if you have not used a hormonal contraceptive in the past month. In the meantime, use an additional method of contraception (eg, male condoms, spermicide).
  *Following delivery or second-trimester abortion:* Start using the vaginal ring 4 weeks after delivery if you are not breastfeeding. If you are breastfeeding, use another method of contraception (eg, male condoms, spermicide) until the child is weaned. Start using the vaginal ring 4 weeks after a second-trimester abortion. If you begin using the vaginal ring postpartum and have not yet had a period, consider the possibility of ovulation and conception occurring prior to starting the vaginal ring and use an additional method of contraception (eg, male condoms, spermicide) for the first 7 days.
- One vaginal ring is inserted in the vagina by the patient. This ring is to remain in place continuously for 3 weeks. It is removed for a 1-week break, during which a withdrawal bleed usually occurs. A new ring is inserted 1 week after the last ring was removed on the same days of the week as it was inserted in the previous cycle. The withdrawal bleed usually starts on day 2 to 3 after removal of the ring and may not have finished before the next ring is inserted. In order to maintain contraceptive effectiveness, insert a new ring 1 week after the previous one was removed even if menstrual bleeding has not finished.
- *Insertion:* The patient can choose the insertion position that is most comfortable for her, for example, standing with one leg up, squatting, or lying down. Compress the ring and insert into the vagina. The exact position of the contraceptive vaginal ring inside the vagina is not critical for its function. Insert the contraceptive vaginal ring on the appropriate day and leave in place for 3 consecutive weeks.
- *Removal:* The ring is removed 3 weeks later on the same day of the week as it was inserted and at about the same time. Remove the vaginal ring by hooking the index finger under the forward rim or by grasping the rim between the index and middle finger and pulling it out.

## Guidelines for Use: (cont.)

- *Removal:* (cont.)
  Place the used ring in the sachet (foil pouch) and discard in a waste receptacle out of the reach of children and pets. Do not flush in the toilet.
- *Inadvertent removal, expulsion, or prolonged ring-free interval:* The vaginal ring can be accidentally expelled when it has not been inserted properly, or while removing a tampon, moving the bowels, straining, or with severe constipation. If the vaginal ring has been out during the 3-week use period, rinse with cool to lukewarm (not hot) water and reinsert as soon as possible, at the latest within 3 hours. If the ring has been out of the vagina for more than 3 hours, contraceptive effectiveness may be reduced. Use an additional method of contraception (eg, male condoms, spermicide) until the vaginal ring has been used continuously for 7 days. Consider the possibility of pregnancy if the ring-free interval has lasted more than one week. Use an additional method of contraception (eg, male condoms, spermicide) until the vaginal ring has been used continuously for 7 days. If the vaginal ring is expelled and lost, insert a new ring and continue the regimen without alteration.
- *Prolonged use:* If the vaginal ring has been left in place for up to 1 extra week (ie, up to 4 weeks total), remove it and insert a new ring after a 1-week ring-free interval. Rule out pregnancy if the vaginal ring has been left in place for more than 4 weeks. Use an additional method of contraception (eg, male condoms, spermicide) until the vaginal ring has been used continuously for 7 days.
- *Missed menstrual period:* If you have not followed the prescribed instructions and you miss a period, consider the possibility of pregnancy. Stop using the vaginal ring if pregnancy is confirmed.
- Notify your doctor immediately if you experience sharp chest pain, coughing blood, sudden shortness of breath, pain in the calf, crushing chest pain or heaviness in the chest, sudden severe headache or vomiting, dizziness, fainting, problems with vision or speech, weakness or numbness in an arm or leg, severe pain, swelling, or tenderness in the abdomen, breast lumps, irregular vaginal bleeding or spotting that happens in more than 1 menstrual cycle or lasts for more than a few days, swelling of the fingers or ankles, difficulty in sleeping, weakness, lack of energy, fatigue, changes in contact lens tolerance, or yellowing of the skin or eyes, especially with fever, tiredness, loss of appetite, dark-colored urine, or light-colored bowel movements.
- The vaginal ring does not protect against HIV or any other sexually transmitted diseases.
- The vaginal ring may not be suitable for women with conditions that make the vagina more susceptible to vaginal irritation or ulceration.
- Some women are aware of the vaginal ring at random times during the 21 days of use or during intercourse. During intercourse, some sexual partners may feel the ring in the vagina. This is not cause for concern.
- The vaginal ring may interfere with the correct placement and position of a diaphragm. Therefore, a diaphragm is not recommended as a backup method with vaginal ring use.
- Store up to 4 months at room temperature (59° to 86°F). Avoid heat and direct sunlight.

*If you have any questions, consult your doctor, pharmacist, or health care provider.*

| | Brand Name Examples | Estrogen (mcg) | Progestin (mg) |
|---|---|---|---|
| Rx | **Monophasic** | | |
| | Necon 1/50, Nelova 1/50M, Norinyl 1+50, Ortho-Novum 1/50 | 50 mestranol | 1 norethindrone |
| | Ovcon 50 | 50 ethinyl estradiol | 1 norethindrone |
| | Demulen 1/50, Zovia 1/50E | 50 ethinyl estradiol | 1 ethynodiol diacetate |
| | Ovral | 50 ethinyl estradiol | 0.5 norgestrel |
| | Necon 1/35, Nelova 1/35E, Norethindrone and Ethinyl Estradiol, Norinyl 1+35, Ortho-Novum 1/35 | 35 ethinyl estradiol | 1 norethindrone |
| | Brevicon, Modicon, Necon 0.5/35, Nelova 0.5/35E, Norethindrone and Ethinyl Estradiol | 35 ethinyl estradiol | 0.5 norethindrone |
| | Ovcon 35 | 35 ethinyl estradiol | 0.4 norethindrone |
| | Ortho-Cyclen | 35 ethinyl estradiol | 0.25 norgestimate |
| | Demulen 1/35, Zovia 1/35E | 35 ethinyl estradiol | 1 ethynodiol diacetate |
| | Loestrin 1.5/30, Loestrin Fe 1.5/30[1] | 30 ethinyl estradiol | 1.5 norethindrone acetate |
| | Lo/Ovral, Low-Ogestrel | 30 ethinyl estradiol | 0.3 norgestrel |
| | Levlen, Levora, Nordette | 30 ethinyl estradiol | 0.15 levonor-gestrel |
| | Apri, Desogen, Desogestrel and Ethinyl Estra-diol, Ortho-Cept | 30 ethinyl estradiol | 0.15 desogestrel |
| | Loestrin 1/20, Loestrin Fe 1/20[1] | 20 ethinyl estradiol | 1 norethindrone acetate |
| | Alesse, Levlite | 20 ethinyl estradiol | 0.1 levonorgestrel |

|     | Brand Name Examples | Estrogen (mcg) | Progestin (mg) |
| --- | --- | --- | --- |
| Rx | **Biphasic** | | |
|  | *Jenest, Necon 10/11, Nelova 7/14, Nelova 10/11, Norethindrone and Ethinyl Estradiol (7/14), Norethindrone and Ethinyl Estradiol (10/11), Ortho-Novum 10/11* | | |
|  | Phase 1 | 35 ethinyl estradiol | 0.5 norethindrone |
|  | Phase 2 | 35 ethinyl estradiol | 1 norethindrone |
|  | *Mircette* | | |
|  | Phase 1 | 20 ethinyl estradiol | 0.15 desogestrel |
|  | Phase 2 | 10 ethinyl estradiol | |
| Rx | **Triphasic** | | |
|  | *Tri-Norinyl* | | |
|  | Phase 1 | 35 ethinyl estradiol | 0.5 norethindrone |
|  | Phase 2 | 35 ethinyl estradiol | 1 norethindrone |
|  | Phase 3 | 35 ethinyl estradiol | 0.5 norethindrone |
|  | *Ortho-Novum 7/7/7* | | |
|  | Phase 1 | 35 ethinyl estradiol | 0.5 norethindrone |
|  | Phase 2 | 35 ethinyl estradiol | 0.75 norethindrone |
|  | Phase 3 | 35 ethinyl estradiol | 1 norethindrone |
|  | *Ortho Tri-Cyclen* | | |
|  | Phase 1 | 35 ethinyl estradiol | 0.18 norgestimate |
|  | Phase 2 | 35 ethinyl estradiol | 0.215 norgestimate |
|  | Phase 3 | 35 ethinyl estradiol | 0.25 norgestimate |
|  | *Tri Levlen, Triphasil, Trivora* | | |
|  | Phase 1 | 30 ethinyl estradiol | 0.05 levonorgestrel |
|  | Phase 2 | 40 ethinyl estradiol | 0.075 levonorgestrel |
|  | Phase 3 | 30 ethinyl estradiol | 0.125 levonorgestrel |

| | Brand Name Examples | Estrogen (mcg) | Progestin (mg) |
|---|---|---|---|
| Rx | **Triphasic (cont.)** | | |
| | Estrostep, Estrostep Fe[1] | | |
| | Phase 1 | 20 ethinyl estradiol | 1 norethindrone acetate |
| | Phase 2 | 30 ethinyl estradiol | 1 norethindrone acetate |
| | Phase 3 | 35 ethinyl estradiol | 1 norethindrone acetate |
| Rx | **Progestin Only** | | |
| | Micronor, Nor-QD | none | 0.35 norethin-drone |
| | Ovrette [2] | none | 0.075 norgestrel |

[1] Seven tablets in the 28-day package contain 75 mg ferrous fumarate (iron) per tablet.
[2] Contains tartrazine.

All of the products listed in the table are oral contraceptives; however, they are not interchangeable. For example, Lo/Ovral cannot be used for Ortho-Novum. Daily doses may vary depending on individual needs. Do not adjust the dose without consulting your pharmacist or doctor.

## Type of Drug:

Oral contraceptives. Birth-control pills, "the pill." POPs, "mini-pill" (progestin only).

## How the Drug Works:

There are two different types of birth-control pills: Combination pills and progestin-only pills (POPs).

The combination pill contains the hormones estrogen and progestin. It prevents pregnancy by preventing ovulation, altering cervical mucous to inhibit sperm and decrease the chances of fertilization if an egg is released, and altering the lining of the uterus to prevent implantation of a fertilized egg.

There are three kinds of combination pills. The monophasic pill has the same dose of estrogen and progestin in each pill. The biphasic and triphasic pills have varying amounts of hormones. This produces an effect that more closely resembles the normal hormone cycle of the body. All of the biphasic pills (except Mircette) contain the same amount of estrogen in each pill. The progestin present is lower in the first half of the menstrual cycle than during the second half. The triphasic pill may contain differing amounts of both estrogen and progestin in the monthly cycle.

POPs contain only progestin. They appear to prevent pregnancy by causing changes in the cervical mucus and the inner lining of the uterus. These changes inhibit sperm from fertilizing the egg and prevent implantation should fertilization occur. POPs prevent ovulation in some women.

## Uses:

To prevent pregnancy. Oral contraceptives are highly effective. Less than 1 of 100 women taking the oral contraceptives for 1 year become pregnant. Some of the pregnancies are not due to failure of the pill but to a failure of the user to take the pill properly (eg, missed doses). Approximately 3 of 100 women taking POPs for 1 year become pregnant.

Because of an association between estrogen use and the risk of blood clots, the estrogen dose in the combination pill should be as low as possible. Women should discuss this matter with their doctors.

*Ortho Tri-Cyclen* — Also indicated for the treatment of moderate acne in women 15 years of age or older who have no known contraindications to oral contraceptive therapy, desire contraception, have had their first menstruation, and are unresponsive to topical anti-acne medications.

*Unlabeled Use(s):* Occasionally doctors may prescribe oral contraceptives as a postcoital contraceptive or "morning-after" pill. See the Emergency Contraceptives monograph in this chapter.

## Precautions:

*Do not use in the following situations:*

allergy to the oral contraceptive or any of its ingredients
angina pectoris (chest pain)
blood clots in the deep veins of the legs, active or history of
blood clotting disorder
cancer of breast, cervix, uterus, or vagina; known or suspected
cerebrovascular disease
coronary artery disease
estrogen-dependent growths, known or suspected
heart attack, history of
jaundice (yellowing of skin or eyes) during pregnancy or during previous use of oral contraceptives
liver disease or tumors
pregnancy, known or suspected
stroke, history of
thromboembolic disorders, active or history of
vaginal bleeding, undiagnosed or abnormal

*Use with caution in the following situations:*

abnormal breast x-ray or mammogram
breast nodules
depression, history of
diabetes or prediabetes
epilepsy
fibroids
gallbladder disease
headaches
heart disease
high blood pressure
hyperlipidemia (increased cholesterol or triglycerides)
kidney disease
menstrual flow, absent or irregular, history of
migraine
porphyria
smoker, current
surgery

*Risk factors:* All of the following are considered risk factors. The likelihood of side effects from oral contraceptives multiplies with each additional risk factor.

coronary artery disease, family history of
diabetes
high blood pressure
high cholesterol or triglycerides
jaundice, active or history of
older than 35 years of age
long term use (over 10 years)
smoking 15 or more cigarettes/day

*Increased risk:* Use of oral contraceptives is associated with an increased risk of the following:

blood clots
cerebral hemorrhage
decreased glucose tolerance
depression
fluid retention
gallbladder disease
headache
heart attack
high blood pressure
liver tumors
menstrual bleeding irregularities
stroke
vascular disease
visual disorders

*Cigarette smoking:* Cigarette smoking increases the risk of serious cardio-vascular side effects from oral contraceptive use. The risk increases with age and with heavy smoking (15 or more cigarettes/day) and is quite marked in women over 35 years of age. Women who use oral contraceptives should not smoke.

*Contact lens wearers:* If you develop changes in vision or lens tolerance, contact your eye-care specialist. Consider temporarily or permanently stopping contact lens wear.

*Diabetics:* Oral contraceptives may cause decreased glucose tolerance. Monitor blood sugar closely and report changes to your doctor.

*Eye problems:* Discontinue use and notify your doctor if you experience double vision, unexplained loss of vision, or other vision changes.

*Side effects:* Side effects noted during initial cycles are usually related to the potency of the estrogen or progestin in the product and may be transient. If side effects continue, discuss changing products (different estrogen/progestin potency) with your doctor.

*Use preceding pregnancy:* Women who discontinue oral contraceptives with the intent of becoming pregnant should use an alternate form of contraception for approximately 3 months before attempting to conceive.

*Pregnancy:* Do not use during pregnancy. The risk of use in a pregnant woman clearly outweighs any possible benefit.

*Breastfeeding:* Oral contraceptives appear in breast milk. They may decrease both the quantity and quality of breast milk. Do not use until the infant is weaned.

*Children:* Safety and effectiveness have been established in women of reproductive age. Safety and effectiveness are expected to be the same for postpubertal adolescents 16 years of age or younger. Use of this product before the first menstruation is not indicated.

*Tartrazine:* Some of these products may contain the dye tartrazine (FD&C Yellow No. 5), which can cause allergic reactions in certain individuals. Check package label when available or consult your pharmacist or doctor.

## Drug Interactions:

Tell your doctor or pharmacist if you are taking or planning to take any over-the-counter or prescription medications or dietary supplements with oral contraceptives. Doses of one or both drugs may need to be modified or a different drug may need to be prescribed. The following drugs and drug classes interact with oral contraceptives:

antibiotics (eg, penicillins, tetracyclines)
anticoagulants (eg, warfarin)
azole antifungal agents (eg, fluconazole, itraconazole)
barbiturates (eg, phenobarbital)
benzodiazepines
  (eg, diazepam)
beta blockers (eg, propranolol)
caffeine
carbamazepine (eg, *Tegretol*)
corticosteroids (eg, prednisone)
felbamate (*Felbatol*)
griseofulvin (eg, *Grisfulvin*)
hydantoins (eg, phenytoin)
penicillin V (eg, *Beepen-VK*)
phenylbutazone (not available
  in the US)
primidone (eg, *Mysoline*)
protease inhibitors
  (eg, nelfinavir, ritonavir)
rifampin (eg, *Rifadin*)
selegiline (eg, *Eldepryl*)
tetracyclines (eg, doxycycline)
theophyllines (eg, amino-
  phylline)
troleandomycin (*Tao*)

## Side Effects:

Every drug is capable of producing side effects. Many oral contraceptive users experience no, or minor, side effects. The frequency and severity of side effects depend on many factors including dose, duration of therapy, and individual susceptibility. Possible side effects include:

*Serious:* Blood clots; stroke; high blood pressure; heart attack; gall-bladder disease; liver problems; changes in vision.

*Urinary and Reproductive Tract:* Change in menstrual flow; vaginal bleeding at abnormal times; absence of menstrual bleeding; spotting; temporary infertility after discontinuing drug; unusual vaginal secretions; vaginal fungal infection; change in cervical erosion or secretion.

*Digestive Tract:* Nausea; vomiting; stomach cramps; bloating.

*Nervous System:* Migraine; depression; headache; dizziness.

*Skin:* Spotty skin discoloration; rash; light sensitivity.

*Other:* Breast changes, tenderness, or enlargement; breast secretions; decrease in breast milk when given after childbirth; contact lens intolerance; change in corneal curvature; fluid retention; weight changes; reduced tolerance to carbohydrates; elevated blood sugar (diabetic patients); yellowing of skin or eyes; hypertriglyceridemia.

## Guidelines for Use:

- Carefully read the patient package insert available with the product.
- Your doctor or health care provider will take a medical and family history and examine you before prescribing oral contraceptives. The physical examination may be delayed to another time if you request it and your doctor believes that it is a good medical practice to postpone it. You should be reexamined at least once a year while taking oral contraceptives.
- Take exactly as directed at intervals not greater than 24 hours. Take regularly with a meal or at bedtime. Strictly adhere to the dosage schedule for maximum effectiveness.
- Notify your doctor immediately if you experience pain in the groin or calves; sharp or crushing chest pain; heaviness in the chest; sudden shortness of breath; abnormal vaginal bleeding; missed menstrual period or suspected pregnancy; lumps in the breast; sudden severe headache, dizziness, or fainting; vision or speech disturbances; weakness or numbness in an arm or leg; severe stomach pain or tenderness in the stomach area; yellowing of the skin or eyes (especially if accompanied by fever, fatigue, loss of appetite, dark-colored urine, or light-colored bowel movements); severe depression; contact lens intolerance; coughing up blood; vomiting; sudden partial or complete loss of vision; difficulty sleeping; weakness; lack of energy; fatigue; or mood changes.
- Notify your doctor if you miss 2 consecutive menstrual periods. Oral contraceptive use should be discontinued until pregnancy is ruled out.
- If you experience vomiting or diarrhea, your oral contraceptive may not be as effective. Use a backup contraceptive method (eg, condoms, spermicide) until you speak with your doctor or pharmacist.
- May cause spotting, breakthrough bleeding, or nausea, especially during the first months of therapy. If this continues past the second month, notify your doctor.
- Fluid retention caused by oral contraceptives may aggravate seizure disorders; migraine; asthma; and heart, liver, or kidney disease. Use with caution in these situations.
- Report side effects to your doctor. Numerous combinations of oral contraceptives are available. Changes may be necessary to find the best one for you.
- If you have trouble remembering to take your oral contraceptive, talk to your doctor about how to make pill-taking easier or about using another method of contraception.
- Use an additional form of birth control for at least the first week after you begin taking oral contraceptives.
- *Diabetic patients* — Glucose tolerance may be decreased. Monitor blood sugar closely and report changes to your doctor.
- Oral contraceptives do not protect against HIV (the virus that causes AIDS) or any other sexually transmitted diseases.
- Lab tests may be required to monitor therapy. Be sure to keep appointments.
- Store at room temperature (59° to 77°F).

## Guidelines for Use (cont.):

- *How to take the combination pill —*

  *Sunday-Start packaging:* If the instructions recommend starting the regimen on Sunday, take the first tablet on the first Sunday after menstruation begins. If menstruation begins on Sunday, take the first tablet on that day.

  *21-Day regimen:* For day 1 start, count the first day of menstrual bleeding as day 1. Take 1 tablet daily for 21 days, then no tablets are taken for 7 days; whether bleeding has stopped or not, start a new course of 21 days followed by 7 days off. Withdrawal flow will normally occur approximately 3 days after the last tablet is taken. Follow the schedule whether flow occurs as expected, or whether spotting or breakthrough bleeding occurs during the cycle.

  *28-Day regimen:* To eliminate the need to count the days between cycles, some products contain 7 inert or iron-containing tablets to permit continuous daily dosage during the entire 28-day cycle. Take the 7 inert or iron-containing tablets on the last 7 days of the cycle.

  *Biphasic and triphasic pills:* Follow the instructions on the dispensers or packs; these are clearly marked (ususally with arrows), indicating where to start on the regimen and in what order to take the pills, along with the appropriate week numbers. If there is any question, detailed instructions are provided in the specific package insert. As with the monophasic pills, 1 tablet is taken each day; however, as the color or shape of the tablet changes, the strength of the tablet also changes (ie, the estrogen/progestin ratio varies).

- *Missed dose: Combination pill —* Although ovulation is not likely to occur if only 1 tablet is missed, the possibility of spotting or bleeding is increased. The possibility of ovulation occurring increases each day that tablets are missed, especially if 2 or more consecutive tablets are missed. Any time 1 or more active tablets are missed, use an additional method of contraception until tablets have been taken for 7 consecutive days. If you forget to take 1 or more tablets, the following is suggested:

  *One tablet:* Take it as soon as remembered, or take 2 tablets the next day; alternatively, take 1 tablet, discard the other missed tablet, and continue as scheduled and use another form of contraception until menstruation.

  *Two consecutive tablets:* Take 2 tablets as soon as remembered with the next pill at the usual time, or take 2 tablets daily for the next 2 days, then resume the regular schedule. Use an additional method of contraception for the 7 days after pills are missed, preferably for the remainder of the cycle. If 2 active pills are missed in a row in the third week and you are a Sunday starter, 1 pill should be taken every day until Sunday. On Sunday, the rest of the pack should be discarded and a new pack of pills started that same day. If 2 active pills are missed in a row in the third week and you are a day 1 starter, the rest of the pill pack should be discarded and a new pack started that same day. Menstruation may not occur this month, but this is expected. However, if menstruation does not occur 2 months in a row, contact your doctor or health care professional to discuss the possibility of pregnancy.

## Guidelines for Use (cont.):

- *Missed dose: Combination Pills* (cont.)
  *Three consecutive tablets:* If you are a Sunday starter, you should continue taking 1 pill every day until Sunday. On Sunday, the rest of the pack should be discarded and a new pack of pills started that same day. If you are a day 1 starter, the rest of the pill pack should be discarded and a new pack started that same day. Menstruation may not occur this month, but that is expected. However, if menstruation does not occur 2 months in a row, contact your doctor or health care professional to discuss the possibility of pregnancy. Pregnancy may result from sexual intercourse during the 7 days after the pills are missed. Use another form of contraception (eg, condoms, spermicide) as a backup method for those 7 days.

- *How to take POPs* — Take 1 tablet every day at the same time. Administration is continuous, with no interruption between pill packs. Every time a pill is taken late, and especially if a pill is missed, pregnancy is more likely.

- *Missed dose: POPs* — If you are more than 3 hours late or miss 1 or more tablet, take the missed pill as soon as you remember, then go back to taking the pill at the regular time, but be sure to use a backup method (eg, condom, spermicide) every time you have sexual intercourse for the next 48 hours.

- *Switching pills* — If you are switching from the combination pills to POPs, take the first POP the day after the last active combination pill is taken. Do not take any of the 7 inactive pills from the combination pill pack. Many women have irregular periods after switching to POPs. This is normal. If you are switching from POPs to the combination pills, take the first active combination pill on the first day of menstruation, even if the POP pack is not finished. If you are switching to another brand of POP, start the new brand at any time.

- *Missed menstruation* — If prescribed dosage regimen has not been followed, consider possible pregnancy. Stop taking the drug until pregnancy has been ruled out. If the prescribed regimen has been followed and 2 consecutive periods are missed, rule out the possibility of pregnancy before continuing the regimen. After several months of treatment, the menstrual flow may reduce to a point of virtual absence. This may occur as a result of medication and is not an indication of pregnancy.

*If you have any questions, consult your doctor, pharmacist, or health care provider.*

| Generic Name<br>*Brand Name Examples* | Supplied As | Generic<br>Available |
|---|---|---|
| *Rx* **Ethinyl Estradiol/ Levonorgestrel** | | |
| *Preven* | **Tablets**: 50 mcg ethinyl estra-diol, 0.25 mg levonorgestrel | No |
| *Rx* **Levonorgestrel** | | |
| *Plan B* | **Tablets**: 0.75 mg | No |

## Type of Drug:

Sex hormones; emergency contraceptives; emergency contraceptive pills (ECPs).

## How the Drug Works:

The exact mechanism of action is not known. ECPs may prevent pregnancy by inhibiting ovulation, altering transport of sperm or eggs to prevent fertilization, or altering the uterine environment to prevent implantation should fertilization occur.

## Uses:

For the prevention of pregnancy following unprotected intercourse or a known or suspected contraceptive failure. Use of the ECPs should begin as soon as possible, but within 72 hours of intercourse.

## Precautions:

*Do not use in the following situations:*
*Preven and Plan B —*
allergy to the drug or any of its ingredients
pregnancy, known or suspected
vaginal bleeding, abnormal or undiagnosed

*Preven only —*
blood clots in the deep leg veins, current or history of
blood clots in the lungs, current or history of
breast cancer, history of
breast cancer, known or suspected
cerebrovascular accidents, history of
diabetes with vascular involvement
headaches, severe (including migraine)
heart disease, ischemic
heavy smoking (more than 15 cigarettes/day) and more than 35 years of age
high blood pressure, severe
liver disease, active
liver tumors
major surgery with prolonged immobilization
stroke, current or history of
valvular heart disease with complications

*Use with caution in the following situations:*
diabetes
headaches
high blood pressure

*Pregnancy:* Do not use during pregnancy. The risk of use in a pregnant woman clearly outweighs any possible benefit.

*Breastfeeding:* Levonorgestrel and ethinyl estradiol appear in breast milk. Consult your doctor before you begin breastfeeding.

*Children:* Safety and effectiveness have been established in women of reproductive age. Safety and effectiveness are expected to be the same for postpubertal adolescents 16 years of age or younger. Use of this product before the onset of first menstruation is not indicated.

## Drug Interactions:
Tell your doctor or pharmacist if you are taking or planning to take any over-the-counter or prescription medications or dietary supplements while taking emergency contraceptives. Doses of one or both drugs may need to be modified or a different drug may need to be prescribed. The following drugs and drug classes interact with emergency contraceptives:

barbiturates (eg, phenobarbital)
carbamazepine (eg, *Tegretol*)
hydantoins (eg, phenytoin)
griseofulvin (eg, *Grisactin*)
rifampin (eg, *Rifadin*)

primidone (eg, *Mysoline*)
protease inhibitors
 (eg, nelfinavir)
selegiline (eg, *Eldepryl*)

## Side Effects:
Every drug is capable of producing side effects. Many emergency contraceptive users experience no, or minor, side effects. The frequency and severity of side effects depend on many factors including dose, duration of therapy, and individual susceptibility. Possible side effects include:

*Digestive Tract:* Nausea; vomiting; stomach pain or cramps.

*Other:* Headaches; dizziness; menstrual irregularities; breast tenderness; fatigue.

## Guidelines for Use:

- Carefully read the patient package insert available with this product.
- Emergency contraceptives can be used at any time during the menstrual cycle.
- Take 1 (*Plan B)* or 2 (*Preven*) tablets as soon as possible, but no later than 72 hours after unprotected intercourse. Take the second dose of 1 (*Plan B)* or 2 (*Preven*) tablets 12 hours after the first dose.
- If vomiting occurs within 1 hour of taking either dose of the medication, notify your doctor to discuss whether to repeat that dose and whether to take an antinausea medication before taking the dose again.
- Nausea occurs frequently. It is usually mild and stops within a few hours, but may continue for up to 1 or 2 days.
- *Preven* — The *Preven* emergency contraceptive kit contains a pregnancy test. This test can be used to verify an existing pregnancy resulting from intercourse that occurred earlier in the current menstrual cycle or the previous cycle. If a positive pregnancy test is obtained, contact your doctor and do not take the pills in the kit.
- Notify your doctor immediately if you experience sharp or crushing chest pain, coughing up blood, sudden shortness of breath, pain in a calf, heaviness in the chest, sudden severe headache, vomiting, dizziness, fainting, vision or speech disturbance, weakness, numbness in an arm or leg, sudden partial or complete loss of vision, or severe pain or tenderness in the stomach area.
- Emergency contraceptives are not to be used for ongoing pregnancy protection and should not be used as a woman's routine form of contraception.
- Taking more emergency contraceptive pills than prescribed does not further reduce the risk of pregnancy, but does increase the risk of nausea and vomiting.
- Emergency contraceptives do not protect against HIV (the virus that causes AIDS) or any other sexually transmitted diseases.
- A 3-week follow-up visit with your doctor or health care provider is recommended.
- Store at controlled room temperature (59° to 86°F).

*If you have any questions, consult your doctor, pharmacist, or health care provider.*

| Generic Name Brand Name Example | Supplied As | Generic Available |
|---|---|---|
| Rx **Progesterone** | | |
| *Progestasert* | **Intrauterine System**: 38 mg reservoir | No |

## Type of Drug:
Progestin-containing intrauterine birth-control device; IUD.

## How the Drug Works:
The exact mechanism of action is not known. It is believed that the system inhibits sperm and alters the uterine environment to prevent implantation should fertilization occur.

## Uses:
To prevent pregnancy for up to 1 year in women who have had at least one child, are in a stable, mutually monogamous relationship, and have no history of pelvic inflammatory disease (PID).

*Unlabeled Use(s):* Occasionally doctors may prescribe IUDs for excessive and prolonged menstrual bleeding.

## Precautions:
*Do not use in the following situations:*

abnormal pap smear
cervical cancer, known or suspected
ectopic pregnancy, predisposal to or history of
genital actinomycosis
incomplete involution of uterus following abortion or childbirth
increased susceptibility to infections (eg, leukemia, diabetes, steroid therapy, immunosuppression)
infected abortion
inflammation of the cervix
inflammation of the vagina
IUD still in place
IV drug abuse
multiple sexual partners, either partner
pelvic inflammatory disease, history or presence of, or predisposing factors to
pelvic surgery, history of
postpartum endometritis (inflammation of uterine lining)
pregnancy, known or suspected
sexually transmitted disease, history or presence of
shunt, systemic pulmonary
uterine cancer, known or suspected
uterine cavity distortion
vaginal bleeding, undiagnosed abnormal

*Use with caution in the following situations:*

anemia
anticoagulant therapy, concurrent
blood clotting disorder
congenital heart condition
excessive or prolonged menstrual bleeding, history of

*Continuation of pregnancy:* If pregnancy occurs while the IUD is in place and the pregnancy is continued without removing the IUD, there may be an increased risk of birth defects, miscarriage, infection, or premature labor and delivery. During pregnancy, report any of the following to your doctor immediately: Flu-like symptoms, fever, chills, stomach cramps and pain, vaginal bleeding or discharge.

*Ectopic pregnancy:* Although the IUD acts to prevent normal pregnancy, it does not prevent ovulation or ectopic pregnancy. Therefore, a pregnancy that occurs with an IUD in place is more likely to be ectopic. Ectopic pregnancies are potentially fatal and have been associated with complications leading to loss of fertility. Discuss symptoms of ectopic pregnancy with your doctor.

*Pelvic inflammatory disease (PID):* An increased risk of PID associated with IUD use has been reported. The highest rate occurs shortly after insertion and up to 4 months thereafter. PID can result in tubal damage, affect fertility, or cause predisposition to ectopic pregnancy. Discuss symptoms of PID and ectopic pregnancy with your doctor.

*Embedment:* Partial penetration or lodging of an IUD in the uterine lining has occurred. This can result in difficult removal or IUD fragmentation that may require surgical removal.

*Pregnancy:* Long-term effects on the fetus are unknown. If pregnancy is suspected, consult your doctor. Risks of an infected abortion may be increased if pregnancy occurs with a system in place. This is more likely to occur in the second trimester. If pregnancy occurs with the system in place, the system must be removed and termination of the pregnancy must be considered.

*Breastfeeding:* Oral progestins appear in breast milk. It is not known if the IUD affects breast milk or breastfeeding. Consult your doctor before you begin breastfeeding.

## Drug Interactions:

Tell your doctor or pharmacist if you are taking or if you are planning to take any over-the-counter or prescription medications or dietary supplements with IUDs. Doses of one or both drugs may need to be modified or a different drug may need to be prescribed. Anticoagulants (eg, warfarin) increase the risk of bleeding from the IUD insertion site.

## Side Effects:

Every drug is capable of producing side effects. Many IUD users experience no, or minor, side effects. The frequency and severity of side effects depend on many factors including duration of therapy, and individual susceptibility. Possible side effects include:

*Urinary and Reproductive Tract:* Inflammation of the uterine lining; miscarriage; septic abortion; perforation of uterus and cervix; pelvic infection; cervical erosion; inflammation of the vagina; vaginal discharge; ectopic pregnancy; uterine embedment; difficult removal; complete or partial expulsion of the IUD; vaginal bleeding at abnormal times; prolonged menstrual bleeding; lack of or delayed menstrual bleeding; pelvic pain and cramping; painful menstruation; difficult or painful intercourse; fragmentation of IUD; tuboovarian abscess; tubal damage; fetal damage; birth defects; intrauterine pregnancy.

*Digestive Tract:* Perforation into the abdomen followed by peritonitis; abdominal adhesions; stomach pain; intestinal penetration; intestinal obstruction; local inflammatory reaction with abscess formation and erosion of adjacent organs; cystic masses in the pelvis.

*Circulatory System:* Decreased heart rate during insertion or removal; blood poisoning; anemia.

*Other:* Fainting during insertion or removal; backache.

---

## Guidelines for Use:

- The patient information leaflet must be read and each section initialed by the patient.
- The Informed Choice Statement must be signed by the patient and by her doctor.
- A complete medical history and examination, including tests for chlamydia and gonorrhea, is required prior to insertion. The IUD should not be inserted immediately following childbirth or abortion.
- To prevent insertion in the presence of pregnancy, the system should be inserted during or shortly following menstruation.
- Reexamination is necessary within 3 months after the first postinsertion menstrual period and at 12 months for removal of the system. Normal pregnancy can occur after system removal, unless another system is inserted or other forms of contraception are started.
- Bleeding and cramps may occur during the first few weeks after insertion. Notify your doctor if symptoms continue or are severe.
- Notify your doctor immediately if you suspect you may be pregnant.
- Notify your doctor if you experience unusual, abnormal, or excessive vaginal bleeding; unusual or odorous vaginal discharge; fever; flu-like symptoms; genital sores; delayed or missed menstruation; pain during sexual intercourse; chills; pelvic pain or tenderness associated with fainting or the urge to defecate; unexplained shoulder pain; or stomach pain, cramping, or tenderness.
- If you notice the threads attached to the IUD, notify your doctor. Do not pull on the threads.
- Intrauterine progesterone does not protect against HIV (the virus that causes AIDS) or any other sexually transmitted diseases.

---

*If you have any questions, consult your doctor, pharmacist, or health care provider.*

| Generic Name<br>*Brand Name Example* | Supplied As | Generic<br>Available |
|---|---|---|
| *Rx* **Levonorgestrel** | | |
| *Norplant System* | **Implants:** 6 each containing<br>36 mg (216 mg total) | No |

## Type of Drug:

Long-term (less than 5 years), reversible birth-control system; progestin-containing contraceptive system.

## How the Drug Works:

Levonorgestrel appears to prevent pregnancy by preventing ovulation. It also causes changes in the inner lining of the uterus, preventing implantation should fertilization occur.

## Uses:

To prevent pregnancy for up to 5 years. The implants should be removed by the end of the fifth year; new implants may be inserted at that time if continuing contraceptive protection is desired. Approximately 0.2 (patients weighing less than 110 lbs) to 8.5 (patients weighing 154 lbs or more) of 100 women using levonorgestrel implants become pregnant. The effectiveness of this method is not dependent on proper use, but does appear to vary in accordance with body weight.

## Precautions:

*Do not use in the following situations:*

allergy to levonorgestrel or any of its ingredients
blood clotting disorder
breast cancer, known or suspected
idiopathic intracranial hypertension, history of
liver disease, acute
liver tumors, benign or malignant
pregnancy, known or suspected
vaginal bleeding, undiagnosed abnormal

*Use with caution in the following situations:*

depression, history of
diabetes or prediabetes
hyperlipidemia (increased cholesterol or triglycerides)

*Contact lens wearers:* If you develop changes in vision or lens tolerance, contact your eye care specialist. Consider temporarily or permanently stopping contact lens wear.

*Delayed follicular atresia:* If the development of an ovarian follicle occurs, growth beyond the size attained in a normal cycle may occur. These enlarged follicles cannot be distinguished clinically from ovarian cysts. Usually they will spontaneously disappear; rarely, they may twist or rupture, possibly requiring surgery.

*Ectopic pregnancy:* Ectopic pregnancies have occurred among levonorgestrel implant users, although studies have shown no increase in the rate per year as compared with users of no method of contraception or of intrauterine progesterone (IUDs). The risk may increase with duration of use and possibly with the increased weight of the user.

*Impaired liver function:* If jaundice (yellowing of skin or eyes) develops, removal of the implants should be considered. Steroid hormones may be poorly metabolized in patients with impaired liver function.

*Fluid retention:* Steroid contraceptives may cause fluid retention. Therefore, they should be used with caution in patients with conditions that might be aggravated by fluid retention (eg, high blood pressure, heart failure).

*Pregnancy:* Do not use during pregnancy. The risk of use in a pregnant woman clearly outweighs any possible benefit.

*Breastfeeding:* Levonorgestrel appears in breast milk. Consult your doctor before you begin breastfeeding.

*Children:* Safety and effectiveness have been established in women of reproductive age. Safety and effectiveness are expected to be the same for postpubertal adolescents 16 years of age or younger. Use of this product before the onset of first menstruation is not indicated.

## Drug Interactions:
Tell your doctor or pharmacist if you are taking or if you are planning to take any over-the-counter or prescription medications or dietary supplements with levonorgestrel implants. Doses of one or both drugs may need to be modified or a different drug may need to be prescribed. The following drugs and drug classes interact with levonorgestrel implants:

> carbamazepine (eg, *Tegretol*)
> phenytoin (eg, *Dilantin*)
> rifampin (eg, *Rifadin*)

## Side Effects:
Every drug is capable of producing side effects. Many levonorgestrel implant users experience no, or minor, side effects. The frequency and severity of side effects depend on many factors including duration of therapy and individual susceptibility. Possible side effects include:

*Insertion site reactions:* Pain; swelling; bruising; infection; blistering; ulceration; itching; skin sloughing; excessive scarring; discoloration; arm pain; numbness and tingling; nerve injury; removal difficulties; vein inflammation.

*Urinary and Reproductive Tract:* Change (typically a decrease) in menstrual flow; spotting; lack of menstrual bleeding; breast pain; breast discharge; inflammation of the vagina or cervix; vaginal discharge; enlarged ovarian follicles; prolonged, frequent, or irregular menstrual bleeding.

*Digestive Tract:* Nausea; vomiting; appetite changes; stomach ache.

*Nervous System:* Headache; anxiety; depression; nervousness; dizziness.

*Other:* Acne; skin inflammation; weight gain; excessive hair growth; scalp hair loss; abnormal lab tests; pain; fluid retention; rash; idiopathic intracranial hypertension; adnexal enlargement.

Also consider all side effects for combination (estrogen/progestin) oral contraceptives when using levonorgestrel implant. See the Oral Contraceptives monograph in this chapter.

## Guidelines for Use:

- Carefully read the patient package insert available with this product.
- Capsules will be inserted beneath the skin of the upper arm.
- Capsules should be implanted or removed only by a health care professional thoroughly instructed in the insertion and removal technique.
- Pregnancy must be ruled out prior to insertion. Conduct pregnancy tests whenever pregnancy is suspected. If pregnancy occurs, the implants must be removed.
- Insertion of the levonorgestrel implants should be performed during the first 7 days after the beginning of menstruation or immediately following an abortion. If performed at any other time during the cycle, a non-hormonal contraceptive method (eg, condom, diaphragm) should be used for the remainder of that cycle. Insertion is not recommended until 6 weeks after childbirth in breastfeeding women.
- Removal of the implants should be considered in women who will be immobilized for a prolonged period of time due to surgery or illness.
- Implants must be removed at the end of the 5-year period. If new implants are not inserted at the same time, the patient's previous level of fertility will return and pregnancy can occur at any time.
- Some change in menstruation patterns can be expected, especially during the first year.
- Notify your doctor if you experience stomach or pelvic pain, persistent headache, visual disturbances, depression, or yellowing of the skin or eyes.
- *Diabetic patients* — Levonorgestrel implants may alter glucose tolerance. Monitor your blood glucose closely.
- Bruising may occur at the implant site during insertion or removal. Darkening of the skin over the implant site may occur in some women but is usually reversible upon removal.
- Levonorgestrel implants do not protect against HIV infection (the virus that causes AIDS) or any other sexually transmitted diseases.

*If you have any questions, consult your doctor, pharmacist, or health care provider.*

| Generic Name<br>*Brand Name Example* | Supplied As | Generic<br>Available |
|---|---|---|
| *Rx* **Levonorgestrel** | | |
| *Mirena* | **Intrauterine system**: T-shaped unit containing a reservoir of 52 mg levonorgestrel covered by a silicone membrane | No |

## Type of Drug:

Levonorgestrel-releasing intrauterine system (LRIS).

## How the Drug Works:

How LRIS works to prevent pregnancy is not fully understood. The system may inhibit ovulation, alter the transport of sperm or eggs to prevent fertilization, or alter the lining of the uterus to prevent egg implantation should fertilization occur.

## Uses:

For intrauterine contraception for up to 5 years. Thereafter, if continued contraception is desired, the system should be replaced or alternative forms of contraception used.

LRIS is recommended for women who have had at least 1 child, are in a stable, mutually monogamous relationship, have no history of pelvic inflammatory disease (PID), and have no history of ectopic pregnancy or condition that would predispose to ectopic pregnancy.

## Precautions:

*Do not use in the following situations:*

abnormal, unresolved Pap smear

allergy to the intrauterine system or any of its components

breast cancer, known or suspected

cervical cancer, known or suspected

cervicitis or vaginitis, untreated (including bacterial vaginosis or other lower genital tract infections until infection is controlled)

conditions associated with increased susceptibility to infections (eg, leukemia, AIDS, IV drug abuse)

ectopic pregnancy, history of or predisposition to

genital actinomycosis

genital bleeding of unknown etiology

infected abortion in the previous 3 months

intrauterine device already in place

liver disease, acute

liver tumor, benign or malignant

multiple sexual partners, patient or patient's partner

pelvic inflammatory disease (PID), acute or a history of unless there has been a subsequent intrauterine pregnancy

postpartum endometriosis in the past 3 months

pregnancy or suspicion of pregnancy

uterine irregularity (including fibroids if they distort the uterine cavity)

uterine cancer, known or suspected

*Use with caution in the following situations:*

anticoagulant therapy, concurrent coagulopathy (bleeding disorder)

congenital heart disease
diabetes
valvular heart disease

*Intrauterine pregnancy:* If a patient becomes pregnant with the LRIS in place, and if the LRIS cannot be removed or the patient chooses not to have it removed, she should be warned that failure to remove the LRIS increases the risk of miscarriage, sepsis, premature labor, and premature delivery. She should be monitored closely and advised to report immediately any flu-like symptoms, fever, chills, cramping, pain, bleeding, vaginal discharge, or leakage of fluid. When pregnancy continues with the LRIS in place, long-term effects on the offspring are unknown. Congenital anomalies have occurred infrequently when the LRIS has been in place during pregnancy.

*Irregular bleeding and amenorrhea:* LRIS can alter the bleeding pattern. During the first 3 to 6 months of LRIS use, the number of bleeding and spotting days may be increased and bleeding patterns may be irregular. Thereafter, the number of bleeding and spotting days usually decreases, but bleeding patterns may remain irregular. If bleeding irregularities develop during prolonged treatment, appropriate diagnostic measures should be taken to rule out other causes.

Amenorrhea (absence of menstrual flow) develops in approximately 20% of LRIS users by 1 year. The possibility of pregnancy should be considered if menstruation does not occur within 6 weeks of the onset of previous menstruation. Once pregnancy has been excluded, repeated pregnancy tests are not necessary in amenorrheic subjects unless indicated by other signs of pregnancy or by pelvic pain.

*Pelvic inflammatory disease (PID):* Use of IUDs had been associated with an increased risk of PID. All women who choose the LRIS must be informed prior to insertion about the possibility of PID and that PID can cause tubal damage leading to ectopic pregnancy or infertility, or in infrequent cases can necessitate hysterectomy, or can cause death. Women who have ever had PID are at an increased risk for a recurrence or reinfection. Symptoms of PID include the development of menstrual disorders (eg, prolonged or heavy bleeding), unusual vaginal discharge, stomach or pelvic pain or tenderness, pain during sexual intercourse, chills, and fever. The highest risk of PID occurs shortly after insertion (usually within the first 20 days thereafter). A decision to use the LRIS must include consideration of the risks of PID.

*Pregnancy:* Do not use during pregnancy. The risk of use in a pregnant woman outweighs any possible benefit.

*Breastfeeding:* Levonorgestrel appears in the breast milk of women using LRIS. There is an increased risk of intrauterine perforation in women who are lactating. Consult your doctor before you begin breastfeeding.

*Children:* Safety and effectiveness have been established in women of reproductive age. Use of LRIS before the onset of menstruation is not indicated.

*Lab tests* and exams will be required before and during therapy. Tests include a pelvic examination, Pap smear, tests for genital disease (eg, gonorrhea, chlamydia), and a pregnancy test.

## Drug Interactions:

Tell your doctor or pharmacist if you are taking or planning to take any over-the-counter or prescription medications or dietary supplements with LRIS. Doses of one or both drugs may need to be modified or a different drug may need to be prescribed. To date, there have been no drug interactions reported.

## Side Effects:

Every drug is capable of producing side effects. Many LRIS users experience no, or minor, side effects. The frequency and severity of side effects depend on many factors including dose, duration of therapy, and individual susceptibility. Possible side effects include:

*Circulatory System:* Fainting or abnormal heartbeat during insertion or removal; high blood pressure.

*Nervous System:* Headache; depression; nervousness; migraine.

*Skin:* Acne; skin disorder; hair loss; eczema.

*Digestive Tract:* Stomach pain; nausea; vomiting.

*Urinary and Reproductive Tract:* Enlarged follicles; ectopic pregnancy; septic abortion; PID; irregular or prolonged bleeding; spotting; cramping; absence of menstruation; perforation; partial penetration or embedment; ovarian cysts; vaginal discharge; vaginal inflammation; painful menstruation; abnormal Pap smear; cervical inflammation.

*Other:* Upper respiratory tract infection; sinus inflammation; sepsis; back or breast pain; weight gain; decreased sex drive; failed insertion; anemia; pain during sexual intercourse.

## Guidelines for Use:

- Read the patient package insert provided before insertion of the LRIS.
- A complete medical history and examination will be required before LRIS insertion. A follow-up examination is required within 3 months of insertion.
- LRIS must be replaced every 5 years because contraceptive effectiveness after 5 years has not been established.
- Some vaginal bleeding, such as irregular or prolonged bleeding or spotting, or cramps may occur during the first few weeks after insertion. Notify your doctor if your symptoms continue or are severe.
- Notify your doctor immediately if you experience abnormal vaginal bleeding or pain, odorous vaginal discharge, fever, genital lesions or sores, migraine with or without vision loss, exceptionally severe headaches, yellowing of the skin or eyes, or increased blood pressure.
- Notify your doctor immediately if you suspect you may be pregnant.
- Women who currently have or have had breast cancer should not use hormonal contraception because breast cancer is a hormone-sensitive tumor.
- Patients with diabetes should closely monitor their blood glucose. Levonorgestrel may affect glucose tolerance.
- To check the location of the LRIS, reach to the top of the vagina with a clean finger after each menstrual period and feel the threads. Do not pull on the threads. If you feel more of the LRIS than just the threads or if you cannot feel the threads at all, the LRIS may not be in the right place, Contact your doctor immediately.
- Contraceptive effectiveness of the LRIS is lost if the system is displaced or expelled.
- Tampons can be used safely while the LRIS is in place.
- LRIS does not protect against HIV (the virus that causes AIDS) or any other sexually transmitted diseases.
- About 8 out of 10 women who wish to become pregnant conceive within 12 months after removal of the LRIS.
- Lab tests and exams will be required before and during therapy. Be sure to keep appointments.

*If you have any questions, consult your doctor, pharmacist, or health care provider.*

| Generic Name<br>*Brand Name Example* | Supplied As | Generic<br>Available |
|---|---|---|
| *Rx* **Norelgestromin/ Ethinyl Estradiol** | | |
| *Ortho Evra* | **Transdermal patch**: 20 cm$^2$/ 6 mg norelgestromin, 0.75 mg ethinyl estradiol | No |

## Type of Drug:

Combination contraceptive drug.

## How the Drug Works:

Norelgestromin is the active form of the progestin norgestimate found in some oral contraceptives. Ethinyl estradiol is an estrogen. Together, norelgestromin and ethinyl estradiol inhibit ovulation, change cervical mucus, and alter the endothelium (uterine lining).

## Uses:

To prevent pregnancy.

## Precautions:

*Do not use in the following situations:*

abnormal genital bleeding
allergy to norelgestromin/ethinyl estradiol or any of its ingredients
artery disease
breast cancer
cerebrovascular disease (stroke)
chest pain
diabetes with kidney, eye, nerve, or blood vessel complications
emergency contraception use
estrogen-dependent neoplasia
headaches with neurological symptoms
heart disease
high blood pressure, severe
jaundice
liver disease
pregnancy
prolonged bed rest following major surgery
thromboembolic disorders
thrombophlebitis (blood clots in legs, lungs, or eyes)

*Use with caution in the following situations:*

cigarette smoking
conditions made worse by edema (fluid retention)
depression
lipid disorders

*Combination hormonal contraceptive risks:* Women who use combination hormonal contraceptives have an increased risk of several serious conditions including myocardial infarction, thromboembolism, stroke, liver tumors, cancer, and gallbladder disease.

*Pregnancy:* Do not use during pregnancy. The risk of use in a pregnant woman clearly outweighs any possible benefit.

*Breastfeeding:* Norelgestromin/ethinyl estradiol appears in breast milk. Do not breastfeed while taking this medicine.

*Children:* Safety and effectiveness in children younger than 16 years of age have not been established.

## Drug Interactions:

Tell your doctor or pharmacist if you are taking or planning to take any over-the-counter or prescription medications or dietary supplements while using norelgestromin/ethinyl estradiol. Doses of one or both drugs may need to be modified or a different drug may need to be prescribed. The following drugs and drug classes interact with norelgestromin/ethinyl estradiol:

acetaminophen (eg, *Tylenol*)
antibiotics (eg, ampicillin)
anticonvulsants (eg, phenytoin)
antifungals (eg, griseofulvin)
atorvastatin (eg, *Lipitor*)
barbiturates (eg, phenobarbital)
carbamazepine (eg, *Tegretol*)
clofibric acid
cyclosporine (eg, *Sandimmune*)
felbamate (eg, *Felbatol*)

morphine (eg, *MSIR*)
oxcarbazepine (eg, *Trileptal*)
prednisolone (eg, *Prelone*)
protease inhibitors
 (eg, saquinavir)
rifampin (eg, *Rifadin*)
salicylic acid
St. John's wort
theophylline (eg, *Theo-Dur*)
topiramate (eg, *Topamax*)

## Side Effects:

Every drug is capable of producing side effects. Many norelgestromin/ethinyl estradiol users experience no, or minor, side effects. The frequency and severity of side effects depend on many factors including dose, duration of therapy, and individual susceptibility. Possible side effects include:

*Digestive Tract:* Nausea; vomiting; cramps; bloating.

*Circulatory System:* Thrombophlebitis (leg clots); venous thrombosis; arterial thromboembolism; myocardial infarction (heart attack); increased blood pressure.

*Nervous System:* Stroke; brain clots; depression; emotional instability.

*Urinary and Reproductive Tract:* Breakthrough bleeding; spotting; change in menstrual flow; temporary infertility after discontinuation of treatment; vaginal fungal infections; menstrual cramps.

*Other:* Gallbladder disease; pulmonary embolism (lung clots); liver tumors; retinal thrombosis; mesenteric thrombosis; swelling of legs; patchy pigmentation of skin; breast tenderness or enlargement; nipple discharge; weight changes; jaundice; migraine; rash; decreased carbohydrate tolerance; intolerance to contact lenses; application site reaction; upper respiratory infection.

## Guidelines for Use:

- Use exactly as prescribed.
- This medicine does not protect against HIV or any other sexually transmitted disease.
- A woman is not protected from pregnancy if she has more than 7 patch-free days. Use backup contraception (eg, condoms, spermicides, diaphragm) for the first week of the new cycle.
- Contact lens wearers may develop visual changes or changes in lens tolerance. See your doctor.
- The system uses a 28-day cycle. Apply a new patch each week for 3 weeks (21 total days). Week 4 is patch-free.
- Every patch should be applied on the same day of the week.
- Apply the patch to clean, dry, healthy skin on buttock, abdomen, upper outer arm, or upper torso.
- If a patch is partially or completely detached for 24 hours or more, or if the woman doesn't know how long the patch was detached, she may not be protected from pregnancy. Remove the old patch and start a new cycle by applying a new patch. Use backup contraception (eg, condoms, spermicides, diaphragm) for the first week of the new cycle.
- Do not apply makeup, creams, lotions, or powders to the skin where the patch is or will be placed.
- Lab tests may be required. Be sure to keep appointments.
- Store at room temperature.

*If you have any questions, consult your doctor, pharmacist, or health care provider.*

| Generic Name<br>*Brand Name Example* | Supplied As | Generic<br>Available |
|---|---|---|
| *Rx* **Choriogonadotropin Alfa** | | |
| *Ovidrel* | **Powder for injection:** 250 mcg | No |

## Type of Drug:

Fertility drug.

## How the Drug Works:

Choriogonadotropin alfa contains some of the same proteins that are in the naturally occurring hormones human chorionic gonadotropin (hCG), follicle stimulating hormone (FSH), and luteinizing hormone (LH).

## Uses:

For use in women in assisted reproductive technology (ART) programs. Choriogonadotropin alfa is given when monitoring indicates that the follicles have developed adequately. Choriogonadotropin alfa induces ovulation.

To bring about ovulation and pregnancy in infertile patients with irregular cycles.

## Precautions:

*Do not use in the following situations:*

abnormal uterine bleeding of undetermined origin
adrenal dysfunction, uncontrolled
allergy to choriogonadotropin alfa or any of its ingredients
allergy to hCG preparations
kidney disease
liver disease
ovarian cyst
ovarian enlargement
pituitary tumor
pregnancy
primary ovarian failure
thyroid dysfunction, uncontrolled
tumors (sex hormone dependent tumors of reproductive tract and accessory organs)

*Ovarian enlargement/hyperstimulation:* Choriogonadotropin alfa may cause ovarian enlargement or ovarian hyperstimulation syndrome (OHSS). OHSS can develop rapidly (within 24 hours to several days) and can become a serious medical event. Contact your doctor immediately if you experience severe pelvic pain, nausea, vomiting, and weight gain.

*Multiple births:* Choriogonadotropin alfa treatment has been associated with multiple births. Consult your doctor.

*Pregnancy:* Do not use during pregnancy. The risk of use in a pregnant woman clearly outweighs any possible benefit.

*Breastfeeding:* It is not known if choriogonadotropin alfa appears in breast milk. Do not breastfeed while taking this medicine.

*Children:* Safety and effectiveness in children have not been established.

*Lab tests* will be required to monitor therapy.

## Drug Interactions:

Tell your doctor or pharmacist if you are taking or planning to take any over-the-counter or prescription medications or dietary supplements while taking choriogonadotropin alfa. Doses of one or both drugs may need to be modified or a different drug may need to be prescribed.

## Side Effects:

Every drug is capable of producing side effects. Many choriogonadotropin alfa users experience no, or minor, side effects. The frequency and severity of side effects depend on many factors including dose, duration of therapy, and individual susceptibility. Possible side effects include:

*Digestive Tract:* Stomach pain; nausea; vomiting.

*Other:* Injection site pain; bruising; post-operative pain.

---

### Guidelines for Use:

- This medicine is injected subcutaneously (SC; under the skin). Use exactly as prescribed.
- Follow the injecting procedure taught to you by your health care provider.
- Visually inspect the solution. Do not use if discolored or contains particles.
- Overstimulation of the ovary may occur (ovarian hyperstimulation syndrome; OHSS). Contact your doctor immediately if you experience severe pelvic pain, nausea, vomiting, or weight gain.
- Use immediately after reconstitution. Discard unused solution.
- Lab tests will be required to monitor therapy. Be sure to keep appointments.
- Store vials at controlled room temperature (68° to 77°F) or refrigerate (36° to 46°F). Protect from light.

---

*If you have any questions, consult your doctor, pharmacist, or health care provider.*

| Generic Name<br>*Brand Name Examples* | Supplied As | Generic<br>Available |
|---|---|---|
| *Rx* **Chorionic Gonadotropin** | | |
| *Pregnyl*[1] | **Powder for injection:**<br>10,000 units/vial | Yes |
| *Profasi*[1] | **Powder for injection:**<br>2000 units/vial; 5000 units/<br>vial; 10,000 units/vial | No |

[1] Contains benzyl alcohol.

## Type of Drug:

HCG (human chorionic gonadotropin); hormone that stimulates the ovaries and testes.

## How the Drug Works:

This hormone is produced by the human placenta. Its action is identical to the luteinizing hormone (LH) secreted from the pituitary gland. It also has a small degree of follicle stimulating hormone (FSH) activity. HCG has different uses in men and women. In men, HCG stimulates sex glands, specifically the cells in the testicles, to stimulate their growth and development and produce androgens (eg, testosterone). HCG also causes the development of secondary sex characteristics and may cause the testicles to drop. In women, HCG stimulates the ovaries to produce progesterone.

## Uses:

*Men:* To stimulate testicular descent in prepubescent males whose testicles have not dropped or descended. Usually given to males between 4 and 9 years of age.

For selected cases of hypogonadism caused by pituitary deficiency.

To assist in the development of secondary sex characteristics in cases of hormone deficiency.

*Women:* To promote ovulation. HCG is used in combination with other medications.

## Precautions:

*Do not use in the following situations:*

allergy to chorionic gonadotropin
 or any of its ingredients
early puberty
pregnancy

prostate cancer
some types of cancers
 (eg, androgen dependent)

*Use with caution in the following situations:*

asthma
epilepsy
heart disease

kidney disease
migraine

*Early puberty:* In young males using HCG to cause the testes to drop, early puberty can occur. Discontinue use if signs of early puberty (eg, enlargement of penis or testes, development of pubic hair, aggressive behavior) occur.

*Multiple births:* Pregnancies following therapy with HCG and menotropins resulted in 80% single births and 15% twin births; 5% of pregnancies resulted in 3 or more fetuses.

*Fluid retention:* Since androgens may cause fluid retention, use HCG with caution in patients with epilepsy, migraine, asthma, heart, or kidney disease.

*Pregnancy:* Do not use during pregnancy. The risk of use in a pregnant women clearly outweighs any possible benefit.

*Breastfeeding:* It is not known if chorionic gonadotropin appears in breast milk. Consult your doctor before you begin breastfeeding.

*Children:* Safety and effectiveness in children younger than 4 years of age have not been established.

*Lab tests* may be required to monitor treatment.

## Drug Interactions:

Tell your doctor or pharmacist if you are taking or planning to take any over-the-counter or prescription medications or dietary supplements with chorionic gonadotropin. Doses of one or both drugs may be modified or a different drug may need to be prescribed.

## Side Effects:

Every drug is capable of producing side effects. Many chorionic gonadotropin users experience no, or minor, side effects. The frequency and severity of side effects depend on many factors including dose, duration of therapy, and individual susceptibility. Possible side effects include:

*Men only:* Acne; enlargement or redness of penis or testes; early growth of pubic hair; rapid increase in height; breast tenderness or swelling.

*Women only:* Stomach pain; pelvic pain; multiple births.

*Nervous System:* Headache; irritability; restlessness; depression; fatigue; aggressive behavior.

*Other:* Fluid retention (edema); pain at injection site; redness; rash; hives; stroke; difficulty breathing; shortness of breath.

## Guidelines for Use:

- Dosage is individualized. Take exactly as prescribed.
- Do not change the dose or stop taking, unless directed by your doctor.
- HCG has not been demonstrated to be effective in the treatment of obesity. HCG has no known effect on fat mobilization, appetite, sense of hunger, or body fat distribution.
- Inject intramuscularly (IM; into a muscle) only.
- If a dose is missed, inject it as soon as possible. If several hours have passed or it is nearing time for the next dose, do not double the dose to catch up, unless advised to do so by your doctor. If more than one dose is missed or it is necessary to establish a new dosage schedule, contact your doctor or pharmacist.
- Visually inspect solution for particles or discoloration before use.
- Lab tests may be required to monitor therapy. Be sure to keep appointments.
- Store dry powder at room temperature (59° to 86°F). After reconstitution (mixing), refrigerate at 36° to 46°F and use within 60 days.
- *Women —*
  HCG must be given following menotropins when tests indicate mature follicles are present (changes in vaginal smear or in cervical mucus, urinary estrogen test).
  Ovulation is confirmed by testing for progesterone production (rise in basal temperature, change in cervical mucus, etc).
  The couple should have intercourse daily, beginning on the day prior to HCG administration, until ovulation occurs. Take care to ensure insemination.
  During treatment with menotropins and HCG and for 2 weeks after treatment, patients must be examined by a doctor at least every other day.
  Monitor for signs of pregnancy. If pregnancy is suspected, contact your doctor.
  Multiple pregnancy is possible and poses potential hazards.
- *Men —*
  HCG is first used alone. Then menotropins and HCG are used together to stimulate sperm production.

*If you have any questions, consult your doctor, pharmacist, or health care provider.*

| Generic Name<br>*Brand Name Examples* | Supplied As | Generic<br>Available |
|---|---|---|
| *Rx* **Urofollitropin** | | |
| *Bravelle, Fertinex* | **Injection:** 75 IU FSH activity | No |
| *Fertinex* | **Injection:** 150 IU FSH activity | No |

## Type of Drug:
Gonadotropin; hormone that stimulates the ovaries.

## How the Drug Works:
Stimulates eggs in the ovaries to fully develop before ovulation.

## Uses:
Used with human chorionic gonadotropin (HCG) to induce ovulation.

Urofollitropin and HCG may be used to stimulate the development of multiple eggs in patients participating in assisted reproductive programs.

## Precautions:
*Do not use in the following situations:*

adrenal disorders, uncontrolled
allergy to the drug or any of its ingredients
bleeding, abnormal
infertility (other than not ovulating)
intracranial lesion (eg, hypothalamus or pituitary tumor)
ovarian cysts or enlargement not due to polycystic ovary syndrome
ovary failure, primary
pregnancy
thyroid disorder, uncontrolled
tumor (eg, ovary, breast, uterus)

*Before therapy:* Women must have a thorough pelvic exam and testing of the endocrine glands. A cervical dilation and curettage (D and C) must be done before beginning therapy if there is abnormal uterine bleeding or other signs of endometriosis. The partner's fertility potential must also be evaluated by a doctor.

*Ovarian enlargement:* Mild to moderate uncomplicated ovarian enlargement, which may be accompanied by abdominal bloating or pain, occurs in approximately 20% of patients treated with urofollitropin and HCG. It usually regresses without treatment within 2 to 3 weeks. If significant ovarian enlargement occurs after ovulation, do not engage in sexual intercourse.

*Pregnancy:* Do not use during pregnancy. The risk of use in a pregnant women clearly outweighs any possible benefit.

*Breastfeeding:* It is not known if urofollitropin is excreted in breast milk. Consult your doctor before you begin breastfeeding.

*Children:* Not indicated for use in children.

*Lab tests* may be required to monitor therapy. Tests include estradiol levels and ultrasonography.

## Side Effects:

Every drug is capable of producing side effects. Many patients experience no, or minor, side effects. The frequency and severity of side effects depend on many factors including dose, duration of therapy, and individual susceptibility. Possible side effects include:

*Digestive Tract:* Nausea; vomiting; diarrhea; stomach cramps.

*Urinary and Reproductive Tract:* Bloating; severe pelvic pain; bleeding into the pelvic area (hemoperitoneum); ovarian hyperstimulation syndrome (OHSS); vaginal bleeding; ovarian enlargement; ovarian cysts.

*Skin:* Rash, pain, swelling, or irritation at injection site; dry skin; hair loss; hives; itching; facial swelling.

*Other:* Headache; breast tenderness; pain; multiple births; hot flashes; enlarged abdomen; intravascular thrombosis and embolism (blood clots in the legs or lungs, lung damage, stroke, death).

### Guidelines for Use:

- Dosage is individualized. Use exactly as prescribed.
- Do not stop taking or change the dose, unless instructed by your doctor.
- Inject *Bravelle* subcutaneously (SC; beneath the skin) or intramuscularly (IM; into a muscle). Inject *Fertinex* SC.
- Visually inspect solution for discoloration or particles. Use immediately after reconstitution (mixing). Discard any unused portion.
- If a dose is missed, inject it as soon as possible. If several hours have passed or it is nearing time for the next dose, do not double the dose to catch up, unless instructed by your doctor. If more than one dose is missed or it is necessary to establish a new dosage schedule, contact your doctor or pharmacist.
- Discontinue use and contact your doctor immediately if you experience severe pelvic pain, bloating, nausea, vomiting, diarrhea, weight gain, difficulty breathing, or decreased urination.
- HCG must be given following urofollitropin when tests indicate mature follicles are present (ie, changes in vaginal smear or cervical mucus, urinary estrogen test).
- Ovulation is confirmed by testing for progesterone production (ie, rise in basal temperature, change in cervical mucus).
- A couple should have intercourse daily, beginning on the day prior to HCG administration, until ovulation occurs. Take care to ensure insemination. However, intercourse should be prohibited in patients in whom significant ovarian enlargement occurs after ovulation.
- Monitor for signs of pregnancy. If pregnancy is suspected, contact your doctor.
- Multiple pregnancy is possible and poses potential hazards.
- Lab tests may be required to monitor therapy. Be sure to keep appointments.
- Store refrigerated or at room temperature (37° to 77°F). Protect from light.

*If you have any questions, consult your doctor, pharmacist, or health care provider.*

| Generic Name Brand Name Example | Supplied As | Generic Available |
|---|---|---|
| Rx **Follitropin Alfa** | | |
| *Gonal-F* | **Powder for injection:** 37.5 IU,[1] 75 IU,[1] 150 IU[1] | No |

[1] Contains 30 mg sucrose.

## Type of Drug:

Gonadotropin; hormone that stimulates the ovaries; fertility drug.

## How the Drug Works:

Follitropin alfa stimulates the ovaries to produce eggs.

## Uses:

For the induction of ovulation and pregnancy in women whose ovaries still work but cannot form eggs (ovulate), and as a result, are not fertile (unable to become pregnant).

To stimulate the development of mutiple follicles in ovulatory patients undergoing Assisted Reproductive Therapy (ART) (eg, in vitro fertilization).

## Precautions:

*Do not use in the following situations:*

adrenal dysfunction, uncontrolled

allergy to follitropin alfa or any of its ingredients

follicle stimulating hormone, high levels of

lesion, organic intracranial (eg, pituitary tumor)

ovarian cyst or enlargement

pregnancy

thyroid disease, uncontrolled

tumors, sex hormone dependent

uterine bleeding, abnormal

*Multiple births:* Reports of multiple births have been associated with follitropin alfa treatment. Discuss this with your doctor before starting therapy.

*Overstimulation of the ovary:* Mild to moderate ovarian enlargement, with or without bloating or stomach pain, may occur and generally goes away within 2 or 3 weeks after discontinuing this medicine. All patients who experience bloating or stomach pain should be examined for ovarian enlargement. If significant ovarian enlargement occurs after ovulation, do not engage in sexual intercourse.

*Respiratory complications:* Serious respiratory conditions (eg, difficulty breathing, worsening of asthma) and blood clotting have been reported.

*Pregnancy:* Do not use during pregnancy. The risk of use in a pregnant woman clearly outweighs any possible benefit.

*Breastfeeding:* It is not known if follitropin alfa appears in breast milk. Consult your doctor before you begin breastfeeding.

*Children:* Safety and effectiveness in children have not been established.

*Lab tests* will be required during treatment. Tests may include blood hormone levels, ultrasound, and body temperature measurement.

## Side Effects:

Every drug is capable of producing side effects. Many follitropin alfa users experience no, or minor, side effects. The frequency and severity of side effects depend on many factors including dose, duration of therapy, and individual susceptibility. Possible side effects include:

*Digestive Tract:* Stomach pain; nausea; gas; diarrhea; vomiting; indigestion; enlarged stomach; loss of appetite; thirst.

*Nervous System:* Headache; dizziness; drowsiness; anxiety; nervousness.

*Respiratory System:* Upper respiratory infection; congested or runny nose; sore throat; difficulty breathing; coughing; sinus headache; head congestion.

*Urinary and Reproductive Tract:* Bleeding between periods; ovarian cyst; breast pain; ovarian hyperstimulation; painful menstruation; ovarian disorder; cervix lesion; menstrual disorder; pelvic pain; unusual vaginal discharge; vaginal bleeding; urinary tract infection; genital fungal infection; genital itching.

*Other:* Back pain; muscle pain; flu-like symptoms; fever; acne; unstable emotions; injection site pain; weight gain; abnormal skin sensations; fatigue; low blood pressure.

---

## Guidelines for Use:

- Dosage is individualized. Take exactly as prescribed.
- Carefully follow the preparation and administration techniques taught to you by your health care provider.
- Visually inspect the solution for discoloration or particles. Use immediately after reconstitution (mixing). Discard any unused portion.
- For subcutaneous (beneath the skin) injection only.
- Treatment with this drug requires close monitoring for overstimulation of the ovary. Contact your doctor immediately if you experience difficulty breathing, severe pelvic pain, nausea, vomiting, weight gain, stomach pain or bloating, diarrhea, or infrequent urination.
- The couple should have sexual intercourse daily, beginning on the day prior to human chorionic gonadotropin (HCG) administration, until ovulation occurs. Take care to ensure insemination. However, intercourse should be prohibited in patients in whom significant ovarian enlargement occurs after ovulation.
- Multiple pregnancy is possible and poses potential hazards.
- Other causes of infertility, as well as pregnancy, will be excluded before this medicine is used.
- Monitor signs of pregnancy. If pregnancy is suspected, contact your doctor.
- Lab tests will be required to monitor treatment. Be sure to keep appointments.
- Store in refrigerator or at room temperature (36° to 77°F). Protect from light.

---

*If you have any questions, consult your doctor, pharmacist, or health care provider.*

| Generic Name<br>*Brand Name Example* | Supplied As | Generic<br>Available |
|---|---|---|
| Rx **Follitropin Beta** | | |
| *Follistim[1]* | **Powder for injection:**<br>75 IU | No |

[1] Contains 25 mg sucrose.

## Type of Drug:
Gonadotropin; hormone that stimulates the ovaries; fertility drug.

## How the Drug Works:
Follitropin beta stimulates the ovaries to produce eggs.

## Uses:
For the induction of ovulation and pregnancy in women whose ovaries still work but cannot form eggs (ovulate) and as a result, are not fertile (unable to become pregnant).

To stimulate the development of mutiple follicles in ovulatory patients undergoing Assisted Reproductive Therapy (ART) (eg, in vitro fertilization).

## Precautions:
*Do not use in the following situations:*

adrenal dysfunction, uncontrolled
allergy to follitropin beta or any
of its ingredients
follicle stimulating hormone, high
levels
ovarian cyst or enlargement

pregnancy
thyroid disease, uncontrolled
tumors of the ovary, breast,
uterus, hypothalamus, or pituitary gland
uterine bleeding, irregular or
heavy of unknown cause

*Multiple births:* Reports of multiple births have been associated with follitro-pin beta treatment. Discuss this with your doctor before starting therapy.

*Ovarian Hyperstimulation Syndrome (OHSS):* Mild to moderate ovarian enlargement, with or without bloating or stomach pain, may occur and generally goes away within 2 or 3 weeks after discontinuing this medi-cine. All patients who experience bloating or stomach pain should be examined for ovarian enlargement. If significant ovarian enlargement occurs after ovulation, do not engage in sexual intercourse.

*Respiratory complications:* Serious respiratory conditions (eg, difficulty breathing, worsening of asthma) and blood clotting have been reported.

*Pregnancy:* Do not use during pregnancy. The risk of use in a pregnant woman clearly outweighs any possible benefit.

*Breastfeeding:* It is not known if follitropin beta appears in breast milk. Con-sult your doctor before you begin breastfeeding.

*Children:* Safety and effectiveness in children have not been established.

*Lab tests* will be required during treatment. Tests may include blood hormone levels, ultrasound, and body temperature measurement.

## Side Effects:

Every drug is capable of producing side effects. Many follitropin beta users experience no, or minor, side effects. The frequency and severity of side effects depend on many factors including dose, duration of therapy, and individual susceptibility. Possible side effects include:

*Digestive Tract:* Stomach pain; bloating; nausea; vomiting; diarrhea.

*Urinary and Reproductive Tract:* Miscarriage; ovarian hyperstimulation; ectopic pregnancy; ovarian cyst; pelvic pain; breast tenderness; heavy or irregular vaginal bleeding; infrequent urination.

*Skin:* Dry skin; rash; hair loss; hives.

*Other:* Rapid heart beat; fast or difficult breathing; headache; dizziness; muscle or joint pain; aches; body discomfort; fever; chills; flu-like symptoms; injection site pain; weight gain.

---

### Guidelines for Use:

- Dosage is individualized. Take exactly as prescribed.
- Visually inspect the solution for discoloration or particles. Use immediately after reconstitution (mixing). Discard any unused portion.
- Carefully follow the preparation and administration technique taught to you by your health care provider.
- For subcutaneous (beneath the skin) or intramuscular (into a muscle) injection only.
- Treatment with this drug requires close monitoring for overstimulation of the ovary. Contact your doctor immediately if you experience difficulty breathing, severe pelvic pain, nausea, vomiting, weight gain, stomach pain or bloating, diarrhea, or infrequent urination.
- The couple should have intercourse daily, beginning on the day prior to human chorionic gonadotropin (HCG) administration, until ovulation occurs. Take care to ensure insemination. However, intercourse should be prohibited in patients in whom significant ovarian enlargement occurs after ovulation.
- Multiple pregnancy is possible and poses potential hazards.
- Other causes of infertility will be excluded before this medicine is used.
- Monitor for signs of pregnancy before and during treatment. If pregnancy is suspected, contact your doctor.
- Lab tests will be required to monitor treatment. Be sure to keep appointments.
- Store in refrigerator or at room temperature (36° to 77°F). Protect from light.

---

*If you have any questions, consult your doctor, pharmacist, or health care provider.*

| Generic Name<br>*Brand Name Examples* | Supplied As | Generic<br>Available |
|---|---|---|
| Rx **Clomiphene Citrate** | | |
| *Clomid, Serophene* | **Tablets:** 50 mg | Yes |

## Type of Drug:

Ovulation stimulant.

## How the Drug Works:

Clomiphene produces a "false signal" that estrogen levels are low. The body responds by increasing the secretion of hormones (eg, gonadotropins) from the pituitary gland. These hormones stimulate the ovaries, causing the ovarian follicle to mature, resulting in ovulation (release of the egg). Clomiphene is not a steroid.

Effectiveness is documented but unpredictable. In clinical trials, pregnancy occurred in approximately 30% of women with ovulation problems who received clomiphene.

## Uses:

To treat female ovulatory dysfunction (infertility) when the patient desires pregnancy, the sexual partner is fertile and potent, and the patient has normal liver function and normal estrogen levels.

Ovulatory dysfunction due to thyroid or adrenal conditions will not respond to clomiphene.

*Unlabeled Use(s):* Occasionally doctors may prescribe clomiphene citrate for male infertility.

## Precautions:

*Do not use in the following situations:*

adrenal disorders, uncontrolled
allergy to the drug or any of its ingredients
bleeding disorder, undiagnosed
intracranial lesion (eg, pituitary tumor)
liver disease, history of
ovarian cyst or enlargement not due to polycystic ovarian syndrome
pregnancy
thyroid disorders, uncontrolled
uterine bleeding, abnormal

*Before therapy:* A complete pelvic examination is mandatory prior to treatment and repeated before each course. Clomiphene is not used in the presence of an ovarian cyst; further enlargement may occur. Other lab tests may also be required.

*Multiple births:* The risk of a multiple pregnancy is increased approximately 6 times when clomiphene is given. In 2369 pregnancies associated with clomiphene therapy, 92.1% were single and 6.9% were twins. The remainder resulted in triplets or more. Of the multiple pregnancies, 96% to 99% were live births.

*Eyes:* Blurring or other visual symptoms, such as spots or flashes may occur. Use caution while driving or operating machinery, especially in variable light. If visual symptoms occur, discontinue treatment and call your doctor about a complete eye evaluation.

*Overstimulation of the ovary:* The lowest effective dose is used to reduce the risk of abnormal ovarian enlargement. Mild to moderate ovarian enlargement, with or without bloating or stomach pain, may occur and generally goes away within 2 or 3 weeks after discontinuing this medicine. All patients who experience bloating or stomach pain should be examined for ovarian enlargement. If significant ovarian enlargement occurs after ovulation, do not engage in sexual intercourse.

*Pregnancy:* Do not use during pregnancy. The risk of use in a pregnant woman clearly outweighs any possible benefit. Consult your doctor if pregnancy is suspected. Clomiphene may be linked to birth defects.

*Breastfeeding:* It is not known if clomiphene appears in breast milk. However, it may reduce lactation. Consult your doctor before you begin breastfeeding.

## Side Effects:

Every drug is capable of producing side effects. Many patients experience no, or minor, side effects. The frequency and severity of side effects depend on many factors including dose, duration of therapy, and individual susceptibility. Possible side effects include:

*Eyes or Ocular:* Blurred vision; spots or flashes of light; sensitivity to light; double vision.

*Digestive Tract:* Nausea; vomiting; diarrhea; stomach pain.

*Nervous System:* Headache; dizziness; light-headedness; nervousness; feeling of whirling motion (vertigo); sleeplessness.

*Other:* Multiple pregnancy; tubal pregnancy; hot flushes; flushing; abnormal uterine bleeding; breast tenderness; ovarian enlargement; pelvic discomfort; distention or bloating; weight gain.

## Guidelines for Use:

- Dosage is individualized. Use exactly as prescribed.
- Do not stop taking or change the dose, unless instructed by your doctor.
- If a dose is missed, take it as soon as possible. If several hours have passed or it is nearing time for the next dose, do not double the dose to catch up, unless instructed by your doctor. If more than one dose is missed or it is necessary to establish a new dosage schedule, contact your doctor or pharmacist.
- Each course of clomiphene should be started on or about the fifth day of the menstrual cycle. Wait 30 days between courses.
- Properly timed intercourse is important for good results.
- Intercourse should be prohibited in patients in whom significant ovarian enlargement occurs after ovulation.
- Notify your doctor immediately if you experience bloating, stomach or pelvic pain, blurred vision, weight gain, yellowing of skin or eyes, hot flushes, breast discomfort, headache, difficulty breathing, decreased urination, nausea, or vomiting.
- May cause dizziness, light-headedness, and visual disturbances. Use caution while driving or performing tasks requiring alertness, coordination, or physical dexterity, particularly in variable lighting.
- Multiple pregnancy is possible and poses potential hazards.
- The likelihood of conception diminishes with each succeeding course of therapy. If pregnancy has not been achieved after three courses of treatment, further treatment is not recommended. Long-term cyclic therapy is not recommended.
- Do not use this medicine if you are pregnant or think you might be pregnant. A reliable pregnancy test should be administered before starting therapy to avoid taking this medicine during early pregnancy.
- Lab tests will be required to monitor therapy. Be sure to keep appointments.
- Store at room temperature (59° to 86°F) away from heat, light, and moisture.

*If you have any questions, consult your doctor, pharmacist, or health care provider.*

| Generic Name<br>*Brand Name Examples* | Supplied As | Generic<br>Available |
|---|---|---|
| *Rx* **Menotropins** | | |
| *Pergonal, Repronex* | **Injection:** 75 IU FSH activity<br>and 75 IU LH activity/amp,<br>150 IU FSH activity and 150 IU<br>LH activity/amp | No |

## Type of Drug:

Gonadotropins; hormones that stimulate the ovaries and testes.

## How the Drug Works:

Menotropins are a combination of follicle stimulating hormone (FSH) and luteinizing hormone (LH). In women, menotropins stimulate the ovaries to produce mature eggs. Human chorionic gonadotropin (HCG) is given after menotropins to stimulate ovulation. Menotropins stimulate sperm formation (spermatogenesis) in men who have a low sperm count due to decreased function of the pituitary gland.

## Uses:

To induce ovulation in women who do not ovulate due to hormone problems. Menotropins are used in combination with HCG.

Menotropins and HCG may be used to stimulate the development and release of multiple eggs in patients participating in an in vitro fertilization program.

To increase sperm count in men who have low sperm count due to hormone problems. Menotropins are used in combination with HCG.

## Precautions:

*Do not use in the following situations:*
Women —

| | |
|---|---|
| adrenal disorders, uncontrolled | intracranial lesion (eg, pituitary |
| allergy to the drug or any of | tumor) |
| its ingredients | ovarian cysts or enlargement |
| bleeding, abnormal | ovary failure, primary |
| infertility (other than not | pregnancy |
| ovulating) | thyroid disorders, uncontrolled |

Men —

| | |
|---|---|
| allergy to the drug or any of its | pituitary function, normal |
| ingredients | testicular failure, primary |
| infertility (other than low sperm | |
| count) | |

*Before therapy:* Women must have a thorough pelvic exam and testing of the endocrine glands. A cervical dilation and curettage (D and C) must be done before beginning therapy if there is abnormal uterine bleeding or other signs of endometrial disorders. The partner's fertility potential must also be evaluated by a doctor. Men should have their pituitary gland function evaluated.

*Multiple births:* Pregnancies following therapy with HCG and menotropins resulted in 80% single births, 15% twin births, and 5% of pregnancies resulted in 3 or more babies.

*Overstimulation of the ovary:* Mild to moderate ovarian enlargement, with or without bloating or stomach pain, may occur and generally goes away within 2 or 3 weeks after discontinuing this medicine. All patients who experience bloating or stomach pain should be examined for ovarian enlargement. If significant ovarian enlargement occurs after ovulation, do not engage in sexual intercourse.

*Respiratory complications:* Serious respiratory complications (eg, difficulty breathing) and blood clotting have been reported.

*Pregnancy:* Do not use during pregnancy. The risk of use in a pregnant woman clearly outweighs any possible benefit.

*Breastfeeding:* It is not known if menotropins appear in breast milk. Consult your doctor before you begin breastfeeding.

*Children:* Safety and effectiveness have not been established.

## Drug Interactions:

Tell your doctor or pharmacist if you are taking or planning to take any over-the-counter or prescription medications or dietary supplements while taking this drug. Drug doses may need to be modified or a different drug prescribed.

## Side Effects:

Every drug is capable of producing side effects. Many patients experience no, or minor, side effects. The frequency and severity of side effects depend on many factors including dose, duration of therapy, and individual susceptibility. Possible side effects include:

*Digestive Tract:* Nausea; vomiting; diarrhea; stomach pain or cramps; bloating.

*Urinary and Reproductive Tract:* Vaginal bleeding; pelvic pain; ovarian cysts; ectopic pregnancy; multiple births.

*Other:* Fever; chills; breast enlargement or pain (men); rash; muscle and joint pain; pain, rash, swelling, or irritation at injection site; headache; dizziness; excitation; difficult or quick, shallow breathing; rapid heartbeat; general body discomfort; swelling of the lower legs.

## Guidelines for Use:

- Dosage is individualized. Use exactly as prescribed.
- Carefully follow the storage, preparation, administration, and disposal techniques taught to you by your health care provider.
- Visually inspect the solution for discoloration or particles. Use immediately after reconstitution (mixing). Discard any unused portion.
- If a dose is missed, inject it as soon as possible. If several hours have passed or it is nearing time for the next dose, do not double the dose to catch up, unless instructed by your doctor. If more than one dose is missed or it is necessary to establish a new dosage schedule, contact your doctor or pharmacist.
- Discontinue use and contact your doctor immediately if you experience severe pelvic pain, bloating, nausea, vomiting, diarrhea, weight gain, difficulty breathing, or decreased urination.
- Store refrigerated or at room temperature (37° to 77°F). Protect from light.
- *Women* —
  HCG must be given following menotropins when tests indicate mature eggs are present (ie, changes in vaginal smear or cervical mucus, urinary estrogen test).
  Ovulation is confirmed by testing for progesterone production (ie, rise in basal temperature, change in cervical mucus).
  The couple should have intercourse daily, beginning on the day prior to HCG administration, until ovulation occurs. Take care to ensure insemination.
  Intercourse should be prohibited in patients in whom significant ovarian enlargement occurs after ovulation.
  During treatment with menotropins and HCG and for 2 weeks after treatment, patients must be examined by a doctor at least every other day.
  Multiple pregnancy is possible and poses potential hazards.
- *Men* —
  HCG is first used alone prior to treatment with both menotropins and HCG.

*If you have any questions, consult your doctor, pharmacist, or health care provider.*

| Generic Name  *Brand Name Example* | Supplied As | Generic Available |
|---|---|---|
| Rx **Nafarelin Acetate** | | |
| *Synarel* | **Solution, nasal:** 2 mg/mL | No |

## Type of Drug:

Synthetic hormone.

## How the Drug Works:

Nafarelin is similar to natural gonadotropin releasing hormone. It stimulates the release of the pituitary hormones, luteinizing hormone (LH), and follicle stimulating hormone (FSH). These hormones stimulate the ovaries to produce estrogen and progestogen. Stimulation of the pituitary gland decreases over time.

Tissues and organs dependent on secretion of gonadal hormones (estrogen and progestogen) to function, including the uterine lining (endometrium), will become less active after about 4 weeks of twice daily therapy. This causes a decrease in the symptoms of endometriosis (eg, pelvic pain, menstrual cramps, painful intercourse).

## Uses:

For the management of endometriosis in women 18 years of age and older for a period not to exceed 6 consecutive months of therapy.

Also used for the treatment of central precocious puberty (CPP) in children of both sexes.

## Precautions:

*Do not use in the following situations:*

allergy to the drug, any of its ingredients, or to gonadotropin releasing hormone-type drugs breastfeeding

pregnancy vaginal bleeding, undiagnosed abnormal

*Use with caution in the following situations:*

alcohol or tobacco use, chronic drug therapy that can reduce bone mass (eg, anticonvulsant, corticosteroid), current hypoestrogenism

menstruation osteoporosis, family history of polycystic ovarian disease runny nose, chronic

*Pregnancy:* Do not use during pregnancy. The risk of use in a pregnant woman clearly outweighs any possible benefit.

*Breastfeeding:* It is not known if nafarelin acetate appears in breast milk. Use in nursing mothers is not recommended.

## Drug Interactions:

Tell your doctor or pharmacist if you are taking or planning to take any over-the-counter or prescription medications or dietary supplements while taking this drug. Drug doses may need to be modified or a different drug prescribed. Topical nasal decongestants (eg, *Afrin*) interact with this drug.

## Side Effects:

Every drug is capable of producing side effects. Many patients experience no, or minor, side effects. The frequency and severity of side effects depend on many factors including dose, duration of therapy, and individual susceptibility. Possible side effects include:

*Nervous System:* Depression; headache; sleeplessness; emotional instability.

*Respiratory System:* Shortness of breath; chest pain; runny nose; nasal irritation.

*Skin:* Acne; body odor; excessive pubic or other hair growth; excessively oily skin; rash; hives; itching.

*Urinary and Reproductive Tract:* Vaginal dryness; change in breast size; change in sex drive; vaginal bleeding; lack of menstruation; white or brownish vaginal discharge; ovarian cysts.

*Other:* Weight changes; fluid retention (edema); hot flashes; muscle pain; possible elevation of serum triglycerides and cholesterol; abnormal lab tests.

## Guidelines for Use:

- Dosage is individualized. Use exactly as prescribed.
- Do not stop taking or change the dose, unless instructed by your doctor.
- Avoid sneezing during or immediately following administration.
- Tilt head back slightly while administering this medicine.
- If using more than 1 spray in each nostril, wait 30 seconds between sprays.
- If the use of a topical nasal decongestant is necessary during treatment with nafarelin, do not use the decongestant until at least 2 hours after taking nafarelin.
- If a dose is missed, inhale it as soon as possible. If several hours have passed or it is nearing time for the next dose, do not double the dose to catch up, unless instructed by your doctor. If more than one dose is missed or it is necessary to establish a new dosage schedule, contact your doctor or pharmacist.
- Store upright at room temperature (68° to 77°F). Protect from light.
- *For endometriosis —*
  Treatment should begin between the 2nd and 4th day of the menstrual period.
  Usual dose is 1 spray (about 200 mcg) into one nostril in the morning and 1 spray into the other nostril in the evening.
  When used regularly at the recommended dose, nafarelin usually inhibits ovulation and stops menstruation. However, use of the drug should not be considered a reliable form of contraception. Nonhormonal contraceptive measures (eg, condom, diaphragm) should be used during therapy.
  Do not use if pregnancy is suspected, if you are breastfeeding, or if you are experiencing undiagnosed vaginal bleeding.
  May cause breakthrough bleeding if doses are missed. However, if regular menstruation persists, notify your doctor.
  The usual course of therapy is 6 months. Retreatment is not recommended.
- *For CCP —*
  Usual dose is 2 sprays (about 400 mcg) into each nostril in the morning (4 sprays total) and 2 sprays into each nostril in the evening (4 sprays total).
  During the first month of treatment, some signs of puberty may occur. If this does not resolve within the first 2 months of treatment, contact your doctor.

*If you have any questions, consult your doctor, pharmacist, or health care provider.*

| Generic Name<br>*Brand Name Example* | Supplied As | Generic<br>Available |
|---|---|---|
| *Rx* **Danazol** | | |
| *Danocrine* | **Capsules:** 50 mg, 100 mg,<br>200 mg | Yes |

## Type of Drug:
Synthetic hormone; synthetic androgen.

## How the Drug Works:
Danazol blocks the release of gonadotropin, a hormone secreted from the pituitary gland. The result of this blocking effect is to depress the output of two other hormones, FSH (follicle stimulating hormone) and LH (luteinizing hormone). FSH and LH are important in many functions of the sex glands, including ovulation.

## Uses:
To treat endometriosis (an abnormal condition involving the inner lining of the uterus).

To treat fibrocystic breast disease (cysts or lumps in the breast).

To treat hereditary angioedema (swelling of the abdominal organs and tissue, extremities, throat, and airway).

*Unlabeled Use(s):* Occasionally doctors may prescribe danazol for early puberty, development of breasts (in males), and heavy menstrual flow. It has also been studied for the treatment of anemia.

## Precautions:
*Do not use in the following situations:*

breastfeeding
genital bleeding, undiagnosed
 or abnormal
heart disease, severe
kidney disorders, severe
liver disorders, severe
porphyria
pregnancy

*Use with caution in the following situations:*

breast cancer
epilepsy
migraine

*Diabetes:* Insulin requirements may increase. Abnormal glucose (sugar) tolerance tests may occur. Monitor urine and blood sugar levels.

*Fluid retention:* Danazol can cause fluid retention, which may aggravate epilepsy, migraine, or heart or kidney disease. Use with caution.

*Women:* Women taking danazol may experience masculinizing effects, including acne, edema (fluid retention), increased hair growth, decrease in breast size, deepening of the voice, oily skin or hair, weight gain, and enlargement of the clitoris. These effects may not go away when the drug is stopped.

*Pregnancy:* Do not use during pregnancy. The risk of use in a pregnant woman clearly outweighs any possible benefit. Masculinization of a female fetus may occur.

*Breastfeeding:* Do not use if you are breastfeeding.

*Children:* Safety and effectiveness have not been established.

*Lab tests* may be required to monitor treatment. Tests include urine and blood sugar levels.

## Drug Interactions:

Tell your doctor or pharmacist if you are taking or planning to take any over-the-counter or prescription medications or dietary supplements while taking this drug. Drug doses may need to be modified or a different drug prescribed. The following drugs and drug classes interact with this drug:

carbamazepine (eg, *Tegretol*)
insulin
warfarin (eg, *Coumadin*)

## Side Effects:

Every drug is capable of producing side effects. Many patients experience no, or minor, side effects. The frequency and severity of side effects depend on many factors including dose, duration of therapy, and individual susceptibility.

If you experience any effects different from those listed, do not hesitate to contact your doctor or pharmacist. It could be a sign of a rare or unusual side effect that requires treatment. Possible side effects include:

*Masculinizing Androgenic Effects* – Acne; fluid retention (edema); decrease in breast size; deepening of the voice; mild abnormal growth of fine body hair; oily skin or hair; weight gain; menstrual changes or pain; hair loss; hoarseness; sore throat.

*Signs of Low Estrogen Levels* – Flushing; sweating; vaginitis (itching, dryness, burning, and vaginal bleeding); nervousness; emotional instability.

*Men* – Reduction in sperm count; semen changes (decreased volume and viscosity).

*Miscellaneous* – Liver dysfunction; yellowing of the skin; abnormal lab tests; severe headache (intracranial hypertension); nausea; vomiting; vision disturbances; hives; itching; rash; blood clots; fatigue; sleep disorder; anxiety, constipation; joint pain.

## Guidelines for Use:

- Dosage is individualized. Take exactly as prescribed.
- Do not stop taking or change the dose, unless instructed by your doctor.
- If a dose is missed, take it as soon as possible. If several hours have passed or it is nearing time for the next dose, do not double the dose to catch up, unless instructed by your doctor. If more than one dose is missed or it is necessary to establish a new dosage schedule, contact your doctor or pharmacist.
- Notify your doctor if you experience masculinizing effects (eg, abnormal growth of facial or fine body hair, deepening of the voice).
- Notify your doctor if you experience headache, breast swelling, nausea, vomiting, visual disturbances, or yellowing of the skin or eyes.
- *Females —*
  Begin treatment during menstruation.
  Use nonhormonal contraceptive measures (eg, condom, diaphragm) during therapy. Discontinue use if pregnancy is suspected.
  It is essential that therapy for endometriosis continues uninterrupted for 3 to 6 months, but it may be extended to 9 months.
- Lab tests may be required to monitor treatment. Be sure to keep appointments.
- Store in a tightly closed container at room temperature (68° to 77°F).

*If you have any questions, consult your doctor, pharmacist, or health care provider.*

# POSTERIOR PITUITARY HORMONES — DESMOPRESSIN ACETATE

218

| Generic Name<br>*Brand Name Examples* | Supplied As | Generic<br>Available |
|---|---|---|
| Rx **Desmopressin Acetate** | | |
| *DDAVP* | **Tablet:** 0.1 mg, 0.2 mg | No |
| *DDAVP, Stimate* | **Nasal Solution:** 0.1 mg/mL, 1.5 mg/mL | No |
| *DDAVP* | **Injection:** 4 mcg/mL | Yes |

## Type of Drug:
Human antidiuretic hormone (ADH).

## How the Drug Works:
A hormone which makes the kidneys reabsorb (retain) water and increases the concentration/activity of certain blood factors necessary for normal blood clotting.

## Uses:
*DDAVP:* As antidiuretic hormone replacement therapy in the management of central cranial diabetes insipidus and for temporary excessive urination and excessive thirst following head injury or surgery in the pituitary region. This will allow return to a more normal lifestyle with decreased urinary frequency and nighttime urination.

To treat nighttime bed-wetting (nasal solution only). May be used alone or in combination with behavioral conditioning or other nonmedicinal intervention.

To control bleeding in hemophilia A patients during and after surgery, and to stop spontaneous or trauma-induced bleeding in hemophilia A patients (injection only).

To control bleeding in patients with mild to moderate von Willebrand disease (Type I) during and after surgery, and to stop spontaneous or trauma-induced bleeding in patients with von Willebrand disease (injection only).

*Stimate:* To stop spontaneous or trauma-induced bleeding in patients with hemophilia A or mild to moderate von Willebrand disease (Type I).

*Unlabeled Use(s):*

*Nasal solution* – To treat chronic autonomic failure (eg, nighttime bed-wetting, over-night weight loss and morning dizziness or lightheadedness when rising from a sitting or lying position).

## Precautions:
*Do not use in the following situations:* allergy to this medicine.

*Use with caution in the following situations:*

blood clots
coronary artery insufficiency
fluid electrolyte imbalance (eg,
  cystic fibrosis)
hemophilia A, severe

high blood pressure
nasal blockage/obstruction
  (nasal solution only)
von Willebrand disease (Type
  I), severe

*Water intoxication:* Very young and elderly patients should drink only enough fluids to satisfy thirst in order to decrease the potential occurrence of water intoxication (over-load) and salt depletion in the blood.

*Long-term use:* There have been reports of reduced responsiveness or duration of effect in patients using the drug for more than 6 months. Consult your doctor if such changes occur.

*Pregnancy:* Studies in pregnant women or in animals have been judged not to show a risk to the fetus. However, no drug should be used during pregnancy unless clearly needed.

*Breastfeeding:* It is not known if desmopressin acetate appears in breast milk. Consult your doctor before you begin breastfeeding.

*Children:* Infants and children need careful fluid intake restrictions to prevent possible salt depletion in the blood and water intoxication (overload). Nasal solution has been used safely and is modestly effective for short-term use (4 to 8 weeks) in children 6 years of age and older for the treatment of nighttime bed-wetting. Do not use injection in children under 3 months of age or the nasal solution in children under 11 months of age in the treatment of hemophilia A or von Willebrand disease. Safety and effectiveness have not been established in children under 12 years of age (injection) or under 3 months of age (nasal solution) with diabetes insipidus. Desmopressin tablets have been used safely in children 4 years of age and older for periods of up to 44 months.

*Lab tests* may be necessary to monitor therapy. Be sure to keep appointments.

## Drug Interactions:

Tell your doctor or pharmacist if you are taking or if you are planning to take any over-the-counter or prescription medications or dietary supplements while taking this medicine. Doses of one or both drugs may need to be modified or a different drug may need to be prescribed. The following drugs and drug classes interact with this medicine.

blood pressure elevating agents (eg, epinephrine )
carbamazepine (eg, *Tegretol*)
chlorpropamide (*Diabinese*)

## Side Effects:

Every drug is capable of producing side effects. Many patients experience no, or minor, side effects. The frequency and severity of side effects depend on many factors including dose, duration of therapy and individual susceptibility. Possible side effects include:

*DDAVP nasal solutions* – Headache; runny nose; nausea; stomach cramps; vaginal pain; high blood pressure; facial flushing; nosebleed; sore throat; cough; difficulty breathing.

*DDAVP injection* – Redness, swelling or burning at injection site; headache; runny nose; nausea; stomach cramps; vaginal pain; high blood pressure; facial flushing.

*Stimate nasal solution* – Sleepiness; dizziness; itchy or light-sensitive eyes; sleeplessness; chills; warm feeling; pain; chest pain; palpitations (pounding in the chest); fast heartbeat; indigestion; fluid retention; vomiting; agitation; genital inflammation; difficulty breathing.

---

### Guidelines for Use:

- Read and follow patient instructions carefully and use exactly as prescribed.
- If a dose is missed, take or use it as soon as possible. If several hours have passed or if it is nearing time for the next dose, do not double the dose in order to "catch up" (unless advised to do so by your doctor). If more than one dose is missed or it is necessary to establish a new dosage schedule, contact your doctor or pharmacist.
- If bleeding is not controlled or worsens, contact your doctor.
- Contact your doctor if headache, shortness of breath, heartburn, nausea, stomach cramps or vaginal pain occurs.
- *Nasal solutions* — For nasal use only. Use one spray per nostril. If used before surgery, administer 2 hours before the scheduled procedure.
- *Stimate* —
  Spray pump must be primed before the first use. To prime the pump, press down 4 times. The pump will stay primed for 1 week if refrigerated. Reprime the pump after 1 week if not used.
  Discard any solution remaining after 25 doses since the amount delivered thereafter may be less than the required dose. Do not transfer the remaining solution to another bottle.
- *Storage* —
  Refrigerate nasal solutions and injection at 36° to 46°F. When travelling, closed nasal solution containers may be kept at room temperature (72°F) for up to 3 weeks.
  Store tablets at room temperature (59° to 86°F) protected from heat and light.

---

*If you have any questions, consult your doctor, pharmacist, or health care provider.*

| Generic Name<br>*Brand Name Examples* | Supplied As | Generic<br>Available |
|---|---|---|
| *Rx* **Somatrem** | | |
| *Protropin* | **Injection:** 5 mg (approx. 15 IU),<br>10 mg (approx. 30 IU) | No |

## Type of Drug:
Growth Hormone.

## How the Drug Works:
Mimics actions of naturally occurring growth hormone; stimulates growth of bone, tissues, blood cells and internal organs.

## Uses:
For the long-term treatment of children who have growth failure due to a lack of adequate endogenous growth hormone secretion.

## Precautions:
*Do not use in the following situations:*
closed epiphyses (end of growth of arm and leg bones)
tumor growth
allergy to benzyl alcohol

*Use with caution in the following situations:*
glucose intolerance          intracranial hypertension
brain lesion                 scoliosis
endocrine problems (diabetes)

*Benzyl alcohol* is used in the diluent of this product as a preservative and has been associated with toxicity in newborns. When administering somatrem to newborns, reconstitute with sterile water for injection.

*Pregnancy:* Adequate studies have not been done in pregnant women; animal studies may have shown a risk to the fetus. Use only if clearly needed and if potential benefits outweigh the possible hazards to the fetus.

*Breastfeeding:* It is not known if somatrem appears in breast milk. Consult your doctor before you begin breastfeeding.

*Lab tests* and examinations will be required periodically to monitor treatment. Be sure to keep appointments. Tests may include eye examinations and thyroid function tests. In addition, testing for antibodies to human growth hormone may be performed in patients not responding to therapy.

## Drug Interactions:
Tell your doctor or pharmacist if you are taking or planning to take any over-the-counter or prescription medications or dietary supplements while taking this medicine. Doses of one or both drugs may need to be modified or a different drug may need to be prescribed. The following drugs and drug classes interact with this medicine: Glucocorticoids (eg, prednisone).

## Side Effects:

Every drug is capable of producing side effects. Many patients experience no, or minor, side effects. The frequency and severity of side effects depend on many factors including dose, duration of therapy and individual susceptibility. Possible side effects include: Injection site reactions; swelling; carpal tunnel syndrome.

---

### Guidelines for Use:

- Take as directed by your doctor. The weekly dose varies depending on individual needs. Do not adjust the dose or stop taking the medication without consulting your pharmacist or doctor.
- Follow the preparation and injection procedure taught to you by your healthcare provider if you choose to administer the medicine at home. Rotate injection sites.
- Dispose of used equipment (eg, needles and syringes) in an appropriate container as instructed. Do not reuse needles or syringes.
- Patient instructions for use are enclosed with each package; follow instructions exactly.
- If local or systemic allergic reactions occur, contact your doctor.
- Report these symptoms to your physician: Limping; hip or knee pain; injection site reactions.
- Glucocorticoid therapy may inhibit the growth promoting effect of somatrem; if this therapy is required the doses must be carefully adjusted.
- Benzyl alcohol as a preservative in Bacteriostatic Water for Injection has been associated with toxicity in newborns. When administering somatrem to newborns, reconstitute with Sterile Water for Injection.
- Lab tests or exams will be required periodically to monitor treatment. These may include eye examinations and thyroid function tests. In addition, tests for antibodies to human growth hormone may be carried out in patients failing to respond to therapy.
- Store somatrem before and after reconstitution under refrigeration (36° to 46°F). Use reconstituted solution within 14 days. Avoid freezing. Do not use if cloudy.

---

*If you have any questions, consult your doctor, pharmacist, or health care provider.*

| Generic Name<br>*Brand Name Examples* | Supplied As | Generic<br>Available |
|---|---|---|
| *Rx* **Somatropin** | | |
| *Genotropin*[1] | **Powder for Injection,<br>lyophilized:**<br>1.5 mg (≈ 4 IU/mL)<br>5.8 mg (≈ 15 IU/mL)<br>13.8 mg (≈ 36 IU/mL) | No |
| *Norditropin* | **Powder for Injection,<br>lyophilized:**<br>4 mg (≈ 12 IU)/vial<br>8 mg (≈ 24 IU)/vial | No |
| *Nutropin*[2] | **Powder for Injection,<br>lyophilized:**<br>5 mg (≈ 15 IU)/vial<br>10 mg (≈ 30 IU)/vial | No |
| *Humatrope*[3] | **Powder for Injection,<br>lyophilized:**<br>5 mg (15 IU)/vial | No |
| *Serostim* | **Powder for Injection,<br>lyophilized:**<br>5 mg (≈ 15 IU)/vial<br>6 mg (≈18 IU)/vial | No |
| *Nutropin AQ* | **Injection:** 10 mg (≈ 30 IU)/<br>vial | No |

[1] Contains m-cresol in diluent.
[2] Contains benzyl alcohol in diluent.
[3] Contains m-cresol and glycerin in diluent.

## Type of Drug:
Growth hormone.

## How the Drug Works:
Mimics actions of naturally occuring growth hormone; stimulates growth of bone, tissues, blood cells and internal organs.

## Uses:
Growth failure associated with chronic kidney insufficiency until time of transplantation (*Nutropin, Nutropin AQ*).

Growth failure (except *Serostim*).

Turner syndrome (*Nutropin* only).

AIDS wasting or cachexia (*Serostim* only).

Somatotropin deficiency syndrome (*Humatrope* only).

*Unlabeled Use(s):* Occasionally doctors may prescribe growth hormones for short children due to intrauterine growth retardation.

## Precautions:

*Do not use in the following situations:*

active tumor growth (discontinue therapy if this develops)

allergy to benzyl alcohol (diluent supplied with *Nutropin*)

allergy to growth hormone and constituents

allergy to m-cresol or glycerin in certain formulations

closed epiphyses (end of growth of arm and leg bones)

*Use with caution in the following situations:*

acute pancreatitis

brain injury or tumor

carpal tunnel syndrome (*Serostim*)

diabetes mellitus

ear disorders (*Nutropin*)

glucose intolerance (except *Norditropin, Humatrope*)

hip problems, hip or knee pain

HIV infection

hypothyroidism

intracranial hypertension

kidney transplant or insufficiency

scoliosis or other skeletal abnormalities

skin lesions

swelling of hands and feet (*Serostim*)

*Pregnancy:*

*Serostim, Genotropin* – Studies in pregnant women or in animals have been judged not to show a risk to the fetus. However, no drug should be used during pregnancy unless clearly needed.

*Nutropin, Nutropin AQ, Humatrope, Norditropin* – Adequate studies have not been done in pregnant women; animal studies may have shown a risk to the fetus. Use only if clearly needed and potential benefits outweigh the possible hazards to the fetus.

*Breastfeeding:* It is not known if somatropin appears in breast milk. Consult your doctor before you begin breastfeeding.

*Children:*

*Serostim* – Safety and effectiveness in children with AIDS have not been established.

*Benzyl alcohol* – Benzyl alcohol as a preservative in bacteriostatic Water for Injection, USP has been associated with toxicity in newborns. When administering somatropin to newborns, reconstitute with sterile Water for Injection.

## Drug Interactions:

Tell your doctor or pharmacist if you are taking or planning to take any over-the-counter or prescription medications or dietary supplements while taking this medicine. Doses of one or both drugs may need to be modified or a different drug may need to be prescribed. The following drugs and drug classes interact with this medicine:

Glucocorticoid therapy (except *Serostim*)

Corticosteroids (eg, cortisone)

Sex steroids

Anticonvulsants (eg, phenytoin)

Cyclosporine (eg, *Sandimmune*)

## Side Effects:

Every drug is capable of producing side effects. Many patients experience no, or minor, side effects. The frequency and severity of side effects depend on many factors including dose, duration of therapy and individual susceptibility. Possible side effects include: High blood pressure; headache; high sugar in blood; antibody development; muscle pain; weakness; glucose in urine; swelling; swelling in arms and legs; breast growth; joint pain; nausea; stomach pain; vomiting; injection site reactions; leukemia.

*Nutropin* – Eye pain; visual changes; injection site pain; carpal tunnel syndrome; wrist pain.

*Genotropin* – Loss of skin fat; blood in urine.

*Humatrope* – Abnormal skin sensation; pain; runny nose; back pain; acne; joint disorder; flu syndrome; increased cough; decreased sensitivity to touch; respiratory disorder; sore throat.

*Serostim* – Musculoskeletal discomfort; fever; swelling of hands or feet; diarrhea; nerve disease; increased sweating; appetite loss; fast heartbeat; tiredness; abnormal blood counts; protein in urine; lymph node swelling; sleeplessness; carpal tunnel syndrome.

### Guidelines for Use:

- Take as directed by your doctor. The daily dose varies depending on individual needs. Do not adjust the dose without consulting your pharmacist or doctor.
- Follow injection procedure taught to you by your healthcare provider. Follow instructions on patient information insert. Rotate injection sites.
- Report these symptoms to the doctor: Limping; hip or knee pain; headache; weakness; muscle pain; swelling; injection site reactions.
- If local or systemic allergic reactions occur, contact your doctor.
- Lab tests and examinations will include: Blood sugar; eye exams; thyroid function tests; antibody testing; nutritional tests (*Serostim* only). Keep appointments.
- Storage:
  *Serostim:* Store unopened vials at room temperature (59° to 86°F) and reconstituted solution under refrigeration for no longer than 24 hours.
  *Genotropin, Humatrope, Nutropin:* Store unopened vials/cartridges under refrigeration (36° to 46°F); store reconstituted solutions under refrigeration (36° to 46°F) for up to 14 days except 1.5 mg cartridge of *Genotropin* which must be used within 24 hours.
  *Nutropin AQ:* Store under refrigeration (36° to 46°F). Must be used within 28 days once opened.
  Avoid freezing.
- Do not use if cloudy.

*If you have any questions, consult your doctor, pharmacist, or health care provider.*

| Generic Name<br>*Brand Name Examples* | Supplied As | Generic<br>Available |
|---|---|---|
| Rx **Repository Corticotropin<br>(ACTH)** | | Yes |
| *H.P. Acthar Gel* | **Repository injection:** 80 units/mL | |
| Rx **Cosyntropin** | | No |
| *Cortrosyn* | **Powder for injection, lyophi-<br>lized:** 0.25 mg/vial | |

## Type of Drug:

Natural (corticotropin, ACTH) and synthetic (cosyntropin) adrenocortico-
tropic hormone.

## How the Drug Works:

Corticotropin (ACTH) is secreted by the pituitary gland. It stimulates the
adrenal cortex to produce and secrete adrenocortical hormones (corticosteroids, glucocorticoids). A functioning adrenal gland is necessary for
corticotropin to work.

## Uses:

*Corticotropin and cosyntropin:* Diagnostic testing of adrenal gland
function.

*Corticotropin:* Although corticosteroid (eg, prednisone) therapy is the treatment of choice, ACTH may be used instead in the following disorders:
Thyroid gland inflammation; high blood calcium levels due to cancer;
acute worsening of multiple sclerosis; tuberculosis meningitis; trichinosis with brain or heart involvement; and treatment of glucocorticoid-re-
sponsive rheumatic, collagen, skin, allergic, kidney, eye, respiratory,
blood, digestive tract disorders, and cancer.

*Unlabeled Use(s):* Occasionally ACTH is used to treat infantile spasms.

## Precautions:

*Do not use in the following situations:*

*Corticotropin –*
adrenocortical hyperfunction
allergy to pork
congestive heart failure (CHF)
fungal infection, systemic
herpes simplex infection in the
  eye
high blood pressure (IV administration)
live virus vaccine (eg, MMR),
  concurrent

osteoporosis (brittle bones)
primary adrenocortical insufficiency
scleroderma (hardened or thickened skin)
surgery, recent
trauma
ulcer, presence or history

*Cosyntropin –*
allergy to cosyntropin

*Use with caution in the following situations:*

| | |
|---|---|
| abscess | liver disease |
| cirrhosis | myasthenia gravis |
| diabetes | psychological problems |
| diverticulitis | thyroid function, decreased |
| infection | tuberculosis, history |
| kidney disease | |

*Diabetes:* The requirement for insulin or oral sulfonylureas may be increased in diabetic patients receiving corticotropin.

*Electrolytes:* Corticotropin can increase blood pressure, potassium and calcium excretion, and cause salt and water retention. Dietary salt restriction and potassium supplements may be necessary.

*Pregnancy:* There are no adequate and well-controlled studies in pregnant women. Use only if clearly needed and potential benefits to the mother outweigh the possible hazards to the fetus.

*Breastfeeding:* It is not known if corticotropin or cosyntropin appears in breast milk. Consult your doctor before you begin breastfeeding.

*Children:* Prolonged use of corticotropin in children inhibits skeletal bone growth. If use is necessary, the drug should be given intermittently at the lowest effective dose and the child should be closely watched.

## Drug Interactions:

Tell your doctor or pharmacist if you are taking or if you are planning to take any over-the-counter or prescription medications or dietary supplements with adrenal cortical steroids. Doses of one or both drugs may need to be modified or a different drug may need to be prescribed. The following drugs and drug classes interact with adrenal cortical steroids.

| | |
|---|---|
| amphotericin B (eg, *Fungizone*) | aspirin |
| antidiabetic agents (eg, insulin, glyburide) | diuretics (eg, hydrochlorothiazide) |

## Side Effects:

Every drug is capable of producing side effects. Many corticotropin users experience no, or minor, side effects. The frequency and severity of side effects depend on many factors including dose, duration of therapy, and individual susceptibility. Possible side effects of corticotropin include:

*Fluid and Electrolyte Disturbances:* Sodium and fluid retention; potassium and calcium loss; hypokalemic alkalosis.

*Digestive Tract:* Nausea; vomiting; ulceration of esophagus; inflammation of the pancreas; peptic ulcer; stomach bloating.

*Nervous System:* Vertigo (feeling of whirling motion); headache; euphoria; sleeplessness; mood swings; depression; seizures; dizziness; psychic symptoms; increased intracranial pressure with papilledema.

*Circulatory System:* High blood pressure; congestive heart failure.

*Skin:* Impaired wound healing; increased sweating; excessive pigmentation of skin; thin, fragile skin; facial redness; acne; excessive body hair growth; rash; unusual bruising; suppression of skin test reactions; facial swelling; small red spots under the skin.

*Other:* Infection; menstrual irregularities; suppression of growth in children; cataracts; glaucoma; muscle weakness; loss of muscle mass; osteoporosis (brittle bones); abscess; increased intraocular pressure; shock; aseptic necrosis of femoral and humeral heads; vertebral compression fractures; pathologic fracture of long bones; secondary adrenocortical and pituitary unresponsiveness (particularly in times of stress, as in trauma, surgery, or illness); decreased carbohydrate tolerance; manifestations of latent diabetes mellitus; development of cushingoid state; increased requirements for insulin or blood-sugar-lowering agents in diabetic patients; protrusion of one or both eyeballs; negative nitrogen balance due to protein breakdown.

## Guidelines for Use:

*Corticotropin —*

- Dosage will be individualized according to the condition being treated and the general medical condition of the patient. The usual dosage of repository corticotropin is 40 to 80 units given intramuscularly (IM) or subcutaneously (SC) every 24 to 72 hours. In the treatment of multiple sclerosis, daily IM doses of 80 to 120 units for 2 to 3 weeks may be administered.
- For IM or SC use only; intravenous (IV) administration is contra-indicated.
- If self-administering, carefully follow the preparation, administration, and disposal techniques taught to you by your health care provider.
- Warm to room temperature before using.
- Treatment for acute gouty arthritis should be limited to a few days. Since rebound attacks may occur when corticotropin is discontinued, conventional concomitant antigout therapy should be administered during corticotropin treatment and for several days after it is stopped.
- Corticotropin may mask signs of infection. There may be decreased resistance and inability to localize infection when corticotropin is used.
- *Diabetics:* Insulin or oral blood-sugar-lowering agent requirements may increase.
- Notify your doctor if marked fluid retention, muscle weakness, abdominal pain, seizures, headache, dizziness, nausea, vomiting, shock, or skin reactions occur.
- Avoid immunization with live vaccines (eg, MMR) when receiving corticotropin.
- Sudden withdrawal after prolonged use may lead to recurrent disease symptoms which make it difficult to withdraw the medication. It may be necessary to slowly lower the dose and increase the injection interval to gradually discontinue the medication.
- Lab tests or exams may be required to monitor therapy. Be sure to keep appointments.
- Store in the refrigerator (36° to 46°F).

*Cosyntropin —*

- Cosyntropin will be administered by your health care provider. It is for IV or IM use only as a diagnostic agent.

*If you have any questions, consult your doctor, pharmacist, or health care provider.*

| Generic Name<br>*Brand Name Examples* | Supplied As | Generic<br>Available |
|---|---|---|
| *Rx* **Betamethasone** | | |
| *Celestone* | **Tablets:** 0.6 mg | No |
| *Celestone[1]* | **Syrup:** 0.6 mg/5 mL | No |
| *Rx* **Betamethasone Sodium Phosphate** | | |
| *Celestone Phosphate [2]* | **Injection:** 4 mg/mL | No |
| *Rx* **Betamethasone Sodium Phosphate and Betametha-sone Acetate** | | |
| *Celestone Soluspan* | **Injection:** 3 mg betametha-sone acetate and 3 mg betamethasone sodium phosphate/mL | No |
| *Rx* **Cortisone Acetate** | **Tablets:** 5 mg, 10 mg, 25 mg | Yes |
| *Rx* **Dexamethasone** | | |
| *Decadron, Dexameth* | **Tablets:** 0.25 mg, 0.5 mg, 0.75 mg, 1 mg, 1.5 mg, 2 mg, 2.5 mg, 4 mg, 6 mg | Yes |
| *Dexameth[1]* | **Elixir:** 0.5 mg/5 mL | Yes |
| *Dexamethasone* | **Oral solution:** 0.5 mg/5 mL | Yes |
| *Dexamethasone Intensol[1]* | **Oral solution:** 1 mg/mL | Yes |
| *Rx* **Dexamethasone Acetate** | | |
| *Cortastat LA,[2] Dalalone D.P.,[2] Dalalone L.A.,[2] Decaject-L.A.,[2] Solurex-LA* | **Injection:** 8 mg/mL, 16 mg/mL | Yes |
| *Rx* **Dexamethasone Sodium Phosphate** | | |
| *Cortastat,[2] Cortastat 10,[2] Dal-alone,[2] Decadron Phosphate,[2] Decaject,[2] Solurex* | **Injection:** 4 mg/mL, 10 mg/mL, 20 mg/mL, 24 mg/mL | Yes |
| *Rx* **Hydrocortisone (Cortisol)** | | |
| *Cortef, Hydrocortone* | **Tablets:** 5 mg, 10 mg, 20 mg | Yes |
| *Cortenema* | **Retention enema:** 100 mg/60 mL | Yes |
| *Rx* **Hydrocortisone Acetate** | **Injection:** 50 mg/mL | Yes |
| *Cortifoam* | **Aerosol (intrarectal foam):** 90 mg/applicatorful | No |

| Generic Name *Brand Name Examples* | Supplied As | Generic Available |
|---|---|---|
| Rx **Hydrocortisone Cypionate** | | |
| *Cortef* | **Oral suspension**: 10 mg/5 mL | No |
| Rx **Hydrocortisone Sodium Phosphate** | | |
| *Hydrocortone Phosphate[2]* | **Injection:** 50 mg/mL | No |
| Rx **Hydrocortisone Sodium Succinate** | | |
| *Solu-Cortef[3]* | **Injection:** 100 mg/vial, 250 mg/vial, 500 mg/vial, 1000 mg/vial | No |
| Rx **Methylprednisolone** | | |
| *Medrol* | **Tablets:** 2mg, 4mg, 8mg, 16 mg, 24 mg, 32 mg | Yes |
| Rx **Methylprednisolone Acetate** | | |
| *depMedalone 40, depMedalone 80, Depoject-40, Depoject-80, Depo-Medrol, Depopred, Methacort 40, Methacort 80* | **Injection:** 20 mg/mL, 40 mg/mL, 80 mg/mL | Yes |
| Rx **Methylprednisolone Sodium Succinate** | | |
| *Solu-Medrol[3]* | **Injection:** 40 mg/vial, 125 mg/vial, 500 mg/vial, 1000 mg/vial, 2000 mg/vial | No |
| Rx **Prednisone** | **Oral solution:** 5 mg/5 mL | Yes |
| *Deltasone, Meticorten, Sterapred* | **Tablets:** 1 mg, 2.5 mg, 5 mg, 10 mg, 20 mg, 50 mg | Yes |
| *Prednisone Intensol Concentrate[1]* | **Oral solution:** 5 mg/mL | Yes |
| Rx **Prednisolone** | **Tablets:** 5 mg | Yes |
| *Prelone[1]* | **Syrup:** 5 mg/5 mL, 15 mg/5 mL | Yes |
| Rx **Prednisolone Acetate** | | |
| *Key-Pred, Predalone 50* | **Injection:** 25 mg/mL, 40 mg/mL, 50 mg/mL, 100 mg/mL | Yes |
| Rx **Prednisolone Sodium Phosphate** | | |
| *Pediapred* | **Oral solution:** 5 mg/5 mL | No |

| Generic Name<br>*Brand Name Examples* | Supplied As | Generic<br>Available |
|---|---|---|
| Rx **Triamcinolone** | | |
| *Aristocort* | **Tablets:** 1 mg, 2 mg, 4 mg, 8 mg | No |
| Rx **Triamcinolone Acetonide** | | |
| *Clinalog, Kenaject, Kenalog-10, Kenalog-40, Triam-A, Triamonide 40* | **Injection:** 10 mg/mL, 40 mg/mL | Yes |
| Rx **Triamcinolone Diacetate** | | |
| *Aristocort Forte[3], Aristocort Intralesional, Clinacort, Triamcin, Triam Forte, Tristoject* | **Injection:** 25 mg/mL, 40 mg/mL | Yes |
| Rx **Triamcinolone Hexacetonide** | | |
| *Aristospan Intralesional, Aristospan Intra-articular* | **Injection:** 5 mg/mL, 20 mg/mL | No |

[1] Contains alcohol.
[2] Contains sulfites.
[3] Contains benzyl alcohol.

## Type of Drug:

Adrenal cortical steroids; glucocorticoids; anti-inflammatory steroids; corticosteroids.

## How the Drug Works:

The naturally occurring adrenal cortical steroids have both anti-inflammatory (glucocorticoid) and salt-retaining (mineralocorticoid) activity. The synthetic adrenal cortical steroids have much greater anti-inflammatory (glucocorticoid) than salt-retaining activity. The glucocorticoids cause varied effects, including modifying the body's immune response.

The naturally occurring compounds, hydrocortisone and cortisone, are used as replacement therapy when the adrenal cortex is not functioning properly. The synthetic compounds can also be used as replacement therapy in adrenocortical deficiency states, but are more often used for their potent anti-inflammatory action.

## Uses:

To treat primary or secondary adrenal cortex insufficiency (lack of function). Hydrocortisone or cortisone are the drugs of choice. Synthetic agents may be used in combination with mineralocorticoids.

To treat hypercalcemia (high calcium levels) associated with cancer.

To treat rheumatic disorders (eg, bursitis, tenosynovitis, gouty arthritis, rheumatoid arthritis, osteoarthritis). Use must be short term and supplemental with strict medical supervision for acute episodes or recurrences.

To treat selected connective tissue (collagen) disease (eg, systemic lupus erythematosus).

To treat certain skin diseases (eg, psoriasis, Stevens-Johnson syndrome, hives, dermatitis).

To treat certain allergic conditions not responding to standard treatment (eg, serum sickness, bronchial asthma, allergic rhinitis).

To treat certain eye conditions of an allergic or inflammatory nature (eg, allergic inflammation of the conjunctiva, optic nerve, or eyelids; corneal ulcers; herpes infection of the eye).

To treat certain respiratory disorders (eg, berylliosis, sarcoidosis).

To treat serious blood disorders (eg, various anemias, platelet disorders).

To treat certain cancers (eg, leukemias, lymphomas) (used in combination with other therapy).

To treat certain digestive tract diseases (eg, ulcerative colitis, regional enteritis).

To treat certain edematous states (eg, proteinuria in the nephrotic syndrome).

To treat tuberculosis meningitis when used concurrently with appropriate antituberculosis chemotherapy.

To treat trichinosis with brain or heart involvement.

To treat certain diseases of the nervous system (eg, to assist short term in treating a sudden worsening of multiple sclerosis).

To treat brain swelling associated with brain tumors, brain surgery, or heart injury. (dexamethasone only)

The injectable forms of the various glucocorticoids may be used to treat additional conditions.

*Unlabeled Use(s):* Occasionally doctors may prescribe glucocorticoids for some types of shock, vomiting, respiratory distress in premature infants, diagnosis of depression, acute mountain sickness, COPD, alcoholic hepatitis, spinal cord injury, and abnormal hair growth.

## Precautions:

*Do not use in the following situations:*

allergy to the medicine or any of its ingredients
fungal infections, systemic
idiopathic thrombocytopenic purpura (intramuscular [IM] injections only)

ileocolostomy during immediate or early postoperative period (enemas only)
live virus vaccines (eg, smallpox)

*Use with caution in the following situations:*

amebiasis
congestive heart failure
diverticulitis
emotional instability
hepatitis B
herpes simplex in the eye
high blood pressure
infections, active (eg, acute glomerulonephritis, thrombophlebitis)
intestinal anastomosis, recent
kidney disease
liver disease

myasthenia gravis
myocardial infarction, recent
osteoporosis
peptic ulcer
psychotic tendencies
seizure disorders
stress, unusual
*Strongyloides* (threadworm)
  infestation, known or suspected
tuberculosis
ulcer, history of
ulcerative colitis, nonspecific
underactive thyroid

*Diabetes:* Glucocorticoids decrease carbohydrate tolerance. Diabetics may require increased doses of insulin or oral diabetes (hypoglycemic) medications to control blood sugar levels.

*Infection:* Glucocorticoids may mask signs of infection, and new infections may appear during use. Glucocorticoids may decrease resistance to an infection.

*Prolonged use:* Prolonged use may produce cataracts, glaucoma, and may enhance the establishment of secondary eye infections due to fungi or viruses.

*Immunizations:* Immunosuppressive (high) doses of glucocorticoids may reduce the effectiveness of inactivated bacterial and viral vaccines. Use of live virus vaccines is also contraindicated.

*Osteoporosis:* Corticosteroids increase the risk of osteoporosis. Adequate calcium and vitamin D intake may help reduce this problem.

*Pregnancy:* Adequate studies have not been done in pregnant women. Use only if clearly needed and potential benefits to the mother outweigh the possible hazards to the fetus.

*Breastfeeding:* Corticosteroids appear in breast milk. This could cause growth suppression in the infant. Mothers taking these drugs should not breastfeed.

*Children:* Growth and development of infants and children on prolonged therapy must be closely monitored by a doctor. Some of the injectable medications contain benzyl alcohol, which had been associated with the potentially fatal "gasping syndrome" in premature infants. Consult your doctor.

*Elderly:* Lower doses may be needed because of body changes caused by aging (such as loss of muscle mass).

*Sulfites:* Some of these products may contain sulfite preservatives that can cause allergic reactions in certain individuals. Check package label when available or consult your doctor or pharmacist.

## Drug Interactions:

Tell your doctor or pharmacist if you are taking or if you are planning to take any over-the-counter or prescription medications or dietary supplements with glucocorticoids. Doses of one or both drugs may need to be modified or a different drug may need to be prescribed. The following drugs and drug classes interact with glucocorticoids.

anticholinesterases (eg, neostigmine)
barbiturates (eg, phenobarbital)
bile acid sequestrants (eg, cholestyramine, colestipol)
contraceptives, oral (eg, *Ortho-Novum*)
estrogens (eg, ethinyl estradiol)
hydantoins (eg, phenytoin)
interferon alfa (eg, *Intron A*)

ketoconazole (eg, *Nizoral*)
macrolide antibiotics (eg, erythromycin)
potassium-depleting diuretics (eg, furosemide)
rifamycins (eg, rifampin)
salicylates (eg, aspirin)
vaccines, live virus (eg, smallpox)

## Side Effects:

Every drug is capable of producing side effects. Many glucocorticoid users experience no, or minor, side effects. The frequency and severity of side effects depend on many factors including dose, duration of therapy, and individual susceptibility. Possible side effects include:

*Cushing's Syndrome (long-term use)* – Appearance of "moonface"; enlargement of some fat pad areas; the appearance of obesity in the midsection; muscle wasting and weakness; abnormal fat deposits; general obesity; high blood pressure; diabetes; osteoporosis; thinning of skin; easy bruising.

*Too Rapid Withdrawal of Therapy* – Nausea; fatigue; loss of appetite; difficulty breathing; lowered blood pressure; joint and muscle aches; fever; dizziness; fainting; fever; general body discomfort; joint and muscle pain.

*Injectables only* – Skin pigment changes; abscess; joint damage; injection-site reaction; pain or tenderness at injection site; skin inflammation or hardening; delayed pain or soreness.

*Digestive Tract:* Nausea; vomiting; increased appetite; weight gain; heartburn; bloating; inflammation of the pancreas; peptic ulcer; stomach pain; rectal bleeding, local pain, or burning with enemas.

*Nervous System:* Convulsions; increased pressure in the brain; feeling of whirling motion; headache; behavior changes; sleeplessness; hiccups; mood swings; depression; psychotic manifestations; clumsiness; exaggerated sense of well being; seizures.

*Circulatory System:* Heart failure; high blood pressure; clot formation.

*Skin:* Impaired wound healing; thin skin and loss of fat under the skin; changes in pigmentation of skin; acne; excessive body hair growth; rash; hives; easy bruising; facial flushing; abnormal skin sensations; increased sweating.

*Other:* Salt and water retention; general body discomfort; potassium loss; abnormally low calcium; muscle weakness; loss of muscle mass; osteoporosis; bone fractures; menstrual irregularities; growth suppression in children; decreased carbohydrate tolerance; increased blood sugar levels; cataracts; glaucoma; aggravation or masking of an infection; rare instances of blindness; tendon rupture; suppressed reaction to skin tests; Kaposi's sarcoma; hip or shoulder bone degradation; secondary adrenocortical and pituitary unresponsiveness; increased intraocular pressure; bulging eyes; muscle twitching; rapid eye movement.

## Guidelines for Use:

- Dosage will be individualized based on the condition being treated and patient response.
- Injectable glucocorticoids are used when oral therapy is not feasible. They will be prepared and administered by your health care professional.
- Do not change the dose or stop taking unless advised to do so by your doctor.
- May cause stomach upset. Take oral dose forms with meals or snacks. Take single daily or alternate day doses in the morning prior to 9 a.m. Take multiple doses at evenly spaced intervals throughout the day or as advised by your doctor.
- *Alternate day therapy* — Used to retain beneficial drug effects while lowering the risk of side effects. Twice the usual daily dose may be given every other day in the morning before 9 a.m. The benefits of alternate day therapy are obtained when using intermediate-acting agents (eg, prednisone, prednisolone, triamcinolone, methylprednisolone). Alternate day therapy is common if steroid therapy is to be long term. Consult your doctor.
- *Intensol solution* — Mix with liquid or semi-solid food (eg, water, juice, soda-like beverage, applesauce). Use calibrated dropper to measure prescribed dose and then squeeze into liquid or food. Stir until mixed and consume entire amount. Do not store for future use.
- Patients on long-term steroid therapy should wear or carry identification noting that glucocorticoids are being taken.
- Notify your doctor if you experience unusual weight gain; swelling of the lower extremities; muscle weakness; black, tarry stools; vomiting of blood; puffing of the face; prolonged sore throat; fever; cold; or infection.
- *High dose or long-term therapy (longer than 1 month)* — Avoid sudden discontinuation of therapy. Follow a dosage tapering regimen prescribed by your doctor.
- Notify your doctor promptly if these symptoms occur following dosage reduction or withdrawal of therapy: Fatigue, appetite loss, nausea, vomiting, diarrhea, weight loss, weakness, dizziness, low blood sugar, fever, general body discomfort, and joint and muscle pain.
- If you are on immunosuppressant (high) doses of corticosteroids, avoid exposure to chickenpox or measles. If you are exposed, notify your doctor immediately.
- These drugs may cause an elevation in blood pressure and salt and water retention and increased potassium loss. Dietary salt restriction and potassium supplements may be necessary.
- Glucocorticoids cause calcium loss and can promote development of osteoporosis. Take adequate calcium and vitamin D supplements.
- Avoid any type of live virus vaccines, especially for smallpox, while taking this medicine.
- Lab tests and doctor visits will be required during therapy. Be sure to keep appointments.

*If you have any questions, consult your doctor, pharmacist, or health care provider.*

| Generic Name<br>*Brand Name Examples* | Supplied As | Generic<br>Available |
|---|---|---|
| *Rx* **Alclometasone Dipropionate** | | |
| *Aclovate* | **Ointment:** 0.05% | No |
| *Aclovate* | **Cream:** 0.05% | No |
| *Rx* **Amcinonide** | | |
| *Cyclocort* | **Ointment:** 0.1% | No |
| *Cyclocort* | **Cream:** 0.1% | No |
| *Cyclocort* | **Lotion:** 0.1% | No |
| *Rx* **Betamethasone Dipropionate** | | |
| *Alphatrex, Diprolene, Diprosone, Maxivate* | **Ointment:** 0.05% | Yes |
| *Alphatrex, Diprolene AF, Diprosone, Maxivate* | **Cream:** 0.05% | Yes |
| *Alphatrex, Diprolene, Diprosone, Maxivate* | **Lotion:** 0.05% | Yes |
| *Diprosone* | **Aerosol/Spray:** 0.1% | No |
| *Diprolene* | **Gel**: 0.05% | No |
| *Rx* **Betamethasone Valerate** | | Yes |
| *Beta-Val, Betatrex* | **Ointment:** 0.1% | Yes |
| *Beta-Val, Betatrex* | **Cream:** 0.01%, 0.1% | Yes |
| *Beta-Val, Betatrex* | **Lotion:** 0.1% | Yes |
| *Rx* **Clobetasol Propionate** | | |
| *Temovate* | **Ointment:** 0.05% | Yes |
| *Temovate, Temovate E* | **Cream:** 0.05% | Yes |
| *Temovate* | **Gel**: 0.05% | Yes |
| *Temovate* | **Scalp application (solution):** 0.05% | No |
| *Rx* **Clocortolone Pivalate** | | |
| *Cloderm* | **Cream:** 0.1% | No |
| *Rx* **Desonide** | | |
| *DesOwen, Tridesilon* | **Ointment:** 0.05% | Yes |
| *DesOwen* | **Cream:** 0.05% | Yes |
| *DesOwen* | **Lotion:** 0.05% | No |

| Generic Name<br>*Brand Name Examples* | Supplied As | Generic<br>Available |
|---|---|---|
| **Rx Desoximetasone** | | |
| *Topicort* | **Ointment:** 0.25% | Yes |
| *Topicort, Topicort LP* | **Cream:** 0.05%, 0.25% | Yes |
| *Topicort* | **Gel:** 0.05% | Yes |
| **Rx Diflorasone Diacetate** | | |
| *Florone, Maxiflor, Psorcon* | **Ointment:** 0.05% | Yes |
| *Florone, Florone E, Maxi-flor, Psorcon E* | **Cream:** 0.05% | Yes |
| **Rx Fluocinolone Acetonide** | | |
| *Synalar* | **Ointment:** 0.025% | Yes |
| *Synalar, Synemol* | **Cream:** 0.025% | Yes |
| *Fluonid, Synalar* | **Solution:** 0.01% | Yes |
| **Rx Fluocinonide** | | |
| *Lidex* | **Ointment:** 0.05% | Yes |
| *Lidex, Lidex-E* | **Cream:** 0.05% | Yes |
| *Lidex* | **Solution:** 0.05% | Yes |
| *Lidex* | **Gel:** 0.05% | Yes |
| **Rx Flurandrenolide** | | |
| *Cordran* | **Ointment:** 0.025%, 0.05% | No |
| *Cordran SP* | **Cream:** 0.025%, 0.05% | No |
| *Cordran* | **Lotion:** 0.05% | Yes |
| *Cordran* | **Tape:** 4 mcg/cm$^2$ | No |
| **Rx Fluticasone Propionate** | | |
| *Cutivate* | **Ointment:** 0.005% | No |
| *Cutivate* | **Cream:** 0.05% | No |
| **Rx Halcinonide** | | |
| *Halog* | **Ointment:** 0.1% | No |
| *Halog, Halog-E* | **Cream:** 0.025%, 0.1% | No |
| *Halog* | **Solution:** 0.1% | No |
| **Rx Halobetasol Propionate** | | |
| *Ultravate* | **Ointment:** 0.05% | No |
| *Ultravate* | **Cream:** 0.05% | No |

| Generic Name<br>*Brand Name Examples* | Supplied As | Generic<br>Available |
|---|---|---|
| *Rx/* **Hydrocortisone**<br>*otc[1]* | | |
| *otc* *Cortizone-5, Cortizone-10, Cortaid Maximum Strength,* | **Ointment:** 0.5%, 1% | Yes |
| *otc* *Cortaid Intensive Therapy, Cortaid Maximum Strength, Cortaid Sensitive Skin with Aloe, Cortizone-5, Cortizone-10, Cortizone-10 External Anal Itch Relief, Cortizone-10 Plus, Cortizone for Kids, KeriCort-10, Preparation H Anti-Itch, Summer's Eve* | **Cream:** 0.5%, 1% | Yes |
| *Rx* *Ala-Cort, Dermacort, Hytone, Penecort, Procto-Cream-HC 2.5%* | **Cream:** 1%, 2.5% | Yes |
| *Rx* *Ala-Scalp, Cetacort, Dermacort, Hytone, Nutracort* | **Lotion:** 1%, 2%, 2.5% | Yes |
| *Rx* *Penecort* | **Solution:** 1% | No |
| *Rx* *Penecort* | **Gel:** 1% | No |
| *otc* *CortaGel, CortiCool* | **Gel:** 1% | No |
| *otc* *Cortizone-10 Quick Shot* | **Aerosol/Spray:** 1% | No |
| *Rx/* **Hydrocortisone Acetate**<br>*otc[1]* | | |
| *otc* *LanaCort 5* | **Ointment:** 0.5% | No |
| *otc* *Gynecort 5, LanaCort 5* | **Cream:** 0.5% | No |
| *otc* *Caldecort, Gynecort 10, LanaCort 10, LanaCort Cool, Nupercainal* | **Cream:** 1% | No |
| *otc* *Anusol HC-1, LanaCort 10* | **Ointment:** 1% | No |
| *Rx* **Hydrocortisone Probutate** | | |
| *Pandel* | **Cream:** 0.1% | No |
| *Rx* **Hydrocortisone Valerate** | | |
| *Westcort* | **Ointment:** 0.2% | Yes |
| *Westcort* | **Cream:** 0.2% | Yes |

| Generic Name<br>*Brand Name Examples* | Supplied As | Generic<br>Available |
|---|---|---|
| *Rx* **Mometasone Furoate** | | |
| *Elocon* | **Ointment:** 0.1% | No |
| *Elocon* | **Cream:** 0.1% | No |
| *Elocon* | **Lotion:** 0.1% | No |
| *Rx* **Triamcinolone Acetonide** | | |
| *Aristocort A, Kenalog* | **Ointment:** 0.025%, 0.1%, 0.5% | Yes |
| *Aristocort A, Kenalog,*<br>*Triderm* | **Cream:** 0.025%, 0.1%, 0.5% | Yes |
| *Kenalog* | **Lotion:** 0.025%, 0.1% | Yes |
| *Kenalog* | **Aerosol/Spray:** 2 seconds of<br>spray delivers ≈ 0.2 mg | No |

[1] Products are available *otc* or *Rx* depending on product labeling.

## Type of Drug:

Topical anti-inflammatory, anti-itching agents; anti-inflammatory steroids.

## How the Drug Works:

Topical adrenocortical steroids reduce skin inflammation (ie, redness, swelling), itching, and irritation. The exact manner in which the drug works is not fully understood. The effectiveness of the drug depends on many factors, including: The extent of absorption of the drug, the potency of the drug, the size of the area treated, and the doseform (eg, cream, ointment).

## Uses:

To treat inflammation and itching caused by corticosteroid-responsive skin disorders.

*OTC hydrocortisone:* To treat minor skin irritation, itching, and rashes due to eczema; insect bites; poison ivy, oak, or sumac; allergic inflammation from soaps, detergents, cosmetics, or jewelry; itchy genital and anal areas; psoriasis; seborrheic dermatitis; or other minor skin irritations.

## Precautions:

*Do not use in the following situations:*

acne
allergy to corticosteroids or any
 of their ingredients
bacterial infections of the skin,
 single therapy for
cellulitus

facial, groin, or armpit areas
 (high potency agents only)
prolonged use near eyes or eyelids
rosacea

*Use with caution in the following situations:*

blistered, raw, or oozing areas of skin
diaper dermatosis
skin infection

*Absorption into the body:* Absorption into the body of topical corticosteroids has produced manifestations of Cushing's syndrome, reversible hypothalamic-pituitary-adrenal (HPA) axis suppression, and increased blood and urine sugar. This is more likely to occur with application to large body surfaces, use of occlusive dressings, and with the more potent steroids. Patients at higher risk include young children.

Side effects may include growth retardation, delayed weight gain, low plasma cortisol levels and absence of response to ACTH stimulation, including bulging "soft spots," headaches, and bilateral papilledema.

*Alcohol-containing preparations:* Alcohol-containing preparations may cause drying, burning, or irritation of open lesions.

*Formulations:* Corticosteroids are specially formulated to maximize their release and potency. Mixing these products with other products is discouraged because it may affect potency and effectiveness.

*Occlusive vehicles:* A transparent plastic wrap or other vehicles that will not allow air to pass through to the treated area will enhance absorption at least 10 times. These kinds of dressings are not generally recommended (eg, when using clobetasol or halobetasol, when treating children).

Greasy ointment bases are more occlusive and are preferred for dry, scaly lesions. Gels are less occlusive. The aerosols, lotions and solutions are best suited for hairy areas.

*Skin atrophy:* Skin atrophy may occur in 3 to 4 weeks if the most potent corticosteroids are employed. Skin atrophy occurs most readily at sites where absorption through the skin is highest.

*Pregnancy:* There are no adequate and well-controlled studies in pregnant women. Use only if clearly needed and the potential benefits to the mother outweigh the possible hazards to the fetus. Do not use large doses or for prolonged periods of time if you are pregnant.

*Breastfeeding:* It is not known if topical corticosteroids appear in breast milk. Oral corticosteroids appear in breast milk. Consult your doctor before you begin breastfeeding.

*Children:* Limit therapy to the lowest possible dosage because children may be more susceptible to topical corticosteroid-induced side effects. Safety and effectiveness of alclometasone in children less than 1 year of age have not been established. Clobetasol is not recommended in children less than 12 years of age. Safety and effectiveness of hydrocortisone probutate in children less than 18 years of age have not been established.

*Lab tests* may be required to monitor therapy. Tests may include urinary-free cortisol, ACTH stimulation, and early morning plasma cortisol tests.

## Side Effects:

Every drug is capable of producing side effects. Many topical corticosteroid users experience no, or minor, side effects. The frequency and severity of side effects depend on many factors including dose, duration of therapy, and individual susceptibility. Possible side effects include:

*Skin:* Burning; itching; irritation; redness; dryness; allergic inflammation; acne; decreased pigmentation in the area being treated; streaks in skin; skin atrophy; infection; stinging; cracking; rash; tingling; scalp pustules (scalp application only); unusual hair growth.

*Other:* Elevated blood or urine sugar; cataracts and glaucoma (prolonged use near eyes); numbness of fingers; worsening of condition being treated.

Also consider all side effects for oral corticosteroids. See the Glucocorticoids monograph in this chapter.

## Guidelines for Use:

- Dosage is individualized.
- Application frequency and duration of therapy are dependent on the condition treated, its location, the potency of the drug, and the vehicle employed. For assistance in product-specific drug selection and dosage guidelines, consult your doctor or pharmacist.
- Wash hands before and after application.
- Wash or soak the affected area before application. This may increase drug penetration.
- Apply sparingly as a thin film. Rub in lightly until the medication disappears.
- For external use only. Avoid contact with the eyes.
- Avoid prolonged use, especially near the eyes, on the face, on genital and rectal areas, and in skin folds.
- The treated area should not be bandaged, covered, or wrapped to be occlusive, unless advised to do so by your doctor.
- Do not use tight-fitting diapers or plastic pants on children treated with topical corticosteroids in the diaper area. Such garments function as occlusive dressings.
- Skin infections may worsen. It may be necessary to stop the corticosteroid and treat the infection.
- Do not use these agents to treat acne, the lesions of rosacea, skin inflammation near the mouth, or for any disorder other than that for which it was prescribed.
- Allergic reactions may occur. Contact your doctor if the condition being treated worsens or irritation, burning, redness, swelling, or stinging persists. Do not reapply the drug.
- If you do not notice improvement within 2 weeks (or 1 week when using OTC hydrocortisone), consult your doctor.
- *Aerosol/Spray* — Take care to cover the eyes while spraying close to the face. Avoid inhalation. Spray the affected area for 3 seconds or less at a time and at a distance of at least 6 inches between the nozzle and skin.
- *Scalp application* — Apply to the affected scalp areas twice daily, once in the morning and once at night.
  Do not use more than 50 mL/week.
  Treatment must be limited to 2 consecutive weeks.
- *Tape* — Skin should be clean and dry before the tape is applied. Tape should always be cut, never torn.
  Replacement of the tape every 12 hours produces the lowest incidence of side effects, but it may be left in place for 24 hours if it is well-tolerated and adheres well. When replacing the tape, cleanse the skin and allow to dry for 1 hour before applying new tape.
  When necessary, the tape may be used at night only and removed during the day.
  If the ends of the tape loosen prematurely, they may be trimmed off and replaced with fresh tape.
- Lab tests may be required to monitor therapy. Be sure to keep appointments.
- Store at controlled room temperature (59° to 86°F). Protect solutions and lotions from freezing.

*If you have any questions, consult your doctor, pharmacist, or health care provider.*

| Brand Name Examples | Hydrocortisone % | Other |
|---|---|---|
| Rx  Ala-Quin Cream | 0.5 | 3% iodochlor-hydroxyquin |
| Rx  Analpram-HC Cream 2.5%[1], Pramosone Cream 2.5%[1,2] | 2.5 | 1% pramoxine HCl |
| Rx  Zone-A Forte Lotion | 2.5 | 1% pramoxine HCl |
| Rx  Analpram-HC Cream, Pramosone Cream[1,2] | 1 | 1% pramoxine HCl |
| Rx  Epifoam Aerosol Foam, ProctoFoam-HC Aerosol Foam | 1 | 1% pramoxine HCl |
| Rx  Carmol HC Cream[3] | 1 | 10% urea |
| otc  HC Derma-Pax Liquid | 0.5 | 0.5% diphen-hydramine HCl |
| Rx  Mantadil Cream | 0.5 | 2% chlorcyclizine HCl |
| Rx  Vanoxide-HC Lotion | 0.5 | 5% benzoyl per-oxide |
| Rx  Vytone Cream | 1 | 1% iodoquinol |

[1] Also available in same strength as a lotion.
[2] Also available in same strength as an ointment.
[3] Contains sodium bisulfite.

## Type of Drug:

Topical anti-inflammatory, anti-itching agents.

## Uses:

To treat a variety of corticosteroid-responsive skin conditions. Some of these include eczema; insect bites; poison ivy, oak, or sumac; external anal itching; and allergic inflammation from soaps, detergents, cosmetics, or jewelry.

*Vanoxide-HC* is used to treat acne.

Components of these topical corticosteroid combinations include:

*Hydrocortisone* is used for its anti-inflammatory, anti-itch, and vasoconstrictive (blood vessel narrowing) effects.

*Iodochlorhydroxyquin* and *iodoquinol* are used for their antifungal, antibacterial, and antieczematous effects.

*Pramoxine HCl* is used for its local anesthetic effects.

*Urea* is a mild keratolytic and hydrates dry skin.

*Diphenhydramine* and *chlorcyclizine* are antihistamines used to treat itching.

*Benzoyl peroxide* is used for its peeling and drying effects.

## Precautions:

*Do not use in the following situations:*

allergy to the medicine or any of its ingredients

lesions of the eye (*Ala-Quin* only)

most viral skin lesions (eg, vaccinia, varicella, herpes simplex) (*Ala-Quin* and *Mantadil* only)

systemic bacterial infection without concomitant antibacterial therapy

tuberculosis of the skin (*Ala-Quin* and *Mantadil* only)

*Use with caution in the following situations:*

use of more potent steroids

children

occlusive dressing use

prolonged use

use over large surface areas

*Pregnancy:* There are no adequate and well-controlled studies in pregnant women. Topical corticosteroids should be used during pregnancy only if the potential benefits to the mother outweigh the possible risks to the fetus.

*Breastfeeding:* It is not known whether topical corticosteroids appear in breast milk. Consult your doctor before you begin breastfeeding.

*Children:* Pediatric patients may demonstrate greater susceptibility to topical corticosteroid-induced hypothalamic-pituitary-adrenal (HPA) axis suppression and Cushing's syndrome than adult patients because of a larger skin surface area to body weight ratio. Administration of topical corticosteroids to children should be limited to the least amount compatible with an effective therapeutic regimen. Chronic corticosteroid therapy may interfere with the growth and development of children.

*Lab tests* may be required to monitor long-term or high-dose therapy. Tests may include urinary free cortisol or ACTH stimulation tests.

*Sulfites:* Some of these products may contain sulfite preservatives that can cause allergic reactions in certain individuals. Check package label when available or consult your doctor or pharmacist.

## Drug Interactions:

Tell your doctor or pharmacist if you are taking or if you are planning to take any over-the-counter or prescription medications or dietary supplements with topical corticosteroid combinations. Doses of one or both drugs may need to be modified or a different drug may need to be prescribed.

## Side Effects:

Every drug is capable of producing side effects. Many topical corticosteroid combination users experience no, or minor, side effects. The frequency and severity of side effects depend on many factors including dose, duration of therapy, and individual susceptibility. Possible side effects include:

*Skin:* Burning; itching; rash; irritation; dryness; inflammation of hair follicles; excessive hair growth; acne; hypopigmentation; skin irritation around the mouth; allergic contact dermatitis; tearing of the skin; secondary infection; skin atrophy; stretch marks; plugged or inflamed sweat follicles.

*Other:* Reversible hypothalamic-pituitary-adrenal (HPA) axis suppression; manifestations of Cushing's syndrome; high blood sugar; sugar in the urine; abnormal thyroid tests (*iodochlorhydroxyquin-containing products only*); false-positive ferric chloride test for phenylketonuria (PKU) (*iodochlorhydroxyquin-containing products only*).

## Guidelines for Use:

- For external use only.
- Avoid contact with the eyes.
- *ProctoFoam-HC Aerosol* is for anal or perianal use only.
- Topical corticosteroids are generally applied to the affected area as a thin film and rubbed in gently 3 or 4 times daily depending on the severity of the condition. See individual product information for specific instructions.
- Washing or soaking the affected area and then drying it before application is encouraged, as this may increase drug penetration.
- The treated skin should not be bandaged or otherwise covered or wrapped so as to be occlusive unless directed to do so by your doctor.
- Occlusive dressings may be used for the management of psoriasis or recalcitrant conditions. Discontinue the use of occlusive dressings and notify your doctor if symptoms worsen or an infection develops.
- *HC Derma-Pax* is most effective when used as a wet dressing.
- Avoid prolonged use, especially near the eyes, on the face, on genital and rectal areas, and in skin folds.
- Do not use tight-fitting diapers or plastic pants on children being treated with topical corticosteroids in the diaper area. Such garments function as occlusive dressings.
- Skin infections may worsen. It may be necessary to stop the corticosteroid and treat the infection.
- Allergic reactions may occur. If the condition being treated worsens or irritation, burning, redness, pain, swelling, or stinging persists, discontinue use and contact your doctor.
- Iodochlorhydroxyquin may interfere with thyroid function tests. Tell your doctor if you are using this medicine.
- Benzoyl peroxide may bleach hair or clothing.
- Aerosol containers should never be inserted into the vagina or anus.
- Lab tests may be required to monitor therapy. Be sure to keep appointments.
- Store at room temperature (59° to 86°F) in a tightly closed container.
- Aerosol foams are in pressurized containers. Do not puncture, incinerate, or expose to high heat. Store upright at room temperature (59° to 86°F). Do not refrigerate.

*If you have any questions, consult your doctor, pharmacist, or health care provider.*

| Generic Name Brand Name Examples | Supplied As | Generic Available |
|---|---|---|
| Rx **Fludrocortisone Acetate** | | |
| *Florinef Acetate* | **Tablets:** 0.1 mg | No |

## Type of Drug:

Adrenal cortical steroid.

## How the Drug Works:

The mineralocorticoid, fludrocortisone, acts on the kidney to preserve sodium. It increases potassium and hydrogen loss in the urine.

## Uses:

To treat insufficient secretion of steroids from the adrenal cortex in Addison disease. Used in conjunction with glucocorticoid therapy.

To treat excessive salt loss.

*Unlabeled Use(s):* Occasionally doctors may prescribe fludrocortisone for severe orthostatic hypotension (dizziness or lightheadedness that occurs when rising quickly from a lying or sitting position).

## Precautions:

*Do not use in the following situations:*

allergy to fludrocortisone acetate or any of its ingredients
immunization, concurrent
smallpox vaccination, concurrent
systemic fungal infection

*Use with caution in the following situations:*

cirrhosis
diverticulitis
heart disease
herpes simplex, ocular
high blood pressure
hypothyroidism
immunosuppression
infection, active
intestinal anastomoses, fresh
kidney disease
liver disease
myasthenia gravis
osteoporosis
patients who have not had chickenpox or measles
peptic ulcer, active or latent
salicylates (eg, aspirin) use in hypoprothombinemic patients
stress (eg, trauma, surgery, severe illness)
tuberculosis, active
ulcerative colitis, non-specific

*Pregnancy:* Adequate studies have not been done in pregnant women. Use only if clearly needed and potential benefits to the mother outweigh the possible hazards to the fetus.

*Breastfeeding:* Corticosteroids appear in breast milk. Consult your doctor before you begin breastfeeding.

*Children:* Safety and effectiveness in children have not been established. Monitor growth and development of infants and children on prolonged therapy.

*Lab tests* may be required. Tests may include serum electrolyte levels and blood pressure monitoring.

## Drug Interactions:

Tell your doctor or pharmacist if you are taking or if you are planning to take any over-the-counter or prescription medications or dietary supplements with fludrocortisone acetate. Doses of one or both drugs may need to be modified or a different drug may need to be prescribed. The following drugs and drug classes interact with fludrocortisone.

amphotericin B (eg, *Fungizone*)
anabolic steroids (eg, oxy-metholone, methandrosateno-lone, norethandrolone)
anticoagulants, oral (eg, warfarin)
antidiabetics (eg, insulin)
barbiturates (eg, phenobarbital)
cardiac glycosides (eg, digoxin)
cholinesterase inhibitors (eg, neostigmine)
estrogen (eg, *Premarin*)

hydantoins (eg, phenytoin)
immunosuppressive agents (eg, cyclosporine)
potassium-depleting diuretics (eg, benzothiadiazines, furosemide)
rifabutin (*Mycobutin*)
rifampin (eg, *Rifadin*)
salicylates (eg, aspirin)
vaccines (eg, influenza virus vaccine)

## Side Effects:

Every drug is capable of producing side effects. Many mineralocorticoid users experience no, or minor, side effects. The frequency and sever-ity of side effects depend on many factors including dose, duration of therapy, and individual susceptibility. Severe side effects may occur if the dose is too high, if the mineralocorticoid is given for a long time, or if it is withdrawn too fast. Fludrocortisone may cause side effects similar to glucocorticoids. Possible side effects include:

*Circulatory System:* High blood pressure; heart failure; heart enlargement.

*Muscular System:* Muscle weakness; steroid-induced muscle disease; loss of muscle mass; osteoporosis (brittle bones); compression fractures of the spine; hip bone or shoulder bone degradation; fracture of long bones due to diseases; spontaneous fractures.

*Digestive Tract:* Peptic ulcer with possible perforation and bleeding; pancre-atitis; abdominal distention; inflammation of the esophagus.

*Skin:* Impaired wound healing; thin, fragile skin; bruising; small red spots under skin; unusual bruising; increased sweating; subcutaneous fat atrophy; red or purple spots or patches under the skin; stretch marks; excessive pigment in the skin and nails; abnormal hairiness or increased hair growth; acne-like eruptions; hives; rash; facial skin redness; itching.

*Nervous System:* Convulsions; increased intracranial pressure with fluid accumulation at the optic disc (pseudotumor cerebri) usually after treat-ment; feeling of a whirling motion; headache; severe mental distur-bances.

*Eyes or Ocular:* Posterior subcapsular cataracts; increased intraocular pressure (glaucoma with possible damage to the optic nerve); eye infections.

*Other:* Fluid retention; unusual weight gain; potassium loss; hypokalemic alkalosis; allergic reaction; high blood sugar; negative nitrogen balance due to protein catabolism; necrotizing angiitis; inflammation of the veins with clot formation; aggravation or masking of infections; sleeplessness; fainting; menstrual irregularities; development of the cushingoid state (eg, buffalo hump obesity, general obesity, high blood pressure, diabetes, osteoporosis); suppression of growth in children; secondary adrenocortical and pituitary unresponsiveness particularly in times of stress (eg, trauma, surgery, illness); decreased carbohydrate tolerance; manifestations of latent diabetes mellitus; increased requirements for insulin or oral hypoglycemic agents in diabetic patients; calcium loss; euphoria; mood swings; personality changes; depression; emotional instability; psychotic tendencies; glucose in the urine.

## Guidelines for Use:

- Because of its marked effect on sodium retention, the use of fludrocortisone in the treatment of conditions other than those indicated is not advised.
- Dosage depends on the severity of the disease and the response of the patient.
- *Addison Disease* — Administer with a glucocorticoid (eg, 10 to 37.5 mg daily of cortisone or 10 to 30 mg daily of hydrocortisone, both in divided doses). The usual dose is 0.1 mg. Doses ranging from 0.1 to 0.2 mg daily have been used. If blood pressure increases, the dose may be decreased to 0.05 mg daily.
- *Salt-Losing Adrenogenital Syndrome* — The recommended dose is 0.1 mg to 0.2 mg daily.
- Carefully monitor salt intake in order to avoid developing high blood pressure, swelling, or weight gain.
- Higher doses may be required in times of stress (eg, trauma, surgery, severe illness) both during and 1 year after treatment with fludrocortisone.
- If a dose is missed, take it as soon as possible. If several hours have passed or it is nearing time for the next dose, do not double the dose in order to catch up, unless advised to do so by your doctor. If more than one dose is missed or if it is necessary to establish a new dosage schedule, contact your doctor or pharmacist.
- Do not stop taking the medicine suddenly.
- Corticosteroids may mask some signs of infection, and new infections may appear during their use. There may be decreased resistance and difficulty in reducing the spread of an infection when used. If an infection occurs during therapy, notify your doctor immediately.
- Dietary salt restriction and potassium supplementation may be necessary. All corticosteroids increase calcium secretion.
- Prolonged use of corticosteroids may produce cataracts, glaucoma with possible damage to optic nerves, and ocular infections.
- *Chickenpox and Measles* — Patients are more susceptible to infections such as chickenpox and measles. These infections can have a more serious or even fatal course in children. Avoid exposure to infections due to fungi or viruses.
- Carry medical identification indicating dependence on steroids and possibly carry an adequate supply of medicine for use in emergencies.
- Notify your doctor if dizziness, severe headaches, joint pain, extreme weakness, swelling of feet or lower legs, or unusual weight gain occurs.
- Lab tests may be needed to determine blood pressure and sodium and potassium levels in the blood. Regular follow-up visits will also be crucial in checking progress. Be sure to keep appointments.
- Store at room temperature (59° to 86°F). Avoid excessive heat.

*If you have any questions, consult your doctor, pharmacist, or health care provider.*

| Generic Name<br>*Brand Name Examples* | Supplied As | Generic<br>Available |
|---|---|---|
| *Rx* **Aminoglutethimide** | | |
| *Cytadren* | **Tablets:** 250 mg | No |

## Type of Drug:
Adrenal steroid inhibitor.

## How the Drug Works:
Aminoglutethimide inhibits the synthesis of adrenal steroids such as glucocorticoids, mineralocorticoids, estrogens and androgens.

## Uses:
To suppress the adrenal gland functions in selected patients with Cushing syndrome.

*Unlabeled Use(s):* Occasionally doctors may prescribe aminoglutethimide to treat breast cancer in postmenopausal patients or to treat patients with metastatic prostate cancer.

## Precautions:
*Do not use in the following situations:* allergy to aminoglutethimide or glutethimide, serious

*Use with caution in the following situations:*

| | |
|---|---|
| illness, acute | low blood pressure |
| long-term use (more than | surgery |
| 3 months) | trauma |

*Pregnancy:* Studies have shown a potential adverse effect on the fetus. Use only if clearly needed and potential benefits outweigh the possible risks.

*Breastfeeding:* It is not known if aminoglutethimide appears in breast milk. Consult your doctor before you begin breastfeeding.

*Children:* Safety and effectiveness in children have not been established.

*Lab tests* will be required to monitor therapy. Be sure to keep appointments. Tests may include:Thyroid function test; adrenal function tests; blood pressure monitoring; serum electrolytes.

## Drug Interactions:
Tell your doctor or pharmacist if you are taking or planning to take any over-the-counter or prescription medications or dietary supplements while taking this medicine. Doses of one or both drugs may need to be modified or a different drug may need to be prescribed. The following drugs and drug classes interact with this medicine.

| | |
|---|---|
| alcohol | digitoxin |
| anticoagulants, oral | medroxyprogesterone (*Depo-* |
| (eg, warfarin) | *Provera*) |
| dexamethasone (eg, *Decadron*) | theophylline (eg, *Theo-Dur*) |

## Side Effects:

Every drug is capable of producing side effects. Most patients experience side effects. The frequency and severity of side effects depend on many factors including dose, duration of therapy and individual susceptibility. Possible side effects include:

*Digestive Tract:* Nausea; appetite loss; vomiting.

*Nervous System:* Drowsiness; headache; dizziness.

*Circulatory System:* Low blood pressure (occasionally causing dizziness or lightheadedness when rising from sitting or lying); fast heartbeat.

*Skin:* Rash; itching.

*Other:* Muscle pain; fever; reduced adrenal function; underactive thyroid (eg, weight gain); abnormal blood counts.

---

### Guidelines for Use:

- Use exactly as prescribed.
- The usual dose is 250 mg four times daily, every 6 hours.
- If a dose is missed, take it as soon as possible. If several hours have passed or if it is nearing time for the next dose, do not double the dose in order to "catch up" (unless advised to do so by your doctor). If more than one dose is missed or it is necessary to establish a new dosage schedule, contact your doctor or pharmacist.
- May cause dizziness, lightheartedness or fainting, especially when rising quickly from a sitting or lying. If these symptoms should occur, sit or lie down and contact your doctor. Use caution while driving or performing hazardous tasks requiring alertness, coordination or physical dexterity.
- If severe rash, extreme drowsiness, yellowing of skin or eyes, fainting, weakness or headache occur, contact your doctor immediately.
- Nausea and loss of appetite may occur during the first 2 weeks of therapy. Contact you doctor if these do not go away.
- Contraceptive measures (birth control) are recommended during treatment to avoid birth defects. Contact your doctor if pregnancy is suspected.
- Store at room temperature (below 86°F) in a tightly sealed container. Protect from light.

---

*If you have any questions, consult your doctor, pharmacist, or health care provider.*

| Generic Name<br>*Brand Name Examples* | Supplied As |
|---|---|
| *otc* **Insulin Injection (Regular Insulin)** | |
| *Regular Iletin II* | **Injection**: 100 units/mL, purified pork |
| *Novolin R* | **Injection**: 100 units/mL, human insulin (rDNA) |
| *Velosulin BR* | **Injection**: 100 units/mL, human insulin (rDNA) |
| *Novolin R PenFill* | **Cartridges**: 100 units/mL, human insulin (rDNA). Use with *NovoPen* and *Novolin Pen* |
| *Novolin R Prefilled* | **Injection**: 100 units/mL, human insulin (rDNA) |
| *Humulin R* | **Injection**: 100 units/mL, regular insulin (rDNA) |
| *Rx* **Insulin Injection Concentrated** | |
| *Humulin R Regular U-500 (Concentrated)* | **Injection**: 500 units/mL, human insulin (rDNA) |
| *otc* **Insulin Zinc Suspension (Lente Insulin)** | |
| *Lente Iletin I* | **Injection** 100 units/mL, beef and pork |
| *Lente Iletin II* | **Injection**: 100 units/mL, purified pork |
| *Humulin L, Novolin L* | **Injection**: 100 units/mL, human insulin (rDNA) |
| *otc* **Insulin Zinc Suspension, Extended (Ultralente Insulin)** | |
| *Humulin U Ultralente* | **Injection**: 100 units/mL, human insulin (rDNA) |
| *otc* **Isophane Insulin Suspension (NPH Insulin)** | |
| *NPH Iletin I* | **Injection**: 100 units/mL, beef and pork |
| *NPH Iletin II* | **Injection**: 100 units/mL, purified pork |
| *Humulin N, Novolin N* | **Injection**: 100 units/mL, human insulin (rDNA) |

| Generic Name<br>*Brand Name Examples* | **Supplied As** |
|---|---|
| *Novolin N PenFill* | **Cartridges**: 100 units/mL, human insulin(rDNA). Use with *NovoPen* and *Novolin Pen* |
| *Novolin N Prefilled* | **Injection**: 100 units/mL, human insulin (rDNA) |
| *otc* **Isophane Insulin Suspension (NPH) and Regular Insulin Injection Combined** | |
| *Humulin 50/50* | **Injection**: 150 units NPH and 50 units regular insulin/mL, human insulin (rDNA) |
| *Humulin 70/30, Novolin 70/30* | **Injection**: 70 units NPH and 30 units regular insulin/mL, human insulin (rDNA) |
| *Novolin 70/30 PenFill* | **Cartridges**: 70 units NPH and 30 units regular insulin/mL, human insulin (rDNA) |
| *Novolin 70/30 Prefilled* | **Injection**: 70 units NPH and 30 units regular insulin/mL, human insulin (rDNA) |
| *Rx* **Insulin Analog Injection** | |
| *Humalog* | **Injection**: 100 units/mL, human insulin lispro (rDNA) |
| *Humalog Mix 50/50* | **Injection**: 50 units insulin lispro protamine and 50 units insulin lispro/mL, human insulin lispro (rDNA) |
| *Humalog Mix 75/25* | **Injection**: 75 units insulin lispro protamine and 25 units insulin lispro/mL, insulin lispro (rDNA) |
| *NovoLog* | **Injection**: 100 units/mL, human insulin aspart (rDNA) |
| *Rx* **Insulin Glargine Injection** | |
| *Lantus* | **Injection**: 100 IU (3.6378 mg) |

Beef insulin: Obtained from the pancreas gland of a cow.
Pork insulin: Obtained from the pancreas gland of a pig.
Human insulin (rDNA): Synthesized in a special laboratory.

## Type of Drug:

Hormone; antidiabetic agent.

## How the Drug Works:

Insulin, normally produced in the pancreas gland, is the major hormone that regulates glucose (sugar) use in the body. Without insulin, sugar is trapped in the bloodstream and cannot enter the cells of the body where it can be utilized for energy, so blood sugar levels increase, resulting in diabetes. In type 1 (insulin-dependent) and advanced type 2 (non-insulin-dependent) diabetes, the pancreas is not able to make enough insulin to control sugar levels.

Insulin must be injected. If taken by mouth, it would be digested by the acids and enzymes in the stomach.

## Uses:

To treat type 1 (insulin-dependent) diabetes mellitus.

To treat type 2 (non-insulin-dependent) diabetes mellitus that cannot be properly controlled by diet, exercise, or weight reduction.

Used in a hospital setting to treat dangerously high blood levels of potassium.

## Precautions:

*Diet and exercise:* It is important to follow the diet and exercise regimen prescribed by your doctor in order to effectively control diabetes. Do not change this regimen unless advised to do so by your doctor.

*High blood pressure:* High blood pressure in combination with diabetes increases the risk for other health problems (eg, eye or kidney problems, heart attack, stroke). Blood pressure should be monitored frequently. Regular checkups and eye examinations are important.

*Smoking:* Avoid tobacco products. If you are a smoker and stop, your dose of insulin may need to be reduced.

*Brand interchange:* Do not change from one insulin product to another unless advised to do so by your doctor. Insulins vary by strength, brand, onset, maximum effect, and duration of activity (see the following table). Become familiar with how the products you are using affect your blood sugar levels.

## Pharmacokinetics and Compatibility of Various Insulins

| Insulin Preparations | | Onset (hrs) | Peak (hrs) | Duration (hrs) | Compatible mixed with |
|---|---|---|---|---|---|
| Rapid-Acting | Insulin Injection (Regular) | 0.5 to 1 | variable depending on product | 8 to 12 | All |
| | Prompt Insulin Zinc Suspension (semilente) | 1 to 1.5 | 5 to 10 | 12 to 16 | Lente |
| | Insulin Lispro Solution | 0.25 | 0.5 to 1.5 | 6 to 8 | Ultralente, NPH |
| | Insulin Aspart Solution | 0.25 | 1 to 3 | 3 to 5 | NPH |
| Inter-mediate-Acting | Isophane Insulin Suspension (NPH) | 1 to 1.5 | 4 to 12 | 24 | Regular |
| | Insulin Zinc Suspension (Lente) | 1 to 2.5 | 7 to 15 | 24 | Regular, semilente |
| | Insulin Glargine Solution | 1.1 | $5^1$ | $24^2$ | None |
| Long-Acting | Protamine Zinc Insulin Suspension (PZI) | 4 to 8 | 14 to 24 | 36 | Regular |
| | Extended Insulin Zinc Suspension (Ultralente) | 4 to 8 | 10 to 30 | 28 | Regular, semilente |

[1] No pronounced peak; small amounts of insulin glargine are slowly released resulting in a relatively constant concentration/time profile over 24 hours.
[2] Studies only conducted up to 24 hours.

*Insulin mixtures:* Patients stabilized on mixtures should have a consistent response. Unexpected responses are most likely to occur when switching from separate injections to mixtures (or vice versa). When mixing 2 types of insulin, always draw the clear regular insulin into the syringe first. To avoid dosage errors, do not alter the order of mixing insulins or change the model or brand of syringe or needle.

It is recommended to use the self-prepared mixtures within the first 5 minutes after mixing. If this is not possible, clarify with your doctor, pharmacist, or health care provider the instructions on how to store these mixtures.

NPH/regular mixtures of insulin are available in premixed formulations of 70% NPH and 30% regular, and of 50% NPH and 50% regular. Insulin lispro NPH/regular mixtures are available in premixed formulations of 75% NPH and 25% regular and of 50% NPH and 50% regular. These mixtures are stable and are absorbed as if injected separately.

*High blood sugar:* In patients with type 1 diabetes mellitus, high blood sugar levels (hyperglycemia) that are not treated properly with insulin can develop into diabetic ketoacidosis, a life-threatening condition requiring prompt diagnosis and treatment (see the following table for symptoms). Close monitoring and control of blood sugar levels are required to prevent high blood sugar levels from developing.

| Symptoms of Hypoglycemia vs Ketoacidosis | | |
|---|---|---|
| **Reaction** | **Onset** | **Symptoms** |
| Hypoglycemia Too little sugar in the blood (Insulin reaction) | sudden | **Mild to Moderate Hypoglycemia**<br><br>sweating<br>tremor<br>rapid heart rate<br>pounding in the chest<br>anxiety<br>irritability<br>personality changes<br>slurred speech<br>abnormal behavior<br>inability to concentrate<br>drowsiness<br>headache<br>hunger<br>restlessness<br>tingling in the hands, feet, lips, or tongue<br>vision changes |
| | | **Severe Hypoglycemia**<br><br>disorientation<br>unconsciousness<br>seizures<br>death |
| Ketoacidosis Too much sugar and acid in the blood (Diabetic coma) | slow (hours to days) | drowsiness<br>flushed face<br>thirst<br>fruity breath odor<br>rapid breathing<br>stomach ache<br>appetite loss<br>large amounts of sugar and acetone in the urine |

*Low blood sugar:* Insulin use has the potential to cause hypoglycemia, or low blood sugar (refer to the preceding table for symptoms). Hypoglycemia may be due to taking too much insulin, exercising or working more than usual, not eating enough food, or not eating at the appropriate times. Eating sugar or a sugar-sweetened product will often correct the condition and prevent more serious symptoms. Establish a plan with your doctor on how best to treat hypoglycemic reactions. All diabetic patients should carry a source of rapid-acting sugar (eg, candy mints, glucose tablets) to take if symptoms of low blood sugar develop. Commercial products containing 40% glucose are available, such as *B-D Glucose* tablets. Close self-monitoring of blood glucose is necessary to determine when blood sugar levels are too low. Notify your doctor immediately if you experience ongoing symptoms of low blood sugar.

All patients using insulin should also have a *Glucagon* emergency kit available, so that family members, coworkers, or friends can administer the *Glucagon* to raise blood sugar levels in an unconscious patient with diabetes (see the Glucose Elevating Agents — Glucagon monograph in this chapter). Make sure these people know how to prepare and administer *Glucagon*.

*Pregnancy:* If you are using insulin and become pregnant, management of your diabetes will require a greater effort and you should self-monitor blood glucose and ketones more often. Rigid control of blood sugar and avoidance of ketones in the blood are desired throughout pregnancy. Insulin requirements may drop immediately following delivery, then increase to pre-pregnancy levels over time.

*Breastfeeding:* Insulin appears in breast milk, but is destroyed in the stomach of the infant and not absorbed. Breastfeeding women may require adjustments in insulin dose and diet.

*Lab tests* may be required to monitor therapy. Tests may include blood glucose, urine ketones, and glycohemoglobin tests.

## Drug Interactions:

Tell your doctor or pharmacist if you are taking or if you are planning to take any over-the-counter or prescription medications or dietary supplements while taking insulin. Doses of one or both drugs may need to be modified or a different drug may need to be prescribed. The following drugs and drug classes interact with insulin:

*Decrease the glucose-lowering effect of insulin —*

acetazolamide (eg, *Diamox*)
AIDS antivirals (eg, saquinavir)
albuterol (eg, *Proventil*)
asparaginase (*Elspar*)
calcitonin (eg, *Calcimar*)
clonidine (eg, *Catapres*)
contraceptives, oral (eg, *Ortho-Novum*)
corticosteroids (eg, prednisone)
cyclophosphamide (eg, *Cytoxan*)
danazol (eg, *Danocrine*)
dextrothyroxine (*Choloxin*)
diazoxide (*Proglycem*)
diltiazem (eg, *Cardizem*)
dobutamide (eg, *Dobutrex*)
epinephrine (eg, *Adrenalin Chloride*)
estrogens (eg, *Premarin*)
isoniazid (eg, *Nydrazid*)
lithium carbonate (eg, *Eskalith*)
loop diuretics
 (eg, furosemide)
morphine sulfate (eg, *MS Contin*)
niacin (vitamin $B_3$; nicotinic acid)
nicotine
phenothiazines (eg, promethazine)
phenytoin (eg, *Dilantin*)
somatropin (eg, *Genotropin*)
terbutaline (eg, *Brethine*)
thiazide diuretics (eg, hydrochlorothiazide)
thyroid hormone
 (eg, levothyroxine)

*Increase the glucose-lowering effect of insulin —*

ACE inhibitors (eg, ramipril)
alcohol
antidiabetic products, oral (eg, glipizide)
beta blockers (eg, propranolol)
clofibrate (*Atromid-S*)
disopyramide (eg, *Norpace*)
fluoxetine (eg, *Prozac*)
lithium carbonate (eg, *Eskalith*)
MAOIs (eg, phenelzine)
propoxyphene (eg, *Darvon-N*)
salicylates (eg, aspirin)
somatostatin analog (eg, octreotide)
sulfonamides (eg, trimethoprim and sulfamethoxazole)
tetracyclines (eg, oxytetracycline)

## Side Effects:

Every drug is capable of producing side effects. Many insulin users experience no, or minor, side effects. The frequency and severity of side effects depend on many factors including dose, duration of therapy, and individual susceptibility. Possible side effects include:

*Skin:* Rash, itching, redness, or other allergic symptoms at injection site; skin puckering at injection site; skin depression at injection site; skin thickening at injection site; fatty lumps at injection site. For symptoms of high blood sugar and low blood sugar, see Precautions.

## Guidelines for Use:

- Read the package inserts of the insulin and understand all aspects of its use.
- Carefully follow the storage, preparation, and injection techniques taught to you by your doctor or diabetes educator.
- Participate in a thorough diabetes education program so that you understand diabetes and all aspects of its treatment, including diet, exercise, personal hygiene, and how to self-monitor blood glucose.
- Become familiar with the specific type of insulin that you are using and how your blood sugar levels are affected by each dose. Do not switch types, brands, strengths, doses, or the order of mixing your insulin without first consulting your doctor or diabetes educator. Overdosage could result in insulin shock.
- Wear an ID tag (eg, Medic Alert) so appropriate treatment can be given if an emergency occurs away from home.
- Always keep an extra supply of insulin, as well as a spare syringe and needle, on hand.
- Visually inspect the solution/suspension before administration.
- Rotate injection sites to prevent scarring and other possible complications.
- Do not switch the model and brand of syringe or needle without first consulting your doctor or diabetes educator.
- Monitor blood glucose and urine for glucose and ketones as prescribed. Keep track of the results so that adjustments in your treatment can be made more easily.
- Contact your doctor if you experience symptoms of hypoglycemia or ketoacidosis (see table in Precautions for symptoms).
- Insulin requirements may change when you are ill (eg, vomiting, fever), under stress, or exercising. Stay on your regular diet, if possible. Establish a "sick day" plan with your doctor. A "sick day" plan provides directions for what to do when you are sick and cannot keep food down or are having difficulty eating. The plan should include advice on when to call your doctor or seek emergency care.
- To avoid possible transmission of disease, do not share syringes, needles, or cartridges with anyone else.
- Consult your doctor about your insulin schedule if you will be traveling across 2 or more time zones. You may need to make adjustments in your insulin schedule.
- Be sure to have regular physical and eye examinations. The frequency of these exams will be determined by your regular doctor and your eye doctor.
- Lab tests may be required to monitor therapy. Be sure to keep appointments.
- *Regular insulin* — Do not use if solution is cloudy, colored, thickened, or if particles are seen.

## Guidelines for Use (cont.):

- *Lente and NPH insulins* — Gently mix well before using. Do not use if clumps are seen or if white material (the insulin) remains at the bottom of the insulin bottle.
- Store at room temperature (up to 30 days), away from light and heat. If you buy extra bottles of insulin, store the bottles that you are not using in the door of the refrigerator. Do not freeze insulin. Do not use the bottles after the expiration date stamped on the label or if the insulin has been frozen.

*If you have any questions, consult your doctor, pharmacist, or health care provider.*

| Generic Name<br>*Brand Name Example* | Supplied As | Generic<br>Available |
|---|---|---|
| *Rx* **Acarbose** | | |
| *Precose* | **Tablets:** 25 mg, 50 mg, 100 mg | No |
| *Rx* **Miglitol** | | |
| *Glyset* | **Tablets:** 25 mg, 50 mg, 100 mg | No |

## Type of Drug:
Oral antidiabetic.

## How the Drug Works:
Acarbose and miglitol delay the digestion of ingested carbohydrates; this slows the absorption of glucose and results in a smaller rise in blood sugar levels following meals. May be used alone, as an adjunct to diet, or in combination with a sulfonylurea (eg, glyburide) when diet plus antidiabetic agents or sulfonylureas do not result in adequate blood sugar control. Acarbose may be used in combination with metformin or insulin. Miglitol may also be used in combination with insulin.

## Uses:
To help decrease blood sugar levels. Acarbose and miglitol are only prescribed for patients with type 2 diabetes mellitus who are not capable of managing blood sugar levels by diet and exercise alone.

## Precautions:
*Do not use in the following situations:*
allergy to the drug or any of its ingredients
cirrhosis (liver disease, severe) (acarbose only)
colonic ulceration (rectal bleeding)
conditions that may worsen as a result of increased gas formation in the intestine
diabetic ketoacidosis
inflammatory bowel disease
intestinal disease, chronic
intestinal obstruction, current or predisposition to

*Use with caution in the following situations:*
kidney disease
insulin or sulfonylurea use (may increase risk of low blood sugar)
liver disease

*Loss of control of blood glucose:* When diabetic patients are exposed to stress (eg, fever, trauma, infection, surgery) a temporary loss of control of blood glucose may occur. At such times, temporary insulin therapy may be needed.

*Pregnancy:* There are no adequate and well-controlled studies in pregnant women. Use only if clearly needed and potential benefits to the mother outweigh the possible hazard to the fetus.

*Breastfeeding:* It is not known if acarbose appears in breast milk. Miglitol appears in breast milk. Acarbose and miglitol should not be used while breastfeeding. Consult your doctor before you begin breastfeeding.

*Children:* Safety and effectiveness for use in children have not been established.

*Lab tests* are required to monitor therapy. Tests include blood glucose or hemoglobin level tests.

## Drug Interactions:

Tell your doctor or pharmacist if you are taking or planning to take any over-the-counter or prescription medications or dietary supplements while taking this medicine. Doses of one or both drugs may need to be modified or a different drug may need to be prescribed. The following drugs and drug classes interact with alpha-glucosidase inhibitors:

calcium channel blockers (eg, diltiazem) (acarbose only)
corticosteroids (eg, triamcinolone) (acarbose only)
digestive enzymes (eg, amylase)
digoxin (eg, *Lanoxin*)
estrogens (eg, *Premarin*) (acarbose only)
glyburide (eg, *Micronase*) (miglitol only)
insulin
intestinal adsorbents (eg, charcoal)

phenothiazines (eg, perphenazine) (acarbose only)
phenytoin (eg, *Dilantin*) (acarbose only)
propranolol (eg, *Inderal*) (miglitol only)
ranitidine (eg, *Zantac*) (miglitol only)
sulfonylureas (eg, glipizide) (miglitol only)
thiazide diuretics (eg, hydrochlorothiazide) (acarbose only)
thyroid supplements (acarbose only)

## Side Effects:

Every drug is capable of producing side effects. Many patients experience no, or minor, side effects. The frequency and severity of side effects depend on many factors including dose, duration of therapy, and individual susceptibility. Possible side effects include:

*Digestive Tract:* Stomach pain; diarrhea; gas.

*Other:* Abnormal blood or liver function tests; rash (miglitol only).

## Guidelines for Use:

- Dosage will be individualized on the basis of both effectiveness and tolerance. Take exactly as prescribed. Do not exceed the maximum recommended dosage of 100 mg 3 times daily or stop taking, unless advised by your doctor.
- Start with a low dose and increase gradually to reduce side effects and to identify the minimum dose needed for adequate glycemic control.
- Take 3 times daily at the start (with the first bite) of each main meal.
- Do not take a dose if you are going to skip a meal. If more than one dose is missed, contact your doctor or pharmacist.
- If side effects occur, they usually develop during the first few weeks of therapy. Side effects are commonly mild to moderate gastrointestinal (eg, diarrhea, gas, stomach pain) and generally diminish in frequency and intensity with time.
- Be sure to follow the diet, exercise, urine, and blood glucose testing programs prescribed by your doctor.
- This medicine alone does not cause low blood sugar levels, but it may increase the lowering of blood sugar caused by sulfonylureas or insulin. Because this medicine prevents the breakdown of table (cane) sugar, be sure to use glucose, not table sugar or fruits, to treat symptoms of low blood sugar (eg, fatigue, numbness in arms and legs). Contact your doctor if these symptoms occur.
- Lab tests will be required to monitor therapy. Be sure to keep appointments.
- Store acarbose below 77°F in a tightly closed container. Protect from moisture. Store miglitol between 59° and 86°F.

*If you have any questions, consult your doctor, pharmacist, or health care provider.*

| Generic Name<br>*Brand Name Example* | Supplied As | Generic<br>Available |
|---|---|---|
| Rx **Pioglitazone HCl** | | |
| *Actos* | **Tablets:** 15 mg, 30 mg, 45 mg | No |
| Rx **Rosiglitazone Maleate** | | |
| *Avandia* | **Tablets:** 2 mg, 4 mg, 8 mg | No |

## Type of Drug:

Oral antidiabetic (blood sugar lowering) agent used in the management of type 2 diabetes (adult-onset; non-insulin-dependent diabetes mellitus [NIDDM]) not adequately controlled with diet and exercise.

## How the Drug Works:

The thiazolidinedione hypoglycemic agents appear to lower blood sugar (glucose) by improving target cell response or sensitivity to insulin. They also decrease glucose output from the liver and increase insulin-dependent glucose disposal in skeletal muscle. They do not stimulate insulin production but lower tissue resistance (ie, increase sensitivity) to insulin.

## Uses:

Used alone or as an adjunct to diet and exercise to treat type 2 diabetes or in combination with a sulfonylurea or insulin, or metformin to improve glycemic control when diet, exercise, and a single diabetic drug do not accomplish adequate control of blood glucose levels.

## Precautions:

*Do not use in the following situations:*

allergy to a thiazolidinedione or any of its ingredients
diabetic ketoacidosis
liver disease, active
NYHA class III and IV cardiac status
type 1 diabetes mellitus

*Use with caution in the following situations:*

congestive heart failure
edema (fluid retention)
liver disease, history of
liver function test abnormalities, history of

*Pregnancy:* There are no adequate and well-controlled studies in pregnant women. Use only if clearly needed and potential benefits to the mother outweigh the possible hazard to the fetus. Most experts recommend that insulin be used to control diabetes during pregnancy.

*Breastfeeding:* It is not known if thiazolidinediones appear in breast milk. Do not administer to a nursing woman.

*Children:* Safety and effectiveness in patients under 18 years of age have not been established.

*Lab tests* will be required to monitor therapy. Tests may include blood glucose, glycosylated hemoglobin, and liver function.

## Drug Interactions:

Tell your doctor or pharmacist if you are taking or planning to take any over-the-counter or prescription medications or dietary supplements while taking thiazolidinediones. Doses of one or both drugs may need to be modified or a different drug may need to be prescribed. Insulin interacts with thiazolidinediones. The following drugs and drug classes interact with pioglitazone only:

azole antifungals (eg, ketocona-zole)

calcium channel blockers (eg, diltiazem)

contraceptives, oral (eg, *Ortho-Novum*) (pioglitazone only)

corticosteroids

cyclosporine (eg, *Neoral*)

erythromycin (eg, *E-Mycin*)

HMG-CoA reductase inhibitors (eg, lovastatin)

tacrolimus (*Prograf*)

triazolam (*Halcion*)

trimetrexate (*Neutrexin*)

## Side Effects:

Every drug is capable of producing side effects. Many thiazolidinedione users experience no, or minor, side effects. The frequency and severity of side effects depend on many factors including dose, duration of therapy, and individual susceptibility. Possible side effects include:

*Digestive Tract:* Nausea; diarrhea; weight gain.

*Other:* Headache; runny nose; sore throat; muscle or back pain; fluid retention; upper respiratory tract infection; elevated liver enzymes; dark urine; anemia; blood sugar changes; abnormal blood tests.

## Guidelines for Use:

- Dosage will be individualized. Take exactly as prescribed.
- Do not change the dose or stop taking unless advised by your doctor. This could have serious consequences.
- Take pioglitazone once daily without regard to meals.
- Take rosiglitazone as a single dose or divided into 2 doses. May be taken without regard to meals.
- Dietary restriction, weight loss (if obese), and exercise are essential to optimal management of diabetes and help improve insulin sensitivity. Follow your prescribed diet and exercise program closely.
- During periods of stress such as fever, trauma, infection, or surgery, medication requirements may change. Consult your doctor.
- Insulin, a sulfonylurea, or a metformin dose may need to be reduced if hypoglycemia occurs when starting a thiazolidinedione.
- Notify your doctor immediately if you experience nausea, vomiting, stomach pain, fatigue, appetite loss, dark urine, yellowing of skin or eyes.
- Talk to your doctor about low blood sugar risks, predisposing conditions, symptoms (eg, numbness, fatigue, hunger, sweating, rapid pulse, confusion) and treatment (administration of sugar-containing beverage or food) associated with combination therapy with insulin or other oral antidiabetic agents.
- Thiazolidinediones may cause ovulation in nonovulating premenopausal women. Talk to your doctor about adequate contraception.
- Pioglitazone may reduce the effectiveness of oral contraceptives (eg, *Ortho-Novum*). Talk to your doctor about an oral contraceptive with higher levels of estrogen and progestin or an alternative method of contraception.
- Lab tests will be required to monitor therapy. Be sure to keep appointments.
- Store at room temperature (59° to 86°F) in a tightly closed container. Protect from light and moisture.

*If you have any questions, consult your doctor, pharmacist, or health care provider.*

| Generic Name<br>*Brand Name Examples* | Supplied As | Generic<br>Available |
|---|---|---|
| *Rx* **Acetohexamide** | **Tablets:** 250 mg, 500 mg | Yes |
| *Rx* **Chlorpropamide** | | |
| *Diabinese* | **Tablets:** 100 mg, 250 mg | Yes |
| *Rx* **Glimepiride** | | |
| *Amaryl* | **Tablets:** 1 mg, 2 mg, 4 mg | No |
| *Rx* **Glipizide** | | |
| *Glucotrol* | **Tablets:** 5 mg, 10 mg | Yes |
| *Glucotrol XL* | **Tablets, extended release:**<br>2.5 mg, 5 mg, 10 mg | No |
| *Rx* **Glyburide<br>(Glibenclamide)** | | |
| *DiaBeta, Micronase* | **Tablets:** 1.25 mg, 2.5 mg, 5 mg | Yes |
| *Glynase PresTab* | **Tablets, micronized:** 1.5 mg,<br>3 mg, 4.5 mg, 6 mg | Yes |
| *Rx* **Tolazamide** | | |
| *Tolinase* | **Tablets:** 100 mg, 250 mg,<br>500 mg | Yes |
| *Rx* **Tolbutamide** | | |
| *Orinase* | **Tablets:** 500 mg | Yes |

All of the products listed on this table are sulfonylureas; however, they are not interchangeable. For example, glipizide cannot be used for tolazamide. Daily dose may vary depending on individual needs. Do not change the dose without consulting your doctor, pharmacist, or health care provider.

## Type of Drug:

Oral antidiabetic agents for use only as an adjunct to diet and exercise in the management of type 2 (non-insulin-dependent) diabetes mellitus.

## How the Drug Works:

The sulfonylurea hypoglycemic agents appear to decrease blood sugar by stimulating the release of insulin from the pancreas. Sulfonylureas may also decrease the amount of sugar that is dumped into the blood from the liver and may increase the sensitivity of fat and muscle tissue to the action of insulin. By increasing the amount of insulin or the effectiveness of insulin, blood sugar levels are lowered. Sulfonylureas do not work in type 1 (insulin-dependent) diabetes mellitus in which the pancreas is not capable of manufacturing or releasing insulin.

## Uses:

As an adjunct to diet and exercise to lower the blood glucose in patients with type 2 diabetes mellitus whose hyperglycemia cannot be controlled by diet and exercise alone. They may be used alone or combined with other blood sugar lowering medicines (eg, thiazolidinediones, metformin, insulin).

*Unlabeled Use(s):* Occasionally doctors may prescribe chlorpropamide for the treatment of neurogenic diabetes insipidus.

## Precautions:

*Do not use in the following situations:*

allergy to sulfa drugs
allergy to sulfonylureas or any of their ingredients
diabetes complicated by pregnancy

diabetes complicated by ketoacidosis (with or without coma)
insulin-dependent (type 1) diabetes, sole therapy

*Use with caution in the following situations:*

debilitation
elderly
gastrointestinal disease (glipizide extended-release only)

kidney disease
liver disease
malnutrition

*Alcohol:* A reaction may occur, including facial flushing, changes in blood sugar, and breathlessness, when alcohol is ingested. This occurs most often in patients taking chlorpropamide.

*Diet and exercise:* Diet and exercise are the primary management of type 2 diabetes. Sulfonylureas are used with, not as a substitute for, diet and exercise.

*Hyperglycemia (high blood sugar levels):* Hyperglycemia is a major risk factor in the development of diabetes complications. Maintaining blood sugar levels as close to normal as possible is important. Symptoms of hyperglycemia include excessive thirst or urination, nausea, and stomach upset.

*Hypoglycemia (low blood sugar levels):* Patients with kidney or liver problems or patients taking more than 1 blood glucose lowering medicine may be at higher risk for the development of medication-induced hypoglycemia. Symptoms include shaking, dizziness, faintness, headache, irritability, confusion, fatigue, excessive hunger, profuse sweating, numbness of arms or legs, and rapid pulse. May lead to convulsions or coma if extremely severe.

    To prevent hypoglycemia:
1. Understand the symptoms of low blood sugar levels.
2. Maintain an adequate diet. Do not miss meals.
3. Frequently monitor blood glucose levels.
4. Keep a source of quick-acting sugar with you at all times.
5. Know how exercise, alcohol, and other drugs affect your blood sugar level.

    Hypoglycemia is more of a problem with chlorpropamide than with other medications in this class. Discuss the expected results of your sulfonylurea therapy with your doctor, pharmacist, or diabetes educator. Know the onset of action, peak activity, and total duration of activity.

*Heart disease:* Long-term use of sulfonylureas has been associated with increased risk for development of heart problems compared with diet alone or diet plus insulin.

| Sulfonylureas | Doses/day | Onset (hrs) | Duration (hrs) |
|---|---|---|---|
| Acetohexamide | 1 to 2 | 1 | 12 to 24 |
| Chlorpropamide | 1 | 1 | 24 to 60 |
| Glimepiride | 1 | 2 to 3 | 24 |
| Glipizide | 1 to 2 | 1 to 3 | 10 to 24 |
| Glyburide, micronized | 1 to 2 | 1 | 12 to 24 |
| Glyburide, nonmicronized | 1 to 2 | 2 to 4 | 16 to 24 |
| Tolazamide | 1 | 4 to 6 | 12 to 24 |
| Tolbutamide | 2 to 3 | 1 | 6 to 12 |

*Pregnancy:* There are no adequate and well-controlled studies in pregnant women. Use only if clearly needed. In general, avoid sulfonylureas in pregnancy. They will not provide good control in patients whose blood glucose levels cannot be controlled by diet alone. Insulin is recommended to treat pregnant patients with diabetes to maintain blood glucose levels as close to normal as possible.

*Breastfeeding:* Chlorpropamide is excreted in breast milk. It is not known if other sulfonylureas appear in breast milk. Because of the potential for hypoglycemia in nursing infants, decide whether to discontinue nursing or discontinue the drug. Consult your doctor before you begin breastfeeding.

*Children:* Safety and effectiveness in children have not been established.

*Elderly:* Elderly, debilitated, or malnourished patients may be particularly sensitive to sulfonylureas. If there is a tendency toward hypoglycemia (low blood sugar levels), dosage will be reduced or therapy discontinued by your doctor. Use with caution.

*Lab tests* will be required to monitor therapy. Tests may include blood glucose, glycosylated hemoglobin, and kidney and liver function tests.

## Drug Interactions:
Tell your doctor or pharmacist if you are taking or if you are planning to take any over-the-counter or prescription medications or dietary supplements while taking sulfonylureas. Doses of one or both drugs may need to be modified or a different drug may need to be prescribed. The following drugs and drug classes interact with sulfonylureas:

| Decreased Glucose Lowering Effects | Increased Glucose Lowering Effects |
|---|---|
| calcium channel blockers (eg, verapamil) charcoal cholestyramine (eg, *Questran*) contraceptives, oral (eg, *Ortho-Novum*) corticosteroids (eg, prednisone) diazoxide (eg, *Proglycem*) estrogens (eg, oral contraceptives, estradiol) glucocorticoids (eg, prednisone) hydantoins (eg, phenytoin) isoniazid (eg, *Laniazid*) nicotinic acid (eg, *Nicobid*) phenothiazines (eg, chlorpromazine) rifampin (eg, *Rifadin*) sympathomimetics (eg, epinephrine) thiazide diuretics (eg, hydrochlorothiazide) thyroid agents (eg, levothyroxine sodium) urinary alkalinizers (eg, sodium bicarbonate) | androgens (eg, testosterone) anticoagulants, oral (eg, warfarin) azole antifungals (eg, ketoconazole) beta adrenergic blockers (eg, propranolol) chloramphenicol (eg, *Chloromycetin*) clofibrate (eg, *Atromid-S*) fenfluramine (*Pondimin*) gemfibrozil (*Lopid*) histamine $H_2$ antagonists (eg, cimetidine) magnesium salts (eg, *Magonate*) MAOIs (eg, phenelzine) methyldopa (eg, *Aldomet*) probenecid (eg, *Benemid*) salicylates, large doses (eg, aspirin) sulfinpyrazone (eg, *Anturane*) sulfonamides (eg, sulfisoxazole) tricyclic antidepressants (eg, doxepin HCl) urinary acidifiers (eg, ammonium chloride) |

Other: Digitalis glycosides (eg, digoxin); ciprofloxacin (eg, *Cipro*); ethanol; barbiturates (eg, phenobarbital).

## Side Effects:

Every drug is capable of producing side effects. Many sulfonylurea users experience no, or minor, side effects. The frequency and severity of side effects depend on many factors including dose, duration of therapy, and individual susceptibility. Possible side effects include:

*Digestive Tract:* Nausea; heartburn; feeling of fullness; diarrhea; vomiting; appetite loss; taste alteration (tolbutamide only); gas; constipation; stomach pain; indigestion; hunger.

*Nervous System:* Weakness; dizziness; headache; abnormal skin sensations; drowsiness; nervousness; tremor; sleeplessness; anxiety; depression; decreased sensitivity to stimulation; confusion.

*Skin:* Yellowing of the skin or eyes; rash; hives; dry, red skin; itching; sensitivity to sunlight; sweating.

*Other:* Abnormal blood counts and blood tests; pain; dark urine; leg cramps; fainting; joint or muscle pain; runny nose; blurred vision; excessive urination; low blood sugar.

## Guidelines for Use:

- Dosage is individualized. Do not change dose or stop taking this medicine unless advised to do so by your doctor.
- Follow the diet and exercise program and personal hygiene and infection avoidance regimens exactly as prescribed by your doctor.
- May be taken with food if stomach upset occurs. Always take immediate-release glipizide 30 minutes prior to a meal to increase effectiveness.
- Avoid alcohol. It can cause flushing, breathlessness, and changes in blood sugar.
- Avoid aspirin in large doses.
- Get specific instructions from your doctor on how to examine your feet for complications of diabetes. In addition, obtain equipment for and learn the correct process of home glucose monitoring.
- Monitor blood sugar levels as recommended by your doctor. Notify your doctor if you experience low blood sugar symptoms (eg, fatigue, excessive hunger, profuse sweating, numbness of arms or legs, rapid pulse, confusion) or high blood sugar symptoms (eg, bad breath, excessive thirst or urination).
- Diet and exercise are the primary managements of type 2 diabetes. These medications should be used with, not as a substitute for, diet and exercise.
- *To prevent hypoglycemia* — Understand the symptoms of low blood sugar levels. Maintain an adequate diet. Do not miss meals. Know how exercise, alcohol, and other drugs affect blood sugar levels.
- During periods of stress such as fever, trauma, infection, or surgery, medication requirements may change. Consult your doctor.
- Long-term use of sulfonylureas may be associated with increased heart problems when compared with diet treatment alone, or diet plus insulin. Patients with heart problems or concern about heart problems should consult their doctor.
- *Glipizide, extended-release* — Do not crush, chew, or divide tablets. Do not be alarmed if the tablet shell appears in the stool. This drug is designed to slowly release the medicine and then expel the empty shell from the body.
- May cause sensitivity to sunlight. Avoid prolonged exposure to the sun. Use sunscreens and wear protective clothing until tolerance is determined.
- May cause drowsiness or dizziness. Use caution while driving or performing other tasks requiring alertness, coordination, or physical dexterity.
- Lab tests will be required to monitor therapy. Be sure to keep appointments.
- Store at controlled room temperature. Protect from moisture.

*If you have any questions, consult your doctor, pharmacist, or health care provider.*

| Generic Name<br>*Brand Name Examples* | Supplied As | Generic<br>Available |
|---|---|---|
| Rx **Nateglinide** | | |
| *Starlix* | **Tablets**: 60 mg, 120 mg | No |
| Rx **Repaglinide** | | |
| *Prandin* | **Tablets:** 0.5 mg, 1 mg, 2 mg | No |

## Type of Drug:

Oral nonsulfonylurea blood-glucose-lowering drugs for management of type 2 diabetes mellitus (previously known as non-insulin-dependent diabetes mellitus [NIDDM]).

## How the Drug Works:

Meglitinides lower blood glucose levels by stimulating the release of insulin from functioning beta cells of the pancreas.

## Uses:

To treat high blood glucose, in addition to diet and exercise, in patients with type 2 diabetes mellitus whose blood sugar cannot be controlled by diet and exercise alone.

To treat high blood glucose in combination with metformin (*Glucophage*) when blood sugar cannot be controlled by exercise, diet, and either a meglitinide or metformin alone.

## Precautions:

*Do not use in the following situations:*

allergy to the meglitinide or any of its ingredients
diabetic ketoacidosis with or without coma
type 1 diabetes (previously known as insulin-dependent diabetes)

*Use with caution in the following situations:*

adrenal or pituitary insufficiency
debilitation or malnourishment
liver disease, moderate to severe
loss of blood sugar control
low blood sugar

*Diet and exercise:* Diet and exercise are the primary managements of type 2 diabetes. Meglitinides are used with, not as a substitute for, diet and exercise.

*Heart problems:* Meglitinides may increase the risk of heart problems, compared with treatment with diet alone or diet plus insulin.

*Pregnancy:* There are no adequate and well-controlled studies in pregnant women. Use only if clearly needed and the potential benefits to the mother outweigh the possible hazards to the fetus.

*Breastfeeding:* It is not known if meglitinides appear in breast milk. Consult your doctor before you begin breastfeeding.

*Children:* Safety and effectiveness in children have not been established.

*Lab tests* will be required during treatment. Tests may include blood glucose and glycosylated hemoglobin $HbA_{1c}$ levels.

## Drug Interactions:

Tell your doctor or pharmacist if you are taking or planning to take any over-the-counter or prescription medications or dietary supplements while taking a meglitinide. Doses of one or both drugs may need to be modified, or a different drug may need to be prescribed. The following drugs and drug classes interact with meglitinides:

antibacterial agents (eg, chlor-amphenicol, erythromycin, isoniazid, rifampin, sulfon-amides)

antifungal agents (eg, ketocona-zole, miconazole)

barbiturates (eg, phenobarbital)

beta-adrenergic blocking agents (eg, atenolol)

calcium channel blockers (eg, verapamil)

carbamazepine (eg, *Tegretol*)

corticosteroids (eg, hydrocorti-sone, prednisone)

coumarin derivatives (eg, warfarin)

diuretics (eg, thiazides)

estrogens (eg, oral contracep-tives, estradiol)

MAO inhibitors (eg, phenelzine)

NSAIDs (eg, ibuprofen)

phenothiazines (eg, *Thorazine*)

phenytoin (eg, *Dilantin*)

probenecid

salicylates (eg, aspirin)

sympathomimetics (eg, pseudo-ephedrine)

thyroid agents

## Side Effects:

Every drug is capable of producing side effects. Many meglitinide users experience no, or minor, side effects. The frequency and severity of side effects depend on many factors including dose, duration of therapy, and individual susceptibility. Possible side effects include:

*Digestive Tract:* Nausea; diarrhea; constipation; vomiting; indigestion.

*Respiratory System:* Chest or head congestion; bronchitis; sinus inflammation; upper respiratory tract infection; cough.

*Other:* Abnormal skin sensations; changes in blood sugar; joint, chest, or back pain; headache; urinary tract infection; flu-like symptoms; dizziness; accidental trauma; heart problems (eg, high blood pressure, abnormal heart rhythm, pounding in the chest).

## Guidelines for Use:

- Dosage is individualized. Take exactly as prescribed.
- Do not change the dose or stop taking this medicine unless advised to do so by your doctor.
- Take nateglinide 1 to 30 minutes before a meal. Take repaglinide 15 to 30 minutes before a meal.
- Meglitinides stimulate pancreatic insulin secretion within 20 to 30 minutes of oral administration. Peak insulin levels are attained about 1 hour after dosing and return to baseline within about 4 hours after dosing.
- When a meglitinide is used to replace therapy with another oral hypoglycemic agent, it may be started the day after the final dose is given. Closely monitor for hypoglycemia because of a potential overlapping drug effect (particularly with long-acting sulfonylureas [eg, chlorpropamide]).
- Treatment may need to be adjusted. Your doctor will monitor your treatment for the first few weeks of therapy.
- Patients who skip a meal (or add an extra meal) should skip (or add) a dose for that meal. Contact your doctor or pharmacist if you miss a dose.
- Repaglinide may be taken in combination with metformin. One or both dosages may need to be adjusted.
- Follow the diet and exercise program exactly as prescribed by your doctor.
- Diabetic patients may experience loss of glucose control. Be prepared to monitor blood sugar more often.
- Monitor blood glucose levels daily. Notify your doctor if symptoms of hypoglycemia occur (eg, fatigue, excessive hunger, profuse sweating, numbness of extremities) or if blood glucose is below 60 mg/dL. Notify your doctor if symptoms of hyperglycemia occur (eg, bad breath, excessive thirst or urination) or if blood glucose is consistently above 200 mg/dL.
- Lab tests are required to monitor treatment. Be sure to keep appointments.
- Store below 77°F. Protect from moisture. Keep in tightly closed container.

*If you have any questions, consult your doctor, pharmacist, or health care provider.*

| Generic Name<br>*Brand Name Examples* | **Supplied As** | Generic<br>Available |
|---|---|---|
| *Rx* **Metformin HCl** | | |
| *Glucophage* | **Tablets**: 500 mg, 850 mg, 1000 mg | No |
| *Glucophage XR* | **Tablets, extended-release**: 500 mg | No |

## Type of Drug:

Oral nonsulfoylurea antidiabetic agent used in the treatment of type 2 diabetes mellitus (previously referred to as non-insulin-dependent diabetes mellitus [NIDDM]).

## How the Drug Works:

Metformin reduces the amount of glucose produced by the liver and the amount of glucose absorbed by the intestines, and enhances insulin sensitivity by increasing peripheral glucose uptake and utilization.

## Uses:

Used as monotherapy along with diet and exercise to treat type 2 diabetes mellitus. May also be prescribed for use with a sulfonylurea, meglitinide, or insulin.

## Precautions:

*Do not use in the following situations:*

allergy to metformin or any of its ingredients
congestive heart failure
diabetic ketoacidosis
kidney disease or dysfunction
metabolic acidosis, acute or chronic
radiologic studies involving "dyes"

*Use with caution in the following situations:*

alcohol use
elderly
heart disease
infections
liver disease
stroke
surgery
vitamin $B_{12}$, decreased levels

*Lactic acidosis:* Lactic acidosis is a rare but serious side effect that can occur when taking this medication, particularly if kidney function is impaired. Stop taking this medicine and contact your doctor immediately if you experience general body discomfort, muscle pain, difficulty breathing, drowsiness, stomach pain, chills, dizziness, lightheadedness, or slow heartbeat.

*Diet and exercise:* Diet and exercise are the primary managements of type 2 diabetes. Metformin is used with, not as a substitute for, diet and exercise.

*Heart problems:* This medicine may increase the risk of heart problems compared to treatment with diet alone or diet plus insulin.

*Pregnancy:* There are no adequate and well-controlled studies in pregnant women. Pregnant women with diabetes should be treated with insulin. Metformin is not recommended for control of blood sugar levels in pregnant women.

*Breastfeeding:* It is not known if metformin appears in breast milk. Consult your doctor before you begin breastfeeding.

*Children:* Safety and effectiveness for use of metformin tablets in patients under 10 years of age and metformin extended-release tablets in patients under 17 years of age have not been established.

*Elderly:* Elderly and debilitated patients are more likely to develop hypoglycemia (low blood sugar levels). Use with caution.

*Lab tests* will be required to monitor therapy. Tests include blood glucose, glycosylated hemoglobin ($HbA_{1c}$), and kidney function tests.

## Drug Interactions:

Tell your doctor or pharmacist if you are taking or planning to take any over-the-counter or prescription medications or dietary supplements while taking metformin. Doses of one or both drugs may need to be modified or a different drug may need to be prescribed. The following drugs and drug classes interact with metformin:

alcohol (acute or chronic use)
amiloride (*Midamor*)
calcium channel blockers
 (eg, nifedipine)
cimetidine (eg, *Tagamet*)
corticosteroids (eg, prednisone)
digoxin (eg, *Lanoxin*)
diuretics (eg, thiazides)
estrogens (eg, oral contraceptives, estradiol)
furosemide (eg, *Lasix*)
iodinated contrast material
 (eg, x-ray dye)
isoniazid
morphine (eg, *Duramorph*)
nicotinic acid (eg, *Niacor*)
phenothiazines (eg, chlorpromazine)
phenytoin (eg, *Dilantin*)
procainamide (eg, *Pronestyl*)
quinidine (eg, *Quinora*)
quinine
ranitidine (eg, *Zantac*)
sympathomimetics (eg, epinephrine)
thyroid products
triamterene (*Dyrenium*)
trimethorprim (eg, *Trimpex*)
vancomycin (eg, *Vancocin*)

## Side Effects:

Every drug is capable of producing side effects. Many metformin users experience no, or minor, side effects. The frequency or severity of side effects depend on many factors including dose, duration of therapy, and individual susceptibility. Possible side effects include:

*Digestive Tract:* Diarrhea; nausea; vomiting; stomach bloating or pain; gas; constipation; indigestion; abnormal stools; heartburn.

*Nervous System:* Light-headedness; headache; weakness; dizziness.

*Other:* Changes in taste perception; rash; difficulty breathing; increased sweating; low blood pressure; muscle pain; upper respiratory infection; chest discomfort; chills; flu-like symptoms; flushing; palpitations (pounding in the chest).

## Guidelines for Use:

- Dosage is individualized. Take exactly as prescribed. May be taken with other antidiabetic medication.
- Tablets are usually taken twice daily with the morning and evening meals. Extended-release tablets are usually taken once daily with the evening meal.
- Follow the diet and exercise program exactly as prescribed by your doctor.
- If a dose is missed, take it as soon as possible. If several hours have passed or it is nearing time for the next dose, do not double the dose to catch up, unless advised to do so by your doctor. If more than one dose is missed or it is necessary to establish a new dosage schedule, contact your doctor or pharmacist.
- Contact your doctor immediately if you experience difficulty breathing, muscle pain, general body discomfort, drowsiness, dizziness, light-headedness, slow heartbeat, stomach pain, or chills.
- Nausea, vomiting, diarrhea, gas, and appetite loss generally stop with continued use. If they continue, contact your doctor immediately.
- Avoid drinking alcohol while undergoing therapy with metformin.
- The effectiveness of this medicine may decrease over time. If you feel that it is losing its effectiveness, contact your doctor.
- Patients switched from metformin tablets to extended-release tablets do not appear to require dosage adjustments, but glycemic control should be closely monitored when switches occur.
- Lab tests will be required to monitor therapy. Be sure to keep appointments.
- Store at room temperature (59° to 86°F).

*If you have any questions, consult your doctor, pharmacist, or health care provider.*

| Generic Name<br>*Brand Name Example* | Supplied As | Generic<br>Available |
|---|---|---|
| *Rx* **Glyburide/Metformin HCl** | | |
| *Glucovance* | **Tablets**: 1.25 mg/250 mg,<br>2.5 mg/500 mg, 5 mg/500 mg | No |

## Type of Drug:

Combination oral antidiabetic agent used in the treatment of type 2 diabetes mellitus (previously referred to as non-insulin-dependent diabetes mellitus [NIDDM]).

## How the Drug Works:

Glyburide stimulates the release of insulin from the pancreas acutely and lowers glucose chronically by unknown mechanisms. Metformin reduces the amount of sugar produced by the liver and the amount absorbed by the intestines and enhances insulin sensitivity.

## Uses:

Used as initial therapy, along with diet and exercise, to treat type 2 diabetes. Also used as second-line therapy when diet, exercise, and initial treatment with a sulfonylurea or metformin used alone is not sufficient.

## Precautions:

*Do not use in the following situations:*

allergy to glyburide, metformin, or any of their ingredients
congestive heart failure
diabetic ketoacidosis
kidney disease or dysfunction
metabolic acidosis, acute or chronic
radiologic studies involving "dyes"

*Use with caution in the following situations:*

alcohol use
elderly
heart disease
infections
liver disease
stroke
surgery
vitamin $B_{12}$, decreased levels

*Lactic acidosis:* Lactic acidosis is a rare but serious side effect that can occur when taking this medication, particularly if kidney function is impaired. Stop taking this medicine and contact your doctor immediately if you experience general body discomfort, muscle pain, difficulty breathing, drowsiness, stomach pain, chills, dizziness, lightheadedness, or slow heartbeat.

*Diet and exercise:* Diet and exercise are the primary managements of type 2 diabetes. Glyburide/metformin is used with, not as a substitute for, diet and exercise.

*Heart problems:* This medicine may increase the risk of heart problems compared to treatment with diet alone or diet plus insulin.

*Pregnancy:* There are no adequate and well-controlled studies in pregnant women. Pregnant women with diabetes should be treated with insulin. Glyburide/metformin is not recommended for control of blood sugar levels in pregnant women.

*Breastfeeding:* It is not known if glyburide/metformin appears in breast milk. Consult your doctor before you begin breastfeeding.

*Children:* Safety and effectiveness in children have not been established.

*Elderly:* Elderly and debilitated patients are more likely to develop hypoglycemia (low blood sugar levels). Use with caution.

*Lab tests* will be required to monitor therapy. Tests include blood glucose, glycosylated hemoglobin ($HbA_{1c}$), and kidney function tests.

## Drug Interactions:

Tell your doctor or pharmacist if you are taking or planning to take any over-the-counter or prescription medications or dietary supplements while taking glyburide/metformin. Doses of one or both drugs may need to be modified or a different drug may need to be prescribed. The following drugs and drug classes interact with glyburide/metformin:

alcohol (acute or chronic use)
amiloride (*Midamor*)
beta-adrenergic blocking agents
(atenolol)
calcium channel blockers
(eg, nifedipine)
chloramphenicol (eg, *Chloromycetin*)
cimetidine (eg, *Tagamet*)
ciprofloxacin (*Cipro*)
clofibrate (eg, *Atromid-S*)
corticosteroids (eg, prednisone)
coumarin derivatives
(eg, warfarin)
diazoxide (eg, *Proglycem*)
digoxin (eg, *Lanoxin*)
diuretics (eg, thiazides)
estrogens (eg, oral contraceptives, estradiol)
furosemide (eg, *Lasix*)
iodinated contrast material
(eg, x-ray dye)
isoniazid
MAO inhibitors (eg, phenelzine)
miconazole (eg, *Monistat*)
morphine (eg, *Duramorph*)
nicotinic acid (eg, *Niacor*)
NSAIDs (eg, ibuprofen)
phenothiazines (eg, chlorpromazine)
phenylbutazones (eg, oxyphenbutazone)
phenytoin (eg, *Dilantin*)
probenecid
procainamide (eg, *Pronestyl*)
quinidine (eg, *Quinora*)
quinine
ranitidine (eg, *Zantac*)
rifampin (eg, *Rifadin*)
salicylates (eg, aspirin)
sulfonamides (eg, sulfisoxazole)
sympathomimetics
(eg, epinephrine)
thyroid products
triamterene (*Dyrenium*)
trimethorprim (eg, *Trimpex*)
vancomycin (eg, *Vancocin*)

## Side Effects:

Every drug is capable of producing side effects. Many glyburide/metformin users experience no, or minor, side effects. The frequency or severity of side effects depend on many factors including dose, duration of therapy, and individual susceptibility. Possible side effects include:

*Nervous System:* Chills; drowsiness; light-headedness; headache; dizziness; shakiness.

*Digestive Tract:* Diarrhea; nausea; vomiting; stomach pain.

*Other:* Upper respiratory infection; difficulty breathing; muscle pain; rash; changes in taste perception; low blood pressure; sweating; hunger.

## Guidelines for Use:

- Dosage is individualized. Take exactly as prescribed.
- Take with meals.
- Follow the diet and exercise program exactly as prescribed by your doctor.
- If a dose is missed, take it as soon as possible. If several hours have passed or it is nearing time for the next dose, do not double the dose to catch up, unless advised to do so by your doctor. If more than one dose is missed or it is necessary to establish a new dosage schedule, contact your doctor or pharmacist.
- Contact your doctor immediately if you experience difficulty breathing, muscle pain, general body discomfort, drowsiness, dizziness, light-headedness, slow heartbeat, stomach pain, or chills.
- Nausea, vomiting, and diarrhea generally stop with continued use. If they continue, contact your doctor immediately.
- Avoid drinking alcohol while undergoing therapy with glyburide/metformin.
- The effectiveness of this medicine may decrease over time. If you feel that it is losing its effectiveness, contact your doctor.
- Lab tests will be required to monitor therapy. Be sure to keep appointments.
- Store below 77°F. Protect from light.

*If you have any questions, consult your doctor, pharmacist, or health care provider.*

| Generic Name<br>*Brand Name Examples* | Supplied As | Generic<br>Available |
|---|---|---|
| *Rx* **Glucagon (rDNA Origin)** | | |
| *Glucagon Diagnostic Kit,*<br>*Glucagon Emergency Kit* | **Injection**: 1 mg (1 unit) | Yes |

## Type of Drug:
A blood glucose (sugar) elevating agent.

## How the Drug Works:
Glucagon is a natural hormone that is released from the pancreas. It elevates blood sugar in a variety of ways (eg, inhibition of glucogen synthesis, enhanced formation of glucose from noncarbohydrates and fat, increased hydrolysis of glucogen to glucose).

## Uses:
Used to treat severe hypoglycemia (low blood glucose levels). Because patients with type 1 diabetes may have less of an increase in blood glucose levels compared with a stable type 2 diabetes patient, a supplementary carbohydrate should be given as soon as possible, especially to a pediatric patient.

Used as a diagnostic aid in the x-ray examination of the stomach, duodenum, small intestine, and colon when decreased intestinal motility is desired.

*Unlabeled Use(s):* Occasionally doctors may prescribe glucagon for treatment of an overdose of propranolol and in cardiovascular emergencies (eg, severely reduced heart rates).

## Precautions:
*Do not use in the following situations:* Allergy to glucagon or any of its ingredients.

*Use with caution in the following situations:*
      pheochromocytoma, active or history of
      tumor of the pancreas, history of

*Hypoglycemia (low blood sugar levels):* Although glucagon may be used for emergency treatment of low blood sugar levels, notify your doctor so that adjustments in insulin dose and dietary factors can be made. In addition, patients should be given food after they become conscious and alert. Frequently self monitor blood glucose so that blood sugar levels are not allowed to get too low.

*Pregnancy:* There are no adequate and well-controlled studies in pregnant women. Use only if clearly needed and the potential benefits to the mother outweigh the possible hazards to the fetus.

*Breastfeeding:* It is not known if glucagon appears in breast milk. Consult your doctor before you begin breastfeeding.

*Children:* Safety and effectiveness for use in the treatment of hypoglycemia in children have been established.

*Lab tests* will be required to monitor therapy. Tests include blood glucose levels.

## Drug Interactions:

Tell your doctor or pharmacist if you are taking or planning to take any over-the-counter or prescription medications or dietary supplements while taking glucagon. Doses of one or both drugs may need to be modified or a different drug may need to be prescribed. Oral anticoagulants (eg, warfarin) interact with glucagon.

## Side Effects:

Every drug is capable of producing side effects. Many glucagon users experience no, or minor, side effects. The frequency and severity of side effects depend on many factors including dose, duration of therapy, and individual susceptibility. Possible side effects include: Nausea; vomiting; hives; low blood pressure; difficulty breathing.

---

### Guidelines for Use:

- Carefully read the patient instructions provided with the product.
- All patients with diabetes should have a *Glucagon Emergency Kit.*
- *Low blood sugar (conscious patient)* — Consume fast-acting sugars (eg, *B-D Glucose, Glutose*).
- *Low blood sugar (unconscious patient)* — Intravenous (IV; into a vein) glucose use is encouraged, if available and feasible. If not, glucagon is the treatment of choice. Instruct friends, coworkers, and family members of patients with diabetes how to administer glucagon. Prompt treatment is essential.
- The patient will usually awaken within 15 minutes of glucagon use. If not, repeat the dose. Upon awakening, give the patient food (ie, a carbohydrate) as soon as possible and follow the usual dietary regimen.
- The glucagon emergency kit has a diluting fluid in a unit (one) dose syringe. This diluting fluid is injected into a vial of the glucagon crystals. The vial is then shaken and the contents brought back into the syringe. The glucagon crystals now in the diluting fluid are given IV, intramuscularly (IM; into a muscle), or subcutaneously (SC; under the skin).
- Notify your doctor if you experience a hypoglycemic reaction so that your treatment regimen may be adjusted if necessary.
- Lab tests will be required. Be sure to keep appointments.
- Store at controlled room temperature (68° to 77° F) before mixing with the diluting fluid.
- Use glucagon immediately after it has been mixed with the diluting fluid because the drug is stable for only a short time. Discard any unused portion.

---

*If you have any questions, consult your doctor, pharmacist, or health care provider.*

| Generic Name<br>*Brand Name Examples* | Supplied As | Generic<br>Available |
|---|---|---|
| *Rx* **Methimazole** | | |
| *Tapazole* | **Tablets**: 5 mg, 10 mg | Yes |
| *Rx* **Propylthiouracil (PTU)** | **Tablets**: 50 mg | Yes |
| *Rx* **Sodium Iodide I 131** | **Capsules**: 0.75 to 100 mCi | Yes |
| | **Solution, oral**: 3.5 to 150 mCi | Yes |
| *Iodotope* | **Capsules**: 1 to 130 mCi | No |
| *Iodotope* | **Solution, oral**: 7.05 mCi | No |

## Type of Drug:
Antithyroid drugs.

## How the Drug Works:
The oral antithyroid drugs inhibit the formation of thyroid hormones.

## Uses:
To treat hyperthyroidism (overactive thyroid gland). To treat or prepare the overactive thyroid for surgery or radioactive iodine therapy. Sodium iodide I 131 preparations may be used to treat certain forms of thyroid cancer.

*Unlabeled Use(s):* Occasionally doctors may prescribe propylthiouracil to treat liver disease due to alcoholism.

## Precautions:
*Do not use in the following situations:*
allergy to the antithyroid agent or any of its ingredients
breastfeeding

*Pregnancy:* Studies have shown a potential adverse effect to the fetus. Use only if clearly needed and the potential benefits to the mother outweigh the possible hazards to the fetus. These agents, if used carefully, are effective in treating hyperthyroidism complicated by pregnancy. Dose must be adequate but not excessive. These drugs cross the placenta and could induce goiter or even cretinism (congenital lack of thyroid secretion which can stop physical and mental development) in the fetus. Propylthiouracil is less likely than methimazole to cross the placenta.

*Breastfeeding:* Patients receiving antithyroid preparations should not breastfeed.

*Children:* Safety and effectiveness of sodium iodide I 131 in children have not been established. Sodium iodide I 131 is not usually used for treatment of hyperthyroidism in patients under 30 years of age unless circumstances preclude other methods of treatment.

*Lab tests* will be required to monitor therapy. Tests include blood counts, bone marrow function, and thyroid function.

## Drug Interactions:

Tell your doctor or pharmacist if you are taking or planning to take any over-the-counter or prescription medications or dietary supplements while taking an antithyroid agent. Doses of one or both drugs may need to be modified or a different drug may need to be prescribed. The following drugs or drug classes interact with antithyroid agents:

anticoagulants (eg, warfarin)  
beta-adrenergic blocking agents (eg, atenolol)

digoxin (eg, *Lanoxin*)  
theophylline (eg, *Slo-Phyllin*)

## Side Effects:

Every drug is capable of producing side effects. Many antithyroid agent users experience no, or minor, side effects. The frequency and severity of side effects depend on many factors including dose, duration of therapy, and individual susceptibility. Possible side effects include:

*Digestive Tract:* Nausea; vomiting; stomach upset or pain; loss of taste sensation; swelling of salivary glands.

*Nervous System:* Abnormal skin sensations; headache; drowsiness; depression; feeling of whirling motion; hyperactivity.

*Skin:* Unusual bleeding or bruising; rash; itching; hives; excessive skin pigmentation; yellowing of skin or eyes; abnormal hair loss.

*Other:* Joint or muscle pain; fever; fluid retention (edema); swollen lymph glands; abnormal blood counts; kidney disease; lung disease; liver disease; low blood sugar.

*Other: Sodium iodide I 131 only:* Radiation sickness (eg, nausea, vomiting); anemia; chromosomal abnormalities; tenderness and swelling of the neck; pain on swallowing; sore throat; cough; temporary thinning of hair.

## Guidelines for Use:

- Dosage is individualized. Take exactly as prescribed.
- Do not change the dose or stop taking this medicine unless advised to do so by your doctor.
- Take methimazole or propylthiouracil at regular intervals around the clock (usually every 8 hours), unless directed otherwise by your doctor.
- Notify your doctor if fever, sore throat, hay fever, unusual bleeding or bruising, headache, general body discomfort, rash, yellowing of the skin, vomiting, itching, appetite loss, skin surface changes, or pain in the upper right side of your body occurs.
- If a dose of methimazole or propylthiouracil is missed, take it as soon as possible. If several hours have passed or it is nearing time for the next dose, do not double the dose to catch up, unless advised to do so by your doctor. If more than one dose is missed or it is necessary to establish a new dosage schedule, contact your doctor or pharmacist.
- Lab tests will be required to monitor therapy. Be sure to keep appointments.
- Store methimazole or propylthiouracil at room temperature (59° to 86°F). Store sodium iodide I 131 at room temperature controlled in compliance with government regulations.

*If you have any questions, consult your doctor, pharmacist, or health care provider.*

| Generic Name<br>*Brand Name Examples* | Supplied As | Generic<br>Available |
|---|---|---|
| *Rx* **Iodine Products** | | |
| *Strong Iodine Solution*<br>*(Lugol's Solution)* | **Solution**: 5% iodine and 10% potassium iodide | No |
| *Thyro-Block*[1] | **Tablets**: 130 mg potassium iodide | No |

[1] Available only to state and federal agencies.

## Type of Drug:
Iodine drugs.

## How the Drug Works:
Iodine intake is necessary for normal thyroid function and the synthesis of thyroid hormones levothyroxine ($T_4$) and liothyronine ($T_3$). Adequate iodine is generally consumed with a balanced diet.

Extremely large doses of iodine may, however, decrease the synthesis and release of the thyroid hormones. This effect forms the basis for using large doses of iodine to treat an overactive thyroid gland (hyperthyroidism).

## Uses:
For use with an antithyroid drug in hyperthyroid patients prior to thyroid surgery or to treat an overactive thyroid gland.

To block the thyroid gland during a radiation emergency (eg, radioactive fallout).

*Unlabeled Use(s):* Occasionally, doctors may prescribe potassium iodide with topical steroids to treat Sweet disease (acute febrile neutrophilic dermatosis), to treat lymphocutaneous sporotrichosis (a fungus that infects the skin and lymphatic system), or as an expectorant for cough.

## Precautions:
*Do not use in the following situations:* Allergy to the iodine product or any of its ingredients.

*Pregnancy:* Studies have shown a potential risk to the fetus. Use only if clearly needed and the potential benefits to the mother outweigh the possible hazards to the fetus.

*Breastfeeding:* Iodine products appear in breast milk. Consult your doctor before you begin breastfeeding.

## Drug Interactions:
Tell your doctor or pharmacist if you are taking or planning to take any over-the-counter or prescription medications or dietary supplements while taking an iodine product. Doses of one or both drugs may need to be modified or a different drug may need to be prescribed. Lithium (eg, *Eskalith*) interacts with iodine products.

## Side Effects:

Every drug is capable of producing side effects. Many iodine product users experience no, or minor, side effects. The frequency and severity of side effects depend on many factors including dose, duration of therapy, and individual susceptibility. Possible side effects include:

*Digestive Tract:* Swelling of the salivary glands; metallic taste; burning mouth and throat; sore teeth and gums; upset stomach; diarrhea.

*Respiratory System:* Symptoms of a head cold; shortness of breath.

*Other:* Rash; fever; joint pain; swelling of parts of the face and body.

---

### Guidelines for Use:

- Use exactly as prescribed.
- *Strong iodine solution*— Dilute with water or fruit juice to improve taste.
- *Thyroid surgery*— Oral iodine-containing products are usually given for 10 days prior to surgery.
- Discontinue use and notify your doctor if fever, skin rash, metallic taste, swelling of the throat, burning of the mouth and throat, sore teeth and gums, head cold symptoms, severe stomach distress, diarrhea, shortness of breath or enlargement of the thyroid gland (goiter) occurs.
- If a dose is missed, take it as soon as possible. If several hours have passed or if it is nearing time for the next dose, do not double the dose in order to "catch up" (unless advised to do so by your doctor). If more than one dose is missed or if it is necessary to establish a new dosage schedule, contact your doctor or pharmacist.
- *Recommended Dietary Allowances (RDA)* — Adults: 150 mcg.
- If crystals are present in the solution, dissolve by warming the solution and shaking gently.
- Discard solution if it becomes discolored (eg, brownish yellow).
- Store at room temperature in a tight container. Do not freeze.

---

*If you have any questions, consult your doctor, pharmacist, or health care provider.*

| Generic Name<br>*Brand Name Examples* | Supplied As | Generic<br>Available |
|---|---|---|
| Rx **Thyroid Desiccated**<br>*Armour Thyroid, Thyrar,*<br>*Thyroid Strong* | **Tablets:** 15 mg, 30 mg, 60 mg,<br>90 mg, 120 mg, 180 mg,<br>240 mg, 300 mg | Yes |
| *Thyroid Strong* | **Tablets, sugar coated:** 30 mg,<br>60 mg, 120 mg, 180 mg | No |
| *S-P-T* | **Capsules:** 60 mg, 120 mg,<br>180 mg, 300 mg | No |
| Rx **Levothyroxine Sodium**<br>**($T_4$; L-thyroxine)**<br>*Eltroxin, Levothroid,*<br>*Levoxyl, Levo-T, Synthroid* | **Tablets:** 0.025 mg, 0.05 mg,<br>0.075 mg, 0.088 mg, 0.1 mg,<br>0.112 mg, 0.125 mg, 0.137 mg,<br>0.15 mg, 0.175 mg, 0.2 mg,<br>0.3 mg | Yes |
| *Levothroid, Levoxine,*<br>*Synthroid* | **Injection:** 200 mcg/vial,<br>500 mcg/vial | Yes |
| Rx **Liothyronine Sodium**<br>**($T_3$)**<br>*Cytomel* | **Tablets:** 5 mcg, 25 mcg,<br>50 mcg | Yes |
| *Triostat* | **Injection:** 10 mcg/vial | No |
| Rx **Liotrix**<br>*Thyrolar* | **Tablets:** 15 mg, 30 mg, 60 mg,<br>120 mg, 180 mg | No |

*Note:* 16 mg equals grain; 32 mg equals grain; 65 mg equals 1 grain.

## Type of Drug:

Thyroid hormones.

## How the Drug Works:

The natural thyroid hormone products (eg, desiccated thyroid and thyro-globulin) are obtained from beef and pork. They are economical, but standardization of iodine content is difficult. The synthetic products, including levothyroxine ($T_4$), liothyronine ($T_3$) and liotrix ($T_3$ and $T_4$), are generally preferred due to more uniform potency.

Thyroid hormones increase the metabolic rate of body tissues. This involves many varied functions such as oxygen use, respiratory rate, body temperature, heart rate, metabolism of foods, enzyme activity and growth and development of the skeletal and nervous system. Thyroid hormones influence every organ system of the body.

## Uses:

To treat hypothyroidism (low thyroid hormone production).

To treat thyroid nodules, chronic lymphocytic thyroiditis (Hashimoto disease), multinodular goiter and thyroid cancer.

To treat thyrotoxicosis (excessive thyroid hormone production). Used with an antithyroid drug to prevent hypothyroidism.

## Precautions:

*Do not use in the following situations:*
> allergy to thyroid hormones
> heart attack, recent
> obesity, treatment
> thyroid deficiency (hypothyroidism) and hypoadrenalism (Addison disease) together
> thyroid gland, overactive (thyrotoxicosis)

*Use with caution in the following situations:*

| | |
|---|---|
| Addison disease | heart disease |
| angina (chest pain) | infertility |
| diabetes insipidus | kidney disease |
| diabetes mellitus | myxedema (swelling due to |
| elderly | hypothroidism) |

*Pregnancy:* This drug appears to be safe for use during pregnancy. Do not discontinue thyroid replacement therapy in hypothyroid (decreased thyroid activity) women during pregnancy.

*Breastfeeding:* Very small amounts of thyroid hormones appear in breast milk. Use with caution during breastfeeding. The mother and nursing infant should be checked periodically.

*Children:* Thyroid replacement therapy in children may lead to partial hair loss in the first few months of therapy. This is a temporary condition. Normal hair growth and distribution returns.

*Lab tests* will be required to monitor therapy. Be sure to keep appointments.

*Tartrazine:* Some of these products may contain the dye tartrazine (FD&C Yellow No. 5) which can cause allergic reactions in certain individuals. Check package label when available or consult your doctor or pharmacist.

## Drug Interactions:

Tell your doctor or pharmacist if you are taking or if you are planning to take any over-the-counter or prescription medications or dietary supplements while taking this medicine. Doses of one or both drugs may need to be modified or a different drug may need to be prescribed. The following drugs and drug classes interact with this medicine:

| | |
|---|---|
| anticoagulants, oral (eg, *Coumadin*) | colestipol (*Colestid*) |
| | digoxin (eg, *Lanoxin*) |
| beta blockers (eg, propranolol) | estrogens (eg, *Premarin*) |
| cholestyramine (eg, *Questran*) | theophyllines (eg, *Theo-Dur*) |

## Side Effects:

Every drug is capable of producing side effects. Many patients experience no, or minor, side effects. The frequency and severity of side effects depend on many factors including dose, duration of therapy and individual susceptibility.

Side effects other than those indicating too much thyroid due to excessive dosage or too rapid dosage increase are rare. Symptoms of too much thyroid include:

*Digestive Tract:* Diarrhea; vomiting.

*Nervous System:* Tremors; headache; nervousness; sleeplessness.

*Circulatory System:* Increased heart rate; palpitations (pounding in the chest); irregular heartbeat; angina (chest pain); cardiac arrest.

*Other:* Weight loss; menstrual irregularities; sweating; heat intolerance; fever.

---

### Guidelines for Use:

- Use exactly as prescribed.
- Take as a single daily dose on an empty stomach, preferably before breakfast.
- *Brand interchange* — Do not change from one brand of this drug to another without consulting your pharmacist or doctor. Products manufactured by different companies may not be equally effective.
- Replacement therapy is usually taken for life.
- Do not discontinue medication except on advice of your doctor.
- Notify your doctor if headache, nervousness, sleeplessness diarrhea, excessive sweating, heat intolerance, chest pain, increased heart rate, irregular heartbeat or any unusual event occurs.
- Partial loss of hair may be experienced by children in the first few months of thyroid therapy, but this is usually only temporary.
- Do not use this medication to treat obesity. Thyroid hormones are not effective for weight reduction. Large doses of thyroid medications may produce serious or even life-threatening conditions, especially when taken with appetite suppressants.
- If a dose is missed, take it as soon as possible. If several hours have passed or if it is nearing time for the next dose, do not double the dose in order to "catch up" (unless advised to do so by your doctor). If more than one dose is missed or it is necessary to establish a new dosage schedule, contact your doctor or pharmacist.
- Dosage is individualized to approximate the deficit in thyroid secretion. Your response is evaluated by your doctor with lab tests.
- Store at room temperature away from moisture and light.

---

*If you have any questions, consult your doctor, pharmacist, or health care provider.*

| Generic Name<br>*Brand Name Examples* | Supplied As | Generic<br>Available |
|---|---|---|
| *Rx* **Calcitonin-Salmon** | | |
| *Calcimar, Miacalcin,*<br>*Osteocalcin* | **Injection:** 200 IU/mL | Yes |
| *Miacalcin* | **Nasal spray:** 200 IU/activation | No |

## Type of Drug:
Hormone.

## How the Drug Works:
Calcitonin is a hormone secreted by specialized cells of the thyroid gland. It plays a major role in calcium and bone metabolism and has direct actions on the kidneys and digestive tract.

## Uses:
To treat moderate to severe Paget disease (injection only), a condition of abnormal and accelerated bone formation and calcium uptake.

For early treatment in high calcium emergencies when a rapid decrease in serum calcium is required, until a more specific treatment can be done. It can also be added to existing therapies for high calcium levels (injection only).

To treat postmenopausal osteoporosis. May prevent the progressive loss of bone mass. Use nasal spray only in patients who cannot take estrogen.

## Precautions:
*Do not use in the following situations:* Allergy to calcitonin-salmon.

*Use with caution in the following situations:*
>  low calcium levels
>  osteogenic sarcoma (eg, bone cancer)

*Pregnancy:* Adequate studies have not been done in pregnant women, or animal studies may have shown a risk to the fetus. Use only if clearly needed and potential benefits outweigh the possible hazards to the fetus.

*Breastfeeding:* It is not known if calcitonin appears in breast milk. Consult your doctor before you begin breastfeeding.

*Children:* Bone disorders in children (juvenile Paget disease) have been reported rarely. There are no data to support use in children.

*Lab tests* or exams may be necessary to monitor treatment. Be sure to keep appointments. Tests may include: Nasal examinations; skin tests for allergy (prior to treatment); blood calcium levels.

## Side Effects:

Every drug is capable of producing side effects. Many patients experience no, or minor, side effects. The frequency and severity of side effects depend on many factors including dose, duration of therapy and individual susceptibility. Possible side effects include:

*Digestive Tract:* Nausea; vomiting; appetite changes; gas; abdominal pain and discomfort; salty taste.

*Nervous System:* Headache/migraine; sleeplessness; anxiety; vertigo (feeling of a whirling motion); nerve pain; agitation.

*Circulatory System:* Fast heartbeat; palpitation (pounding in the chest); heart attack or block; anemia; stroke; inflammation of the veins.

*Respiratory System:* Nasal congestion; nasal symptoms (eg, irritation, redness, sores); difficulty breathing; sore throat; pneumonia; bronchitis; coughing; distorted sense of smell.

*Skin:* Inflammation at the injection site; flushing of face or hands; itching of ear lobes; swelling of feet; rashes; skin ulcers; eczema; hair loss; sweating.

*Senses:* Eye pain; blurred vision; eye floaters (black or white spots); ringing in the ears; earache; hearing loss.

*Other:* Back, muscle or joint pain; nosebleed; increased urination at night; feverish sensation; weight increase; stiffness; taste distortion; overactive thyroid (eg, weight loss); inflammation of kidney or pelvis; blood in urine; gallstone formation; thirst; yellowing of skin or eyes.

## Guidelines for Use:

- Patient instructions for use are enclosed in each package.
- Follow the injection procedure taught to you by your health care provider.
- Doses vary according to the condition being treated. Do not adjust dose without consulting your doctor.
- If a dose is missed, inject or inhale it as soon as possible. If several hours have passed or if it is nearing time for the next dose, do not double the dose in order to "catch up" (unless advised to do so by your doctor). If more than one dose is missed or it is necessary to establish a new dosage schedule, contact your doctor or pharmacist.
- *Nasal spray* — To activate (prime) the pump, hold the bottle upright and depress the two white side arms toward the bottle six times until a faint spray is emitted. The pump is activated once the first faint spray has been emitted. At this point, firmly place the nozzle into the nostril with the head in the upright position, and depress the pump toward the bottle. It is not necessary to reactivate the pump before each daily dose.
- Nausea, vomiting and flushing tend to decrease with continued use. Administration at bedtime may be helpful.
- Supplemental vitamin D and calcium should be considered in those receiving calcitonin to treat postmenopausal osteoporosis.
- Contact your doctor if any of the following occurs: Allergic reaction to the drug (eg, shortness of breath, difficult breathing, hives, rash), significant nasal irritation or persistent nausea and vomiting.
- *Storage—*
  *Injection:* Store in the refrigerator between 36° and 43° F.
  *Nasal spray:* Store unopened bottle in the refrigerator between 36° and 46° F. Once the pump has been activated, store at room temperature.

*If you have any questions, consult your doctor, pharmacist, or health care provider.*

| Generic Name<br>*Brand Name Examples* | Supplied As | Generic<br>Available |
|---|---|---|
| Rx **Alendronate Sodium** | | |
| *Fosamax* | **Tablets**: 5 mg, 10 mg, 35 mg,<br>40 mg, 70 mg | No |
| Rx **Etidronate Disodium** | | |
| *Didronel*[1] | **Tablets**: 200 mg, 400 mg | No |
| Rx **Pamidronate Disodium** | | |
| *Aredia* | **Powder for injection**: 30 mg,<br>90 mg | No |
| Rx **Risedronate** | | |
| *Actonel* | **Tablets**: 5 mg, 30 mg | No |
| Rx **Tiludronate Disodium** | | |
| *Skelid* | **Tablets**: 200 mg | No |
| Rx **Zoledronic Acid** | | |
| *Zometa* | **Powder for injection**: 4.26 mg<br>zoledronic acid monohydrate<br>(equiv. to 4 mg zoledronic acid<br>anhydrous) | No |

[1] Also available as an intravenous injection.

## Type of Drug:

Bisphosphonates.

## How the Drug Works:

Bisphosphonates help preserve bone mass by inhibiting normal and abnormal bone loss due to resorption (bone tissue loss). Some of these drugs also help control the balance of calcium in bones and blood in certain cancers.

## Uses:

To treat Paget disease of bone (alendronate, etidronate, pamidronate, risedronate, tiludronate only).

To treat osteolytic bone metastases of breast cancer and osteolytic bone lesions of multiple myeloma in conjuction with standard antineoplastic therapy (pamidronate only).

To treat high calcium blood levels in combination with adequate hydration (pamidronate, zoledronic acid only) and bone lesions (pamidronate only) caused by cancer.

To treat osteoporosis in men and postmenopausal women; to prevent osteoporosis in postmenopausal women; to treat glucocorticoid-induced osteoporoses in men and women (alendronate, risedronate only).

To prevent and treat heterotopic ossification (unwanted bone calcification) following total hip replacement or due to spinal cord injury (oral etidronate only).

*Unlabeled Use(s):* To treat osteoporosis in postmenopausal women (etidronate, pamidronate, risedronate only). To prevent osteoporosis in postmenopausal women (risedronate, etidronate only). To treat hyperparathyroidism, high calcium blood levels associated with immobilization; to reduce bone pain in patients with prostatic cancer (pamidronate only). To prevent glucocorticoid-induced osteoporosis (etidronate, pamidronate only).

## Precautions:

*Do not use in the following situations:*

allergy to the bisphosphonate or any of its ingredients
clinically overt bone softening (osteomalacia) (etidronate only)
esophagus abnormalities (alendronate only)
inability to stand or sit upright for at least 30 minutes (alendronate, risedronate only)

kidney disease, severe (alendronate, residronate, tiludronate only)
low blood calcium levels (alendronate, risedronate only)

*Use with caution in the following situations:*

asthma
bone fractures
digestive system disorders
kidney disease

liver disease (zoledronic acid only)
low calcium blood levels

*Pregnancy:* There are no adequate or well-controlled studies in pregnant women. Use only if clearly needed and the potential benefits to the mother outweigh the possible hazards to the fetus.

*Breastfeeding:* It is not known if these drugs appear in breast milk. Consult your doctor before you begin breastfeeding.

*Children:* Safety and effectiveness in children have not been established.

*Lab tests* will be required periodically during treatment. Tests may include blood exams and kidney function tests.

## Drug Interactions:

Tell your doctor or pharmacist if you are taking or planning to take any over-the-counter or prescription medications or dietary supplements with a bisphosphonate. Doses of one or both drugs may need to be modified or a different drug may need to be prescribed. The following drugs and drug classes interact with bisphosphonates:

aminoglycosides (eg, gentamicin sulfate) (zoledronic acid only)
antacids (alendronate, etidronate, tiludronate only)
aspirin (alendronate, tiludronate only)
calcium supplements (alendronate, etidronate, risedronate, tiludronate only)

food (alendronate, etidronate, risedronate, tiludronate only)
indomethecin (eg, *Indocin*) (tiludronate only)
loop diuretics (eg, furosemide) (zoledronic acid only)
warfarin (eg, *Coumadin*) (etidronate only)

## Side Effects:

Every drug is capable of producing side effects. Many bisphosphonate users experience no, or minor, side effects. The frequency or severity of side effects depend on many factors including dose, duration of therapy, and individual susceptibility. Possible side effects include:

*Digestive Tract:* Inflammation of the stomach, nausea; vomiting; diarrhea; constipation; gas; heartburn; indigestion; ulcers; stomach pain; acid regurgitation; difficulty swallowing; bloating; appetite loss; stomach bleeding; taste changes; dental disorder; mouth sores; inflammation of the colon.

*Circulatory System:* High blood pressure; fainting; rapid heartbeat; irregular heartbeat; anemia; decreased white blood cell and platelet count; abnormal blood tests.

*Nervous System:* Headache; fatigue; dizziness; drowsiness; weakness; vertigo (feeling of whirling motion); confusion; anxiety; nervousness; sleep disorders; sleeplessness; hallucinations; amnesia; depression; convulsions.

*Respiratory System:* Difficulty breathing; runny nose; sore throat; sinus infection; coughing; bronchitis; upper respiratory infections.

*Skin:* Rash; itching; redness, swelling, hardness, or pain at injection site (pamidronate, zoledronic acid only); fungal infections; sweating; flushing; hair loss.

*Other:* Urinary tract infection; flu-like symptoms; infection; fracture; vitamin D deficiency; fever; general swelling; joint, muscle, chest, neck, leg, back, or bone pain; involuntary muscle contractions; muscle or leg cramps; abnormal skin sensations (eg, burning, prickling, tingling); cataracts; glaucoma; eye inflammation.

## Guidelines for Use:

- Pamidronate and zoledronic acid are prepared and administered by your health care provider in a medical setting.
- Dosage is individualized. Take exactly as prescribed.
- Do not stop taking or change the dose unless directed by your doctor.
- If a dose is missed, take it as soon as possible. If several hours have passed or it is nearing time for the next dose, do not double the dose to catch up, unless advised to do so by your doctor. If more than one dose is missed or it is necessary to establish a new dosage schedule, contact your doctor or pharmacist.
- These medications may cause upset stomach, nausea, or diarrhea.
- Take supplemental calcium and vitamin D as advised by your doctor if dietary intake is inadequate.
- Avoid nicotine and alcohol, which deplete calcium from the bones.
- Consider weight-bearing exercises to increase the calcium density of bones.
- Lab tests will be required to monitor therapy. Be sure to keep appointments.
- Store tablets at controlled room temperature (59° to 86°F) in a tightly sealed container. Do not remove tiludronate tablets from foil strip until they are to be used.
- *Alendronate and risedronate —*
  Take each tablet first thing in morning with a full glass of water (6 to 8 oz) at least 30 minutes before the first food, beverage, or medication of the day.
  Taking with mineral water, fruit juices, or coffee can decrease its effectiveness.
  Do not lie down for at least 30 minutes following administration and until after the first food of the day.
  Discontinue use and notify your physician if you experience new or worsening heartburn or difficult or painful swallowing.
- *Etidronate —*
  Take tablets with a full glass of water (6 to 8 oz) on an empty stomach, at least 2 hours before meals.
  Take tablets as a single dose. If stomach upset occurs, divide the dose.
  Do not eat foods (such as milk or dairy products), vitamins, mineral supplements, or antacids that are high in calcium within 2 hours of taking.
- *Tiludronate —*
  Take with a full glass of water (6 to 8 oz), at least 2 hours before or after meals.
  Do not take calcium supplements, aspirin, or indomethacin 2 hours before or after taking this medication.
  If needed, take aluminum- or magnesium-containing antacids at least 2 hours after taking this medication.

*If you have any questions, consult your doctor, pharmacist, or health care provider.*

| Generic Name<br>*Brand Name Example* | Supplied As | Generic<br>Available |
|---|---|---|
| *Rx* **Imiglucerase** | | |
| *Cerezyme* | **Injection**: 200 units/vial,<br>400 units/vial | No |

## Type of Drug:
Enzyme replacement therapy.

## How the Drug Works:
An enzyme used long-term to break down glucocerebroside into glucose and ceramide. This prevents the accumulation of glucocerebroside in Gaucher disease.

## Uses:
For long-term enzyme replacement therapy for type I Gaucher disease that results in one or more of the following problems: anemia, low platelet counts, bone disease and deterioration, enlargement of the liver or spleen.

## Precautions:
*Do not use in the following situations:* Allergy to imiglucerase or any of its ingredients.

*Use with caution in the following situations:* Pulmonary hypertension.

*Hypersensitivity:* Approximately 15% of patients have developed IgG antibodies reactive with imiglucerase during the first year of therapy. Approximately 46% of those patients experienced allergic reactions.

*Pregnancy:* There are no adequate and well-controlled studies in pregnant women. Use only if clearly needed and the potential benefits to the mother outweigh the possible hazards to the fetus.

*Breastfeeding:* It is not known if imiglucerase appears in breast milk. Consult your doctor before you begin breastfeeding.

## Side Effects:
Every drug is capable of producing side effects. Many imiglucerase users experience no, or minor, side effects. The frequency and severity of side effects depend on many factors including dose, duration of therapy, and individual susceptibility. Possible side effects include:

*Nervous System:* Headache; fever; chills; fatigue; dizziness.

*Other:* Nausea; vomiting; stomach discomfort; diarrhea; back pain; chest discomfort; swelling; difficulty breathing; low blood pressure; rapid heart rate; injection site burning, itching, and swelling; rash; itching; flushing; skin discoloration.

## Guidelines for Use:

- This drug is prepared and administered intravenously (IV; into a vein) by your health care provider in a medical setting.
- Dosage is individualized and may be administered as frequently as 3 times per week or as infrequently as once every 2 weeks depending on disease severity.
- Contact your doctor immediately if you experience any symptoms of allergic reaction (eg, rash, difficulty breathing).

*If you have any questions, consult your doctor, pharmacist, or health care provider.*

**Diuretics**
Carbonic Anhydrase Inhibitors, 305
Loop Diuretics, 309
Potassium-Sparing Diuretics, 312
Thiazides and Related Diuretics, 315
Combinations, 319
Nonprescription Diuretics, 321

**Cardiac Glycosides,** 322

**Inamrinone Lactate,** 326

**Milrinone Lactate,** 328

**Antianginals**
Nitrates, 330

**Vasodilators**
Bosentan, 336

**Antiarrhythmics**
Amiodarone, 338
Disopyramide, 341
Dofetilide, 344
Flecainide, 347
Mexiletine, 349
Moricizine, 351
Procainamide, 354
Propafenone, 356
Quinidine, 358
Tocainide, 361

**Calcium Channel Blocking Agents,** 363

**Peripheral Vasodilators**
Epoprostenol, 370
Isoxsuprine, 372
Papaverine, 374

**Beta-Adrenergic Blocking Agents,** 376

**Antihypertensives**
Alpha-1-Adrenergic Blockers, 382
Angiotensin Converting Enzyme Inhibitors, 385
Angiotensin II Receptor Antagonists, 390
Clonidine, 394
Guanabenz Acetate, 398
Guanadrel Sulfate, 400
Guanethidine Monosulfate, 402
Guanafacine, 405
Hydralazine, 407
Carvedilol, 410
Labetalol, 413
Mecamylamine, 416
Methyldopa, 418
Minoxidil, 421
Reserpine, 424
Combinations, 427
Selective Aldosterone Receptor Antagonists, 432

**Antihyperlipidemics**
Bile Acid Sequestrants, 434
Ezetimibe, 438
Fenofibrate, 440
Gemfibrozil, 443
HMG-CoA Reductase Inhibitors, 446
Combinations, 450

| Generic Name<br>*Brand Name Examples* | Supplied As | Generic<br>Available |
|---|---|---|
| *Rx* **Acetazolamide** | | |
| *Diamox* | **Tablets:** 125 mg, 250 mg | Yes |
| *Diamox Sequels* | **Capsules, sustained release:** 500 mg | No |
| *Diamox* | **Powder for injection:** 500 mg/vial | Yes |
| *Rx* **Dichlorphenamide** | | |
| *Daranide* | **Tablets:** 50 mg | No |
| *Rx* **Methazolamide** | | |
| *Neptazane* | **Tablets:** 25 mg, 50 mg | No |

## Type of Drug:

Diuretics (water pills); antiglaucoma agents.

## How the Drug Works:

Carbonic anhydrase inhibitors block the activity of the enzyme carbonic anhydrase. This reduces the rate of fluid formation in the inner eye, resulting in reduced pressure within the eye. These drugs also cause increased amounts of electrolytes (sodium, potassium, bicarbonate) and water to be excreted by the kidneys (diuretic effect) and slows abnormal nerve conduction in the brain (anticonvulsant effect).

## Uses:

To treat chronic simple (open-angle) glaucoma and secondary glaucoma, and to lower intraocular pressure preoperatively for acute closed-angle glaucoma.

*Acetazolamide* — To prevent mountain sickness in climbers who are attempting to climb rapidly and in climbers who climb gradually, but who are prone to developing mountain sickness. Also used to treat fluid accumulation and swelling due to congestive heart failure or drugs and to treat some forms of epilepsy (eg, petit mal seizures).

## Precautions:

*Do not use in the following situations:*

adrenocortical insufficiency (eg, Addison disease)
allergy to these medicines or any of their ingredients
cirrhosis
electrolyte imbalance (eg, low potassium or sodium levels)

glaucoma, chronic noncongestive angle-closure
hyperchloremic acidosis
kidney disease, severe
liver disease, severe
lung obstruction, severe

*Use with caution in the following situations:*
allergy to sulfa drugs
(eg, *Bactrim*)
aspirin use, high-dose,
concurrent

emphysema
lung obstruction

*Large doses:* Taking larger than recommended doses does not increase the diuretic (water pill) activity of the drug. However, it will increase the risk of side effects.

*Pregnancy:* There are no adequate and well-controlled studies in pregnant women. Use only if potential benefits to the mother outweigh potential risks to the fetus.

*Breastfeeding:* Acetazolamide may appear in breast milk. It is not known if all carbonic anhydrase inhibitors appear in breast milk. Consult your doctor before you begin breastfeeding.

*Children:* Safety and effectiveness in children have not been established.

*Lab tests* may be required during treatment. Tests may include electrolyte levels (eg, potassium) and blood counts.

## Drug Interactions:
Tell your doctor or pharmacist if you are taking or if you are planning to take any over-the-counter or prescription medications or doetary supplements with carbonic anhydrase inhibitors. Doses of one or both drugs may need to be modified or a different drug may need to be prescribed. The following drugs interact with carbonic anhydrase inhibitors.

cyclosporine (eg, *Sandimmune*)
salicylates (eg, aspirin, *Arthropan*, *Doan's*, *Tusal*)

salsalate (eg, *Disalcid*)
steroid therapy (eg, prednisone)

## Side Effects:
Every drug is capable of producing side effects. Many carbonic anhydrase inhibitor users experience no, or minor, side effects. The frequency and severity of side effects depend on many factors including dose, duration of therapy, and individual susceptibility. Possible side effects include:

*Digestive Tract:* Appetite loss; nausea; vomiting; diarrhea; sore throat; taste changes.

*Nervous System:* Drowsiness; confusion; ringing in the ears; impaired coordination; headache; tingling in the hands or feet.

*Skin:* Rash; itching; unusual bleeding or bruising; sensitivity to light; red or purple spots under the skin.

*Urinary and Reproductive Tract:* Flank or loin pain; excessive urination; crystals in urine; kidney stones.

*Other:* Fever; weight loss; nearsightedness when decreasing or discontinuing the drug; abnormal blood counts; hearing dysfunction; severe allergic reaction.

## Guidelines for Use:

*All:*
- If stomach upset occurs, take with food.
- Drink plenty of water and other fluids.
- May cause drowsiness. Use caution while driving or performing other tasks requiring alertness, coordination, or physical dexterity.
- Notify your doctor if sore throat, fever, unusual bleeding or bruising, tingling or tremors in the hands or feet, flank or loin pain, or skin rash occurs.
- May cause sensitivity to sunlight. Avoid prolonged exposure to the sun or ultraviolet (UV) light (eg, tanning beds).
- Store tablets, capsules, and injection at room temperature (59° to 86°F).

*Acetazolamide:*
- Tablets can be crushed and mixed with sweet foods to mask bitter taste.
- Do not crush or chew sustained release capsules. Capsules can be opened and contents sprinkled on food, if necessary.
- *Acute Mountain Sickness* — Dosage is 500 to 1000 mg daily, in divided doses, using tablets or sustained release capsules as appropiate. The higher dose level of 1000 mg is recommended with rapid ascent (eg, rescue or military operations). Dose should be initiated 24 to 48 hours before ascent and continued for 48 hours while at high altitude, or as long as necessary, to control symptoms.
  Gradual ascent is desirable to avoid acute moutain sickness. If rapid ascent is undertaken and acetazolamide used, prompt descent is still necessary if severe forms of altitude sickness (eg, lung edema or cerebral swelling) occur.
- *Congestive Heart Failure* — Starting dose is usually 250 to 375 mg once daily (5 mg/kg) in the morning. If the initial response fails, do not increase the dose, but allow the kidney to recover by skipping the medicine for a day.
- Acetazolamide yields the best diuretic results when given on alternate days or given for 2 days alternating with a day of rest.
- *Drug-Induced Edema* — Recommended dosage is 250 to 375 mg once a day for 1 to 2 days, alternating with a day of rest.
- *Epilepsy* — Suggested total daily dose is 8 to 30 mg/kg in divided doses. Optimum range appears to be from 375 to 1000 mg daily. When given in combination with other anticonvulsants, starting dose should be 250 mg once daily in addition to existing medicines.
- *Glaucoma* — Acetazolamide is used as an adjunct to the usual therapy. When using capsules, dosage is 500 mg (1 capsule) 2 times a day, usually given as 1 capsule in the morning and 1 capsule in the evening. Dosage for chronic simple (open-angle) glaucoma ranges from 250 to 1000 mg per 24 hours. Daily doses over 250 mg are usually taken in divided doses.
  For secondary glaucoma and in preoperative treatment of acute congestive (closed-angle) glaucoma, the preferred dosage is 250 mg every 4 hours.
- Doses larger than 1000 mg per 24 hours do not increase the effect and may increase drowsiness and other side effects.

## Guidelines for Use (cont.):

*Methazolamide:*
- Effective therapeutic dose varies from 50 to 100 mg 2 to 3 times daily.
- May be used with miotic (eg, *Pilocarpine*) and osmotic (eg, mannitol) agents.

*Dichlorphenamide:*
- Usually given in conjunction with topical ocular antiglaucoma agents.
- In acute angle-closure glaucoma, it may be used together with miotic and osmotic agents in an attempt to reduce internal pressure rapidly. If this is not relieved quickly, surgery may be mandatory.
- Dose must be adjusted carefully to each individual.
- A usual initial dose is 100 to 200 mg (2 to 4 tablets), followed by 100 mg (2 tablets) every 12 hours until the desired response has been obtained.
- Recommended maintenance dosage for adults is 25 to 50 mg (½ to 1 tablet) 1 to 3 times daily.

*If you have any questions, consult your doctor, pharmacist, or health care provider.*

| Generic Name<br>*Brand Name Examples* | Supplied As | Generic<br>Available |
|---|---|---|
| *Rx* **Bumetanide** | | |
| *Bumex* | **Tablets:** 0.5 mg, 1 mg, 2 mg | No |
| *Bumex* | **Injection:** 0.25 mg/mL | Yes |
| *Rx* **Ethacrynic Acid** | | |
| *Edecrin* | **Tablets:** 25 mg, 50 mg | No |
| *Edecrin* | **Powder for injection:** 50 mg<br>(as ethacrynate sodium)/vial | No |
| *Rx* **Furosemide** | | |
| *Lasix* | **Tablets:** 20 mg, 40 mg, 80 mg | Yes |
| *Lasix* | **Oral solution:** 10 mg/mL,<br>40 mg/5 mL | Yes |
| *Lasix* | **Injection:** 10 mg/mL | Yes |
| *Rx* **Torsemide** | | |
| *Demadex* | **Tablets:** 5 mg, 10 mg, 20 mg,<br>100 mg | No |
| *Demadex* | **Injection:** 10 mg/mL | No |

## Type of Drug:

Diuretics or "water pills."

## How the Drug Works:

Loop diuretics cause electrolytes (especially sodium and chloride) to be excreted in the urine. Water is excreted with the electrolytes.

## Uses:

To treat edema (fluid retention and swelling) due to congestive heart failure, liver disease (eg, cirrhosis), and kidney disease.

*Furosemide and torsemide* — To treat hypertension (high blood pressure) alone or with other high blood pressure medicine.

*Ethacrynic acid* — To treat fluid accumulation in the abdomen (ascites) due to cancer, liver failure, and other conditions, and to treat fluid accumulation in children due to congenital heart or kidney disease.

## Precautions:

*Do not use in the following situations:*

allergy to loop diuretics or any
  of their ingredients
allergy to sulfa drugs
allergy to thiazides

electrolyte loss, severe
inability to urinate
infants (ethacrynic acid only)

*Use with caution in the following situations:*

| | |
|---|---|
| diabetes | heart disease |
| digoxin therapy | kidney disease |
| elderly | liver disease |
| gout | systemic lupus erythematosus |

*Loop diuretics:* Loop diuretics are potent diuretics which can lead to profound increase in urine excretion with water and electrolyte depletion when given in large amounts. Careful medical supervision is required. The dose and dose schedule must be adjusted to the individual patient's needs.

*Pregnancy:* There are no adequate and well-controlled studies in pregnant women. Use only if clearly needed and potential benefits to the mother outweigh the possible hazards to the fetus.

*Breastfeeding:* Furosemide appears in breast milk. It is not known if other loop diuretics appear in breast milk. Consult your doctor before you begin breastfeeding.

*Children:* Safety and effectiveness for use of bumetanide in children younger than 18 years of age have not been established. Safety and effectiveness for use of ethacrynic acid in infants have not been established. Furosemide is indicated for use in pediatric patients. Safety and effectiveness for use of torsemide in children have not been established.

*Lab tests* may be required during therapy. Tests may include electrolytes (eg, sodium, potassium, calcium, magnesium), blood counts, blood glucose (sugar), uric acid, urea nitrogen, creatinine, and cholesterol.

## Drug Interactions:

Tell your doctor or pharmacist if you are taking or planning to take any over-the-counter or prescription medications or dietary supplements with loop diuretics. Doses of one or both drugs may need to be modified or a different drug may need to be prescribed. The following drugs and drug classes interact with loop diuretics:

| | |
|---|---|
| ACE inhibitors (eg, benazepril) | digitalis glycosides (eg, digoxin) |
| aminoglycosides (eg, gentamicin) | hydantoins (eg, phenytoin) |
| | lithium (eg, *Eskalith*) |
| cholestyramine (eg, *Questran*) | NSAIDs (eg, ibuprofen) |
| cisapride (*Propulsid*) | thiazide diuretics (eg, hydrochlorothiazide) |
| cisplatin (eg, *Platinol*) | |
| colestipol (*Colestid*) | |

Do not combine furosemide with ethacrynic acid.

## Side Effects:

Every drug is capable of producing side effects. Many loop diuretic users experience no, or minor, side effects. The frequency and severity of side effects depend on many factors including dose, duration of therapy, and individual susceptibility. Possible side effects include:

*Symptoms of Electrolyte Loss:* Weakness; dizziness; confusion; appetite loss; nausea; vomiting; muscle cramps; limb heaviness.

*Digestive Tract:* Difficulty swallowing; diarrhea (including sudden watery diarrhea); irritation of mouth or stomach; constipation; stomach pain; appetite loss; indigestion; bloating.

*Nervous System:* Restlessness; tingling or numbness of hands or feet; apprehension; nervousness; headache; insomnia.

*Circulatory System:* Irregular heartbeat; weak pulse; chest pain; orthostatic hypotension (dizziness or lightheadedness when rising too quickly from a seated or lying position).

*Senses:* Ringing in the ears; hearing loss (usually reversible).

*Skin:* Sweating; itching; rash, hives; jaundice (yellowing of skin or eyes); sensitivity to sunlight; unusual bleeding or bruising.

*Other:* Blood in the urine; dehydration; joint pain; fever; chills; breathing difficulties; yellow vision; blurred vision; premature ejaculation; impotence; difficulty maintaining an erection; dry mouth; excessive urination; rectal bleeding; fluid retention; muscle pain; cold; cough; sore throat; decreased potassium levels; elevated blood sugar.

---

## Guidelines for Use:

- Dosage is individualized.
- If a dose is missed, take it as soon as possible. If several hours have passed or it is nearing time for the next dose, do not double the dose to catch up, unless advised to do so by your doctor. If more than one dose is missed or it is necessary to establish a new dosage schedule, contact your doctor or pharmacist. Use exactly as prescribed.
- Take ethacrynic acid after meals, if necessary.
- Drug will increase urination. Take early in the day to avoid sleep disruption.
- Notify your doctor if muscle weakness, cramps, nausea or dizziness occurs.
- Orthostatic hypotension (dizziness or lightheadedness when arising from a seated or lying position) may occur. Get up slowly.
- *Diabetes mellitus patients* — May increase blood glucose (sugar) levels.
- Photosensitivity (sensitivity to sunlight) may occur. Use sunscreens and wear protective clothing until tolerance is determined.
- Additional potassium may be required while taking loop diuretics.
- Patients with high blood pressure should avoid medications that may increase blood pressure, including nonprescription decongestant products for cold symptoms and stimulant weight-control products.
- Weight should be monitored throughout treatment with loop diuretics. Loss of fluid should not be excessive within a narrow band of time.
- Lab tests will be required. Be sure to keep appointments.
- Store at room temperature (59° to 86°F) in well closed, light-resistant container. Do not freeze.

---

*If you have any questions, consult your doctor, pharmacist, or health care provider.*

| Generic Name<br>*Brand Name Examples* | Supplied As | Generic<br>Available |
|---|---|---|
| Rx **Amiloride HCl** | | |
| *Midamor* | **Tablets:** 5 mg | Yes |
| Rx **Spironolactone** | | |
| *Aldactone* | **Tablets:** 25 mg, 50 mg, 100 mg | Yes |
| Rx **Triamterene** | | |
| *Dyrenium* | **Capsules:** 50 mg, 100 mg | No |

## Type of Drug:
Diuretics or "water pills."

## How the Drug Works:
Potassium-sparing diuretics increase the amount of water and sodium being excreted by the kidneys, but reduce the amount of potassium being excreted by the kidneys.

## Uses:
To treat edema (fluid accumulation and swelling) due to congestive heart failure, cirrhosis of the liver, and in certain kidney conditions.

To treat high blood pressure, usually in combination with other drugs.

To prevent or treat low potassium levels due to use of other medications (eg, other diuretics).

*Spironolactone:* To diagnose and treat primary hyperaldosteronism (an abnormality of electrolyte metabolism). To treat edema in children.

*Triamterene:* To treat edema due to secondary hyperaldosteronism (an abnormality of electrolyte metabolism).

## Precautions:
*Do not use in the following situations:*

allergy to potassium-sparing diuretics
anuria (eg, inability to urinate)
liver disease, severe (triamterene only)
potassium levels, increased
potassium supplement use

*Use with caution in the following situations:*

diabetes (amiloride and triamterene)
elderly (amiloride and triamterene)
congestive heart failure
kidney disease
kidney stone formation, history (triamterene only)
liver disease

*High potassium levels (hyperkalemia):* Occasionally hyperkalemia may occur when these agents are used without diuretics. Symptoms include abnormal skin sensations (burning, tingling), muscle weakness, impaired movement and irregular heartbeat.

*Pregnancy: Amiloride* and *triamterene* — Studies in pregnant women have not shown a risk to the fetus; however, no drug should be used during pregnancy unless clearly needed.

*Spironolactone* may cross the placenta. Use only if clearly needed and potential benefits outweigh the possible risks.

*Breastfeeding:* Spironolactone appears in breast milk. However, it is not known if triamterene or amiloride are excreted in breast milk. Safety for use in breastfeeding has not been established. These drugs can cause serious side effects in a nursing infant. Do not breastfeed while taking these drugs.

*Children:* Safety and effectiveness of triamterene and amiloride in children have not been established.

*Lab tests* should be performed periodically for serum electrolytes, creatinine, BUN and serum potassium. Periodic blood tests should also be performed.

## Drug Interactions:

Tell your doctor or pharmacist if you are taking or planning to take any over-the-counter or prescription medications or dietary supplements with potassium-sparing diuretics. Doses of one or both drugs may need to be modified or a different drug may need to be prescribed. The following drugs and drug classes interact with potassium-sparing diuretics:

ACE inhibitors (eg, captopril)
anesthetics (general)
antihypertensives (spironolactone and triamterene only)
chlorpropamide (eg, *Diabinese*)
  (triamterene only)
digoxin (eg, *Lanoxin*) (spironolactone only)
indomethacin (eg, *Indocin*)
  (spironolactone and triamterene
  only)

lithium (eg, *Eskalith*) (amiloride
  and triamterene only)
nonsteroidal anti-inflammatory
  agents (eg, aspirin) (amiloride and triamterene only)
potassium supplements
  (eg, *Kaon*)
salt substitutes
skeletal muscle relaxants (triamterene only)

## Side Effects:

Every drug is capable of producing side effects. Many potassium-sparing diuretic users experience no, or minor, side effects. The frequency and severity of side effects depend on many factors including dose, duration of therapy, and individual susceptibility. Possible side effects include:

*Digestive Tract:* Stomach or intestinal cramps or pain; nausea; vomiting; thirst; diarrhea; constipation; gas; appetite changes (loss of appetite).

*Nervous System:* Weakness, fatigue; drowsiness; confusion; tingling or numbness of hands or feet; headache; dizziness; lack of coordination.

*Circulatory System:* Irregular pulse; chest pain.

*Respiratory System:* Shortness of breath; cough.

*Skin:* Rash; hives; excessive body hair growth; yellowing of the skin or eyes; sensitivity to sunlight; unusual bleeding or bruising.

*Other:* Deepening of the voice, breast enlargement in males (spirono-lactone only); menstrual abnormalities; fever; muscle weakness or cramping; inability to achieve or maintain an erection; difficult urination; dry mouth; allergic reaction.

## Guidelines for Use:

- *Amiloride* — May cause stomach upset. Take with food.
  Notify your doctor if any of the following occurs: Muscular weakness, irregular heartbeat, shortness of breath, rash, fatigue or muscle cramps.
  May cause dizziness, headache or visual disturbances. Use caution while driving or performing other tasks requiring alertness.
  Avoid large quantities of potassium-rich food.
- *Spironolactone* — May cause drowsiness, lack of coordination and men-tal confusion. Use caution while driving or performing other tasks requir-ing alertness.
  May cause stomach cramping, diarrhea, lethargy, thirst, headache, skin rash, menstrual abnormalities, deepening of the voice and breast enlargement (in males). Notify your doctor if these effects occur.
- *Triamterene* — May cause stomach upset. Take after meals.
  May cause weakness, headache, nausea, vomiting and dry mouth.
  Notify your doctor if these become severe or persistent.
  Notify your doctor if fever, sore throat, mouth sores, or unusual bleed-ing or bruising occurs.
  Avoid prolonged exposure to sunlight. Photosensitivity (sensitivity to sunlight) may occur. Take protective measures (eg, sunscreens, protec-tive clothing) against exposure to ultraviolet light or sunlight.
  If single daily dose is prescribed, take in morning to avoid disruption of sleep because of frequent urination.
- Do not use dietary potassium supplements, potassium-containing medi-cations, low-salt milk or salt substitutes.
- If a dose is missed, take it as soon as possible. If several hours have passed or it is nearing time for the next dose, do not double the dose to catch up, unless advised by your doctor. If more than one dose is missed, contact your doctor or pharmacist.
- Occasionally hyperkalemia (high potassium levels) may occur when these agents are used. Symptoms include abnormal skin sensations (burning, tingling), muscle weakness, fatigue, loss of arm and leg move-ment, irregular heartbeat and shock.
- Patients being treated for high blood pressure often feel tired and run-down for a few weeks after beginning therapy. Continue taking your medication even though you may not feel quite "normal." Contact your doctor or pharmacist about any new symptoms.
- Store below 77°F. Protect from light, moisture, freezing and excessive heat.

*If you have any questions, consult your doctor, pharmacist, or health care provider.*

All of the products listed in the table below are diuretics; however, they are not interchangeable. For example, metolazone cannot be used for hydrochlorothiazide. Daily dose may vary depending on individual needs. Do not adjust the dose without consulting your pharmacist or doctor.

| Generic Name<br>*Brand Name Examples* | Supplied As | Generic<br>Available |
|---|---|---|
| Rx **Bendroflumethiazide** | | |
| *Naturetin* | **Tablets:** 5 mg, 10 mg | No |
| Rx **Benzthiazide** | | |
| *Exna[1]* | **Tablets:** 50 mg | No |
| Rx **Chlorothiazide** | | |
| *Diurigen, Diuril* | **Tablets:** 250 mg, 500 mg | Yes |
| *Diuril[2]* | **Oral suspension:** 250 mg/5 mL | No |
| Rx **Chlorthalidone** | | |
| *Hygroton, Thalitone* | **Tablets:** 15 mg, 25 mg, 50 mg, 100 mg | Yes |
| Rx **Hydrochlorothiazide (HCTZ)** | | |
| *Esidrix, Ezide, HydroDI-URIL, Hydro-Par, Oretic* | **Tablets:** 25 mg, 50 mg, 100 mg | Yes |
| *Hydrochlorothiazide* | **Solution:** 50 mg/5 mL | No |
| *Hydrochlorothiazide* | **Intensol solution:** 100 mg/mL | No |
| Rx **Hydroflumethiazide** | | |
| *Diucardin, Saluron* | **Tablets:** 50 mg | Yes |
| Rx **Indapamide** | | |
| *Lozol* | **Tablets:** 1.25 mg, 2.5 mg | No |
| Rx **Methyclothiazide** | | |
| *Aquatensen, Enduron* | **Tablets:** 2.5 mg, 5 mg | Yes |
| Rx **Metolazone** | | |
| *Mykrox, Zaroxolyn* | **Tablets:** 0.5 mg, 2.5 mg, 5 mg, 10 mg | No |
| Rx **Polythiazide** | | |
| *Renese* | **Tablets:** 1 mg, 2 mg, 4 mg | No |
| Rx **Quinethazone** | | |
| *Hydromox* | **Tablets:** 50 mg | No |
| Rx **Trichlormethiazide** | | |
| *Diurese, Metahydrin[1], Naqua* | **Tablets:** 2 mg, 4 mg | Yes |

[1] Contains the dye tartrazine.
[2] Contains alcohol. *Diuril* is also available as an injection.

## Type of Drug:

Diuretics or "water pills."

## How the Drug Works:

Thiazides and related diuretics reduce water in the body and increase urine flow.

## Uses:

To treat high blood pressure, either alone or in combination with other high blood pressure medications.

To treat edema (excess fluid accumulation in the tissues) associated with congestive heart failure, kidney problems and during estrogen or corticosteroid therapy.

*Unlabeled Use(s):* Occasionally doctors may prescribe thiazide diuretics for calcium kidney stones, osteoporosis and diabetes insipidus (not diabetes mellitus).

## Precautions:

*Do not use in the following situations:*
>> allergy to thiazides, oral diabetic drugs (eg, *Diabinese)* or sulfa drugs (eg, *Gantrisin)*
>> kidney disease (inability to urinate)

*Use with caution in the following situations:*

| | |
|---|---|
| allergy or history of bronchial asthma | kidney impairment |
| | liver disease |
| diabetes | lupus erythematosus |
| gout | |

*Diabetes:* Thiazide diuretics may increase blood sugar levels. Insulin requirements may need to be adjusted.

*Gout* attacks may occur in patients with or without a history of gout.

*Potassium loss:* By increasing urine production, thiazide diuretics may cause an increased loss of electrolytes, especially potassium. (See Side Effects.)

Low potassium levels may be prevented or treated by eating foods and drinking liquids high in potassium content (eg, citrus juice, bananas, dates, raisins, melons and tomatoes). If dietary changes do not increase potassium to a normal level, it may be necessary for your doctor to prescribe a potassium supplement medication to replace lost potassium.

*Pregnancy:* Thiazides cross the placenta. Use only when clearly needed and when potential benefits outweigh the possible hazards to the fetus.

*Breastfeeding:* Thiazides appear in breast milk. Stop nursing if thiazide diuretics are necessary. Consult your doctor before you begin breastfeeding.

*Children:* Metolazone is not currently recommended for use in children. Safety and effectiveness have not been established for hydroflumethiazide or trichlormethiazide.

*Tartrazine:* Some of these products may contain the dye tartrazine (FD&C Yellow No. 5) which can cause allergic reactions in certain individuals. Check package label when available or consult your pharmacist or doctor if you are sensitive to tartrazine.

## Drug Interactions:

Tell your doctor or pharmacist if you are taking or planning to take any over-the-counter or prescription medications with your diuretic. Doses of one or both drugs may need to be modified or a different drug may need to be prescribed. The following drugs and drug classes interact with thiazide diuretics.

cholestyramine *(Questran)*
colestipol *(Colestid)*
corticosteroids
  (eg, hydrocortisone)
cough, cold, sinus or hayfever
  medications

diazoxide *(Proglycem)*
digoxin (eg, *Lanoxin)*
furosemide (eg, *Lasix)*
lithium (eg, *Eskalith)*
oral diabetic drugs (eg, *Orinase)*

## Side Effects:

Every drug is capable of producing side effects. Many thiazide diuretic users experience no, or minor, side effects. The frequency and severity of side effects depend on many factors including dose, duration of therapy, and individual susceptibility. Possible side effects include:

*Potassium loss:* Dry mouth; thirst; irregular heartbeat; confusion and mood changes; nausea; vomiting; unusual tiredness; weakness; weak pulse; muscle cramps; joint pain or spasms; heaviness in limbs.

*Digestive Tract:* Loss of appetite; stomach upset; bloating; diarrhea; constipation.

*Nervous System:* Dizziness; lightheadedness; headache; tingling of toes and fingers; yellow or blurred vision; depression; nervousness; sleeplessness.

*Circulatory System:* Orthostatic hypotension (fall in blood pressure upon standing which may cause dizziness, fainting and blurred vision); chest pain.

*Skin:* Sensitivity to sun; rash; hives; itching; dry skin; flushing; yellowing of skin or eyes; unusual bruising.

*Respiratory System:* Cough; sinus congestion; sore throat; difficult or painful breathing.

*Other:* Frequent urination; impotence; reduced sexual drive; electrolyte (eg, potassium) imbalance; blood sugar imbalance; muscle cramps; joint pain; fever; chills; weight loss; bloody nose; gout attack.

## Guidelines for Use:

- Take exactly as prescribed.
- If a dose is missed, take it as soon as possible. If several hours have passed or if it is nearing time for the next dose, do not double the dose to catch up, unless advised to do so by your doctor. If more than one dose is missed or it is necessary to establish a new dosage schedule, contact your doctor or pharmacist.
- Increases urination, therefore take early in the day.
- May cause stomach upset. May be taken with food or milk.
- May cause loss of potassium. If signs of potassium loss occur (weakness, cramps, nausea, dizziness, etc), contact your doctor. Ask your doctor about foods containing potassium.
- May increase blood sugar levels in diabetics.
- May cause gout attacks. Contact your doctor if significant sudden joint pain occurs.
- Do not take other medications without your doctor's approval. This includes nonprescription medicines for appetite control, asthma, colds, cough, hayfever or sinus.
- Diuretics are usually given as a single daily dose in the morning. Take as directed by your doctor. The daily dose varies depending on individual needs. Do not adjust the dose without consulting your pharmacist or doctor.

*If you have any questions, consult your doctor, pharmacist, or health care provider.*

| Generic Name<br>*Brand Name Examples* | Supplied As | Generic<br>Available |
|---|---|---|
| *Rx* **Amiloride and Hydrochlorothiazide** | | |
| *Moduretic* | **Tablets:** 5 mg amiloride HCl and 50 mg hydrochlorothiazide | Yes |
| *Rx* **Spironolactone and Hydrochlorothiazide** | | |
| *Aldactazide, Spirozide* | **Tablets:** 25 mg spironolactone and 25 mg hydrochlorothiazide | Yes |
| *Aldactazide* | **Tablets:** 50 mg spironolactone and 50 mg hydrochlorothiazide | No |
| *Rx* **Triamterene and Hydrochlorothiazide** | | |
| *Maxzide-25MG* | **Tablets:** 37.5 mg triamterene and 25 mg hydrochlorothiazide | Yes |
| *Dyazide* | **Capsules:** 50 mg triamterene and 25 mg hydrochlorothiazide | Yes |
| *Maxzide* | **Tablets:** 75 mg triamterene and 50 mg hydrochlorothiazide | Yes |

## Type of Drug:

Diuretic or "water pill"; combination of two diuretics.

## How the Drug Works:

Combination diuretics provide additional diuretic activity (increased water excreted by kidneys) and blood-pressure-lowering effects. They minimize the possibility of potassium loss from the body because they contain a potassium-sparing diuretic.

For complete information on hydrochlorothiazide, see the Diuretics-Thiazides and Related Diuretics monograph in this chapter. For complete information on amiloride HCl, spironolactone, and triamterene, see the Diuretics-Potassium-Sparing Diuretics monograph in this chapter.

## Guidelines for Use:

- Increases urination, therefore, take early in the day.
- May cause stomach upset. Take with food or milk.
- May cause a sensitivity to sunlight. Take protective measures (eg, sunscreens, protective clothing) until sensitivity is determined.
- If a dose is missed, take it as soon as possible. If several hours have passed or it is nearing time for the next dose, do not double the dose to catch up, unless advised by your doctor. If more than one dose is missed, contact your doctor or pharmacist.
- Patients being treated for low blood pressure often feel tired and run down for a few weeks after beginning therapy. It takes time for the body to adjust to lowered blood pressure. Continue taking your medicine and check with your doctor.
- Diuretics are usually given as a single daily dose in the morning. Take as directed by your doctor. The daily dose varies depending on individual needs. Do not adjust the dose without consulting your pharmacist or doctor.
- May increase blood sugar levels if you are diabetic.

*If you have any questions, consult your doctor, pharmacist, or health care provider.*

| Brand Name Examples | Supplied As | Generic Available |
|---|---|---|
| otc Aqua·Ban | **Tablets, enteric coated:** 325 mg ammonium Cl, 100 mg caffeine | No |
| otc Aqua·Ban Plus | **Tablets, enteric coated:** 650 mg ammonium, 200 mg caffeine and 6 mg iron | No |

## Type of Drug:

Over-the-counter (*otc*) diuretics or "water pills."

## How the Drug Works:

*Ammonium chloride* alone has limited value in promoting urine flow. Its use in combination with caffeine is effective since the diuretic actions are additive. Doses up to 3 g/day may be given in divided doses 3 to 4 times daily for up to 6 days. Large doses (4 to 12 g/day) may cause nausea and vomiting, headache, hyperventilation, drowsiness and confusion.

*Caffeine* increases urination. It may lessen the mental and physical fatigue associated with water retention. Caffeine is effective for relief of premenstrual and menstrual symptoms in doses of 100 to 200 mg every 3 to 4 hours. For more information on caffeine, see monograph.

## Uses:

Nonprescription diuretics may lessen menstrual discomfort. When taken 4 to 6 days before onset of a period, they may help relieve symptoms related to water retention, including: Excess water weight, bloating, painful breasts, cramps and tension.

## Guidelines for Use:

- *Ammonium chloride* — Do not use if you have impaired kidney or liver function.
- *Caffeine* — May cause sleeplessness when taken within 4 hours of bedtime. Consider this when drinking coffee, tea, or colas, and when taking products containing caffeine. Doses above 100 mg may cause stomach upset.

*If you have any questions, consult your doctor, pharmacist, or health care provider.*

| Generic Name<br>*Brand Name Examples* | Supplied As | Generic<br>Available |
|---|---|---|
| *Rx* **Digoxin** | | |
| *Digitek, Lanoxin* | **Tablets**: 0.125 mg, 0.25 mg | Yes |
| *Lanoxicaps*[1] | **Capsules**: 0.05 mg, 0.1 mg, 0.2 mg | No |
| *Lanoxin Pediatric*[1] | **Elixir**: 0.05 mg/mL | Yes |
| *Lanoxin*[1] | **Injection**: 0.25 mg/mL, 0.5 mg/2 mL | Yes |
| *Lanoxin Pediatric*[1] | **Injection**: 0.1 mg/mL | No |

[1] Contains alcohol.

## Type of Drug:

Digitalis; cardiac glycoside; heart medications which act on the heart muscle and heart conduction system.

## How the Drug Works:

Cardiac glycosides work on the heart to increase the force with which the heart pumps blood through the body (heart tonic). This increases the amount of blood the heart pumps and improves the blood circulation in patients in whom the heart is not pumping strong enough (eg, congestive heart failure). This may also help reduce fluid retention and swelling due to congestive heart failure. Cardiac glycosides also help slow and steady the heart rhythm in situations in which the heart is beating too fast or in an irregular manner (eg, atrial fibrillation).

## Uses:

To treat congestive heart failure.

To treat certain types of abnormal heart rhythms (arrhythmias) in which the heart is beating too fast or too irregularly to function normally (eg, atrial fibrillation).

## Precautions:

*Do not use in the following situations:*

allergy to the cardiac glycoside or any of its ingredients
digitalis toxicity, possibility of

some types of irregular or fast heartbeats (eg, ventricular fibrillation, ventricular tachycardia)

*Use with caution in the following situations:*

acute myocardial infarction
electrolyte disorder (eg, low blood magnesium levels, low blood potassium levels, high blood calcium levels)
hyperdynamic states (eg, hyperthyroidism, hypoxia, arteriovenous shunt)
hypermetabolic state (eg, hyperthyroidism)
hypothyroidism (underactive thyroid)

idiopathic hypertrophic subaortic stenosis
incomplete AV block, preexisting
kidney disease
paroxysmal atrial fibrillation or flutter and a coexisting accessory AV pathway (Wolff-Parkinson-White syndrome)
preserved left ventricular systolic function
sinus node disease, preexisting

*Pregnancy:* There are no adequate and well-controlled studies in pregnant women. Use only if clearly needed and the potential benefits to the mother outweigh the possible hazards to the fetus.

*Breastfeeding:* Digoxin appears in breast milk. No adverse effects to the infant have been reported. Consult your doctor before you begin breastfeeding.

*Children:* Newborns vary considerably in their tolerance and sensitivity to these medications. Premature and immature infants are particularly sensitive to the effects of digoxin, and the dosage of the drug must not only be reduced but must be individualized according to their degree of maturity. Digitalis glycosides are a significant cause of accidental poisoning in children. Use with caution.

*Elderly:* Elderly patients must be dosed carefully. Changes in weight, kidney function, and other physical changes that occur normally with aging can affect dosing. Frequent electrocardiograph monitoring is important in elderly patients.

*Lab tests* may be required to monitor therapy. Alterations in potassium, magnesium, calcium, and other electrolyte or mineral levels can affect therapy. Tests may be required to ensure that these levels are normal. It may also be necessary to perform electrocardiograph monitoring, liver and kidney function tests, and digoxin blood level determinations.

## Drug Interactions:

Tell your doctor or pharmacist if you are taking or planning to take any over-the-counter or prescription medications or dietary supplements with a cardiac glycoside. Doses of one or both drugs may need to be modified or a different drug may need to be prescribed. The following drugs and drug classes interact with cardiac glycosides:

*Increase digoxin blood levels (possibly increasing therapeutic and toxic effects of digoxin)* —

aminoglycosides, oral (eg, neomycin)
amiodarone (*Cordarone*)
alprazolam (*Xanax*)
azole antifungal agents (eg, itraconazole)

bepridil (*Vascor*)
cyclosporine (eg, *Sandimmune*)
diphenoxylate (eg, *Lomotil*)
indomethacin (eg, *Indocin*)
macrolide antibiotics (eg, erythromycin)

propafenone (*Rythmol*)
quinidine (eg, *Quinora*)
quinine (eg, *Quinamm*)
spironolactone (eg, *Aldactone*)
tetracyclines (eg, doxycycline)

thioamines (eg, methimazole,
propylthiouracil)
tolbutamide (eg, *Orinase*)
verapamil (eg, *Calan*)

*Decrease digoxin blood levels (possibly decreasing the therapeutic effects of digoxin)* —

acarbose (*Precose*)
aminoglycosides, oral
(eg, neomycin)
antacids (eg, *Maalox*)
antineoplastics (eg, bleomycin)
charcoal
cholestyramine (eg, *Questran*)

colestipol (*Colestid*)
diets high in fiber
hydantoins (eg, phenytoin)
metoclopramide (eg, *Reglan*)
penicillamine (eg, *Depen*)
rifampin (eg, *Rifadin*)
sulfasalazine (eg, azulfidine)

*Other* —

loop diuretics (eg, furosemide)
propantheline (*Pro-Panthine*)
succinylcholine (eg, *Anectine*)
thiazide diuretics (eg, hydrochlorothiazide)

thyroid hormones
(eg, *Synthroid)*

## Side Effects:

Every drug is capable of producing side effects. Many cardiac glycoside users experience no, or minor, side effects. The frequency and severity of side effects depend on many factors including dose, duration of therapy, and individual susceptibility. Possible side effects include:

*Digestive Tract:* Loss of appetite; diarrhea; nausea; vomiting.

*Circulatory System:* Heart block; heart rhythm disturbances (unusually slow or fast pulse); abnormal heartbeats; pounding in chest (palpitations); ECG changes.

*Nervous System:* Weakness; headache; depression; delirium; restlessness; drowsiness; confusion; hallucinations; dizziness; apathy; anxiety.

*Other:* Visual disturbances (eg, blurred, yellow vision); rash; itching.

## Guidelines for Use:

- *Digoxin* — Dosage is individualized based on age, kidney function, weight, and heart condition. Usual adult maintenance doses range from 0.125 mg to 0.5 mg once daily. A loading dose is sometimes used to achieve a fast response. The loading dose is given in several portions at 6- to 8-hour intervals with careful assessment of the response before each additional portion.

- The injectable doseform will be prepared and administered by your health care provider in a medical setting.

- *Lanoxicaps* have greater bioavailability than standard digoxin tablets. Therefore, the 0.2 mg capsule is equivalent to the 0.25 mg digoxin tablet, the 0.1 mg capsule is equivalent to 0.125 mg tablet, and the 0.05 mg capsule is equivalent to the 0.0625 mg tablet.

- *Pediatric Elixir* — Dosage will be individualized. Divided daily dosing is usually used for infants and children younger than 10 years of age. Use calibrated dropper to carefully withdraw the prescribed dose.

- *Tablets and Capsules* — Individualize dosage for infants and children. Divided daily dosing is recommended for infants and young children under 10 years of age. Children over 10 years of age require adult dosages in proportion to their body weight.

- Do not change the dose or stop taking medication without first consulting your doctor.

- May be taken without regard to meals. Taking with meals high in bran fiber may reduce the amount of medication absorbed.

- If a dose is missed, take it as soon as possible. If several hours have passed or if it is nearing time for the next dose, do not double the dose to catch up, unless advised by your doctor. If more than one dose is missed or it is necessary to establish a new dosage schedule, contact your doctor or pharmacist.

- Avoid nonprescription antacids, cough, cold, allergy, and diet drugs, except on professional advice.

- Notify your doctor if loss of appetite, lower stomach pain, nausea, vomiting, diarrhea, unusual tiredness or weakness, drowsiness, headache, blurred or yellow vision, rash, itching, hives, depression, or a change in heart rate or pulse (eg, slowing, racing) occurs.

- *Brand and doseform interchange* — Do not change from one brand or doseform of this drug to another without consulting your pharmacist or doctor. Products manufactured by different companies may not be equally effective. Different doseforms provide different amounts of medication, requiring dose modification.

- Digitalis glycosides can cause poisoning in children due to accidental ingestion. Keep out of reach of children.

- Lab tests or exams may be required to monitor therapy. Be sure to keep appointments.

- Store tablets and capsules at room temperature (59° to 86°F). Protect from light and moisture.

*If you have any questions, consult your doctor, pharmacist, or health care provider.*

| Generic Name | Supplied As | Generic Available |
|---|---|---|
| Rx **Inamrinone Lactate** | **Injection**: 5 mg/mL (as lactate)[1] | Yes |

[1] Contains metabisulfite.

## Type of Drug:

Heart medication that strengthens heart muscle action and improves blood circulation.

## How the Drug Works:

Inamrinone works on the heart to increase the force with which the heart pumps blood through the body (heart tonic). This increases the amount of blood the heart pumps and improves blood circulation in patients in whom the heart is not pumping enough blood (eg, congestive heart failure).

## Uses:

For the short-term treatment of symptoms of congestive heart failure in patients who have not responded to standard therapy.

## Precautions:

*Do not use in the following situations:*
>     allergy to bisulfites
>     allergy to inamrinone or any of its ingredients
>     heart attack, acute

*Use with caution in the following situations:*

| | |
|---|---|
| decreased platelet counts | kidney disease |
| diuretic therapy, vigorous | liver disease |
| heart rhythm disturbances | low blood pressure |
| hypertrophic subaortic stenosis | |

*Pregnancy:* There are no adequate and well-controlled studies in pregnant women. Use only if clearly needed and the potential benefits to the mother outweigh possible hazards to the fetus.

*Breastfeeding:* It is not known if inamrinone appears in breast milk. Consult your doctor before you begin breastfeeding.

*Children:* Safety and effectiveness in children have not been established.

*Lab tests* and exams will be required to monitor therapy. Tests will include kidney and liver function tests, and fluid and electrolyte, blood pressure, blood tests, and heart rate monitoring.

*Sulfites:* Inamrinone contains sodium metabisulfite, a sulfite preservative that can cause potentially life-threatening allergic reactions in certain individuals. Consult your doctor or pharmacist.

## Drug Interactions:

Tell your doctor or pharmacist if you are taking or planning to take any over-the-counter or prescription medications or dietary supplements while taking inamrinone. Doses of one or both drugs may need to be modified or a different drug may need to be prescribed. Disopyramide (eg, *Norpace*) interacts with inamrinone.

## Side Effects:

Every drug is capable of producing side effects. Many inamrinone users experience no, or minor, side effects. The frequency and severity of side effects depend on many factors including dose, duration of therapy, and individual susceptibility. Possible side effects include:

*Circulatory System:* Irregular heartbeat; low blood pressure; decreased blood platelets.

*Other:* Nausea.

### Guidelines for Use:

- Dosage is individualized. Use exactly as prescribed.
- Solutions will be prepared and administered by your health care provider. Dosage will be determined by your doctor. Do not change, adjust, or manipulate the infusion device.
- Visually inspect solution for particles or discoloration before use.
- Duration of therapy will depend on patient responsiveness.
- Because of limited experience and potential for serious side effects, inamrinone should only be used in patients who can be closely monitored and who have not responded adequately to digitalis, diuretics, or vasodilators.
- During intravenous (IV; into a vein) therapy with inamrinone, blood pressure and heart rate should be monitored and the rate of infusion slowed or stopped in patients showing excessive decreases in blood pressure.
- Notify your doctor if you experience an abnormal heartbeat.
- Furosemide should not be administered in IV lines containing inamrinone.
- Lab tests and exams will be required to monitor therapy.

*If you have any questions, consult your doctor, pharmacist, or health care provider.*

| Generic Name<br>*Brand Name Example* | Supplied As | Generic<br>Available |
|---|---|---|
| *Rx* **Milrinone Lactate** | | |
| *Primacor* | **Injection:** 0.2 mg/mL, 1 mg/mL | No |

## Type of Drug:

A vasodilator; a heart medication that acts on the heart muscle to increase the strength of contraction.

## How the Drug Works:

Milrinone works on the heart to increase the force with which the heart pumps blood through the body (heart tonic). This increases the amount of blood the heart pumps and improves blood circulation in a patient whose heart is not pumping strongly enough (eg, congestive heart failure).

## Uses:

For the short-term intravenous (IV; into a vein) treatment of acute decompensated heart failure.

## Precautions:

*Do not use in the following situations:* Allergy to milrinone or any of its ingredients.

*Use with caution in the following situations:*

| | |
|---|---|
| arrythmia (irregular heart rhythm) | hypokalemia (low potassium levels) |
| heart attack, acute | valvular heart disease, untreated |

*Pregnancy:* There are no adequate and well-controlled studies in pregnant women. Use only if clearly needed and the potential benefits to the mother outweigh the possible hazards to the fetus.

*Breastfeeding:* It is not known if milrinone appears in breast milk. Consult your doctor before you begin breastfeeding.

*Children:* Safety and effectiveness in children have not been established.

*Lab tests* will be required to monitor therapy. Tests may include fluid and electrolyte levels and kidney function. Blood pressure, heart rate, and electrocardiogram will also be monitored during treatment.

## Drug Interactions:

Tell your doctor or pharmacist if you are taking or planning to take any over-the-counter or prescription medications or dietary supplements while taking milrinone. Doses of one or both drugs may need to be modified or a different drug may need to be prescribed. Furosemide (eg, *Lasix*) interacts with milrinone when given through the same IV line.

## Side Effects:

Every drug is capable of producing side effects. Many milrinone users experience no, or minor, side effects. The frequency and severity of side effects depend on many factors including dose, duration of therapy, and individual susceptibility. Possible side effects include:

*Nervous System:* Headache.

*Circulatory System:* Irregular heartbeat; chest pain; low blood pressure.

---

### Guidelines for Use:

- This medicine will be prepared and administered IV by your health care provider in a medical setting.
- Lab tests will be required to monitor therapy.

---

*If you have any questions, consult your doctor, pharmacist, or health care provider.*

| Generic Name<br>*Brand Name Examples* | Supplied As | Generic<br>Available |
|---|---|---|
| Rx **Isosorbide Dinitrate** | | |
| *Isordil Titradose, Sorbitrate* | **Tablets**: 5 mg, 10 mg, 20 mg, 30 mg, 40 mg | Yes |
| *Sorbitrate* | **Tablets, chewable**: 5 mg, 10 mg | No |
| *Isordil, Sorbitrate* | **Tablets, sublingual**: 2.5 mg, 5 mg, 10 mg | Yes |
| *Dilatrate-SR* | **Capsules, sustained release**: 40 mg | Yes |
| Rx **Isosorbide Mononitrate** | | |
| *Monoket* | **Tablets**: 10 mg | No |
| *Ismo, Monoket* | **Tablets**: 20 mg | Yes |
| *Imdur* | **Tablets, extended release**: 30 mg, 60 mg, 120 mg | Yes |
| Rx **Nitroglycerin**[1] | | |
| *NitroQuick, Nitrostat, NitroTab* | **Tablets, sublingual**: 0.3 mg, 0.4 mg, 0.6 mg | No |
| *Nitro-Time* | **Capsules, sustained release**: 2.5 mg, 6.5 mg, 9 mg | Yes |
| *Nitro-Bid* | **Ointment, topical**: 2% in a lanolin-petrolatum base | Yes |
| *Nitrolingual* | **Aerosol spray, translingual**: 0.4 mg/metered dose | No |
| *Nitrogard* | **Tablets, buccal, extended release**: 1 mg, 2 mg, 2.5 mg, 3 mg, 5 mg | No |

[1] Also available as an intravenous injection.

| Rx | Nitroglycerin Transdermal Systems (Patches) Brand Name Examples | Release Rate (mg/hr) | Surface Area (cm$^2$) | Total NTG content (mg) |
|---|---|---|---|---|
| | Minitran | 0.1 | 3.3 | 9 |
| | Nitro-Dur | 0.1 | 5 | 20 |
| | Transderm-Nitro | 0.1 | 5 | 12.5 |
| | Nitroglycerin Trans-dermal | 0.2 | 6-10[1] | 16-62.5[1] |
| | Minitran | 0.2 | 6.7 | 18 |
| | Nitrek | 0.2 | 8 | 22.4 |
| | Nitrodisc | 0.2 | 8 | 16 |
| | Nitro-Dur | 0.2 | 10 | 40 |
| | Transderm-Nitro | 0.2 | 10 | 25 |
| | Deponit | 0.2 | 16 | 16 |
| | Nitrodisc | 0.3 | 12 | 24 |
| | Nitro-Dur | 0.3 | 15 | 60 |
| | Nitroglycerin Trans-dermal | 0.4 | 13-20[1] | 32-125[1] |
| | Minitran | 0.4 | 13.3 | 36 |
| | Nitrek | 0.4 | 16 | 44.8 |
| | Nitrodisc | 0.4 | 16 | 32 |
| | Nitro-Dur | 0.4 | 20 | 80 |
| | Transderm-Nitro | 0.4 | 20 | 50 |
| | Deponit | 0.4 | 32 | 32 |
| | Nitroglycerin Trans-dermal | 0.6 | 20-30[1] | 75-187.5[1] |
| | Minitran | 0.6 | 20 | 54 |
| | Nitrek | 0.6 | 24 | 67.2 |
| | Nitro-Dur | 0.6 | 30 | 120 |
| | Transderm-Nitro | 0.6 | 30 | 75 |
| | Nitro-Dur | 0.8 | 40 | 160 |

[1] Various generic systems have the same release rates but variable surface areas and NTG contents.

## Type of Drug:
Angina drugs; nitroglycerin, nitro, NTG.

## How the Drug Works:

Nitrates relax blood vessels, allowing them to dilate (widen). This allows more blood to flow through the vessels and reduces the workload of the heart. It also reduces the oxygen demand of the heart and improves blood flow to the heart.

## Uses:

To treat and prevent angina attacks. These drugs may be taken before events or activities that are likely to provoke an angina attack.

To treat an acute angina attack.

*Unlabeled Use(s):* Occasionally doctors may prescribe sublingual and topical nitroglycerin and oral nitrates for reducing the workload on the heart in patients with a history of heart attacks or congestive heart failure. Doctors may also prescribe nitroglycerin ointment with other medications for treatment of Raynaud disease.

## Precautions:

*Do not use in the following situations:*

allergy to nitrates or any of their ingredients
anemia, severe
congestive heart failure
enlarged heart
glaucoma, angle closure
head trauma, bleeding, hemorrhage
heart attack (isosorbide mononitrate, nitroglycerin only)
hypotension (low blood pressure)

*Excessive dosages:* Excessive dosages may produce severe headaches. Lower doses and pain medications can help control this problem. Headaches tend to become less severe or disappear as therapy continues.

*Isosorbide mononitrate:* Do not avoid headaches by altering the schedule of drug treatment, since headaches are a marker of the activity of the drug. Aspirin or acetaminophen are helpful in relieving headaches without affecting the action of isosorbide.

*Tolerance:* Tolerance to the effects of nitroglycerin may develop with other nitrates. The effectiveness of nitrate therapy may decrease over time. If this occurs, therapy should be reevaluated by your doctor. Tolerance may be reversed with short periods (8 to 24 hours) of withdrawal. Tolerance may be minimized by using the smallest effective dose, by using intermittent dosing, or by alternating with other vasodilators. Administering isosorbide dinitrate 2 or 3 times daily instead of 4, or using nitroglycerin transdermal patches for only 12 hours during the day, may reduce the possibility of tolerance developing. Nitrates that appear least likely to be associated with tolerance are the short-acting formulations (eg, sublingual, translingual spray). The transmucosal form also appears to be associated with minimal tolerance.

*Transient dizziness or weakness:* Transient dizziness or weakness (orthostatic hypotension) can occur when arising from a seated or lying position. Alcohol can worsen this side effect. Recovery can be hastened by positions in which the head is lower than the heart, deep breathing, and movements of the arms and legs.

*Pregnancy:* There are no adequate and well-controlled studies in pregnant women. Use only if clearly needed and the potential benefits to the mother outweigh the possible hazards to the fetus.

*Breastfeeding:* It is not known if nitrates appear in breast milk. Discontinue nursing during nitrate therapy.

*Children:* Safety and effectiveness have not been established.

## Drug Interactions:

Tell your doctor or pharmacist if you are taking or if you are planning to take any over-the-counter or prescription medications or dietary supplements with nitrates. Doses of one or both drugs may need to be modified or a different drug may need to be prescribed. The following drugs and drug classes interact with nitrates:

alcohol
calcium channel blockers
 (eg, verapamil)
ergot alkaloids (eg, dihydroergotamine)

heparin (eg, *Liquaemin*)
sildenafil citrate (*Viagra*)
vasodilators (eg, papaverine)

## Side Effects:

Every drug is capable of producing side effects. Many nitrate users experience no, or minor, side effects. The frequency and severity of side effects depend on many factors including dose, duration of therapy, and individual susceptibility. Possible side effects include:

*Digestive Tract:* Nausea; vomiting; diarrhea; stomach pain; appetite loss; dry mouth.

*Nervous System:* Persistent or severe headache; apprehension; restlessness; agitation; anxiety; flushing; dizziness; muscle twitching; weakness; lightheadedness.

*Circulatory System:* Abnormally slow or fast pulse; chest pain; palpitations (pounding in the chest); low blood pressure; fainting; irregular heartbeat.

*Skin:* Rash or itching (nitroglycerin patches); flushing; excessive sweating; cold sweat; local burning or tingling (sublingual or buccal tablets).

*Other:* Visual disturbances; fever; involuntary passing of urine or feces.

## Guidelines for Use:

- *Brand interchange* — Do not change from one brand of this drug to another without consulting your pharmacist or doctor. Products manufactured by different companies may not be equally effective.
- Avoid alcohol while undergoing nitrate therapy.
- May cause headache, dizziness, or flushing. Notify your doctor if blurred vision, dry mouth, or persistent headache occurs.
- Take oral nitrates on an empty stomach with a glass of water.
- Keep tablets and capsules in original container. Keep container closed tightly.
- *Sublingual tablets* —
  Dissolve tablet under tongue. Do not crush or chew. Do not swallow. A lack of burning or stinging sensation does not indicate a loss of potency.
  Use when seated. Take at the first sign of an anginal attack (chest pain) before severe pain develops. If angina is not relieved in 5 minutes, dissolve a second tablet under the tongue. If pain is not relieved within another 5 minutes, dissolve a third tablet. If pain continues or intensifies, notify your doctor immediately or report to the nearest hospital emergency room.
  Absorption is dependent on saliva secretion. Dry mouth (including drug-induced dry mouth) decreases absorption.
  Keep in the original container. Store at room temperature. Protect from moisture. Traditionally, unused tablets should be discarded 6 months after the original bottle is opened. Specific manufacturers may have different recommendations.
- *Translingual spray* —
  Do not shake. Spray onto or under tongue. Do not inhale spray.
  At the onset of attack, spray 1 or 2 doses onto oral mucosa. No more than 3 doses are recommended within 15 minutes. If chest pain persists, seek prompt medical attention.
  May be used 5 to 10 minutes prior to engaging in activities that might precipitate an acute attack.
- *Transmucosal tablets* —
  Place tablet between lip and gum above front teeth or between cheek and gum.
  Permit to dissolve slowly over a 3 to 5 hour period.
  Do not chew or swallow tablets. Release of nitroglycerin begins immediately upon contact with the mucosa and will continue until the tablet dissolves. Rate of dissolution is increased by touching tablet with tongue or drinking hot liquids.
- *Sustained-release nitroglycerin* —
  Swallow whole. Do not chew or crush. Not for sublingual use.
- *Topical ointment* —
  Patient instructions are available with products.
  Spread a thin layer on skin using applicator or dose-measuring paper. Do not use fingers. Do not rub or massage. Keep tube tightly closed. When applying ointment, spread at least a 2 × 3 inch area in a thin, uniform layer. The ointment may be applied to the chest or back.
  Rotate application sites to prevent contact dermatitis.

## Guidelines for Use (cont.):

- *Transdermal nitroglycerin patches —*
Patient instructions are available with products.
Patches are not for immediate relief of chest pain. Occasional use of sublingual preparations may be necessary.
Apply pad once each day to a skin site free of hair and excessive movement. Do not apply to the forearms or below the knees. Avoid cuts or irritations.
Change the application site slightly each time to avoid undue skin irritation.
Dispose of used patches carefully. Discarded patches contain significant amounts of nitroglycerin and can be harmful to children or pets.

*If you have any questions, consult your doctor, pharmacist, or health care provider.*

| Generic Name<br>*Brand Name Example* | Supplied As | Generic<br>Available |
|---|---|---|
| *Rx* **Bosentan** | | |
| *Tracleer* | **Tablets:** 62.5 mg, 125 mg | No |

## Type of Drug:
Endothelin receptor antagonist; pulmonary artery vasodilator.

## How the Drug Works:
Endothelin-1 is a hormone that attaches to the blood vessels in the lung and causes them to constrict (narrow). This constriction causes blood pressure in the lungs to increase (pulmonary artery hypertension). Bosentan interferes with the attachment of endothelin-1 and results in a lowering of the elevated blood pressure in the lungs.

## Uses:
For the treatment of pulmonary arterial hypertension in patients with WHO Class III or IV symptoms, to improve exercise ability and decrease the rate of clinical worsening.

## Precautions:
*Do not use in the following situations:*
allergy to the drug or any of its ingredients
cyclosporine A (eg, *Neoral*) therapy, current
glyburide (eg, *Micronase*) therapy, current
liver impairment, preexisting, moderate to severe
pregnancy

*Use with caution in the following situations:* Mild, preexisting liver impairment.

*Pregnancy:* Do not use during pregnancy. The risk of use in a pregnant woman clearly outweighs any possible benefit. Effective contraception must be used in women of child-bearing potential.

*Breastfeeding:* It is not known if bosentan appears in breast milk. Consult your doctor before you begin breastfeeding.

*Children:* Safety and effectiveness have not been established.

*Lab tests* will be required during treatment. Tests include liver enzymes, urine or serum pregnancy tests, or hemoglobin level tests.

## Drug Interactions:

Tell your doctor or pharmacist if you are taking or planning to take any over-the-counter or prescription medications or dietary supplements while taking this drug. Drug doses may need to be modified or a different drug prescribed. The following drugs and drug classes interact with this drug:

cyclosporine A (eg, *Neoral*)
glyburide (eg, *Micronase*)
HMG-CoA reductase inhibitors
(eg, lovastatin)

hormonal contraceptives (eg,
*Ortho-Novum*)
ketoconazole (eg, *Nizoral*)
warfarin (eg, *Coumadin*)

## Side Effects:

Every drug is capable of producing side effects. Many patients experience no, or minor, side effects. The frequency and severity of side effects depend on many factors including dose, duration of therapy, and individual susceptibility. Possible side effects include: nasal and throat inflammation; flushing; abnormal liver function; swelling; low blood pressure; itching; headache; fatigue; indigestion; anemia; pounding in the chest (palpitations).

---

### Guidelines for Use:

- Read the medication guide provided before starting therapy.
- Dosage is individualized. Take exactly as prescribed.
- Do not stop taking or change the dose, unless instructed by your doctor.
- May be taken with or without food. Take with food if stomach upset occurs.
- If a dose is missed, take it as soon as possible. If several hours have passed or it is nearing time for the next dose, do not double the dose to catch up, unless instructed by your doctor. If more than one dose is missed or it is necessary to establish a new dosage schedule, contact your doctor or pharmacist.
- Stop taking and notify your doctor immediately if you experience fever, persistent stomach pain, nausea, vomiting, yellowing of the skin or eyes, or unusual lethargy or fatigue.
- Contraceptive measures (birth control) are recommended during treatment to prevent pregnancy. Taking this medicine while pregnant can result in severe birth defects. Contact your doctor immediately if pregnancy is suspected.
- Lab tests may be required to monitor therapy. Be sure to keep appointments.
- Store at room temperature (59° to 86°F).

---

*If you have any questions, consult your doctor, pharmacist, or health care provider.*

| Generic Name Brand Name Examples | Supplied As | Generic Available |
|---|---|---|
| Rx **Amiodarone**[1] | | |
| *Cordarone, Pacerone* | **Tablets**: 200 mg | Yes |
| *Pacerone* | **Tablets**: 400 mg | No |

[1] This product is also available as an injection.

## Type of Drug:

A drug used for specific types of severe irregular heartbeats.

## How the Drug Works:

Amiodarone corrects and prevents the occurrence of various types of irregular heart rhythms that may lead to life-threatening situations.

## Uses:

To treat certain life-threatening heart rhythm disturbances (ie, recurrent ventricular fibrillation, recurrent hemodynamically unstable ventricular tachycardia) that are not affected by other antiarrhythmics or when other drugs are not tolerated.

*Unlabeled Use(s):* Sometimes used to treat refractory sustained or paroxysmal atrial fibrillation and paroxysmal supraventricular tachycardia, and symptomatic atrial flutter. May improve left ventricular ejection fraction, exercise tolerance, and ventricular arrhythmias in patients with congestive heart failure.

## Precautions:

*Do not use in the following situations:*

allergy to amiodarone or any of its ingredients

fainting episodes caused by bradycardia (without pacemaker)

heart block, second- and third-degree

sinus-node dysfunction, severe

*Use with caution in the following situations:*

electrolyte imbalance (eg, potassium)

liver disease

lung disease

thyroid dysfunction

*Potentially fatal toxicities:* Amiodarone has caused pulmonary toxicity (ie, hypersensitivity pneumonitis or interstitial/alveolar pneumonitis). Overt liver disease has been reported, resulting in a few deaths. Significant heart block or sinus bradycardia has also been reported.

*Heart effects:* A worsening of heart rhythm irregularities is unusual while under treatment but can occur. Amiodarone can also cause slow heart rates or occasional pauses in the heart rhythm.

*Sensitivity to sunlight:* Amiodarone has caused sensitivity of the skin to sunlight and to ultraviolet light. During long-term treatment, exposed skin may appear blue-gray. Risk is increased in patients with a fair complexion and in those with excessive exposure to the sun. Use sunscreens and wear protective clothing.

*Pregnancy:* Amiodarone can cause fetal harm when administered to a pregnant woman. There have been some reports of congenital goiter/hypothyroidism and hyperthyroidism. Use only if clearly needed and potential benefits to the mother outweigh the possible hazards to the fetus.

*Breastfeeding:* Amiodarone appears in breast milk. Mothers should discontinue breastfeeding during therapy.

*Children:* Safety and effectiveness have not been established. Benzyl alcohol, contained in some of these products as a preservative, has been associated with a fatal gasping syndrome in premature infants. Amiodarone is not recommended in children.

*Lab tests* and physical examinations will be required during treatment with amiodarone. Tests may include chest x-rays; blood tests; electrocardiograms; liver, thyroid, and pulmonary function tests; and eye exams.

## Drug Interactions:

Tell your doctor or pharmacist if you are taking or if you are planning to take any over-the-counter or prescription medications or dietary supplements with amiodarone. Doses of one or both drugs may need to be modified or a different drug may need to be prescribed. The following drugs and drug classes interact with amiodarone:

antiarrhythmics, other
 (eg, procainamide)
anticoagulants (eg, warfarin)
calcium channel blockers
 (eg, verapamil)
cimetidine (eg, *Tagamet*)
cyclosporine (eg, *Neoral*)
digoxin (eg, *Lanoxin*)

disopyramide (eg, *Norpace*)
fentanyl (eg, *Sublimaze*)
flecainide (*Tambocor*)
methotrexate (eg, *Rheumatrex*)
hydantoins (eg, phenytoin)
quinidine (eg, *Quinora*)
quinolones (eg, sparfloxacin)
ritonavir (*Norvir*)

## Side Effects:

Every drug is capable of producing side effects. Many amiodarone users experience no, or minor, side effects. The frequency and severity of side effects depend on many factors including dose, duration of therapy, and individual susceptibility. Possible side effects include:

*Eyes or Ocular:* Appearance of halos around lights; sensitivity to light; blurred or spotty vision; dry eyes; sensitivity to light; permanent blindness; eye discomfort; fluid accumulation at the optic disc; other vision disturbances; eye degeneration; optic nerve disease.

*Digestive Tract:* Nausea; vomiting; constipation; diarrhea; loss of appetite; stomach pain.

*Nervous System:* Tremors; twitches; fatigue; loss of coordination; unsteady walking; dizziness; numbness and tingling in hands and feet; difficulty sleeping; headache; general discomfort; abnormal gait.

*Circulatory System:* Slowing of heartbeat (rhythm); worsening of irregular heart rhythm; decrease in blood pressure; decrease in blood platelets; coagulation abnormalities; heart failure; heart block.

*Respiratory System:* Difficulty breathing (shortness of breath); coughing; abnormal x-ray or biopsy; fibrosis.

*Skin:* Sensitivity to sunlight; blue-gray skin color; rash; dermatitis; unexplained bruising; hair loss; flushing; abnormal skin sensations (eg, burning, prickling, tingling).

*Other:* Disturbances in thyroid, respiratory, kidney and liver function (cirrhosis, hepatitis); abnormal taste and smell; edema (fluid retention); abnormal salivation; loss of sex drive; abnormal blood tests.

---

### Guidelines for Use:

- Dosage is individualized. Take exactly as prescribed.
- Do not change the dose or stop taking unless advised by your doctor.
- High doses of amiodarone are usually required for the first 1 to 3 weeks of treatment.
- Take with meals, especially if stomach upset occurs.
- If a dose is missed, take it as soon as possible. If several hours have passed or it is nearing time for the next dose, do not double the dose to catch up, unless advised by your doctor. If more than one dose is missed, or it is necessary to establish a new dosage schedule, contact your doctor or pharmacist.
- Inform your doctor if you are pregnant, become pregnant, planning to become pregnant, or are breastfeeding before beginning therapy.
- May cause photosensitivity (sensitivity to sunlight). Use sunscreen and wear protective clothing until tolerance is determined.
- Shortness of breath, coughing and abnormal diagnostic tests (eg, chest x-ray, lung biopsy) can occur. Report changes in breathing or vision, or any coughing to your doctor and have a routine chest x-ray.
- Loss of vision can occur. Inform your doctor if your vision changes or your peripheral vision decreases.
- Store at room temperature (59° to 86°F). Keep in a tight container away from light.

---

*If you have any questions, consult your doctor, pharmacist, or health care provider.*

| Generic Name<br>*Brand Name Examples* | Supplied As | Generic<br>Available |
|---|---|---|
| Rx **Disopyramide**<br>**Phosphate** | | |
| *Norpace* | **Capsules**: 100 mg, 150 mg | Yes |
| *Norpace CR* | **Capsules, extended release**:<br>100 mg, 150 mg | Yes |

## Type of Drug:

A drug used for specific types of irregular heartbeats.

## How the Drug Works:

Disopyramide slows the rate at which nerve impulses are conducted through the heart and reduces the tendency of the heart to beat irregularly.

## Uses:

To treat documented life-threatening heart rhythm disturbances.

*Unlabeled Use(s):* Occasionally doctors may prescribe disopyramide for certain types of rapid heart rate.

## Precautions:

*Do not use in the following situations:*

allergy to disopyramide or any
 of its ingredients
cardiogenic shock

congenital QT prolongation
heart block (without pacemaker),
 second- or third-degree

*Use with caution in the following situations:*

abnormal heart conduction
antiarrhythmic therapy,
 concomitant
arrhythmias, ventricular
asymptomatic ventricular premature contractions
atrial rhythm disturbances
bundle branch block
congestive heart failure

enlarged prostate
glaucoma
heart block, first-degree
kidney disease
liver disease
low blood pressure
myasthenia gravis
potassium imbalance
urinary retention

*Low blood sugar:* Occasionally low blood glucose (sugar) levels occur with disopyramide therapy. Contact your doctor if symptoms (eg, increased heart rate, sweating, chills, tremor) develop.

*Pregnancy:* There are no adequate and well-controlled studies in pregnant women. Disopyramide has been found in human fetal blood, and may stimulate contractions of the pregnant uterus. Use only if clearly needed and the potential benefits to the mother outweigh the possible hazards to the fetus.

*Breastfeeding:* Disopyramide appears in breast milk. A decision should be made whether to discontinue nursing or discontinue the drug, taking into account the importance of the drug to the mother. Consult your doctor.

*Lab tests* may be required during treatment with disopyramide. Tests may include: blood tests and electrocardiograms.

## Drug Interactions:

Tell your doctor or pharmacist if you are taking or planning to take any over-the-counter or prescription medications or dietary supplements with disopyramide. Doses of one or both drugs may need to be modified or a different drug may need to be prescribed. The following drugs and drug classes interact with disopyramide:

antiarrhythmics, other (eg, procainamide, lidocaine)
beta-blockers (eg, propranolol)
clarithromycin (*Biaxin*)
erythromycin (eg, *E-Mycin*)

hydantoins (eg, phenytoin)
quinidine (eg, *Cardioquin*)
rifampin (eg, *Rifadin*)
verapamil (eg, *Calan*)

## Side Effects:

Every drug is capable of producing side effects. Many disopyramide users experience no, or minor, side effects. The frequency and severity of side effects depend on many factors including dose, duration of therapy, and individual susceptibility. Possible side effects include:

*Digestive Tract:* Constipation; nausea; vomiting; stomach pain; bloating and gas; appetite loss; diarrhea.

*Nervous System:* Headache; nervousness; dizziness; fatigue; difficulty sleeping.

*Circulatory System:* Chest pain; irregular heartbeat; low blood pressure; heart conduction disturbances; congestive heart failure.

*Skin:* Rash; itching; hives.

*Urinary and Reproductive Tract:* Urinary retention, hesitancy, frequency, or urgency; impotence; painful urination.

*Other:* Shortness of breath; edema (fluid retention); weight gain; blurred vision; dry mouth; dry nose, eyes, and throat; aches and pains; fainting; general body discomfort; muscle weakness; decreased potassium level; increased cholesterol and triglyceride blood levels; decreased blood sugar level.

## Guidelines for Use:

- Hospitalization is required when starting this medication.
- Dosage is individualized. Take exactly as prescribed.
- Do not change the dose or stop taking before consulting your doctor. Do not exceed recommended dosage.
- If a dose is missed, take it as soon as possible. If several hours have passed or if it is nearing time for the next dose, do not double the dose to catch up, unless advised by your doctor. If more than one dose is missed, or it is necessary to establish a new dosage schedule, contact your doctor or pharmacist.
- Swallow sustained release capsules whole. Do not break or chew.
- May cause rash, chest pain, dry mouth, dizziness, difficulty breathing, difficult urination, constipation, or blurred vision. Notify your doctor if these symptoms persist.
- Consult your doctor immediately if you experience symptoms of low blood sugar (increased heart rate, sweating, chills, tremors).
- Inform your doctor if you are pregnant, become pregnant, planning to become pregnant, or are breastfeeding before beginning therapy.
- Lab tests may be required to monitor blood counts and heart function. Be sure to keep appointments.
- Store at controlled room temperature (68° to 77°F).

*If you have any questions, consult your doctor, pharmacist, or health care provider.*

| Generic Name<br>*Brand Name Example* | Supplied As | Generic<br>Available |
|---|---|---|
| *Rx* **Dofetilide** | | |
| *Tikosyn* | **Capsules**: 125 mcg, 250 mcg,<br>500 mcg | No |

## Type of Drug:

Antiarrhythmic drug.

## How the Drug Works:

Dofetilide delays cardiac cell electrical activity, normalizing cardiac activity and maintaining normal sinus rhythm.

## Uses:

For the conversion of atrial fibrillation and atrial flutter to normal sinus rhythm.

For maintaining normal sinus rhythm in patients with atrial fibrillation and atrial flutter.

*Unlabeled Use(s):* Dofetilide has been used for ventricular arrhythmias.

## Precautions:

*Do not use in the following situations:*

allergy to dofetilide or any of its ingredients
concominant use of verapamil, cimetidine, trimethoprim, ketoconazole, prochlorperazine, or megestrol
congenital or acquired long QT syndromes
heart rate of less than 50 bpm
kidney impairment, severe
QT baseline interval or QTc greater than 440 msec

*Use with caution in the following situations:*

hypokalemia
hypomagnesemia
kidney disease, mild to moderate
liver disease
torsade de pointes type ventricular tachycardia
QT prolongation

*Gender:* Dofetilide was associated with a greater risk of torsade de pointes in female patients than in male patients.

*Pregnancy:* There are no adaquate and well-controlled studies in pregnant women. Use only if clearly needed and the potential benefits to the mother outweigh the possible hazards to the fetus.

*Breastfeeding:* It is not known if dofetilide appears in breast milk. Consult your doctor before you begin breastfeeding.

*Children:* The safety and efficacy of use in children younger than 18 years of age have not been established.

*Lab tests* will be required during treatment. Tests may include ECG monitoring, QTc levels, kidney function, and liver function.

## Drug Interactions:

Tell you doctor or pharmacist if you are taking or if you a planning to take any over-the-counter or prescription medications or dietary supplements with dofetilide. Doses of one or both drugs may need to be modified or a different drug may need to be prescribed. The following drugs and drug classes interact with dofetilide:

amiloride (*Midamor*)
antiarrhythmic agents (Class I
 or Class III) (eg, moricizine)
bepridil (*Vascor*)
cimetidine (eg, *Tagamet*)
CYP3A4 isoenzyme inhibitors
 (eg, ketoconazole)
digoxin (*Lanoxin*)
megestrol (*Megace*)
metformin (*Glucophage*)
phenothiazines
 (eg, chlorpromazine)
potassium-depleting diuretics
prochlorperazine
 (eg, *Compazine*)
tricyclic antidepressants
 (eg, amitriptyline)
triamterene (*Dyrenium*)
trimethoprim (eg, *Proloprim*)
trimethoprim/sulfamethoxazole
 (eg, *Bactrim*)
verapamil (eg, *Calan*)

## Side Effects:

Every drug is capable of producing side effects. Many dofetilide users experience no, or minor, side effects. The frequency and severity of side effects depend on many factors including dose, duration of therapy, and individual susceptibility. Possible side effects include:

*Circulatory System:* Rapid heart beat; slow heart beat; various cardiac rhythm disturbances; pounding in the chest; heart block; heart arrest; stroke.

*Nervous System:* Headache; chest pain; dizziness; stomach pain; back pain; joint pain; muscle limpness; weakness; anxiety; fainting; muscle dysfunction.

*Skin:* Rash; hives; sweating; abnormal skin sensations (eg, burning, prickling, tingling).

*Other:* Respiratory tract infection; difficulty breathing; nausea; vomiting; thirst; appetite loss; flu syndrome; sleeplessness; accidental injury; diarrhea; urinary tract infection; fluid retention; cough; migraine; dizziness; fainting; liver damage.

## Guidelines for Use:

- Dosage is individualized. Take exactly as prescribed.
- Do not change the dose or stop taking unless advised by your doctor.
- Dofetilide is only available to hospitals and prescribers who have received appropriate dosing and treatment initiation education.
- Compliance with the dosing schedule and periodic heart and kidney function tests is important for minimizing the risk of developing serious abnormal heart rhythm.
- Notify your health care provider of any change in over-the-counter or prescription medication, or dietary supplement use.
- Inform your health care provider if you are hospitalized or prescribed a new medication for any condition.
- Inform your doctor if you are pregnant, become pregnant, planning to become pregnant, or are breastfeeding before beginning therapy.
- Notify your doctor immediately of symptoms associated with altered electrolyte balance, such as excessive or prolonged diarrhea, sweating, vomiting, appetite loss, thirst, or diuretic use.
- If a dose is missed, take it as soon as possible. If several hours have passed or if it is nearing time for the next dose, do not double the dose to catch up, unless advised by your doctor. If more than one dose is missed or it is necessary to establish a new dosage schedule, contact your doctor or pharmacist.
- Store at controlled room temperature (59° to 86°F) in a tight container. Protect from moisture and humidity.

*If you have any questions, consult your doctor, pharmacist, or health care provider.*

| Generic Name Brand Name Example | Supplied As | Generic Available |
|---|---|---|
| **Flecainide Acetate** | | |
| Rx  Tambocor | **Tablets:** 50 mg, 100 mg, 150 mg | No |

## Type of Drug:

Drug used for specific types of irregular heartbeats.

## How the Drug Works:

Flecainide corrects and prevents the occurrence of various types of irregular heartbeats that lead to serious life-threatening situations.

## Uses:

To treat life-threatening heart rhythm disturbances.

## Precautions:

*Do not use in the following situations:*

allergy to flecainide
cardiogenic shock
heart block (without a pacemaker)
specific types of irregular heartbeats

*Use with caution in the following situations:*

heart attack, recent
heart disease (eg, congestive heart failure, sick sinus syndrome)
heart rate, occasional slowing or pausing
kidney disease
liver disease
pacemaker, permanent
potassium imbalance

*Heart rhythm disturbances:* New or worsened heart rhythm disturbances can result. The likelihood of heart rhythm disturbances occurring as a result of using flecainide is greater at high doses or in patients with heart disease. Therefore, the dose of flecainide should not be changed unsupervised.

*Pregnancy:* Adequate studies have not been done in pregnant women. Use only if clearly needed and potential benefits outweigh the possible hazards to the fetus.

*Breastfeeding:* Flecainide appears in breast milk. Because of the potential for serious side effects in nursing infants, decide whether to discontinue nursing or the drug, taking into account the importance of the drug to the mother. Consult your doctor.

*Children:* Safety and effectiveness in children younger than 18 years of age have not been established.

*Lab tests* may be required during treatment with flecainide. Tests may include monitoring of blood levels.

## Drug Interactions:

Tell your doctor or pharmacist if you are taking or planning to take any over-the-counter or prescription medications or dietary supplements with flecainide. Doses of one or both drugs may need to be modified or a different drug may need to be prescribed. The following drugs and drug classes interact with flecainide:

amiodarone *(Cordarone)*
cimetidine (eg, *Tagamet)*
digoxin (eg, *Lanoxin)*
disopyramide (eg, *Norpace)*
propranolol (eg, *Inderal)*

urinary acidifiers (eg, ammonium chloride)
urinary alkalinizers (eg, sodium bicarbonate)
verapamil (eg, *Calan*)

## Side Effects:

Every drug is capable of producing side effects. Many flecainide users experience no, or minor, side effects. The frequency and severity of side effects depend on many factors including dose, duration of therapy, and individual susceptibility. Possible side effects include:

*Digestive Tract:* Nausea; vomiting; constipation; indigestion; appetite loss; diarrhea; stomach pain.

*Nervous System:* Dizziness; numbness and tingling of toes and fingers; tremor; headache; depression; sleeplessness; paralysis; fatigue; weakness; incoordination; vertigo (feeling of whirling motion); anxiety.

*Circulatory System:* New or worsened heart rhythm disturbances; heart rate changes; chest pain; palpitations (pounding in the chest).

*Skin:* Rash; flushing; sweating.

*Other:* Edema (fluid retention); blurred vision; difficulty focusing eyes; spots in front of eyes; double vision; ringing in the ears; difficulty breathing; fever; general body discomfort; fainting.

---

**Guidelines for Use:**
- Take as prescribed by your doctor. Serious heartbeat disturbances can result from missing any doses and serious side effects can result from increasing or decreasing doses without supervision.
- Blood tests for flecainide levels may be required to monitor your therapy.

---

*If you have any questions, consult your doctor, pharmacist, or health care provider.*

| Generic Name<br>*Brand Name Example* | Supplied As | Generic<br>Available |
|---|---|---|
| *Rx* **Mexiletine** | | |
| *Mexitil* | **Capsules:** 150 mg, 200 mg, 250 mg | No |

## Type of Drug:

A drug used for specific types of irregular heartbeats.

## How the Drug Works:

Mexiletine reduces the tendency of the heart to beat irregularly.

## Uses:

To treat documented life-threatening heart rhythm disturbances.

*Unlabeled Use(s):* Occasionally doctors may prescribe mexiletine to reduce the incidence of irregular heartbeats during heart attacks. It may also be used to reduce pain, impaired sense of touch and abnormal sensations associated with diabetic neuropathy.

## Precautions:

*Do not use in the following situations:*
cardiogenic shock
heart block (without pacemaker)

*Use with caution in the following situations:*

certain heart disorders
congestive heart failure, severe
heart block (with pacemaker)

liver disease
low blood pressure
seizures, history

*Heart rhythm disturbances:* Worsened heart rhythm disturbances can result from taking mexiletine. Close monitoring and careful dosage adjustment will be required.

*Pregnancy:* Mexiletine crosses the placenta. Adequate studies have not been done in pregnant women. Use only if clearly needed and potential benefits outweigh the possible hazards to the fetus.

*Breastfeeding:* Mexiletine appears in breast milk. Discontinue nursing if mexiletine therapy is needed.

*Children:* Safety and effectiveness have not been established.

## Drug Interactions:

Tell your doctor or pharmacist if you are taking or planning to take any over-the-counter or prescription medications or dietary supplements with mexiletine. Doses of one or both drugs may need to be modified or a different drug may need to be prescribed. The following drugs and drug classes interact with mexiletine:

aluminum-magnesium hydroxide (eg, *Maalox)*
atropine
caffeine
cimetidine *(Tagamet)*
hydantoins (eg, phenytoin)
metoclopramide (eg, *Reglan)*

narcotics (eg, codeine)
rifampin (eg, *Rifadin)*
theophylline (eg, *Theo-Dur)*
urinary acidifiers (eg, potassium acid phosphate)
urinary alkalinizers (eg, potassium citrate)

## Side Effects:

Every drug is capable of producing side effects. Many mexiletine users experience no, or minor, side effects. The frequency and severity of side effects depend on many factors including dose, duration of therapy, and individual susceptibility. Possible side effects include:

*Digestive Tract:* Nausea; vomiting; heartburn; stomach pain, cramps or discomfort; constipation; diarrhea; changes in appetite.

*Nervous System:* Dizziness; tremor; lightheadedness; nervousness; confusion; incoordination;headache; numbness; abnormal sensations; changes in sleep habits; weakness; fatigue; depression.

*Circulatory System:* Palpitations (pounding in the chest); chest pain; increased irregular heartbeats.

*Other:* Joint pain; blurred vision; vision problems; ringing in the ears; speech difficulties; rash; dry mouth; difficulty breathing; edema (fluid retention); fever.

---

### Guidelines for Use:

- Take medication with food or an antacid.
- Notify your doctor if unexplained general tiredness, yellowing of the skin, fever or sore throat occurs.
- Side effects such as nausea, vomiting, heartburn, diarrhea, constipation, dizziness, tremor, nervousness, in-coordination, changes in sleep habits, headache, visual disturbances, tingling/numbness, weakness, ringing in the ears and palpitations/chest pain may occur. Notify your doctor if they become bothersome.
- Avoid changes in diet that could drastically acidify or alkalinize the urine.
- Hospitalization is required when starting this medication.

---

*If you have any questions, consult your doctor, pharmacist, or health care provider.*

| Generic Name<br>*Brand Name Example* | Supplied As | Generic<br>Available |
|---|---|---|
| *Rx* **Moricizine** | | |
| *Ethmozine* | **Tablets:** 200 mg, 250 mg, 300 mg | No |

## Type of Drug:
A drug used for specific types of irregular heartbeats.

## How the Drug Works:
Moricizine prevents the occurrence of certain types of heart disturbances involving the ventricle of the heart that lead to serious life-threatening situations.

## Uses:
To treat life-threatening heart rhythm disturbances. Because of certain effects of this drug, moricizine use should be reserved for patients in whom the benefits of treatment outweigh the risks.

*Unlabeled Use(s):* Occasionally doctors may prescribe moricizine for certain other heart rhythm disturbances.

## Precautions:
*Do not use in the following situations:*
    allergy to moricizine
    cardiogenic shock
    heart block

*Use with caution in the following situations:*

| | |
|---|---|
| congestive heart failure | kidney disease |
| electrolyte imbalances | liver disease |
| (eg, potassium, magnesium) | sick sinus syndrome |
| heart conduction abnormalities, preexisting | |

*Heart Rhythm Disturbances:* New or worsened heart rhythm disturbances can result from taking moricizine, especially in patients with serious or advanced heart disease. Close monitoring and careful dosage adjustment will be required.

*Pregnancy:* Adequate studies have not been done in pregnant women. Use only if clearly needed and potential benefits outweigh the possible hazards to the fetus.

*Breastfeeding:* Moricizine appears in breast milk. Because of the potential for serious adverse effects, a decision should be made whether to discontinue nursing or the drug, taking into account the importance of the drug to the mother. Consult your doctor.

*Children:* Safety and effectiveness in children under 18 have not been established.

*Lab tests* may be required during treatment with moricizine. Tests may include: Electrocardiograms; kidney and liver function tests.

## Drug Interactions:

Tell your doctor or pharmacist if you are taking or planning to take any over-the-counter or prescription medications or dietary supplements with moricizine. Doses of one or both drugs may need to be modified or a different drug may need to be prescribed. The following drugs and drug classes interact with moricizine:

| | |
|---|---|
| cimetidine (eg, *Tagamet)* | propranolol (eg, *Inderal*) |
| digoxin (eg, *Lanoxin)* | theophylline (eg, *Theo-Dur*) |

## Side Effects:

Every drug is capable of producing side effects. Many moricizine users experience no, or minor, side effects. The frequency and severity of side effects depend on many factors including dose, duration of therapy, and individual susceptibility. Possible side effects include:

*Digestive Tract:* Nausea; vomiting; diarrhea; stomach pain; indigestion; appetite loss; gas; bitter taste; intestinal blockage.

*Nervous System:* Dizziness; drowsinesss; headache; fatigue; nervousness; restlessness; sleep disturbances; vertigo (feeling of whirling motion); abnormal coordination or movement; tremor; anxiety; depression; confusion; seizures; coma; hallucinations; memory loss; euphoria (exaggerated sense of well being); agitation; abnormal gait; weakness.

*Circulatory System:* Palpitations (pounding in the chest); chest pain; changes in heart rate and blood pressure; heart rhythm disturbances; heart failure; heart attack or stroke.

*Respiratory System:* Difficult, accelerated or cessation of breathing; asthma; cough; sore throat; inflamed sinuses.

*Urinary and Reproductive Tract:* Urinary retention, frequency or incontinence; kidney pain; difficult or painful urination.

*Skin:* Rash; dry skin; itching; hives; abnormal or decreased sensation; sweating. *Senses:* Blurred vision; double vision; involuntary eye movements; eye pain; ringing in the ears; difficulty speaking.

*Other:* Dry mouth; difficulty swallowing; swollen lips and tongue; decreased sex drive; impotence; abnormally low body temperature or fever; edema (fluid retention) around the eye socket; muscle and bone pain; fainting; temperature intolerance.

## Guidelines for Use:

- Take exactly as prescribed by your doctor. Serious heartbeat disturbances can result from taking too much or too little of this drug. Dosage changes must be supervised by your doctor.
- Contact your doctor immediately if you develop chest pain or discomfort, palpitations (pounding in the chest), irregular heartbeat or fever.
- Unless instructed otherwise by your doctor, if a dose is missed, take it as soon as possible. If several hours have passed or it is nearing time for the next dose, do not double the dose to catch up, unless advised to do so by your doctor. If more than one dose is missed or it is necessary to establish a new dosage schedule, contact your doctor or pharmacist. Use exactly as prescribed.
- Hospitalization is required when starting on this medication.

*If you have any questions, consult your doctor, pharmacist, or health care provider.*

| Generic Name<br>*Brand Name Examples* | Supplied As | Generic<br>Available |
|---|---|---|
| Rx **Procainamide**[1] | | |
| *Pronestyl* | **Capsules:** 250 mg, 375 mg, 500 mg | Yes |
| *Pronestyl*[2] | **Tablets:** 250 mg, 375 mg, 500 mg | Yes |
| *Procan SR, Pronestyl-SR* | **Tablets, sustained release:** 250 mg, 500 mg, 750 mg, 1000 mg | Yes |

[1] Some of these products are also available as an injection.
[2] Contains the dye tartrazine.

## Type of Drug:

A drug used for specific types of irregular heartbeats.

## How the Drug Works:

Procainamide slows the rate at which nerve impulses are conducted through the heart and reduces the tendency of the heart to beat irregularly.

## Uses:

To treat documented life-threatening heart rhythm disturbances.

## Precautions:

*Do not use in the following situations:*

| allergies to procainamide, pro-caine or procaine-like anesthetics | heart block<br>lupus erythematosus<br>torsade de pointes |
|---|---|

*Use with caution in the following situations:*

| bone marrow failure, preexisting congestive heart failure cytopenia digitalis intoxication | heart disease<br>kidney disease<br>myasthenia gravis |
|---|---|

*Lupus erythematosus-like syndrome:* A syndrome similar to systemic lupus erythematosus may occur (see Side Effects). Contact your doctor if symptoms develop.

*Pregnancy:* Procainamide crosses the placenta. Adequate studies have not been done in pregnant women. Use only if clearly needed and potential benefits outweigh the possible hazards to the fetus.

*Breastfeeding:* Procainamide is excreted in breast milk. Because of the potential for adverse effects, a decision should be made whether to discontinue nursing or the drug, taking into account the importance of the drug to the mother. Contact your doctor.

*Children:* Safety and effectiveness have not been established.

*Lab tests* may be required during treatment with procainamide. Tests may include: Electrocardiograms, procainamide blood levels and blood counts.

*Tartrazine:* Some of these products may contain the dye tartrazine (FD&C Yellow No. 5) which can cause allergic reactions in certain individuals. Check package label when available or consult your doctor or pharmacist.

## Drug Interactions:

Tell your doctor or pharmacist if you are taking or if you are planning to take any over-the-counter or prescription medications with procainamide. Doses of one or both drugs may need to be modified or a different drug may need to be prescribed. The following drugs and drug classes interact with procainamide.

alcohol
beta-blockers (eg, propranolol)
histamine $H_2$ antagonists
 (eg, cimetidine)

lidocaine (eg, *Xylocaine*)
quinidine (eg, *Quinora*)
succinylcholine (eg, *Sucostrin*)
trimethoprim (eg, *Proloprim*)

## Side Effects:

Every drug is capable of producing side effects. Many procainamide users experience no, or minor, side effects. The frequency and severity of side effects depend on many factors including dose, duration of therapy and individual susceptibility. Possible side effects include:

*Lupus Erythematosus-like Syndrome:* Joint pain or stiffness; skin lesions; muscle aches; chest pain with breathing; fever; chills; abdominal pain.

*Digestive Tract:* Appetite loss; nausea; vomiting; diarrhea; abdominal pain.

*Nervous System:* Depression; dizziness; weakness; giddiness; hallucinations.

*Skin:* Rash; itching; hives; flushing.

*Other:* Irregular heartbeat; fibrillation; bitter taste.

---

### Guidelines for Use:

- Notify your doctor of any drug allergies, especially to procaine, other local anesthetic agents or aspirin, and report any history of kidney disease, congestive heart failure, myasthenia gravis, liver disease or lupus erythematosus.
- Notify your doctor promptly of the following symptoms: joint or muscle pain, fever, chills, rash, easy bruising, sore throat or mouth, infections, dark urine, yellowing of skin or eyes, wheezing, muscular weakness, chest or abdominal pain, palpitations, nausea, vomiting, appetite loss, diarrhea, hallucinations, dizziness or depression.
- Do not break or chew sustained-release tablets.

---

*If you have any questions, consult your doctor, pharmacist, or health care provider.*

| Generic Name Brand Name Example | Supplied As | Generic Available |
|---|---|---|
| Rx **Propafenone HCl** | | |
| *Rythmol* | **Tablets:** 150 mg, 300 mg | No |

## Type of Drug:

Drug used for specific types of irregular heartbeats.

## How the Drug Works:

Propafenone reduces the tendency of the heart to beat irregularly. It stabilizes the activity of the heart muscle under certain conditions.

## Uses:

To treat documented life-threatening heart rhythm disturbances. Because of certain effects of this drug, propafenone use should be reserved for patients in whom the benefits of treatment outweigh the risks.

*Unlabeled Use(s):* Occasionally doctors may prescribe propafenone for heart rhythm disturbances associated with Wolff-Parkinson-White syndrome.

## Precautions:

*Do not use in the following situations:*

allergy to propafenone
cardiogenic shock
congestive heart failure
 (uncontrolled)
decreased blood pressure,
 marked
decreased heart rate
electrolyte imbalance
heart disorders, certain
 (without pacemaker)
lung disorders

*Use with caution in the following situations:*

bronchospasm, nonallergic
kidney disease
liver disease
pacemakers

*Heart rhythm disturbances:* New or worsened heart rhythm disturbances can result. Therefore, periodic electrocardiograms (EKGs) will be required prior to, and during, treatment with propafenone.

*Pregnancy:* Adequate studies have not been done in pregnant women. Use only if clearly needed and potential benefits outweigh the possible hazards to the fetus.

*Breastfeeding:* It is not known if propafenone appears in breast milk. A decision should be made whether to discontinue nursing or the drug, taking into account the importance of the drug to the mother. Consult your doctor.

*Children:* Safety and effectiveness have not been established.

*Elderly:* Use with caution. The usual adult dose may need to be lowered in these patients.

*Lab tests* may be required during treatment with propafenone. These tests may include electrocardiograms (EKGs); blood counts; liver and kidney function tests.

## Drug Interactions:

Tell your doctor or pharmacist if you are taking or planning to take any over-the-counter or prescription medications or dietary supplements with propafenone. Doses of one or both drugs may need to be modified or a different drug may need to be prescribed. The following drugs and drug classes interact with propafenone:

anesthetics, local (eg, benzo-caine)
anticoagulants (eg, warfarin)
beta-blockers (eg, propranolol)
cimetidine (eg, *Tagamet*)

cyclosporine (eg, *Sandimmune*)
digoxin (eg, *Lanoxin*)
quinidine (eg, *Quinora*)
rifampin (eg, *Rifadin*)

## Side Effects:

Every drug is capable of producing side effects. Many propafenone users experience no, or minor, side effects. The frequency and severity of side effects depend on many factors including dose, duration of therapy, and individual susceptibility. Possible side effects include:

*Digestive Tract:* Nausea; vomiting; constipation; diarrhea; gas; appetite loss; indigestion; stomach pain; abdominal cramping; dry mouth; unusual taste.

*Nervous System:* Dizziness; headache; fatigue; anxiety; sleeplessness; drowsiness; incoordination; tremor.

*Circulatory System:* Congestive heart failure; chest pain; palpitations (pounding in the chest); irregular heartbeats (rhythm); decrease in blood pressure.

*Other:* Blurred vision; rash; difficulty breathing; edema (fluid retention); joint pain; sweating; weakness; fainting.

---

## Guidelines for Use:

- Unless instructed otherwise by your doctor, if a dose is missed, take it as soon as possible. If several hours have passed or it is nearing time for the next dose, do not double the dose to catch up, unless advised to do so by your doctor. If more than one dose is missed, or it is necessary to establish a new dosage schedule, contact your doctor or pharmacist. Take this medication at evenly spaced intervals around the clock.
- Palpitations (pounding in the chest), chest pain, blurred or abnormal vision, or difficulty breathing may occur. Notify your doctor if these symptoms become bothersome.
- Notify your doctor if you develop any signs of infection such as fever, sore throat, chills or unusual bleeding or bruising.
- Watch for signs of overdose or toxicity, such as lowered blood pressure, excessive drowsiness, slowed heart rate or abnormal heartbeat.

---

*If you have any questions, consult your doctor, pharmacist, or health care provider.*

| Generic Name<br>*Brand Name Examples* | Supplied As | Generic<br>Available |
|---|---|---|
| Rx **Quinidine Gluconate**[1] | | |
| *Quinalan* | **Tablets, sustained release:** 324 mg | Yes |
| Rx **Quinidine Polygalacturonate** | | |
| *Cardioquin* | **Tablets:** 275 mg (equiv. to 200 mg sulfate) | No |
| Rx **Quinidine Sulfate** | | |
| *Quinora* | **Tablets:** 200 mg, 300 mg | Yes |
| *Quinidex Extentabs* | **Tablets, sustained release:** 300 mg | No |

[1] Some of these products are also available as an injection.

## Type of Drug:
Drugs used to treat irregular heartbeats.

## How the Drug Works:
Quinidine reduces excitability of the heart muscle, slows the rate at which nerve impulses are conducted through the heart and reduces the ability of the heart to contract.

## Uses:
To treat abnormal heart rhythms.

*Injection:* To treat *Plasmodium falciparum* malaria when oral therapy is not feasible or when a rapid effect is required.

## Precautions:
*Do not use in the following situations:*

allergy to quinidine
certain heart rate or rhythm
 disturbances
digitalis intoxication

discoloration or "bruising"
 associated with quinidine,
 history
heart block
myasthenia gravis

*Use with caution in the following situations:*

heart disease
heart flutters or fibrillations

kidney disease
liver disease

*Pregnancy:* Adequate studies have not been done in pregnant women. Quinidine crosses the placenta and is found in fetal blood. Use only if clearly needed and potential benefits outweigh the possible hazards to the fetus.

*Breastfeeding:* Quinidine appears in breast milk. Consult your doctor before you begin breastfeeding.

*Children:* Safety and effectiveness have not been established.

*Lab tests* may be required during treatment with quinidine. Tests may include: Electrocardiograms; potassium and quinidine blood levels; kidney and liver function tests.

## Drug Interactions:

Tell your doctor or pharmacist if you are taking or planning to take any over-the-counter or prescription medications or dietary supplements with quinidine. Doses of one or both drugs may need to be modified or a different drug may need to be prescribed. The following drugs and drug classes interact with quinidine:

acetazolamide (eg, *Diamox*)
amiodarone (*Cordarone*)
antacids (eg, *Tums*)
anticholinergics
  (eg, diphenhydramine)
anticoagulants, oral
  (eg, warfarin)
barbiturates (eg, phenobarbital)
beta-blockers
  (eg, propranolol)
cholinergic drugs (eg, pilo-carpine)
cimetidine (eg, *Tagamet*)
dichlorphenamide (*Daranide*)
digitoxin (eg, *Crystodigin*)
digoxin (eg, *Lanoxin*)
disopyramide (*Norpace*)
hydantoins (eg, phenytoin)
methazolamide (*Neptazane*)
nifedipine (eg, *Procardia*)
procainamide (*Pronestyl*)
propafenone (*Rythmol*)
rifampin (eg, *Rifadin*)
sucralfate (*Carafate*)
succinylcholine (eg, *Quelicin*)
tricyclic antidepressants
  (eg, amitriptyline)
urinary alkalinizers (eg, potas-sium citrate)
verapamil (eg, *Calan*)

## Side Effects:

Every drug is capable of producing side effects. Many quinidine users experience no, or minor, side effects. The frequency and severity of side effects depend on many factors including dose, duration of therapy, and individual susceptibility. Possible side effects include:

*Quinidine Overdose:* Ringing in the ears; hearing loss; headache; nausea; dizziness; vertigo (feeling of whirling motion); lightheadedness; disturbed vision. These may appear after a single dose.

*Digestive Tract:* Nausea; vomiting; stomach pain; diarrhea; appetite loss.

*Nervous System:* Headache; confusion; excitement; apprehension; vertigo (feeling of whirling motion); incoordination, depression; dementia; delirium.

*Circulatory System:* Low blood pressure; changes in heart rate or rhythm; heart flutter.

*Respiratory System:* Respiratory distress; asthma (allergic reaction).

*Skin:* Rash; itching; hives; sensitivity to sunlight; flushing; eczema; psoriasis; abnormal pigmentation.

*Eyes or Ocular:* Blurred vision; disturbed color perception; decreased visual field; double vision; night blindness; blind or dark spot in visual field; sensitivity to light.

*Other:* Hepatitis; lupus erythematosus; hearing disturbances; abnormal blood counts; fainting; fever; joint or muscle pain.

---

### Guidelines for Use:
- Do not discontinue medication unless instructed by your doctor.
- May cause stomach upset. Take with food.
- Notify your doctor if ringing in the ears, visual disturbances, dizziness, headache, nausea, rash, or difficulty breathing occurs.
- Do not crush or chew sustained release tablets.
- Hospitalization is sometimes required when starting on this medication.

---

*If you have any questions, consult your doctor, pharmacist, or health care provider.*

| Generic Name<br>*Brand Name Example* | Supplied As | Generic<br>Available |
|---|---|---|
| *Rx* **Tocainide** | | |
| *Tonocard* | **Tablets:** 400 mg, 600 mg | No |

## Type of Drug:

A drug for specific types of irregular heartbeats.

## How the Drug Works:

Tocainide reduces the tendency of the heart to beat irregularly.

## Uses:

To treat life-threatening heart rhythm disturbances.

*Unlabeled Use(s):* Occasionally doctors may prescribe tocainide for the treatment of myotonic dystrophy and trigeminal neuralgia.

## Precautions:

*Do not use in the following situations:*
    allergy to tocainide or to amide-type local anesthetics
    heart block (without ventricular pacemaker)

*Use with caution in the following situations:*
    bone marrow failure, preexisting cytopenia
    heart disease, certain types (eg, heart failure)
    kidney disease, severe
    liver disease, severe

*Heart rhythm disturbances:* Worsened heart rhythm disturbances can result from taking tocainide. Close monitoring and careful dosage adjustment will be required.

*Pregnancy:* Adequate studies have not been done in pregnant women. Use only if clearly needed and potential benefits outweigh the possible hazards to the fetus.

*Breastfeeding:* Tocainide appears in breast milk. Because of the potential for adverse effects, a decision should be made whether to discontinue nursing or the drug, taking into account the importance of the drug to the mother. Consult your doctor.

*Children:* Safety and effectiveness have not been established.

*Lab tests* may be required during treatment with tocainide. Tests may include: Electrocardiograms; potassium levels; blood counts and chest x-rays, especially during the first 3 months of therapy. Report any unusual bruising or bleeding, signs of infection (fever, sore throat, chills) painful or difficult breathing, coughing or wheezing to your doctor.

## Drug Interactions:

Tell your doctor or pharmacist if you are taking or planning to take any over-the-counter or prescription medications or dietary supplements with tocainide. Doses of one or both drugs may need to be modified or a different drug may need to be prescribed. The following drugs and drug classes interact with tocainide:

cimetidine (eg, *Tagamet*)
metoprolol (*Lopressor*)
rifampin (*eg, Rifadin*)

## Side Effects:

Every drug is capable of producing side effects. Many tocainide users experience no, or minor, side effects. The frequency and severity of side effects depend on many factors including dose, duration of therapy, and individual susceptibility. Possible side effects include:

*Digestive Tract:* Appetite loss; nausea; vomiting; diarrhea; loose stools.

*Nervous System:* Dizziness; vertigo (feeling of whirling motion); drowsiness; tremor; confusion; disorientation; hallucinations; change in mood or awareness; incoordination; unsteadiness; walking disturbances; anxiety; headache; abnormal sensations.

*Circulatory System:* Irregular heartbeats; palpitations (pounding in the chest); decreased blood pressure; chest pain; congestive heart failure.

*Other:* Blurred vision; visual disturbances; ringing in the ears; hearing loss; sweating; hot/cold feelings; rash; skin lesion/disorder; joint or muscle pain.

---

### Guidelines for Use:

- Notify your doctor if any of the following occurs: painful or difficult breathing; cough; wheezing; tremor; palpitations; rash; easy bruising or bleeding; fever; sore throat; soreness and ulcers in the mouth; or chills.
- May cause drowsiness or dizziness. Observe caution while driving or performing other tasks requiring alertness.
- May cause nausea, vomiting or diarrhea. Notify your doctor if these persist or become severe.

---

*If you have any questions, consult your doctor, pharmacist, or health care provider.*

| Generic Name<br>*Brand Name Examples* | Supplied As | Generic<br>Available |
|---|---|---|
| *Rx* **Amlodipine** | | |
| *Norvasc* | **Tablets**: 2.5 mg, 5 mg, 10 mg | No |
| *Rx* **Bepridil HCl[1]** | | |
| *Vascor* | **Tablets**: 200 mg, 300 mg,<br>400 mg | No |
| *Rx* **Diltiazem HCl[2]** | **Capsules, extended-release**:<br>60 mg, 90 mg | Yes |
| *Tiamate* | **Tablets, extended-release**:<br>120 mg, 180 mg, 240 mg | No |
| *Cardizem[1]* | **Tablets**: 30 mg, 60 mg, 90 mg,<br>120 mg | Yes |
| *Cardizem SR* | **Capsules, sustained-release**:<br>60 mg, 90 mg | Yes |
| *Cardizem CD, Cardizem<br>SR, Dilacor XR, Tiazac* | **Capsules, sustained-release**:<br>120 mg | Yes |
| *Cardizem CD, Dilacor XR,<br>Tiazac* | **Capsules, sustained-release**:<br>180 mg, 240 mg | No |
| *Cardizem CD, Tiazac* | **Capsules, sustained-release**:<br>300 mg | No |
| *Cartia XT, Diltia XT,<br>Tiazac* | **Capsules, extended-release**:<br>120 mg, 180 mg, 240 mg | Yes |
| *Cartia XT* | **Capsules, extended-release**:<br>300 mg | No |
| *Cardizem CD, Tiazac* | **Capsules, extended-release**:<br>360 mg | No |
| *Tiazac* | **Capsules, extended-release**:<br>420 mg | No |
| *Rx* **Felodipine** | | |
| *Plendil[1]* | **Tablets, sustained-release**:<br>2.5 mg, 5 mg, 10 mg | No |
| *Rx* **Isradipine** | | |
| *DynaCirc CR* | **Tablets, controlled-release**:<br>5 mg, 10 mg | No |
| *DynaCirc[1]* | **Capsules**: 2.5 mg, 5 mg | No |
| *Rx* **Nicardipine HCl[2]** | | |
| *Cardene* | **Capsules**: 20 mg, 30 mg | Yes |
| *Cardene SR[1]* | **Capsules, sustained-release**:<br>30 mg, 45 mg, 60 mg | No |

| Generic Name<br>*Brand Name Examples* | Supplied As | Generic<br>Available |
|---|---|---|
| *Rx* **Nifedipine** | | |
| *Nifedical XL* | **Tablets, extended-release**:<br>30 mg, 60 mg | No |
| *Adalat CC*[1], *Procardia XL* | **Tablets, sustained-release**:<br>30 mg, 60 mg, 90 mg | Yes |
| *Adalat, Procardia* | **Capsules**: 10 mg[3], 20 mg | Yes |
| *Rx* **Nimodipine** | | |
| *Nimotop*[1] | **Capsules**: 30 mg | No |
| *Rx* **Nisoldipine** | | |
| *Sular* | **Tablets, extended-release**:<br>10 mg, 20 mg, 30 mg, 40 mg | No |
| *Rx* **Verapamil HCl**[2] | **Capsules, extended-release**:<br>120 mg, 180 mg, 240 mg | Yes |
| *Calan*[1] | **Tablets**: 40 mg, 80 mg, 120 mg | Yes |
| *Calan SR, Isoptin SR* | **Tablets, sustained-release**:<br>120 mg, 180 mg, 240 mg | Yes |
| *Covera-HS* | **Tablets, extended-release**:<br>180 mg, 240 mg | No |
| *Verelan* | **Capsules, sustained-release**:<br>120 mg, 180 mg, 240 mg,<br>360 mg | Yes |
| *Verelan PM* | **Capsules, sustained-release**:<br>100 mg, 200 mg, 300 mg | No |

[1] Contains lactose.
[2] Also available as an injection.
[3] Contains saccharin.

## Type of Drug:

Calcium channel blockers (ie, slow channel blockers, calcium ion antagonists); drugs that inhibit the movement of calcium across the cell membrane of cardiac muscle and vascular smooth muscle.

## How the Drug Works:

Calcium is involved in blood vessel and heart muscle contraction, nerve
impulse transmission and energy storage, and energy use in the heart.
Calcium channel blocking agents dilate arteries of the heart and other
arteries, may increase or decrease heart rate, may decrease heart contraction, slow ability of the heart to contract, and slow the rate at which
nerve impulses are conducted through the heart.

## Uses:

To treat angina due to coronary artery spasm (Prinzmetal angina) (amlodipine, nifedipine, nifedipine sustained-release, verapamil).

To treat chronic stable (stress-associated) angina in patients who cannot tolerate or are unresponsive to beta-adrenergic blockers or nitrates (amlodipine, bepridil, diltiazem, nicardipine, nifedipine, nifedipine sustained-release, verapamil only).

To treat unstable angina (verapamil only).

To treat arrhythmias (irregular heartbeats) at rest and during stress in association with digitalis (verapamil only).

To treat high blood pressure (amlodipine, diltiazem sustained-release, felodipine, isradipine, nicardipine, nifedipine sustained-release, nisoldipine, verapamil only).

To improve neurological deficiencies caused by spasms following subarachnoid hemorrhage (SAH) (ruptured vessels in the brain). Therapy must begin within 96 hours and continue for 21 days (nimodipine only).

*Unlabeled Use(s):* Occasionally doctors may prescribe diltiazem to treat unstable angina, Raynaud syndrome, and tardive dyskinesia, and to prevent certain types of heart attack.

Isradipine may be useful in the treatment of chronic stable angina.

Nicardipine may be useful in the treatment of congestive heart failure and in combination with aminocaproic acid for SAH.

Occasionally doctors may prescribe nifedipine to lower blood pressure in hypertensive emergencies; to prevent or treat migraine headaches; and to treat primary pulmonary (lung) and pregnancy-associated hypertension, asthma, preterm labor, disorders of the esophagus, certain types of heart disorders, coronary artery disease, congestive heart failure, Raynaud syndrome, biliary and renal colic, and cardiomyopathy.

Nimodipine appears to be beneficial in some patients with common and classic migraine and chronic cluster headache.

Occasionally doctors may prescribe verapamil to prevent migraine headache, cluster headache, and exercise-induced asthma; to treat manic-depressive states, night leg cramps, and hypertrophic cardiomyopathy. Verapamil has also been used for paroxysmal supraventricular tachycardia.

## Precautions:

*Do not use in the following situations:*

allergy to calcium channel block-ing agents or their ingredients

aortic stenosis, advanced (nicar-dipine only)

arrhythmias, serious, history of (bepridil only)

atrial flutter or atrial fibrillation and an accessory bypass tract (eg, Wolff-Parkinson-White, Lown-Ganong-Levine syndromes) (verapamil only)

AV block, second or third degree, except with functioning pacemaker (bepridil, diltia-zem, verapamil only)

cardiac insufficiency, uncompen-sated (bepridil only)

cardiogenic shock (verapamil only)

congenital QT interval prolonga-tion (bepridil only)

drugs that prolong QT interval, (eg, antiarrhythmics), concurrent use (bepridil only)

low blood pressure (bepridil, diltiazem, verapamil only)

myocardial infarction, acute (diltiazem only)

severe left ventricular dysfunc-tion (verapamil only)

sick sinus syndrome, without pacemaker (bepridil, diltiazem, verapamil only)

*Use with caution in the following situations:*

agranulocytosis

beta-blocker withdrawal (nifedi-pine, nicardipine only)

bradycardia, transient (verapamil only)

chest pain (nicardipine, nifedi-pine only)

congestive heart failure

coronary artery disease (nisol-dipine only)

Duchenne muscular dystrophy (verapamil only)

edema (felodipine, nifedipine only)

heart attack

heart conduction problems

hypertrophic cardiomyopathy (enlarged heart) (verapamil only)

hypokalemia (bepridil only)

kidney disease

left bundle branch block (bepridil only)

liver disease

low blood pressure

sinus bradycardia (bepridil only)

*New serious arrhythmias:* Bepridil has been associated with the occur-rence of new serious arrhythmias. Use should be limited to patients in whom other antianginal drugs have failed.

*Pregnancy:* There are no adaquate and well-controlled studies in preg-nant women. Use only if clearly needed and the potential benefits to the mother outweigh the possible hazards to the fetus.

*Breastfeeding:* Bepridil, diltiazem, nifedipine, and verapamil appear in breast milk. It is not known if amlodipine, felodipine, isradipine, nicardi-pine, nimodipine, or nisoldipine appear in breast milk. Decide whether to discontinue nursing or the drug, taking into account the importance of the drug to the mother. Consult your doctor.

*Children:* Safety and effectiveness have not been established in children.

*Elderly:* Felodipine, nifedipine, and verapamil may result in a greater low-ering of blood pressure than in younger patients.

*Lab tests* may be required periodically during treatment. Tests may include electrocardiograms, serum potassium levels, liver and kidney function tests, blood pressure, and blood and platelet counts.

## Drug Interactions:

Tell your doctor or pharmacist if you are taking or planning to take any over-the-counter or prescription medications or dietary supplements with calcium channel blocking agents. Doses of one or both drugs may need to be modified or a different drug may need to be prescribed.The following drugs and drug classes interact with calcium channel blocking agents:

alcohol (verapamil only)

anesthetics

antiarrhythmics (eg, flecainide) (verapamil only)

antihistamines, nonsedating (eg, loratadine) (bepridil only)

antihypertensives (eg, diuretics) (verapamil only)

azole antifungals (eg, ketoconazole, itraconazole) (felodipine, nisoldipine only)

barbiturates (eg, phenobarbital) (felodipine, nifedipine only)

benzodiapines (eg, midazolam) (diltiazem only)

beta-blockers (eg, propranolol)

calcium salts (verapamil only)

carbamazepine (eg, *Tegretol*) (diltiazem, felodipine, verapamil only)

cardiac glycosides (eg, digoxin) (bepridil only)

cimetidine (eg, *Tagamet*)

cyclosporine (eg, *Neoral*) (diltiazem, nicardipine, verapamil only)

digoxin (eg, *Lanoxin*)

diltiazem (eg, *Cardizem*) (nifedipine only)

encainide (*Enkaid*) (diltiazem only)

erythromycin (eg, *E-Mycin*) (felodipine only)

fentanyl (eg, *Duragesic*)

grapefruit juice (felodipine, nifedipine, nisoldipine only)

HMG-CoA reductase inhibitors (eg, lovastatin) (diltiazem, verapamil only)

lithium (eg, *Eskalith*) (verapamil only)

neuromuscular blockers (eg, atracurium) (verapamil only)

nifedipine (eg, *Procardia*) (diltiazem only)

nondepolarizing muscle relaxants (eg, pancuronium) (verapamil only)

phenytoin (eg, *Dilantin*) (felodipine, nisoldipine only)

prazosin (eg, *Minipress*) (verapamil only)

primidone (eg, *Mysoline*) (nifedipine only)

procainamide (eg, *Pronestyl*) (bepridil only)

quinidine (eg, *Quinora*) (bepridil, nisoldipine, verapamil only)

rifampin (eg, *Rifadin*) (diltiazem, isradipine, nifedipine, verapamil only)

tacrolimus (*Prograf*) (diltiazem only)

theophyllines (eg, aminophylline) (diltiazem, verapamil only)

tricyclic antidepressants (eg, amitriptyline) (bepridil only)

## Side Effects:

Every drug is capable of producing side effects. Many calcium channel blocking agent users experience no, or minor, side effects. The frequency and severity of side effects depend on many factors including dose, duration of therapy, and individual susceptibility. Possible side effects include:

*Nervous System:* Headache; dizziness; giddiness (felodipine only); lightheadedness; fainting; weakness; fatigue; nervousness; anxiety; tremor; general body discomfort; impaired movement; excessive movement (nicardipine only); confusion; irritability; drowsiness; sleep disturbances; difficulty sleeping; abnormal dreams; psychiatric disturbances (eg, depression, amnesia, paranoia, psychosis).

*Digestive Tract:* Nausea; vomiting; diarrhea; constipation; gas; stomach pain or cramps; indigestion; changes in taste perception; dry mouth; swollen gums (felodipine only); appetite changes (bepridil only).

*Respiratory System:* Congestion; runny nose; sinus infection; cough; shortness of breath; wheezing; sore throat; sneezing; bronchitis; fluid retention in lungs.

*Circulatory System:* Fluid retention; low blood pressure; high blood pressure; anemia; pounding in the chest; chest pain; decreased heart rate; increased heart rate; abnormal heart rhythm; abnormal electrocardiogram readings; myocardial infarction; AV block; congestive heart failure.

*Skin:* Rash; skin irritation; flushing; sweating; acne (nimodipine only); itching; hives; abnormal skin sensations (eg, burning, prickling, tingling); hair loss.

*Other:* Fever; chills; flu-like symptoms; muscle cramps or pain; joint stiffness or pain; back pain (felodipine only); weight loss; weight gain; nosebleed; ringing in ears; pain; blurred vision; difficult urination; painful urination; frequent urination; sexual difficulties; infection (nicardipine only).

---

### Guidelines for Use:

- Dosage is individualized. Take exactly as prescribed.
- Do not change the dose or stop taking this medicine unless advised to do so by your doctor. Abrupt withdrawal may result in increased angina attacks.
- All of the products listed are calcium channel blockers; however, they are not interchangeable. For example, diltiazem cannot be used for nimodipine.
- *Extended- or sustained-release* — Swallow whole; do not chew, crush, or divide. An empty tablet may appear in stool; this is no cause for concern.
- *Amlodipine, felodipine, isradipine, nicardipine* — May be taken with or without food. Do not take felodipine with grapefruit juice.
- *Verapamil* — Verapamil extended-release is usually taken at bedtime with or without food. Take verapamil sustained-release with food in the morning. If heart failure is not severe or rate-related, use digitalis and diuretics before verapamil.

## Guidelines for Use (cont.):

- *Diltiazem sustained-release* — The usual dose is taken in the morning on an empty stomach.
- *Bepridil* — If stomach upset occurs, take with meals or at bedtime. Notify any doctor who treats that you are taking bepridil, as well as any other medications you may be taking. Bepridil use has been associated with the occurrence of new arrhythmias. Use should be limited to patients in whom other antianginal drugs have failed.
- *Nimodipine* — Take preferably less than 1 hour before or 2 hours after meals. Therapy to improve neurological deficiencies caused by spasms following SAH must begin within 96 hours and continue for 21 days. If capsule cannot be swallowed (eg, time of surgery, unconsciousness), a hole can be made in both ends of the capsule with an 18 gauge needle, and the contents extracted into a syringe for oral administration.
- *Nisoldipine* — Do not take with grapefruit juice or with high-fat meals.
- *Adalat CC* — Take once daily on an empty stomach.
- *Felodipine* — May cause swollen or bleeding gums. Good dental hygiene decreases incidence and severity of this condition.
- Calcium channel blockers may interfere with normal blood-clotting mechanisms. Contact your doctor if unusual bleeding or bruising of the skin occurs.
- Low blood pressure may occur, but is usually well tolerated. It is more likely to occur in patients who are also taking beta-blockers (eg, propranolol).
- Beta-blockers should be tapered slowly rather than stopped abruptly before starting nicardipine or nifedipine therapy. When starting nicardipine therapy, taper beta-blockers over 8 to 10 days with coadministration.
- Maintain use of potassium supplementation or potassium-sparing diuretics.
- If a dose is missed, take it as soon as possible. If several hours have passed or it is nearing time for the next dose, do not double the dose to catch up, unless advised to do so by your doctor. If more than one dose is missed or it is necessary to establish a new dosage schedule, contact your doctor or pharmacist.
- Notify your doctor if you experience irregular heartbeat, increased frequency or severity of angina, shortness of breath, swelling of hands and feet, dizziness, constipation, nausea, or low blood pressure (eg, lightheadedness).
- Notify your doctor if you experience symptoms of an allergic reaction (eg, itching, rash, hives, difficulty breathing).
- Inform your doctor if you are pregnant, become pregnant, plan on becoming pregnant, or are breastfeeding.
- Lab tests may be required to monitor therapy. Be sure to keep appointments.
- Store at controlled room temperature (59° to 77°F) in a tightly sealed container. Keep away from light and moisture. Protect nimodipine from freezing.

*If you have any questions, consult your doctor, pharmacist, or health care provider.*

| Generic Name<br>*Brand Name Example* | Supplied As | Generic<br>Available |
|---|---|---|
| *Rx* **Epoprostenol Sodium** | | |
| *Flolan* | **Injection (powder for reconstitution)**: 0.5 mg, 1.5 mg | No |

## Type of Drug:
Peripheral vasodilator.

## How the Drug Works:
Epoprostenol relaxes pulmonary and arterial blood vessels, allowing them to dilate (widen). This allows more blood to flow through the vessels and improves heart function in patients with pulmonary hypertension.

## Uses:
For the long-term treatment of primary pulmonary hypertension in NYHA Class III and Class IV patients who do not adequately respond to conventional therapy.

## Precautions:
*Do not use in the following situations:*
>> allergy to the drug or any of its ingredients
>> congestive heart failure due to severe left ventricular systolic dysfunction (chronic use)
>> pulmonary edema during dose initiation

*Pregnancy:* There are no adequate and well-controlled studies in pregnant women. Use only if clearly needed and the potential benefits outweigh the possible risks to the fetus.

*Breastfeeding:* It is not known if this drug appears in breast milk. Consult your doctor before you begin breastfeeding.

*Children:* Safety and effectiveness have not been established.

*Elderly:* In general, dose selection should be cautious, reflecting the greater frequency of decreased liver, kidney, or heart function and of concomitant disease or other drug therapy.

## Drug Interactions:
Tell your doctor or pharmacist if you are taking or planning to take any over-the-counter or prescription medications or dietary supplements while taking this drug. Drug doses may need to be modified or a different drug prescribed. The following drugs and drug classes interact with this drug:

| | |
|---|---|
| antihypertensive agents (eg, ACE inhibitors) | diuretics (eg, hydrochlorothiazide) |
| antiplatelet agents (eg, anticoagulants) | vasodilators (eg, nitrates) |

## Side Effects:

Every drug is capable of producing side effects. Many patients experience no, or minor, side effects. The frequency and severity of side effects depend on many factors including dose, duration of therapy, and individual susceptibility. Possible side effects include:

*Circulatory System:* Low blood pressure; chest pain; abnormal heart rhythm; changes in heartbeat; heart failure; fainting; pounding in the chest (palpitations).

*Nervous System:* Headache; anxiety; nervousness; agitation; dizziness; tremor; confusion; convulsions; depression; sleeplessness; stroke.

*Skin:* Flushing; sweating; abnormal skin sensations; itching; rash; pallor; bluish skin.

*Digestive Tract:* Nausea; vomiting; stomach pain; indigestion; diarrhea; appetite loss; constipation; fluid in the abdomen.

*Other:* Muscle, back, jaw, or bone pain; difficulty breathing; local infection; pain at the injection site; chills; fever; flu-like symptoms; shock; deficiency of oxygen to body tissues (hypoxia); bleeding; swelling (edema); low blood calcium levels; weight changes; increased cough; nosebleed; abnormal vision; weakness; abnormal blood counts.

---

### Guidelines for Use:

- This drug is administered by continuous intravenous (IV; into a vein) infusion via a central venous catheter using an ambulatory infusion pump. Therapy requires commitment to drug reconstitution (mixing), administration, and care of the catheter for a prolonged period, possibly years. Brief interruptions in therapy may result in rapid deterioration.
- Dosage is individualized. Take exactly as prescribed.
- Do not stop taking or change the dose, unless instructed by your doctor.
- Abrupt withdrawal of the drug may result in symptoms associated with pulmonary hypertension, including difficulty breathing, dizziness, and weakness.
- Store unopened vials at 59° to 77°F. Protect from light.
- Refrigerate reconstituted solution at 36° to 46°F for not more than 40 hours; discard any solution that has been refrigerated for more than 48 hours. Do not freeze; discard any solution that has been frozen. Protect from light.
- A single reservoir of reconstituted solution can be administered at room temperature for a duration of 8 hours or it can be used with a cold pouch and administered for 24 hours or less with the use of 2 frozen 6 oz gel packs. Insulate solution from temperatures higher than 77°F and lower than 32°F. Do not expose to direct sunlight.

---

*If you have any questions, consult your doctor, pharmacist, or health care provider.*

| Generic Name<br>*Brand Name Example* | Supplied As | Generic<br>Available |
|---|---|---|
| *Rx* **Isoxsuprine HCl** | | |
| *Vasodilan* | **Tablets:** 10 mg, 20 mg | Yes |

## Type of Drug:

Peripheral vasodilator (relaxes blood vessels in skeletal muscles).

## How the Drug Works:

Isoxsuprine increases blood flow in skeletal muscle by relaxing and dilating (widening) blood vessels in these muscles.

## Uses:

"Possibly effective" to relieve symptoms of disorders related to inadequate blood flow or blood supply to the brain and extremities (arms and legs). These disorders include: Vascular disease, Buerger disease, and Raynaud disease.

*Unlabeled Use(s):* Occasionally doctors may provide isoxsuprine for painful menstrual periods and premature labor.

## Precautions:

*Do not use in the following situations:*
    arterial bleeding
    immediately after childbirth

*Pregnancy:* Safety in pregnancy has not been established. Risks of fluid accumulation in lungs in pregnant women is increased. Lower amounts of calcium and glucose in the blood, lower blood pressure and poorly functioning intestines in newborns have resulted. Consult your doctor.

## Drug Interactions:

Tell your doctor or pharmacist if you are taking or planning to take any over-the-counter or prescription medications or dietary supplements with isoxsuprine. Doses of one or both drugs may need to be modified or a different drug may need to be prescribed.

## Side Effects:

Every drug is capable of producing side effects. Many isoxsuprine users experience no, or minor, side effects. The frequency and severity of side effects depend on many factors including dosage, duration of therapy, and individual susceptibility. Possible side effects include:

*Circulatory System:* Decreased blood pressure; orthostatic hypotension (dizziness or lightheadedness when arising from a seated or lying position); rapid heartbeat; pounding in the chest (palpitations); chest pain.

*Other:* Severe rash; dizziness; nausea; vomiting; stomach pain.

### Guidelines for Use:

- Take exactly as prescribed.
- Do not stop taking this medicine or change the dosage without checking with your doctor; this could have serious adverse effects.
- Pounding sensation in chest (palpitations) and skin rash can occur. Notify your doctor if these symptoms persist.
- Dizziness or weakness may occur after sudden changes in posture (eg, when rising from a lying position). This can usually be avoided by rising slowly or sitting upright for a few minutes before standing.
- Store at controlled room temperature (59° to 86°F). Protect from moisture.

*If you have any questions, consult your doctor, pharmacist, or health care provider.*

| Generic Name<br>*Brand Name Examples* | Supplied As | Generic<br>Available |
|---|---|---|
| Rx **Papaverine HCl** | | |
| *Pavabid Plateau Caps* | **Capsules, timed release:**<br>150 mg | Yes |

## Type of Drug:
Peripheral vasodilator (relaxes blood vessels in skeletal muscles).

## How the Drug Works:
Papaverine relaxes and dilates (widens) blood vessels to increase blood flow.

## Uses:
To treat problems associated with blood vessel constriction or spasm in the brain, heart, arms and legs.

## Precautions:
*Do not use in the following situations:*
> allergy to papaverine
> irregular heartbeats, history of

*Use with caution in the following situations:*
> glaucoma                          heart beat irregularities
> heart attack, history of          liver disease

*Heart:* Large doses can produce serious arrhythmias (irregular heartbeats).

*Liver sensitivity* has been reported with intestinal symptoms, yellowing of the skin and eyes and altered liver function tests. Discontinue medication if these symptoms occur.

*Pregnancy:* Adequate studies have not been done in pregnant women or animal studies may have shown a risk to the fetus. Use only if clearly needed and potential benefits outweigh the possible hazards to the fetus.

*Breastfeeding:* It is not known if papaverine appears in breast milk. Consult your doctor before you begin breastfeeding.

*Children:* Safety and effectiveness have not been established.

## Drug Interactions:
Tell your doctor or pharmacist if you are taking or planning to take any over-the-counter or prescription medications or dietary supplements with papaverine. Doses of one or both drugs may need to be modified or a different drug may need to be prescribed. Levodopa (eg, *Larodopa*) interacts with papaverine.

## Side Effects:

Every drug is capable of producing side effects. Many papaverine users experience no, or minor, side effects. The frequency and severity of side effects depend on many factors including dosage, duration of therapy, and individual susceptibility. Possible side effects include:

*Digestive Tract:* Nausea; stomachache; appetite loss; constipation; diarrhea.

*Nervous System:* Headache; dizziness; drowsiness; feeling of whirling motion.

*Circulatory System:* Increased heart rate; increased blood pressure.

*Skin:* Yellowing of skin or eyes; sweating; flushing of face; rash.

*Other:* Fatigue and general body aches; increase in depth of respirations; abnormal liver tests.

---

### Guidelines for Use:

- May cause drowsiness or dizziness. Use caution when driving or performing tasks requiring alertness. Alcohol may intensify these effects.
- May cause flushing, sweating, headache, tiredness, jaundice, rash, nausea, appetite loss, abdominal distress, constipation or diarrhea. Notify your doctor if these effects become pronounced.
- Take at evenly spaced intervals throughout the day.
- Store at controlled room temperature (59° to 86°F). Protect from moisture.

---

*If you have any questions, consult your doctor, pharmacist, or health care provider.*

| Generic Name<br>*Brand Name Examples* | Supplied As | Generic<br>Available |
|---|---|---|
| *Rx* **Acebutolol HCl** | | |
| *Sectral* | **Capsules**: 200 mg, 400 mg | Yes |
| *Rx* **Atenolol**[1] | | |
| *Tenormin* | **Tablets**: 25 mg, 50 mg, 100 mg | Yes |
| *Rx* **Betaxolol HCl** | | |
| *Kerlone* | **Tablets**: 10 mg, 20 mg | No |
| *Rx* **Bisoprolol Fumarate** | | |
| *Zebeta* | **Tablets**: 5 mg, 10 mg | Yes |
| *Rx* **Carteolol HCl** | | |
| *Cartrol* | **Tablets**: 2.5 mg, 5 mg | No |
| *Rx* **Metoprolol**[1] | | |
| *Toprol XL* | **Tablets, extended release**:<br>25 mg, 50 mg, 100 mg, 200 mg | No |
| *Lopressor* | **Tablets**: 50 mg, 100 mg | No |
| *Rx* **Nadolol** | | |
| *Corgard* | **Tablets**: 20 mg, 40 mg, 80 mg,<br>120 mg, 160 mg | Yes |
| *Rx* **Penbutolol Sulfate** | | |
| *Levatol* | **Tablets**: 20 mg | No |
| *Rx* **Pindolol** | | |
| *Visken* | **Tablets**: 5 mg, 10 mg | Yes |
| *Rx* **Propranolol HCl**[1] | **Tablets**: 90 mg | Yes |
| | **Solution, oral**:[2] 4 mg/mL<br>8 mg/mL | Yes |
| *Inderal* | **Tablets**: 10 mg, 20 mg, 40 mg,<br>60 mg, 80 mg | Yes |
| *Inderal LA* | **Capsules, sustained release**:<br>60 mg, 80 mg, 120 mg, 160 mg | Yes |
| *Propranolol Intensol*[2] | **Solution, concentrated oral**:<br>80 mg/mL | No |
| *Rx* **Sotalol HCl** | | |
| *Betapace, Sorine* | **Tablets**: 80 mg, 120 mg,<br>160 mg, 240 mg | Yes |
| *Betapace AF* | **Tablets**: 80 mg, 120 mg,<br>160 mg | No |
| *Rx* **Timolol Maleate** | | |
| *Blocadren* | **Tablets**: 5 mg, 10 mg, 20 mg | Yes |

[1] Also available as an injection.       [2] Sugar free.

All of the products listed in the above table are beta-blockers; however, they are not interchangeable. For example, atenolol cannot be used for nadolol.

## Type of Drug:

Beta-blockers; antihypertensives; drugs used to lower high blood pressure; antianginal drugs; antiarrhythmic drugs.

## How the Drug Works:

Beta-adrenergic blocking agents interfere with the action of adrenalin and similar chemicals on heart muscle contraction (heart may beat with less force and pump out less blood) and nerve conduction in the heart (heart may beat more slowly and regularly). Beta-adrenergic blocking agents reduce the amount of work the heart has to do (reduces angina chest pain) and the amount of blood the heart pumps out (lowers elevated blood pressure) and stabilize heart rhythm in conditions in which the heart is beating too fast or irregularly (antiarrhythmic effects).

## Uses:

| Beta-Adrenergic Blocking Agents | | | | | | | | | | | | |
|---|---|---|---|---|---|---|---|---|---|---|---|---|
| Indications<br>✔ = labeled<br>x = unlabeled | Acebutolol | Atenolol | Betaxolol | Bisoprolol | Carteolol | Metoprolol[1] | Nadolol | Penbutolol | Pindolol | Propranolol[1] | Sotalol | Timolol |
| Hypertension | ✔ | ✔ | ✔ | ✔ | ✔ | ✔ | ✔ | ✔ | ✔ | ✔ | | ✔ |
| Angina pectoris | x | ✔ | | x | | ✔ | ✔ | | | ✔ | | |
| Cardiac arrhythmias | | | | | | | | | | | | |
| Supraventricular arrhythmias/tachycardias | | | | | | | | | | ✔ | | |
| Ventricular arrhythmias/tachycardias | | | | | | | | | | ✔ | ✔[2] | |
| Premature ventricular contractions (PVCs) | ✔ | | | | | | | | | ✔ | | |
| Digitalis-induced tachyarrhythmias | | | | | | | | | | ✔ | | |
| Resistant tachyarrhythmias (during anesthesia) | | | | | | | | | | ✔ | | |
| Atrial ectopy | | | | | | x | | | | | | |
| Maintenance of normal sinus rhythm | | | | | | | | | | | ✔[3] | |
| Myocardial Infarction | | ✔ | | | | ✔[4] | | | | ✔ | | ✔ |
| CHF (stable)[5] | | | | x | | ✔[6] | | | | | | |
| Pheochromocytoma | | | | | | | | | | ✔ | | |
| Migraine prophylaxis | | x | | | | x | x | | | ✔ | | ✔ |
| Hypertrophic subaortic stenosis | | | | | | | | | | ✔ | | |
| Parkinsonian tremors | | | | | | | | x | | x[7] | | |
| Akathisia, antipsychotic-induced | | | | | | | x | | | x | | |

## Beta-Adrenergic Blocking Agents

| Indications<br>✔= labeled<br>x = unlabeled | Acebutolol | Atenolol | Betaxolol | Bisoprolol | Carteolol | Metoprolol[1] | Nadolol | Penbutolol | Pindolol | Propranolol[1] | Sotalol | Timolol |
|---|---|---|---|---|---|---|---|---|---|---|---|---|
| Variceal bleeding in portal hypertension, prevention of | | x | | | | x | x | | | x | | x |
| Atrial fibrillation | | | | | | | | | | | | |
|   Rapid heart rate control | | | | | | x | | | | | | |
|   Maintenance heart rate control | | | | | | x | | | | | | |
| Generalized anxiety disorder | | | | | | | | | | x | | |
| Angina, unstable | | x | | | | x | | | | | | |
|   Stable | x | | | x | | | | | | | | |
|   Unstable | | x | | | | x | | | | | | |
| Essential Tremor | | | | | | | | | | ✔ | | |

[1] Includes long-acting formulation.
[2] Not *Betapace AF*.
[3] Not *Betapace*.
[4] Immediate-release tablets only.
[5] See Precautions.
[6] *Toprol-XL* only.
[7] Sustained-release only.

## Precautions:

*Do not use in the following situations:*

allergy to beta-blockers or any of their ingredients
bronchial asthma, broncho-spasm, or severe chronic obstructive pulmonary diseases (eg, emphysema, bronchitis)
cardiac failure, moderate to severe (metoprolol only)
cardiac failure, uncontrolled
cardiac shock
heart block, greater than first degree
long QT syndromes, congenital or acquired (sotalol only)
low blood pressure, less than 100 mmHg (metoprolol only)
renal impairment, severe (sotalol only)
slow heart rate, severe

*Use with caution in the following situations:*

acute myocardial infarction, recent
adrenal gland tumor
anesthesia for major surgery
AV block, first block
bronchospastic diseases
calcium channel blocker therapy, concurrent
congestive heart failure, controlled
diabetes
electrolyte disturbances (eg, potassium, magnesium)
kidney disease
liver disease
low blood pressure
low blood sugar
low heart rate
overactive thyroid
peripheral vascular disease
sick sinus syndrome
Wolff-Parkinson-White syndrome

*Discontinuing therapy:* When discontinuing these medications, slowly reduce the dose over 1 to 2 weeks. Sudden discontinuation of these drugs has caused worsening of angina (chest pain), heart attacks, irregular heartbeats, and death. Other serious withdrawal symptoms include: sweating, palpitations (pounding in the chest), headache, tremulousness, discomfort, and allergy to catecholamines. If discontinued suddenly, beta-blockers may mask the signs of hyperthyroidism (overactive thyroid). If thyroid patients stop taking these medications too suddenly, symptoms of hyperthyroidism (eg, a rapid pulse) may occur.

*Diabetes:* These products can mask some of the signs of hypoglycemia (low blood sugar) such as rapid heart rate and tremors, and alter blood sugar levels. It may be necessary for your doctor to alter your dose of diabetic medications while taking beta-blockers.

*Proarrhythmia: Betapace AF* can cause or worsen ventricular arrhythmias, a different type of heartbeat that can be dangerous and even cause death. To minimize the risk of this heartbeat, patients should be placed in a medical facility that can provide cardiac resuscitation, continuous ECG monitoring, and calculations of creatinine clearance for a minimum of 3 days when starting or restarting therapy.

*Allergic reaction:* Patients with a history of allergic reactions to various allergens may be unresponsive to the usual doses of epinephrine used to treat the allergic reaction.

*Pregnancy:* There are no adequate or well-controlled studies in pregnant women. Use only if clearly needed and the potential benefits to the mother outweigh the possible hazards to the fetus.

*Atenolol, acebutolol, and sotalol* – Acebutolol crosses the placenta; reduced birth weight and decreased blood pressure and heart rate have occurred.

*Breastfeeding:* Acebutolol, atenolol, betaxolol, metoprolol, nadolol, pindolol, propranolol, sotalol, and timolol appear in breast milk. It is not known if carteolol, bisoprolol, or penbutolol appear in breast milk. Discontinue nursing when taking any beta-blockers.

*Children:* Safety and effectiveness have not been established.

## Drug Interactions:

Tell your doctor or pharmacist if you are taking or planning to take any over-the-counter or prescription medications or dietary supplements with beta-blockers. Doses of one or both drugs may need to be modified or a different drug may need to be prescribed. The following drugs and drug classes interact with beta-blockers:

antacids (eg, aluminum carbonate)
antiarrhythmics (eg, quinidine)
antidiabetic drugs, oral (eg, glipizide)
barbiturates (eg, phenobarbital)
calcium channel blockers (eg, verapamil)

cimetidine (eg, *Tagamet*)
clonidine (eg, *Catapres*)
colestipol (eg, *Colestid*)
contraceptives, oral (eg, *Ortho-Novum*)
cyclosporine (eg, *Neoral*)
epinephrine (eg, *Adrenalin*)
ergot alkaloids (eg, ergotamine)

hydantoins (eg, phenytoin)
hydralazine (eg, *Apresoline*)
insulin
lidocaine (eg, *Xylocaine*)
NSAIDs (eg, ibuprofen)
penicillins (eg, ampicillin)
phenothiazines (eg, chlorpromazine )

prazosin (eg, *Minipress*)
propafenone (eg, *Rythmol*)
rifamycins (eg, rifampin)
selective serotonin reuptake
  inhibitors (eg, paroxetine)
theophyllines (eg, amino-
  phylline)
thioamines (eg, methimazole)

## Side Effects:

Every drug is capable of producing side effects. Many beta-blocker users
experience no, or minor, side effects. The frequency and severity of side
effects depend on many factors including dose, duration of therapy, and
individual susceptibility. Possible side effects include:

*Digestive Tract:* Nausea; vomiting; stomach pain; gas; bloating; diarrhea;
constipation; heartburn; indigestion; stomach cramping; appetite
changes; dry mouth; colon or rectal problems.

*Nervous System:* Depression; anxiety; nervousness; disorientation; confusion; fainting; weakness; dizziness; catatonia; vertigo (feeling of whirling motion); lightheadedness; fatigue; sleeplessness; drowsiness;
lethargy; sleep disturbances; nightmares; abnormal, vivid dreams; hallucinations; short-term memory loss; decreased concentration; sedation;
headache; emotional lability; mood changes; behavior changes; slurred
speech.

*Circulatory System:* Changes in heart rate; decreased heart rate; irregular
heart rate; heart rhythm abnormalities; chest pain; palpitations (pounding in the chest); cold extremities; changes in blood pressure; heart
arrest; heart block; congestive heart failure; abnormal ECG; decreased
blood platelets; decreased white blood cells; blood clot; vein inflammation; stroke.

*Respiratory System:* Shortness of breath or difficulty breathing; cough;
nasal congestion; wheezing; upper respiratory infection; sinus infection; fluid in the lungs; bronchitis; asthma; bronchospasm; sore or
inflamed throat; throat spasms.

*Skin:* Rash; swelling; flushing or paleness; abnormal skin sensations (eg,
burning, prickling, tingling); increased or decreased skin sensitivity to
stimulation; itching and irritation; hair loss; sweating; dry skin; numbness
of the hands.

*Muscular System:* Aching or painful joints and muscles; back pain; limb
pain; shoulder pain; muscle weakness; muscle cramps or twitching;
tremor.

*Urinary and Reproductive Tract:* Painful urination; inability to urinate; frequent urination; urinary tract infection; excessive urination at night;
sexual problems; decreased sex drive; impotence.

*Senses:* Blurred vision; dry, burning, or irritated eyes; eye inflammation;
visual disturbances; ringing in the ears; earache; taste changes; eye
pain; abnormal tearing.

*Other:* Fever; weight changes; changes in blood sugar levels; infection; swelling of arms and legs; general body discomfort; decreased exercise tolerance; gout; cold- or flu-like symptoms.

## Guidelines for Use:

- Dosage is individualized. Take exactly as prescribed.
- Do not stop taking or change the dose unless directed by your doctor. Abrupt withrawal has resulted in worsening of angina and ventricular arrhythmias and can cause myocardial infarction and death.
- If a dose is missed, take it as soon as possible. If several hours have passed or it is nearing time for the next dose, do not double the dose to catch up, unless advised to do so by your doctor. If more than one dose is missed or it is necessary to establish a new dosage schedule, contact your doctor or pharmacist.
- Do not chew or crush sustained-release or extended-release products.
- *Diabetes* — May mask some signs of low blood sugar (eg, rapid heart rate, tremors) or alter blood glucose levels.
- *Glaucoma* — May reduce intraocular pressure and interfere with the glaucoma screening test.
- Consult your pharmacist or doctor before using dietary supplements or other prescription or nonprescription products including nasal decongestants, diet aids, and nonprescription cold preparations.
- May cause drowsiness, dizziness, lightheadedness, or blurred vision. Use caution while driving or performing other tasks requiring alertness, coordination, or physical dexterity.
- Notify your doctor if you experience difficulty breathing (especially on exertion or when lying down), night cough, swelling of the extremities, slow pulse rate, dizziness, light-headedness, fainting, confusion, depression, rash, fever, sore throat, unusual bleeding or bruising, fatigue with exertion, cough, fast heartbeat, severe diarrhea, or unusual bleeding.
- Inform your doctor or dentist of therapy before any type of surgery.
- Inform your doctor if you are pregnant, become pregnant, plan on becoming pregnant, or are breastfeeding.
- *Brand interchange* — Do not change from one brand of this drug to another without consulting your pharmacist or doctor. For example, *Betapace* and *Betapace AF* are not interchangeable.
- *Nadolol, pindolol, acebutolol, atenolol, carteolol, bisoprolol, betaxolol, and penbutolol* — May be taken without regard to meals.
- *Metoprolol and propranolol* — Take consistently with or without food at the same time each day.
- *Propranolol Intensol* — Mix prescribed dose with liquid or semi-solid food such as water, juices, soda or soda-like beverages, applesauce, or pudding. Use calibrated dropper to measure dose. Administer entire amount of mixture immediately after mixing. Do not store mixture after mixing.
- *Sotalol* — Food may reduce absorption. Take on an empty stomach.
- *Sotalol* — To reduce the risk of induced arrhythmias, patients should be placed in a medical facility that can provide cardiac resuscitation, continuous ECG monitoring, and calculations of creatine clearance for a minimum of 3 days when starting or restarting therapy.
- Store at room temperature (59° to 86°F). Avoid excessive heat. Protect from light, moisture, and freezing.

*If you have any questions, consult your doctor, pharmacist, or health care provider.*

| Generic Name<br>*Brand Name Example* | Supplied As | Generic<br>Available |
|---|---|---|
| *Rx* **Doxazosin Mesylate** | | |
| *Cardura* | **Tablets (as base)**: 1 mg, 2 mg,<br>4 mg, 8 mg | Yes |
| *Rx* **Prazosin HCl** | | |
| *Minipress* | **Capsules (as base)**: 1 mg,<br>2 mg, 5 mg | Yes |
| *Rx* **Tamsulosin HCl** | | |
| *Flomax* | **Capsules:** 0.4 mg | No |
| *Rx* **Terazosin HCl** | | |
| *Hytrin* | **Capsules (as base)**: 1 mg,<br>2 mg, 5 mg, 10 mg | Yes |

## Type of Drug:
Antihypertensives; drugs used to lower high blood pressure.

## How the Drug Works:
Alpha-1-adrenergic blockers dilate both veins and arteries to reduce resistance against which the blood must flow. This lowers blood pressure. Alpha-1-adrenergic blockers also relax the muscles around the urethra and improve symptoms of benign prostatic hyperplasia.

## Uses:
*Doxazosin, prazosin, terazosin:* To treat high blood pressure alone or in combination with other blood pressure-lowering medications (eg, diuretics).

*Doxazosin, tamsulosin, terazosin:* For the treatment symptoms of benign prostatic hyperplasia (BPH).

*Unlabeled Use(s):* Occasionally doctors may prescribe prazosin for treatment of benign prostatic hypertrophy.

## Precautions:
*Do not use in the following situations:* Allergy to the drug or any of its ingredients.

*Use with caution in the following situations:*
    liver disease (doxazosin only)          prostate cancer

*"First dose" effect:* Dizziness, fainting, and falling are possible because of lowered blood pressure, especially early in therapy. These symptoms are more likely to occur when rising quickly from a seated or lying position, if the dose is increased, if the therapy is stopped and then started again, or if more than one antihypertensive drug is being taken. To lessen the chances of problems, the first dose should be given at bedtime. Sit or lie down if you feel light-headed.

*Priapism:* A painful penile erection that sustains for hours occurs rarely. Contact your doctor if you experience symptoms of this condition.

*Pregnancy:* There are no adequate and well-controlled studies in pregnant women. Use only if clearly needed and potential benefits outweigh the possible hazards to the fetus. Tamsulosin is not indicated for use in women.

*Breastfeeding:* Prazosin appears in breast milk. It is not known if doxazosin or terazosin appear in breast milk. Tamsulosin is not indicated for use in women. Consult your doctor before you begin breastfeeding.

*Children:* Safety and effectiveness in children have not been established. Tamsulosin is not indicated for use in children.

*Lab tests* and blood pressure testing may be required to monitor treatment.

## Drug Interactions:
Tell your doctor or pharmacist if you are taking or planning to take any over-the-counter or prescription medications or dietary supplements while taking this drug. Drug doses may need to be modified or a different drug prescribed. The following drugs and drug classes interact with this drug:

beta-adrenergic blockers
(eg, propranolol) (prazosin only)
cimetidine (eg, *Tagamet*)
(tamsulosin only)

clonidine (eg, *Catapres*)
(prazosin only)
verapamil (eg, *Calan*) (terazosin
only)

## Side Effects:
Every drug is capable of producing side effects. Many patients experience no, or minor, side effects. The frequency and severity of side effects depend on many factors including dose, duration of therapy, and individual susceptibility. Possible side effects include:

*Digestive Tract:* Nausea; vomiting; stomachache; indigestion; diarrhea; constipation; gas.

*Nervous System:* Depression; dizziness; incoordination; feeling of whirling motion (vertigo); nervousness; anxiety; drowsiness; fatigue; sleeplessness; headache; abnormal skin sensations; lack of energy; fainting.

*Circulatory System:* Pounding in the chest (palpitations); dizziness or lightheadedness when rising quickly from a sitting or lying position (orthostatic hypotension); rapid or irregular pulse; low blood pressure.

*Respiratory System:* Difficulty breathing; nasal congestion; sore throat; runny nose; inflamed sinuses; cold symptoms; bronchitis; increased cough; nosebleed; flu symptoms.

*Skin:* Rash; itching; sweating; flushing.

*Other:* Painful erections; sexual problems; swelling of arms and legs (edema); facial swelling; dry mouth; ringing in the ears; weight gain; loss of bladder control; frequent urination; abnormal or blurred vision; eye pain or irritation; fever; urinary tract infections; gout; muscle cramps or spasms; neck, shoulder, back, chest, joint, muscle, or general body pain or discomfort; red eyes; infection; weakness; tooth disorder.

## Guidelines for Use:

- Dosage is individualized. Take exactly as prescribed.
- Do not stop taking or change dose, unless instructed by your doctor.
- If a dose is missed, take it as soon as possible. If several hours have passed or it is nearing time for the next dose, do not double the dose to catch up, unless instructed by your doctor. If more than one dose is missed or it is necessary to establish a new dosage schedule, contact your doctor or pharmacist.
- Patients being treated for high blood pressure often feel tired and run down for a few weeks after beginning therapy. It takes time for the body to adjust to lowered blood pressure. Continue taking your medication even though you may not feel quite normal. Check with your doctor or pharmacist during this time regarding any new symptoms that occur to ensure that these new feelings are a normal consequence of changes in blood pressure.
- Take the first dose at bedtime in order to reduce the risk of dizziness and light-headedness which may occur early in therapy. Take doxazosin, prazosin, and terazosin without regard to food. Take tamsulosin about 30 minutes after the same meal each day.
- Do not crush, chew, or open tamsulosin capsules.
- Medication will be started at a low dose and then slowly increased until maximum benefit is achieved.
- If therapy is stopped for several days, therapy should be restarted at the low dose and then slowly increased.
- May cause drowsiness, dizziness, light-headedness, or blurred vision. Use caution when driving or performing other tasks requiring alertness, coordination, or physical dexterity. Avoid engaging in any hazardous tasks for at least 12 to 24 hours after taking the first dose of these medications, missing several doses, increasing the dose, or taking other high blood pressure medications with these products. Sit or lie down if you feel light-headed.
- Dizziness or light-headedness may also occur following alcohol ingestion, standing for long periods of time, exercise, or during exposure to extreme heat.
- Use caution when rising from a sitting or lying position. If dizziness, light-headedness, or pounding in the chest (palpitations) become bothersome, notify your doctor.
- Stop taking and contact your doctor immediately if you experience a painful penile erection lasting for hours and not relieved by intercourse or masturbation.
- Do not take any other prescription or OTC medication or dietary supplements without first consulting your pharmacist or doctor.
- Inform your doctor if you are pregnant, become pregnant, plan on becoming pregnant, or are breastfeeding.
- Tamsulosin is not indicated for use in women or children.
- Lab tests and blood pressure testing may be required to monitor therapy. Be sure to keep appointments.
- Store at room temperature (68° to 86°F). Protect from light and moisture.

*If you have any questions, consult your doctor, pharmacist, or health care provider.*

| Generic Name<br>*Brand Name Examples* | Supplied As | Generic Available |
|---|---|---|
| Rx **Benazepril HCl** | | |
| *Lotensin* | **Tablets:** 5 mg, 10 mg, 20 mg, 40 mg | No |
| Rx **Captopril** | | |
| *Capoten* | **Tablets:** 12.5 mg, 25 mg, 50 mg, 100 mg | Yes |
| Rx **Enalapril** | | |
| *Vasotec* | **Tablets:** 2.5 mg, 5 mg, 10 mg, 20 mg | Yes |
| Rx **Fosinopril Sodium** | | |
| *Monopril* | **Tablets:** 10 mg, 20 mg, 40 mg | No |
| Rx **Lisinopril** | | |
| *Prinivil, Zestril* | **Tablets**: 2.5 mg, 5 mg, 10 mg, 20 mg, 40 mg | Yes |
| *Zestril* | **Tablets**: 30 mg | Yes |
| Rx **Moexipril HCl** | | |
| *Univasc* | **Tablets:** 7.5 mg, 15 mg | No |
| Rx **Perindopril Erbumine** | | |
| *Aceon* | **Tablets:** 2 mg, 4 mg, 8 mg | No |
| Rx **Quinapril HCl** | | |
| *Accupril* | **Tablets:** 5 mg, 10 mg, 20 mg, 40 mg | No |
| Rx **Ramipril** | | |
| *Altace* | **Capsules**: 1.25 mg, 2.5 mg, 5 mg, 10 mg | No |
| Rx **Trandolapril** | | |
| *Mavik* | **Tablets**: 1 mg, 2 mg, 4 mg | No |

## Type of Drug:

Angiotensin converting enzyme inhibitors (ACEIs); drugs used to lower blood pressure.

## How the Drug Works:

Angiotensin converting enzyme (ACE) is involved in certain chemical reactions that constrict (narrow) blood vessels and cause sodium and fluid retention by the kidney. This can cause an increase in blood pressure. ACEIs lower blood pressure by interfering with ACE, which causes blood vessels to relax (widen). Blow flows more freely and at a lower pressure. ACEIs also increase the heart's ability to pump blood in some types of heart failure.

## Uses:

To treat high blood pressure alone or in combination with other blood pressure-lowering medications.

*Captopril, enalapril, fosinopril, lisinopril, quinapril, ramipril, trandolapril:* To treat certain types congestive of heart failure, usually in combination with other medications (eg, diuretics, digitalis).

*Captopril:* To treat diabetic nephropathy (kidney damage) in patients with Type I (insulin-dependent) diabetes mellitus and retinopathy.

*Lisinopril:* To improve survival in patients who have had a heart attack within 24 hours.

*Unlabeled Use(s):* Occasionally, doctors may prescribe captopril for the management of specific types of hypertensive crises or neonatal and childhood hypertension, treatment of rheumatoid arthritis, certain types of edema, Bartter and Raynaud syndromes, and diagnosis of primary aldosteronism and certain kidney disorders. Enalapril has been used to treat diabetic nephropathy.

## Precautions:

*Do not use in the following situations:*
> allergy to the drug or any of its ingredients
> angioedema, history of
> pregnancy, second and third trimester

*Use with caution in the following situations:*

| | |
|---|---|
| agranulocytosis | low blood pressure |
| anesthesia, surgical | lupus erythematosus, systemic |
| aortic stenosis | neutropenia (low white blood cell |
| diabetes mellitus | count) |
| heart disease | pregnancy, first trimester |
| hemodialysis | proteinuria (protein in the urine) |
| high blood potassium levels | (captopril only) |
| kidney disease | renal artery stenosis |
| liver disease (fosinopril, quina- | |
| pril, ramipril only) | |

*Low blood pressure:* Dizziness and fainting due to lowered blood pressure may occur early in therapy. This effect is more likely to occur with concurrent diuretic treatment and when arising from a seated or lying position, but can occur at any time early in therapy. This effect can also occur if several doses are missed and then the medicine is restarted, if the dosage is increased rapidly, or if other blood pressure medications are added.

*Potassium:* Elevated serum potassium levels have occurred. Use with caution in the presence of kidney disease, diabetes, and with potassium-containing products (eg, salt substitutes, potassium supplements).

*Cough:* A persistent, dry, nonproductive cough can be caused by ACEIs. The cough is more likely to occur in women and at low doses. Recovery is rapid and complete in 1 to 4 days when the drug has been discontinued.

*Race:* ACEIs may not be as effective in black patients.

*Pregnancy:* Report pregnancy or suspected pregnancy to your doctor immediately.

*First trimester* – Fetal exposure to ACEIs only during the first trimester usually causes no problems, but the drug should be stopped as soon as possible. Continue use only if clearly needed and potential benefits outweigh the possible hazards to the fetus.

*Second and third trimesters* – Studies have shown a potential adverse effect on the fetus. When used during the second and third trimesters, ACEIs can cause fetal harm or even death. Discontinue the drug as soon as possible.

*Breastfeeding:* Several ACEIs appear in breast milk. It is not known if lisinopril, moexipril, perindopril, or ramipril appear in breast milk. Do not take fosinopril, ramipril, or trandolapril while breastfeeding. Consult your doctor before you begin breastfeeding.

*Children:* Safety and effectiveness have not been established. There is limited experience with the use of captopril in children. Unpredictable decreases in blood pressure and associated complications have occurred. Use catopril in children only when other measures for controlling blood pressure have not been effective.

*Lab tests* will be required periodically during treatment. Tests include urine protein, liver function, kidney function, blood cell counts, and sodium and potassium levels.

## Drug Interactions:

Tell your doctor or pharmacist if you are taking or planning to take any over-the-counter or prescription medications or dietary supplements while taking these drugs. Drug doses may need to be modified or a different drug prescribed. The following drugs and drug classes interact with these drugs:

allopurinol (eg, *Zyloprim*) (captopril only)
antacids (eg, *Maalox*)
capsaicin (eg, *Capsin*)
diuretics (eg, furosemide)
lithium (eg, *Eskalith*)
NSAIDs (eg, indomethacin)
phenothiazines (eg, promethazine)
potassium-containing salt substitutes (eg, *Nu-Salt*)

potassium-sparing diuretics (eg, triamterene)
potassium supplements (eg, potassium chloride)
probenecid (captopril only)
rifampin (eg, *Rifadin*) (enalapril only)
tetracyclines (eg, oxytetracyline) (quinapril only)

## Side Effects:

Every drug is capable of producing side effects. Many patients experience no, or minor, side effects. The frequency and severity of side effects depend on many factors including dose, duration of therapy, and individual susceptibility. Possible side effects include:

*Digestive Tract:* Stomach pain or ache; nausea; vomiting; diarrhea; constipation; indigestion; ulcers; appetite changes; gas; tongue swelling; difficulty swallowing; taste changes; mouth ulcer; dry mouth.

*Nervous System:* Depression; headache; dizziness; nervousness; sleeping difficulties; drowsiness; sleeplessness; fatigue; feeling of whirling motion; abnormal skin sensations; weakness.

*Circulatory System:* Chest pain; pounding in the chest; rapid or irregular heart beat; lowered blood pressure; dizziness or light-headedness when rising quickly from a sitting or lying position (orthostatic hypotension); fainting; heart attack.

*Respiratory System:* Difficulty breathing or shortness of breath; cough; sore throat; runny nose; sinus irritation; pneumonia; upper respiratory infection; bronchitis.

*Skin:* Rash; itching; flushing; hair loss.

*Other:* Fluid retention; pain in arms or legs; back, joint, muscle, neck, or shoulder pain; menstrual disorder; decreased or increased urination; protein in urine; fever; general body discomfort; flu syndrome; cold symptoms; ringing in the ears; ear infection; urinary tract infection; sexual problems; impotence; low serum sodium levels; elevated serum uric acid; elevated serum potassium levels.

## Guidelines for Use:

- Dosage is individualized. Take exactly as prescribed.
- Do not stop taking or change the dose, unless instructed by your doctor.
- Take captopril, moexipril, and quinapril 1 hour before meals or 2 hours after meals if possible. Take other ACEIs without regard to meals.
- *Ramipril* — Ramipril capsules are usually swallowed whole. However, the capsules may be opened and the contents sprinkled on approximately 4 oz of applesauce or mixed in 4 oz of apple juice or water. Consume the entire mixture. Mixtures and be prepared ahead of time and stored for up to 24 hours at room temperature or for up to 48 hours under refrigeration.
- If a dose is missed, take it as soon as possible. If several hours have passed or it is nearing time for the next dose, do not double the dose to catch up, unless instructed by your doctor. If more than one dose is missed, or it is necessary to establish a new dosage schedule, contact your doctor or pharmacist.
- Inform your doctor if you are pregnant, become pregnant, or are planning to become pregnant. ACEIs can cause injury to and even death of a developing fetus.
- Inform your doctor if you intend to breastfeed or are breastfeeding.
- Notify your doctor if you experience sore throat, fever, swelling of hands or feet, irregular heartbeat, chest pain, or yellowing of the skin or eyes.
- Stop taking and notify your doctor immediately if you experience swelling of the face, eyes, lips, or tongue, hoarseness, or difficulty swallowing or breathing.
- Excessive perspiration, inadequate fluid intake, dehydration, vomiting, or diarrhea may lead to a fall in blood pressure while taking this medicine.
- May cause dizziness, fainting, or light-headedness, especially after the first dose or during the first days of therapy; avoid sudden changes in posture. If actual fainting occurs, stop taking your medicine until you talk to your doctor. Heart failure patients should avoid rapid increases in physical activity. Sit or lie down if you feel light-headed.
- May cause skin rash or impaired taste perception. Notify your doctor if these persist.
- A persistent dry cough may occur and usually does not go away unless the medication is stopped. Notify your doctor if a cough develops and becomes bothersome.
- Do not use potassium supplements or salt substitutes containing potassium without consulting your doctor.
- May cause sensitivity to sunlight. Avoid prolonged exposure to the sun or other forms of ultraviolet light (UV) light (eg, tanning beds). Use sunscreens and wear protective clothing until tolerance is determined.
- Do not take any other prescription or OTC medications or dietary supplements without first consulting your doctor or pharmacist.
- Lab tests and follow-up visits will be required to monitor therapy. Be sure to keep appointments.
- Store in a tight, light-resistant container at room temperature (59° to 86°F). Protect from moisture.

*If you have any questions, consult your doctor, pharmacist, or health care provider.*

| Generic Name<br>*Brand Name Example* | Supplied As | Generic<br>Available |
|---|---|---|
| *Rx* **Candesartan Cilexetil** | | |
| *Atacand* | **Tablets:** 4 mg, 8 mg, 16 mg,<br>32 mg | No |
| *Rx* **Eprosartan Mesylate** | | |
| *Teveten* | **Tablets:** 400 mg, 600 mg | No |
| *Rx* **Irbesartan** | | |
| *Avapro* | **Tablets:** 75 mg, 150 mg,<br>300 mg | No |
| *Rx* **Losartan Potassium** | | |
| *Cozaar* | **Tablets:** 25 mg, 50 mg, 100 mg | No |
| *Rx* **Olmesartan Medoxomil** | | |
| *Benicar* | **Tablets:** 5 mg, 20 mg, 40 mg | No |
| *Rx* **Telmisartan** | | |
| *Micardis* | **Tablets:** 20 mg, 40 mg, 80 mg | No |
| *Rx* **Valsartan** | | |
| *Diovan* | **Tablets:** 40 mg, 80 mg,<br>160 mg, 320 mg | No |

## Type of Drug:

Antihypertensive; blood pressure-lowering agent.

## How the Drug Works:

Angiotensin II is a chemical transmitter that combines with chemical receptors in blood vessels and other tissues and causes blood vessels to constrict (narrow) and the kidneys to retain sodium and fluids. Angiotensin II receptor antagonists inhibit the action of angiotensin II and allow the blood vessels to dilate (widen) and the kidneys to eliminate extra sodium and fluids. These actions combine to help lower elevated blood pressure.

## Uses:

To lower blood pressure. May be used alone or in combination with other antihypertensive agents.

*Irbesartan, losartan:* To treat diabetic nephropathy (kidney damage) in patients with type 2 diabetes and hypertension.

*Valsartan:* To treat heart failure in patients who cannot tolerate angiotensin-converting enzyme (ACE) inhibitors.

## Precautions:

*Do not use in the following situations:*
> allergy to the drug or any of its ingredients
> pregnancy (second and third trimesters)

*Use with caution in the following situations:*
> diuretic use, concurrent
> kidney disease
> liver disease
> volume or salt-depletion (eg, dehydration) from diarrhea, vomiting, or excessive sweating

*Race:* Angiotensin II receptor antagonists may not be as effective in black patients.

*Pregnancy:*

> *First trimester* – When pregnancy is detected, the patient should discontinue use as soon as possible. Use only if clearly needed and the potential benefits outweigh the possible risks to the fetus.

> *Second and third trimesters* – Studies have shown a potential adverse effect on the fetus.

*Breastfeeding:* It is not known if angiotensin II receptor antagonists are excreted in breast milk. Because of the potential for adverse effects, a decision should be made whether to discontinue nursing or discontinue the drug, taking into account the importance of the drug to the mother. Consult your doctor before you begin breastfeeding.

*Children:* Safety and effectiveness of irbesartan in children younger than 6 years of age have not been established. Safety and effectiveness of other agents in children younger than 18 years of age have not been established.

*Elderly:* Older patients may be more sensitive to the blood pressure-lowering effects of these agents.

*Lab tests* may be required to monitor therapy. Tests include blood pressure readings, kidney function tests, liver function tests, and blood tests for electrolytes (eg, potassium).

## Drug Interactions:

Tell your doctor or pharmacist if you are taking or planning to take any over-the-counter or prescription medications or dietary supplements while taking these drugs. Drug doses may need to be modified or a different drug prescribed. The following drugs and drug classes interact with these drugs:

> digoxin (eg, *Lanoxin*) (telmisartan only)
> indomethacin (eg, *Indocin*) (losartan only)
> potassium-containing salt substitutes
> potassium-sparing diuretics (eg, spironolactone)
> potassium supplements (eg, *K-Dur*)

## Side Effects:

Every drug is capable of producing side effects. Many patients experience no, or minor, side effects. The frequency and severity of side effects depend on many factors including dose, duration of therapy, and individual susceptibility. Possible side effects include:

*Digestive Tract:* Indigestion; diarrhea; nausea; heartburn; stomach pain; vomiting.

*Nervous System:* Headache; dizziness; fatigue; nervousness; anxiety; sleeplessness; depression.

*Respiratory System:* Upper respiratory tract infection; cough; nasal congestion; sinus irritation; runny nose; sore throat; bronchitis.

*Other:* Rapid heartbeat; changes in blood pressure; chest, muscle, back, leg, or joint pain; muscle cramps; viral infection; swelling (fluid retention); trauma; weakness; flu; urinary tract infection; rash; protein in the urine; dizziness when rising from a sitting or lying position (orthostatic hypotension).

## Guidelines for Use:

- Dosage is individualized. Take exactly as prescribed.
- Do not stop taking or change the dose, unless instucted by your doctor.
- May be taken without regard to food. Take with food if stomach upset occurs.
- *Telmisartan* — Do not remove tablets from blister pack until just before taking.
- May be taken with other blood pressure-lowering agents prescribed by your doctor.
- Maximum blood pressure-lowering effect is generally attained after 2 to 4 weeks.
- If a dose is missed, take it as soon as possible. If several hours have passed or it is nearing time for the next dose, do not double the dose to catch up, unless instructed by your doctor. If more than one dose is missed or it is necessary to establish a new dosage schedule, contact your doctor or pharmacist.
- May cause dizziness or drowsiness. Use caution while driving or performing other tasks requiring alertness, coordination, or physical dexterity until tolerance is determined.
- Dehydration (eg, excess sweating, vomiting, diarrhea) may increase the blood pressure-lowering effect, causing dizziness or fainting. Notify your doctor if dizziness develops.
- A low dose of a diuretic may be added by your doctor if blood pressure is not controlled.
- Inform your doctor immediately if you are pregnant, become pregnant, are planning to become pregnant, or are breastfeeding.
- Lifestyle changes (eg, stop smoking, lose weight, exercise, limit salt in diet) also help to reduce blood pressure.
- Lab tests may be required to monitor therapy. Be sure to keep appointments.
- Store at room temperature (68° to 77°F for eprosartan and olmesartan; 59° to 86°F for other agents) in a tightly closed container. Protect from light and moisture.

*If you have any questions, consult your doctor, pharmacist, or health care provider.*

| Generic Name Brand Name Examples | Supplied As | Generic Available |
|---|---|---|
| Rx **Clonidine HCl** | | |
| Catapres | **Tablets:** 0.1 mg, 0.2 mg, 0.3 mg | Yes |
| Catapres-TTS-1, Catapres-TTS-2, Catapres-TTS-3 | **Transdermal patches:** 0.1 mg/day, 0.2 mg/day, 0.3 mg/day | No |
| Duraclon | **Injection:** 100 mcg/mL in 10 mL vials, 500 mcg/mL in 10 mL vials | No |

## Type of Drug:
Antihypertensive; blood pressure-lowering agent.

## How the Drug Works:
Clonidine lowers blood pressure primarily by relaxing and dilating (widening) blood vessels.

## Uses:
*Tablets and patches:* To treat high blood pressure. Used either alone or in combination with other blood pressure-lowering drugs.

*Injection:* Used in combination with narcotic pain relievers for the treatment of severe pain in cancer patients.

*Unlabeled Use(s):* Occasionally, doctors may prescribe clonidine for atrial fibrillation, attention deficit hyperactivity disorder, kidney damage from cyclosporine, excessive sweating, mania, restless legs syndrome, psychosis, alcohol withdrawal, growth delay in children, diabetic diarrhea, Tourette syndrome, hypertensive "urgencies," menopausal flushing, methadone/opiate detoxification, postherpetic neuralgia, reduction of inflammatory reactions in patients with asthma, smoking cessation, ulcerative colitis, and diagnosing pheochromocytoma.

## Precautions:
*Do not use in the following situations:* Allergy to clonidine or any of its ingredients, including adhesive on patch.

*Use with caution in the following situations:*

| | |
|---|---|
| coronary artery disease | heart rhythm disturbances |
| depression, history of | kidney disease, chronic |
| heart attack, recent | stroke, history of |
| heart disease, severe | |

*Tolerance:* Tolerance may develop. Clonidine's effectiveness may decrease over time. If this occurs, therapy will have to be reevaluated by your doctor.

*Withdrawal reaction:* Stopping clonidine suddenly can sometimes cause a sudden, intense increase in blood pressure. Symptoms may include nervousness, agitation, headache, and tremors. Do not stop taking clonidine without consulting your doctor.

*Pregnancy:* There are no adequate or well-controlled studies in pregnant women. Use only if clearly needed and the potential benefits outweigh the possible risks to the fetus.

*Breastfeeding:* Clonidine appears in breast milk. Consult your doctor before you begin breastfeeding.

*Children:* Safety and effectiveness in children younger than 12 years of age have not been established.

*Lab tests* may be required to monitor therapy. Tests include eye examinations and blood pressure monitoring.

## Drug Interactions:

Tell your doctor or pharmacist if you are taking or planning to take any over-the-counter or prescription medications or dietary supplements with this drug. Drug doses may need to be modified or a different drug prescribed. The following drugs and drug classes interact with this drug:

alcohol
barbiturates (eg, phenobarbital)
beta blockers
 (eg, propranolol)
calcium channel blockers
 (eg, verapamil)
digitalis (eg, digoxin)

levodopa (eg, *Dopar*)
prazosin (eg, *Minipress*)
sedative drugs (eg, tranquilizers, sleeping pills, antihistamines)
tricyclic antidepressants
 (eg, amitriptyline)

## Side Effects:

Every drug is capable of producing side effects. Many patients experience no, or minor, side effects. The frequency and severity of side effects depend on many factors including dose, duration of therapy, and individual susceptibility. Possible side effects include:

*Patches only:* Redness; itching; blisters; skin discoloration; swelling; sores; burning; pain; bruising; pale skin; throbbing; skin inflammation at application site.

*Digestive Tract:* Constipation; nausea; vomiting; decreased appetite; weight gain; dry mouth or throat.

*Nervous System:* Drowsiness; depression; headache; nervousness; sedation; dizziness; agitation; fatigue; sleeplessness; confusion.

*Other:* Impotence; loss of sex drive; general body discomfort; excessive urination at night; dizziness or unsteadiness after rising from a lying or sitting position (orthostatic hypotension); low blood pressure; weakness; slow heartbeat.

## Guidelines for Use:

- Take this medication exactly as directed, have your blood pressure checked regularly, and keep your appointments with your doctor even if you feel well. Most patients with high blood pressure do not feel sick.
- If dry mouth occurs, take frequent sips of water, suck on ice chips or sugarless hard candy, or chew sugarless gum.
- Patients being treated for high blood pressure often feel tired or run down for a few weeks after beginning therapy. Continue taking your medication even though you may not feel quite normal. Contact your doctor or pharmacist about any new symptoms.
- This medicine may cause drowsiness or dizziness. Use caution while driving or performing other tasks requiring alertness, coordination, or physical dexterity until tolerance is determined.
- Avoid alcohol and other mental depressants (eg, tranquilizers) while you are taking this medicine. They may cause excessive drowsiness.
- *Tablets —*
  Usually taken in 2 divided doses (morning and bedtime).
  If a dose is missed, take it as soon as possible. If several hours have passed or it is nearing time for the next dose, do not double the dose to catch up, unless instructed by your doctor. If more than one dose is missed or it is necessary to establish a new dosage schedule, contact your doctor or pharmacist.
  Do not stop taking this medicine suddenly. If your doctor discontinues this drug, the dose must be gradually reduced over at least 2 to 4 days in order to avoid a rapid increase in blood pressure, nervousness, agitation, or headache.
  Store tablets below 86°F. Keep container closed and protect from light.
- *Patches —*
  Patient instructions are included with each box of patches.
  Apply to a hairless area on the upper-outer arm or chest once every 7 days.
  Do not apply over any abnormal or damaged skin. Do not shave skin before applying.
  Use a different skin site from the previous application. If the patch loosens during the 7-day wearing, apply the white adhesive overlay directly over the patch to ensure good adhesion.
  Tell your doctor if an allergic reaction or skin irritation extends beyond the local patch area.
  It may take 2 to 3 days after the first patch application before blood pressure is reduced.
  Doctors will occasionally have patients wear more than 1 patch at a time to adjust the dose. Apply patches at different locations.
  If mild skin irritation occurs during the 7-day wearing, remove and discard the patch and apply a new patch in another area.
  Usual exposure to water (eg, showering, bathing, swimming) should not affect the patch.
  After removal, fold used patch in half with sticky sides together and dispose of carefully.
  Store patches below 86°F. Do not open pouch until ready to apply.

**Guidelines for Use (cont.):**

- *Injection* —
  Frequently inspect infusion pump and catheter. Notify your doctor immediately if pump stops running or catheter becomes plugged or comes loose.
  Carefully follow catheter care and pump instructions provided by your doctor.

*If you have any questions, consult your doctor, pharmacist, or health care provider.*

| Generic Name<br>*Brand Name Example* | Supplied As | Generic<br>Available |
|---|---|---|
| Rx **Guanabenz Acetate** | | |
| *Wytensin* | **Tablets:** 4 mg, 8 mg | No |

## Type of Drug:
Antihypertensive; blood pressure-lowering agent.

## How the Drug Works:
Guanabenz acetate lowers blood pressure, primarily by relaxing and dilating (widening) blood vessels. Blood flows more freely at a lower pressure.

## Uses:
To treat high blood pressure alone or in conjunction with a diuretic (water pill).

## Precautions:
*Do not use in the following situations:* Allergy to the drug or any of its ingredients.

*Use with caution in the following situations:*

| | |
|---|---|
| coronary insufficiency | liver disease, severe |
| heart attack, recent | stroke, history of |
| kidney disease, severe | |

*Discontinuing treatment:* Do not stop taking this medicine without consulting your doctor. Abrupt withdrawal of treatment may result in high blood pressure.

*Pregnancy:* There are no adequate studies and well-controlled studies in pregnant women. Use only if clearly needed and the potential benefits outweigh the possible risks to the fetus.

*Breastfeeding:* It is not known if guanabenz acetate appears in breast milk. Consult your doctor before you begin breastfeeding.

*Children:* Safety and effectiveness have not been established.

## Drug Interactions:
Tell your doctor or pharmacist if you are taking or planning to take any over-the-counter or prescription medications or dietary supplements while taking this drug. Drug doses may need to be modified or a different drug prescribed.

## Side Effects:
Every drug is capable of producing side effects. Many patients experience no, or minor, side effects. The frequency and severity of side effects depend on many factors including dose, duration of therapy, and individual susceptibility. Possible side effects include:

*Digestive Tract:* Nausea; vomiting; stomach pain; diarrhea; constipation; dry mouth.

*Nervous System:* Depression; sleep disturbances; dizziness; drowsiness; headache; anxiety; taste disturbances; blurred vision; weakness.

*Circulatory System:* Irregular heartbeat; chest pain; pounding in the chest.

*Respiratory System:* Difficulty breathing; nasal congestion.

*Other:* Edema (fluid retention); muscle pain in arms and legs; breast growth in males; impotenc;, decreased sex drive; urinary frequency; rash; itching.

## Guidelines for Use:

- Dosage is individualized. Take exactly as prescribed.
- Take twice a day. Do not exceed 32 mg twice daily.
- If a dose is missed, take it as soon as possible. If several hours have passed or it is nearing time for the next dose, do not double the dose to catch up, unless advised to do so by your doctor. If more than one dose is missed or it is necessary to establish a new dosage schedule, contact your doctor or pharmacist.
- Take this medication daily as directed, have your blood pressure checked regularly, and keep your appointments with your doctor even if you feel well. Most patients with high blood pressure do not feel sick.
- Do not stop taking this medicine suddenly or without consulting your doctor. Abrupt withdrawal of treatment may result in high blood pressure.
- Patients being treated for high blood pressure often feel tired or run-down for a few weeks after beginning therapy. Continue taking your medication even though you may not feel quite "normal." Contact your doctor or pharmacist about any new symptoms.
- This medicine may cause drowsiness or dizziness. Use caution while driving or performing other tasks requiring alertness, coordination, or physical dexterity.
- Avoid alcohol and other mental depressants (eg, tranquilizers) while you are taking this medicine. They may cause excessive drowsiness.
- Lab tests may be required to monitor therapy. Keep appointments.
- Store at room temperature (68° to 77°F) in a tightly closed container. Protect from light.

*If you have any questions, consult your doctor, pharmacist, or health care provider.*

| Generic Name<br>*Brand Name Example* | Supplied As | Generic<br>Available |
|---|---|---|
| Rx **Guanadrel Sulfate** | | |
| *Hylorel* | **Tablets:** 10 mg, 25 mg | No |

## Type of Drug:
Drug used to lower high blood pressure.

## How the Drug Works:
Guanadrel allows blood vessels to relax and dilate (widen), decreasing the resistance of the blood vessels to blood flow and resulting in lower blood pressure.

## Uses:
To treat high blood pressure in conjunction with a diuretic ("water pill").

## Precautions:
*Do not use in the following situations:*

allergy to this medication
congestive heart failure
MAO inhibitor antidepressant use (eg, phenelzine), within 1 week
pheochromocytoma (tumor of the adrenal gland)

*Use with caution in the following situations:*

asthma
kidney disease
peptic ulcer
surgery
tricyclic antidepressant use
vascular disease

*Pregnancy:* Studies in pregnant women or in animals have been judged not to show a risk to the fetus. However, no drug should be used during pregnancy unless clearly needed.

*Breastfeeding:* It is not known if guanadrel appears in breast milk. Consult your doctor before you begin breastfeeding.

*Children:* Safety and effectiveness have not been established.

## Drug Interactions:
Tell your doctor or pharmacist if you are taking or planning to take any over-the-counter or prescription medications or dietary supplements while taking this medicine. Doses of one or both drugs may need to be modified or a different drug may need to be prescribed. The following drugs and drug classes interact with this medicine:

alpha-blocking agents (eg, prazosin)
beta blockers (eg, propanolol)
ephedrine
MAOIs (eg, phenelzine)
norepinephrine
phenothiazines (eg, promethazine)
phenylpropanolamine (eg, *Propagest*)
reserpine
tricyclic antidepressants (eg, amitriptyline)
vasodilators (eg, hydralazine)

## Side Effects:

Every drug is capable of producing side effects. Many patients experience no, or minor, side effects. The frequency and severity of side effects depend on many factors including dose, duration of therapy, and individual susceptibility. Possible side effects include:

*Digestive Tract:* Nausea; vomiting; increased bowel movements; stomach pain; constipation; gas; indigestion; appetite loss; weight changes; dry mouth or throat; swollen tongue.

*Nervous System:* Headache; sleep disturbances; confusion; drowsiness; fatigue; fainting; depression; psychological problems; tingling or numbness.

*Circulatory System:* Chest pain; pounding in the chest.

*Respiratory System:* Shortness of breath; cough.

*Other:* Vision problems; swelling in hands and feet; impotence; back or neck ache; leg cramps and aches; joint pain or inflammation; urination frequency; urine retention; increased urination at night; blood in urine; ejaculation disturbances.

---

### Guidelines for Use:

- Use exactly as prescribed.
- Usual adult daily dose is 20 to 75 mg, taken in two divided doses.
- If a dose is missed, take it as soon as possible. If several hours have passed or it is nearing time for the next dose, do not double the dose to catch up, unless advised to do so by your doctor. If more than one dose is missed or it is necessary to establish a new dosage schedule, contact your doctor or pharmacist.
- Take this medicine daily as directed, have your blood pressure checked regularly and keep your appointments with your doctor even if you feel well. Most patients do not feel sick.
- Do not stop taking this medicine suddenly or without consulting your doctor.
- Patients being treated for high blood pressure often feel tired or run-down for a few weeks after beginning therapy. Continue taking your medication even though you may not feel quite "normal." Contact your doctor or pharmacist about any new symptoms.
- This medicine may cause dizziness, lightheadedness, blurred vision or fainting, especially when rising or standing. This condition is worsened by alcohol use, fever, hot weather, prolonged standing or exercise. If these symptoms should occur, sit or lie down and contact your doctor.
- This medicine may cause drowsiness. Use caution while driving or performing other tasks requiring alertness, coordination or physical dexterity.
- Do not take any prescription or over-the-counter medications, especially for colds, allergy or asthma, without the advice of your doctor or pharmacist.
- Store at controlled room temperature (59° to 86°F).

---

*If you have any questions, consult your doctor, pharmacist, or health care provider.*

| Generic Name<br>*Brand Name Example* | Supplied As | Generic<br>Available |
|---|---|---|
| *Rx* **Guanethidine Monosulfate** | | |
| *Ismelin* | **Tablets:** 10 mg, 25 mg | No |

## Type of Drug:

Drug used to lower high blood pressure.

## How the Drug Works:

Guanethidine lowers blood pressure by relaxing and dilating (widening) blood vessels. Blood flows more freely at a lower pressure.

## Uses:

To treat moderate and severe high blood pressure, either alone or in conjuction with a diuretic ("water pill").

To treat high blood pressure caused by certain kidney diseases.

## Precautions:

*Do not use in the following situations:*

| | |
|---|---|
| allergy to this medicine | MAOI (eg, phenelzine), use |
| congestive heart failure, not due to hypertension | pheochromocytoma (adrenal gland tumor) |

*Use with caution in the following situations:*

| | |
|---|---|
| asthma | heart failure |
| cerebral vascular disease (stroke) | kidney disease |
| | nitrogen retention |
| coronary insufficiency | peptic ulcers |
| fever | surgery |
| heart attack, recent | |

*Pregnancy:* Adequate studies have not been done in pregnant women, or animal studies may have shown a risk to the fetus. Use only if clearly needed and potential benefits outweigh the possible hazards to the fetus.

*Breastfeeding:* Guanethidine appears in breast milk. Contact your doctor before you begin breastfeeding.

*Children:* Safety and effectiveness in children have not been established.

## Drug Interactions:

Tell your doctor or pharmacist if you are taking or planning to take any over-the-counter or prescription medications or dietary supplements while taking this medicine. Doses of one or both drugs may need to be modified or a different drug may need to be prescribed. The following drugs and drug classes interact with this medicine:

alcohol
appetite suppressants
 (eg, amphetamines)
barbiturates (eg, phenobarbital)
blood sugar lowering medications (eg, insulin)
contraceptives, oral (eg, *Ortho-Novum*)
digoxin (eg, *Lanoxin*)
haloperidol (eg, *Haldol*)
MAO inhibitor antidepressants
 (eg, phenelzine)

maprotiline (*Ludiomil*)
methylphenidate (eg, *Ritalin*)
minoxidil (eg, *Loniten*)
phenylthiazine (eg, *Compazine*)
rauwolfia derivatives
 (eg, reserpine)
sympathomimetics (eg, ephedrine)
thioxanthenes (eg, thiothixene)
tricyclic antidepressants
 (eg, amitriptyline)

## Side Effects:

Every drug is capable of producing side effects. Many patients experience no, or minor, side effects. The frequency and severity of side effects depend on many factors including dose, duration of therapy, and individual susceptibility. Possible side effects include:

*Digestive Tract:* Diarrhea; nausea; vomiting; increased bowel movements; dry mouth.

*Nervous System:* Dizziness; weakness; depression; fainting; drowsiness; blurred vision; tiredness.

*Circulatory System:* Slowed heart rate; chest pain or numbness.

*Respiratory System:* Nasal congestion; difficulty breathing; asthma.

*Other:* Hair loss; impotence; muscle tremors or aches; edema (fluid retention); increased urination at night; loss of bladder control; drooping eyelids; skin inflammation; ejaculation problems; scalp hair loss.

## Guidelines for Use:

- Use exactly as prescribed.
- Usual adult dose is 25 to 50 mg taken once daily.
- If a dose is missed, take it as soon as possible. If several hours have passed or it is nearing time for the next dose, do not double the dose to catch up, unless advised to do so by your doctor. If more than one dose is missed or it is necessary to establish a new dosage schedule, contact your doctor or pharmacist.
- Take this medication daily as directed, have your blood pressure checked regularly and keep your appointments with your doctor even if you feel well. Most patients with high blood pressure do not feel sick.
- Do not stop taking this medicine suddenly or abruptly.
- Patients being treated for high blood pressure often feel tired or run-down for a few weeks after beginning therapy. Continue taking your medication even though you may not feel quite "normal." Contact your doctor or pharmacist about any new symptoms.
- Dizziness or lightheadedness may occur if you stand up too fast from a lying or sitting position. If this occurs, get up slowly and avoid sudden changes in posture.
- This medicine can cause dizziness. Use caution while driving or performing other tasks requiring alertness, coordination or physical dexterity.
- Contact your doctor if severe diarrhea, nausea, vomiting, frequent dizziness or fainting occurs.
- This medicine may interfere with ejaculation.
- Avoid alcohol while you are taking this medicine, as it aggravates the orthostatic hypotensive effects (dizziness or lightheadedness when rising quickly from a sitting or lying position) of this medicine.
- Do not take any prescription or over-the-counter medications, especially for colds, allergy or asthma, without consulting with your doctor or pharmacist.
- Store below 86°F in a tightly closed container.

*If you have any questions, consult your doctor, pharmacist, or health care provider.*

| Generic Name Brand Name Example | Supplied As | Generic Available |
|---|---|---|
| Rx **Guanfacine HCl** | | |
| *Tenex* | **Tablets:** 1 mg, 2 mg | No |

## Type of Drug:

Drug used to lower high blood pressure.

## How the Drug Works:

Guanfacine lowers blood pressure by relaxing and dilating (widening) blood vessels. Blood flows more freely at a lower pressure.

## Uses:

To treat high blood pressure. May be used alone or in conjunction with other blood pressure lowering drugs, especially a thiazide diuretic ("water pill").

*Unlabeled Use(s):* Occasionally doctors may prescribe guanfacine for heroin withdrawal, to reduce the frequency of migraine headaches or to reduce nausea and vomiting.

## Precautions:

*Do not use in the following situations:* Allergy to guanfacine or any of its ingredients.

*Use with caution in the following situations:*

| | |
|---|---|
| cerebrovascular disease (stroke) | kidney disease, chronic |
| coronary insufficiency, severe | liver disease, chronic |
| heart attack, recent | |

*Drug withdrawal reaction:* Do not stop taking this medicine without consulting with your doctor. Abrupt withdrawal may result in high blood pressure.

*Pregnancy:* Studies in pregnant women or in animals have been judged not to show a risk to the fetus. However, no drug should be used during pregnancy unless clearly needed.

*Breastfeeding:* It is not known if guanfacine appears in breast milk. Consult your doctor before you begin breastfeeding.

*Children:* Safety and effectiveness in children under 12 years of age have not been established.

## Drug Interactions:

Tell your doctor or pharmacist if you are taking or planning to take any over-the-counter or prescription medications or dietary supplements while taking this medicine. Doses of one or both drugs may need to be modified or a different drug may need to be prescribed. The following drugs and drug classes interact with this medicine:

| | |
|---|---|
| barbiturates (eg, phenobarbital) | tricyclic antidepressants |
| phenytoin (eg, *Dilantin*) | (eg, amitriptyline) |

## Side Effects:

Every drug is capable of producing side effects. Many patients experience no, or minor, side effects. The frequency and severity of side effects depend on many factors including dose, duration of therapy, and individual susceptibility. Possible side effects include:

*Digestive Tract:* Nausea; constipation; dry mouth; stomach pain; diarrhea; indigestion; difficulty swallowing.

*Nervous System:* Dizziness; headache; drowsiness; weakness; sleeplessness; memory loss; confusion; depression; numbness or tingling; paralysis.

*Circulatory System:* Slow heartbeat; pounding in the chest; chest pain.

*Respiratory System:* Nasal congestion; difficulty breathing.

*Skin:* Inflammation; itching; hives; sweating.

*Other:* Impotence; decrease in sexual desire; problems with testicles; changes in taste or vision; ringing in the ears; eye inflammation or infection; leg cramps, tremors; loss of bladder control; general body discomfort; decreased mobility or activity; unusual bleeding.

---

### Guidelines for Use:

- Use exactly as prescribed.
- Usual adult dose is 1 mg daily. Take at bedtime to decrease daytime drowsiness.
- If a dose is missed, take it as soon as possible. If several hours have passed or it is nearing time for the next dose, do not double the dose to catch up, unless advised to do so by your doctor. If more than one dose is missed or it is necessary to establish a new dosage schedule, contact your doctor or pharmacist.
- Take this medication daily as directed, have your blood pressure checked regularly and keep your appointments with your doctor even if you feel well. Most patients with high blood pressure do not feel sick.
- Do not stop taking this medicine suddenly. If your doctor discontinues this drug, the dose must be gradually reduced in order to avoid a rapid increase in blood pressure, nervousness or agitation.
- Patients being treated for high blood pressure often feel tired or run-down for a few weeks after beginning therapy. Continue taking your medication even though you may not feel quite "normal." Contact your doctor or pharmacist about any new symptoms.
- This medicine may cause drowsiness or dizziness. Use caution while driving or performing other tasks requiring alertness, coordination or physical dexterity.
- Avoid alcohol and other mental depressants (eg, tranquilizers) while you are taking this medicine. They may cause excessive drowsiness.
- Store at controlled room temperature (59° to 86°F) in a tight, light-resistant container.

---

*If you have any questions, consult your doctor, pharmacist, or health care provider.*

| Generic Name<br>*Brand Name Example* | Supplied As | Generic<br>Available |
|---|---|---|
| *Rx* **Hydralazine HCl** | | |
| *Apresoline*[1] | **Tablets:** 10 mg, 25 mg, 50 mg, 100 mg | Yes |
| *Apresoline* | **Injection:** 20 mg/mL | Yes |

[1] 100 mg tablet contains the dye tartrazine.

## Type of Drug:
Drug used to lower high blood pressure.

## How the Drug Works:
Hydralazine lowers blood pressure by relaxing and dilating (widening) the blood vessels. Blood flows more freely at a lower pressure.

## Uses:
To treat high blood pressure alone or in conjunction with other blood pressure lowering medications.

*Unlabeled Use(s):* Occasionally doctors may prescribe hydralazine for the treatment of congestive heart failure, severe aortic insufficiency and after heart valve replacement.

## Precautions:
*Do not use in the following situations:*
>allergy to this medicine
>coronary artery disease
>mitral valvular rheumatic heart disease

*Use with caution in the following situations:*
>kidney disease, advanced          stroke

*Systemic lupus erythematosus:* Hydralazine may produce symptoms similar to lupus (joint pain, fever, chest pain, continued general body discomfort, enlarged spleen, skin problems). Symptoms usually go away when the drug is discontinued.

*Pregnancy:* Adequate studies have not been done in pregnant women, or animal studies may have shown a risk to the fetus. Use only if clearly needed and potential benefits outweigh the possible hazards to the fetus.

*Breastfeeding:* Hydralazine appears in breast milk. Consult your doctor before you begin breastfeeding.

*Children:* Safety and effectiveness have not been established.

*Lab tests* may be required to monitor therapy. Tests may include blood tests. Be sure to keep appointments.

*Tartrazine:* Some of these products may contain the dye tartrazine (FD&C yellow No. 5) which can cause allergic reactions in certain individuals. Check package label when available or consult your doctor or pharmacist.

## Drug Interactions:

Tell your doctor or pharmacist if you are taking or planning to take any over-the-counter or prescription medications or dietary supplements while taking this medicine. Doses of one or both drugs may need to be modified or a different drug may need to be prescribed. The following drugs and drug classes interact with this medicine:

beta blockers (eg, propranolol)          MAO inhibitor antidepressants
diazoxide (*Hyperstat IV*)                (eg, phenelzine)
indomethacin (eg, *Indocin*)

## Side Effects:

Every drug is capable of producing side effects. Many patients experience no, or minor, side effects. The frequency and severity of side effects depend on many factors including dose, duration of therapy, and individual susceptibility. Possible side effects include:

*Digestive Tract:* Nausea; vomiting; diarrhea; appetite loss; constipation.

*Nervous System:* Headache; dizziness; tremors; depression; anxiety; disorientation; drowsiness.

*Circulatory System:* Chest pain; palpitations (pounding in the chest); increased heart beat; fainting.

*Respiratory System:* Difficulty breathing; nasal congestion.

*Skin:* Rash; itching; flushing; hives.

*Other:* Muscle pain or cramps; joint pain; difficult urination; red, swollen, puffy, infected, watery eyes; numbness or tingling in the hands or feet; fever; chills; fluid retention (edema); flushing.

## Guidelines for Use:

- Use exactly as prescribed.
- Usual adult tablet dose is 50 mg taken four times daily.
- Take with meals.
- If a dose is missed, take it as soon as possible. If several hours have passed or it is nearing time for the next dose, do not double the dose to catch up, unless advised to do so by your doctor. If more than one dose is missed or it is necessary to establish a new dosage schedule, contact your doctor or pharmacist.
- Take this medication daily as directed. Have your blood pressure checked regularly and keep your appointments with your doctor even if you feel well. Most patients with high blood pressure do not feel sick.
- Patients being treated for high blood pressure often feel tired or run-down for a few weeks after beginning therapy. Continue taking your medication even though you may not feel quite "normal." Contact your doctor or pharmacist about any new symptoms.
- This medicine may cause dizziness or drowsiness. Use caution while driving or performing other tasks requiring alertness, coordination or physical dexterity.
- Contact your doctor if rash, joint pain, fever, chest pain or prolonged tiredness or general body discomfort occurs.
- Lab tests may be required to monitor therapy. Be sure to keep appointments.
- *Injection* — Follow the injection procedure taught to you by your health care provider.
  Visually inspect solution for particles or discoloration before use.
- Store tablets below 86°F in a tight, light-resistant container.

*If you have any questions, consult your doctor, pharmacist, or health care provider.*

| Generic Name<br>*Brand Name Example* | Supplied As | Generic<br>Available |
|---|---|---|
| *Rx* **Carvedilol** | | |
| *Coreg* | **Tablets:** 6.25 mg, 12.5 mg,<br>25 mg | No |

## Type of Drug:

Drug used to lower high blood pressure; antihypertensive; alpha/beta-adrenergic blocking agent.

## How the Drug Works:

Carvedilol lowers blood pressure by dilating blood vessels, thereby decreasing blood pressure and pulse rate.

## Uses:

For the management of high blood pressure. It can be used alone or in combination with other antihypertensive drugs such as thiazide diuretics ("water pills").

*Unlabeled Use(s):* Occasionally doctors may prescribe carvedilol for congestive heart failure, chest pain (angina pectoris) or idiopathic cardiomyopathy.

## Precautions:

*Do not use in the following situations:*

allergy to this medicine
bronchial asthma (or related
  bronchial conditions)
heart problems, severe (eg, slow
  heartbeat or shock)
liver disease, severe

*Use with caution in the following situations:*

anesthesia/surgery
heart failure
hyperthyroidism (overactive
  thyroid)
hypoglycemia (low blood sugar)
peripheral vascular disease
  (hardening of the arteries)

*Diabetes:* These products can mask signs of hypoglycemia (low blood sugar) and alter blood sugar levels. It may be necessary for your doctor to alter your dose of diabetic medications while you are taking this medicine.

*Bronchospasm, nonallergic (eg, chronic bronchitis, emphysema):* In general, patients with bronchospastic disease should not take carvedilol. However, carvedilol may be used with caution in patients who do not respond to or cannot tolerate other high blood pressure drugs. Use the lowest possible dose in these cases.

*Pregnancy:* Adequate studies have not been done in pregnant women, or animal studies may have shown a risk to the fetus. Use only if clearly needed and potential benefits outweigh the possible hazards to the fetus.

*Breastfeeding:* It is not known if carvedilol appears in breast milk. Consult your doctor before you begin breastfeeding.

*Children:* Safety and effectiveness in children under 18 years of age have not been established.

## Drug Interactions:

Tell your doctor or pharmacist if you are taking or planning to take any over-the-counter or prescription medications while taking this medicine. Doses of one or both drugs may need to be modified or a different drug may need to be prescribed. The following drugs and drug classes interact with this medicine:

calcium channel blockers
 (eg, nifedipine)
catecholamine-depleting agents
 (eg, reserpine, MAOIs)
cimetidine (eg, *Tagamet*)
clonidine (eg, *Catapres*)

digoxin (eg, *Lanoxin*)
insulin
oral hypoglycemics
 (eg, sulfonylureas)
rifampin (eg, *Rifadin*)

## Side Effects:

Every drug is capable of producing side effects. Many patients experience no, or minor, side effects. The frequency and severity of side effects depend upon many factors including dose, duration of therapy, and individual susceptibility. Possible side effects include:

*Digestive Tract:* Stomach pain; diarrhea.

*Nervous System:* Dizziness; sleeplessness; drowsiness; fatigue.

*Circulatory System:* Slow heart rate; postural hypotension (dizziness or lightheadedness when rising from a sitting or lying position); swelling of the lower legs.

*Other:* Runny nose; sore throat; difficulty breathing; back pain; infections; unusual bleeding or bruising.

## Guidelines for Use:

- Use exactly as prescribed.
- Take with food to reduce lightheadedness when rising or standing.
- If a dose is missed, take it as soon as possible. If several hours have passed or it is nearing time for the next dose, do not double the dose to catch up, unless advised to do so by your doctor. If more than one dose is missed or it is necessary to establish a new dosage schedule, contact your doctor or pharmacist.
- Do not stop taking this medicine or change the dose without checking with your doctor; this could cause serious adverse effects.
- May cause drowsiness, dizziness, lightheadedness or fainting (especially when rising or standing). If these symptoms should occur, sit or lie down and contact your doctor. Use caution when driving or performing other tasks requiring alertness, coordination or physical dexterity.
- Patients being treated for high blood pressure often feel tired and run down for a few weeks after beginning therapy. It takes time for the body to adjust to lowered blood pressure. The full effect may take 7 to 14 days. Continue taking your medication even though you may not feel quick "normal." Check with your doctor or pharmacist during this time regarding any new symptoms that occur to assure that these new feelings are a normal consequence of changes in blood pressure.
- If itching, dark urine, appetite loss, yellowing of skin or eyes, pain in the upper right side or flu-like symptoms occur, contact your doctor immediately.
- Dose adjustments may be required after checking blood pressure. Be sure to keep appointments.
- Contact lens wearers may notice decreased tearing (dry eyes).
- Store at room temperature (59° to 86° F) away from moisture and light.

*If you have any questions, consult your doctor, pharmacist, or health care provider.*

| Generic Name<br>*Brand Name Examples* | Supplied As | Generic<br>Available |
|---|---|---|
| *Rx* **Labetalol HCl** | | |
| *Normodyne, Trandate* | **Tablets:** 100 mg, 200 mg,<br>300 mg | No |
| *Normodyne, Trandate* | **Injections:** 5 mg/mL | No |

## Type of Drug:

Drug used to lower high blood pressure; antihypertensive; alpha/beta blocker.

## How the Drug Works:

Labetalol lowers blood pressure alone and prevents blood pressure and pulse rate from increasing during exercise.

## Uses:

To treat high blood pressure alone or with other blood pressure lowering drugs, such as thiazide diuretics (water pills).

*Unlabeled Use(s):* Occasionally doctors may prescribe labetalol for pheochromocytoma and for clonidine withdrawal.

## Precautions:

*Do not use in the following situations:*

allergy to this medicine
bronchial asthma
heart problems, severe (eg, slow heartbeat or shock)

*Use with caution in the following situations:*

anesthesia/surgery
bronchitis, chronic
congestive heart failure, history
emphysema
hypoglycemia (low blood sugar
liver disease
pheochromocytoma (tumor)

*Diabetes:* These products can mask signs of hypoglycemia (low blood sugar) and alter blood sugar levels. It may be necessary for your doctor to alter your dose of diabetic medications while you are taking labetalol.

*Discontinuing therapy:* Do not suddenly discontinue labetalol without consulting your doctor. Angina (chest pain) or blood pressure may worsen.

*Pregnancy:* Adequate studies have not been done in pregnant women, or animal studies may have shown a risk to the fetus. Use only if clearly needed and potential benefits outweigh the possible hazards to the fetus.

*Breastfeeding:* Labetalol appears in breast milk. Consult your doctor before you begin breastfeeding.

*Children:* Safety and effectiveness have not been established.

*Lab tests* may be required to monitor therapy. Be sure to keep appointments.

## Drug Interactions:

Tell your doctor or pharmacist if you are taking or planning to take any over-the-counter or prescription medications or dietary supplements while taking this medicine. Doses of one or both drugs may need to be modified or a different drug may need to be prescribed. The following drugs and drug classes interact with this medicine:

alkalines (eg, furosemide)
 (*Normodyne* injection only)
beta-adrenergic agonists
 (eg, albuterol)
cimetidine (eg, *Tagamet*)

halothane anesthesia
nitroglycerin (eg, *Nitro-Bid*)
tricyclic antidepressants
 (eg, imipramine)
verapamil (eg, *Isoptin*)

## Side Effects:

Every drug is capable of producing side effects. Many patients experience no, or minor, side effects. The frequency and severity of side effects depend on many factors including dose, duration of therapy, and individual susceptibility. Possible side effects include:

*Digestive Tract:* Nausea; vomiting; indigestion.

*Nervous System:* Dizziness; headache; fatigue; drowsiness; abnormal skin sensations; tingling of scalp or skin; weakness; yawning; numbness; feeling of whirling motion.

*Circulatory System:* Postural hypotension (dizziness or lightheadedness when rising from a sitting or lying position); slow heartbeat.

*Skin:* Itching; rash; yellowing of skin or eyes; hair loss.

*Other:* Difficulty breathing; wheezing; nasal congestion; swelling of lower legs; visual disturbances; taste changes; muscle cramps; sexual difficulty; urinary problems.

## Guidelines for Use:

- Use exactly as prescribed.
- Usually taken twice a day. Tablets may be taken with or without food, but should be taken the same way each time.
- Do not stop taking this medicine without contacting your doctor; this could cause serious adverse effects.
- If a dose is missed, take it as soon as possible. If several hours have passed or it is nearing time for the next dose, do not double the dose to catch up, unless advised to do so by your doctor. If more than one dose is missed or it is necessary to establish a new dosage schedule, contact your doctor or pharmacist.
- Patients being treated for high blood pressure often feel tired and run down for a few weeks after beginning therapy. It takes time for the body to adjust to lowered blood pressure. Continue taking your medication even though you may not feel quite "normal." Check with your doctor or pharmacist during this time regarding any new symptoms that occur to assure that these new feelings are a normal consequence of changes in blood pressure.
- May cause dizziness or fainting, especially when rising or standing. If these symptoms should occur, sit or lie down and contact your doctor. Use caution when driving or performing other tasks requiring alertness, coordination or physical dexterity.
- Temporary scalp tinging may occur, especially at the start of treatment.
- Contact your doctor if any of the following occurs: Difficulty breathing; chest pain; slowed heartbeat; swelling of the lower legs; itching; dark urine; appetite loss; stomach pain; flu-like symptoms; yellowing of skin or eyes; upper right side pain.
- Diabetics may require adjustments in the dose of their antidiabetic medicine.
- Lab tests/exams will be required. Be sure to keep appointments.
- Store at room temperature (36° to 86° F) away from light and moisture. Do not freeze.

*If you have any questions, consult your doctor, pharmacist, or health care provider.*

| Generic Name<br>*Brand Name Example* | Supplied As | Generic<br>Available |
|---|---|---|
| Rx **Mecamylamine HCl** | | |
| *Inversine* | **Tablets:** 2.5 mg | No |

## Type of Drug:
Drug used to lower high blood pressure.

## How the Drug Works:
Mecamylamine lowers blood pressure primarily by relaxing and dilating (widening) blood vessels. Blood flows more freely at a lower pressure.

## Uses:
To treat moderately severe to severe high blood pressure or uncomplicated malignant hypertension.

## Precautions:
*Do not use in the following situations:*

| | |
|---|---|
| allergy to this medicine | kidney disease |
| antibiotic use | pyloric stenosis |
| coronary insufficiency | sulfonamide use |
| glaucoma | noncompliant patients |
| heart attack, recent | uremia |
| high blood pressure, mild,<br>  moderate or labile | |

*Use with caution in the following situations:*

| | |
|---|---|
| arteriosclerosis (hardening of<br>  the arteries) | prostate enlargement |
| urination difficulties | stroke, recent |

*Discontinuing treatment:* Do not discontinue this medicine without consulting your doctor. Abrupt withdrawal may result in a sudden return of high blood pressure and may result in a stroke or heart failure.

*Action of mecamylamine* may be increased by: Excessive heat; fever; infection; hemorrhage; pregnancy; anesthesia; surgery; vigorous exercise; other high blood pressure drugs; alcohol; salt depletion from diminished intake or increased excretion due to diarrhea, vomiting, excessive sweating or diuretics. Do not restrict sodium ingestion during therapy.

*Pregnancy:* Adequate studies have not been done in pregnant women, or animal studies may have shown a risk to the fetus. Use only if clearly needed and potential benefits outweigh the possible hazards to the fetus.

*Breastfeeding:* Because of the potential for serious adverse reactions in nursing infants, either discontinue nursing or discontinue the drug. Consult your doctor before you begin breastfeeding.

## Side Effects:
Every drug is capable of producing side effects. Many patients experience no, or minor, side effects. The frequency and severity of side effects depend on many factors including dose, duration of therapy, and individual susceptibility. Possible side effects include:

*Digestive Tract:* Nausea; vomiting; constipation; appetite loss; tongue inflammation; dry mouth; intestinal obstruction.

*Nervous System:* Convulsions; lightheadedness; weakness; drowsiness; fainting and dizziness when rising from a sitting or lying position; low blood pressure when standing; tremors; abnormal involuntary movements; abnormal mental state.

*Other:* Dilated pupils; blurred vision; shortness of breath; urinary retention; impotence; decreased sexual desire; tingling or numbness.

## Guidelines for Use:

- Use exactly as required.
- Usual adult dose is 25 mg, taken in three divided daily doses. Take after meals.
- The timing of doses in relation to meals should be consistent. Take the largest dose at noontime or in the evening. The smallest dose should be in the morning.
- Do not restrict dietary salt. Depleted salt states may increase the action of this medicine. Loss of salt can occur through sweating, vomiting, diarrhea or dehydration.
- If a dose is missed, take it as soon as possible. If several hours have passed or it is nearing time for the next dose, do not double the dose to catch up, unless advised to do so by your doctor. If more than one dose is missed or it is necessary to establish a new dosage schedule, contact your doctor or pharmacist.
- May cause dizziness, lightheadedness or fainting, especially when rising from a lying or sitting position. This effect may be increased by alcoholic beverages, exercise or during hot weather.
- Take this medication daily as directed, have your blood pressure checked regularly and keep your appointments with your doctor even if you feel well. Most patients with high blood pressure do not feel sick.
- Do not stop taking this medicine suddenly. If your doctor discontinues this drug, the dose must be gradually reduced in order to avoid a rapid increase in blood pressure and may result in a stroke or heart failure.
- Patients being treated for high blood pressure often feel tired or run-down for a few weeks after beginning therapy. Continue taking your medication even though you may not feel quite "normal." Contact your doctor or pharmacist about any new symptoms.
- Stop taking this medicine and contact your doctor immediately if tremors, diarrhea, bloating, decreased stomach rumbling or signs of bowel obstruction occur.
- This medicine may cause drowsiness. Use caution while driving or performing other tasks requiring alertness, coordination or physical dexterity.
- Avoid alcohol while you are taking this medicine. It may cause excessive drowsiness.
- Store at room temperature in a tight, light-resistant container.

*If you have any questions, consult your doctor, pharmacist, or health care provider.*

| Generic Name<br>*Brand Name Example* | Supplied As | Generic<br>Available |
|---|---|---|
| *Rx* **Methyldopa HCl** | | |
| *Aldomet* | **Tablets:** 125 mg, 250 mg, 500 mg | Yes |
| *Aldomet*[1] | **Oral Suspension:** 250 mg/5 mL | Yes |
| *Aldomet*[2] | **Injection:** 250 mg/5 mL | Yes |

[1] Contains sulfites and alcohol.
[2] Contains sulfites.

## Type of Drug:
Drug used to lower high blood pressure.

## How the Drug Works:
Methyldopa lowers blood pressure by relaxing and dilating (widening) blood vessels. Blood flows more freely at a lower pressure.

## Uses:
To treat high blood pressure alone or in conjunction with other blood pressure lowering drugs.

## Precautions:
*Do not use in the following situations:*

allergy to any component of this medicine
blood vessel disease
cirrhosis, active
hepatitis, active
MAOI (eg, phenelzine), use

*Use with caution in the following situations:*

anemia or other blood disorders
anesthetics
kidney disease
liver disease, history

*Pregnancy:*

*Tablets, oral suspension* – Studies in pregnant women have not shown a risk to the fetus. However, no drug should be used during pregnant unless clearly needed.

*Injection* – Adequate studies have not been done in pregnant women or animal studies may have shown a risk to the fetus. Use only if clearly needed and potential benefits outweigh the possible hazards to the fetus.

*Breastfeeding:* Methyldopa appears in breast milk. Contact your doctor before you begin breastfeeding.

*Elderly:* Dizziness and lightheadedness in older patients may be related to an increased sensitivity and to the patient's physical condition. Lower doses may need to be prescribed.

*Lab tests* may be required to monitor treatment. Tests may include Coombs test, liver function tests, hemoglobin, hematocrit, white and red cell counts. Be sure to keep appointments.

*Sulfites:* The oral suspension and injection contain sulfite preservatives which can cause allergic reactions in certain individuals (eg, asthmatics).

## Drug Interactions:

Tell your doctor or pharmacist if you are taking or planning to take any over-the-counter or prescription medications or dietary supplements while taking this medicine. Doses of one or both drugs may need to be modified or a different drug may need to be prescribed. The following drugs and drug classes interact with this medicine:

barbiturates (eg, phenobarbital)
beta blockers
 (eg, propranolol)
haloperidol (eg, *Haldol*)
levodopa (eg, *Larodopa*)
lithium (eg, *Eskalith*)
MAOIs (eg, phenelzine)

phenothiazines (eg, trifluoperazine)
sulfonylureas (eg, tolbutamide)
sympathomimetics
 (eg, ephedrine)
tricyclic antidepressants
 (eg, amitriptyline)

## Side Effects:

Every drug is capable of producing side effects. Many patients experience no, or minor, side effects. The frequency and severity of side effects depend on many factors including dose, duration of therapy, and individual susceptibility. Possible side effects include:

*Digestive Tract:* Nausea; vomiting; diarrhea; constipation; gas; colitis; bloating; dry mouth; inflammation of salivary glands; sore or black tongue; weight gain; mouth sores; stomach pain.

*Nervous System:* Dizziness; weakness; lightheadedness; drowsiness; headache; depression; decreased concentration; nightmares; tingling or numbness; unusual body movements; fainting.

*Circulatory System:* Slow heart rate; chest pain; congestive heart failure.

*Respiratory System:* Nasal congestion; sore throat; difficulty breathing.

*Skin:* Rash; yellowing of skin or eyes; easy bruising or bleeding.

*Other:* Joint or muscle pain; edema (fluid retention); fever; absence of menstruation; impotence; decrease sexual desire; breast swelling; breast secretions; anemia; dark or amber urine; breast growth in males; pancreatitis; liver or blood disorders; abnormal liver functions tests; Parkinsonism; Bell palsy.

## Guidelines for Use:

• Take exactly as prescribed.

• Usual adult dose of tablets and suspension is 500 mg to 2 g in two to four divided daily doses.

• If a dose is missed, take it as soon as possible. If several hours have passed or it is nearing time for the next dose, do not double the dose to catch up, unless advised to do so by your doctor. If more than one dose is missed or it is necessary to establish a new dosage schedule, contact your doctor or pharmacist.

• Take this medication daily as directed, have your blood pressure checked regularly and keep your appointments with your doctor even if you feel well. Most patients with high blood pressure do not feel sick.

• Do not stop taking this medicine suddenly. If your doctor discontinues this drug, the dose must be gradually reduced over 2 to 4 days in order to avoid a rapid increase in blood pressure.

• Patients being treated for high blood pressure often feel tired or run-down for a few weeks after beginning therapy. Continue taking your medication even though you may not feel quite "normal." Contact your doctor or pharmacist about any new symptoms.

• Dizziness or lightheadedness may occur if you stand up too fast from a lying or sitting position. If this occurs, get up slowly and avoid sudden changes in posture.

• This medicine may cause drowsiness. Use caution while driving or performing other tasks requiring alertness, coordination or physical dexterity.

• Avoid alcohol and other mental depressants (eg, tranquilizers) while you are taking this medicine. They may cause excessive drowsiness.

• Notify your doctor if prolonged general tiredness, edema (fluid retention), shortness of breath, involuntary movements, fever, mouth sores, sore throat or yellowing of skin or eyes occurs.

• Tolerance may occur, usually between the second or third month of therapy. Your doctor may increase the dosage of methyldopa or add a diuretic (water pill).

• When urine is exposed to air, it may darken. This is not a problem.

• *Injection* — Usual adult dose is 250 to 500 mg every 6 hours. Follow the injection procedure taught to you by a health care provider. Visually inspect solution for particles or discoloration before use.

• Lab tests may be required to monitor treatment. Be sure to keep appointments.

• *Storage* — Store tablets at room temperature in a tight, light-resistant container.
Store suspension below 78°F in a light, light-resistant container. Do not freeze.

*If you have any questions, consult your doctor, pharmacist, or health care provider.*

| Generic Name<br>*Brand Name Example* | Supplied As | Generic<br>Available |
|---|---|---|
| *Rx* **Minoxidil** | | |
| *Loniten* | **Tablets:** 2.5 mg, 10 mg | Yes |

## Type of Drug:

Drug used to lower high blood pressure.

## How the Drug Works:

Minoxidil lowers blood pressure by relaxing and dilating (widening) the arteries. Blood flows more freely at a lower pressure.

## Uses:

To treat severe elevations of blood pressure. It is always used in combination with other blood pressure lowering agents (eg, beta blockers, diuretics).

*Unlabeled Use(s):* Occasionally doctors may prescribe topical minoxidil to treat male pattern baldness. See the Miscellaneous-Minoxidil monograph in the Topical Products chapter.

## Precautions:

*Do not use in the following situations:*

allergy to any component of this medicine
aortic aneurysm, dissecting
heart attack, acute
pheochromocytoma (tumor of the adrenal gland)

*Use with caution in the following situations:*

angina
circulation, compromised
cryoglobulinemia
guanethidine use (*Ismelin*)
heart attack, recent
hypertension, severe
kidney dialysis
kidney failure

*Doctor supervision:* Minoxidil may produce serious side effects. Use of this drug must be closely supervised by your doctor. Minoxidil is given with other blood pressure medications. Take all medications exactly as prescribed. Notify your doctor if any of the following occur: Increased heart rate; rapid weight gain (over 5 pounds); unusual swelling of face, hands, ankles or abdomen; breathing difficulty; chest pain; severe indigestion; dizziness; lightheadedness or fainting.

*Fluid and electrolyte balance* and body weight must be monitored. Diuretics alone, or with restricted salt intake, usually minimize fluid retention. Fluid retention rarely may require discontinuation of minoxidil. Under close medical supervision, it may be possible to discontinue the drug for 1 or 2 days and then resume treatment in conjunction with diuretic therapy.

*Increased hair growth:* 80% of patients who are taking this medicine develop elongation, thickening and enhanced pigmentation of fine body hair within 3 to 6 weeks after starting therapy. It is usually first noticed on the temples, between the eyebrows, between the hairline and eyebrows or in the sideburn area of the upper cheek, later extending to the back, arms, legs and scalp. Upon discontinuation of the drug, new hair growth stops, but 1 to 6 months may be required for restoration to pretreatment appearance. Unwanted hair can be controlled by a hair remover or by shaving. For further information on minoxidil as a treatment for male pattern baldness, see the Miscellaneous-Minoxidil monograph in the Topicals chapter.

*Lab tests:* Your doctor may require lab tests at 1 to 3 month intervals in the beginning of minoxidil therapy, and at 6 to 12 month intervals later. Some of the tests that may be required include: Urine tests, kidney function tests, echocardiograms, electrocardiograms and chest x-rays.

*Pregnancy:* Adequate studies have not been done in pregnant women, or animal studies may have shown a risk to the fetus. Use only if clearly needed and potential benefits outweigh the possible hazards to the fetus.

*Breastfeeding:* Minoxidil appears in breast milk. It should not be given to nursing women. Contact your doctor before beginning breastfeeding.

*Children:* Experience in children is limited. Doses must be adjusted very carefully. Consult your doctor.

## Drug Interactions:

Tell your doctor or pharmacist if you are taking or planning to take any over-the-counter or prescription medications or dietary supplements while take this medicine. Doses of one or both drugs may need to be modified or a different drug may need to be prescribed. Guanethidine (eg, *Ismelin*) interacts with this medicine.

## Side Effects:

Many patients experience side effects. The frequency and severity of side effects depend on many factors including dose, duration of therapy and individual susceptibility. Possible side effects include:

*Digestive Tract:* Nausea; vomiting; severe indigestion.

*Circulatory System:* Chest pain; rapid pulse.

*Respiratory System:* Shortness of breath; difficulty breathing.

*Skin:* Rash; increased hair growth and darkening of fine body hair.

*Other:* Weight gain or swelling of arms, legs, face or abdomen; dizziness.

## Guidelines for Use:

- Use exactly as prescribed.
- Usual adult dose (patients over 12 years of age) is 10 to 40 mg as a single daily dose. Do not exceed 100 mg per day.
- Minoxidil is usually taken with at least two other antihypertensive drugs (a beta blocker and a diuretic). Take all medications as prescribed.
- If a dose is missed, take it as soon as possible. If several hours have passed or it is nearing time for the next dose, do not double the dose to catch up, unless advised to do so by your doctor. If more than one dose is missed or it is necessary to establish a new dosage schedule, contact your doctor or pharmacist.
- A low salt diet should be closely followed.
- Take this medication daily as directed, have your blood pressure checked regularly and keep your appointments with your doctor even if you feel well. Most patients with high blood pressure do not feel sick.
- Do not stop taking this medicine suddenly. If your doctor discontinues this drug, the dose must be gradually reduced in order to avoid a rapid increase in blood pressure, nervousness, agitation or headache.
- Patients being treated for high blood pressure often feel tired or run-down for a few weeks after beginning therapy. Continue taking your medication even though you may not feel quite "normal." Contact your doctor or pharmacist about any new symptoms.
- This medicine may cause dizziness or drowsiness. Use caution while driving or performing other tasks requiring alertness, coordination or physical dexterity.
- Notify your doctor if any of the following occurs: Increased heart rate; rapid weight gain of more than 5 pounds; unusual swelling of hands, feet, face or abdomen; breathing difficulty, especially when lying down; new or aggravated angina symptoms (chest, arm or shoulder pain); severe indigestion; dizziness; lightheadedness or fainting.
- Enhanced growth and darkening of fine body hair occurs in most patients. This may become bothersome. However, do not discontinue medication without consulting your doctor. Unwanted hair can be controlled by a hair remover or by shaving.
- Lab tests may be required to monitor treatment. Be sure to keep appointments.
- Store at controlled room temperature (59° to 86°F).

*If you have any questions, consult your doctor, pharmacist, or health care provider.*

| Generic Name | Supplied As | Generic Available |
|---|---|---|
| *Rx* Reserpine | **Tablets:** 0.1 mg, 0.25 mg | Yes |

## Type of Drug:

Antihypertensive; drug used to lower high blood pressure.

## How the Drug Works:

Reserpine (a rauwolfia alkaloid) lowers blood pressure by altering nerve function and decreasing the heart rate. It also has sedative and tranquilizing properties.

## Uses:

To treat mild high blood pressure. May be used with other blood pressure lowering drugs to treat serious high blood pressure.

To relieve symptoms in agitated mental states (eg, schizophrenia).

## Precautions:

*Do not use in the following situations:*

allergy to rauwolfia derivatives
depression, history of
electroshock therapy
peptic ulcer, active
ulcerative colitis

*Use with caution in the following situations:*

anesthetics, surgical
gallstones
kidney disease
peptic ulcer, history
ulcerative colitis, history

*Depression:* Reserpine may cause mental depression. Contact your doctor at the first sign of extreme sadness, early morning sleeplessness, loss of appetite, impotence, or low self-esteem.

*Pregnancy:* Adequate studies have not been done in pregnant women, or animal studies may have shown a potential hazard to the fetus. Use only if clearly needed and potential benefits outweigh the possible hazards to the fetus.

*Breastfeeding:* Reserpine appears in breast milk. Consult your doctor before you begin breastfeeding.

*Children:* Safety and effectiveness have not been established.

*Lab tests* may be required to monitor therapy. Be sure to keep appointments.

## Drug Interactions:

Tell your doctor or pharmacist if you are taking or planning to take any over-the-counter or prescription medications or dietary supplements while taking this medicine. Drug doses may need to be modified or a different drug prescribed. The following drugs and drug classes interact with this medicine:

amphetamines
anesthesia, general
digoxin (eg, *Lanoxin*)
isoproterenol (eg, *Isuprel*)
MAO inhibitor antidepressant
  use (eg, phenelzine)

quinidine (eg, *Quinidex*)
sympathomimetics (eg, ephedrine)
tricyclic antidepressants
  (eg, amitriptyline)

## Side Effects:

Every drug is capable of producing side effects. Many patients experience no, or minor, side effects. The frequency and severity of side effects depend on many factors including dose, duration of therapy, and individual susceptibility. Possible side effects include:

*Digestive Tract:* Nausea; vomiting; diarrhea; appetite loss; increased stomach acid; dry mouth; black or bloody stools.

*Nervous System:* Depression; dizziness; headache; nervousness; anxiety; nightmares; drowsiness; tremors; involuntary movements.

*Circulatory System:* Irregular pulse; chest pain; slow pulse; swelling of the lower legs.

*Respiratory System:* Shortness of breath; difficult or painful breathing; congestion.

*Skin:* Rash; itching.

*Other:* Dulling of the senses; deafness; breast secretions; breast swelling in men; changes in sex drive; muscle aches; weight gain; glaucoma, inflammation and redness of eyes, blurred vision, or other eye problems; difficulty urinating; fainting; nosebleeds.

## Guidelines for Use:

- Dosage is individualized. Take exactly as prescribed.
- Do not stop taking or change the dose, unless instructed by your doctor.
- May cause stomach upset. Take with food or milk.
- Do not take this medication for any disorder other than for which it was prescribed.
- If a dose is missed, take it as soon as possible. If several hours have passed or it is nearing time for the next dose, do not double the dose to catch up, unless instructed by your doctor. If more than one dose is missed or it is necessary to establish a new dosage schedule, contact your doctor or pharmacist.
- Patients being treated for high blood pressure often feel tired and run down for a few weeks after beginning therapy. It takes time for the body to adjust to lowered blood pressure. Continue taking your medication even though you may not feel quite "normal." Check with your doctor or pharmacist during this time regarding any new symptoms that occur to assure that these new feelings are a normal consequence of changes in blood pressure.
- This medicine may cause drowsiness, dizziness, or blurred vision. Use caution when driving or performing other tasks requiring alertness, coordination, or physical dexterity.
- Notify your doctor of continued or severe stomach pain, mental depression, early-morning sleeplessness, appetite loss, impotence, nausea, vomiting, chest pain, nervousness, dizziness, breast enlargement, or changes in mood or sleep habits.
- Avoid tyramine-containing foods (eg, yogurt, cheddar cheese, raisins). See the Antidepressants-Monoamine Oxidase Inhibitors monograph in the CNS Drugs chapter for a more complete list of foods.
- Check with your doctor before using a nonprescription cold, flu, or weight loss medication.
- Store at room temperature (59° to 86°F). Protect from heat and light.

*If you have any questions, consult your doctor, pharmacist, or health care provider.*

| Generic Name<br>*Brand Name Examples* | Diuretic | Other |
|---|---|---|
| *Rx* **Thiazide Diuretics and Hydralazine** | | |
| *Hydra-Zide Capsules* | 25 mg hydrochlorothiazide | 25 mg hydralazine |
| *Hydra-Zide Capsules* | 50 mg hydrochlorothiazide | 50 mg hydralazine |
| *Hydra-Zide Capsules* | 50 mg hydrochlorothiazide | 100 mg hydralazine |
| *Rx* **Thiazide Diuretics and Beta-Blockers** | | |
| *Tenoretic 50 Tablets* | 25 mg chlorthalidone | 50 mg atenolol |
| *Tenoretic 100 Tablets* | 25 mg chlorthalidone | 100 mg atenolol |
| *Corzide 40/5 Tablets* | 5 mg bendroflumethiazide | 40 mg nadolol |
| *Corzide 80/5 Tablets* | 5 mg bendroflumethiazide | 80 mg nadolol |
| *Timolide Tablets* | 25 mg hydrochlorothiazide | 10 mg timolol maleate |
| *Inderide LA Capsules* | 50 mg hydrochlorothiazide | 80 mg propranolol HCl |
| *Inderide LA Capsules* | 50 mg hydrochlorothiazide | 120 mg propranolol HCl |
| *Inderide LA Capsules* | 50 mg hydrochlorothiazide | 160 mg propranolol HCl |
| *Inderide Tablets* | 25 mg hydrochlorothiazide | 40 mg propranolol HCl |
| *Inderide Tablets* | 25 mg hydrochlorothiazide | 80 mg propranolol HCl |
| *Lopressor HCT 50/25 Tablets* | 25 mg hydrochlorothiazide | 50 mg metoprolol tartrate |
| *Lopressor HCT 100/25 Tablets* | 25 mg hydrochlorothiazide | 100 mg metoprolol tartrate |
| *Lopressor HCT 100/50 Tablets* | 50 mg hydrochlorothiazide | 100 mg metoprolol tartrate |
| *Ziac Tablets* | 6.25 mg hydrochlorothiazide | 2.5 mg bisoprolol fumarate |
| *Ziac Tablets* | 6.25 mg hydrochlorothiazide | 5 mg bisoprolol fumarate |
| *Ziac Tablets* | 6.25 mg hydrochlorothiazide | 10 mg bisoprolol fumarate |

| Generic Name<br>*Brand Name Examples* | Diuretic | Other |
|---|---|---|
| *Rx* **Thiazide Diuretics and Methyldopa** | | |
| *Aldoril 15 Tablets* | 15 mg hydrochlorothiazide | 250 mg methyldopa |
| *Aldoril 25 Tablets* | 25 mg hydrochlorothiazide | 250 mg methyldopa |
| *Aldoril D30 Tablets* | 30 mg hydrochlorothiazide | 500 mg methyldopa |
| *Aldoril D50 Tablets* | 50 mg hydrochlorothiazide | 500 mg methyldopa |
| *Rx* **Thiazide Diuretics and Angiotensin Converting Enzyme Inhibitors (ACEIs)** | | |
| *Lotensin HCT Tablets* | 6.25 mg hydrochlorothiazide | 5 mg benazepril |
| *Lotensin HCT Tablets* | 12.5 mg hydrochlorothiazide | 10 mg benazepril |
| *Lotensin HCT Tablets* | 12.5 mg hydrochlorothiazide | 20 mg benazepril |
| *Lotensin HCT Tablets* | 25 mg hydrochlorothiazide | 20 mg benazepril |
| *Capozide 25/15 Tablets* | 15 mg hydrochlorothiazide | 25 mg captopril |
| *Capozide 25/25 Tablets* | 25 mg hydrochlorothiazide | 25 mg captopril |
| *Capozide 50/15 Tablets* | 15 mg hydrochlorothiazide | 50 mg captopril |
| *Capozide 50/25 Tablets* | 25 mg hydrochlorothiazide | 50 mg captopril |
| *Vaseretic Tablets* | 12.5 mg hydrochlorothiazide | 5 mg enalapril maleate |
| *Vaseretic Tablets* | 25 mg hydrochlorothiazide | 10 mg enalapril maleate |
| *Monopril-HCT 10/12.5 Tablets* | 12.5 mg hydrochlorothiazide | 10 mg fosinopril sodium |
| *Monopril-HCT 20/12.5 Tablets* | 12.5 mg hydrochlorothiazide | 20 mg fosinopril sodium |
| *Prinzide Tablets, Zestoretic Tablets* | 12.5 mg hydrochlorothiazide | 10 mg lisinopril |
| *Prinzide Tablets, Zestoretic Tablets* | 12.5 mg hydrochlorothiazide | 20 mg lisinopril |
| *Prinzide Tablets, Zestoretic Tablets* | 25 mg hydrochlorothiazide | 20 mg lisinopril |

| Generic Name<br>*Brand Name Examples* | Diuretic | Other |
| --- | --- | --- |
| **Thiazide Diuretics and Angiotensin Converting Enzyme Inhibitors (ACEIs) (cont.)** | | |
| *Uniretic Tablets* | 12.5 mg hydrochlorothiazide | 7.5 mg moexipril HCl |
| *Uniretic Tablets* | 12.5 mg hydrochlorothiazide | 15 mg moexipril HCl |
| *Uniretic Tablets* | 25 mg hydrochlorothiazide | 15 mg moexipril HCl |
| *Accuretic Tablets* | 12.5 mg hydrochlorothiazide | 10 mg quinapril |
| *Accuretic Tablets* | 12.5 mg hydrochlorothiazide | 20 mg quinapril |
| *Accuretic Tablets* | 25 mg hydrochlorothiazide | 20 mg quinapril |
| *Rx* **Thiazide Diuretics and Clonidine** | | |
| *Clorpres 0.1 Tablets* | 15 mg chlorthalidone | 0.1 mg clonidine HCl |
| *Clorpres 0.2 Tablets* | 15 mg chlorthalidone | 0.2 mg clonidine HCl |
| *Clorpres 0.3 Tablets* | 15 mg chlorthalidone | 0.3 mg clonidine HCl |
| *Rx* **Thiazide Diuretics and Angiotensin II Receptor Antagonists** | | |
| *Atacand HCT 16/12.5 Tablets* | 12.5 mg hydrochlorothiazide | 16 mg candesartan cilexetil |
| *Atacand HCT 32/12.5 Tablets* | 12.5 mg hydrochlorothiazide | 32 mg candesartan cilexetil |
| *Avalide Tablets* | 12.5 mg hydrochlorothiazide | 150 mg irbesartan |
| *Avalide Tablets* | 12.5 mg hydrochlorothiazide | 300 mg irbesartan |
| *Hyzaar Tablets* | 12.5 mg hydrochlorothiazide | 50 mg losartan potassium |
| *Hyzaar Tablets* | 25 mg hydrochlorothiazide | 100 mg losartan potassium |
| *Micardis HCT Tablets* | 12.5 mg hydrochlorothiazide | 40 mg telmisartan |
| *Micardis HCT Tablets* | 12.5 mg hydrochlorothiazide | 80 mg telmisartan |
| *Diovan HCT Tablets* | 12.5 mg hydrochlorothiazide | 80 mg valsartan |

| **Generic Name** *Brand Name Examples* | **Diuretic** | **Other** |
|---|---|---|
| *Rx* **Thiazide Diuretics and Angiotensin II Receptor Antagonists (cont.)** | | |
| *Diovan HCT Tablets* | 12.5 mg hydrochlorothiazide | 160 mg valsartan |
| *Diovan HCT Tablets* | 25 mg hydrochlorothiazide | 160 mg valsartan |
| *Rx* **Miscellaneous Antihypertensives†** | | |
| *Lotrel Capsules* | — | 2.5 mg amlodipine, 10 mg benazepril |
| *Lotrel Capsules* | — | 5 mg amlodipine, 10 mg benazepril |
| *Lotrel Capsules* | — | 5 mg amlodipine, 20 mg benazepril |
| *Lotrel Capsules* | — | 10 mg amlodipine, 20 mg benazepril |
| *Lexxel Extended-Release Tablets* | — | 5 mg enalapril maleate, 2.5 mg felodipine |
| *Lexxel Extended-Release Tablets* | — | 5 mg enalapril maleate, 5 mg felodipine |
| *Tarka Extended-Release Tablets* | — | 2 mg trandolapril, 180 mg verapamil |
| *Tarka Extended-Release Tablets* | — | 1 mg trandolapril, 240 mg verapamil |
| *Tarka Extended-Release Tablets* | — | 2 mg trandolapril, 240 mg verapamil |
| *Tarka Extended-Release Tablets* | — | 4 mg trandolapril, 240 mg verapamil |

† Products do not contain a diuretic.

For more information on the ingredients in these combinations, see the individual drug monographs in this chapter.

## Type of Drug:

Antihypertensives; drugs used to lower high blood pressure.

## Uses:

To treat high blood pressure. Used with other drugs when adequate control is not achieved by a single drug.

## Guidelines for Use:

- Dosage is individualized. Take exactly as prescribed.
- Do not stop taking or change the dose, unless instructed by your doctor.
- May cause stomach upset. Check with your doctor or pharmacist to see if your medicine can be taken with food or milk.
- Diuretics may increase urination. Take combinations containing diuretics early in the day.
- If a dose is missed, take it as soon as possible. If several hours have passed or it is nearing time for the next dose, do not double the dose to catch up, unless instructed by your doctor. If more than one dose is missed or it is necessary to establish a new dosage schedule, contact your doctor or pharmacist.
- ACEIs may cause a persistent dry cough. Recovery is rapid when the medicine is stopped.
- Dizziness, fainting, or light-headedness is most likely to occur after the first dose or in the first days of therapy. Avoid sudden changes in posture. If dizziness persists, contact your doctor.
- Do not take other prescription or OTC medications, dietary supplements, or salt substitutes unless instructed by your doctor or pharmacist.
- May cause sensitivity to sunlight. Avoid prolonged exposure to the sun and ultraviolet (UV) light (eg, tanning beds). Use sunscreens and wear protective clothing until tolerance is determined.
- Diuretics may increase blood sugar levels in diabetics.
- Many of these medications cause drowsiness or dizziness. Use caution while driving or performing other tasks requiring alertness, coordination, or physical dexterity until tolerance is determined.
- Contact your doctor if significant, sudden joint pain occurs while taking combinations containing hydralazine
- Inform your doctor if you are pregnant, become pregnant, are planning to become pregnant or if you are breastfeeding.
- Lab tests may be required to monitor therapy. Be sure to keep appointments.
- Store at room temperature in a tightly sealed container away from light.

*If you have any questions, consult your doctor, pharmacist, or health care provider.*

| Generic Name Brand Name Examples | Supplied As | Generic Available |
|---|---|---|
| Rx **Eplerenone** | | |
| *Inspra* | **Tablets**: 25 mg, 50 mg, 100 mg | No |

## Type of Drug:

Antihypertensive; renin angiotensin system antagonist.

## How the Drug Works:

Eplerenone lowers blood pressure by blocking aldosterone from binding to mineralocorticoid receptors.

## Uses:

For the treatment of high blood pressure alone or in combination with other antihypertensive agents.

## Precautions:

*Do not use in the following situations:*

allergy to the drug or any of its ingredients
creatinine clearance less than 50 mL/min
CYP-450 3A4 inhibitor (eg, keto-conazole) therapy, current
potassium supplement or potas-sium-sparing diuretic therapy, current
serum creatinine greater than 2 mg/dL in males or greater than 1.8 mg/dL in females
serum potassium greater than 5.5 mEq/L
type 2 diabetes with microalbuminuria

*Use with caution in the following situations:* Severe liver disease.

*Pregnancy:* There are no adequate and well-controlled studies in preg-nant women. Use only if clearly needed and the potential benefits out-weigh the possible risks to the fetus.

*Breastfeeding:* It is not known if eplerenone is excreted in breast milk. Con-sult your doctor before you begin breastfeeding.

*Children:* Safety and effectiveness have not been established.

*Lab tests* may be required to monitor treatment. Tests include serum potas-sium level monitoring.

## Drug Interactions:

Tell your doctor or pharmacist if you are taking or planning to take any over-the-counter or prescription medications or dietary supplements with this drug. Drug doses may need to be modified or a different drug pre-scribed. The following drugs and drug classes interact with this drug:

ACE inhibitors (eg, lisinopril)
angiotensin II receptor antago-nists (eg, losartan)
CYP-450 3A4 inhibitors (eg, erythromycin, ketoconazole, saquinavir, verapamil)
lithium (eg, *Eskalith*)
NSAIDs (eg, ibuprofen)
potassium supplements or potassium-sparing diuretics (eg, amiloride, triamterene)
St. John's wort

## Side Effects:

Every drug is capable of producing side effects. Many patients experience no, or minor, side effects. The frequency and severity of side effects depend on many factors including dose, duration of therapy, and individual susceptibility. Possible side effects include:

*Urinary and Reproductive Tract:* Albumin in the urine; abnormal vaginal bleeding; breast enlargement or pain.

*Other:* Diarrhea; stomach pain; abnormal blood tests; dizziness; coughing; fatigue; flu-like symptoms; headache.

---

### Guidelines for Use:

- Dosage is individualized. Take exactly as prescribed.
- Do not stop taking or change the dose, unless instructed by your doctor.
- Do not take potassium supplements or salt substitutes containing potassium while taking this drug.
- Lab tests may be required to monitor therapy. Be sure to keep appointments.
- Store at room temperature (59° to 86°F).

---

*If you have any questions, consult your doctor, pharmacist, or health care provider.*

| Generic Name<br>*Brand Name Examples* | Supplied As | Generic Available |
|---|---|---|
| *Rx* **Cholestyramine** | | |
| *LoCHOLEST* | **Powder:** 4 g cholestyramine resin/9 g powder | No |
| *Questran* | **Powder:** 4 g cholestyramine resin/9 g powder | Yes |
| *Questran Light* | **Powder:** 4 g cholestyramine resin/6.4 g powder | Yes |
| *LoCHOLEST Light[1]* | **Powder:** 4 g cholestyramine resin/5.7 g powder | No |
| *Prevalite* | **Powder:** 4 g cholestyramine resin/5.5 g powder | No |
| *Rx* **Colesevelam HCl** | | |
| *Welchol* | **Tablets:** 625 mg | No |
| *Rx* **Colestipol HCl** | | |
| *Colestid* | **Tablets:** 1 g colestipol HCl | No |
| *Colestid* | **Granules:** 5 g packets, 300 g bottle, 500 g bottle | No |
| *Flavored Colestid[1]* | **Granules:** 7.5 g packets, 450 g bottle | No |

[1] Contains phenylalanine.

## Type of Drug:

Drugs used as adjunctive therapy to diet and exercise to lower the level of LDL cholesterol and total cholesterol in the blood.

## How the Drug Works:

Bile acid sequestrants increase the removal of bile acids from the body. As the body loses bile acids, it replaces them by converting cholesterol from the blood to bile acids. This causes the blood level of cholesterol to decrease.

High blood levels of cholesterol may increase the risk of developing heart, coronary artery, or other vascular disease.

## Uses:

To lower high levels of cholesterol in the blood alone or in conjunction with proper diet, exercise, and possibly other lipid-lowering drugs.

*Cholestyramine:* To relieve itching associated with partial biliary obstruction.

*Unlabeled Use(s):* Occasionally doctors may prescribe cholestyramine to bind the toxins produced by *Clostridium difficile,* the organism which causes antibiotic-induced pseudomembranous colitis. Cholestyramine has also been used for treatment of chlordecone *(Kepone)* pesticide poisoning, bile salt-mediated and postvagotomy diarrhea, and thyroid hormone overdose. Cholestyramine and colestipol have both been used to treat digitalis toxicity.

## Precautions:

*Do not use in the following situations:*

allergy to a bile acid sequestrant or any of its ingredients
bowel obstruction
complete biliary obstruction

gallstones or other obstructive
gallbladder diseases
phenylketonuria (*Questran Light*
only)

*Use with caution in the following situations:*

constipation
dysphagia
gastrointestinal motility disorder
(*Questran Light* only)

gastrointestinal surgery, recent
swallowing disorder

*Before treatment:* Before treatment with a bile acid sequestrant, a vigorous attempt should be made to control cholesterol with appropriate diet, exercise, and weight reduction (in obese people).

Diseases that may increase cholesterol and must be treated before beginning treatment with bile acid sequestrants include:

diabetes mellitus
hypothyroidism
nephrotic syndrome (kidney)

obstructive liver disease
protein in the blood

*Phenylketonuria:* Some of these products contain phenylalanine. Consult your doctor or pharmacist.

*Supplementation:* Treatment with bile acid sequestrants may require supplementation with vitamins A , E, and D, oral vitamin K, or folic acid.

*Pregnancy:* Safety for use during pregnancy has not been established. These agents are not absorbed systemically, and are not expected to cause fetal harm when administered during pregnancy in recommended doses. Use only when clearly needed the potential benefits to the mother outweigh the possible hazards to the fetus.

*Breastfeeding:* Use caution when breastfeeding. The possible lack of proper vitamin absorption may have an effect on nursing infants. Consult your doctor.

*Children:* Dosage schedules have not been established. The effects of long-term use and effectiveness in maintaining lowered cholesterol levels are unknown.

*Lab tests* will be required periodically during treatment with bile acid sequestrants. Tests may include blood counts, triglycerides, and cholesterol levels.

## Drug Interactions:

Tell your doctor or pharmacist if you are taking or planning to take any over-the-counter or prescription medications or dietary supplements while taking bile acid sequestrants. Doses of one or both drugs may need to be modified or a different drug may need to be prescribed. The following drugs and drug classes interact with bile acid sequestrants:

diclofenac (eg, *Cataflam*)
dicumarol
digoxin (eg, *Lanoxin*)
divalproex sodium (eg, *Depakote*)
furosemide (eg, *Lasix*)
hydrocortisone (eg, *Cortef*)
piroxicam (eg, *Feldene*)

sulindac (eg, *Clinoril*)
thiazide diuretics (eg, hydrochlorothiazide)
thyroid hormones (eg, levothyroxine sodium)
valproic acid (eg, *Depakene*)
warfarin (eg, *Coumadin*)

## Side Effects:

Every drug is capable of producing side effects. Many patients experience no, or minor, side effects. The frequency and severity of side effects depend on many factors including dose, duration of therapy, and individual susceptibility. Possible side effects include:

*Digestive Tract:* Severe constipation or other persistent stomach problems; gastrointestinal bleeding or irritation; fatty or black stools; loose stools; occasional stomach pain; gas; indigestion; ulcer attack; bloating; belching; nausea; vomiting; heartburn; aggravated hemorrhoids; appetite loss; difficulty swallowing; diarrhea.

*Nervous System:* Headache; leg pain; anxiety; feeling of whirling motion; dizziness; fatigue; insomnia; drowsiness; fainting.

*Respiratory System:* Asthma; wheezing; shortness of breath.

*Skin:* Rash; itching; hives; abnormal skin sensations.

*Other:* Unusual bruising or bleeding (eg, gums, rectum); hiccups; sour taste; weight loss or gain; difficulty swallowing; muscle pain; anemia, backache; chest pain; arthritis; ringing in the ears; blood in urine; painful urination; increased urination; burnt urine odor; fluid retention; tingling or numbness in legs and arms; swelling of hands or feet; inflammation of the uveal tract; inflammation of the pancreas or gall bladder; gallstones; increased libido; deficiencies of fat-soluble vitamins (eg, A and D).

## Guidelines for Use:

- Dosage is individualized. Take exactly as prescribed.
- Do not stop taking or change the dose, unless instructed by your doctor.
- *Granules, powder* — Mix with liquid (water or noncarbonated drinks), very liquid soups or cereals, or pulpy fruits (applesauce or crushed pineapple). Do not take the dry powder or granules alone.
- *Tablets* — Take with food and liquids.
- *Cholestyramine tablets* — May be taken with meals. Swallowing tablets is easier if you drink plenty of fluid as you swallow each tablet.
- *Cholestyramine powder* — Mix the contents of 1 powder packet or 1 level scoopful with 2 to 6 fl oz water or noncarbonated beverage. Avoid accidental inhalation. Do not take dry.
- *Colestipol granules* — Add the prescribed amount to a glass (3 oz or more) of liquid. Stir until completely mixed. Colestipol will not dissolve. May also mix with carbonated beverages, slowly stirred in a large glass. After taking, rinse glass with a small amount of additional beverage and swallow to ensure that all the medication is taken.
- If a dose is missed, take it as soon as possible. If several hours have passed or it is nearing time for the next dose, do not double the dose to catch up, unless instructed by your doctor. If more than one dose is missed or it is necessary to establish a new dosage schedule, contact your doctor or pharmacist.
- May interfere with the effects of other drugs taken at the same time. Take other drugs 1 hour before or 4 to 6 hours after bile acid sequestrants.
- Contact your doctor if you experience unusual bleeding (eg, gums, rectum).
- May cause constipation, gas, nausea, or heartburn. These effects usually disappear with continued use, but contact your doctor if these effects continue and are bothersome.
- Most effective when used with a diet that decreases the intake of cholesterol and saturated fats.
- Lab tests may be required to monitor therapy. Be sure to keep appointments.
- Store at room temperature (59° to 86°F) in a dry place.

*If you have any questions, consult your doctor, pharmacist, or health care provider.*

| Generic Name<br>*Brand Name Example* | Supplied As | Generic<br>Available |
|---|---|---|
| *Rx* **Ezetimibe** | | |
| *Zetia* | **Tablets**: 10 mg | No |

## Type of Drug:

Antihyperlipidemic; cholesterol-lowering drug.

## How the Drug Works:

Ezetimibe lowers blood cholesterol levels by blocking the absorption of cholesterol from the small intestine.

## Uses:

As adjunctive therapy to lifestyle changes for the reduction of elevated total cholesterol, LDL ("bad") cholesterol, and apolipoprotein B in patients with high cholesterol. May be used in combination with other cholesterol-lowering drugs.

## Precautions:

*Do not use in the following situations:*
allergy to the drug or any of its ingredients
liver disease, active (when used in combination with HMG-CoA reductase inhibitors)
liver disease, moderate to severe
pregnant and nursing women (when used in combination with HMG-CoA reductase inhibitors)

*Use with caution in the following situations:* Current HMG-CoA reductase inhibitor (eg, lovastatin) use.

*Pregnancy:* There are no adequate and well-controlled studies in pregnant women. Use only if clearly needed and potential benefits outweigh the possible risks to the fetus.

*Breastfeeding:* It is not known if ezetimibe appears in breast milk. Consult your doctor before you begin breastfeeding.

*Children:* Safety and effectiveness in children younger than 10 years of age have not been established.

*Lab tests* will be required during treatment. Tests include cholesterol levels and liver function tests.

## Drug Interactions:

Tell your doctor or pharmacist if you are taking or planning to take any over-the-counter or prescription medications or dietary supplements with this drug. Drug doses may need to be modified or a different drug prescribed. The following drugs and drug classes interact with this drug:

bile acid sequestrants (eg, cholestyramine)
cyclosporine (eg, *Neoral*)
fenofibrate (eg, *Tricor*)
gemfibrozil (eg, *Lopid*)
HMG-CoA reductase inhibitors (eg, lovastatin)

## Side Effects:

Every drug is capable of producing side effects. Many patients experience no, or minor, side effects. The frequency and severity of side effects depend on many factors, including dose, duration of therapy, and individual susceptibility. Possible side effects include:

*Digestive Tract:* Stomach pain; diarrhea.

*Respiratory System:* Sore throat; sinus infection; cough; upper respiratory tract infection.

*Other:* Fatigue; chest, back, muscle, and joint pain; dizziness; headache.

## Guidelines for Use:

- Dosage is individualized. Use exactly as prescribed.
- Do not stop taking or change the dose, unless instructed by your doctor.
- May be taken without regard to food.
- Take 2 or more hours before or 4 or more hours after a bile acid sequestrant (eg, cholestyramine).
- Continue to follow a cholesterol-lowering diet while taking ezetimibe. Ask your doctor if you need diet information.
- If a dose is missed, take it as soon as possible. If several hours have passed or it is nearing time for the next dose, do not double the dose to catch up, unless instructed by your doctor. If more than one dose is missed, or it is necessary to establish a new dosage schedule, contact your doctor or pharmacist.
- Inform your doctor if you are pregnant, become pregnant, are planning to become pregnant, or are breastfeeding.
- Notify your doctor if you experience persistent stomach pain or tiredness or unexplained muscle pain, tenderness, or weakness.
- Lab tests will be required to monitor therapy. Be sure to keep appointments.
- Store at 59° to 86°F. Protect from moisture.

*If you have any questions, consult your doctor, pharmacist, or health care provider.*

| Generic Name<br>*Brand Name Example* | Supplied As | Generic<br>Available |
|---|---|---|
| Rx **Fenofibrate** | | |
| *Tricor* | **Tablets:** 54 mg, 160 mg | No |

## Type of Drug:
Triglyceride- and cholesterol-lowering agent.

## How the Drug Works:
Fenofibrate decreases triglyceride and cholesterol blood levels by increasing the elimination of these fat-like substances from the body.

## Uses:
Used in addition to diet to treat hypercholesterolemia (increased blood cholesterol) and mixed dyslipidemia (Fredrickson types IIa and IIb) (increased blood triglycerides).

## Precautions:
*Do not use in the following situations:*

allergy to the drug or any of its ingredients
biliary cirrhosis, primary
breastfeeding
gallbladder disease, preexisting
kidney disease, severe
liver disease
liver function abnormalities, persistent

*Use with caution in the following situations:*

anticoagulant (eg, warfarin) use, current
HMG-CoA reductase inhibitor (eg, atorvastatin) use, current

*Pregnancy:* There are no adequate and well-controlled studies in pregnant women. Use only if clearly needed and the potential benefits outweigh the possible risks to the fetus.

*Breastfeeding:* Breastfeeding mothers should not use fenofibrate. A decision should be made whether to discontinue breastfeeding or discontinue the drug, taking into account the importance of the drug to the mother. Consult your doctor before you begin breastfeeding.

*Children:* Safety and effectiveness have not been established.

*Elderly:* Dosage may need to be lowered, depending on kidney function.

*Lab tests* will be required to monitor therapy. Tests may include kidney and liver function tests, blood counts, and triglyceride and cholesterol levels.

## Drug Interactions:

Tell your doctor or pharmacist if you are taking or planning to take any over-the-counter or prescription medications or dietary supplements while taking this drug. Drug doses may need to be modified or a different drug prescribed. The following drugs and drug classes may interact with this drug:

anticoagulants (eg, warfarin)
bile acid sequestrants
(eg, cholestyramine)

cyclosporine (eg, *Sandimmune*)
HMG-CoA reductase inhibitors
(eg, atorvastatin)

## Side Effects:

Every drug is capable of producing side effects. Many patients experience no, or minor, side effects. The frequency and severity of side effects depend on many factors including dose, duration of therapy, and individual susceptibility. Possible side effects include:

*Digestive Tract:* Belching; gas; nausea; vomiting; constipation; appetite loss; heartburn; stomach pain; diarrhea; indigestion; dry mouth.

*Nervous System:* Dizziness; fatigue; headache; sleeplessness; anxiety.

*Skin:* Itching; rash.

*Other:* Muscle aches, tenderness, or weakness with or without fever or malaise (general feeling of discomfort); infections; flu-like symptoms; pain; eye floaters; eye irritation; decreased sex drive; runny nose; back, joint, or chest pain; abnormal liver function; abnormal blood tests; decreased blood pressure; increased blood sugar; weight changes; swelling of legs; eye disorder.

## Guidelines for Use:

- Dosage is individualized. Take exactly as prescribed.
- Do not stop taking or change dose, unless instructed by your doctor.
- Take with meals to increase effectiveness.
- Continue the diet regimen prescribed by your doctor while taking fenofibrate.
- If a dose is missed, take it as soon as possible. If several hours have passed or it is nearing time for the next dose, do not double the dose to catch up, unless instructed by your doctor. If more than one dose is missed, contact your doctor or pharmacist.
- Fenofibrate is not a replacement for diet and exercise. Every effort should be made to control triglyceride and cholesterol levels with diet, exercise, weight loss (if appropriate), and control of any medical problems such as diabetes mellitus or hypothyroidism.
- Notify your doctor immediately if you experience muscle pain, tenderness, or weakness, especially if accompanied by fever or general body discomfort. This could be a sign of a serious medical complication.
- Notify your doctor if you develop abdominal pain, which may vary from mild to severe and may be felt in the back, chest, or sides. This could be a sign of pancreatis, a serious medical complication.
- Discontinue use at first appearance of rash or other signs of allergic reaction (eg, difficulty breathing).
- Take fenofibrate at least 1 hour before or 4 to 6 hours after taking a bile acid sequestrant (eg, cholestyramine).
- If not effective after 2 months of treatment, your doctor may discontinue therapy with fenofibrate.
- Do not take fenofibrate while breastfeeding.
- Lab tests will be required. Be sure to keep appointments.
- Store at room temperature (59° to 86°F). Protect from moisture.

*If you have any questions, consult your doctor, pharmacist, or health care provider.*

| Generic Name<br>*Brand Name Example* | Supplied As | Generic<br>Available |
|---|---|---|
| *Rx* **Gemfibrozil** | | |
| *Lopid* | **Tablets:** 600 mg | Yes |

## Type of Drug:
Antihyperlipidemic; fibric acid derivative.

## How the Drug Works:
Gemfibrozil decreases the blood level of triglycerides and some types of cholesterol (LDL) by reducing the production of these items by the liver. It also increases blood levels of HDL cholesterol. High levels of LDL cholesterol and triglycerides may block blood vessels, increasing the risk of heart or blood vessel disease (arteriosclerosis).

## Uses:
As an adjunct to diet to lower elevated triglyceride levels (Types IV and V hyperlipidemia) in adult patients at risk for pancreatitis and who are unable to control triglyceride levels by diet and exercise alone.

As an adjunct to diet to reduce risk of developing coronary artery disease in adult patients with low HDL cholesterol levels and elevated LDL cholesterol and triglycerides (Type IIb hyperlipidemia) and who have not responded to weight loss, diet, exercise, and other lipid-lowering drugs.

## Precautions:
*Do not use in the following situations:*

allergy to the drug or any of its ingredients
cirrhosis
gallbladder disease, preexisting kidney disease
liver disease

*Use with caution in the following situations:*

alcohol use, chronic or excessive
anticoagulant (eg, warfarin) use, current
diabetes
estrogen therapy
HMG-CoA reductase inhibitor (eg, atorvastatin) use, current
underactive thyroid (hypothyroidism)

*Before treatment:* Before starting treatment with gemfibrozil, an attempt should be made to control high LDL cholesterol and triglycerides with appropriate diet, exercise, and weight reduction (in obese people), and to control any medical problems such as diabetes mellitus or hypothyroidism that are contributing to the lipid abnormalities.

*Pregnancy:* There are no adequate and well-controlled studies in pregnant women. Use only if clearly needed and the potential benefits outweigh the possible hazards to the fetus.

*Breastfeeding:* It is not known if gemfibrozil appears in breast milk. Consult your doctor before you begin breastfeeding.

*Children:* Safety and effectiveness have not been established.

*Lab tests* may be required during treatment. Tests may include blood counts, cholesterol and triglycerides, liver and kidney function tests.

## Drug Interactions:

Tell your doctor or pharmacist if you are taking or planning to take any over-the-counter or prescription medications or dietary supplements with gemfibrozil. Doses of one or both drugs may need to be modified or a different drug may need to be prescribed. The following drugs and drug classes interact with gemfibrozil:

> anticoagulants (eg, warfarin)
> HMG-CoA reductase inhibitors (eg, lovastatin)

## Side Effects:

Every drug is capable of producing side effects. Many gemfibrozil users experience no, or minor, side effects. The frequency and severity of side effects depend on many factors including dose, duration of therapy, and individual susceptibility. Possible side effects include:

*Digestive Tract:* Indigestion; stomach pain; vomiting; nausea; diarrhea; constipation; acute appendicitis.

*Nervous System:* Headache; dizziness; vertigo (feeling of whirling motion); fatigue.

*Skin:* Rash; itching; hives; inflamed or irritated skin; abnormal skin sensations (eg, burning, prickling, tingling); abnormal sensitivity to touch, pain, or other stimuli.

*Other:* Muscle pain or weakness; changes in taste perception; blurred vision.

## Guidelines for Use:

- Dosage is individualized. Take exactly as prescribed.
- Do not change the dose or stop taking this medicine unless advised to do so by your doctor.
- Take this drug 30 minutes before the morning and evening meal.
- Most effective when used with a diet that reduces the intake of cholesterol and saturated fats, and an exercise program.
- If a dose is missed, take it as soon as possible. If several hours have passed or it nearing time for the next dose, do not double the dose to catch up, unless advised to do so by your doctor. If more than one dose is missed or it is necessary to establish a new dosage schedule contact your doctor or pharmacist.
- Avoid alcohol while taking this medicine.
- Inform your doctor if you are pregnant, become pregnant, plan on becoming pregnant, or are breastfeeding.
- May cause dizziness or blurred vision. Use caution when driving or performing other tasks requiring alertness, coordination, or physical dexterity.
- Notify your doctor immediately if you experience muscle pain, tenderness, or weakness.
- May cause stomach pain, diarrhea, nausea, or vomiting. Contact your doctor if these effects become particularly bothersome or severe.
- Lab tests may be required to monitor therapy. Be sure to keep appointments.
- Store below 86°F in a tightly sealed container.

*If you have any questions, consult your doctor, pharmacist, or health care provider.*

| Generic Name<br>*Brand Name Examples* | Supplied As | Generic<br>Available |
|---|---|---|
| Rx **Atorvastatin Calcium** | | |
| *Lipitor* | **Tablets**: 10 mg, 20 mg, 40 mg, 80 mg | No |
| Rx **Fluvastatin Sodium** | | |
| *Lescol* | **Capsules**: 20 mg, 40 mg | No |
| *Lescol XL* | **Tablets, extended-release**: 80 mg | No |
| Rx **Lovastatin** | | |
| *Mevacor* | **Tablets**: 10 mg, 20 mg, 40 mg | No |
| Rx **Pravastatin Sodium** | | |
| *Pravachol* | **Tablets**: 10 mg, 20 mg, 40 mg | No |
| Rx **Simvastatin** | | |
| *Zocor* | **Tablets**: 5 mg, 10 mg, 20 mg, 40 mg, 80 mg | No |

## Type of Drug:

Drugs used to lower high blood levels of certain types of lipids or fats (eg, LDL cholesterol, triglycerides) in the blood.

## How the Drug Works:

HMG-CoA reductase inhibitors lower the blood levels of triglycerides and LDL ("bad") cholesterol by reducing their production by the liver. They also increase blood levels of HDL ("good") cholesterol.

## Uses:

As an adjunct to diet for reducing elevated total and LDL cholesterol, apo-B, and triglyceride levels; and to increase HDL cholesterol in patients with primary hypercholesterolemia and mixed dyslipidemia (Fredrickson IIa and IIb).

*Atorvastatin:* As an adjunct to other lipid-lowering treatments to reduce total and LDL cholesterol in patients with homozygous familial hypercholesterolemia; to treat primary dysbetalipoproteinemia (Fredrickson type III); and to lower elevated serum triglyceride levels (Fredrickson type IV).

*Fluvastatin:* To slow the progression of coronary atherosclerosis in patients with coronary heart disease.

*Lovastatin:* To slow the progression of coronary atherosclerosis in patients with coronary heart disease; to reduce the risk of heart attack, unstable angina, or the chance of coronary revascularization procedures (eg, angioplasty) in patients without symptomatic cardiovascular disease, average to moderately elevated total and LDL cholesterol, and below average HDL cholesterol.

*Pravastatin:* To reduce the risk of myocardial infarction, stroke and stroke/transient ischemic attack, cardiovascular mortality, or the chance of coronary revascularization procedures (eg, angioplasty) in patients with clinically evident coronary heart disease; to slow the progression of coronary atheroclerosis; to treat primary dysbetalipoproteinemia (Fredrickson type III); to lower elevated serum triglyceride levels (Fredrickson type IV).

*Simvastatin:* To reduce the risk of heart attack, stroke or transient ischemic attack, cardiovascular mortality, or the chance of coronary revascularization procedures (eg, angioplasty) in patients with clinically evident coronary heart disease; as an adjunct to other lipid-lowering treatments to reduce total and LDL cholesterol; to lower elevated serum triglyceride levels (Fredrickson type IV); to treat primary dysbetalipoproteinemia (Fredrickson type III).

*Unlabeled Use(s):* Occasionally doctors may prescribe atorvastatin or fluvastatin to lower elevated total cholesterol levels in patients with heterozygous familial hypercholesterolemia and diabetic dyslipidemia in type 2 diabetic patients.

Lovastatin may be useful to treat diabetic dyslipidemia, nephrotic hyperlipidemia, neck artery disease, familial dysbetalipoproteinemia, and familial combined hyperlipidemia.

Pravastatin and Simvastatin can lower elevated cholesterol levels in patients with heterozygous familial hypercholesterolemia, familial combined hyperlipidemia, diabetic dyslipidemia in type 2 diabetic patients, hyperlipidemia secondary to the nephrotic syndrome, and homozygous familial hypercholesterolemia in patients with reduced LDL receptors.

## Precautions:

*Do not use in the following situations:*

allergy to HMG-CoA reductase inhibitors or any of their ingredients
breastfeeding
elevated liver function tests, unexplained and persistent
liver disease, active
pregnancy

*Use with caution in the following situations:*

alcohol use, concurrent
electrolyte, hormone, or metabolic disorders
endocrine dysfunction
high creatine phosphokinase levels
immunosuppressant therapy, concurrent
infection, severe and acute
kidney disease
lipid-lowering therapy, concurrent
liver disease, history of
low blood pressure
ophthalmic disorders
seizures, uncontrolled
surgery, major
trauma

*Pregnancy:* Do not use during pregnancy. The risk to the fetus clearly outweighs any possible benefit to the mother. Women of childbearing age should use only if it is highly unlikely that they will become pregnant and they have been informed of the potential hazards. If you become pregnant while taking one of these drugs, discontinue use immediately and consult your doctor.

*Breastfeeding:* Fluvastatin and pravastatin appear in breast milk. It is not known if atorvastatin, lovastatin, or simvastatin appear in breast milk. Do not breastfeed while taking these drugs.

*Children:* Safety and effectiveness in children younger than 18 years of age have not been established. Treatment is not recommended.

*Elderly:* Lower starting doses of lovastatin and pravastatin may be considered in patients older than 70 years of age.

*Lab tests* will be required to monitor therapy. Tests may include cholesterol levels, eye exams, liver and kidney function tests, and liver (transaminase) and muscle (creatine phosphokinase) enzymes.

## Drug Interactions:

Tell your doctor or pharmacist if you are taking or planning to take any over-the-counter or prescription medications or dietary supplements with HMG-CoA reductase inhibitors. Doses of one or both drugs may need to be modified or a different drug may need to be prescribed. The following drugs and drug classes interact with HMG-CoA reductase inhibitors:

antacids (atorvastatin only)
azole antifungals (eg, ketoconazole, itraconazole)
bile acid sequestrants
  (eg, cholestyramine)
cimetidine (eg, *Tagamet*)
  (fluvastatin only)
cyclosporine (eg, *Sandimmune*)
diltiazem (eg, *Cardizem*)
gemfibrozil (eg, *Lopid*)
grapefruit juice
isradipine (*DynaCirc*)
macrolide antibiotics
  (eg, erythromycin)

nefazodone (*Serzone*)
niacin (eg, *Nicobid*)
omeprazole (*Prilosec*)
  (fluvastatin only)
protease inhibitors
  (eg, ritonavir)
ranitidine (eg, *Zantac*)
  (fluvastatin only)
rifampin (eg, *Rifadin*)
  (fluvastatin only)
verapamil (eg, *Calan*)
warfarin (eg, *Coumadin*)

## Side Effects:

Every drug is capable of producing side effects. Many HMG-CoA reductase inhibitor users experience no, or minor, side effects. The frequency and severity of side effects depend on many factors including dose, duration of therapy, and individual susceptibility. Possible side effects include:

*Digestive Tract:* Nausea; vomiting; diarrhea; stomach pain; constipation; gas; indigestion; heartburn.

*Nervous System:* Headache; dizziness; weakness; fatigue; sleeplessness.

*Respiratory System:* Cold or flu-like symptoms; cough; congestion; upper respiratory tract infection; sore throat; sinus infection; runny nose.

*Other:* Muscle pain or cramps; urinary abnormality; abnormal blood tests; blurred vision; accidental trauma; tooth disorders; localized pain; urinary tract infection; chest, leg, back, or joint pain; joint inflammation; swelling of arms and legs; infection; rash.

## Guidelines for Use:

- Exercise and a diet that reduces the intake of cholesterol and saturated fats should accompany HMG-CoA reductase inhibitor treatment.
- Dosage is individualized. Take exactly as prescribed.
- Do not change the dose or stop taking this medicine unless advised to do so by your doctor.
- *Atorvastatin, fluvastatin, simvastatin* — Take once daily in the evening with or without food.
- *Lovastatin* — Take with evening meals.
- *Pravastatin* — Take once daily with or without food.
- If a dose is missed, take it as soon as possible. If several hours have passed or it is nearing time for the next dose, do not double the dose to catch up, unless advised to do so by your doctor. If more than one dose is missed or it is necessary to establish a new dosage schedule, contact your doctor or pharmacist.
- If taken in conjunction with cholestyramine or colestipol, take HMG-CoA reductase inhibitors either 1 hour before or at least 4 hours after the cholestyramine or colestipol.
- Inform your doctor if you are pregnant, become pregnant, plan on becoming pregnant, or are breastfeeding.
- Notify your doctor immediately if you experience unexplained headache, muscle pain, tenderness or weakness, nausea, vomiting, or diarrhea, particularly if accompanied by fever or general body discomfort.
- Lab tests will be required to monitor therapy. Be sure to keep appointments.
- Store between 41° and 86°F. Protect from light and moisture.

*If you have any questions, consult your doctor, pharmacist, or health care provider.*

| Generic Name<br>Brand Name Example | Supplied As | Generic Available |
|---|---|---|
| Rx **Niacin (extended-release) and lovastatin**<br>*Advicor* | **Tablets**: 500 mg/20 mg,<br>750 mg/20 mg, 1000 mg/20 mg | No |

## Type of Drug:

Antihyperlipidemic; lipid-lowering combination drug.

## How the Drug Works:

The exact mechanism of action of niacin is not known, but may involve partial inhibition of the release of free fatty acids from adipose tissue and increased removal of triglycerides from plasma. Lovastatin inhibits an enzyme in the biosynthetic pathway for cholesterol.

## Uses:

To treat high cholesterol and other lipid disorders in patients who require further lipid-lowering than can be achieved with either drug alone.

## Precautions:

*Do not use in the following situations:*

allergy to niacin, lovastatin, or any component of this medication

arterial bleeding
liver disease, active
peptic ulcer disease, active

*Use with caution in the following situations:*

angina, unstable
diabetes
gout
jaundice, history of

kidney disease
liver disease
peptic ulcer disease, history of

*Pregnancy:* Do not use during pregnancy. The risk of use in a pregnant woman clearly outweighs any possible benefit.

*Breastfeeding:* It is not known if niacin/lovastatin appears in breast milk. Consult your doctor before you begin breastfeeding.

*Children:* Safety and effectiveness in children younger than 18 years of age have not been established.

## Drug Interactions:

Tell your doctor or pharmacist if you are taking or planning to take any over-the-counter or prescription medications or dietary supplements with this drug. Drug doses may need to be modified or a different drug prescribed. The following drugs and drug classes interact with this drug:

anticoagulants (eg, warfarin)
azole antifungals (eg, ketoconazole)
bile acid sequestrants (eg, cholestyramine)
cyclosporine (eg, *Neoral*)
diltiazem (eg, *Cardizem*)

gemfibrozil (eg, *Lopid*)
grapefruit juice
isradipine (*DynaCirc*)
macrolide antibiotics (eg, erythromycin)
verapamil (eg, *Calan*)

## Side Effects:

Every drug is capable of producing side effects. Many patients experience no, or minor, side effects. The frequency and severity of side effects depend on many factors including dose, duration of therapy, and individual susceptibility. Possible side effects include:

*Digestive Tract:* Diarrhea; upset stomach; nausea; vomiting; stomach pain.

*Skin:* Itching; rash.

*Other:* Headache; infection; muscle, back, or joint pain; increased blood glucose; flushing.

## Guidelines for Use:

- Dosage is individualized. Take exactly as prescribed.
- Do not stop taking or change the dose, unless instructed by your doctor.
- Do not break, crush, or chew. Take tablets whole.
- If a dose is missed, take it as soon as possible. If several hours have passed or it is nearing time for the next dose, do not double the dose to catch up, unless instructed by your doctor. If more than one dose is missed or if it is necessary to establish a new dosage schedule, contact your doctor or pharmacist.
- Take this medicine at bedtime with a low-fat snack. Do not take this medicine with grapefruit juice.
- Contact your doctor immediately if you experience unexplained muscle pain, tenderness, or weakness.
- This medicine may cause dizziness. Use caution while driving or performing other tasks requiring alertness, coordination, or physical dexterity until tolerance is determined.
- Flushing is a common side effect of niacin and may last for several hours after taking a dose. Flushing usually subsides after several weeks of regular use. Aspirin or another NSAID like ibuprofen taken up to 30 minutes before taking this drug may minimize flushing.
- Avoid alcohol or hot drinks to minimize flushing.
- Inform your doctor if you are pregnant, become pregnant, plan to become pregnant, or are breastfeeding.
- Store at room temperature (68° to 77°F).

*If you have any questions, consult your doctor, pharmacist, or health care provider.*

**Bronchodilators**
Sympathomimetics, 455
Xanthine Derivatives, 461

**Leukotriene Receptor Antagonists/Formation Inhibitors,** 467

**Inhalants**
Corticosteroids, 470
Cromolyn Sodium, 474
Ipratropium Bromide, 477
Ipratropium Bromide/Albuterol
  Sulfate, 480
Mucolytics, 484
Nedocromil Sodium, 487

**Intranasal Steroids,** 489

**Antihistamines,** 493

**Nasal Decongestants,** 500

**Antitussives**
Narcotic, 506
Nonnarcotic, 509

**Expectorants,** 513

**Upper Respiratory Combinations,** 517

| Generic Name<br>*Brand Name Examples* | Supplied As | Generic<br>Available |
|---|---|---|
| *Rx* **Albuterol Sulfate** | | |
| *Proventil, Proventil HFA, Ventolin* | **Aerosol:** 90 mcg/actuation | Yes |
| *Proventil* | **Tablets:** 2 mg, 4 mg | Yes |
| *Proventil Repetabs, Volmax* | **Tablets, extended release:** 4 mg, 8 mg | No |
| *Proventil, Ventolin* | **Syrup:** 2 mg/5 mL | Yes |
| *Airet, Proventil, Ventolin Nebules* | **Solution for inhalation:** 0.083% (in unit dose containers) | Yes |
| *Proventil, Ventolin* | **Solution for inhalation:** 0.5% | Yes |
| *Ventolin Rotocaps* | **Capsules for inhalation:** 200 mcg microfine (as sulfate) | No |
| *Rx* **Bitolterol Mesylate** | | |
| *Tornalate* | **Solution for inhalation:** 0.2% | No |
| *Tornalate* | **Aerosol:** 0.8% (0.37 mg/ actuation) | No |
| **Ephedrine Sulfate** | | |
| *otc Ephedrine Sulfate* | **Capsules:** 25 mg | Yes |
| *Rx Ephedrine Sulfate* | **Injection:** 50 mg/mL | Yes |
| **Epinephrine** | | |
| *Rx Adrenalin Chloride*[1] | **Solution for inhalation:** 1:100 epinephrine solution | No |
| *otc microNefrin*[1]*, Nephron*[1]*, S-2*[1] | **Solution for inhalation:** 2.25% racepinephrine (1.125% epinephrine base) | No |
| *otc AsthmaHaler Mist, Primatene Mist* | **Aerosol:** 0.22 mg epinephrine/ spray | No |
| *Rx Adrenalin Chloride*[1]*, Ana-Guard*[1] | **Injection:**1:1000 (1 mg/mL as HCl) solution | Yes |
| *Rx* **Isoetharine HCl**[1] | **Solution for inhalation:** 1% | Yes |
| *Rx* **Isoproterenol**[1] | **Injection:** 1:50,000 (0.02 mg/ mL) | Yes |
| *Isuprel*[1] | **Injection:** 1:5000 (0.2 mg/mL) | Yes |
| *Rx* **Levalbuterol HCl** | | |
| *Xopenex* | **Solution for inhalation:** 0.063 mg/3 mL, 1.25 mg/3 mL | No |

| Generic Name<br>*Brand Name Examples* | Supplied As | Generic Available |
|---|---|---|
| Rx **Metaproterenol Sulfate** | **Tablets:** 10 mg, 20 mg | Yes |
| | **Syrup:** 10 mg/5 mL | Yes |
| *Alupent* | **Solution for inhalation:** 0.4% (in unit dose containers), 0.6%, 5% (in unit dose containers) | Yes |
| *Alupent* | **Aerosol:** 75 mg as micronized powder (0.65 mg/dose; 100 inhalations) | No |
| *Alupent* | **Aerosol:** 150 mg as micronized powder (0.65 mg/dose; 200 inhalations) | No |
| Rx **Pirbuterol Acetate** | | |
| *Maxair Autohaler* | **Aerosol:** 0.2 mg/actuation | No |
| Rx **Salmeterol Xinafoate** | | |
| *Serevent* | **Aerosol:** 25 mcg base/actuation | No |
| *Serevent Diskus* | **Powder for inhalation:** 50 mcg | No |
| Rx **Terbutaline Sulfate** | | |
| *Brethine* | **Tablets:** 2.5 mg, 5 mg | No |
| *Brethine* | **Injection:** 1 mg/mL | No |

[1] Contains sulfites.

All of the products listed in this table are bronchodilators; however, they are not interchangeable. For example, albuterol cannot be used for epinephrine, and salmeterol cannot be used for albuterol. Daily dose may vary depending on individual needs. Do not adjust the dose or change products without consulting your pharmacist or doctor.

## Type of Drug:

Bronchodilators; "rescue" medicines. Drugs that make breathing easier by opening breathing tubes (bronchial tubes) of the lung.

## How the Drug Works:

Sympathomimetics dilate (open) the bronchioles (air tubes) of the lung by relaxing the smooth muscle around the bronchioles. They are also used to prevent spasms or contractions of the smooth muscles around the bronchioles. This allows easier airflow into and out of the lungs. This may also assist in removing (expectorating) mucus and other debris causing congestion in the lungs.

## Uses:

To treat and prevent reversible bronchospasm associated with bronchial and nocturnal (nighttime) asthma, chronic bronchitis, emphysema, exercise-induced bronchospasm, and other obstructive airway diseases of the lungs.

To treat serious allergic reactions (epinephrine injection only).

## Precautions:

*Do not use in the following situations:*

allergy to a sympathomimetic or any of its ingredients

asthma (acute, significantly worsening, or deteriorating) (salmeterol only)

asthma, manageable with occasional short use of short-acting, inhaled beta$_2$-agonists (bronchodilators) (salmeterol only)

asthma attack, once it has begun (salmeterol only)

glaucoma, narrow angle (ephedrine and epinephrine injection only)

heart rhythm disturbances associated with a rapid heart rate (metaproterenol only)

substitute for inhaled or oral corticosteroids (salmeterol only)

*Use with caution in the following situations:*

abnormal heart rhythm

bronchospasm, life threatening (salmeterol only)

diabetes mellitus

elderly (epinephrine only)

heart disease

high blood pressure

hyperthyroidism

pregnancy, labor, and delivery

prostate enlargement (ephedrine and epinephrine only)

psychoneurosis (eg, obsessions, phobias) (epinephrine only)

seizures, history of

sensitivity to sympathomimetics

*Pregnancy:* There are no adequate and well-controlled studies in pregnant women. Use only if clearly needed and the potential benefits to the mother outweigh the possible risks to the fetus.

*Breastfeeding:* It is not known if these drugs appear in breast milk. Consult your doctor before you begin breastfeeding.

*Children:*

*Aerosol* – Safety and effectiveness for use of albuterol, bitolterol, metaproterenol, pirbuterol, salmeterol, and terbutaline in children younger than 12 years of age (younger than 4 years of age for *Ventolin*) have not been established. Consult a doctor about the use of epinephrine in children younger than 4 years of age.

*Oral doseforms* – Safety and effectiveness of albuterol have not been established for children younger than 2 years (syrup) and younger than 6 years (tablets and extended-release tablets) of age. Ephedrine is rarely used alone in children. Metaproterenol is not recommended for use in children younger than 6 years of age. Terbutaline is not recommended for use in children younger than 12 years of age.

*Powder for inhalation* – Safety and effectiveness of albuterol and salmeterol have not been established in children younger than 4 years of age.

*Solution for inhalation* – Safety and effectiveness of albuterol, bitolterol, epinephrine, isoetharine, and levalbuterol have not been established in children younger than 12 years of age (younger than 2 years of age for *Ventolin*). Safety and effectiveness of metaproterenol have not been established in children younger than 6 years of age.

*Sulfites:* Some of these products may contain sulfite preservatives, which can cause allergic reactions in certain individuals. Check package label when available or consult your doctor or pharmacist.

## Drug Interactions:

Tell your doctor or pharmacist if you are taking or planning to take any over-the-counter or prescription medications or dietary supplements while taking sympathomimetics. Doses of one or both drugs may need to be modified or a different drug may need to be prescribed. The following drugs and drug classes interact with sympathomimetics:

beta blocking agents (eg, propranolol)

digoxin (eg, *Lanoxin)*

diuretics, non-potassium sparing (eg, loop diuretics, thiazide)

ergot alkaloids (eg,*Hydergine)* (epinephrine only)

furazolidone*(Furoxone)* (ephedrine only)

guanethidine (eg, *Ismelin)* (ephedrine and epinephrine only)

methyldopa (eg, *Aldomet)* (ephedrine and epinephrine only)

MAO inhibitors (eg, phenelzine)

phenothiazines (eg, chlorpromazine) (epinephrine only)

rauwolfia alkaloids (eg, reserpine) (ephedrine and epinephrine only)

tricyclic antidepressants (eg, amitriptyline)

urinary acidifiers (eg, ammonium chloride) (ephedrine only)

urinary alkalinizers (eg, sodium bicarbonate) (ephedrine only)

## Side Effects:

Every drug is capable of producing side effects. Many sympathomimetic bronchodilator users experience no, or minor, side effects. The frequency and severity of side effects depend on many factors including dose, duration of therapy, and individual susceptibility. Possible side effects include:

*Digestive Tract:* Nausea; vomiting; appetite changes; heartburn; diarrhea; stomach pain; dry mouth; indigestion; constipation; mouth fungal infection; mouth or throat irritation; gastrointestinal distress; belching; gas.

*Nervous System:* Vertigo (feeling of whirling motion); dizziness; lightheadedness; headache; anxiety; tension; tremor; drowsiness; weakness; fatigue; nervousness; unstable emotions; aggressive behavior; restlessness; excitement; hyperactivity; sleeplessness; agitation; nightmares; irritability; shakiness.

*Circulatory System:* Changes in heart rate or rhythm; changes in blood pressure; chest pain or discomfort; pounding in the chest; irregular pulse.

*Respiratory System:* Breathing problems; bronchospasm; respiratory infections; nasal congestion; lower respiratory infections; bronchitis; increased mucous or phlegm discharge; cough; wheezing; nosebleed; sinus headache; hoarseness (especially in children); worsening of asthma; chest discomfort; runny nose; viral infection; sneezing.

*Skin:* Flushing; pallor; sweating; hives; rash; pain at the injection site (injections only); eczema; skin inflammation.

*Other:* Muscle cramps, stiffness, or soreness; unusual or bad taste; tooth pain or discoloration; painful menstruation; general body discomfort; joint, arm, neck, chest, shoulder, or back pain; low potassium levels; localized aches and pains; urinary tract infection; flu-like symptoms; allergic reaction; fever; decreased sensitivity to stimulation; accidental injury; pain; migraine; leg cramps; chills; abnormal lab tests; fainting; abnormal skin sensations; eye itch; sweating; eye inflammation.

## Guidelines for Use:

- Read and follow the patient instructions provided with the products.
- Dosage will be individualized. Do not use more frequently or at higher doses than recommended by your doctor.
- Do not crush or chew extended-release tablets. Swallow whole with liquids. The outer coating of the tablet may not be absorbed and may be noticeable in the stool.
- *Brand interchange* — Do not change from one brand of these drugs to another without consulting your pharmacist or doctor.
- While you are using a sympathomimetic bronchodilator, take other inhaled drugs and asthma medications only as directed by your doctor.
- If asthma attack continues or worsens, discontinue use and contact your doctor.
- *Salmeterol* — Do not use once an asthma attack begins. Use a quick-acting bronchodilator (eg, albuterol) instead. This medicine is not a substitute for inhaled or oral corticosteroids.
- If a dose is missed, take it as soon as possible. If several hours have passed or it is nearing time for the next dose, do not double the dose to catch up, unless advised to do so by your doctor. If several doses are missed, contact your doctor or pharmacist.
- May cause dizziness or drowsiness. Use caution while driving or performing other tasks requiring alertness, coordination, or physical dexterity.
- May cause nervousness, restlessness, or sleeplessness. Notify your doctor if the effects continue.
- Notify your doctor if palpitations, fast heartbeat, chest pain, muscle tremors, dizziness, headache, flushing, or difficulty in urination occurs, or if difficulty breathing persists.
- *Oral doseforms* — Do not exceed recommended dosage. If stomach upset occurs, take with food.
- *Nebulizer* — Mix medication as directed. Do not use if solution is brown or cloudy. Dilute concentrated solution (0.5%) before use.
  Do not mix different types of medication, unless advised to do so by your doctor.
  Assemble mask or mouthpiece. Administer treatment while sitting in a comfortable, upright position. Take slow, deep breaths until medication canister is empty. Wash mask or mouthpiece and medication container with hot water. Allow to air dry.

## Guidelines for Use (cont.):

• *Pressurized aerosol* — Follow administration, storage, and disposal instructions exactly.

Shake aerosol canister before each use.

Use of a spacing device (eg, *Aerochamber*) will enhance effectiveness and decrease side effects.

Protect from heat and light.

Do not stop or adjust the dose unless directed by your doctor. Overuse may result in the drug losing its effectiveness.

Breathe out fully through the mouth, expelling as much air from the lungs as possible. Place the mouthpiece of the inhaler (or spacer) into your mouth and, while breathing deeply and slowly through the mouth, activate the medication canister. Hold your breath for 3 to 5 seconds and then breathe out.

If more than 1 inhalation per dose is necessary, wait at least 1 full minute between doses. (Administer second inhalation at 3 to 5 minutes for albuterol and epinephrine; 10 minutes for metaproterenol).

If a previously effective dosage regimen fails to provide the usual relief, consult your doctor immediately. This may be a sign of seriously worsening asthma, which requires reassessment of therapy. Consult your doctor.

If any of the following occurs with the use of a short-acting beta$_2$-agonist (eg, albuterol, bitolterol, pirbuterol, terbutaline), contact your doctor: Use of 4 or more inhalations daily for more than 2 consecutive days; use of more than 1 canister in an 8-week period (ie, canister with 200 inhalations); sudden need for increased inhalations.

Do not interchange medication canisters and adapters (plastic colored sleeves) from different aerosol products.

*If you have any questions, consult your doctor, pharmacist, or health care provider.*

| Generic Name<br>*Brand Name Examples* | Supplied As | Generic<br>Available |
|---|---|---|
| *Rx* **Aminophylline**<br>**(Theophylline**<br>**Ethylenediamine)** | **Tablets:** 100 mg, 200 mg | Yes |
| | **Liquid:** 105 mg/5 mL | Yes |
| | **Suppositories:** 250 mg, 500 mg | Yes |
| | **Injection:** 250 mg/10 mL | Yes |
| *Rx* **Dyphylline**<br>**(Dihydroxypropyl**<br>**Theophylline)** | | |
| *Dilor, Dilor-400, Lufyllin,*<br>*Lufyllin-400* | **Tablets:** 200 mg, 400 mg | Yes |
| *Dilor, Lufyllin* | **Elixir:** 100 mg/15 mL,<br>160 mg/15 mL | No |
| *Dilor* | **Injection:** 250 mg/mL | No |
| *Rx* **Oxtriphylline (Choline**<br>**Theophyllinate)** | | |
| *Choledyl SA* | **Tablets, extended release (8 to**<br>**12 hours):** 400 mg, 600 mg | No |
| *Rx* **Theophylline** | **Oral solution:** 80 mg/15 mL | Yes |
| *Quibron-T Accudose,*<br>*Slo-Phyllin, Theolair* | **Tablets:** 100 mg, 125 mg,<br>200 mg, 250 mg, 300 mg | Yes |
| *Theochron* | **Tablets, extended release:**<br>100 mg, 200 mg, 300 mg | No |
| *Quibron-T/SR Accu-*<br>*dose, Respbid, Theo-*<br>*lair-SR, T-Phyl* | **Tablets, sustained release (8 to**<br>**12 hours):** 200 mg, 250 mg,<br>300 mg, 500 mg | No |
| *Theo-Dur* | **Tablets, extended release (8 to**<br>**24 hours):** 100 mg, 200 mg,<br>300 mg, 450 mg | No |
| *Theo-X* | **Tablets, extended release (12 to**<br>**24 hours):** 100 mg, 200 mg, 300<br>mg | No |
| *Uniphyl* | **Tablets, extended release**<br>**(24 hours):** 400 mg, 600 mg | No |
| *Theo-24* | **Capsules, extended release**<br>**(24 hours):** 100 mg, 200 mg,<br>300 mg, 400 mg | No |
| *Elixophyllin* | **Elixir:** 80 mg/15 mL | Yes |
| *Slo-Phyllin* | **Syrup:** 80 mg/15 mL | No |

All of the products listed in the table are bronchodilators; however, they are not all equivalent on a weight basis and cannot be interchanged without adjusting the dose. For example, oxtriphylline cannot be used for theophylline without adjusting the dose. Daily dose may vary depending on individual needs. Do not adjust the dose or change products without consulting your pharmacist or doctor.

| Theophylline Content and Equivalent Dose of Various Theophylline Salts | | |
|---|---|---|
| Theophylline salts | Theophylline % | Equivalent dose |
| Theophylline anhydrous | 100 | 100 mg |
| Aminophylline anhydrous | 86 | 116 mg |
| Aminophylline dihydrate | 79 | 127 mg |
| Oxtriphylline | 64 | 156 mg |

## Type of Drug:

Bronchodilators; theophylline products; drugs that make breathing easier by relaxing and widening certain breathing passages (bronchial tubes) of the lung.

## How the Drug Works:

The xanthine derivatives directly relax the smooth muscle surrounding the bronchial tubes (air passages) of the lungs, allowing the tubes to widen, making breathing easier. These drugs may improve contraction of the diaphragm (the major breathing muscle) in patients with chronic obstructive airway disease.

## Uses:

To prevent and relieve symptoms of bronchial asthma. Not for use by themselves in an acute attack (status asthmaticus).

To treat bronchospasm (spasm in breathing tubes) associated with chronic bronchitis and emphysema.

*Unlabeled Use(s):* Occasionally doctors may prescribe xanthine bronchodilators for other breathing problems and slow heart rates in premature infants.

## Precautions:

*Do not use in the following situations:*

allergy to any xanthine compounds (eg, caffeine, chocolate) or any of their ingredients
allergy to ethylenediamine (aminophylline only)
irritation or infection of the rectum or lower colon (aminophylline suppositories only)

peptic ulcer disease, active
seizure disorder, underlying (unless receiving anticonvulsants)
xanthine use, concurrent

*Use with caution in the following situations:*

abnormal heart rhythm
alcoholism (some liquid forms)
congestive heart failure
dehydration
elderly (particularly males with chronic lung disease)
heart disease, severe
high blood pressure
high fever, sustained
hyperthyroidism
hypothyroidism
hypoxemia (deficient oxygenation of the blood)
influenza vaccine
kidney function, impaired (infants younger than 3 months of age)
liver function, impaired (except dyphylline)
low blood pressure
myocardial injury, acute
newborns and infants younger than 1 year of age
peptic ulcer disease, history
pregnancy, third trimester
pulmonary edema, acute
sepsis with multiple organ failure
smoking (decreases theophylline levels)
status asthmaticus (oral products act too slowly)
viral infection

*Acute asthma attacks (status asthmaticus)* are a medical emergency and are not rapidly responsive to usual doses of conventional bronchodilators. Therapy frequently requires IV medication and close monitoring. These products alone are not appropriate treatment for an acute asthma attack.

*Pregnancy:* There are no adequate and well-controlled studies in pregnant women. Use only if clearly needed and potential benefits outweigh the possible hazards to the fetus.

*Breastfeeding:* Xanthines appear in breast milk. Because of the potential for serious adverse reactions in nursing infants, decide whether to discontinue nursing or to discontinue the drug, taking into account the importance of the drug to the mother. Consult your doctor before you begin breastfeeding.

*Children:* Safety and effectiveness of aminophylline and theophylline for use in children younger than 1 year of age have not been established. Caution should be exercised for younger children who cannot complain of side effects. If used in children younger than 1 year of age, strict attention should be directed at dosing and monitoring of serum levels. However, some dosage forms of theophylline are not recommended for certain age groups. Please check individual dosing and administration in package inserts. Oxtriphylline is not recommended for children younger than 6 years of age. Dyphylline is not recommended for children.

*Elderly:* Reduced theophylline elimination has been documented in patients older than 55 years of age, particularly in males with chronic lung disease, congestive heart failure, or liver disease. It is important to consider reduction of dosage and frequent measurement of serum theophylline levels in these individuals, as they may experience toxicity more easily.

*Lab tests* may be necessary. High blood levels of xanthine bronchodilators may cause severe side effects. Therapy is monitored with lab tests to maintain nontoxic levels of medication, as serious toxicity is not reliably preceded by less severe side effects. Lung function measurements before and after a period of treatment may also be necessary to determine therapy effectiveness. Note that dyphylline is not converted to theophylline; thus, theophylline blood levels cannot be used to monitor its use.

## Drug Interactions:

Tell your doctor or pharmacist if you are taking or planning to take any over-the-counter or prescription medications or dietary supplements while taking xanthine bronchodilators. Doses of one or both drugs may need to be modified or a different drug may need to be prescribed. The following drugs and drug classes interact with xanthine bronchodilators:

These drugs *decrease* the effectiveness of xanthine bronchodilators:

aminoglutethimide (*Cytadren)*
barbiturates (eg, phenobarbital)
carbamazepine (eg, *Tegretol)*[1]
charcoal
hydantoins (eg, phenytoin)
moricizine (*Ethmozine*)
rifampin (eg, *Rifadin)*
ritonavir (*Norvir*)
smoking (cigarettes and marijuana)
sucralfate (*Carafate*)
sulfinpyrazone (eg, *Anturane*)

These drugs *increase* the effects of xanthine bronchodilators (increasing side effects):

alcohol
allopurinol (eg, *Zyloprim*)
beta blockers (nonselective) (eg, propranolol)
carbamazepine (eg, *Tegretol)*[1]
cimetidine (eg, *Tagamet*)
clarithromycin (*Biaxin*)
contraceptives, oral estrogen-containing (eg, *Ortho-Novum*)
corticosteroids (eg, hydrocortisone)
disulfiram *(Antabuse)*
ephedrine (eg, *Sudafed*)
erythromycin (eg, *Eryc)*
fluoroquinolones (eg, ciprofloxacin, enoxacin, norfloxacin, ofloxacin)
fluvoxamine (*Luvox*)
influenza vaccine (eg, *Fluzone)*
interferon, human recombinant alpha-A
isoniazid (eg, *Laniazid)*[1]
methotrexate (eg, *Rheumatrex)*
mexiletine *(Mexitil)*
pentoxifylline (*Trental*)
propafenone (*Rythmol*)
propranolol (eg, *Inderal*)
tacrine (*Cognex*)
thiabendazole *(Mintezol)*[1]
thyroid hormones (eg, levothyroxine)
ticlopidine (*Ticlid*)
troleandomycin *(Tao)*
verapamil (eg, *Verelan*)

Other drugs which xanthine bronchodilators affect:

adenosine (*Adenocard*)
benzodiazepines (eg, diazepam)
beta agonists
halothane (eg, *Fluothane)*
ketamine (*Ketalar)*
lithium (eg, *Eskalith*)
nondepolarizing muscle relaxants (eg, metocurine iodide)
probenecid (dyphylline only)
tetracyclines (eg, *Sumycin)*

[1]May increase or decrease effects.

## Side Effects:

Every drug is capable of producing side effects. Many xanthine bronchodilator users experience no, or minor, side effects, particularly if serum theophylline levels are less than 20 mcg/mL. The frequency and severity of side effects depend on many factors including dose, duration of therapy, and individual susceptibility. High blood levels (generally higher than 30 mcg/mL) of these medications will cause serious side effects, although high blood levels and serious toxicity are not always preceded by side effects. Possible side effects include:

*Digestive Tract:* Stomach pain; nausea; vomiting; vomiting of blood; diarrhea; gastroesophageal reflux (nocturnal).

*Nervous System:* Seizures; headache; sleeplessness; irritability; restlessness; muscle twitching; reflex hyperexcitability; agitation.

*Circulatory System:* Decreased blood pressure; abnormal heart beat; pounding in the chest (palpitations); fast heartbeat.

*Skin:* Flushing; rash; hair loss.

*Other:* Increased urination; high blood sugar; rectal irritation or bleeding (suppository only); muscle tremors or twitching.

---

### Guidelines for Use:

- Take exactly as prescribed. Individual doses are determined by response (decrease in symptoms) and blood levels (except with dyphylline). Do not take a different dose, take the drug more often, or for a longer time than prescribed.
- *Immediate Release Tablets and Liquids:*
  Take at regular intervals around the clock.
  If a dose is missed, take it as soon as possible. If several hours have passed or if it is nearing time for the next dose, do not double the dose in order to catch up, unless advised to do so by your doctor. If more than one dose is missed or it is necessary to establish a new dosage schedule, contact your doctor or pharmacist.
- *Sustained, Extended, or Controlled Release Products:*
  Take 8- to 12-hour release products at regular intervals (8 or 12 hours) around the clock. Try to take at the same time each day.
  Take 12- to 24-hour release products generally every 12 hours. However, a few patients may be able to take once a day.
  Take 24-hour release products once daily, preferably in the morning. Try to take at the same time each day.
  Although normally given once daily, patients who require very large doses may be asked to split the dose and take 2 doses per day. In this event, the second dose should be taken 10 to 12 hours after the first dose and before the evening meal.
  If a dose is missed, take the next dose at the usually scheduled time. Do not make up the missed dose.

## Guidelines for Use (cont.):

• *Brand interchange* — Do not change from one brand of this drug to another without consulting your pharmacist or doctor. Products are not equivalent on a weight basis and cannot be interchanged without adjusting the dose.

• If stomach upset occurs with liquid preparations or non-sustained release forms, take with food.

• Do not crush or chew enteric coated or sustained, extended, or controlled release tablets or capsules.

• Taking theophylline immediately after a high-fat meal or a fasting period may alter its rate of absorption.

• Do not use for an acute episode of bronchospasm.

• If rash, nausea, vomiting, restlessness, irregular heartbeat, or convulsions occur, contact your doctor immediately.

• Inform your doctor of bothersome side effects such as headache, stomach pain, sleeplessness, or jitteriness.

• Notify your doctor if respiratory symptoms return repeatedly near the end of the dosing interval.

• Avoid large amounts of caffeine-containing beverages, such as tea, coffee, cocoa, and cola drinks, or eating large amounts of chocolate. These products may increase side effects.

• Tell your doctor if you are a smoker. Smoking increases the clearance rate of theophylline and may decrease overall effect. Nicotine replacement therapy (NRT) used in smoking cessation programs does not adversely affect theophylline clearance.

• *Uniphyl, Theolair SR* — Take this drug consistently with respect to food, either with meals or fasting (at least 2 hours pre- or 2 hours post-meals).

• *Theo-24* — In patients receiving once-daily doses of 900 mg or more, avoid eating a high-fat morning meal or take at least 1 hour before eating. If you cannot comply with this regimen, talk to your doctor about alternative therapy.

• Lab tests will be required. Be sure to keep appointments. Blood levels must be checked regularly to avoid underdosing and overdosing.

• Store oral dosage forms at room temperature (59° to 86°F) in a tightly closed container. Store suppositories between 36° to 46°F (refrigerated).

*If you have any questions, consult your doctor, pharmacist, or health care provider.*

| Generic Name<br>*Brand Name Examples* | How Supplied | Generic<br>Available |
|---|---|---|
| Rx **Montelukast Sodium** | | |
| *Singulair* | **Tablets**: 10 mg | No |
| *Singulair*[1] | **Tablets, chewable**: 4 mg, 5 mg | No |
| Rx **Zafirlukast** | | |
| *Accolate* | **Tablets**: 10 mg, 20 mg | No |
| Rx **Zileuton** | | |
| *Zyflo Filmtabs* | **Tablets**: 600 mg | No |

[1] Contains phenylalanine.

## Type of Drug:
Anti-asthma drug.

## How the Drug Works:
Zileuton inhibits the formation of certain chemicals (leukotrienes) that are responsible for causing some forms of asthma. Montelukast and zafirlukast block the action of certain chemicals (leukotrienes) that are responsible for causing some forms of asthma.

These drugs are useful for controlling or preventing some forms of asthma but do not help during an acute asthma attack.

## Uses:
For the prevention and chronic treatment of asthma in adult and children 2 years of age and older (montelukast), 7 years of age and older (zafirlukast), and 12 years of age and older (zileuton).

## Precautions:
*Do not use in the following situations:*
>       allergy to the leukotriene receptor antagonist or any of its ingredients
>       liver disease, active (zileuton only)
>       to treat bronchospasm in acute asthmatic attacks

*Use with caution in the following situations:*
>       alcohol use (zileuton only)
>       elderly (zafirlukast only)
>       liver disease, history of (zileuton only)

*Phenylketonuria:* Montelukast chewable tablets contain phenylalanine. Consult your doctor or pharmacist.

*Pregnancy:* There are no adequate and well-controlled studies in pregnant women. Use only if clearly needed and potential benefits to the mother outweigh the possible hazards to the fetus.

*Breastfeeding:* Zafirlukast appears in breast milk. Do not breastfeed while taking zafirlukast. It is not known if zileuton or montelukast appear in breast milk. Consult your doctor before you begin breastfeeding.

*Children:* Safety and effectiveness for use in children younger than 12 years of age (zileuton), younger than 5 years of age (zafirlukast), and younger than 2 years of age (montelukast) are not established.

*Elderly:* Patients older than 65 years of age are more likely to experience infections while taking zafirlukast. These infections are usually mild to moderate and mostly affect the respiratory tract.

*Lab tests* may be required to monitor therapy. Tests may include breathing tests. Liver enzymes will be monitored with zileuton therapy.

## Drug Interactions:

Tell your doctor or pharmacist if you are taking or planning to take any over-the-counter or prescription medications or dietary supplements while taking a leukotriene receptor antagonist or formation inhibitor. Doses of one or both drugs may need to be modified or a different drug may need to be prescribed. The following drugs and drug classes may interact with leukotriene receptor antagonists or formation inhibitors:

aspirin (zafirlukast only)
calcium channel blockers
 (eg, nifidipine) (zafirlukast and
 zileuton only)
cyclosporine (eg, *Sandimmune*)
 (zafirlukast and zileuton only)
erythromycin (eg, *E-Mycin*)
 (zafirlukast only)

propranolol (eg, *Inderal*)
 (zileuton only)
theophylline (eg, *Theo-Dur*)
 (zafirlukast and zileuton only)
warfarin (eg, *Coumadin*)
 (zafirlukast and zileuton only)

## Side Effects:

Every drug is capable of producing side effects. Many leukotriene receptor antagonist or formation inhibitor users experience no, or minor, side effects. The frequency or severity of side effects depend on many factors including dose, duration of therapy, and individual susceptibility. Possible side effects include:

*Nervous System:* Headache; weakness; dizziness; sleeplessness; nervousness; drowsiness; fatigue.

*Digestive Tract:* Nausea; vomiting; diarrhea; stomach pain; indigestion; gas; constipation.

*Other:* Infection; accidental injury; generalized pain; muscle, chest, joint, leg, or back pain; fever; eye inflammation; stiffness; swollen lymph nodes; general body discomfort; neck pain; itching; urinary tract infection; inflammation of the vagina; flu; cough; nasal congestion; dental pain; rash; laryngitis; sore throat; ear pain or inflammation; sinus inflammation; viral infection; thirst; sneezing; hives; pus in the urine.

## Guidelines for Use:

- Dosage is individualized. Take exactly as prescribed.
- These medicines are used for long-term control or prevention of asthma and should be taken regularly as prescribed, even during symptom-free periods. They should also be continued during acute exacerbations of asthma.
- Do not decrease the dose or stop taking any other asthma medications unless instructed by your doctor.
- Take zafirlukast 2 times a day on an empty stomach, at least 1 hour before or 2 hours after meals.
- Take zileuton 4 times a day with meals and at bedtime.
- Take montelukast once a day in the evening without regard to meals. Take with food if stomach upset occurs.
- If a dose is missed, take it as soon as possible. If several hours have passed or it is nearing time for the next dose, do not double the dose to catch up, unless advised by your doctor. If more than one dose is missed or it is necessary to establish a new dosage schedule, contact your doctor or pharmacist.
- May cause dizziness. Use caution when driving or performing other tasks requiring alertness, coordination or physical dexterity.
- These medicines are not bronchodilators and should not be used as "rescue medicines" to treat acute episodes of asthma.
- Do not breastfeed while taking zafirlukast.
- Contact your doctor if you need your short-acting bronchodilators ("rescue medicines") more often than usual.
- Contact your doctor if you are taking zileuton and experience right upper quadrant pain, nausea, tiredness, unconsciousness, itchiness, yellowing of the skin or the whites of the eyes, "flu-like" symptoms, or unusually dark urine.
- Lab tests may be required to monitor therapy. Be sure to keep appointments.
- Store at controlled room temperature (68° to 77°F). Protect from light and moisture.

*If you have any questions, consult your doctor, pharmacist, or health care provider.*

| Generic Name<br>*Brand Name Examples* | Supplied As | Generic<br>Available |
|---|---|---|
| *Rx* **Beclomethasone Dipropionate** | | |
| *Vanceril* | **Aerosol**: 42 mcg/actuation | No |
| *Vanceril Double Strength* | **Aerosol**: 84 mcg/actuation | |
| *QVAR* | **Aerosol**: 40 mcg/actuation,<br>80 mcg/actuation | No |
| *Rx* **Budesonide** | | |
| *Pulmicort Turbuhaler* | **Inhalation powder**:<br>≈ 160 mcg/actuation | No |
| *Pulmicort Respules* | **Inhalation suspension**:<br>0.25 mg/2 mL, 0.5 mg/2 mL | No |
| *Rx* **Flunisolide** | | |
| *AeroBid, AeroBid-M*[1] | **Aerosol:** ≈ 250 mcg/actuation | No |
| *Rx* **Fluticasone Propionate** | | |
| *Flovent* | **Aerosol:** 44 mcg/actuation,<br>110 mcg/actuation, 220 mcg/<br>actuation | No |
| *Flovent Rotadisk* | **Inhalation powder:** 44 mcg/<br>actuation, 88 mcg/actuation,<br>220 mcg/actuation | No |
| *Rx* **Fluticasone Propionate/Salmeterol** | | |
| *Advair Diskus* | **Inhalation powder**: 93 mcg/<br>45 mcg/actuation, 233 mcg/<br>45 mcg/actuation, 465 mcg/<br>45 mcg/actuation | No |
| *Rx* **Triamcinolone Acetonide** | | |
| *Azmacort*[2] | **Aerosol:** 100 mcg/actuation | No |

[1] Contains menthol
[2] Contains alcohol

## Type of Drug:

Respiratory inhalants; drugs that produce an anti-inflammatory effect in lungs of stable asthma patients; asthma controllers; asthma preventatives.

## How the Drug Works:

Irritation and inflammation (swelling) of the bronchial tubes (air tubes) of the lung is frequently a cause of persistent or recurrent asthma symptoms. These synthetic "anti-inflammatory steroids" decrease the irritation and swelling (inflammation) of the air tubes of the lungs and control or prevent asthma symptoms. These drugs do not directly open the bronchial tubes and do not provide rapid relief. They are useful for controlling or preventing asthma symptoms but do not help during an acute asthma attack. When inhaled into the bronchial tubes, the effect is local and the incidence of side effects is very low when compared to side effects when these medications are given by mouth.

## Uses:

To prevent or reduce the frequency and severity of bronchial asthma attacks in patients requiring chronic (long-term) treatment.

Corticosteroid inhalants are *not* to be used to treat an acute asthma attack or in the treatment of nonasthmatic bronchitis.

*Flovent Rotadisk* — For treatment of chronic asthma attacks in patients 4 years of age and older or for asthma requiring long-term corticosteroid therapy.

Patients using corticosteroid inhalants may also take oral corticosteroid therapy or specific bronchodilator therapy.

## Precautions:

*Do not use in the following situations:*

acute bronchospasm, treatment of

allergy to any ingredient of the formulation

asthma that can be controlled by bronchodilators and other nonsteroidal medicine (beclomethasone aerosol only)

nonasthmatic bronchitis (beclomethasone aerosol only)

systemic corticosteroid treatment, infrequently required (beclomethasone aerosol only)

*Use with caution in the following situations:*

adrenal insufficiency
chicken pox, exposure
herpes infection in the eye
measles, exposure
oral corticosteroid use, chronic

respiratory infections (fungal, bacterial, or viral)
systemic fungal, bacterial, parasitic, or viral infection, untreated
tuberculosis, active or inactive

*Changing from other dosage forms:* Patients who have been on long-term oral corticosteroids may lose their body's natural ability to produce corticosteroid hormones. Switching or lessening current oral doses may cause symptoms of withdrawal (eg, joint or muscle pain, tiredness, depression). Therefore, taper dosage of oral steroid gradually and only with the instruction of a doctor.

*Pregnancy:* There are no adequate and well-controlled studies in pregnant women. Use only if clearly needed and the potential benefits to the mother outweigh the possible hazards to the fetus.

*Breastfeeding:* It is not known if inhaled corticosteroids appear in breast milk. Consult your doctor before you begin breastfeeding.

*Children:* There is insufficient information available to warrant use in children younger than 12 months of age (budesonide suspension), younger than 6 years of age (beclomethasone, budesonide inhalation powder, flunisolide, and triamcinolone), or younger than 12 years of age (fluticasone aerosol). Extended regular use may suppress growth in children and teenagers.

## Drug Interactions:

Tell your doctor or pharmacist if you are taking or planning to take any over-the-counter or prescription medications or dietary supplements with inhaled corticosteroids. Doses of one or both drugs may need to be modified or a different drug may need to be prescribed. Ketoconazole (eg, *Nizoral*) interacts with inhaled corticosteroids.

## Side Effects:

Every drug is capable of producing side effects. Many inhaled corticosteroid users experience no, or minor, side effects. The frequency and severity of side effects depend on many factors including dose, duration of therapy, and individual susceptibility. Possible side effects include:

*Digestive Tract:* Diarrhea; toothache; nausea; vomiting; stomach pain or upset; constipation; gas; oral thrush (white patches in mouth); heartburn; indigestion; changes in appetite.

*Nervous System:* Headache; migraine; fatigue; dizziness; irritability; sleeplessness; fainting; shakiness; nervousness; mental disturbances; depression; agitation; lightheadedness; anxiety; changes in energy level; moodiness; numbness; vertigo (feeling of whirling motion); emotional lability.

*Respiratory System:* Sore throat; flu-like symptoms; head, nasal, or chest congestion; dry or irritated mouth, nose, or throat; hoarseness; voice changes; mouth infections; coughing; wheezing; difficulty breathing; runny nose; sneezing; throat infection; upper respiratory tract infection; loss of voice; nosebleed; sinus inflammation; chest tightness; phlegm; chest tightness; worsening of asthma.

*Skin:* Acne; red, itchy skin; rash; itching; hives; bruising; skin discoloration; sensitivity to sunlight.

*Other:* Fever; urinary tract or vaginal infections; neck pain; back problems; pain; weight gain; unpleasant taste and smell; blurred vision; eye discomfort; speech problems; high blood pressure; rapid heartbeat; ear or eye infection; loss of sense of taste and smell; menstrual problems; bone fracture; palpitations (pounding in the chest); chest pain; suppression of HPA function; weakness; pain; back pain; enlarged lymph nodes; general body discomfort; sweating; swelling of the arms or legs; muscle or joint pain; chills; fever.

---

### Guidelines for Use:

- Read and follow patient instructions provided with the product.
- Use exactly as prescribed. Do not increase recommended dose. Benefits are not immediate and effectiveness requires regular use. Contact your doctor if symptoms do not improve or condition worsens.
- *Aerosol* — Using the inhaler beyond the labeled number of actuations (puffs) will result in ineffective doses of medication and loss of control of asthma.
  Canisters should only be used with their actuator (plastic holder). Administering with a spacing device (eg, *OptiHaler, Aerochamber*) will enhance medication delivery and effectiveness.

## Guidelines for Use (cont.):

- *QVAR* — Prime the aerosol canister before using the first time or if it has not been used for 10 or more days. Activating the aerosol into the air 2 times will prime the canister.
- *Inhalation suspension* — Must be administered by air-driven jet nebulizer. Shake gently before adding to nebulizer canister.
- Do not stop using when you feel better, unless advised by your doctor. These medicines are designed to prevent asthma symptoms and must be used on a daily basis, even when you feel well.
- Rinse mouth thoroughly, without swallowing, after completing inhalations. This reduces the risk of mouth infection.
- Do not use for an acute asthma attack requiring rapid relief. Inhaled corticosteroids are not bronchodilators.
- Avoid spraying in eyes.
- *Bronchodilator inhaler use* — Use the bronchodilator (eg, isoproterenol, albuterol, epinephrine) several minutes before the corticosteroid aerosol. This opens the air tubes and increases penetration of the steroid into the passageways.
- Notify your doctor if you experience oral thrush (white patches in mouth or throat), voice changes, sore throat, sore mouth, mental disturbances, increased bruising, weight gain, cushingoid features, acne, or cataracts.
- Contact your doctor when asthma attacks do not adequately respond to bronchodilators or if you notice a sudden increase in the need for your bronchodilator. Oral or injectable steroids may be required.
- May cause dizziness or lightheadedness. Use caution while driving or performing other tasks requiring alertness, coordination, or physical dexterity.
- May cause photosensitivity (sensitivity to sunlight). Avoid prolonged exposure to the sun and other ultraviolet (UV) light (eg, tanning beds). Use sunscreens and wear protective clothing until tolerance is determined.
- Supplementary oral steroids may be necessary during periods of high stress such as surgery, trauma, infection, or severe asthma attack. Carry a warning card indicating this potential need.
- Notify your doctor immediately if symptoms of steroid withdrawal occur when changing from oral to inhalant therapy (eg, joint or muscle pain, lack of energy, depression, more problems breathing, wheezing, dizziness). Your doctor may increase your oral steroid dose temporarily and then begin decreasing the oral steroid dose more slowly.
- Allergic reactions (eg, rash, hives, difficulty breathing) have occurred following beclomethasone use. These may be immediate or delayed. Contact your doctor if you suspect a reaction.
- Avoid exposure to chicken pox, measles, or other infections involving the respiratory tract. If exposed, consult your doctor immediately.
- Store at room temperature. Use inhalation suspension within 2 weeks of opening foil pouch. Use fluticasone powder within 2 months of opening foil pouch. Use fluticasone/salmeterol powder within 1 month of opening foil pouch.

*If you have any questions, consult your doctor, pharmacist, or health care provider.*

| Generic Name<br>*Brand Name Examples* | Supplied As | Generic<br>Available |
|---|---|---|
| **Cromolyn Sodium** | **Inhalation (for nebulizer only)**: 20 mg/2 mL | Yes |
| *Rx  Intal Inhaler* | **Aerosol**: 800 mcg/spray | No |
| *Rx  Intal Nebulizer Solution* | **Solution (for nebulizer only)**: 20 mg/2 mL amp | No |
| *otc  Nasalcrom*[1] | **Nasal solution**: 5.2 mg/spray | No |
| *otc  Children's Nasalcrom*[1] | **Nasal solution**: 5.2 mg/spray | No |

[1] Contains 0.01% benzalkonium chloride and 0.01% EDTA.

## Type of Drug:

Respiratory inhalant.

## How the Drug Works:

Cromolyn sodium is an antiasthmatic, antiallergic stabilizer of mast cells, which release histamine and slow-reacting substances of anaphylaxis. The decreased release of these and other chemicals assist in preventing constriction (narrowing) of the breathing airways in asthma and allergy attacks.

## Uses:

*Cromolyn Sodium and Intal:* To prevent symptoms in the management of bronchial asthma, exercise-induced bronchospasm (spasm of breathing airways in the lungs), and acute bronchospasm due to environmental pollution and known allergens (chemicals that may produce an asthmatic or allergic reaction).

*Nasalcrom:* To prevent or treat symptoms of allergic rhinitis (eg, runny, itchy, stuffy nose; sneezing).

*Unlabeled Use(s):* Oral use of cromolyn is being evaluated in patients with food allergies, eczema, ulcers, hives (chronic), and postexercise-induced bronchospasms.

## Precautions:

*Do not use in the following situations:*

allergy to cromolyn or any of its ingredients
asthma attack, prolonged and severe
eosinophilic pneumonia (bacterial lung infection)
sinus infection (nasal solution only)
cold symptoms

*Use with caution in the following situations:*

coronary artery disease (aerosol only)
coughing or wheezing
irregular heartbeat (aerosol only)
kidney disease
liver disease

*Pregnancy:* Safety for use during pregnancy has not been established. Use only if clearly needed and potential benefits to the mother outweigh the possible hazards to the fetus.

*Breastfeeding:* It is not known if cromolyn appears in breast milk. Consult your doctor before you begin breastfeeding.

*Children:* Safety and effectiveness for use in children under 6 (nasal solution), 5 (aerosol), or 2 (nebulizer) years of age have not been established.

## Drug Interactions:

Tell your doctor or pharmacist if you are taking or if you are planning to take any over-the-counter or prescription medications or dietary supplements while taking cromolyn. Doses of one or both drugs may need to be modified or a different drug may need to be prescribed. Isoproterenol interacts with this medicine.

## Side Effects:

Every drug is capable of producing side effects. Many patients experience no, or minor, side effects. The frequency and severity of side effects depend on many factors including dose, duration of therapy, and individual susceptibility. Possible side effects include:

*Aerosol:* Dizziness; dry or irritated throat; joint swelling and pain; painful or difficult urination; urinary frequency; hives; skin inflammation; excessive eye tearing; swollen parotid gland.

*Nasal Solution:* Nasal stinging; nasal burning; postnasal drip.

*Nebulizer Solution:* Drowsiness; serum sickness; stomach ache.

*Other:* Headache; nausea; cough; wheezing; nasal irritation; sneezing; nosebleed; bad taste in mouth; rash.

## Guidelines for Use:

- Use exactly as prescribed.
- Not for the treatment of an existing asthma attack. Only use when an asthma attack is under control and you can breathe well.
- Notify your doctor if coughing, wheezing, or other unusual symptoms occur.
- Blow your nose before administering the nasal solution. If congested, use a shortacting topical decongestant before the solution. Nasal solution may cause mild stinging or sneezing, but this rarely requires stopping therapy.
- Instructions for use of inhalation devices accompany each product.
- Use continuously. Effectiveness depends on regularity of use. Do not stop therapy suddenly. Consult your doctor before stopping the drug.
- *To prevent exercise-induced bronchospasm* — Administer no longer than 1 hour before beginning exercise.
- If a dose is missed, inhale it as soon as possible. If several hours have passed or it is nearing time for the next dose, do not double the dose to catch up, unless advised to do so by your doctor. If more than one dose is missed or it is necessary to establish a new dosage schedule, contact your doctor or pharmacist.
- Improvement ordinarily occurs within the first 4 weeks of use. Improvement should be apparent by a decrease in the severity of symptoms and the need for other therapy (eg, oral steroids, inhaled broncho-dilators).
- Long-term use is justified if cromolyn produces a significant reduction in frequency or severity of symptoms, permits reduction of doses or elimination of oral steroids, or improves management of patients experiencing intolerable side effects from other asthma drugs.
- If allergic rhinitis (eg, runny nose) is seasonal, continue treatment throughout exposure period. If it is year-round, continuous use may be necessary. Cromolyn use may decrease or eliminate the need for anti-histamines or decongestants.
- Store nebulizer solution, aerosol, and nasal solution at room temperature, away from light. Do not use nebulizer solution if it is discolored or contains particles. Do not puncture the aerosol container or store near heat, cold, or open flame. Keep away from children.

*If you have any questions, consult your doctor, pharmacist, or health care provider.*

| Generic Name<br>*Brand Name Example* | Supplied As | Generic<br>Available |
|---|---|---|
| *Rx* **Ipratropium Bromide** | | |
| *Atrovent* | **Aerosol**: Delivers 18 mcg/<br>actuation (200 actuations/<br>canister) | No |
| *Atrovent* | **Solution**: 0.02% | Yes |

## Type of Drug:
Respiratory inhalant; bronchodilator.

## How the Drug Works:
Ipratropium bromide blocks the action of the chemical transmitter acetylcholine when inhaled orally. Acetylcholine stimulates the muscles around the bronchial tubes (air passages in the lung) to spasm or constrict. This closes the bronchial tubes and makes it harder to breath. By blocking acetylcholine, ipratropium allows the muscles around the bronchial tubes to relax. This allow the bronchial tubes to open wider (bronchodilation) and makes it easier to breath.

## Uses:
To treat bronchospasms (spasms of air passages) occurring in chronic obstructive pulmonary disease (COPD), including chronic bronchitis, and emphysema.

## Precautions:
*Do not use in the following situations:*
> allergy to ipratropium bromide, atropine, or any of its anticholinergic derivatives
> allergy to soya lecithin or related food products (eg, soybeans, peanuts) (aerosol only)

*Use with caution in the following situations:*
> acute bronchospasm attacks (eg, asthma attacks)
> enlarged prostate
> glaucoma, narrow-angle
> obstruction of the neck of the urinary bladder

*Pregnancy:* There are no adequate and well-controlled studies in pregnant women. Use only if clearly needed and benefits outweigh the possible hazards to the fetus.

*Breastfeeding:* It is not known if ipratropium bromide appears in breast milk. Consult your doctor before you begin breastfeeding.

*Children:* Safety and effectiveness in children younger than 12 years of age have not been established.

**Side Effects:**

Every drug is capable of producing side effects. Many patients experience no, or minor, side effects. The frequency and severity of side effects depend on many factors including dose, duration of therapy, and individual susceptibility. Possible side effects include:

*Digestive Tract:* Nausea; stomach ache.

*Nervous System:* Headache; nervousness; dizziness; sleeplessness.

*Circulatory System:* Increased heart rate or irregular heartbeat; palpitations (pounding in the chest); low blood pressure; increased blood pressure.

*Skin:* Rash; itching; hives; flushing; hair loss.

*Respiratory System:* Cough; difficulty breathing; bronchitis; bronchospasm; increased sputum; upper respiratory tract infection; respiratory disorder; sore throat; dry mouth or throat; hoarseness; sinus infection; nasal irritation or congestion; runny nose; blood-tinged mucus.

*Other:* Worsening of narrow-angle glaucoma with acute eye pain; blurred vision; eye irritation; eye inflammation; ear ringing; tremors; pain; flu-like symptoms; joint, back, or chest pain; general pain; difficult urination; thirst.

## Guidelines for Use:

- Dosage is individualized. Use exactly as prescribed.
- Do not stop taking or change the dose unless directed by your doctor.
- If a dose is missed, inhale it as soon as possible. If several hours have passed or it is nearing time for the next dose, do not double the dose to catch up, unless advised to do so by your doctor. If more than one dose is missed or it is necessary to establish a new dosage schedule, contact your doctor or pharmacist.
- Shake the aerosol canister well before using.
- The pump requires 7 actuations to initiate first dose. If not used for more than 24 hours, the pump will require 2 actuations; if not used for more than 7 days, the pump will require 7 actuations to reprime.
- Use of a spacer (eg, *OptiHaler*) with the aerosol may increase the amount of medicine that gets into the bronchial tubes and its effectiveness.
- The aerosol contains enough medication for 200 inhalations. Discard the canister after you have used 200 inhalations. Use of the aerosol after 200 inhalations will not provide the correct amount of medication.
- The aerosol total daily dose should not exceed 12 inhalations in 24 hours. If the recommended dosage does not provide relief or symptoms become worse, contact your doctor immediately.
- Do not use the aerosol with other inhaled drugs unless directed by your doctor.
- Do not use for the treatment of acute episodes of bronchospasm in which rapid response is required. This medicine is considered maintenance therapy. Drugs with faster action may be preferred for initial therapy in this situation.
- Temporary blurring of vision, causing or worsening of narrow-angle glaucoma, or eye pain may occur if the drug comes into contact with the eye. For the solution form, use of a nebulizer with a mouthpiece (rather than a face mask) may be preferable to reduce the chance of getting the solution in the eyes.
- The solution can be mixed in the nebulizer with albuterol. The combination should then be used within 1 hour.
- Inform your doctor if you are pregnant, become pregnant, are planning to become pregnant, or are breastfeeding.
- *Aerosol* — Store at room temperature (59° to 86°F). Avoid excessive humidity.
- *Solution* — Store at room temperature (59° to 86°F) away from light. Store unused vials in the foil pouch.

*If you have any questions, consult your doctor, pharmacist, or health care provider.*

| Generic Name Brand Name Examples | Supplied As | Generic Available |
|---|---|---|
| Rx **Ipratropium Bromide/ Albuterol Sulfate** | | |
| *Combivent* | **Aerosol**: 18 mcg ipratropium bromide/103 mcg albuterol sulfate per actuation | No |
| *DuoNeb* | **Inhalation solution**: 0.5 mg ipratropium bromide/3 mg albuterol sulfate | No |

## Type of Drug:

Combination respiratory inhalant; anticholinergic bronchodilator (ipratropium) and beta$_2$-adrenergic bronchodilator (albuterol).

## How the Drug Works:

Ipratropium blocks the action of the chemical transmitter acetylcholine. Acetylcholine causes the muscles around the bronchial tubes to spasm and constrict, which makes it harder to breathe. By blocking acetylcholine, ipratropium allows these muscles to relax, widening the bronchial tubes (bronchodilation) and allowing more air into the lungs.

Albuterol dilates (opens) the bronchial tubes of the lungs by relaxing the muscles around the bronchial tubes. This allows for easier air flow into and out of the lungs. It also assists in removing (expectorating) mucus and other debris causing congestion in the lungs.

## Uses:

To treat bronchospasm in patients with chronic obstructive pulmonary disease (COPD) who are on a regular inhalant bronchodilator but continue to have symptoms of bronchial tube spasm.

## Precautions:

*Do not use in the following situations:*

allergy to atropine, sympathomimetic amines, or any other ingredients within the drug

allergy to soya lecithin or related food products (eg, soybeans, peanuts) (aerosol only)

*Use with caution in the following situations:*

abnormal heart rhythm
cardiovascular disorders
 (eg, angina)
diabetes mellitus
enlarged prostate
glaucoma, narrow-angle
high blood pressure
kidney disease

liver disease
low blood potassium
 (hypokalemia)
obstruction of the neck of the urinary bladder
overactive thyroid
 (hyperthyroidism)
seizure disorders

*Do not exceed recommended dose:* Deaths have been reported in association with excessive use of inhaled sympathomimetic drugs in patients with asthma.

*Pregnancy:* There are no adequate and well-controlled studies in pregnant women. Use only if clearly needed and the potential benefits outweigh the possible hazards to the fetus.

*Breastfeeding:* It is not known whether ipratropium/albuterol appears in breast milk. Consult your doctor before you begin breastfeeding.

*Children:* Safety and effectiveness in children have not been established.

## Drug Interactions:

Tell your doctor or pharmacist if you are taking or planning to take any over-the-counter or prescription medications or dietary supplements with this drug. Doses of one or both drugs may need to be modified or a different drug may need to be prescribed. The following drugs and drug classes interact with this drug:

anticholinergic agents (eg, dicyclomine)
beta-adrenergic agents (eg, epinephrine)
beta-receptor blocking agents (eg, propranolol)

diuretics (eg, thiazides)
MAOIs (eg, phenelzine)
tricyclic antidepressants (eg, amitriptyline)

## Side Effects:

Every drug is capable of producing side effects. Many patients experience no, or minor, side effects. The frequency and severity of side effects depend on many factors including dose, duration of therapy, and individual susceptibility. Possible side effects include:

*Digestive Tract:* Nausea; vomiting; indigestion; taste changes; dry mouth; diarrhea.

*Nervous System:* Headache; fatigue; sleeplessness; dizziness; nervousness; tremor.

*Respiratory System:* Runny nose; sore throat; coughing; difficulty breathing; bronchospasm; bronchitis; pneumonia; sinus infection; upper respiratory tract infection; flu-like symptoms; increased mucus.

*Circulatory System:* Abnormal heart rhythm; pounding in the chest (palpitations); rapid heartbeat; high blood pressure.

*Other:* Chest, joint, or general body pain; cramps; swelling of feet, ankles, or hands and fingers (edema); difficulty speaking; abnormal skin sensations (eg, burning, prickling, tingling); urinary tract infection; voice alterations.

## Guidelines for Use:

- Read and follow the patient instructions provided.
- Dosage is individualized. Do not exceed recommended dosage. Take exactly as prescribed.
- Do not stop taking or change the dose unless instructed by your doctor.
- Contact your doctor immediately if your medicine becomes less effective, your breathing symptoms become worse, or if you need to use the medicine more frequently than usual.
- If a dose is missed, take it as soon as possible. If several hours have passed or it is nearing time for the next dose, do not double the dose to catch up, unless instructed by your doctor. If more than one dose is missed or it is necessary to establish a new dosage schedule, contact your doctor or pharmacist.
- Inform your doctor if you are pregnant, become pregnant, plan on becoming pregnant, or are breastfeeding.
- Do not take other inhaled drugs during therapy unless instructed by your doctor.
- *Aerosol —*
  Shake aerosol canister well before each use.
  Test spray 3 times before using the first time or if the aerosol has not been used for longer than 24 hours.
  The recommended dose is 2 inhalations 4 times daily, which should last 4 to 5 hours or longer. Additional inhalations may be taken as required, but do not exceed 12 inhalations in 24 hours.
  Use of a spacing device (eg, *Aerochamber*) will enhance effectiveness and decrease side effects.
  Breathe out fully through the mouth, expelling as much air from the lungs as possible. Place the mouthpiece of the inhaler (or spacer) into your mouth and, while breathing deeply and slowly through the mouth, activate the medication canister. Hold your breath for 3 to 5 seconds and then breathe out.
  Wait at least 5 minutes between doses (puffs).
  Avoid spraying the aerosol into the eyes. Thoroughly wash eyes immediately should this occur. Contact your doctor if you experience blurring vision, eye pain or discomfort, visual halos, or colored images.
  Use aerosol canister with the included actuator only. Do not use actuator with other aerosol medications.
  Discard canister after labeled number of actuations have been used. Each canister contains 200 actuations.
  Aerosol contents are under pressure. Do not puncture canister. Do not use or store near heat or open flame. Exposure to temperatures higher than 120°F may cause bursting. Do not throw canister into a fire or incinerator.
  Store at room temperature (59° to 86°F). Avoid excessive humidity.

## Guidelines for Use (cont.):

- *Inhalation solution* —
  The recommended dose is one 3 mL vial administered 4 times per day via rebulization with up to 2 additional 3 mL doses allowed per day, if needed. Safety and efficacy of additional doses or increased frequency of administration beyond these guidelines has not been studied. Squeeze 1 vial of medication into nebulizer chamber. Sit in a comfortable, upright position. Place the mouthpiece in your mouth or put on the face mask. Turn on the compressor. Breathe in as calmly, deeply, and evenly as possible through your mouth until no more mist is formed in the nebulizer chamber (about 5 to 15 minutes). Clean the nebulizer with hot water. Allow to air dry.
  Store between 36° and 77°F. Vials should be protected from light before use. Keep unused vials in box or foil pouch. Do not use after expiration date.

*If you have any questions, consult your doctor, pharmacist, or health care provider.*

| Generic Name<br>*Brand Name Examples* | Supplied As | Generic<br>Available |
|---|---|---|
| *Rx* **Acetylcysteine** | | |
| *Mucomyst, Mucosil-10* | **Solution**: 10% | Yes |
| *Mucomyst, Mucosil-20* | **Solution**: 20% | Yes |
| *Rx* **Dornase Alfa** | | |
| *Pulmozyme* | **Solution**: 1 mg/mL | No |

## Type of Drug:

Respiratory inhalant; drug that thins mucus.

## How the Drug Works:

Acetylcysteine decreases the thickness and stickiness of mucus secretions of the lung, making them easier to cough up, and therefore promoting removal (expectoration) of this fluid.

Dornase alfa decreases the thickness and stickiness of mucus secretions of cystic fibrosis patients.

## Uses:

*Acetylcysteine:* To treat abnormally thick mucus secretions in chronic emphysema, emphysema with bronchitis, chronic asthmatic bronchitis, tuberculosis, bronchiectasis (chronic dilation of the airways), pneumonia, bronchitis, tacheobronchitis, cystic fibrosis, and other conditions involving excess mucus accumulation in the lung that is significant enough to affect breathing.

To reduce abnormally thick mucus secretion during tracheostomy care and diagnostic bronchial tests (eg, bronchograms, bronchospirometry, bronchial wedge catheterization).

To reduce abnormally thick mucus secretions during anesthesia in or after surgery or chest injuries.

As an emergency oral antidote drug to decrease liver damage after acetaminophen (eg, *Tylenol)* poisoning.

*Dornase alfa:* To reduce frequency of respiratory infections requiring parenteral (injectable) antibiotics and to improve pulmonary function in conjunction with standard therapies for patients with cystic fibrosis.

*Unlabeled Use(s):* Occasionally, doctors may prescribe acetylcysteine as an eye solution to treat severe dry eyes or as an enema to treat bowel obstruction.

## Precautions:

*Do not use in the following situations:* Allergy to acetylcysteine, dornase alfa, Chinese hamster ovary cell products (dornase alfa only), or any other ingredients within the drug.

*Use with caution in the following situations:*
asthma (eg, bronchospasm)
inadequate cough reflex
liver failure

*Prolonged use:* Safety and effectiveness of daily administration of dornase alfa for longer than 12 months have not been established.

*Pregnancy:* There are no adequate or well-controlled studies in pregnant women. Use only if clearly needed and the potential benefits to the mother outweigh the possible hazards to the fetus.

*Breastfeeding:* It is not known if acetylcysteine or dornase alfa appear in breast milk. Consult your doctor before you begin breastfeeding.

*Children:* Safety and effectiveness of dornase alfa in children younger than 5 years of age have not been established.

## Side Effects:
Every drug is capable of producing side effects. Many mucolytic users experience no, or minor, side effects. The frequency and severity of side effects depend on many factors including dose, duration of therapy, and individual susceptibility. Possible side effects include:

*Respiratory System:* Increased mucus; runny nose; sore throat; voice changes; voice loss; cough; difficulty breathing; bronchitis; bronchspasm (spasm of the air tubes); chest tightness.

*Digestive Tract:* Nausea; vomiting; stomach pain; mouth inflammation.

*Other:* Fever; rash; drowsiness; eye inflammation; clamminess.

## Guidelines for Use:

- Dosage is individualized. Take exactly as prescribed.
- Do not stop taking or change the dose unless directed by your doctor.
- If a dose is missed, inhale it as soon as possible. If several hours have passed or it is nearing time for the next dose, do not double the dose to catch up, unless advised to do so by your doctor. If more than one dose is missed or it is necessary to establish a new dosage schedule, contact your doctor or pharmacist.
- Discontinue therapy if symptoms of allergy appear, unless symptoms can be controlled with other drugs and therapy is considered essential.
- Inform your doctor if you are pregnant, become pregnant, plan on becoming pregnant, or are breastfeeding.
- Do not mix other drugs in the nebulizer unless advised to do so by your doctor.
- Only administer with equipment provided by, or recommended by, your doctor.
- *Acetylcysteine* — Follow dilution and administration techniques taught by your doctor.
  When used to treat acetaminophen poisoning, it will be prepared and administered by a health care professional in a medical setting.
  May produce an increased volume of liquified secretions that must be coughed up. Notify your doctor if you have difficulty coughing up these secretions.
  May initially produce a slight disagreeable odor which soon disappears.
  May cause a stickiness on the face after nebulization with a face mask. This can be easily removed by washing with water.
  Color of the solution may change in the opened bottle, but the light purple color does not significantly reduce the drug's safety or effectiveness if used within 96 hours after opening.
  The 20% solution may be diluted with either Normal Saline, Water for Injection, or Sterile Water for inhalation. The 10% solution may be used undiluted.
  Continued nebulization of acetylcysteine with a dry gas results in concentration of the drug in the nebulizer due to evaporation. This may reduce nebulization and drug delivery. Dilute with Sterile Water for Injection as concentration occurs.
  Store unopened vial at controlled room temperature (59° to 86°F). Store unused portion in refrigerator once opened and use within 96 hours.
- *Dornase alfa* — The recommended dose is one 2.5 mg single-use ampule inhaled once daily using a recommended nebulizer. Some patients may benefit from twice daily administration. Use in conjunction with standard therapies for cystic fibrosis.
  Discard solution if it is cloudy or discolored. Dornase alfa contains no preservatives; therefore, once opened, the entire ampule must be used or discarded.
  Do not dilute or mix dornase with other drugs in the nebulizer.
  Store in protective foil pouch under refrigeration (36° to 46°F). Protect from light. Do not use beyond the expiration date.

*If you have any questions, consult your doctor, pharmacist, or health care provider.*

| Generic Name<br>*Brand Name Example* | Supplied As | Generic<br>Available |
|---|---|---|
| Rx **Nedocromil Sodium** | | |
| *Tilade* | **Aerosol:** 1.75 mg/actuation | No |

## Type of Drug:
Respiratory inhalant.

## How the Drug Works:
Nedocromil sodium inhibits the activity of inflammatory cells associated with asthma.

## Uses:
As maintenance therapy in the management of mild to moderate bronchial asthma. Nedocromil sodium is not used to reverse acute bronchospasm.

## Precautions:
*Do not use in the following situations:* Allergy to nedocromil sodium or any ingredient in the product.

*Pregnancy:* Adequate studies have not been done in pregnant women. Use only if clearly needed and potential benefits outweigh the possible hazards to the fetus.

*Breastfeeding:* It is not known if nedocromil sodium appears in breast milk. Consult your doctor before you begin breastfeeding.

*Children:* Safety and effectiveness in children under 12 have not been established.

## Side Effects:
Every drug is capable of producing side effects. Many nedocromil sodium users experience no, or minor, side effects. The frequency and severity of side effects depend on many factors including dose, duration of therapy and individual susceptibility. Possible side effects include:

*Digestive Tract:* Nausea; vomiting; indigestion; diarrhea; stomach pain.

*Nervous System:* Dizziness; headache; fatigue; difficulty speaking.

*Respiratory System:* Coughing; sore throat; congestion; upper respiratory tract infection; increased sputum; bronchitis; difficulty breathing; wheezing.

*Other:* Dry mouth; chest pain; viral infection; unpleasant taste.

## Guidelines for Use:

- Proper inhalation technique is very important. Follow the directions that are in the patient information leaflet that is included with the medicine.
- Use continuously. Effectiveness depends on regularity of use, even during symptom-free periods.
- Notify your doctor if coughing or wheezing occurs.
- Not for the treatment of an existing asthma attack. Nedocromil sodium should generally be continued during an asthma attack though, unless intolerance develops.
- This medicine should be added to your existing treatment therapy. Once a positive response is made to the inhaler, and the asthma is under good control, your doctor may gradually reduce your other medicine usage.

*If you have any questions, consult your doctor, pharmacist, or health care provider.*

| Generic Name<br>*Brand Name*<br>*Examples* | Supplied As | Generic<br>Available |
|---|---|---|
| *Rx* **Beclomethasone Dipropionate** | | |
| *Beconase* | **Aerosol**: 0.042% (42 mcg/actuation) | No |
| *Beconase AQ* | **Spray**: 0.042% (42 mcg/actuation) | No |
| *Vancenase AQ* | **Spray**: 0.084% (84 mcg/actuation) | No |
| *Rx* **Budesonide** | | |
| *Rhinocort* | **Aerosol**: 0.032% (32 mcg/actuation) | No |
| *Rhinocort Aqua* | **Spray**: 0.032% (32 mcg/actuation) | No |
| *Rx* **Flunisolide** | | |
| *Nasalide, Nasarel* | **Spray**: 0.025% (25 mcg/actuation) | Yes |
| *Rx* **Fluticasone Propionate** | | |
| *Flonase* | **Spray**: 0.05% (50 mcg/actuation) | No |
| *Rx* **Mometasone Furoate Monohydrate** | | |
| *Nasonex* | **Spray**: 0.05% (50 mcg/actuation) | No |
| *Rx* **Triamcinolone Acetonide** | | |
| *Nasacort* | **Aerosol**: 0.055% (55 mcg/actuation) | No |
| *Nasacort AQ* | **Spray**: 0.055% (55 mcg/actuation) | No |

## Type of Drug:

Nasal corticosteroids; anti-inflammatory agents.

## How the Drug Works:

Intranasal steroids for inhalation shrink swollen and irritated nasal tissue primarily by reducing inflammation, but also by constricting blood vessels of the nasal mucosa.

## Uses:

To relieve nasal symptoms of seasonal or perennial allergic rhinitis (eg, hay fever), which involves inflammation of the mucous membranes of the nasal passages. Symptoms of allergic rhinitis include itching of the nose and eyes, runny nose, postnasal drip, nasal congestion, and sneezing.

*Budesonide and beclomethasone (spray):* Used to treat nonallergic perennial rhinitis in adults.

*Beclomethasone:* Used to prevent the recurrence of nasal polyps after surgical removal.

## Precautions:

*Do not use in the following situations:*

allergy to the drug or any of its ingredients

infection of the nasal mucous membranes, untreated

*Use with caution in the following situations:*

children (growth suppression),
extended use
chickenpox exposure
herpes simplex eye infection
immunosuppressant (eg, prednisone, methotrexate) use
infections (fungal, bacterial, or
viral), untreated

lesions (sores, injuries) in nasal
tissue (eg, nasal surgery, frequent nosebleed)
measles, exposure
orally inhaled glucocorticoids
use
stress, related to adrenal insufficiency
tuberculosis, active or inactive

*Changing from other dosage forms:* Patients on long-term oral corticosteroids may lose their body's natural ability to produce corticosteroid hormones. Switching or lessening current doses may cause symptoms of
withdrawal (eg, joint or muscle pain, tiredness, depression). Therefore,
taper dosage of oral steroid gradually and only with the instruction of
a doctor.

*Intranasal steroids:* Intranasal steroids are absorbed into the blood stream.
Using higher than recommended doses may interfere with normal adrenal functions.

*Nasal decongestants:* In the presence of excessive nasal congestion, the
drug may fail to reach the site of intended action. In such cases, use a
nasal decongestant spray just before use during the first 2 to 3 days of
therapy. Do not use a nasal decongestant spray for more than 3 consecutive days.

*Pregnancy:* Adequate studies have not been done in pregnant women. Use
only if clearly needed and potential benefits outweigh the possible hazards to the fetus.

*Breastfeeding:* It is not known whether these drugs are excreted in breast
milk. Other corticosteroids do appear in breast milk. Consult your
doctor before you begin breastfeeding.

*Children:* Safety and effectiveness in children under 3 years of age
(mometasone), under 4 years of age (fluticasone), or under 6 years of
age (beclomethasone, budesonide, flunisolide, triamcinolone) have not
been established. Use is not recommended. May suppress growth in
children and teenagers with extended use.

## Drug Interactions:

Tell your doctor or pharmacist if you are taking or planning to take any over-
the-counter or prescription medications or dietary supplements while taking these drugs. Doses of one or both drugs may need to be modified
or a different drug may need to be prescribed. The following drugs or
drug classes interacts with these drugs:

cytochrome P-450 3A4 inhibitors (eg, erythromycin, ketoconazole, ritonavir)

glucocorticoids (eg, prednisone)
immunosuppressants
(eg, methotrexate)

## Side Effects:

Every drug is capable of producing side effects. Many patients experience no, or minor, side effects. The frequency and severity of side effects depend on many factors including dose, duration of therapy, and individual susceptibility. Possible side effects include:

*Nervous System:* Headache; light-headedness; dizziness; nervousness.

*Digestive Tract:* Nausea; vomiting; dry mouth; indigestion; diarrhea; stomach pain.

*Eyes or Ocular:* Watery eyes; eye disorders; eye infection; cataracts; dry or irritated eyes; glaucoma; blurred vision.

*Respiratory System:* Nasal or throat irritation; stinging; burning; dryness; nosebleed; runny nose; sneezing (especially in children); blood in nasal mucus; congestion; asthma; increased cough; sore throat; thrush or sores in nose or throat; nasal pain; difficulty breathing; wheezing.

*Other:* Joint or muscle pain; weakness; depression; sense of smell or taste changes; earache; ringing in ears; painful menstruation; fever; flu-like symptoms; aches and pains; herpes simplex; hoarseness; infection; voice changes; facial swelling; hives; rash; itching.

## Guidelines for Use:

- Dosage is individualized. Take exactly as prescribed.
- Do not stop taking or change the dose, unless instructed by your doctor. Do not exceed the recommended dosage.
- Read and follow patient instructions provided with these products.
- If a dose is missed, take it as soon as possible. If several hours have passed or it is nearing time for the next dose, do not double the dose to catch up, unless instructed by your doctor. If more than one dose is missed, or it is necessary to establish a new dosage schedule, contact your doctor or pharmacist.
- Effects are not immediate. Product requires daily use, and improvement usually occurs in a few days. Improvement time varies with each patient. Consult your doctor if condition does not improve or worsens after 3 weeks of daily use.
- May cause irritation and drying of nasal mucosa. Contact your doctor if symptoms do not improve, if the condition worsens, if sneezing or nasal irritation occurs, or if symptoms do not improve within 3 weeks.
- Report any unusual fever, muscle or joint pain, weakness, sneezing, dizziness, nasal irritation, depression, or fluid retention to your doctor.
- Clear nasal passages prior to use by blowing the nose. If nasal passages are congested or blocked, use a decongestant nasal spray just before use to ensure adequate penetration of the spray. Do not use the decongestant nasal spray for more than 3 consecutive days.
- Shake the nasal inhaler, pump, or spray before using. Keep head upright and close one nostril with a finger. With mouth closed, insert the tip of the device into the open nostril. Sniff in through the nostril while quickly activating the device. Hold breath for a few seconds and exhale out of the mouth. Shake device again and repeat procedure for the other nostril if directed to do so. Rinse the inhaler, pump, or spray tip with hot water and replace the cap on the container.

## Guidelines for Use (cont.):

- Clean outer portion of the nose with a damp tissue and wash hands with soap and water after drug administration.
- Infection of the nose and throat by a fungus (*Candida albicans*) has been associated with chronic use. Such infection (thrush) may require stopping the intranasal steroid to treat the infection.
- Avoid exposure to chickenpox, measles, or other infections. Consult your doctor immediately if exposed.
- *Nasal polyps* — Treatment may have to be continued for several weeks or more before results can be fully assessed. Recurrence of symptoms due to polyps can occur after stopping treatment, depending on the severity of the disease.
- Inform your doctor if you are pregnant, become pregnant, planning to become pregnant, or are breastfeeding.
- Lab tests may be required if you are using this medicine for several months. Be sure to keep appointments.
- *Beclomethasone* — Beneficial effects may decrease when the aerosol canister is cold. This medicine comes in different strengths and dosage forms. Products and use may not be interchangeable.
- *Budesonide* — Store with valve upward. After opening aluminum pouch, use within 6 months. Avoid storage in areas of high humidity.
- *Fluticasone* — Do not exceed more than 2 sprays per nostril per day. Adolescents and children should start at one spray per nostril per day.
- *Mometasone* — In patients with known seasonal allergies, preventive use is recommended 2 to 4 weeks prior to the start of pollen season.
- Store at room temperature (59° to 86°F) in a dry place. Store mometasone at 36° to 77°F. Protect from light and moisture.

*If you have any questions, consult your doctor, pharmacist, or health care provider.*

| Generic Name<br>*Brand Name Examples* | Supplied As | Generic<br>Available |
|---|---|---|
| *Rx* **Azatadine Maleate** | | |
| *Optimine*[1] | **Tablets**: 1 mg | No |
| *Rx* **Azelastine** | | |
| *Astelin* | **Nasal spray**: 137 mcg/spray | No |
| *Rx* **Cetirizine HCl** | | |
| *Zyrtec* | **Tablets**: 5 mg, 10 mg | No |
| *Zyrtec* | **Syrup**: 5 mg/5 mL | No |
| **Chlorpheniramine Maleate** | | |
| *otc* *Chlo-Amine* | **Tablets, chewable**: 2 mg | No |
| *otc* *Allergy*[1] | **Tablets**: 4 mg | Yes |
| *otc* *Chlor-Trimeton Allergy 8-Hour, Chlor-Trimeton Allergy 12-Hour, Efidac 24* | **Tablets, extended release**: 8 mg, 12 mg, 16 mg | Yes |
| **Clemastine Fumarate** | | |
| *otc* *Antihist-1*[1], *Dayhist-1*[1], *Tavist Allergy*[1] | **Tablets**: 1.34 mg | Yes |
| *Rx* *Tavist*[1] | **Tablets**: 2.68 mg | Yes |
| *otc* *Aller-Chlor, Chlor-Trimeton* | **Syrup**: 0.5mg/5 mL | Yes |
| *Rx* **Cyproheptadine HCl** | | |
| *Periactin*[1] | **Tablets**: 4 mg | Yes |
| *Periactin*[2] | **Syrup**: 2 mg/5 mL | Yes |
| *Rx* **Dexchlorpheniramine Maleate** | | |
| *Polaramine*[1] | **Tablets**: 2 mg | No |
| *Polaramine Repetabs* | **Tablets, timed release**: 4 mg, 6 mg | Yes |
| *Polaramine*[2] | **Syrup**: 2 mg/5 mL | Yes |

| Generic Name<br>*Brand Name Examples* | Supplied As | Generic<br>Available |
|---|---|---|
| **Diphenhydramine HCl** | | |
| *otc Banophen[1], Banophen Softgels, Benadryl Dye-Free Allergy Liqui-Gels, Complete Allergy Relief, Diphen, Diphenhist[1], Genahist[1]* | **Capsules**: 25 mg, 50 mg | Yes |
| *Rx Diphenhydramine HCl* | **Capsules**: 25 mg, 50 mg | Yes |
| *otc AllerMax[1], Banophen, Benadryl Allergy Ultratab, Diphenhist Captabs[1]* | **Tablets**: 25 mg, 50 mg | Yes |
| *otc Benadryl Allergy[3]* | **Tablets, chewable**: 12.5 mg | No |
| *otc AllerMax Allergy and Cough Formula[2], Banophen Allergy, Benadryl Allergy, Benadryl Dye-Free Allergy, Diphen AF, Genahist, Scot-Tussin Allergy* | **Liquid**: 6.25 mg/5 mL, 12.5 mg/5 mL | No |
| *otc Diphen Cough[2], Diphenhist[2], Hydramine Cough[2]* | **Syrup**: 12.5 mg/5 mL | Yes |
| *Rx Benadryl, Hyrexin-50* | **Injection**: 50 mg/mL | Yes |
| *Rx* **Fexofenadine HCl** | | |
| *Allegra* | **Tablets**: 30 mg, 60 mg, 180 mg | No |
| *Allegra[1]* | **Capsules**: 60 mg | No |
| *Rx* **Hydroxyzine** | | |
| *Atarax[1]* | **Tablets**: 10 mg, 25 mg, 50 mg (as HCl) | Yes |
| *Atarax 100[1]* | **Tablets**: 100 mg (as HCl) | No |
| *Atarax[1]* | **Syrup**: 10 mg/5 mL (as HCl) | Yes |
| *Vistaril* | **Capsules**: 25 mg, 50 mg, 100 mg (as pamoate) | Yes |
| *Vistaril* | **Suspension, oral**: 25 mg/5 mL (as pamoate) | No |
| *Vistaril* | **Injection**: 25 mg/mL, 50 mg/mL (as HCl) | No |

| Generic Name<br>*Brand Name Examples* | Supplied As | Generic<br>Available |
|---|---|---|
| *Rx* **Loratadine** | | |
| *Claritin*[1] | **Tablets**: 10 mg | No |
| *Claritin* | **Syrup**: 1 mg/mL | No |
| *Claritin Reditabs* | **Tablets, rapidly disintegrating**: 10 mg | No |
| *otc* **Phenindamine Tartrate** | | |
| *Nolahist* | **Tablets**: 25 mg | No |
| *Rx* **Promethazine HCl** | | |
| *Phenergan*[1] | **Tablets**: 12.5 mg, 25 mg, 50 mg | Yes |
| *Phenergan Plain*,[2]<br>*Phenergan Fortis*[2] | **Syrup**: 6.25 mg/5 mL, 25 mg/ 5 mL | Yes |
| *Phenergan* | **Suppositories**: 12.5 mg, 25 mg, 50 mg | Yes |
| *Phenergan*[4] | **Injection**: 25 mg/mL, 50 mg/mL | Yes |

[1] Contains lactose.
[2] Contains alcohol.
[3] Contains aspartame.
[4] Contains sulfites.

## Type of Drug:
Antihistamine; allergy medications.

## How the Drug Works:
Antihistamines block the effects of histamine at $H_1$ receptors in the body. Histamine is one of the chemicals released in the body during an allergic reaction. It causes redness, itching, and irritation of respiratory mucosal tissues, and can cause watery eyes, runny nose, sneezing, itchy nose, eyes, palate, and throat, and hives.

## Uses:
To provide relief of symptoms associated with seasonal and year-round allergies causing runny nose, sneezing, itching of the nose or throat, or watery, itchy eyes; hives; and rash, insect bites, and stings where there is mild to moderate itching and no complications.

*Certizine and fexofenadine:* To treat chronic idiopathic urticaria (hives).

*Diphenhydramine:* To treat or prevent motion sickness, sleeplessness, and parkinsonism. Also used as a suppressant for coughs caused by colds or allergies.

*Promethazine:* To treat or prevent motion sickness, nausea, and vomiting associated with anesthesia and surgery, apprehension, and sleeplessness. Used with pain medication (eg, meperidine) to help control pain following surgery.

*Unlabeled Use(s):* Occasionally doctors may prescribe cyproheptadine to stimulate appetite in underweight people (eg, anorexia nervosa) and to treat cluster headaches.

## Precautions:

*Do not use in the following situations:*

alcohol and other depressants (eg, tranquilizers)
allergy to antihistamines
anesthesia, local
bone marrow depression
breastfeeding
digestive tract obstruction
enlarged prostate
glaucoma, narrow angle
liver disease
MAOI use, concurrent
newborns or premature infants
peptic ulcer
ulcers (promethazine only)
urinary bladder obstruction

*Use with caution in the following situations:*

asthma
hypertension (high blood pressure)
hyperthyroidism (overactive thyroid)
increased pressure in the eye
kidney disease
liver disease
pregnancy
seizures (promethazine only)

*Pregnancy:* Safety for use during pregnancy has not been established. Several possible associations with malformations have been found, but significance is unknown. Use only when clearly needed and the potential benefits outweigh the possible hazards to the fetus. Do not use during the third trimester; newborns and premature infants may have severe reactions (eg, convulsions) to some antihistamines.

*Breastfeeding:* Antihistamines appear in breast milk. Breastfeeding should be discouraged while taking these medications, or antihistamines should be avoided during the breastfeeding months.

*Children:* Antihistamine overdosage in children may cause hallucinations, convulsions, or death. Antihistamines may decrease mental alertness or produce hyperactivity in young children. Consult your pharmacist or product label to determine the appropriate dose of nonprescription drugs to be given to children younger than 12 years of age. Do not give prescription antihistamines to children younger than 12 years of age unless advised by your doctor or approved in the package labeling.

*Elderly:* Elderly patients may require lower doses. Antihistamines are more likely to cause dizziness, sedation, confusion, disorientation, fainting, excitation, and decreased blood pressure.

## Drug Interactions:

Tell your doctor or pharmacist if you are taking or planning to take any over-the-counter or prescription medications or dietary supplements while taking antihistamines. Doses of one or both drugs may need to be modified or a different drug may need to be prescribed. Alcohol, sedatives (sleeping pills), tranquilizers, antianxiety medications, and narcotic pain relievers all are known to interact with antihistamines. The following drugs and drug classes also interact antihistamines:

aluminum- and magnesium-containing antacids (eg, *Maalox*)
anesthesia (promethazine only)
barbiturates (promethazine only)
cimetidine (azelastine only)
epinephrine (eg, *Adrenalin*)
erythromycin (eg, *E-Mycin*) (fexofenadine only)
ketoconazole (eg, *Nizoral*)
MAOIs (eg, phenelzine)
tricyclic antidepressants (eg, *Elavil*)

## Side Effects:

Every drug is capable of producing side effects. Many antihistamine users experience no, or minor, side effects. The frequency and severity of side effects depend on many factors including dose, duration of therapy, and individual susceptibility. Possible side effects include:

*Digestive Tract:* Stomachache; constipation; appetite changes; nausea; vomiting; diarrhea; indigestion; decreased salivation; gas; altered sense of taste; dry mouth.

*Nervous System:* Drowsiness; dizziness; confusion; disorientation; nervousness; restlessness; excitation; tremor; decreased coordination; fatigue; headache; sleeplessness; sedation; irritability; exaggerated sense of well being; fainting; migraine; abnormal skin sensations; feeling of whirling motion; impaired concentration; hallucination; hysteria; amnesia; abnormal thinking; agitation; anxiety; depersonalization; depression; convulsions.

*Circulatory System:* Changes in blood pressure; irregular heartbeat; fast heartbeat; shock; palpitations (pounding in the chest); chest pain.

*Respiratory System:* Dry nose and throat; cough; sore throat; thickening of mucus in respiratory tract; chest tightness; wheezing; nasal stuffiness; hyperventilation; upper respiratory tract infection; laryngitis; bronchospasm; nasal and throat burning; nosebleed; difficulty breathing; sneezing.

*Skin:* Rash; hives; sweating; itching; flushing; dry skin; excessively oily skin; skin inflammation; red or purple patches under the skin; acne; excessive sweating; hair loss.

*Other:* Weight gain; joint pain; muscle pain; sensitivity to light; frequent, abnormal, or difficult urination; urine retention; ringing in the ears; blurred or double vision; itchy, watery eyes; yellowing of skin or eyes; chills; painful menstruation (loratadine and fexofenadine only); thirst; earache; fever; leg cramps; weakness; decreased sensitivity to stimulation; eye pain or abnormality; altered tearing; twitching eyes; tight muscles; breast pain; heavy menstruation; allergic reaction; back pain; "flu-like" symptoms; general body discomfort; pain in extremities; twitching; decreased sex drive; excessive movement; inflammation of the vagina with itching or abnormal discharge; urinary discoloration; distorted sense of smell; hot flashes; anemia.

## Guidelines for Use:
- Dosage is individualized. Use exacty as prescribed.
- If a dose is missed, take it as soon as possible. If several hours have passed or it is nearing time for the next dose, do not double the dose to catch up, unless advised by your doctor. If more than one dose is missed or it is necessary to establish a new dosage schedule, contact your doctor or pharmacist.
- Loratadine tablets and syrup should be taken once daily on an empty stomach (1 hour before or 2 hours after a meal). Loratadine rapidly-disintegrating tablets break down quickly after being placed on the tongue; they may be given with or without water.
- Do not crush or chew sustained-release products.
- May cause drowsiness or dizziness. Avoid alcohol and other sedatives (eg, tranquilizers). Chlorpheniramine, loratadine, cetirizine, and fexofenadine cause the least amount of drowsiness; promethazine and diphenhydramine cause the most. Use caution while driving or performing tasks requiring alertness, coordination, or physical dexterity.
- *Promethazine* — Report any involuntary muscle movements or unusual sensitivity to sunlight.
- Use alone when sneezing and runny nose exist, but nasal congestion is slight. When nasal congestion accompanies sneezing and runny nose, an oral decongestant (eg, pseudoephedrine) may be added.
- Avoid therapy with combination products containing antihistamines, decongestants, anticholinergics, expectorants, pain medication, cough suppressants, caffeine, and vitamins. Deal with symptoms as specifically as possible. Combination products frequently contain some ingredients in ineffective amounts. They increase risk for side effects and drug interactions, and usually cost more than products with fewer ingredients.
- A persistent cough may be a sign of a serious condition. Contact your doctor if cough persists for more than 1 week, tends to recur, or is accompanied by a high fever, rash, or persistent headache.
- Do not take antihistamines for persistent or chronic cough, such as occurs with smoking, asthma, or emphysema or if cough is accompanied by excessive phlegm, unless directed by a doctor. Cough is a protective reflex that helps clear the respiratory tract of mucus and other debris.
- Do not take for 7 days before allergy skin testing.
- Contact your doctor immediately if you experience fainting, dizziness, unusual heartbeats, stomach pain, chest pain, vomiting, or any other unusual symptoms occur,
- If sleeplessness persists continuously for more than 2 weeks, consult your doctor.
- If the medication loses effectiveness with continued use, make sure you are taking it according to directions. Sometimes, loss of effectiveness indicates that your condition has gotten worse. Treatment may require a different medication or dose.
- May rarely cause photosensitivity (sensitivity to sunlight). Avoid prolonged exposure to the sun or other forms of ultraviolet (UV) light (eg, tanning beds). Use sunscreens and wear protective clothing until tolerance is determined.

## Guidelines for Use (cont.):

- *Azelastine* — Prime the nasal spray delivery system before initial use and after storage for 3 or more days. Avoid spraying in the eyes.
- Store at room temperature (59° to 77°F) in a tightly closed container. Protect from heat, light, and moisture. Keep away from children.
- *Suppositories and some syrups* — Store in the refrigerator (36° to 46°F) in a tightly closed container. See individual labels for specific storage information.

*If you have any questions, consult your doctor, pharmacist, or health care provider.*

| Generic Name<br>*Brand Name Examples* | **Supplied As** | Generic<br>Available |
|---|---|---|
| *otc* **Ephedrine Sulfate** | | |
| *Pretz-D Nasal Spray* | **Solution**: 0.25% | No |
| *Rx* **Epinephrine HCl** | | |
| *Adrenalin Chloride*[1] | **Solution**: 0.1% | No |
| *otc* **Naphazoline HCl** | | |
| *Privine Nasal Drops and Spray* | **Solution**: 0.05% | No |
| *otc* **Oxymetazoline HCl** | | |
| *4-Way 12 Hour Nasal Spray, Afrin Extra Moisturizing Nasal Spray, Afrin Original 12 Hour Decongestant Nasal Spray, Afrin Severe Congestion Nasal Spray with Menthol, Afrin Sinus 12 Hour Nasal Spray, Dristan 12-hr Nasal Spray, Duramist Plus Nasal Spray, Duration 12 Hour Nasal Spray, Genasal Nasal Spray, Long-Acting Nasal Relief Spray. Nasal Relief Spray, Neo-Synephrine 12-Hour Extra Moisturizing Nasal Spray, Neo-Synephrine 12-Hour Nasal Spray, Nostrilla 12 Hour Nasal Spray, Twice-A-Day 12 Hour Nasal Spray, Vicks Sinex 12 Hour Nasal Spray and Ultra Fine Mist* | **Solution**: 0.05% | Yes |
| *otc* **Phenylephrine HCl** | | |
| *AH-chew D* | **Tablets, chewable**: 10 mg | No |
| *4-Way Fast Acting Nasal Spray, Neo-Synephrine Extra Strength Nasal Drops and Spray* | **Solution**: 1% | Yes |
| *Neo-Synephrine Regular Strength Nasal Drops and Spray, Vicks Sinex Nasal Spray and Ultra Fine Mist* | **Solution**: 0.5% | No |
| *Afrin Children's Nasal Decongestant Spray, Neo-Synephrine Mild Strength Nasal Spray, Rhinall Nose Drops[1] and Spray[1]* | **Solution**: 0.25% | No |
| *Tur-Bi-Kal Nasal Drops* | **Solution**: 0.17% | No |

| Generic Name<br>*Brand Name Examples* | Supplied As | Generic<br>Available |
|---|---|---|
| *otc* **Pseudoephedrine HCl** | | |
| *Genafed, Medi-First Sinus Deconges-<br>tant, Ridafed, Sudafed, Sudodrin, Sudo-<br>Gest* | **Tablets**: 30 mg | Yes |
| *Children's Sudafed², Triaminic Allergy<br>Congestion Softchews²* | **Tablets,<br>chewable**:<br>15 mg | No |
| *Dimetapp 12 Hour Non-Drowsy<br>Extentabs, Sudafed 12 Hour Caplets,<br>Suphedrine 12 Hour* | **Tablets,<br>extended<br>release**: 120 mg | No |
| *Efidac 24 Pseudoephedrine, Sudafed<br>24 Hour* | **Tablets**:<br>240 mg (60 mg<br>immediate-<br>release,<br>180 mg<br>controlled-<br>release) | No |
| *Dimetapp Decongestant Liqui-Gels* | **Capsules**:<br>30 mg | No |
| *Sinustop* | **Capsules**:<br>60 mg | No |
| *Dimetapp Decongestant Infant Drops,<br>PediaCare Infants' Drops* | **Liquid**:<br>7.5 mg/0.8 mL | Yes |
| *Children's Sudafed, Triaminic AM* | **Liquid**:<br>15 mg/5 mL | No |
| *Children's Decofed, Children's Silfed-<br>rine* | **Liquid**:<br>30 mg/5 mL | Yes |
| *otc* **Pseudoephedrine Sulfate** | | |
| *Drixoral Non-Drowsy 12 Hour Relief* | **Tablets,<br>extended<br>release**: 120 mg | No |
| *Rx* **Tetrahydrozoline HCl** | | |
| *Tyzine Pediatric Nasal Drops* | **Solution**: 0.05% | No |
| *Tyzine Nasal Drops and Spray* | **Solution**: 0.1% | No |
| *otc* **Xylometazoline HCl** | | |
| *Otrivin Pediatric Nasal Drops* | **Solution**: 0.05% | No |
| *Natru-vent Nasal Spray, Otrivin Nasal<br>Drops and Spray* | **Solution**: 0.1% | No |

| Generic Name<br>*Brand Name Examples* | Supplied As | Generic<br>Available |
|---|---|---|
| **Nasal Decongestant Combinations** | | |
| *otc*   *Dristan Fast Acting Formula Nasal Spray* | **Solution**: 0.5% phenylephrine HCl and 0.2% pheniramine maleate | No |
| **Nasal Decongestant Inhalers** | | |
| *otc*   *Benzedrex* | **Inhaler**: 250 mg propylhexedrine | No |
| *otc*   *Vicks Vapor Inhaler* | **Inhaler**: 50 mg levmetamfet-amine | No |
| **Nasal Products** | | |
| *otc*   *Afrin Saline Nasal Spray, Pediamist Nasal Spray, Pretz Irrigation, Pretz Nasal Spray* | **Solution**: Sodium chloride | Yes |
| *otc*   *SalineX Nasal Drops and Spray* | **Solution**: 0.4% sodium chloride | No |
| *otc*   *Ayr Saline Nasal Drops and Spray, Baby Ayr Nasal Drops and Spray, Breathe Free Nasal Spray, Breathe Right Saline Nasal Spray, HuMist Moisturizing Nasal Mist, Little Noses Saline Nasal Drops and Spray, Moisturizing Nasal Spray, Nasal Moist Nasal Spray, NaSal Nasal Drops and Spray, Ocean Nasal Drops and Spray* | **Solution**: 0.65% sodium chloride | Yes |
| *otc*   *Natru-vent Saline Nasal Spray, Simply Saline Nasal Spray* | **Solution**: 0.9% sodium chloride | No |
| *otc*   *Ayr Saline, Little Noses Moisturizing Saline, Nasal Moist* | **Gel**: Sodium chloride | No |

[1] Contains sodium bisulfite.
[2] Contains phenylalanine.

## Type of Drug:

Nasal decongestants.

## How the Drug Works:

Nasal decongestants shrink swollen and congested nasal tissues (mucous membranes) by constricting blood vessels. This should relieve congestion (stuffy feeling), promote drainage of mucus, and improve breathing. Local application (eg, nasal drops, sprays) causes more intense and rapid nasal decongestion than oral drugs (eg, tablets, syrup). Oral drugs generally last longer, cause less local irritation, and are not associated with rebound nasal congestion (rhinitis medicamentosa).

## Uses:

For temporary relief of nasal congestion due to the common cold, hay fever, and other upper respiratory allergies, and sinusitis.

To treat eustachian tube congestion (plugged ears).

To promote nasal or sinus drainage.

To relieve ear pressure and pain in air travel.

*Sodium chloride:* To restore moisture to nasal tissue, thin nasal secretions, and relieve dry, crusted, and inflamed nasal membranes due to colds, low humidity, nasal decongestant overuse, allergies, nosebleeds, sinus infection, and other irritations.

## Precautions:

*Do not use in the following situations:*

allergy to the nasal decongestant or any of its ingredients
high blood pressure, severe (oral doseforms only)
MAOI (eg, phenelzine) use, current or within the previous 14 days

*Use with caution in the following situations:*

angina (chest pain)
bowel obstruction or narrowing (pseudoephedrine extended-release only)
breastfeeding (oral doseforms only)
coronary artery disease (oral doseforms only)
diabetes mellitus
dizziness with previous use
elderly
glaucoma
heart disease
high blood pressure
hyperthyroidism (overactive thyroid)
insomnia (sleeplessness) with previous use
irregular heartbeat with previous use
prostatic hypertrophy (enlarged prostate)
weakness with previous use

*Excessive use:* Excessive use of topical decongestants may cause side effects (eg, nervousness, dizziness, sleeplessness) that are more likely in infants and in the elderly. Long-term high-dose therapy may be habit forming (ie, rebound congestion).

*Hypertension (high blood pressure):* Use these products only with medical advice. You may experience a change in blood pressure because of the increased narrowing of the blood vessels.

*Phenylketonuria patients:* Some of these drugs contains phenylalanine. Consult your doctor or pharmacist.

*Rebound congestion:* Rebound congestion (rhinitis medicamentosa) may occur following several days of regular topical application. Rebound congestion, which is worse than the original symptoms, occurs when the drug wears off. Increasing the amount of drug or frequency of use only worsens rebound congestion and increases the risks of medication toxicity. Talk to your doctor or pharmacist if congestion continues to return when the drug effect wears off.

*Sulfite sensitivity:* Some of these products contain sulfites, which may cause allergic-type reactions (eg, rash, hives, itching, wheezing) in certain susceptible persons. Although the overall prevalence of sensitivity in the general population is probably low, it is seen more frequently in asthmatics or in atopic nonasthmatic persons.

*Treatment for rebound congestion:* A simple but uncomfortable solution is to completely withdraw the topical medication. A more acceptable method is to gradually withdraw therapy by discontinuing the medication in one nostril, followed by total withdrawal. Substituting an oral decongestant for a topical one also may be useful.

*Pregnancy:* There are no adequate and well-controlled studies in pregnant women. Use only if clearly needed and the potential benefits to the mother outweigh the possible hazards to the fetus.

*Breastfeeding:* Consult your doctor before taking an oral decongestant while breastfeeding. It is not known if topical decongestants appear in breast milk. Use caution when administering to a nursing woman.

*Children:* Dosage restrictions may vary according to product instructions; refer to individual product information for dosage and administration.

*Elderly:* Patients 60 years of age and older are more likely to experience side effects. Overdosage may cause hallucinations, convulsions, depression, and death.

## Drug Interactions:

Tell your doctor or pharmacist if you are taking or planning to take any over-the-counter or prescription medications or dietary supplements with nasal decongestants. Doses of one or both drugs may need to be modified or a different drug may need to be prescribed. The following drugs and drug classes interact with nasal decongestants:

furazolidone *(Furoxone)*
guanethidine (*Ismelin*)
MAOIs (eg, phenelzine)
methyldopa (eg, *Aldomet*)

rauwolfia alkaloids (eg, reserpine)
tricyclic antidepressants (eg, amitriptyline)

## Side Effects:

Every drug is capable of producing side effects. Many nasal decongestant users experience no, or minor, side effects. The frequency and severity of side effects depend on many factors including dose, duration of therapy, individual susceptibility, and method of administration. Side effects are more likely to occur with oral nasal decongestants. Oral agents, however, cause less local irritation and are not associated with rebound congestion (rhinitis medicamentosa). Possible side effects include:

*Topical Use:* Burning; stinging; sneezing; dryness; local irritation; rebound congestion; nasal discharge; weakness.

*Digestive Tract:* Nausea; vomiting; appetite loss; indigestion.

*Nervous System:* Anxiety; restlessness; tremor; CNS depression; weakness; tenseness; headache; dizziness; drowsiness; sleeplessness; lightheadedness; nervousness.

*Circulatory System:* Irregular heartbeat; changes in blood pressure; palpitations (pounding in the chest).

*Other:* Sweating; pale skin; chest pain; eye sensitivity to light; painful or difficult urination; rash; hives.

## Guidelines for Use:

- Dosage is individualized. Take exactly as prescribed.
- Do not change the dose or stop taking, unless directed by your doctor.
- Patients with high blood pressure or other cardiovascular diseases, thyroid disease, glaucoma, diabetes mellitus, or enlarged prostate should use these products only with medical advice.
- To prevent pressure pain in air travel or other situations where there is a rapid change in altitude, nose drops and nasal sprays act quickly. Take oral dosage forms 1 to 2 hours prior to a major altitude change.
- Side effects are most likely in the elderly and children. Excessive use (misuse) increases risk for side effects.
- Stop using and contact your doctor if you experience persistent stomach pain or vomiting.
- *Oral* — If symptoms do not improve within 7 days or are accompanied by a high fever, consult your doctor before continuing use. Do not exceed recommended dosage. Higher doses may cause nervousness, irregular heartbeat, dizziness, or sleeplessness. If these occur, stop use and contact your doctor. Do not split, dissolve, crush, or chew extended-release preparations.
- *Topical* — Use only as needed. Avoid excessive use. Stop using and contact your doctor if you experience sleeplessness, dizziness, weakness, tremor, or irregular heartbeat. Do not exceed recommended dosage and do not use longer than 3 days, unless directed by your doctor. Stinging or burning sensations or drying of the nose may occur. This often disappears after a few applications. If rebound congestion occurs from excessive doses and frequent use, withdraw the topical drug gradually. Stop using the medication in one nostril, then both nostrils. An oral decongestant may be used instead. Notify your doctor if symptoms persist.
- *Nasal spray* — Hold head upright, insert nozzle into nostril, spray quickly and firmly and sniff deeply while blocking off other nostril. Wipe nozzle clean after use.
- *Nasal drops* — Recline on a bed and hang your head over the edge. Instill nose drops. Remain in this position for several minutes after using the drops, turning your head from side to side while gently "sniffing" and squezing the nostrils.
- Use of the same container of nasal spray or drops by more than 1 person may spread infection. Do not allow the tip of the container or dropper to touch the nasal passage. Store as directed on package labeling.

*If you have any questions, consult your doctor, pharmacist, or health care provider.*

| Generic Name | Supplied As | Generic Available |
|---|---|---|
| C-II **Codeine Sulfate** | **Tablets**: 15 mg, 30 mg, 60 mg | Yes |
| C-II **Codeine Phosphate**[1] | **Tablets, soluble**: 30 mg, 60 mg | Yes |
| | **Solution, oral**: 15 mg/5 mL | Yes |

[1] Also available as an injection.

*Cough* is a normal, protective reflex. It helps clear mucus, irritants, and other foreign matter from the throat, trachea, and lungs. Caution is advised in attempting to suppress a productive cough (mucus is coughed up). If mucus is not removed from the lungs, it may support growth of bacteria and make breathing more difficult. Moderate cough suppression may be used to reduce discomfort and allow sleep, but do not attempt to completely suppress a productive cough.

The dry, nonproductive cough is a good candidate for therapeutic cough suppression, although increased fluid intake is also appropriate to help produce a productive cough. If such coughs are persistent, bothersome, or sleep disrupting, they may respond well to treatment with codeine.

## Type of Drug:

Cough medicine; cough suppressant; narcotic analgesic (pain reliever).

## How the Drug Works:

Codeine suppresses the "cough center" in the brain. The dose required to suppress coughing is lower than the dose required for pain relief. The risk of dependence is slight if taken as directed.

## Uses:

To suppress cough induced by irritation of the respiratory tract.

To relieve mild to moderate pain.

## Precautions:

*Do not use in the following situations:*

allergy to codeine or any of its ingredients

during labor, premature premature infants

*Use with caution in the following situations:*

abdominal conditions, acute (undiagnosed)
Addison disease
asthma attack
bronchitis, chronic
convulsive disorders
cough, persistent (10 days)
emphysema
enlarged prostate
fever

gastrointestinal or urinary tract surgery, recent
head injury
hypothyroidism (underactive thyroid)
kidney disease
liver disease
respiratory tract diseases
urethra, abnormally narrow
ulcers

*Pregnancy:* There are no adequate and well-controlled studies in pregnant women. Use only if clearly needed and the potential benefits to the mother outweigh the possible hazards to the fetus. Dependence has been reported in newborns whose mothers took narcotics regularly during pregnancy.

*Breastfeeding:* Codeine appears in breast milk. Consult your doctor before you begin breastfeeding.

*Children:* Give to infants and small children only with great caution and carefully monitor dosage. Safety and effectiveness in newborn infants have not been established.

*Elderly:* Use with caution in elderly patients.

## Drug Interactions:

Tell your doctor or pharmacist if you are taking or planning to take any over-the-counter or prescription medications or dietary supplements with codeine. Doses of one or both drugs may need to be modified or a different drug may need to be prescribed. Drugs which have central nervous system depressant activity have additive effects when given with codeine. The following drugs are examples of such agents.

alcohol
anesthetics, general
  (eg, methohexital)
benzodiazepines (eg, diazepam)

phenothiazines
  (eg, chlorpromazine)
tricyclic antidepressants
  (eg, amitriptyline)

Consider all drug interactions reported for narcotic pain relievers (see Analgesics - Narcotic Pain Relievers in the CNS Drugs chapter) when using codeine.

## Side Effects:

Every drug is capable of producing side effects. Many codeine users experience no, or minor, side effects. The frequency and severity of side effects depend on many factors including dose, duration of therapy, and individual susceptibility. Possible side effects include:

*Nervous System:* Sedation; hallucinations; headache; convulsions; euphoria; dizziness; weakness; disorientation; lightheadedness; nervous system depression; shock; restlessness.

*Circulatory System:* Irregular heartbeat; palpitations (pounding heart); circulatory depression; cardiac arrest.

*Other:* Dependency; urine retention; infrequent urination; allergic reaction (eg, itching, hives, rash); respiratory arrest; fainting; visual disturbances; nausea; vomiting; constipation; biliary tract spasm. Consider all side effects reported for narcotic pain relievers (see Analgesics - Narcotic Pain Relievers in the CNS Drugs chapter) when using codeine.

## Guidelines for Use:

- May cause stomach upset. Take with food or milk.
- Do not exceed recommended daily dose.
- May impair mental or physical ability. Use caution when driving or performing other tasks requiring alertness. Use of alcohol, sedatives, hypnotics, tranquilizers, promethazine, and antihistamines may have an additive effect.
- *Injection* — Visually inspect for particulate matter and discoloration prior to administration. Do not use if solution is discolored or contains precipitate.
- May produce orthostatic hypotension (dizziness or lightheadedness when rising from a standing or lying position), dry mouth, and constipation in some patients.
- Do not take for persistent or chronic cough, such as occurs with smoking, asthma, or emphysema, or where cough is accompanied by mucus (productive cough) except under supervision of your doctor. Consult your doctor regarding use of a cough suppressant.
- If a cough continues beyond 7 to 10 days or is accompanied by a fever, consult your doctor.

*If you have any questions, consult your doctor, pharmacist, or health care provider.*

| Generic Name<br>*Brand Name Examples* | Supplied As | Generic<br>Available |
|---|---|---|
| *Rx* **Benzonatate** | | |
| *Tessalon Perles* | **Capsules:** 100 mg | No |
| *otc* **Dextromethorphan HBr** | | |
| *Hold DM, Scot-Tussin DM Cough Chasers, Sucrets 4-hour Cough Suppressant* | **Lozenges:** 2.5 mg, 5 mg | No |
| *Benylin, Benylin Pediatric, Pertussin CS, Pertussin DM[1], Silphen–DM* | **Syrup:** 3.5 mg/5 mL, 7.5 mg/ 5 mL, 10 mg/5 mL, 15 mg/5 mL | No |
| *Delsym* | **Suspension, extended release:** 30 mg/5 mL | No |
| **Diphenhydramine HCl** | | |
| *otc* *Beldin[1], Bydramine Cough[1], Diphen AF, Diphen Cough[1], Hydramine Cough[1]* | **Syrup:** 12.5 mg/5 mL | Yes |
| *Rx* *Tusstat[1]* | **Syrup:** 12.5 mg/5 mL | Yes |
| **Nonnarcotic Antitussive Combinations** | | |
| *otc* *Spec-T Cough Suppressant[2]* | **Lozenges:** 10 mg dextromethorphan HBr and 10 mg benzocaine | No |

[1] Contains alcohol.
[2] Contains the dye tartrazine.

*Cough* is a normal protective reflex. It helps clear mucus, irritants, and other foreign matter from the throat, trachea, and lungs. Caution is advised in attempting to suppress a productive cough (mucus is coughed up). The productive cough is essential to the removal of foreign debris. If mucus is not removed from the lungs, it may support growth of bacteria and make breathing more difficult. Moderate cough suppression may be used to reduce discomfort and allow sleep, but do not attempt to completely suppress a productive cough.

The dry, nonproductive cough is a good candidate for therapeutic cough suppression. If such coughs are persistent, bothersome, or sleep-disrupting, they may respond well to treatment with antitussives.

## Type of Drug:

Cough medicine; cough suppressant.

## How the Drug Works:

Nonnarcotic antitussives depress the cough center in the brain.

*Benzonatate:* Reduces the cough reflex by anesthetizing the nerve receptors in the breathing passages and lungs.

## Uses:

To relieve or suppress nonproductive cough (no mucus production) or cough due to colds or allergy.

## Precautions:

*Do not use in the following situations:*

allergy to the drug or any of its ingredients
newborn or premature infants (diphenhydramine)

*Use with caution in the following situations:*

asthma
bladder obstruction (diphenhydramine)
bronchitis, chronic
chronic cough (smoker, etc)
cough with mucus
CNS stimulants
difficulty urinating (diphenhydramine)
difficulty breathing
emphysema
fever
glaucoma (diphenhydramine)
headache, persistent
MAO inhibitor use (dextromethorphan, diphenhydramine)
nausea or vomiting
prostate gland enlargement
(diphenhydramine)
pulmonary disease, chronic
(diphenhydramine)
pyloroduodenal obstruction
(diphenhydramine)
rash
shortness of breath (diphenhydramine)

*Pregnancy:* Adequate studies have not been done in pregnant women. Use only if clearly needed and potential benefits outweigh the possible hazards to the fetus.

*Breastfeeding:* It is not known if nonnarcotic antitussives appear in breast milk. Consult your doctor before you begin breastfeeding. Nursing women should not use *Tusstat* syrup.

*Children:* Use only as directed by your doctor or pharmacist. Most of these products are not recommended for children under 2 to 12 years of age. Consult individual product information for pediatric dosing.

*Elderly:* Products containing an antihistamine are more likely to cause dizziness, sedation, and hypotension in the elderly.

*Tartrazine:* Some of these products may contain the dye tartrazine (FD&C Yellow No. 5) which can cause allergic reactions in certain individuals. Check package label when available or consult your doctor or pharmacist.

## Drug Interactions:

Tell your doctor or pharmacist if you are taking or planning to take any over-the-counter or prescription medications or dietary supplements with nonnarcotic antitussives. Doses of one or both drugs may need to be modified or a different drug may need to be prescribed. The following drugs and drug classes may interact with nonnarcotic antitussives:

alcohol
MAOIs (eg, isocarboxazid)
sedatives (eg, benzodiazepines)
tranquilizers (eg, perphenazine,
phenobarbital)

## Side Effects:

Every drug is capable of producing side effects. Many nonnarcotic antitussive users experience no, or minor, side effects. The frequency and severity of side effects depend on many factors including dose, duration of therapy, and individual susceptibility. Possible side effects include:

*Circulatory System:* Pounding in chest; rapid heartbeat; low blood pressure; extrasystoles.

*Digestive Tract:* Constipation; nausea; stomach upset; loss of appetite; vomiting.

*Eyes or Ocular:* Burning sensation in eyes; blurred vision; vision problems.

*Nervous System:* Headache; mental confusion; visual hallucinations; sedation; dizziness; excitability in children; neuritis.

*Respiratory System:* Tightness in chest; wheezing; chest numbness; nasal congestion; thick bronchial secretions.

*Skin:* Itching; skin eruptions; abnormal skin sensations.

*Urinary and Reproductive Tract:* Urinary frequency; difficult urination; urinary retention; early menstruation.

*Other:* A vague "chilly" sensation; allergy; shock; sensitivity to light; excessive perspiration; dryness of mouth, nose, and throat; decreased blood platelets; agranulocytosis; incoordination; feeling of whirling motion; ringing in ears; acute labyrinthitis; hysteria; convulsions.

## Guidelines for Use:

- Take only as directed. Do not exceed recommended dose.
- See individual package instructions for dosing information.
- *Pertussin CS, Pertussin DM, and Delsym* — Shake well before use.
- Do not take for persistent or chronic cough, such as occurs with smoking, asthma, chronic bronchitis, emphysema, or where cough is accompanied by excessive phelgm, except under supervision of your doctor.
- Do not use *Spec-T* lozenges for more than 2 days unless directed by your doctor.
- Some products may cause drowsiness, whether they contain alcohol or not. Alcohol, sedatives, and tranquilizers may increase the drowsiness effect. Avoid alcoholic beverages while taking this product and do not take sedatives or tranquilizers without consulting your doctor.
- May cause drowsiness, dizziness, or blurred vision. Use caution while driving or performing other tasks requiring mental alertness, coordination, or physical dexterity.
- A persistent cough may be a sign of a serious condition. If cough persists for more than 1 week, tends to recur, or is accompanied by fever, rash, or persistent headache, notify your doctor.
- Do not use dextromethorphan or diphenhydramine if you are taking an MAO inhibitor or for 2 weeks after stopping MAO inhibitor therapy.
- *Benzonatate* — Do not chew or suck *Tessalon Perles*. Severe hypersensitivity reactions (eg, bronchospasm, laryngospasm, and cardiovascular collapse) have occurred.
- Store at room temperature (59° to 86°F).

*If you have any questions, consult your doctor, pharmacist, or health care provider.*

| Generic Name<br>*Brand Name Examples* | Supplied As | Generic<br>Available |
|---|---|---|
| **Guaifenesin (Glyceryl Guaiacolate)** | | |
| *otc* Gee-Gee, Glytuss, Hytuss | **Tablets:** 100 mg, 200 mg | Yes |
| *Rx* Fenesin, Humibid L.A., Sinumist-SR | **Tablets, sustained release:** 600 mg | No |
| *otc* Breonesin[1], Hytuss 2X | **Capsules:** 200 mg | No |
| *Rx* Humibid Sprinkle | **Capsules, sustained release:** 300 mg | No |
| *otc* Anti-Tuss[2], Genatuss, Guiatuss[1,2,3], Mytussin[2], Robitussin, Scot-tussin[1,3] | **Syrup:** 100 mg/5 mL | Yes |
| *otc* Naldecon Senior EX[1] | **Liquid:** 200 mg/5 mL | No |
| **Iodine Products** | | |
| *Rx* Potassium Iodide, SSKI | **Solution:** 1 g potassium iodide/mL | Yes |
| *Rx* Pima | **Syrup:** 325 mg potassium iodide/5 mL | No |

[1] Sugar free.
[2] Contains alcohol.
[3] Dye free.

Only one expectorant, guaifenesin, is safe and effective for use in nonprescription cough and cold medications to help loosen excessive respiratory secretions, mucus, and other foreign debris, according to a recent standard published by the Food and Drug Administration. No other nonprescription expectorant is considered both safe and effective by the FDA.

## Type of Drug:

Loosens excessive respiratory secretions, mucus, and other foreign debris.

## How the Drug Works:

Expectorants thin mucous secretions in the lungs and make the phlegm less sticky. The mucus is easier to cough up. This reduces chest congestion and makes coughs more productive. The exact mechanism by which expectorants thin mucous secretions in the lung is not known.

## Uses:

*Guaifenesin:* For symptomatic relief of respiratory conditions characterized by dry, nonproductive cough and in the presence of mucus in the respiratory tract.

*Iodine Products:* For symptomatic treatment of lung disease where mucus complicates the condition (eg, emphysema, bronchial asthma, chronic bronchitis, bronchiectasis). Also used as adjunctive treatment in respiratory conditions such as cystic fibrosis, chronic sinusitis, and after surgery to help prevent lung collapse.

## Precautions:

*Do not use in the following situations:*

Guaifenesin —
allergy to guaifenesin or any of
its ingredients

*Potassium iodide* —
Addison disease, untreated
allergy to iodides
bronchitis, acute
dehydration, acute
heat cramps
hyperkalemia
iodine poisoning
kidney disease

*Use with caution in the following situations:*

Guaifenesin —
cough with excessive
secretions
cough (7 to 10 days in
duration)
cough, recurring (eg, asthma,
chronic bronchitis, emphysema,
smoking)
cough with fever, rash, or persistent headache
diabetes
heart disease
high blood pressure
prostate enlargement
thyroid disease

*Potassium iodide* —
cough (7 to 10 days duration)
cystic fibrosis in children
heart disease
hyperthyroidism
iodine-induced goiters
kidney function impairment
myotonia congenita
(hereditary muscle disease)
tuberculosis

*Pregnancy: Guaifenesin* — Adequate studies have not been done in pregnant women. Use only if clearly needed and the benefits outweigh the possible risks.

*Potassium iodide* – Studies have shown a potential risk to the fetus, including abnormal thyroid function and goiter development. Use only if clearly needed and potential benefits outweigh the possible risks.

*Breastfeeding:* It is not known if guaifenesin appears in breast milk. Potassium iodide appears in breast milk and may cause skin rash and thyroid suppression in the infant. Decide whether to discontinue nursing or the drug. Consult your doctor.

*Children:* Safety and effectiveness in children under 2 years of age have not been established for guaifenesin. Safety and effectiveness in children have not been established for potassium iodide.

## Drug Interactions:

Tell your doctor or pharmacist if you are taking, have recently discontinued, or are planning to take any over-the-counter or prescription medications with these expectorants. Doses of one or both drugs may need to be modified or a different drug may need to be prescribed. The following drugs and drug classes may interact with guaifenesin or potassium iodide expectorants.

angiotensin-converting enzyme (ACE) inhibitors (eg, captopril)
antithyroid agents (eg, propylthiouracil (PTU), methimazole)
lithium (eg, *Eskalith)*
monoamine oxidase inhibitors (MAOIs) (eg, phenelzine sulfate)

potassium products (eg, *Slow-K)*
potassium-sparing diuretics (eg, spironolactone, triamterene, amiloride)

## Side Effects:

Every drug is capable of producing side effects. Many expectorant users experience no, or minor, side effects. The frequency and severity of side effects depend on many factors including dose, duration of therapy, and individual susceptibility. Possible side effects include:

*Guaifenesin* — Nausea; vomiting; diarrhea; gas; abnormal urine tests.

*Potassium iodide* —

*Iodism or chronic iodine poisoning:* Sore or burning mouth or throat; severe headache; productive cough; metallic taste; sneezing; eyelid swelling; increased salivation; acneiform skin lesions in oily skin areas; severe skin eruptions.

*Allergic Reactions:* Nerve swelling; skin and mucous membrane bleeding; serum sickness-like symptoms (eg, fever, bloating, lymph node enlargement, joint pain, blood disorder, fluid in lungs).

*Digestive Tract:* Nausea; vomiting; diarrhea; stomach upset or pain; bleeding.

*Nervous System:* Mental confusion; numbness.

*Skin:* Acne; rash; minor skin eruptions.

*Other:* Benign thyroid tumor; goiter; myxedema (hypothyroidism); irregular heartbeat; swelling of salivary glands, neck, or throat; tingling, pain, or weakness in hands or feet; weakness or heaviness of legs; fever; abnormal thyroid tests; unusual tiredness; metallic aftertaste.

## Guidelines for Use:

- Dosage is individualized. Take exactly as prescribed.
- Do not change the dose or stop taking, unless directed by your doctor.
- Do not take these products for persistent or chronic cough such as occurs with smoking, asthma, chronic bronchitis, or emphysema, or when cough is accompanied by excessive phlegm, unless directed by your doctor.
- A persistent cough may be a sign of a serious condition. If cough persists for more than 1 week, tends to recur, or is accompanied by fever, rash, or persistent headache, consult a doctor.
- Guaifenesin is the only expectorant approved by the FDA as safe and effective. It is well tolerated. Iodine-containing products have the potential to produce many adverse effects.
- Drink a glass of water or other fluid with each dose of expectorant. Most authorities believe a well hydrated body (due to fluid intake) is responsible for thinning respiratory tract mucus and may be as valuable as or more so than the expectorant itself.
- Do not cut, crush, or chew sustained-release tablets or capsules.
- *Iodine-containing expectorants* — Stop taking if stomach pain, rash, nausea, vomiting, bloating, gastrointestinal bleeding, or a metallic taste develops.

*If you have any questions, consult your doctor, pharmacist, or health care provider.*

Combination products are frequently used in the therapy of respiratory conditions. These fixed-dose combination products may present two problems: (1) The patient may not need all the components in the product; (2) the patient may need the components, but in different strengths or at different dosing intervals.

*Product Selection Guidelines:* The following guidelines should be employed when choosing a respiratory combination product.

*Symptoms* – Pain, fever, congestion, runny nose, cough (productive or nonproductive).

*Medical history and health* – Age, allergy history, pregnancy, heart disease, high blood pressure, asthma, bronchitis, glaucoma, hyperthyroidism (overactive thyroid), diabetes, depression.

*Drugs you are currently taking* – Other cold or allergy medications; medications for high blood pressure, diabetes, etc.

*Do not exceed the recommended dosage* – Do not take a nonprescription *(otc)* respiratory product for more than 7 days. If symptoms do not improve or are accompanied by fever, consult a doctor.

*Humidification* – Humidification of room air and adequate fluid intake (6 to 8 glasses/day) are important in treating cold symptoms.

*Sulfites and Tartrazine* – Some of these products contain sulfites or tartrazine, which may cause allergic-type reactions (eg, rash, hives, itching, wheezing) in certain susceptible persons. Although the overall prevalence of sensitivity in the general population is probably low, it is seen more frequently in asthmatics or in atopic nonasthmatic persons (sulfites) or in patients who have aspirin allergy (tartrazine).

*Sugar free liquid products* – The small amount of sugar in usual doses of medication is probably insignificant to the well-controlled diabetic. However, consider the effects of alcohol and sympathomimetics in addition to the sugar content of these formulations.

*Sustained release formulations* – Products with identical active ingredients are listed together. Due to formulation differences, do not consider them bioequivalent.

*Groups:* These combination products are presented in groups based on their formulations. Products with identical or similar ingredients are listed next to each other, regardless of therapeutic claims, which may differ even for identical formulas. Pediatric preparations (those products intended mainly or exclusively for children) are grouped together at the end of the main sections.

*Antiasthmatic Combinations* contain xanthine derivatives and sympathomimetics for bronchodilation (widening of air passages). Many products also contain expectorants to facilitate break up and removal of mucus.
Xanthine Combinations
Xanthine-Sympathomimetic Combinations

*Upper Respiratory Combinations* are used primarily for relief of symptoms associated with colds, upper respiratory infections and allergies (eg, inflammation of nose and sinuses, etc). Cough preparations include an antitussive (cough suppressant) or expectorant, but may also contain ingredients for relief of other symptoms.

Decongestant and Analgesic Combinations
Pediatric Decongestant and Analgesic Combinations
Decongestant and Expectorant Combinations
Pediatric Decongestant and Expectorant Combinations
Antihistamine and Analgesic Combinations
Decongestant, Antihistamine, and Expectorant Combinations
Pediatric Decongestant, Antihistamine, and Expectorant Combinations
Decongestants and Antihistamines
Pediatric Decongestants and Antihistamines
Decongestant, Antihistamine, and Analgesic Combinations
Decongestant, Antihistamine, and Anticholinergic Combinations
Pediatric Decongestant, Antihistamine, and Anticholinergic Combinations
Antitussive Combinations
Pediatric Antitussive Combinations
Antitussive and Expectorant Combinations
Pediatric Antitussive and Expectorant Combinations
Antitussives with Expectorants
Pediatric Antitussives with Expectorants
Topical Combinations

*Ingredients:*

*Antihistamines* are used for relief from allergic symptoms (hay fever) including runny nose, sneezing, itching of the nose or throat and itchy, watery eyes. The anticholinergic (drying) effects of antihistamines may cause a thickening of lung secretions; therefore, these agents may not be helpful in respiratory conditions characterized by congestion. Antihistamines may cause drowsiness. Antihistamines can also cause drying of the eyes. This can be a problem for people who wear contact lenses. Appropriate lubricating drops may be indicated.

*Xanthines* primarily theophylline, relieve spasms of the air passages by direct action on the bronchial smooth muscle in asthma and chronic bronchitis. Some xanthine-containing combination products are available over-the-counter, but asthmatic patients should use them only under supervision of a doctor.

*Sympathomimetics* are used for their decongestant or bronchodilator (widening of air passages) effects. Side effects may include nervousness, heart stimulation and high blood pressure if taken orally.

*Decongestants* – Used for temporary relief of nasal congestion due to colds or allergy. Given orally, they are less effective than topical nasal decongestants, and they have a potential for side effects. Frequent or prolonged topical use may lead to local irritation and rebound congestion. Topical decongestants (sprays and drops) should not be used for more than 3 to 5 days in a row. After that, switch to an oral product, or avoid use of decongestants altogether.

*Bronchodilators* – Ephedrine is common in these combinations; however, it may stimulate the heart. Bronchodilation effects may decrease congestion of mucous membranes. Pseudoephedrine is not an effective bronchodilator.

*Narcotic Antitussives* – The antitussive dose is lower than that required for pain relief. Consider general precautions for the use of narcotics, including the potential for abuse, when using these products.

*Nonnarcotic Antitussives* decrease the cough reflex without inducing many of the common characteristics of narcotic preparations. Examples include: Dextromethorphan, diphenhydramine, carbetapentane and caramiphen edisylate.

*Expectorants* may be of limited value in loosening and liquifying respiratory mucus, in soothing the irritated lining of the lungs (bronchial mucosa) and in making coughs more productive. Guaifenesin is the only FDA-recognized safe and effective ingredient for use in *otc* cough and cold medicines to loosen phlegm. Humidification of room air and adequate fluid intake (6 to 8 glasses/day) are importart measures as well.

*Analgesics* (eg, pain relievers, acetaminophen, aspirin, ibuprofen) are frequently included for symptoms of headache, fever, muscle aches and pain.

*Anticholinergics* are included for their drying effects on mucus secretions. This action may be beneficial in acute runny nose; however, drying of respiratory secretions may lead to obstruction. Traditionally, anticholinergics have been avoided in patients with asthma or chronic obstructive pulmonary disease (COPD); however, some patients respond well to these agents. Caution is still advised, particularly among patients with heart disease.
An anticholinergic for oral inhalation is available as a bronchodilator for maintenance of air passage spasms (bronchospasms) associated with COPD, including chronic bronchitis and emphysema.

*Papaverine* relaxes the smooth muscle of the air passageways tree.

*Barbiturates* are included for their sedative effects in combination with xanthines or sympathomimetics which may cause CNS stimulation. The sedative effectiveness of low doses (eg, 8 mg phenobarbital) is questionable. OTC avaiiability of phenobarbital-containing products may be limited according to state laws.

*Caffeine* is included in some combinations for CNS stimulation to counteract antihistamine depression and to enhance the effects of pain relievers.

## Xanthine Combinations

Content given per capsule, tablet, or 15 mL.

| | Brand Name Examples | Xanthine | Expectorant |
|---|---|---|---|
| Rx | Quibron-300 Capsules | 300 mg theophylline | 180 mg guaifenesin |
| Rx | Quibron Capsules | 150 mg theophylline | 90 mg guaifenesin |
| Rx | Slo-Phyllin GG Syrup | | |
| Rx | Theolate Liquid | | |
| Rx | Elixophyllin-GG Liquid | 100 mg theophylline | 100 mg guaifenesin |
| Rx | Elixophyllin-KI Elixir | 80 mg theophylline | 130 mg potassium iodide |
| Rx | Dilor-G Liquid | 300 mg dyphylline | 300 mg guaifenesin |
| Rx | Dy-G Liquid | | |
| Rx | Panfil-G Syrup | 300 mg dyphylline | 150 mg guaifenesin |
| Rx | Dilor-G Tablets | 200 mg dyphylline | 200 mg guaifenesin |
| Rx | Dyflex-G Tablets | | |
| Rx | Lufyllin-GG Tablets | | |
| Rx | Panfil-G Capsules | 200 mg dyphylline | 100 mg guaifenesin |
| Rx | Dyphylline-GG Elixir | 100 mg dyphylline | 100 mg guaifenesin |
| Rx | Lufyllin-GG Elixir | | |
| Rx | Brondelate Elixir | 300 mg oxtriphylline | 150 mg guaifenesin |

### Xanthine-Sympathomimetic Combinations

Content given per tablet.

| | Brand Name Examples | Xanthine | Bronchodilator | Expectorant | Other |
|---|---|---|---|---|---|
| Rx | Lufyllin-EPG Tablets | 100 mg dyphylline | 16 mg ephedrine HCl | 200 mg guaifenesin | 16 mg pheno-barbital |

### Decongestant and Analgesic Combinations

Content given per capsule, tablet, or 5 mL.

| | Brand Name Examples | Decongestant | Analgesic |
|---|---|---|---|
| otc | Alka-Seltzer Plus Cold & Sinus Tablets[1] | 5 mg phenyl-ephrine HCl | 250 mg acetaminophen |
| otc | Cepacol Sore Throat Liquid[2,3] | 10 mg pseudo-ephedrine HCl | 106.7 mg acetaminophen |
| otc | Alka-Seltzer Plus Cold & Sinus Liqui-Gels[3] | 30 mg pseudo-ephedrine HCl | 325 mg acetaminophen |
| otc | Ornex No Drowsi-ness Tablets[3] | | |
| otc | Phenapap Tablets[3] | | |
| otc | Sinutab Sinus Without Drowsiness Regular Strength Tablets | | |
| otc | Sudafed Cold & Sinus Non-Drowsy Liqui-Caps | | |

| | Brand Name Examples | Decongestant | Analgesic |
|---|---|---|---|
| otc | Dristan Cold Non-Drowsy Maximum Strength Tablets | 30 mg pseudo-ephedrine HCl | 500 mg acetaminophen |
| otc | Mapap Sinus Maximum Strength Geltabs | | |
| otc | Nasal Decongestant Sinus Non-Drowsy Tablets | | |
| otc | Ornex No Drowsiness Maximum Strength Tablets | | |
| otc | Sine-Off No-Drowsiness Formula Tablets | | |
| otc | Sinus-Relief Maximum Strength Tablets | | |
| otc | Sinutab Sinus Without Drowsiness Maximum Strength Tablets | | |
| otc | Sudafed Sinus Headache Non-Drowsy Tablets | | |
| otc | SudoGest Sinus Maximum Strength Tablets | | |
| otc | Tavist Sinus Maximum Strength Tablets | | |
| otc | Tylenol Sinus Non-Drowsy Maximum Strength Geltabs, Tablets, and Gelcaps | | |

| | Brand Name Examples | Decongestant | Analgesic |
|---|---|---|---|
| otc | Advil Cold & Sinus Tablets | 30 mg pseudo-ephedrine HCl | 200 mg ibuprofen |
| otc | Advil Flu & Body Ache Tablets | | |
| otc | Dristan Sinus Tablets | | |
| otc | Motrin Sinus Head-ache Tablets | | |
| otc | Aleve Cold & Sinus Tablets | 120 mg pseudo-ephedrine HCl | 220 mg naproxen sodium (200 mg naproxen) |
| otc | Aleve Sinus & Head-ache Tablets[4] | | |

[1] Contains phenylalanine.
[2] Alcohol free.
[3] This product may also be used in children; refer to package labeling.
[4] Extended release.

### Pediatric Decongestant and Analgesic Combinations

Content given per tablet, 5 mL (liquid), or 1 mL (drops).

| | Brand Name Examples | Decongestant | Analgesic |
|---|---|---|---|
| otc | Tylenol Infant's Cold Concen-trated Drops[1] | 9.375 mg/mL pseudoephedrine HCl | 100 mg/mL acetamino-phen |
| otc | Tylenol Chil-dren's Sinus Suspension | 15 mg pseudo-ephedrine HCl | 160 mg acetaminophen |
| otc | Triaminic Soft-chews Allergy Sinus & Head-ache Tablets[2] | | |
| otc | Motrin Chil-dren's Cold Suspension | 15 mg pseudo-ephedrine HCl | 100 mg ibuprofen |

[1] Alcohol free.
[2] Contains phenylalanine.

## Decongestant and Expectorant Combinations

Content given per capsule, tablet, or 5 mL.

| Brand Name Examples | Decongestant | Expectorant |
|---|---|---|
| Rx  *Broncholate Syrup* | 6.25 mg ephedrine HCl | 600 mg guaifenesin |
| Rx  *KIE Syrup*[1] | 8 mg ephedrine HCl | 150 mg potassium iodide |
| otc  *Mini Two-Way Action Tablets* | 12.5 mg ephedrine HCl | 200 mg guaifenesin |
| otc  *Primatene Tablets* | | |
| otc  *Dynafed Asthma Relief Tablets* | 25 mg ephedrine HCl | 200 mg guaifenesin |
| otc  *Mini Two-Way Action Tablets* | | |
| otc  *Bronkaid Dual Action Tablets* | 25 mg ephedrine sulfate | 400 mg guaifenesin |
| otc  *Rescon-GG Liquid*[1,2,5] | 5 mg phenylephrine HCl | 100 mg guaifenesin |
| Rx  *Entex Liquid*[1,2,3,5] | 7.5 mg phenylephrine HCl | 100 mg guaifenesin |
| Rx  *Endal Tablets*[4] | 20 mg phenylephrine HCl | 300 mg guaifenesin |
| Rx  *GFN 600/Phenylephrine 20 Tablets*[1,5] | 20 mg phenylephrine HCl | 600 mg guaifenesin |
| Rx  *Entex LA Tablets*[1,5,6] | 30 mg phenylephrine HCl | 600 mg guaifenesin |
| Rx  *Liquibid-D Tablets*[1] | 40 mg phenylephrine HCl | 600 mg guaifenesin |
| otc  *Guiatuss PE Liquid*[2] | 30 mg pseudoephedrine HCl | 100 mg guaifenesin |
| otc  *Robafen PE Liquid*[1,2] | | |
| otc  *Robitussin PE Liquid*[1] | | |

| Brand Name Examples | Decongestant | Expectorant |
|---|---|---|
| otc *Sudafed Non-Drowsy Non-Drying Sinus Liquid Caps* | 30 mg pseudoephedrine HCl | 120 mg guaifenesin |
| otc *Guaifed Syrup[1,2]* | 30 mg pseudoephedrine HCl | 200 mg guaifenesin |
| otc *Robitussin Severe Congestion Liqui-Gels[1]* | | |
| otc *Severe Congestion Tussin Softgels[1]* | | |
| otc *Sinutab Non-Drying Liquid Caps* | | |
| otc *Robitussin Cold Sinus & Congestion Tablets[1,7]* | 30 mg pseudoephedrine HCl | 200 mg guaifenesin |
| Rx *PanMist-S Syrup[1]* | 45 mg pseudoephedrine HCl | 200 mg guaifenesin |
| Rx *Coldmist JR Tablets[1,6]* | 45 mg pseudoephedrine HCl | 600 mg guaifenesin |
| Rx *PanMist JR Tablets[1,8]* | | |
| Rx *Profen II Tablets[1,8]* | 45 mg pseudoephedrine HCl | 800 mg guaifenesin |
| Rx *Respa-1st Tablets[1,6]* | 58 mg pseudoephedrine HCl | 600 mg guaifenesin |
| Rx *Respaire-60 SR Capsules[1,8]* | 60 mg pseudoephedrine HCl | 200 mg guaifenesin |
| Rx *Guaifed-PD Capsules[1,6]* | 60 mg pseudoephedrine HCl | 300 mg guaifenesin |
| Rx *Versacaps Capsules[1,6]* | | |

| Brand Name Examples | Decongestant | Expectorant |
|---|---|---|
| otc Congestac Tablets[1] | 60 mg pseudoephed-rine HCl | 400 mg guaifenesin |
| otc Refenesen Plus Severe Strength Cough & Cold Medicine Tablets | | |
| Rx Sudal 60/500 Tablets[1,6] | 60 mg pseudoephed-rine HCl | 500 mg guaifenesin |
| Rx Maxifed-G Tablets[1,6] | 60 mg pseudoephed-rine HCl | 550 mg guaifenesin |
| Rx Guaifenesin/ Pseudoephedrine HCl Tablets[1,6] | 60 mg pseudoephed-rine HCl | 600 mg guaifenesin |
| Rx AquatabD Dose Pack Tablets[1,6] | | |
| Rx Deconsal II Tablets[1,6] | | |
| Rx Defen-LA Tablets[1,6] | | |
| Rx Guaifenex PSE 60 Tablets[1,8] | | |
| Rx Iosal II Tablets[1,6] | | |
| Rx Guaifenex-Rx Tablets[8] | Day: 60 mg pseudo-ephedrine HCl | 600 mg guaifenesin |
| | Night: | 600 mg guaifenesin |
| Rx AquatabD Tablets | 60 mg pseudoephed-rine HCl | 1200 mg guaifenesin |
| Rx G/P 1200/60 Tablets[1,6] | | |
| Rx Maxifed Tablets[1] | 80 mg pseudoephed-rine HCl | 700 mg guaifenesin |
| Rx Coldmist LA Tablets[1,8] | 80 mg pseudopehed-rine HCl | 800 mg guaifenesin |
| Rx PanMist LA Tablets[1,8] | | |
| Rx H 9600 SR Tablets[1,5,6] | 90 mg pseudoephed-rine HCl | 600 mg guaifenesin |

| Brand Name Examples | Decongestant | Expectorant |
|---|---|---|
| Rx *Profen Forte Tablets*[1,8] | 90 mg pseudoephed-rine HCl | 800 mg guaifenesin |
| Rx *Dynex Tablets*[1,5,6] | 90 mg pseudoephed-rine HCl | 1200 mg guaifenesin |
| Rx *Guaifed Capsules*[6] | 120 mg pseudoephed-rine HCl | 250 mg guaifenesin |
| Rx *Pseudovent Capsules*[6] | | |
| Rx *Respaire-120 SR Capsules*[8] | | |
| Rx *GP-500 Tablets*[1,3,5,6] | 120 mg pseudoephed-rine HCl | 500 mg guaifenesin |
| Rx *Nasatab LA Tablets*[1,6] | | |
| Rx *Stamoist E Tablets*[1,6] | | |
| Rx *V-Dec-M Tablets*[1,6] | | |
| Rx *Touro LA Tablets*[6] | 120 mg pseudoephed-rine HCl | 525 mg guaifenesin |
| Rx *Duratuss Tablets*[5,6] | 120 mg pseudoephed-rine HCl | 600 mg guaifenesin |
| Rx *Entex PSE Tablets*[1,6] | | |
| Rx *Guaifenex PSE 120 Tablets*[1,5,8] | | |
| Rx *GuaiMAX-D Tablets*[1,8] | | |
| Rx *Guaipax PSE Tablets*[1,6] | | |
| Rx *Guai-Vent/PSE Tablets*[1,6] | | |
| Rx *Miraphen PSE Tablets*[1,8] | | |

| *Brand Name*<br>*Examples* | **Decongestant** | **Expectorant** |
|---|---|---|
| Rx *Duratuss GP*<br>*Tablets*[5,6] | 120 mg pseudoephed-<br>rine HCl | 1200 mg guaifenesin |
| Rx *GFN/PSE*<br>*Tablets*[1,6] | | |
| Rx *Guaifenex GP*<br>*Tablets*[5,8] | | |

[1] This product may also be used in children; refer to package labeling.
[2] Alcohol free.
[3] Sugar free.
[4] Timed release.

[5] Dye free.
[6] Sustained release.
[7] Also contains 325 mg acetaminophen.
[8] Extended release.

## Pediatric Decongestant and Expectorant Combinations

Content given per capsule or 5 mL.

|  | Brand Name Examples | Decongestant | Expectorant |
|---|---|---|---|
| otc | Thera-Hist Expectorant Chest Congestion Liquid | 15 mg pseudo-ephedrine HCl | 50 mg guai-fenesin |
| otc | Triacting Liquid | | |
| otc | Triaminic Chest Congestion Liquid | | |
| Rx | Pseudovent-PED Capsules[1] | 60 mg pseudo-ephedrine HCl | 300 mg guai-fenesin |

[1] Sustained release.

## Anthistamine and Analgesic Combinations

Content given per capsule or tablet.

| | Brand Name Examples | Antihistamine | Analgesic |
|---|---|---|---|
| otc | Coricidin HBP Cold & Flu Tablets[1] | 2 mg chlorphenir- amine maleate | 325 mg acetamino- phen |
| otc | Percogesic Extra Strength Tablets | 12.5 mg diphen- hydramine HCl | 500 mg acetamino- phen |
| otc | Tylenol Severe Allergy Tablets | | |
| otc | Tylenol PM Extra Strength Tablets, Gelcaps, and Geltabs | 25 mg diphenhydra- mine HCl | 500 mg acetamino- phen |
| Rx | Ed-Flex Capsules[1] | 20 mg phenyltolox- amine citrate | 300 mg acetamino- phen, 200 mg salicyl- amide |
| otc | Aceta-Gesic Tablets[1] | 30 mg phenyltolox- amine citrate | 325 mg acetamino- phen |
| otc | Major-gesic Tablets[1] | | |
| otc | Percogesic Tablets[1] | | |
| otc | Phenylgesic Tablets[1] | | |

[1] This product may also be used in children; refer to package labeling.

## Decongestant, Antihistamine, and Expectorant Combinations

Content given per tablet or 5 mL.

| | Brand Name Examples | Decongestant | Antihistamine | Expectorant |
|---|---|---|---|---|
| Rx | Decolate Tablets | 5 mg phenyl-ephrine HCl | 4 mg chlor-pheniramine maleate | 100 mg guai-fenesin |
| Rx | Polaramine Expectorant Liquid[1,2] | 20 mg pseudo-ephedrine sul-fate | 2 mg dexchlor-pheniramine maleate | 100 mg guai-fenesin |

[1] This product may also be used in children; refer to package labeling.
[2] Contains alcohol.

## Pediatric Decongestant, Antihistamine, and Expectorant Combinations

Content given per 1 mL.

| | Brand Name Examples | Decongestant | Antihistamine | Expectorant |
|---|---|---|---|---|
| Rx | Donatussin Drops | 2 mg/mL phenylephrine HCl | 1 mg/mL chlor-pheniramine maleate | 20 mg/mL guai-fenesin |

## Decongestants and Antihistamines

Content given per capsule, tablet, or 5 mL.

| | Brand Name Examples | Decongestant | Antihistamine |
|---|---|---|---|
| otc | Histatab Plus Tablets[1] | 5 mg phenyl-ephrine HCl | 2 mg chlor-pheniramine maleate |
| Rx | Ed A-Hist Liquid[1,2] | 10 mg phenyl-ephrine HCl | 4 mg chlor-pheniramine maleate |
| Rx | Ed A-Hist Tablets[3] | 20 mg phenyl-ephrine HCl | 8 mg chlor-pheniramine maleate |
| Rx | Promethazine HCl and Phenylephrine HCl Syrup[1,2] | 5 mg phenyl-ephrine HCl | 6.25 mg pro-methazine HCl |
| Rx | Phenergan VC Syrup[1,2] | | |
| Rx | Prometh VC Plain Syrup[1,2] | | |
| Rx | Rynatan Tablets | 25 mg phenyl-ephrine HCl | 9 mg chlor-pheniramine tannate |
| Rx | Semprex-D Capsules | 60 mg pseudo-ephedrine HCl | 8 mg acrivas-tine |
| otc | Bromfed Syrup | 30 mg pseudo-ephedrine HCl | 2 mg brom-pheniramine maleate |
| Rx | Brofed Liquid[1] | 30 mg pseudo-ephedrine HCl | 4 mg brom-pheniramine maleate |
| Rx | Rondec Syrup[1] | 45 mg pseudo-ephedrine HCl | 4 mg brom-pheniramine maleate |
| Rx | Brompheniramine Maleate/Pseudoephedrine HCl Syrup[1] | 60 mg pseudo-ephedrine HCl | 4 mg brom-pheniramine maleate |
| Rx | Andehist Syrup[1,4,5] | | |
| Rx | Bromfed Tablets[1] | | |
| Rx | Lodrane Liquid[1,4-6] | | |
| Rx | Touro Allergy Capsules[1,3] | 60 mg pseudo-ephedrine HCl | 5.75 mg brom-pheniramine maleate |
| Rx | Lodrane LD Capsules[1,6] | 60 mg pseudo-ephedrine HCl | 6 mg brom-pheniramine maleate |
| Rx | Respahist Capsules[1,3] | | |

| | Brand Name Examples | Decongestant | Antihistamine |
|---|---|---|---|
| Rx | Histex SR Capsules[7] | 120 mg pseudo-ephedrine HCl | 10 mg brompheniramine maleate |
| Rx | Bromfed Capsules[7] | 120 mg pseudo-ephedrine HCl | 12 mg brompheniramine maleate |
| Rx | Bromfenex Capsules[7] | | |
| Rx | ULTRAbrom Capsules[7] | | |
| Rx | Cardec-S Liquid[1] | 60 mg pseudo-ephedrine HCl | 4 mg carbinoxamine maleate |
| Rx | Rondec Tablets[1] | | |
| Rx | Coldec D Tablets[1] | 90 mg pseudo-ephedrine HCl | 8 mg carbinoxamine maleate |
| Rx | Palgic-D Tablets[1] | | |
| Rx | Rondec-TR Tablets[8] | 120 mg pseudo-ephedrine HCl | 8 mg carbinoxamine maleate |
| Rx | Zyrtec-D 12 Hour Tablets[7] | 120 mg pseudo-ephedrine HCl | 5 mg cetirizine HCl |
| otc | Allerest Maximum Strength Tablets | 30 mg pseudo-ephedrine HCl | 2 mg chlorpheniramine maleate |
| Rx | Deconamine Syrup[1,5,6] | | |
| otc | Scot-Tussin Hayfebrol Liquid[1,4-6] | | |
| Rx | Histex Liquid[1] | | |
| otc | Ryna Liquid[1,4-6] | | |
| Rx | Deconamine Tablets | 60 mg pseudo-ephedrine HCl | 4 mg chlorpheniramine maleate |
| Rx | Kronofed-A Jr. Capsules[3] | | |
| otc | Sudafed Cold & Allergy Maximum Strength Tablets[1] | | |
| Rx | Chlorpheniramine Maleate/Pseudoephedrine HCl ER Capsules[7] | 120 mg pseudo-ephedrine HCl | 8 mg chlorpheniramine maleate |
| Rx | Brexin-L.A. Capsules | | |
| Rx | Colfed-A Capsules[7] | | |
| Rx | Deconamine SR Capsules[3] | | |
| Rx | Deconomed SR Capsules[3] | | |
| Rx | Kronofed-A Capsules[3] | | |
| Rx | N D Clear Capsules[3] | | |
| Rx | Rinade B.I.D. Capsules[6,7] | | |
| Rx | Time-Hist Capsules[3] | | |

| | Brand Name Examples | Decongestant | Antihistamine |
|---|---|---|---|
| Rx | Biohist-LA Tablets[1,3] | 120 mg pseudo-ephedrine HCl | 12 mg chlor-pheniramine maleate |
| Rx | Histade Capsules[3] | | |
| Rx | Rescon 12 Hour Capsules[3] | | |
| otc | Benadryl Allergy & Sinus Fastmelt Dissolving Tablets[9] | 30 mg pseudo-ephedrine HCl | 19 mg diphen-hydramine cit-rate (12.5 mg diphenhydra-mine HCl) |
| otc | Benadryl Allergy & Sinus Liquid[1] | 30 mg pseudo-ephedrine HCl | 12.5 mg diphenhydra-mine HCl |
| otc | Benadryl Allergy & Sinus Tablets | 60 mg pseudo-ephedrine HCl | 25 mg diphen-hydramine HCl |
| Rx | Allegra-D Tablets[7] | 120 mg pseudo-ephedrine HCl | 60 mg fexo-fenadine HCl |
| Rx | Quadra-Hist D Capsules[7] | 80 mg pseudo-ephedrine HCl | 16 mg phenyl-toloxamine cit-rate, 16 mg pyrilamine maleate, 16 mg pheniramine maleate |
| otc | Triprolidine HCl w/Pseudo-ephedrine HCl Syrup[1] | 30 mg pseudo-ephedrine HCl | 1.25 mg triproli-dine HCl |
| otc | Allerfrim Syrup[1] | | |
| otc | Aprodine Syrup[1] | | |
| otc | Silafed Syrup[1] | | |
| otc | Actifed Cold & Allergy Tablets[1] | 60 mg pseudo-ephedrine HCl | 2.5 mg triproli-dine HCl |
| otc | Allerfrim Tablets[1] | | |
| otc | Aprodine Tablets[1] | | |
| otc | Cenafed Plus Tablets[1] | | |
| otc | Genac Tablets[1] | | |
| otc | Sudafed Sinus Nighttime Maximum Strength Tablets[1] | | |
| Rx | Trinalin Repetabs Tablets[3] | 120 mg pseudo-ephedrine sulfate | 1 mg azatadine maleate |
| otc | Chlor-Trimeton Allergy-D 4 Hour Tablets[1] | 60 mg pseudo-ephedrine sulfate | 4 mg chlor-pheniramine maleate |

| | Brand Name Examples | Decongestant | Antihistamine |
|---|---|---|---|
| otc | *Chlor-Trimeton Allergy-D 12 Hour Tablets* | 120 mg pseudo-ephedrine sulfate | 8 mg chlor-pheniramine maleate |
| Rx | *Drixomed Tablets*[3] | 120 mg pseudo-ephedrine sulfate | 6 mg dex-bromphenir-amine maleate |
| otc | *Drixoral Cold & Allergy Tablets* | | |
| Rx | *Claritin-D 12 Hour Tablets*[7] | 120 mg pseudo-ephedrine sulfate | 5 mg loratadine |
| Rx | *Claritin-D 24 Hour Tablets*[7] | 240 mg pseudo-ephedrine sulfate | 10 mg lorata-dine |
| Rx | *C-PHED Tannate Suspension*[1] | 75 mg pseudo-ephedrine tannate | 4.5 mg chlor-pheniramine tannate |
| Rx | *CP-TANNIC Suspension*[1] | | |
| Rx | *Tanafed Suspension* | | |

[1] This product may also be used in children; refer to package labeling.
[2] Contains alcohol.
[3] Sustained release.
[4] Sugar free.
[5] Alcohol free.
[6] Dye free.
[7] Extended release.
[8] Timed release.
[9] Contains phenylalanine.

## Pediatric Decongestants and Antihistamines

Content given per tablet, capsule, 5 mL (liquid), or 1 mL (drops).

| | Brand Name Examples | Decongestant | Antihistamine |
|---|---|---|---|
| Rx | Rhinatate-NF Pediatric Suspension | 5 mg phenyl-ephrine tannate | 4.5 mg chlor-pheniramine tannate |
| Rx | Rynatan Pediatric Suspension[1] | | |
| Rx | Phenylephrine Tannate/ Chlorpheniramine Tannate/Pyrilamine Tannate Pediatric Suspension | 5 mg phenyl-ephrine tannate | 2 mg chlor-pheniramine tannate, 12.5 mg pyrilamine tannate |
| Rx | Rhinatate Pediatric Suspension | | |
| Rx | Triotann Pediatric Suspension | | |
| Rx | Triotann-S Pediatric Suspension | | |
| Rx | Duonate-12 Suspension | 5 mg phenyl-ephrine tannate | 30 mg pyril-amine tannate |
| Rx | R-Tanna 12 Suspension | | |
| Rx | R-Tannic-S A/D Suspension | | |
| Rx | Ryna-12 S Suspension | | |
| otc | Bromanate Elixir[2] | 15 mg pseudo-ephedrine HCl | 1 mg brom-pheniramine maleate |
| otc | Dimaphen Elixir[2,3] | | |
| otc | Dimetapp Cold & Allergy Elixir[2,3] | | |
| Rx | Brompheniramine Maleate/Pseudoephedrine HCl Syrup | 60 mg pseudo-ephedrine HCl | 4 mg brom-pheniramine maleate |
| Rx | Bromfed-PD Capsules[3,4] | 60 mg pseudo-ephedrine HCl | 6 mg brom-pheniramine maleate |
| Rx | Bromfenex PD Capsules[3,4] | | |
| Rx | DALLERGY-JR Capsules[3,4] | | |
| Rx | ULTRAbrom PD Capsules[3,4] | | |
| Rx | Rondec Oral Drops | 15 mg pseudo-ephedrine HCl | 1 mg carbinox-amine maleate |
| Rx | Andehist Drops[2,5] | 15 mg pseudo-ephedrine HCl | 2 mg carbinox-amine maleate |
| Rx | Palgic DS Syrup | | |
| Rx | Pediatex-D Liquid[2,5,6] | | |

| | Brand Name Examples | Decongestant | Antihistamine |
|---|---|---|---|
| Rx | *Carbinoxamine Oral Drops*[2,5] | 25 mg pseudo-ephedrine HCl | 2 mg carbinox-amine maleate |
| Rx | *Cydec Oral Drops* | | |
| Rx | *Carbinoxamine Syrup*[2,3,5] | 60 mg pseudo-ephedrine HCl | 4 mg carbinox-amine maleate |
| otc | *PediaCare Children's Cold & Allergy Liquid*[2] | 15 mg pseudo-ephedrine HCl | 1 mg chlor-pheniramine maleate |
| otc | *Thera-Hist Cold & Allergy Syrup* | | |
| otc | *Tri-Acting Cold & Allergy Syrup*[2] | | |
| otc | *Triacting Cold & Allergy Liquid*[2] | | |
| otc | *Triaminic Cold & Allergy Liquid*[2] | | |
| otc | *Triaminic Softchews Tablets*[7] | | |
| Rx | *Rescon-Jr. Capsules*[3,8] | 60 mg pseudo-ephedrine HCl | 4 mg chlor-pheniramine maleate |
| otc | *Benadryl Children's Allergy & Cold Fastmelt Tablets*[3,7] | 30 mg pseudo-ephedrine HCl | 19 mg diphen-hydramine cit-rate (12.5 mg diphenhydra-mine HCl) |
| otc | *Benadryl Children's Allergy & Sinus Liquid*[2,3,5] | 30 mg pseudo-ephedrine HCl | 12.5 mg diphenhydra-mine HCl |
| Rx | *Quadra-Hist D PED Capsules*[4] | 40 mg pseudo-ephedrine HCl | 8 mg phenyl-toloxamine cit-rate, 8 mg pyrilamine maleate, 8 mg pheniramine maleate |
| Rx | *Chlorpheniramine Tan-nate/Pseudoephedrine Tannate Suspension*[2,5] | 75 mg pseudo-ephedrine tannate | 4.5 mg chlor-pheniramine tannate |

[1] Contains tartrazine dye.
[2] Alcohol free.
[3] This product may also be used in adults; refer to package labeling.
[4] Extended release.
[5] Sugar free.
[6] Dye free.
[7] Contains phenylalanine.
[8] Sustained release.

## Decongestant, Antihistamine, and Analgesic Combinations

Content given per capsule, tablet, packet, or 5 mL.

| | Brand Name Examples | Decongestant | Antihistamine | Analgesic/ Other |
|---|---|---|---|---|
| otc | Alka-Seltzer Plus Cold Medicine Effervescent Tablets[1] | 5 mg phenyl-ephrine HCl | 2 mg chlor-pheniramine maleate | 250 mg aceta-minophen |
| otc | Decodult Tablets | 5 mg phenyl-ephrine HCl | 2 mg chlor-pheniramine maleate | 300 mg aceta-minophen |
| otc | Dristan Cold Multi-Symptom Formula Tablets | 5 mg phenyl-ephrine HCl | 2 mg chlor-pheniramine maleate | 325 mg aceta-minophen |
| otc | Dryphen Multi-Symptom Formula Tablets | | | |
| otc | Scot-Tussin Original Clear 5-Action Cold and Allergy Formula Liquid[2,3-5] | 4.2 mg phenyl-ephrine HCl | 13.3 mg pheni-ramine maleate | 83.3 mg Na citrate, 83.3 mg Na salicylate, 25 mg caffeine citrate |
| otc | Scot-Tussin Original 5-Action Cold and Allergy Formula Syrup[2,4] | | | |
| otc | Comtrex Acute Head Cold & Sinus Pressure Relief, Multi-Symptom Maximum Strength Tablets | 30 mg pseudo-ephedrine HCl | 2 mg brom-pheniramine maleate | 500 mg aceta-minophen |
| otc | Alka-Seltzer Plus Cold Medicine Liqui-Gels[2] | 30 mg pseudo-ephedrine HCl | 2 mg chlor-pheniramine maleate | 325 mg aceta-minophen |
| otc | Kolephrin Tablets[2] | | | |

| | Brand Name Examples | Decongestant | Antihistamine | Analgesic/ Other |
|---|---|---|---|---|
| otc | Actifed Cold & Sinus Maximum Strength Tablets | 30 mg pseudo-ephedrine HCl | 2 mg chlor-pheniramine maleate | 500 mg aceta-minophen |
| otc | Comtrex Allergy-Sinus Treatment, Maximum Strength Tablets | | | |
| otc | Good Sense Maximum Strength Dose Sinus Tablets | | | |
| otc | Good Sense Maximum Strength Pain Relief Allergy Sinus Gelcaps | | | |
| otc | Sine-Off Sinus Medicine Tablets | | | |
| otc | Tylenol Allergy Sinus, Maximum Strength Tablets, Gelcaps, and Geltabs | | | |
| otc | Comtrex Flu Therapy & Fever Relief Day & Night, Multi-Symptom Maximum Strength Tablets | Day: 30 mg pseudoephed-rine HCl | | 500 mg aceta-minophen |
| | | Night: 30 mg pseudoephed-rine HCl | 2 mg chlor-pheniramine maleate | 500 mg aceta-minophen |
| Rx | Simplet Tablets | 60 mg pseudo-ephedrine HCl | 4 mg chlor-pheniramine maleate | 650 mg aceta-minophen |
| otc | Singlet for Adults Tablets | | | |
| otc | TheraFlu Flu and Cold Medicine Original Formula Powder | | | |
| otc | Triaminicin Cold, Allergy, Sinus Medicine Tablets | | | |

| | Brand Name Examples | Decongestant | Antihistamine | Analgesic/ Other |
|---|---|---|---|---|
| otc | TheraFlu Flu & Cold Medicine for Sore Throat, Maximum Strength Powder[1] | 60 mg pseudo-ephedrine HCl | 4 mg chlorpheniramine maleate | 1000 mg acetaminophen |
| otc | TheraFlu Flu & Sore Throat, Maximum Strength Powder | | | |
| otc | TheraFlu Flu & Sore Throat Night Time, Maximum Strength Powder[4] | | | |
| otc | Tavist Allergy/ Sinus/Headache Tablets | 30 mg pseudo-ephedrine HCl | 0.335 mg clemastine fumarate | 500 mg acetaminophen |
| otc | Benadryl Allergy & Cold Tablets | 30 mg pseudo-ephedrine HCl | 12.5 mg diphenhydramine HCl | 500 mg acetaminophen |
| otc | Benadryl Allergy & Sinus Headache Tablets and Gelcaps | | | |

| | Brand Name Examples | Decongestant | Antihistamine | Analgesic/ Other |
|---|---|---|---|---|
| otc | Benadryl Maximum Strength Severe Allergy & Sinus Headache Tablets | 30 mg pseudo-ephedrine HCl | 25 mg diphen-hydramine HCl | 500 mg aceta-minophen |
| otc | Sine-Off Night Time Formula Sinus, Cold, & Flu Medicine Geltabs | | | |
| otc | Sudafed Maximum Strength Sinus Nighttime Plus Pain Relief Tablets | | | |
| otc | Tylenol Allergy Sinus NightTime, Maximum Strength Tablets | | | |
| otc | Tylenol Flu NightTime, Maximum Strength Gelcaps | | | |
| otc | Contac Day & Night Allergy/ Sinus Relief Tablets | *Day:* 60 mg pseudoephed-rine HCl | | 650 mg aceta-minophen |
| | | *Night:* 60 mg pseudoephed-rine HCl | 50 mg diphen-hydramine HCl | 650 mg aceta-minophen |
| otc | Tylenol Sinus NightTime, Maximum Strength Tablets | 30 mg pseudo-ephedrine HCl | 6.25 mg doxyl-amine succi-nate | 500 mg aceta-minophen |
| otc | Coricidin 'D' Cold, Flu, & Sinus Tablets[2] | 30 mg pseudo-ephedrine sul-fate | 2 mg chlor-pheniramine maleate | 325 mg aceta-minophen |
| otc | Drixoral Allergy Sinus Tablets[6] | 60 mg pseudo-ephedrine sul-fate | 3 mg dex-bromphenir-amine maleate | 500 mg aceta-minophen |

[1] Contains phenylalanine.
[2] This product may also be used in children; refer to package labeling.
[3] Sugar free.
[4] Alcohol free.
[5] Dye free.
[6] Extended release.

## Pediatric Decongestant, Antihistamine, and Analgesic Combinations

Content given per tablet or 5 mL.

| | Brand Name Examples | Decongestant | Antihistamine | Analgesic |
|---|---|---|---|---|
| otc | Tylenol Children's Cold Chewable Tablets[1] | 7.5 mg pseudo-ephedrine HCl | 0.5 mg chlor-pheniramine maleate | 80 mg aceta-minophen |
| otc | Tylenol Children's Cold Liquid | 15 mg pseudo-ephedrine HCl | 1 mg chlor-pheniramine maleate | 160 mg aceta-minophen |

[1] Contains phenylalanine.
[2] Alcohol free.

## Decongestant, Antihistamine, and Anticholinergic Combinations

Content given per tablet or 5 mL.

| | Brand Name Examples | Decongestant | Antihistamine | Anticholinergic |
|---|---|---|---|---|
| Rx | Dallergy Syrup[1] | 10 mg phenyl-ephrine HCl | 2 mg chlor-pheniramine maleate | 0.625 mg meth-scopolamine nitrate |
| Rx | AH-chew Tablets[1,2] | 10 mg phenyl-ephrine HCl | 2 mg chlor-pheniramine maleate | 1.25 mg methscopol-amine nitrate |
| Rx | Dehistine Syrup[1,3] | | | |
| Rx | Duradryl Syrup[1] | | | |
| Rx | Extendryl Chewable Tablets[1] | | | |
| Rx | Extendryl Syrup[1] | | | |
| Rx | Ex-Histine Syrup[1] | | | |
| Rx | Dallergy Tablets[1] | 10 mg phenyl-ephrine HCl | 4 mg chlor-pheniramine maleate | 1.25 mg methscopol-amine nitrate |

| | Brand Name Examples | Decongestant | Antihistamine | Anticholinergic |
|---|---|---|---|---|
| Rx | Dallergy Extended Release Tablets[1] | 20 mg phenyl-ephrine HCl | 8 mg chlor-pheniramine maleate | 2.5 mg methscopol-amine nitrate |
| Rx | Extendryl SR Capsules | | | |
| otc | Hista-Vent DA Tablets[1,4] | | | |
| Rx | OMNIhist L.A. Tablets[4] | | | |
| Rx | Pre-Hist-D Tablets[1,4] | | | |
| Rx | Stahist Tablets[4,5] | 25 mg phenyl-ephrine HCl, 40 mg pseudo-ephedrine | 8 mg chlor-pheniramine maleate | 0.19 mg hyoscy-amine sulfate, 0.04 mg atropine sul-fate, 0.01 mg scopol-amine HBr |
| Rx | AlleRx-D Tablets[6] | 120 mg pseudoephed-rine HCl | | 2.5 mg methscopol-amine nitrate |
| Rx | PSE 120/ MSC 2.5 Tablets[4] | | | |
| Rx | Pannaz S Syrup[1] | 15 mg pseudo-ephedrine HCl | 2 mg carbinox-amine maleate | 1.25 mg methscopol-amine nitrate |
| Rx | Respa A.R. Tablets[5,7] | 90 mg pseudo-ephedrine HCl | 8 mg chlor-pheniramine maleate | 0.024 mg belladonna alkaloids (atropine, hyoscyamine, scopolamine) |
| Rx | CPM 8/PSE 90/MSC 2.5 Tablets[1,4] | 90 mg pseudo-ephedrine HCl | 8 mg chlor-pheniramine maleate | 2.5 mg methscopol-amine nitrate |
| Rx | Pannaz Tablets[1,4] | | | |

| | Brand Name Examples | Decongestant | Antihistamine | Anticholinergic |
|---|---|---|---|---|
| Rx | Mescolor Tablets[1,4,5] | 120 mg pseudoephedrine HCl | 8 mg chlorpheniramine maleate | 2.5 mg methscopolamine nitrate |
| Rx | Rescon-MX Tablets[1,4] | | | |
| Rx | Xiral Tablets[1,4,5] | | | |
| Rx | AlleRx Dose Pack Tablets[6] | Day: 120 mg pseudoephedrine HCl | | 2.5 mg methscopolamine nitrate |
| | | Night: | 8 mg chlorpheniramine maleate | 2.5 mg methscopolamine nitrate |

[1] This product may also be used in children; refer to package labeling.
[2] Chewable.
[3] Alcohol free.
[4] Sustained release.
[5] Dye free.
[6] Controlled release.
[7] Sugar free.

### Pediatric Decongestant, Antihistamine, and Anticholinergic Combinations

Content given per capsule.

| | Brand Name Examples | Decongestant | Antihistamine | Anticholinergic |
|---|---|---|---|---|
| Rx | Duradryl JR Capsules | 10 mg phenyl-ephrine HCl | 4 mg chlor-pheniramine maleate | 1.25 mg meth-scopolamine nitrate |
| Rx | Extendryl JR Capsules | | | |

### Antitussive Combinations

Content given per tablet, capsule, packet, pouch, or 5 mL.

| | Brand Name Examples | Anti-tussive | Anti-histamine | Decongestant | Other |
|---|---|---|---|---|---|
| Rx | Tannic-12 Tablets[1] | 60 mg carbeta-pentane tannate | 5 mg chlor-pheniramine tannate | | |
| Rx | Trionate Tablets | | | | |
| Rx | Tussi-12 Tablets | | | | |
| Rx | Quad Tann Tablets | 60 mg carbeta-pentane tannate | 5 mg chlor-pheniramine tannate | 10 mg phenyl-ephrine tan-nate, 10 mg ephedrine tan-nate | |
| Rx | Rynatuss Tablets | | | | |
| c-III | Cycofed Syrup[2] | 20 mg codeine phosphate | | 60 mg pseudo-ephedrine HCl | |
| c-III | Nucofed Syrup[2,3] | | | | |
| c-III | Nucofed Capsules | | | | |
| c-v | Dihistine DH Elixir[2,4] | 10 mg codeine phosphate | 2 mg chlor-pheniramine maleate | 30 mg pseudo-ephedrine HCl | |
| c-v | Decohistine DH Liquid[4] | | | | |
| c-v | Ryna-C Liquid[1,2,3,5] | | | | |

| | Brand Name Examples | Anti-tussive | Anti-histamine | Decongestant | Other |
|---|---|---|---|---|---|
| c-v | Prometh w/Codeine Cough Syrup[2,4] | 10 mg codeine phosphate | 6.25 mg promethazine HCl | | |
| c-v | Promethazine HCl w/Codeine Syrup[2] | | | | |
| c-v | Promethazone VC w/Codeine Cough Syrup[2,4] | 10 mg codeine phosphate | 6.25 mg promethazine HCl | 5 mg phenylephrine HCl | |
| c-v | Prometh VC w/Codeine Cough Syrup[2,4] | | | | |
| c-v | Tricodene Cough & Cold Liquid[2] | 8.2 mg codeine phosphate | 12.5 mg pyrilamine maleate | | |
| c-v | Codimal PH Syrup[2,3] | 10 mg codeine phosphate | 8.33 mg pyrilamine maleate | 5 mg phenylephrine HCl | |
| c-v | Triacin-C Cough Syrup[2,4] | 10 mg codeine phosphate | 1.25 mg triprolidine HCl | 30 mg pseudoephedrine HCl | |
| otc | Robitussin Honey Cough & Cold Liquid | 10 mg dextromethorphan HBr | | 20 mg pseudoephedrine HCl | |
| otc | Top Care Maximum Strength Soothing Cough & Head Congestion Relief D Liquid[2,4] | | | | |
| otc | Vicks 44D Cough & Head Congestion Relief Liquid[2,4] | | | | |
| otc | Robitussin Maximum Strength Cough & Cold Syrup[4] | 15 mg dextromethorphan HBr | | 30 mg pseudoephedrine HCl | |

| | Brand Name Examples | Anti-tussive | Anti-histamine | Decongestant | Other |
|---|---|---|---|---|---|
| otc | 666 Cold Preparation, Maximum Strength Liquid[2] | 3.3 mg dextromethorphan HBr | | 10 mg pseudo-ephedrine HCl | 108.3 mg acetaminophen |
| otc | Vicks DayQuil Multi-Symptom Cold/FLu Relief Liquid[2] | | | | |
| otc | Robitussin Honey Flu Multi-Symptom Liquid | 6.6 mg dextromethorphan HBr | | 20 mg pseudo-ephedrine HCl | 166.6 mg acetaminophen |
| otc | Vicks DayQuil LiquiCaps Multi-Symptom Cold/Flu Relief Capsules[2] | 10 mg dextromethorphan HBr | | 30 mg pseudo-ephedrine HCl | 250 mg acetaminophen |
| otc | Alka-Seltzer Plus Cold & Flu Liqui-Gels[2] | 10 mg dextromethorphan HBr | | 30 mg pseudo-ephedrine HCl | 325 mg acetaminophen |
| otc | Alka-Seltzer Plus Liqui-Gels Flu Medicine[2] | | | | |
| otc | Tylenol Cold Non-Drowsy Formula Gel-caps and Tablets[2] | 15 mg dextromethorphan HBr | | 30 mg pseudo-ephedrine HCl | 325 mg acetaminophen |
| otc | Top Care Multi-Symptom Pain Relief Cold Tablets[2] | | | | |

| | Brand Name Examples | Anti-tussive | Anti-histamine | Decongestant | Other |
|---|---|---|---|---|---|
| otc | Comtrex Multi-Symptom Maximum Strength Non-Drowsy Cold & Cough Relief Tablets | 15 mg dextromethorphan HBr | | 30 mg pseudo-ephedrine | 500 mg acetaminophen |
| otc | TheraFlu Non-Drowsy Formula Maximum Strength Tablets | | | | |
| otc | Tylenol Flu Maximum Strength Non-Drowsy Gelcaps | | | | |
| otc | Sudafed Non-Drowsy Severe Cold Formula Maximum Strength Tablets | | | | |
| otc | Robitussin Honey Flu Non-Drowsy Syrup | 20 mg dextromethorphan HBr | | 60 mg pseudo-ephedrine HCl | 500 mg acetaminophen |
| otc | TheraFlu Non-Drowsy Flu, Cold & Cough Maximum Strength Powder | 30 mg dextromethorphan HBr | | 60 mg pseudo-ephedrine HCl | 1000 mg acetaminophen |
| otc | TheraFlu Severe Cold & Congestion Non-Drowsy, Maximum Strength Powder | | | | |

| | Brand Name Examples | Anti-tussive | Anti-histamine | Decongestant | Other |
|---|---|---|---|---|---|
| Rx | Bromatane DX Syrup[2,4,5] | 10 mg dextromethorphan HBr | 2 mg brompheniramine maleate | 30 mg pseudoephedrine HCl | |
| Rx | Bromfed DM Cough Syrup[2] | | | | |
| Rx | Dimetane-DX Cough Syrup[2,4,5] | | | | |
| otc | Robitussin Allergy & Cough Liquid[1,2,3] | | | | |
| Rx | Alacol DM Syrup[3,5] | 10 mg dextromethorphan HBr | 2 mg brompheniramine maleate | 5 mg phenylephrine HCl | |
| Rx | Carbodex DM Syrup | 15 mg dextromethorphan HBr | 4 mg brompheniramine maleate | 45 mg pseudoephedrine HCl | |
| Rx | Carbofed DM Syrup[2] | | | | |
| Rx | Rondec-DM Syrup[2] | | | | |
| Rx | Andehist-DM Syrup[2,3] | 15 mg dextromethorphan HBr | 4 mg brompheniramine maleate | 60 mg pseudoephedrine HCl | |
| Rx | Coldec DM Syrup[2,3,5] | | | | |
| Rx | Rondamine DM Syrup | | | | |
| Rx | Sildec-DM Syrup[2,3,5] | | | | |
| Rx | Anaplex-DM Liquid[1,2,3,5] | 30 mg dextromethorphan HBr | 4 mg brompheniremine maleate | 60 mg pseudoephedrine HCl | |
| Rx | Balamine DM Syrup[2] | 12.5 mg dextromethorphan HBr | 4 mg carbinoxamine maleate | 60 mg pseudoephedrine HCl | |

| Brand Name Examples | Anti-tussive | Anti-histamine | Decongestant | Other |
|---|---|---|---|---|
| Rx Carbinoxamine Compound Syrup[4] | 15 mg dextromethorphan HBr | 4 mg carbinoxamine maleate | 60 mg pseudoephedrine HCl | |
| Rx Cardec DM Syrup[2,4] | | | | |
| Rx Cydec-DM Syrup[2] | | | | |
| Rx Tussafed Syrup[2,3,5] | | | | |
| otc Tricodene Sugar Free Liquid[2,3,5] | 10 mg dextromethorphan HBr | 2 mg chlorpheniramine maleate | | |
| otc Scot-Tussin DM Liquid[1,2,3,5] | 15 mg dextromethorphan HBr | 2 mg chlorpheniramine maleate | | |
| otc Coricidin HBP Cough & Cold Tablets | 30 mg dextromethorphan HBr | 4 mg chlorpheniramine maleate | | |
| otc Coricidin HBP Maximum Strength Flu Tablets | 15 mg dextromethorphan HBr | 2 mg chlorpheniramine maleate | | 500 mg acetaminophen |
| otc Alka-Seltzer Plus Flu Medicine Effervescent Tablets[6] | 15 mg dextromethorphan HBr | 2 mg chlorpheniramine maleate | | 500 mg aspirin |
| otc Father John's Medicine Plus Liquid[3] | 1.66 mg dextromethorphan HBr | 0.66 mg chlorpheniramine maleate | 1.66 mg phenylephrine HCl | |
| otc Alka-Seltzer Plus Cold & Cough Medicine Effervescent Tablets[6] | 10 mg dextromethorphan HBr | 2 mg chlorpheniramine maleate | 5 mg phenylephrine HCl | |
| otc Rescon-DM Liquid[1,2,3,5] | 10 mg dextromethorphan HBr | 2 mg chlorpheniramine maleate | 30 mg pseudoephedrine HCl | |

| | Brand Name Examples | Anti-tussive | Anti-histamine | Decongestant | Other |
|---|---|---|---|---|---|
| otc | Robitussin Flu Liquid[2,3] | 5 mg dextromethorphan HBr | 1 mg chlorpheniramine maleate | 15 mg pseudoephedrine HCl | 160 mg acetaminophen |
| otc | Vicks 44M Cough, Cold, & Flu Relief Liquid[4] | 7.5 mg dextromethorphan HBr | 1 mg chlorpheniramine maleate | 15 mg pseudoephedrine HCl | 162.5 mg acetaminophen |
| otc | Alka-Seltzer Plus Cold & Cough Liqui-Gels[2] | 10 mg dextromethorphan HBr | 2 mg chlorpheniramine maleate | 30 mg pseudoephedrine HCl | 325 mg acetaminophen |
| otc | Kolephrin/DM Tablets[2] | | | | |
| otc | Top Care Multi-Symptom Pain Relief Cold Tablets[2] | 15 mg dextromethorphan HBr | 2 mg chlorpheniramine maleate | 30 mg pseudoephedrine HCl | 325 mg acetaminophen |
| otc | Tylenol Cold Complete Formula Tablets[2] | | | | |
| otc | Mapap Cold Formula Tablets[2] | | | | |

| | Brand Name Examples | Anti-tussive | Anti-histamine | Decongestant | Other |
|---|---|---|---|---|---|
| otc | Contac Severe Cold & Flu Maximum Strength Tablets | 15 mg dextromethorphan HBr | 2 mg chlorpheniramine maleate | 30 mg pseudoephedrine HCl | 500 mg acetaminophen |
| otc | Comtrex Day & Night Cold & Cough Relief, Multi-Symptom Maximum Strength Tablets | | | | |
| otc | Genacol Maximum Strength Cold & Flu Relief Tablets | | | | |
| otc | Comtrex Cough and Cold Relief, Multi-Symptom Maximum Strength Tablets[2] | | | | |
| otc | Cold Symptoms Relief Maximum Strength Tablets | | | | |
| otc | TheraFlu Maximum Strength NightTime Formula Flu, Cold, & Cough Medicine Tablets | | | | |
| otc | Robitussin Honey Flu Nighttime Syrup | 20 mg dextromethorphan HBr | 4 mg chlorpheniramine maleate | 60 mg pseudoephedrine HCl | 500 mg acetaminophen |
| otc | TheraFlu Flu, Cold & Cough Powder | 20 mg dextromethorphan HBr | 4 mg chlorpheniramine maleate | 60 mg pseudoephedrine HCl | 650 mg acetaminophen |
| otc | TheraFlu Cold & Cough Night Time Powder | | | | |

| | Brand Name Examples | Anti-tussive | Anti-histamine | Decongestant | Other |
|---|---|---|---|---|---|
| otc | TheraFlu Flu, Cold, & Cough and Sore Throat, Maximum Strength Powder[6] | 30 mg dextromethorphan HBr | 4 mg chlorpheniramine maleate | 60 mg pseudoephedrine HCl | 1000 mg acetaminophen |
| otc | TheraFlu Flu & Cough Night Time, Maximum Strength Powder[6] | | | | |
| otc | TheraFlu Flu, Cold, & Cough Night Time, Maximum Strength Powder | | | | |
| otc | TheraFlu Severe Cold & Congestion Night Time, Maximum Strength Powder | | | | |
| otc | Top Care Maximum Strength Flu, Cold, & Cough Medicine Night Time Powder | | | | |
| otc | Contac Day & Night Cold & Flu Tablets | Day: 30 mg dextromethorphan HBr | | 60 mg pseudoephedrine HCl | 650 mg acetaminophen |
| | | Night: | 50 mg diphenhydramine HCl | 60 mg pseudoephedrine HCl | 650 mg acetaminophen |
| otc | Vicks NyQuil Cough Syrup[2,4] | 5 mg dextromethorphan HBr | 2.1 mg doxylamine succinate | | |

| Brand Name Examples | Anti-tussive | Anti-histamine | Decongestant | Other |
|---|---|---|---|---|
| otc *Alka-Seltzer Plus Night-Time Cold Medicine Effervescent Tablets*[6] | 10 mg dextromethorphan HBr | 6.25 mg doxylamine succinate | 5 mg phenylephrine HCl | |
| otc *All-Nite Liquid*[4] | 5 mg dextromethorphan HBr | 2.1 mg doxylamine succinate | 10 mg pseudoephedrine HCl | 167 mg acetaminophen |
| otc *Nite Time Cold Formula for Adults Liquid*[4] | | | | |
| otc *Tylenol Flu NightTime, Maximum Strength Liquid*[2] | | | | |
| otc *Vicks NyQuil Multi-Symptom Cold/Flu Relief Liquid*[4] | | | | |
| otc *Top Care LiquiCaps Nite Time Multi-Symptom Cold/ Flu Relief Capsules* | 10 mg dextromethorphan HBr | 6.25 mg doxylamine succinate | 30 mg pseudoephedrine HCl | 250 mg acetaminophen |
| otc *Vicks NyQuil Multi-Symptom Cold & Flu Relief LiquiCaps Capsules* | | | | |
| otc *Alka-Seltzer Plus NightTime Cold Liqui-Gels*[3] | 10 mg dextromethorphan HBr | 6.25 mg doxylamine succinate | 30 mg pseudoephedrine HCl | 325 mg acetaminophen |
| Rx *Prometh w/Dextromethorphan Syrup*[2,4] | 15 mg dextromethorphan HBr | 6.25 mg promethazine | | |
| Rx *Promethazine w/Dextromethorphan Cough Syrup*[2,4] | | | | |

| | Brand Name Examples | Anti-tussive | Anti-histamine | Decongestant | Other |
|---|---|---|---|---|---|
| otc | Codal-DM Syrup[1,2,3,5] | 10 mg dextromethorphan HBr | 8.33 mg pyrilamine maleate | 5 mg phenylephrine HCl | |
| otc | Codimal DM Syrup[1,2,3,5] | | | | |
| otc | Dicomal-DM Syrup[1,2,3,5] | | | | |
| otc | Robitussin Night Relief Liquid[3] | 5 mg dextromethorphan HBr | 8.3 mg pyrilamine maleate | 10 mg pseudoephedrine HCl | 108.3 mg acetaminophen |
| c-III | Hycodan Tablets[2] | 5 mg hydrocodone bitartrate | | | 1.5 mg homatropine MBr |
| c-III | Hycodan Syrup[2] | | | | |
| c-III | Hydromet Syrup[2] | | | | |
| c-III | Hydromide Syrup[2,4] | | | | |
| c-III | Hydropane Syrup[2] | | | | |
| c-III | Tussigon Tablets[2] | | | | |
| c-III | Detussin Liquid[2,4] | 5 mg hydrocodone bitartrate | | 60 mg pseudoephedrine HCl | |
| c-III | Histussin D Liquid[2] | | | | |
| c-III | P-V-Tussin Tablets | | | | |

| Brand Name Examples | Anti-tussive | Anti-histamine | Decongestant | Other |
|---|---|---|---|---|
| c-III *Anaplex HD Liquid*[1,2,3,5] | 1.7 mg hydro-codone bitartrate | 2 mg brom-pheniramine maleate | 30 mg pseudo-ephedrine HCl | |
| c-III *S-T Forte 2 Liquid*[1,2,3,5] | 2.5 mg hydro-codone bitartrate | 2 mg chlor-pheniramine maleate | | |
| c-III *ED-TLC Liquid*[2] | 1.67 mg hydro-codone bitartrate | 2 mg chlor-pheniramine maleate | 5 mg phenyl-ephrine HCl | |
| c-III *Hydrocodone HD Liquid*[2,3] | | | | |
| c-III *Endagen-HD Liquid*[2] | 1.7 mg hydro-codone bitartrate | 2 mg chlor-pheniramine maleate | 5 mg phenyl-ephrine HCl | |
| c-III *Vanex HD Liquid*[1] | | | | |
| c-III *Hydro-PC Liquid*[2] | 2 mg hydro-codone bitartrate | 2 mg chlor-pheniramine maleate | 5 mg phenyl-ephrine HCl | |
| c-III *Hydro-PC II Liquid*[2] | 2 mg hydro-codone bitartrate | 2 mg chlor-pheniramine maleate | 7.5 mg phenyl-ephrine HCl | |
| c-III *Comtussin HC Syrup*[1,5] | 2.5 mg hydro-codone bitartrate | 2 mg chlor-pheniramine maleate | 5 mg phenyl-ephrine HCl | |
| c-III *Cytuss HC Liquid*[2] | | | | |
| c-III *Histussin HC Syrup*[3,5] | | | | |
| c-III *Hydrocodone CP Syrup*[2,3,5] | | | | |
| c-III *Histinex HC Syrup*[2,3,5] | | | | |

| Brand Name Examples | Anti-tussive | Anti-histamine | Decongestant | Other |
|---|---|---|---|---|
| c-III Atuss HD Liquid[2] | 2.5 mg hydro-codone bitartrate | 4 mg chlor-pheniramine maleate | 10 mg phenyl-ephrine HCl | |
| c-III ED Tuss HC Syrup[2,4] | | | | |
| c-III Maxi-Tuss HC Liquid[2] | | | | |
| c-III Atuss MS Liquid[2] | 5 mg hydro-codone bitartrate | 2 mg chlor-pheniramine maleate | 10 mg phenyl-ephrine HCl | |
| c-III Histinex PV Syrup[2,3,5] | 2.5 mg hydro-codone bitartrate | 2 mg chlor-pheniramine maleate | 30 mg pseudo-ephedrine HCl | |
| c-III Hyphed Liquid[2,4] | | | | |
| c-III P-V-Tussin Syrup[2,4] | | | | |
| c-III Tussend Syrup[2,4] | | | | |
| c-III Hydro-Tussin HC Syrup[1,2,3,5] | 3 mg hydro-codone bitartrate | 2 mg chlor-pheniramine maleate | 15 mg pseudo-ephedrine HCl | |
| c-III Pancof-HC Liquid[1,2,3,5] | | | | |
| c-III Tussend Tablets[2] | 5 mg hydro-codone bitartrate | 4 mg chlor-pheniramine maleate | 60 mg pseudo-ephedrine HCl | |
| c-III Statuss Green Liquid[2,3,5] | 2.5 mg hydro-codone bitartrate | 2 mg chlor-pheniramine maleate, 3.3 mg pyril-amine maleate | 5 mg phenyl-ephrine HCl, 3.3 mg pseudoephed-rine HCl | |
| c-III Tussionex Pennkinetic Suspension[2,3,7] | 10 mg hydrodone (as polis-tirex) | 8 mg chlor-pheniramine (as polistirex) | | |

| Brand Name Examples | Anti-tussive | Anti-histamine | Decongestant | Other |
|---|---|---|---|---|
| c-III *Hydrocodone Bitartrate 5 mg/ Pseudoephed-rine HCl 30 mg/ Carbinoxamine Maleate 2 mg Liquid* | 5 mg hydro-codone bitartrate | 2 mg car-binoxamine maleate | 30 mg pseudo-ephedrine HCl | |
| c-III *Codal-DH Syrup[2]* | 1.66 mg hydro-codone bitartrate | 8.33 mg pyrilamine maleate | 5 mg phenyl-ephrine HCl | |
| c-III *Codimal DH Syrup[2,3]* | | | | |
| c-III *Dicomal-DH Syrup[2]* | | | | |

[1] Dye free.
[2] This product may also be used in children; refer to package labeling.
[3] Alcohol free.

[4] Contains alcohol.
[5] Sugar free.
[6] Contains phenylalanine.
[7] Extended release.

## Pediatric Antitussive Combinations

Content given per tablet, 5 mL (liquid), or 1 mL (drops).

| | Brand Name Examples | Decongestant | Anti-histamine | Anti-tussive | Other |
|---|---|---|---|---|---|
| Rx | Tussi-12 S Suspension[1] | | 4 mg chlor-pheni-ramine tannate | 30 mg car-betapentane tannate | |
| Rx | Tannic-12 Suspension | 5 mg phenyl-ephrine tan-nate | 4 mg chlor-pheni-ramine tannate | 30 mg car-betapentane tannate | |
| Rx | Rynatuss Pediatric Suspension[1] | 5 mg phenyl-ephrine tan-nate, 5 mg ephedrine tan-nate | 4 mg chlor-pheni-ramine tannate | 30 mg car-betapantane tannate | |
| otc | Dimetapp Decongestant Plus Cough Infant Drops[2] | 9.375 mg/mL pseudoephed-rine HCl | | 3.125 mg/mL dextrometh-orphan HBr | |
| otc | Pedia Care Infants' Decon-gestant & Cough Drops[2] | | | | |
| otc | Pedia Relief Decongestant Plus Cough Infants' Drops[2] | | | | |
| otc | Tylenol Infants' Cold Decon-gestant & Fever Reducer Plus Cough Concen-trated Drops[2] | 9.375 mg/mL pseudoephed-rine HCl | | 3.125 mg/mL dextrometh-orphan HBr | 100 mg/mL aceta-minophen |
| otc | Sudafed Chil-dren's Non-Drowsy Cold & Cough Liquid[2-4] | 15 mg pseudo-ephedrine HCl | | 5 mg dextro-methorphan HBr | |

| | Brand Name Examples | Decongestant | Anti-histamine | Anti-tussive | Other |
|---|---|---|---|---|---|
| otc | Dimetapp Children's Non-Drowsy Flu Syrup[2,3] | 15 mg pseudo-ephedrine HCl | | 5 mg dextro-methorphan HBr | 160 mg aceta-minophen |
| otc | Triaminic Throat Pain & Cough Soft-chews Tablets[1,3] | | | | |
| otc | Pedia Care Children's Long-Lasting Cough Plus Cold Liquid[2] | 15 mg pseudo-ephedrine HCl | | 7.5 mg dextrometh-orphan HBr | |
| otc | Robitussin Pediatric Cough & Cold Formula Liquid[2,3] | | | | |
| otc | Triaminic AM Non-Drowsy Cough & Decongestant Liquid[3] | | | | |
| otc | Triaminic Cough & Congestion Liquid[2] | | | | |
| otc | Triaminic Cough & Sore Throat Liquid[2] | 15 mg pseudo-ephedrine HCl | | 7.5 mg dextrometh-orphan HBr | 160 mg aceta-minophen |

| | Brand Name Examples | Decongestant | Anti-histamine | Anti-tussive | Other |
|---|---|---|---|---|---|
| otc | Bromanate DM Cold & Cough Elixir[2,3] | 15 mg pseudo-ephedrine HCl | 1 mg brom-pheni-ramine maleate | 5 mg dextro-methorphan HBr | |
| otc | Children's Elixir DM Cough & Cold Elixir[2,3] | | | | |
| otc | Dimaphen DM Cold & Cough Elixir[2,3] | | | | |
| otc | Dimetapp DM Children's Cold & Cough Elixir[2,3] | | | | |
| otc | Dimetapp Children's Night-time Flu Syrup[2,3] | 15 mg pseudo-ephedrine HCl | 1 mg brom-pheni-ramine maleate | 5 mg dextro-methorphan HBr | 160 mg aceta-minophen |
| Rx | C.P.-DM Drops | 15 mg/mL pseudoephed-rine HCl | 1 mg/mL carbinox-amine maleate | 4 mg/mL dextrometh-orphan HBr | |
| Rx | Carbofed DM Oral Drops[2,4] | | | | |
| Rx | Rondec-DM Oral Drops | | | | |
| Rx | Andehist DM Oral Drops | 15 mg/mL pseudoephed-rine HCl | 2 mg/mL carbinox-amine maleate | 4 mg/mL dextrometh-orphan HBr | |
| Rx | Carbodex DM Drops | | | | |
| Rx | Sildec-DM Oral Drops[2,4] | | | | |
| Rx | Pediatex-DM Liquid[8] | 15 mg pseudo-ephedrine HCl | 2 mg car-binox-amine maleate | 15 mg dextrometh-orphan HBr | |
| Rx | Balamine DM Oral Drops | 25 mg/mL pseudoephed-rine HCl | 2 mg/mL carbinox-amine maleate | 3.5 mg/mL dextrometh-orphan HBr | |

| | Brand Name Examples | Decongestant | Anti-histamine | Anti-tussive | Other |
|---|---|---|---|---|---|
| Rx | Carbinoxamine Compound Drops | 25 mg/mL pseudoephed-rine HCl | 2 mg/mL carbinox-amine maleate | 4 mg/mL dextrometh-orphan HBr | |
| Rx | Cydec-DM Drops | | | | |
| Rx | Balamine DM Syrup[3] | 60 mg pseudo-ephedrine HCl | 4 mg car-binox-amine maleate | 12.5 mg dextrometh-orphan HBr | |
| Rx | Cydec-DM Syrup[3] | 60 mg pseudo-ephedrine HCl | 4 mg car-binox-amine maleate | 15 mg dextrometh-orphan HBr | |
| otc | Tylenol Children's Cold Plus Cough Chewable Tablets | 7.5 mg pseudoephed-rine HCl | 0.5 mg chlor-pheni-ramine maleate | 2.5 mg dextrometh-orphan HBr | 80 mg aceta-minophen |
| otc | All-Nite Children's Cold/ Cough Relief Liquid[2,3] | 10 mg pseudo-ephedrine HCl | 0.67 mg chlor-pheni-ramine maleate | 5 mg dextrometh-orphan HBr | |
| otc | Nite Time Children's Liquid[2,3] | | | | |
| otc | Vicks Children's NyQuil Cold/ Cough Relief Liquid[2,3] | | | | |
| otc | Vicks Pediatric 44M Cough & Cold Relief Liquid[2,3] | | | | |

| Brand Name Examples | Decongestant | Anti-histamine | Anti-tussive | Other |
|---|---|---|---|---|
| otc *Kid Kare Children's Cough/ Cold Liquid[2]* | 15 mg pseudo-ephedrine HCl | 1 mg chlor-pheni-ramine maleate | 5 mg dextro-methorphan HBr | |
| otc *Pedia Care Cough-Cold Liquid[2]* | | | | |
| otc *Pedia Care Multi-Symptom Cold Liquid[2]* | | | | |
| otc *Thera-Hist Cold & Cough Syrup[3]* | | | | |
| otc *Tri-Acting Cold & Cough Syrup[2]* | | | | |
| otc *Triaminic Cold & Cough Liquid[2]* | | | | |
| otc *Triaminic Cold & Cough Soft-chews Tablets[5]* | | | | |
| otc *Triaminic Cough Soft-chews Tablets[3,5]* | | | | |
| otc *Tylenol Children's Cold Plus Cough Suspension[2]* | 15 mg pseudo-ephedrine HCl | 1 mg chlor-pheni-ramine maleate | 5 mg dextro-methorphan HBr | 160 mg aceta-minophen |

| Brand Name Examples | Decongestant | Anti-histamine | Anti-tussive | Other |
|---|---|---|---|---|
| otc Pedia Care NightRest Cough & Cold Liquid[2] | 15 mg pseudo-ephedrine HCl | 1 mg chlor-pheni-ramine maleate | 7.5 mg dextrometh-orphan HBr | |
| otc Robitussin Pediatric Night Relief Cough & Cold Liquid[2] | | | | |
| otc Triaminic Cold & Night Time Cough Liquid[2] | | | | |
| otc Triaminic Cold, Cough & Fever Liquid | 15 mg pseudo-ephedrine HCl | 1 mg chlor-pheni-ramine maleate | 7.5 mg dextrometh-orphan HBr | 160 mg aceta-minophen |
| otc Tylenol Children's Flu Suspension[2] | | | | |

[1] Contains tartrazine.
[2] Alcohol free.
[3] This product may also be used in adults; refer to package labeling.
[4] Sugar free.
[5] Contains phenylalanine.

## Antitussive and Expectorant Combinations

Content given per tablet, 5 mL, or packet.

| | Brand Name Examples | Anti-tussive | Expecto-rant | Deconges-tant | Antihista-mine/Other |
|---|---|---|---|---|---|
| Rx | Levall Liquid[1,2] | 20 mg car-betapantane citrate | 100 mg guaifene-sin | 15 mg phenyl-ephrine HCl | |
| c-v | Dihistine Expectorant Liquid | 10 mg codeine phosphate | 100 mg guaifene-sin | 30 mg pseudo-ephedrine HCl | |
| c-v | Guiatuss DAC Liquid[1,3] | | | | |
| c-v | Halotussin DAC Syrup[1,3,4] | | | | |
| c-v | Mytussin DAC Liquid[1,3,4] | | | | |
| c-v | Novagest Expectorant with Codeine Liquid[1,3] | | | | |
| c-III | Nucofed Expectorant Syrup[1,3] | 20 mg codeine phosphate | 200 mg guaifene-sin | 60 mg pseudo-ephedrine HCl | |
| c-III | Nucotuss Expectorant Syrup[1,3] | | | | |
| c-v | Tussirex Syrup[2,5] | 10 mg codeine phosphate | 83.3 mg sodium citrate | 4.17 mg phenyl-ephrine HCl | 13.33 mg pheni-ramine maleate, 83.33 mg sodium salicylate, 25 mg caffeine citrate |
| c-v | Tussirex Sugar Free Liquid[2,4,5] | | | | |

| | Brand Name Examples | Anti-tussive | Expecto-rant | Deconges-tant | Antihista-mine/ Other |
|---|---|---|---|---|---|
| Rx | Donatussin Syrup[1,2] | 7.5 mg dextromethorphan HBr | 100 mg guaifenesin | 10 mg phenylephrine HCl | 2 mg chlorpheniramine maleate |
| otc | Tussex Cough Syrup[1,2,4] | 10 mg dextromethorphan HBr | 100 mg guaifenesin | 5 mg phenylephrine HCl | |
| otc | Tussafed Ex Syrup[1,2] | 30 mg dextromethorphan HBr | 200 mg guaifenesin | 10 mg phenylephrine HCl | |
| otc | Guiatuss CF Syrup[1,2] | 10 mg dextromethorphan HBr | 100 mg guaifenesin | 30 mg pseudoephedrine HCl | |
| otc | Robafen CF Syrup[1,2] | | | | |
| otc | Robitussin CF Syrup[1,2] | | | | |
| otc | Comtrex Multi-Symptom Deep Chest Cold & Congestion Relief Softgels | 10 mg dextromethorphan HBr | 100 mg guaifenesin | 30 mg pseudoephedrine HCl | 250 mg acetaminophen |
| otc | Robitussin Cold, Multi-Symptom Cold & Flu Softgels | | | | |
| otc | Sudafed Multi-Symptom Cold & Cough Liquid Caps | | | | |
| Rx | Profen II DM Liquid[1,2,4,5] | 10 mg dextromethorphan HBr | 200 mg guaifenesin | 15 mg pseudoephedrine HCl | |

| | Brand Name Examples | Anti-tussive | Expecto-rant | Deconges-tant | Antihista-mine/ Other |
|---|---|---|---|---|---|
| otc | Cold & Cough Tussin Softgels[1] | 10 mg dextromethorphan HBr | 200 mg guaifenesin | 30 mg pseudoephedrine HCl | |
| otc | Robitussin Cold, Cold & Cough Softgels[1] | | | | |
| otc | Robitussin Cold, Cold & Congestion Softgels and Tablets[1] | | | | |
| otc | Robitussin Cold, Multi-Symptom Cold & Flu Tablets[1] | 10 mg dextromethorphan HBr | 200 mg guaifenesin | 30 mg pseudoephedrine HCl | 325 mg acetaminophen |
| Rx | PanMist-DM Syrup[1,2,4,5] | 15 mg dextromethorphan HBr | 100 mg guaifenesin | 45 mg pseudoephedrine HCl | |
| otc | Tylenol Multi-Symptom Cold Severe Congestion Tablets[1] | 15 mg dextromethorphan HBr | 200 mg guaifenesin | 30 mg pseudoephedrine HCl | 325 mg acetaminophen |
| Rx | Z-Cof DM Syrup[1,2,4] | 15 mg dextromethorphan HBr | 200 mg guaifenesin | 40 mg pseudoephedrine HCl | |

| Brand Name Examples | Anti-tussive | Expecto-rant | Deconges-tant | Antihista-mine/ Other |
|---|---|---|---|---|
| otc TheraFlu Maximum Strength Flu & Conges-tion Non-Drowsy Powder[6] | 30 mg dextrometh-orphan HBr | 400 mg guaifene-sin | 60 mg pseudo-ephedrine HCl | 1000 mg aceta-minophen |
| otc TheraFlu Maximum Strength Flu, Cold & Cough Powder[2,6] | | | | |
| Rx Maxifed DM Tablets[1,5,7] | 30 mg dextrometh-orphan HBr | 550 mg guaifene-sin | 60 mg pseudo-ephedrine HCl | |
| Rx Touro CC Tablets[1,5,7] | 30 mg dextrometh-orphan HBr | 575 mg guaifene-sin | 60 mg pseudo-ephedrine HCl | |
| Rx PanMist-DM Tablets[1,8] | 30 mg dextrometh-orphan HBr | 600 mg guaifene-sin | 45 mg pseudo-ephedrine HCl | |
| Rx Protuss DM Tablets[1,5,7] | 30 mg dextrometh-orphan HBr | 600 mg guaifene-sin | 60 mg pseudo-ephedrine HCl | |
| Rx Tussafed-LA Tablets[1,5,7] | | | | |
| Rx Guai-fenex-Rx DM Tablets[8] | Day: | 600 mg guaifene-sin | 60 mg pseudo-ephedrine HCl | |
| | Night: 30 mg dextrometh-orphan HBr | 600 mg guaifene-sin | | |

| | Brand Name Examples | Anti-tussive | Expecto-rant | Deconges-tant | Antihista-mine/ Other |
|---|---|---|---|---|---|
| Rx | MED-Rx DM Tablets[9] | Day: | 600 mg guaifene-sin | 60 mg pseudo-ephedrine HCl | |
| | | Night: 30 mg dextrometh-orphan HBr | 600 mg guaifene-sin | | |
| Rx | Profen II DM Tablets[1,8] | 30 mg dextrometh-orphan HBr | 800 mg guaifene-sin | 45 mg pseudo-ephedrine HCl | |
| Rx | Medent-DM Tablets[1,5,7] | 30 mg dextrometh-orphan HBr | 800 mg guaifene-sin | 60 mg pseudo-ephedrine HCl | |
| Rx | Profen Forte DM Tablets[1,7] | 60 mg dextrometh-orphan HBr | 800 mg guaifene-sin | 90 mg pseudo-ephedrine HCl | |
| Rx | Aquatab C Tablets | 60 mg dextrometh-orphan HBr | 1200 mg guaifene-sin | 120 mg pseudo-ephedrine HCl | |
| Rx | GFN 1200/DM 60/PSE 120 Tablets[5,7] | | | | |
| c-III | Atuss-G Syrup[1] | 2 mg hydro-codone bitar-trate | 100 mg guaifene-sin | 10 mg phenyl-ephrine HCl | |
| c-III | Donatussin DC Syrup[1,2] | 2.5 mg hydrocodone bitartrate | 50 mg guaifene-sin | 7.5 mg phenyl-ephrine HCl | |
| c-III | Tussafed HC Syrup[1,2] | | | | |
| c-III | Entex HC Liquid[1,2,4,5] | 5 mg hydro-codone bitar-trate | 100 mg guaifene-sin | 7.5 mg phenyl-ephrine HCl | |
| c-III | Levall 5.0 Liquid[1,2,4] | 5 mg hydro-codone bitar-trate | 100 mg guaifene-sin | 15 mg phenyl-ephrine HCl | |

| Brand Name Examples | Anti-tussive | Expecto-rant | Deconges-tant | Antihista-mine/ Other |
|---|---|---|---|---|
| c-III ZTuss Expectorant Liquid[1,6] | 2.5 mg hydrocodone bitartrate | 100 mg guaifene-sin | 15 mg pseudo-ephedrine HCl | 2 mg chlor-pheni-ramine maleate |
| c-III Duratuss HD Elixir[1,3] | 2.5 mg hydrocodone bitartrate | 100 mg guaifene-sin | 30 mg pseudo-ephedrine HCl | |
| c-III Hydro-Tussin HD Liquid[1,2] | | | | |
| c-III Su-Tuss HD Elixir[1,3] | | | | |
| c-III Pancof-XP Liquid[1,2,4,5] | 3 mg hydro-codone bitar-trate | 100 mg guaifene-sin | 15 mg pseudo-ephedrine HCl | |
| c-III Protuss-D Liquid[1,2,4,5] | 5 mg hydro-codone bitar-trate | 300 mg potassium guaiacol-sulfonate | 30 mg pseudo-ephedrine HCl | |

[1] This product may also be used in children; refer to package labeling.
[2] Alcohol free.
[3] Contains alcohol.
[4] Sugar free.
[5] Dye free.
[6] Contains phenylalanine.
[7] Sustained release.
[8] Extended release.
[9] Controlled release.

### Pediatric Antitussive and Expectorant Combinations

Content given per 5 mL.

| | Brand Name Examples | Decongestant | Antitussive | Expectorant |
|---|---|---|---|---|
| c-v | Nucofed Pediatric Expectorant Syrup[1,2] | 30 mg pseudoephedrine HCl | 10 mg codeine phosphate | 100 mg guaifenesin |
| c-v | Nucotuss Pediatric Expectorant Syrup[1,2] | | | |
| otc | Robitussin Cough & Cold Infant Drops[1] | 6 mg/mL pseudoephedrine HCl | 2 mg/mL dextromethorphan HBr | 40 mg/mL guaifenesin |

[1] This product may also be used in adults; refer to package labeling.
[2] Contains alcohol.

### Antitussives with Expectorants

Content given per tablet or 5 mL.

| | Brand Name Examples | Antitussive | Expectorant |
|---|---|---|---|
| c-v | Cheracol Cough Syrup[1,2] | 10 mg codeine phosphate | 100 mg guaifenesin |
| c-v | Gani-Tuss NR Liquid[1,3,4] | | |
| c-v | Guiatuss AC Syrup[1,2,3] | | |
| c-v | Halotussin AC Liquid[1,3,4] | | |
| c-v | Mytussin AC Cough Syrup[1,2,3] | | |
| c-v | Romilar AC Liquid[1,3-6] | | |
| c-v | Tussi-Organidin NR Liquid[1] | | |
| c-v | Tussi-Organidin-S NR Liquid[1] | | |
| c-iii | Codeine Phosphate and Guaifenesin Tablets | 10 mg codeine phosphate | 300 mg guaifenesin |

| | Brand Name Examples | Antitussive | Expectorant |
|---|---|---|---|
| otc | Benylin Expectorant Liquid[1,3,4] | 5 mg dextromethorphan HBr | 100 mg guaifenesin |
| otc | Vicks 44E Cough & Chest Congestion Relief Liquid[1,2] | 6.67 mg dextromethorphan HBr | 66.7 mg guaifenesin |
| otc | Cheracol D Cough Formula Syrup[1,2] | 10 mg dextromethorphan HBr | 100 mg guaifenesin |
| otc | Cheracol Plus Liquid[1,2] | | |
| otc | Diabetic Tussin DM Liquid[1,3-6] | | |
| otc | Extra Action Cough Syrup[1] | | |
| Rx | Gani-Tuss-DM NR Liquid[1,3,4] | | |
| otc | Genatuss DM Syrup[1,4] | | |
| otc | Guaifenesin DM Syrup[1,4] | | |
| Rx | Guaifenesin-DM NR Liquid[1,3,4] | | |
| otc | Guiatuss-DM Syrup[1,4] | | |
| otc | Mytussin DM Syrup[1,4] | | |
| otc | Phanatuss DM Cough Syrup[1,3,4] | | |
| otc | Robitussin-DM Liquid[1] | | |
| otc | Robitussin Sugar Free Cough Liquid[1,3-5] | | |

| | Brand Name Examples | Antitussive | Expectorant |
|---|---|---|---|
| otc | Siltussin DM Cough Syrup[1,4] | 10 mg dextro-methorphan HBr | 100 mg guaifenesin |
| otc | Tolu-Sed DM Liquid[1-3] | | |
| Rx | Tussi-Organidin-DM NR Liquid[1] | | |
| otc | Kolephrin GG/DM Liquid[1,4] | 10 mg dextro-methorphan HBr | 150 mg guaifenesin |
| otc | Diabetic Tussin Maximum Strength DM Liquid[3-6] | 10 mg dextro-methorphan HBr | 200 mg guaifenesin |
| otc | Naldecon Senior DX Liquid[3,4] | | |
| otc | Robitussin Cough & Congestion Formula Liquid[1,4] | | |
| otc | Tuss-DM Tablets[1] | | |
| otc | Safe Tussin Liquid[1,3-5] | 15 mg dextro-methorphan HBr | 100 mg guaifenesin |
| otc | Scot-Tussin Senior Clear Liquid[3,4,6] | 15 mg dextro-methorphan HBr | 200 mg guaifenesin |
| Rx | Duratuss DM Elixir[1,2] | 20 mg dextro-methorphan HBr | 200 mg guaifenesin |
| Rx | Hydro-Tussin DM Liquid[1] | | |
| Rx | Maxi-Tuss DM Liquid[1] | | |
| Rx | SU-TUSS DM Liquid[1,2] | | |
| Rx | Respa-DM Tablets[1,5,7] | 28 mg dextro-methorphan HBr | 600 mg guaifenesin |
| Rx | Sudal-DM Tablets[1,5,7] | 30 mg dextro-methorphan HBr | 500 mg guaifenesin |
| Rx | Touro DM Tablets[1,7] | 30 mg dextro-methorphan HBr | 575 mg guaifenesin |

| Brand Name Examples | Antitussive | Expectorant |
|---|---|---|
| Rx Guaifenex DM Tablets[1,8] | 30 mg dextro-methorphan HBr | 600 mg guaifenesin |
| Rx Guiadrine DM Tablets[1,7] | | |
| Rx Humibid DM Tablets[1,7] | | |
| Rx Iobid DM Tablets[1,7] | | |
| Rx Muco-Fen-DM Tablets[1,7] | | |
| Rx Allfen-DM Tablets[1,5,7] | 50 mg dextro-methorphan HBr | 1000 mg guaifenesin |
| Rx Dex GG TR Tablets[1,8] | 60 mg dextro-methorphan HBr | 1000 mg guaifenesin |
| Rx GFN 1000/DM 60 Tablets[7] | | |
| Rx Guaifenesin 1000 mg and Dextro-methorhan HBr 60 mg LA Tablets[1] | | |
| Rx Aquatab DM Tablets | 60 mg dextro-methorphan HBr | 1200 mg guaifenesin |
| Rx GFN 1200/DM 60 Tablets[1,7] | | |
| Rx TUSSI-bid Tablets[1,7] | | |
| C-III Pneumotussin 2.5 Cough Syrup[1,3-5] | 2.5 mg hydro-codone bitartrate | 200 mg guaifenesin |
| C-III Pneumotussin Tablets[1,5] | 2.5 mg hydro-codone bitartrate | 300 mg guaifenesin |

| | Brand Name Examples | Antitussive | Expectorant |
|---|---|---|---|
| C-III | Hydrocodone Bitartrate and Guaifenesin Liquid[1,3-5] | 5 mg hydrocodone bitartrate | 100 mg guaifenesin |
| C-III | Codiclear DH Syrup[1,3-5] | | |
| C-III | Hycosin Expectorant Syrup[1,2] | | |
| C-III | Hycotuss Expectorant Syrup[1,2] | | |
| C-III | Hydrocodone GF Syrup[1,3-5] | | |
| C-III | Kwelcof Liquid[1,3-5] | | |
| C-III | Vitussin Syrup[1,3-5] | | |
| C-III | Atuss EX Syrup[1,3-5] | 2.5 mg hydrocodone bitartrate | 120 mg potassium guaiacolsulfonate |
| C-III | Prolex DH Liquid[1,3,4] | 4.5 mg hydrocodone bitartrate | 300 mg potassium guaiacolsulfonate |
| C-III | Hydron KGS Liquid[1,3,4] | 5 mg hydrocodone bitartrate | 300 mg potassium guaiacolsulfonate |
| C-III | Protuss Liquid[1,3,4] | | |
| C-III | Marcof Expectorant Syrup[1,3-5] | 5 mg hydrocodone bitartrate | 350 mg potassium guaiacolsulfonate |
| C-II | Dilaudid Cough Syrup[2] | 1 mg hydromorphone HCl | 100 mg guaifenesin |

[1] This product may also be used in children; refer to package labeling.
[2] Contains alcohol.
[3] Sugar free.
[4] Alcohol free.
[5] Dye free.
[6] Contains phenylalanine.
[7] Sustained release.
[8] Extended release.

## Pediatric Antitussives with Expectorants

Content given per 5 mL (liquid) or 1 mL (drops).

| | Brand Name Examples | Antitussive | Expectorant |
|---|---|---|---|
| otc | Robitussin DM Infant Drops[1] | 2 mg/mL dextromethorphan HBr | 40 mg/mL guaifenesin |
| otc | Vicks Pediatric 44E Cough & Chest Congestion Relief Liquid[2] | 3.3 mg dextromethorphan HBr | 33.3 mg guaifenesin |

[1] Alcohol free.
[2] This product may also be used in adults; refer to package labeling.

## Topical Combinations

| | Brand Name Examples | Ingredients |
|---|---|---|
| otc | Nose Better Gel | 0.5% allantoin, 0.75% camphor, 0.5% menthol |
| otc | TheraPatch Vapor Patch for Kids Cough Suppressant | 4.7% camphor, 2.6% menthol |
| otc | Triaminic Vapor Patch for Cough | |
| otc | Mentholatum Cherry Chest Rub for Kids | 4.7% camphor, 2.6% menthol, 1.2% eucalyptus oil |
| otc | Tom's of Maine Natural Cough & Cold Rub Cough Suppressant | 4.8% camphor, 2.6% menthol |
| otc | Vicks VapoRub Cream | 5.2% camphor, 2.8% menthol, 1.2% eucalyptus oil |
| otc | Mentholatum Ointment | 9% camphor, 1.3% menthol |
| otc | Breathe Right Children's Colds Nasal Strips | Menthol |
| otc | Breathe Right Colds Nasal Strips | |

*If you have any questions, consult your doctor, pharmacist, or health care provider.*

## CNS Stimulants
Amphetamines, 579
Analeptics, 583
Anorexiants, 587
Dexmethylphenidate, 592
Methylphenidate, 594
Pemoline, 598

## Analgesics
Acetaminophen, 601
Aspirin and Salicylates, 605
Buffered Aspirin, 610
Nonnarcotic Combinations, 612
Diflunisal, 616
Narcotic Pain Relievers, 618
Narcotic Pain Reliever
    Combinations, 626
Butorphanol Tartrate, 633
Pentazocine, 635
Tramadol, 638

## Nonsteroidal Anti-Inflammatory Agents, 640

## Antirheumatic Agents
Gold Compounds, 648
Hydroxychloroquine, 651
Methotrexate, 653

## Agents for Gout
Allopurinol, 657
Colchicine, 660
Probenecid, 664
Sulfinpyrazone, 668

## Agents for Migraine
Migraine Combinations, 670
Serotonin 5-HT$_1$ Receptor
    Antagonists, 673

## Antiemetic/Antivertigo Agents
Anticholinergics, 676
Cannabinoids, 681
5-HT$_3$ Receptor Antagonists, 684
Phenothiazines, 687
Phosphorated Carbohydrate, 693

## Vasopressor/Antihypotensive Agents
Midodrine, 695

## Antianxiety Agents
Benzodiazepines, 698
Buspirone, 703
Hydroxyzine, 706
Meprobamate, 708

## Antidepressants
Bupropion, 711
Nefazodone, 714
Escitalopram, 717
Fluoxetine, 719
Fluvoxamine, 723
Citalopram Hydrobromide, 726
Tetracyclic Compounds, 729
Monoamine Oxidase
    Inhibitors, 732
Paroxetine, 738
Sertraline, 741
Trazodone, 743
Venlafaxine, 746
Tricyclic Antidepressants, 749

## Antipsychotic Agents
Benzisoxazole Derivatives, 758
Dibenzapine Derivatives, 761
Dihydroindolone Derivatives, 765
Phenothiazine Derivatives, 768
Phenylbutylpiperadine
    Derivatives, 776
Quinolone Derivatives, 780
Thioxanthene Derivatives, 782

## Psychotherapeutic Agents
Ergoloid Mesylates, 785
Lithium, 787
Cholinesterase Inhibitors, 791
Psychotherapeutic
    Combinations, 795

## Sedatives
Barbiturates, 800
Hypnotics, 805

**Nonprescription Sleep Aids,** 810

**Anticonvulsants**
Acetazolamide, 813
Carbamazepine, 816
Clonazepam, 820
Felbamate, 824
Gabapentin, 827
Hydantoins, 829
Oxazolidinediones, 834
Oxcarbazepine, 836
Zonisamide, 839
Primidone, 841
Topiramate, 843
Succinimides, 846
Lamotrigine, 849
Tiagabine, 852
Levetiracetam, 855
Valproic Acid and Derivatives, 857

**Muscle Relaxants**
Baclofen, 862
Dantrolene Sodium, 865
Tizanidine, 868
Skeletal Muscle Relaxants, 871
Skeletal Muscle Relaxant
    Combinations, 875

**Antiparkinson Agents**
Anticholinergics, 877
Dopaminergics, 881
Pramipexole, 886
Ropinirole, 889
Pergolide Mesylate, 892
Selegiline, 895
Entacapone, 898

| Generic Name<br>*Brand Name Examples* | Supplied As | Generic<br>Available |
|---|---|---|
| *C-II* **Dextroamphetamine Sulfate** | | |
| *Dexedrine*[1], *DextroStat*[1] | **Tablets**: 5 mg, 10 mg | Yes |
| *Dexedrine Spansules* | **Capsules, sustained release**: 5 mg, 10 mg, 15 mg | Yes |
| *C-II* **Methamphetamine HCl** | | |
| *Desoxyn* | **Tablets**: 5 mg | No |
| *C-II* **Amphetamine Mixtures** | | |
| *Adderall* | **Tablets**: 5 mg, 7.5 mg, 10 mg, 12.5 mg, 15 mg, 20 mg, 30 mg (containing a mixture of amphetamine aspartate, amphetamine sulfate, dextro-amphetamine saccharate, dextroamphetamine sulfate) | Yes |
| *C-II* *Adderall XR* | **Capsules, extended release**: 5 mg, 10 mg, 15 mg, 20 mg, 25 mg, 30 mg (containing a mixture of amphetamine aspar-tate, amphetamine sulfate, dextroamphetamine saccharate, dextroamphetamine sulfate) | No |

[1] Contains tartrazine.

## Type of Drug:

Central nervous system stimulants: "Bennies," "dexies," "speed", or "crystal."

## How the Drug Works:

These synthetic drugs are a stronger form of the natural body stimulant adrenaline. They work by altering natural chemicals (neurotransmitters) in the brain and can affect other body systems (eg, circulatory system) in high doses.

## Uses:

Indicated as an integral part of a total treatment program of attention deficit disorder with hyperactivity that includes other remedial measures (psychological, educational, social) for a stabilizing effect in children 3 to 16 years of age with a behavioral syndrome characterized by moderate to severe distractibility, short attention span, hyperactivity, emotional lability, and impulsivity.

To improve wakefulness in patients with excessive daytime sleepiness associated with narcolepsy.

*Methamphetamine only:* For short-term (eg, a few weeks) use in a weight reduction program based on caloric restriction, for patients who have failed alternative therapy (eg, repeated diets, group programs, other drugs).

*Unlabeled Use(s):* Dextroamphetamine has been used to treat cocaine dependence and autism.

## Precautions:

*Do not use in the following situations:*

agitated states
allergy to amphetamines or any
 of their ingredients
arteriosclerosis (hardening of
 the arteries), advanced
drug abuse, history of
glaucoma

heart disease, symptomatic
high blood pressure, moderate
 to severe
MAOI therapy, concurrent or
 within 2 weeks
overactive thyroid gland

*Use with caution in the following situations:*

high blood pressure
Tourette syndrome

*Abuse:* Amphetamines have a high potential for abuse. Use in weight reduction programs only when alternative therapy (diets, group programs, other drugs) has been ineffective. Use for prolonged periods may lead to drug dependence.

*Attention deficit disorders:* Drug treatment is not indicated in all cases. The decision to use amphetamines depends on the chronicity and severity of the child's symptoms and appropriateness for his/her age. When symptoms are associated with acute stress reactions, treatment with amphetamines is usually not indicated.

*Chronic intoxication:* Severe skin rash, marked sleeplessness, irritability, hyperactivity, personality changes, disorganization of thoughts, poor concentration, hallucinations, and compulsive behavior often occur. The most severe side effect of chronic intoxication is psychosis, often indistinguishable from paranoid schizophrenia.

*Diabetes:* Insulin requirements may be altered with the use of amphetamines and diet restriction.

*Do not use:* Do not use to combat fatigue or to replace rest.

*Drug dependence:* Tolerance, extreme dependence and severe social disability have occurred with amphetamine abuse. Patients may gradually increase the dosage to many times that recommended. Abrupt discontinuation following a long period of using high doses results in extreme fatigue, mental depression, and changes in sleep habits.

*Pregnancy:* Adequate studies have not been done in pregnant women, or animal studies may have shown a risk to the fetus. Birth defects have been reported with amphetamine use in pregnancy. Use only if clearly needed and potential benefits outweigh the possible hazards to the fetus. Infants born to mothers dependent on amphetamines have an increased risk of premature delivery and low birth weight. These infants may experience symptoms of amphetamine withdrawal demonstrated by restlessness including agitation and weakness.

*Breastfeeding:* Amphetamines appear in breast milk. Discontinue nursing or discontinue the drug, taking into account the importance of the drug to the mother. Consult your doctor before you begin breastfeeding.

*Children:* Long-term effects in children have not been well established. Amphetamines are not recommended in children younger than 3 years of age. Do not use methamphetamine as a weight loss medication in children younger than 12 years of age. Extended-release amphetamine mixture capsules are indicated for children 6 years of age and older. Effects of extended-release amphetamine mixture capsules in children 3 to 5 years of age have not been studied. In psychotic children, amphetamines may worsen symptoms of behavior disturbance and thought disorder. Amphetamines may precipitate or worsen Tourette syndrome. Monitor growth during treatment. Chronic administration may be associated with growth inhibition.

*Tartrazine:* Some of these products may contain tartrazine dye (FD&C Yellow No. 5), which can cause allergic reactions in certain individuals. Check package labeling when available or consult your doctor or pharmacist.

## Drug Interactions:

Tell your doctor or pharmacist if you are taking or planning to take any over-the-counter or prescription medications or dietary supplements while taking this medicine. Doses of one or both drugs may need to be modified or a different drug may need to be prescribed. The following drugs and drug classes interact with amphetamines:

antihypertensives (eg, methyl-dopa)
furazolidone (*Furoxone*)
guanethidine (*Ismelin*)
MAOIs (eg, phenelzine)
phenothiazines (eg, chlorpromazine)
selective serotonin reuptake inhibitors (eg, fluoxetine)
urinary acidifiers (eg, ammonium chloride)
urinary alkalinizers (eg, acetazolamide)

## Side Effects:

Every drug is capable of producing side effects. Many amphetamine users experience no, or minor, side effects. The frequency and severity of side effects depend on many factors including dosage, duration of therapy, and individual susceptibility. Possible side effects include:

*Digestive Tract:* Diarrhea; constipation; appetite loss; dry mouth; unpleasant taste sensation; indigestion; nausea; vomiting.

*Nervous System:* Dizziness; sleeplessness; depression; irritability; restlessness; nervousness; headache; tremor; exacerbation of motor and phonic tics and Tourette syndrome; exaggerated sense of well-being (euphoria); overstimulation; difficulty moving; unpleasant feelings; weakness; drowsiness between doses or after stopping medicine.

*Circulatory System:* Pounding in the chest (palpitations); rapid or irregular heartbeat; high blood pressure.

*Other:* Impotence; changes in sex drive; hives; weight loss; suppression of growth in children (long-term use).

## Guidelines for Use:

- Dosage is individualized. Take exactly as prescribed.
- Do not change the dose or stop taking, unless directed by your doctor.
- Do not take more frequently than prescribed. These drugs can be addicting.
- Do not chew or crush sustained- or extended-release products.
- Extended-release amphetamine mixture capsules may be taken whole, or the capsule may be opened and the entire contents sprinkled on applesauce. The sprinkled applesauce should then be consumed immediately; it should not be stored. Take the applesauce with sprinkled beads in its entirety without chewing. The dose of a single capsule should not be divided.
- May cause insomnia. Avoid taking these medications late in the day.
- This medicine may cause dizziness. Use caution while driving or performing other tasks requiring alertness, coordination, or physical dexterity.
- May cause nervousness, restlessness, sleeplessness, dizziness, appetite loss, dry mouth, and digestive tract disturbances. Contact your doctor if these become troublesome.
- If a dose is missed, take it as soon as possible. If several hours have passed or it is nearing time for the next dose, do not double the dose to catch up, unless advised to do so by your doctor. If more than one dose is missed or it is necessary to establish a new dosage schedule, contact your doctor or pharmacist.
- Do not take any prescription or OTC medications or dietary supplements, unless directed by your doctor.
- Inform your doctor if you are pregnant, become pregnant, are planning to become pregnant, or if you are breastfeeding.
- Use of many of these drugs to improve athletic skills, mental alertness, or to stay awake is dangerous and illegal. Never share drugs with others.
- *Attention deficit disorder in children* – Your doctor may occasionally interrupt drug therapy to determine if there is a recurrence of symptoms.
- *Weight control* – Appropriate lifestyle changes (eg, diet and exercise) should be made while on therapy in order to avoid continued use of the drug.
- Store at room temperature (59° to 86°F) in a tight, light-resistant container.

*If you have any questions, consult your doctor, pharmacist, or health care provider.*

| Generic Name Brand Name Examples | Supplied As | Generic Available |
|---|---|---|
| **Caffeine**[1] | | |
| otc *357 HR Magnum, Caffedrine, Keep Alert, Maximum Strength NoDoz, Stay Awake, Vivarin* | **Tablets**: 200 mg | No |
| otc *44 Magnum, Molie* | **Capsules**: 200 mg | No |
| c-iv **Modafinil** | | |
| *Provigil* | **Tablets**: 100 mg, 200 mg | No |

[1] Also available as an injection (caffeine citrate and caffeine/sodium benzoate).

## Type of Drug:

Central nervous system (brain) stimulant; analeptic.

## How the Drug Works:

Caffeine stimulates the brain. It also stimulates the heart, dilates (widens) blood vessels in the body, constricts (narrows) blood vessels in the brain, increases acid secretion in the stomach, and acts as a mild or weak diuretic (water pill).

How modafinil works to stimulate the brain is not completely known. It may act by altering natural chemicals (neurotransmitters) in the brain that affect alertness.

## Uses:

*Caffeine:* As an aid in staying awake and restoring mental alertness.

As an adjuvant (added to) in various pain medications (eg, aspirin, acetaminophen) to increase pain relieving effects.

*Modafinil:* To improve wakefulness in patients with excessive daytime sleepiness associated with narcolepsy.

*Unlabeled Use(s):* Topical treatment with caffeine in a hydrophilic base or hydrocortisone has been used to treat skin rash, hives, redness, scaling, oozing, and itching. In combination with ephedrine, caffeine causes a modest weight loss in obese individuals when energy intake is restricted over an extended period. Caffeine enhances the migraine-treating effects of ergotamine. Caffeine has been used to treat excited or comatose alcoholic patients. Caffeine has eased postprandial (after meal) hypotension in a small number of patients, although its use is strongly discouraged by most doctors.

## Precautions:

*Do not use in the following situations:*
allergy to the analeptic or any of its ingredients

cardiovascular side effects, history of, associated with CNS stimulant use

*Use with caution in the following situations:*

diabetes (caffeine only)
high blood pressure (modafinil only)
kidney disease
liver disease, severe (modafinil only)

myocardial infarction, history of (modafinil only)
psychosis, history of (modafinil only)
unstable angina, history of (modafinil only)

| Caffeine Content from Various Sources | | |
|---|---|---|
| Source | Serving size | Caffeine (mg) |
| *Coffee:*[1] | | |
| Espresso | 2 oz | 120 |
| Regular, brewed | 5 to 8 oz | 40 to 180 |
| Instant | 5 to 8 oz | 30 to 120 |
| Decaffeinated | 5 to 8 oz | 1 to 5 |
| *Tea:*[1] | | |
| Brewed | 5 to 8 oz | 20 to 110 |
| Instant/Bags | 5 to 8 oz | 20 to 50 |
| *Soft drinks:* | | |
| *Mountain Dew* | 12 oz | 55 |
| *Coke* | 12 oz | 47 |
| *Pepsi* | 12 oz | 37 |
| *Slice* | 12 oz | 11 |
| *Chocolate:* | | |
| Baking chocolate | 1 oz | 25 to 58 |
| Milk chocolate | 1 oz | 1 to 15 |
| *Medications, otc:* | | |
| Analgesics | 1 tablet | 32 to 65 |
| Cold combinations | 1 tablet | 30 to 65 |
| Stimulants | 1 tablet | 75 to 200 |
| *Other:* | | |
| Guarana | 1 g | 25 to 50 |

[1] Depending on strength and brew of product.

*Diabetic patients:* Caffeine may cause blood sugar levels to increase in diabetic patients. Monitor blood sugar more closely until effects have been determined.

*Pregnancy:* There are no adequate and well-controlled studies of modafinil in pregnant women. Use only if clearly needed and the potential benefits to the mother outweigh the possible hazards to the fetus. Pregnant patients should minimize their intake of caffeine and caffeine-containing beverages.

*Breastfeeding:* Caffeine appears in breast milk. It is not known if modafinil appears in breast milk. Consult your doctor before you begin breastfeeding.

*Children:* Use of caffeine in children younger than 12 years of age is not recommended. Safety and effectiveness of modafinil in patients younger than 16 years of age have not been established.

*Elderly:* Safety and effectiveness of modafinil in patients older than 65 years of age have not been established. Consider reduced dosages in elderly patients.

*Lab tests* may be required to monitor modafinil therapy. Tests may include blood pressure monitoring.

*Tartrazine:* Some of these products may contain the dye tartrazine (FD&C Yellow No. 5), which can cause allergic reactions in certain individuals. Check package label when available or consult your doctor or pharmacist.

## Drug Interactions:

Tell your doctor or pharmacist if you are taking or if you are planning to take any over-the-counter or prescription medications or dietary supplements while taking analeptics. Doses of one or both drugs may need to be modified or a different drug may need to be prescribed. The following drugs and drug classes interact analeptics:

*caffeine —*
allopurinol (eg, *Zyloprim*)
aspirin
cimetidine (eg, *Tagamet*)
clozapine (eg, *Clozaril*)
contraceptives, oral (eg, *Ortho-Novum*)
disulfiram (eg, *Antabuse*)
fluoroquinolones (eg, ciprofloxacin)
lithium (eg, *Eskalith*)
mexiletine (*Mexitil*)
phenytoin (eg, *Dilantin*)
smoking
theophylline (eg, *Theo-Dur*)

*modafinil —*
alcohol
clomipramine (eg, *Anafranil*)
contraceptives, oral (eg, *Ortho-Novum*)
cyclosporine (eg, *Neoral*)
diazepam (eg, *Valium*)
MAOIs (eg, phenelzine)
methylphenidate (eg, *Metadate*)
phenytoin (eg, *Dilantin*)
SSRIs (eg, fluoxetine)
tricyclic antidepressants (eg, amitriptyline)
warfarin (eg, *Coumadin*)

## Side Effects:

Every drug is capable of producing side effects. Many analeptic users experience no, or minor, side effects. The frequency and severity of side effects depend on many factors including dose, duration of therapy and individual susceptibility. Possible side effects include:

*Digestive Tract:* Nausea; vomiting; diarrhea; stomach pain; dry mouth; appetite loss; mouth ulcer; gum inflammation; thirst.

*Nervous System:* Sleeplessness; restlessness; excitement; nervousness; ringing in the ears; muscle tremor; headache; light-headedness; dizziness; depression; anxiety; muscle weakness; abnormal skin sensations; involuntary movements; confusion; muscle tension; amnesia; emotional instability; stumbling.

*Circulatory System:* Increased heart rate; palpitations (pounding in the chest); changes in blood pressure.

*Skin:* Hives; herpes simplex; dry skin.

*Other:* Abnormal vision; high blood sugar; fainting; abnormal liver function; abnormal urine; urinary retention; abnormal ejaculation; runny nose; sore throat; lung disorder; difficulty breathing; asthma; nosebleed; lazy eye; abnormal blood counts; chest or neck pain; chills; fever; rigid neck; joint disorder.

## Guidelines for Use:

- Dosage is individualized. Take exactly as prescribed.
- Do not change the dose or stop taking, unless directed by your doctor.
- If a dose is missed, take it as soon as possible. If several hours have passed or if it is nearing time for the next dose, do not double the dose in order to catch up, unless advised to do so by your doctor. If more than one dose is missed or it is necessary to establish a new dosage schedule, contact your doctor or pharmacist.
- May cause dizziness, changes in judgment, or abnormal vision. Use caution while driving or performing other tasks requiring alertness, coordination, or physical dexterity.
- Stop taking and notify your doctor immediately if you experience an increased or abnormal heart rate, dizziness, or palpitations.
- Notify your doctor if fatigue or drowsiness persists or recurs, or if you experience rash, hives or other allergic reactions.
- Limit use of caffeine-containing medications, foods, or beverages while taking caffeine tablets or capsules. Too much caffeine may cause nervousness, irritability, sleeplessness, and rapid heart rate.
- Avoid alcohol while taking modafinil.
- Effectiveness of hormonal contraceptives (eg, injectable or implantable birth control, birth control pills) may be reduced by modafinil during treatment and for one month after stopping treatment. Additional or alternative methods of contraception (eg, condoms) should be used.
- Inform your doctor if you are pregnant, are planning to become pregnant, become pregnant, or are breastfeeding.
- Caffeine is not intended for use as a substitute for normal sleep.
- Do not take any other prescription or OTC medications or dietary supplements, unless directed by your doctor.
- Store caffeine products at room temperature (59° to 86°F). Store modafinil at 68° to 77°F.

*If you have any questions, consult your doctor, pharmacist, or health care provider.*

| Generic Name<br>*Brand Name Examples* | Supplied As | Generic<br>Available |
|---|---|---|
| *c-iii* **Benzphetamine HCl** | | |
| *Didrex* | **Tablets**: 50 mg | No |
| *c-iv* **Diethylpropion HCl** | | |
| *Tenuate* | **Tablets**: 25 mg | Yes |
| *Tenuate Dospan* | **Tablets, controlled release**:<br>75 mg | Yes |
| *c-iii* **Phendimetrazine Tartrate** | | |
| *Bontril PDM* | **Tablets**: 35 mg | Yes |
| *Bontril Slow-Release, Mel-<br>fiat-105 Unicelles, Prelu-2* | **Capsules, sustained release**:<br>105 mg | No |
| *c-iv* **Phentermine HCl** | **Capsules**: 30 mg (equiv. to<br>24 mg phentermine base) | Yes |
| *Ionamin* | **Capsules**: 15 mg phentermine<br>resin | Yes |
| *Ionamin* | **Capsules**: 30 mg phentermine<br>resin | No |
| *Adipex-P* | **Capsules**: 37.5 mg (equiv. to<br>30 mg phentermine base) | Yes |
| *Adipex-P* | **Tablets**: 37.5 mg (equiv. to<br>30 mg phentermine base) | Yes |
| *c-iv* **Sibutramine HCl** | | |
| *Meridia* | **Capsules**: 5 mg, 10 mg, 15 mg | No |

## Type of Drug:

Anorectic or anorexigenic drugs.

## How the Drug Works:

Benzphetamine, diethylpropion, phendimetrazine, and phentermine are central stimulants similar to amphetamine. These drugs reduce appetite and may have other central or metabolic effects. Sibutramine prolongs the activity of central neurotransmitters.

## Uses:

For the management of exogenous obesity as a short-term adjunct (a few weeks) in a regimen of weight reduction based on caloric restriction.

## Precautions:

*Do not use in the following situations:*

allergy to the anorexiant or any of its ingredients
allergy to sympathomimetic amines
anorexia nervosa (sibutramine only)

arrythmias (abnormal heart rhythms), history of
arteriosclerosis, advanced
CNS stimulant (eg, amphetamines) therapy, concurrent

congestive heart failure, history of
coronary artery disease, history of
drug abuse, history of
glaucoma
heart disease, symptomatic
high blood pressure, uncontrolled or poorly controlled
highly nervous or agitated state
kidney disease (sibutramine only)
liver disease (sibutramine only)
MAOI (eg, phenelzine) therapy, concurrent or within two weeks
other centrally-acting appetite suppressant drug therapy, concurrent (sibutramine only)
overactive thyroid
pulmonary hypertension
stroke, history of (sibutramine only)

*Use with caution in the following situations:*
diabetes mellitus
high blood pressure, history of
narrow-angle glaucoma (sibutramine only)
seizures, history of
valvular heart disease

*Psychological disturbances:* Psychological disturbances have occurred in patients who received an anorexiant together with a restrictive diet.

*Tolerance:* Tolerance may develop within a few weeks. If tolerance develops, do not exceed the recommended dose to increase the effect; rather, discontinue the drug.

*Pregnancy:* There are no adequate and well-controlled studies in pregnant women. Anorexiant use in pregnancy is not recommended. Do not use benzphetamine in pregnant women.

*Breastfeeding:* Anorexiants are excreted in breast milk. It is not known if sibutramine appears in breast milk. Anorexiants are not recommended for nursing mothers. Consult your doctor before you begin breastfeeding.

*Children:* Safety and effectiveness of diethylpropion, phentermine, and sibutramine in children younger than 16 years of age have not been established. Phendimetrazine and benzphetamine are not recommended for use in children younger than 12 years of age.

   *Phentermine* – Safety and effectiveness of *Adipex-P* have not been established. *Ionamin* is not recommended in children younger than 16 years of age.

*Elderly:* Use sibutramine with caution in elderly patients.

*Lab tests* or exams may be required to monitor treatment. Tests may include blood pressure, pulse rate, and heart rhythm monitoring.

## Drug Interactions:

Tell your doctor or pharmacist if you are taking or if you are planning to take any over-the-counter or prescription medications or dietary supplements with an anorexiant. Doses of one or both drugs may need to be modified or a different drug may need to be prescribed. The following drugs and drug classes interact with anorexiants:

drugs that may raise blood pressure or increase heart rate (eg, certain decongestants; cough, cold, and allergy medications that contains ephedrine or pseudoephedrine)
erythromycin (eg, *E-Mycin*) (sibutramine only)
furazolidone (*Furoxone*)
guanethidine (Ismelin)
insulin
ketoconazole (eg, *Nizoral*) (sibutramine only)

MAOIs (eg, phenelzine)
methyldopa (*Aldomet*)
serotonergic agents (eg, SSRIs, migraine drugs, certain opioids, lithium, tryptophan)
tricyclic antidepressants (eg, amitriptyline)
urinary acidifiers (eg, ammonium chloride)
urinary alkalinizers (eg, acetazolimide)

## Side Effects:

Every drug is capable of producing side effects. Many anorexiant users experience no, or minor, side effects. The frequency and severity of side effects depend on many factors including dose, duration of therapy, and individual susceptibility. Possible side effects include:

*Digestive Tract:* Appetite changes; constipation; nausea; indigestion; vomiting; intestinal inflammation; stomach pain; diarrhea; dry mouth; gas.

*Nervous System:* Headache; migraine; sleeplessness; dizziness; nervousness; anxiety; depression; drowsiness; restlessness; general body discomfort; euphoria; agitation; jitteriness; emotional instability; abnormal involuntary movements; tremor; leg cramps; abnormal thinking.

*Circulatory System:* Increased heart rate; flushing; increased blood pressure; palpitations (pounding in the chest); chest pain; heart rhythm disturbances.

*Respiratory System:* Increased cough; shortness of breath.

*Urinary and Reproductive Tract:* Irregular vaginal bleeding; difficult or painful urination; changes in urinary frequency; impotence; changes in sex drive; increased breast size in males.

*Skin:* Rash; sweating; itching; hair loss; flushing.

*Other:* Abnormal lab tests; muscle, chest, neck, or back pain; joint pain or disorder; taste sensation changes; fever; fluid retention; double vision; weakness; blurred vision; pupil dilation.

## Guidelines for Use:

- If there is a patient package insert available with your prescription, read it before starting therapy and reread it each time your prescription is renewed.
- Dosage is individualized. Take exactly as prescribed.
- Do not change the dose or stop taking, unless directed by your doctor. These drugs can be addicting.
- A single daily dose of benzphetamine is preferably given in the mid-morning or mid-afternoon, according to your eating habits. In an occasional patient, it may be desirable to avoid late afternoon administration.
- Take diethylpropion 1 hour before meals, and in mid-evening if needed to overcome night hunger. Take diethylpropion controlled-release once daily at mid-morning.
- Take immediate-release phendimetrazine 1 hour before meals. Take sustained-release phendimetrazine once daily in the morning, 30 to 60 minutes before the morning meal.
- Take 15 or 37.5 mg phentermine as a single daily dose before breakfast or 10 to 14 hours before bedtime. Take *Adipex-P* capsules and tablets before breakfast or 1 to 2 hours after breakfast; the tablet dosage may be adjusted to the patient's need.
- Swallow *Ionamin* capsules and all sustained-release products whole. Do not crush or chew.
- Take sibutramine once daily with or without food.
- If a dose is missed, take it as soon as possible. If several hours have passed or it is nearing time for the next dose, do not double the dose to catch up, unless advised to do so by your doctor. If more than one dose is missed or it is necessary to establish a new dosage schedule, contact your doctor or pharmacist.
- Wait at least 2 weeks before starting treatment with an anorexiant after stopping MAOIs and before starting MAOIs after stopping an anorexiant.
- Notify your doctor immediately if you experience rash, hives, or other allergic reactions; shortness of breath; chest pain; palpitations (pounding in the chest); nervousness; dizziness; fainting; swelling of the legs; pronounced dry mouth or constipation; deterioration of exercise tolerance; seizures; or sleeplessness.
- Discontinue sibutramine and contact your doctor if seizures occur.
- May cause drowsiness, dizziness, or blurred vision. Use caution while driving or performing other tasks requiring alertness, coordination, or physical dexterity.
- Do not take other medications or dietary supplements without your doctor's approval. This includes nonprescription medicines for appetite control, asthma, colds, cough, hay fever, or sinus problems.
- Avoid alcohol and other mental depressants (eg, narcotics, tranquilizers, antidepressants, hypnotics, antihistamines) while you are taking this medicine unless approved by your doctor.
- Inform you doctor if you are pregnant, become pregnant, are planning to become pregnant, or if you are breastfeeding. Women of childbearing potential should use adequate contraception while taking these drugs.

## Guidelines for Use (cont.):

- Appetite suppressants are not a substitute for proper dieting. Lifestyle changes (eg, diet, exercise) are necessary to lose and then maintain weight loss.
- *Diabetic patients* — Insulin requirements in diabetes mellitus may change in association with the use of anorexiants and the concomitant diet restrictions.
- Avoid taking late in the day because of the possibility of sleeplessness.
- The long-term effects of this medicine are unknown.
- Lab tests or exams may be required to monitor treatment. Be sure to keep appointments.
- Store at controlled room temperature (59° to 86°F) in a tightly closed container. Protect from heat and moisture.

*If you have any questions, consult your doctor, pharmacist, or health care provider.*

| Generic Name<br>*Brand Name Example* | Supplied As | Generic<br>Available |
|---|---|---|
| *Rx* **Dexmethylphenidate HCl** | | |
| *Focalin* | **Tablets**: 2.5 mg, 5 mg,<br>10 mg | No |

## Type of Drug:

Central nervous system stimulant.

## How the Drug Works:

Dexmethylphenidate is thought to block reuptake of norepinephrine and dopamine in the brain, but the exact mechanism of action is not known.

## Uses:

Dexmethylphenidate is indicated for the treatment of attention deficit hyperactivity disorder (ADHD).

## Precautions:

*Do not use in the following situations:*

agitated states or anxiety, marked
allergy to the drug or any of its ingredients
glaucoma
MAOI (eg, phenelzine) use within 14 days
motor tics
Tourette syndrome

*Use with caution in the following situations:*

alcoholism
drug dependence, history of
heart failure
high blood pressure
myocardial infarction, recent
overactive thyroid (hyperthyroidism)
psychosis
seizures

*Drug Dependence:* Dexmethylphenidate should be given cautiously to patients with a history of drug dependence or alcoholism. Chronic, abusive use can lead to marked tolerance and psychological dependence with varying degrees of abnormal behavior. Psychotic episodes can occur.

*Pregnancy:* There are no adequate and well-controlled studies in pregnant women. Use only if clearly needed and the potential benefits outweigh the potential hazards to the fetus.

*Breastfeeding:* It is not known if dexmethylphenidate is excreted in breast milk. Consult your doctor before you begin breastfeeding.

*Children:* Safety and efficacy in children younger than 6 years of age have not been established.

## Drug Interactions:

Tell your doctor or pharmacist if you are taking or planning to take any over-the-counter or prescription medications or dietary supplements while taking this drug. Doses of one or both drugs may need to be modified or a different drug may need to be prescribed. The following drugs drug classes interact with this drug:

anticonvulsants (eg, phenytoin)
antidepressants (eg, amitriptyline, sertraline)
centrally acting alpha-2 agonists (eg, clonidine)
coumarin anticoagulants (eg, warfarin)

dopamine (eg, *Inotrpin*)
epinephrine (eg, *Adrenalin Chloride*)
phenylephrine (eg, *Rhinall*)

## Side Effects:

Every drug is capable of producing side effects. Many patients experience no, or minor, side effects. The frequency and severity of side effects depend on many factors, including dose, duration of therapy, and individual susceptibility. Possible side effects include:

*Digestive Tract:* Nausea; stomach pain; appetite loss.

*Nervous System:* Dizziness; drowsiness; sleeplessness; headache; nervousness; Tourette syndrome; involuntary movements; abnormal thinking or hallucinations.

*Circulatory System:* Irregular heartbeat; pulse increased or decreased; chest pain; pounding in the chest (palpitations); changes in blood pressure.

*Other:* Fever; weight loss; skin rash; joint pain.

---

### Guidelines for Use:

- Dosage is individualized. Take exactly as prescribed.
- Do not take more frequently than prescribed. This drug can be addicting.
- If a dose is missed, take it as soon as possible. If several hours have passed or it is nearing time for the next dose, do not double the dose to catch up, unless instructed by your doctor. If more than one dose is missed or it is necessary to establish a new dosage schedule, contact your doctor or pharmacist.
- May be administered with or without food.
- Tell your doctor if you have ever abused or been dependent on alcohol or drugs, or if you are now abusing or dependent on alcohol or drugs.
- May cause sleeplessness. Avoid taking these medications late in the day.
- Notify your doctor if you experience blurred vision.
- Inform your doctor if you are pregnant, become pregnant, are planning to become pregnant, or are breastfeeding.
- Growth (weight gain and height) will be monitored by a doctor during therapy. Be sure to keep appointments.
- Store at room temperature (59° to 86°F).

---

*If you have any questions, consult your doctor, pharmacist, or health care provider.*

| Generic Name<br>*Brand Name Examples* | Supplied As | Generic<br>Available |
|---|---|---|
| *c-II* **Methylphenidate HCl** | | |
| *Methylin, Ritalin* | **Tablets:** 5 mg, 10 mg, 20 mg | Yes |
| *Concerta* | **Tablets, extended-release:**<br>18 mg, 36 mg, 54 mg | No |
| *Metadate ER, Methylin ER* | **Tablets, extended-release:**<br>10 mg, 20 mg | Yes |
| *Ritalin-SR[1]* | **Tablets, sustained-release:**<br>20 mg | Yes |
| *Metadate CD* | **Capsules, extended-release:**<br>20 mg | No |

[1] Dye free.

## Type of Drug:
Central nervous system stimulant.

## How the Drug Works:
Methylphenidate mildly stimulates the central nervous system.

## Uses:
To aid in treatment of children with behavior problems (attention deficit disorder) characterized by hyperactivity, moderate-to-severe distractibility, short attention span, impulsive behavior, and extreme mood changes that are not stress induced. Stimulants are not for a child who exhibits symptoms due to living conditions or psychiatric disorders, or when symptoms are caused by acute stress reactions.

To treat narcolepsy (sudden or irresistable periods of spontaneous sleep lasting less than 15 minutes that occur during any type of activity).

Do not use methylphenidate for the prevention or treatment of normal fatigue states.

*Unlabeled Use(s):* Occasionally doctors may prescribe methylphenidate to treat depression in elderly patients, poststroke patients, or patients with cancer, brain injury, or HIV infection, or to treat anesthesia-related hiccups.

## Precautions:
*Do not use in the following situations:*
allergy to methylphenidate or
  any of its ingredients
anxiety, agitation, or tension,
  moderate to severe
GI obstruction (*Concerta* only)
glaucoma

MAOI therapy, concurrent or
  within 14 days
motor tics
Tourette syndrome, diagnosed
  or family history of

*Use with caution in the following situations:*

| | |
|---|---|
| alcoholism, history of | emotional instability |
| children with psychosis | high blood pressure |
| drug dependence, history of | seizure disorders |

*Drug dependence:* Chronic abuse of methylphenidate can lead to marked tolerance and psychic dependence with varying degrees of abnormal behavior. Methylphenidate should be given with caution to emotionally unstable patients who may increase the dosage on their own.

*Neuroleptic malignant syndrome:* Neuroleptic malignant syndrome (NMS) is a potentially fatal syndrome which has been rarely associated with methylphenidate use. Symptoms include increased body heat; muscle rigidity; altered mental abilities, including catatonia; irregular pulse and blood pressure; increased heart rate; sweating; and irregular heart rhythm.

*Total treatment program:* Methylphenidate therapy should be a part of a total treatment program that includes psychological, educational, and social measures.

*Pregnancy:* There are no adequate and well-controlled studies in pregnant women. Use only if clearly needed and the potential benefits to the mother outweigh the possible hazards to the fetus.

*Breastfeeding:* Safety for use in the nursing mother has not been established. Consult your doctor before you begin breastfeeding.

*Children:* Do not use in children younger than 6 years of age, since safety and effectiveness have not been established. In psychotic children, the drug may worsen symptoms of behavior disturbance and thought disorder. Aggravation of Tourette syndrome has been reported. Safety and effectiveness of long-term use in children have not been established. Suppression of growth (eg, not gaining height or weight) has been reported with long-term use of stimulants in children. Carefully monitor patients on long-term therapy.

*Lab tests* may be required during therapy. Tests include blood counts, platelet counts, and blood pressure measurements.

## Drug Interactions:

Tell your doctor or pharmacist if you are taking or planning to take any over-the-counter or prescription medications or dietary supplements with methylphenidate. Doses of one or both drugs may need to be modified or a different drug may need to be prescribed. The following drugs and drug classes interact with methylphenidate:

| | |
|---|---|
| anticoagulants, oral (eg, warfarin) | selective serotonin reuptake inhibitors (eg, paroxetine) |
| anticonvulsants (eg, phenobarbital, primidone, phenytoin) | tricyclic antidepressants (eg, imipramine, clomipramine, desipramine) |
| guanethidine (eg, *Ismelin)* | |
| MAOIs (eg, phenelzine) | |
| pressor agents (eg, norepinephrine) | |

## Side Effects:

Every drug is capable of producing side effects. Many methylphenidate users experience no, or minor, side effects. The frequency and severity of side effects depend on many factors including dose, duration of therapy, and individual susceptibility. Possible side effects include:

*Children:* Appetite loss; stomach pain; weight loss during prolonged therapy; sleeplessness; and fast heartbeat occur more frequently in children; however, any of the following side effects may also occur.

*Allergic Reactions:* Rash; hives; fever; joint pain; peeling skin; skin redness; itching.

*Digestive Tract:* Appetite loss; nausea; stomach pain.

*Nervous System:* Nervousness; dizziness; sleeplessness; difficulty moving; drowsiness; Tourette syndrome; headache.

*Circulatory System:* Palpitations (pounding in chest); pulse rate changes; chest pain; fast heartbeat; abnormal heart rhythm; blood pressure changes (usually increased).

*Other:* Weight loss; depression; visual disturbances.

## Guidelines for Use:

- Dosage will be individualized. Take exactly as prescribed.
- Do not stop taking or change the dose, unless directed by your doctor.
- Take regular tablets 30 to 45 minutes before taking other medication, if possible.
- *Children older than 6 years of age:* Methylphenidate will be initiated in small doses, with gradual weekly incremental adjustments.
- *Adults:* Administer regular tablets in divided doses 2 to 3 times daily.
- Patients who are unable to sleep if medication is taken late in the day should take the last dose before 6 PM.
- Sustained-release tablets have a duration of action of approximately 8 hours (12 hours for *Concerta* and *Metadate CD*).
- Do not crush or chew sustained-release tablets.
- If a dose is missed, take it as soon as possible. If several hours have passed or it is nearing time for the next dose, do not double the dose to catch up, unless advised by your doctor. If more than one dose is missed or it is necessary to establish a new dosage schedule, contact your doctor or pharmacist.
- May disguise tiredness, impair physical coordination, or cause dizziness, drowsiness, or blurred vision. Use caution when driving or performing other tasks requiring alertness, coordination, or physical dexterity.
- Notify your doctor if you experience nervousness, sleeplessness, chest pain, palpitations, vomiting, fever, rash, or other unusual, unexplained effects.
- Drug treatment for attention deficit disorders is not indefinite and is usually discontinued after puberty.
- Prolonged use may cause tolerance to the drug. Dose may need to be adjusted. Your doctor may recommend "drug-free days" to evaluate the need for continued use and to re-establish drug potency. Consult your doctor before withdrawing the drug.
- Very rare reports of neuroleptic malignant syndrome have been reported. It is uncertain whether these cases were caused by methylphenidate alone or by some other combination of factors. Notify your doctor if you experience fever, excessive sweating, shortness of breath, urinary incontinence, muscle rigidity, tremors, or unusual muscle movements.
- Inform your doctor if you are pregnant, become pregnant, are planning to become pregnant, or are breastfeeding.
- Lab tests may be required during therapy. Be sure to keep appointments.
- Store at room temperature (59° to 86°F). Protect from moisture and light.

*If you have any questions, consult your doctor, pharmacist, or health care provider.*

| Generic Name<br>*Brand Name Examples* | Supplied As | Generic<br>Available |
|---|---|---|
| *c-iv* **Pemoline** | | |
| *Cylert, PemADD* | **Tablets**: 18.75 mg, 37.5 mg, 75 mg | Yes |
| *Cylert, PemADD CT* | **Tablets, chewable**: 37.5 mg | No |

## Type of Drug:

Central nervous system stimulant.

## How the Drug Works:

Pemoline stimulates the central nervous system. How it does this is not fully understood.

## Uses:

To aid in treatment of children with behavior problems (attention deficit disorder) characterized by hyperactivity, moderate to severe distractibility, short attention span, impulsive behavior, and extreme mood changes.

*Unlabeled Use(s):* Occasionally doctors may prescribe pemoline for narcolepsy (irresistible periods of sleep lasting less than 15 minutes during normal waking hours) and excessive daytime sleepiness.

## Precautions:

*Do not use in the following situations:*
> allergy to pemoline or any of its ingredients
> liver disease, active or history of

*Use with caution in the following situations:*
> children with psychosis          kidney disease
> drug dependence, history of       seizure disorders
> emotional instability            Tourette syndrome

*Drug dependence:* The similarity of pemoline to other brain stimulants with known dependence liability suggests that psychological and physical dependence might also occur. There have been isolated reports of temporary psychotic symptoms occurring in adults following the long-term misuse of excessive doses. Pemoline should be given with caution to emotionally unstable patients who may increase the dosage on their own initiative.

*CNS stimulants:* CNS stimulants, including pemoline, have been reported to precipitate motor and phonic tics, and Tourette syndrome. Therefore, clinical evaluation for tics and Tourette syndrome in children and their families should precede use of stimulant medications.

*Potential liver toxicity:* Report any unexplained appetite loss, nausea, vomiting, general body discomfort, weakness, or yellowing of the skin or eyes to your doctor.

*Total treatment program:* Pemoline therapy should be a part of a total treatment program that includes psychological, educational, and social measures.

*Pregnancy:* There are no adequate and well-controlled studies in pregnant women. Use only if clearly needed and the potential benefits to the mother outweigh the possible hazards to the fetus.

*Breastfeeding:* It is not known if pemoline appears in breast milk. Consult your doctor before you begin breastfeeding.

*Children:* Safety and effectiveness in children less than 6 years of age have not been established. Pemoline use may worsen symptoms of behavior disturbance and thought disorder in psychotic children. Aggravation of Tourette syndrome and seizure disorders have been reported after starting pemoline therapy. Chronic administration of stimulants to children may be associated with growth inihibition. Therefore, growth must be monitored during treatment. Long-term effects in children have not been well established. Treatment is not indicated in all cases of attention deficit disorder with hyperactivity. The decision to prescribe pemoline should depend on the assessment of the severity of the child's symptoms for his or her age, and not depend solely on the presence of one or more of the behavioral characteristics.

*Lab tests* will be required before and during pemoline therapy. Tests may include periodic liver function evaluation.

## Drug Interactions:

Tell your doctor or pharmacist if you are taking or planning to take any over-the-counter or prescription medications or dietary supplements while taking pemoline. Doses of one or both drugs may need to be modified or a different drug may need to be prescribed. Decreased seizure threshold has been reported in patients also taking antiepileptic medications (eg, phenytoin).

## Side Effects:

Every drug is capable of producing side effects. Many pemoline users experience no, or minor, side effects. The frequency and severity of side effects depend on many factors including dose, duration of therapy, and individual susceptibility. Possible side effects include:

*Digestive Tract:* Nausea; stomachache; loss of appetite.

*Nervous System:* Sleeplessness; seizures; hallucinations; dizziness; drowsiness; increased irritability; involuntary movements of tongue, lips, face, arms, and legs; Tourette syndrome; depression; headache; abnormal eye movements.

*Other:* Rash; yellowing of skin or eyes; dark urine; abnormal liver function tests; weight loss; liver dysfunction.

## Guidelines for Use:

- Do not use pemoline until you have discussed with your doctor the risks and benefits of treatment. A written informed consent is required before beginning therapy.
- Dosage is individualized. Take exactly as prescribed. Administer as a single dose each morning.
- Do not stop taking or change the dose unless directed your doctor.
- If a dose is missed, take it as soon as possible. If several hours have passed or it is nearing time for the next dose, do not double the dose to catch up, unless advised by your doctor. If more than one dose is missed or it is necessary to establish a new dosage schedule, contact your doctor or pharmacist.
- Clinical improvement with pemoline is gradual. Significant benefit may not be evident until after 3 to 4 weeks of therapy.
- Because of its association with life-threatening liver failure, pemoline should not ordinarily be considered as first-line drug therapy for attention deficit hyperactivity disorder (ADHD).
- May cause drowsiness or dizziness. Use caution while driving or performing other tasks requiring alertness, coordination, or physical dexterity until tolerance is determined.
- Inform your doctor if you are pregnant, become pregnant, are planning to become pregnant, or are breastfeeding.
- Notify your doctor immediately if you experience darkening of urine, appetite loss, general body discomfort, nausea, vomiting, yellowing of the skin or eyes, or uncontrolled movement.
- Notify your doctor if sleeplessness occurs and is bothersome.
- Chronic use may suppress growth in children.
- Your doctor may interrupt treatment occasionally to determine if there is a recurrence of behavioral symptoms sufficient to require continued therapy.
- Pemoline therapy should be stopped if no benefit is noted after 3 weeks of taking the maximum dose.
- Lab tests will be required to monitor therapy. Be sure to keep appointments.
- Store at room temperature (59° to 86°F).

*If you have any questions, consult your doctor, pharmacist, or health care provider.*

| Generic Name<br>*Brand Name Examples* | **Supplied As** | Generic<br>Available |
|---|---|---|
| *otc* **Acetaminophen** | | |
| *Aceta, Arthritis Pain Formula Aspirin Free, Aspirin Free Anacin Maximum Strength, Aspirin Free Pain Relief, Dapa, Genapap Extra Strength, Genebs, Genebs Extra Strength, Mapap Extra Strength, Mapap Regular Strength, Maranox, Meda Tab, Panadol, Panex, Redutemp, Tapanol Extra Strength, Tylenol Caplets, Tylenol Extra Strength, Tylenol Junior Strength, Tylenol Regular Strength* | **Tablets:** 160 mg, 325 mg, 500 mg, 650 mg | Yes |
| *Apacet, Children's Genapap, Children's Panadol[1], Children's Tylenol, St. Joseph Aspirin-Free for Children, Tylenol Junior Strength* | **Tablets, chewable:** 80 mg, 160 mg | Yes |
| *Dapa Extra Strength, Feverall Sprinkle Caps, Meda Cap* | **Capsules:** 80 mg, 160 mg, 500 mg | Yes |
| *Tylenol Extended Relief* | **Caplets, extended release:** 650 mg | No |
| *Arthritis Foundation Pain Reliever Aspirin Free, Aspirin Free Anacin Maximum Strength, Panadol Junior Strength[1]* | **Caplets:** 160 mg, 500 mg | No |
| *Aspirin Free Anacin Maximum Strength* | **Gel caplets:** 500 mg | No |
| *Snaplets-FR* | **Granules:** 80 mg | No |
| *Aceta[2], Children's Genapap,[3] Children's Mapap[3], Children's Silapap[1,3], Children's Tylenol[3], Dolanex[1,2], Liquiprin, Oraphen-PD[2], Ridenol* | **Elixir:** 80 mg/tsp, 120 mg/tsp, 130 mg/tsp, 160 mg/tsp, 325 mg/tsp | Yes |

| Generic Name<br>*Brand Name Examples* | Supplied As | Generic<br>Available |
|---|---|---|
| *Children's Halenol[3], Children's Panadol[1,3], St. Joseph Aspirin-Free Fever Reducer for Children[1,3], Tylenol Extra Strength[2]* | **Liquid:** 160 mg/tsp, 500 mg/tbsp | Yes |
| *Genapap Infants' Drops[3], Liquiprin Infants' Drops[3], Mapap Infants' Drops[3], Myapap Drops[1,3], Panadol Infants' Drops[1,3], Silapap Infants' Drops[3], St. Joseph Aspirin-Free Infants' Drops[1,3], Tempra Drops[3], Tylenol Infants' Drops[3], Uni-Ace[3]* | **Solution:** 80 mg/0.8 mL, 100 mg/mL, 120 mg/2.5 mL | Yes |
| *Children's Tylenol[3], Tylenol Infants' Drops[3]* | **Suspension:** 80 mg/tsp, 160 mg/tsp | No |
| *Acetaminophen Uniserts, Acephen, Children's Feverall, Infants' Feverall, Neopap, Suppap* | **Suppositories:** 80 mg, 120 mg, 125 mg, 325 mg, 650 mg | Yes |
| *otc* **Acetaminophen, Buffered** | | |
| *Bromo Seltzer* | **Effervescent granules:** 325 mg with 2.781 g sodium bicarbonate and 2.224 g citric acid/¾ capful | No |

[1] Sugar free.
[2] Contains alcohol.
[3] Alcohol free.

## Type of Drug:

Non-aspirin pain reliever and fever reducer. "Tylenol," APAP.

## How the Drug Works:

Acetaminophen reduces fever by increasing the removal of body heat through increased sweating and dilating of the blood vessels. It changes the body's thermostat. It is unclear how it relieves pain. The pain relieving and fever reducing qualities of acetaminophen are similar to aspirin.

## Uses:

To relieve pain.

To reduce fever.

*Unlabeled Use(s):* Occasionally, doctors may use acetaminophen in children receiving DTP vaccination to reduce the chances for fever and injection site pain. A dose given immediately after the vaccination and every 4 to 6 hours for 2 to 3 days is suggested.

## Precautions:

*Do not use in the following situations:* Allergy to acetaminophen.

*Use with caution in the following situations:*
kidney disease
liver disease

*Alcohol use:* Liver toxicity and liver failure have occurred in chronic alcoholics taking normal doses of acetaminophen. Chronic alcoholics should take no more than 2 g of acetaminophen per day.

*Overdosage:* Do not exceed recommended dosage. Even a small amount over the maximum daily dose can cause liver or kidney damage. Maintain adequate food and fluid intake while taking this medicine.

*Pregnancy:* This drug appears to be safe for short-term use during pregnancy. However, no drug should be used during pregnancy unless clearly needed. Long-term use during pregnancy should be avoided.

*Breastfeeding:* Acetaminophen appears in breast milk. Consult your doctor before you begin breastfeeding.

*Children:* Safety and effectiveness in children younger than 3 years of age have not been established.

## Drug Interactions:

Tell your doctor or pharmacist if you are taking or will be taking any over-the-counter or prescription medication or dietary supplements while taking this medicine. Doses of one or both drugs may need to be modified or a different drug may need to be prescribed. The following drugs and drug classes interact with this medicine:

| | |
|---|---|
| alcohol | hydantoins (eg, phenytoin) |
| barbiturates (eg, phenobarbital) | rifampin (eg, *Rifadin*) |
| carbamazepine (eg, *Tegretol*) | sulfinpyrazone (*Anturane*) |
| charcoal | |

## Side Effects:

Every drug is capable of producing side effects. Many patients experience no, or minor, side effects. The frequency and severity of side effects include many factors including dose, duration of therapy, and individual susceptibility. Possible side effects include:

*Allergic reactions:* Difficulty breathing; rash; fever; skin eruptions; hives.

*Other:* Low blood sugar; abnormal blood counts and liver function tests; yellowing of skin or eyes.

**Guidelines for Use:**

- Severe or recurrent pain or high or continued fever may indicate serious illness. If pain persists for more than 5 days, if redness is present or in arthritic and rheumatic conditions affecting children younger than 12 years of age, consult your doctor immediately.
- Do not exceed the recommended dosage. Consult your doctor for use in children younger than 3 years of age or for oral use longer than 5 days (children), 10 days (adults) or 3 days for fever.
- If fever, difficulty breathing, rash, or hives occur, discontinue use and contact your doctor immediately.
- Poisoning or overdose may cause few early symptoms (eg, nausea, vomiting, drowsiness, confusion, liver pain, yellowing of skin or eyes), but requires immediate medical treatment.
- Avoid alcohol while taking this medicine.
- Keep out of reach of children.
- Store at room temperature. Store suppositories at room temperature (59° to 86°F) or in the refrigerator (36° to 46°F).

*If you have any questions, consult your doctor, pharmacist, or health care provider.*

| Generic Name<br>*Brand Name Examples* | Supplied As | Generic<br>Available |
|---|---|---|
| *otc* **Aspirin, Children's** | | |
| *Bayer Children's* | **Chewable tablets:** 81 mg | No |
| **Aspirin** | | |
| *otc Aspergum* | **Gum tablets:** 227.5 mg | No |
| *otc St. Joseph Adult Chewable Aspirin* | **Chewable tablets:** 81 mg | No |
| *otc Arthritis Foundation Pain Reliever,Empirin, Genprin, Genuine Bayer Aspirin Tablets and Caplets, Maximum Bayer Aspirin Tablets and Caplets, Norwich, Norwich Extra Strength* | **Tablets:** 325 mg, 500 mg | Yes |
| *otc Ecotrin Tablets and Caplets, Ecotrin Maximum Strength Tablets and Caplets, Extra Strength Bayer Enteric 500, Halfprin, Halfprin 81, Regular Strength Bayer Enteric Coated Caplets* | **Tablets, enteric coated:** 165 mg, 325 mg, 500 mg, 650 mg | Yes |
| *otc Bayer Low Adult Strength* | **Tablets, delayed release:** 81 mg | No |
| *otc 8-Hour Bayer Caplets* | **Tablets, timed release:** 650 mg | No |
| *otc Adprin-B, Asprimox Extra Protection for Arthritis Pain, Bayer Buffered, Extra Strength Adprin-B, Extra Strength Bayer Plus* | **Tablets, buffered:** 325 mg, 500 mg | No |
| *Rx Eastprin* | **Tablets, enteric coated:** 975 mg | Yes |
| *Rx ZORprin* | **Tablets, controlled release:** 800 mg | No |
| *otc Aspirin* | **Suppositories[1]:** 120 mg, 200 mg, 300 mg, 600 mg | Yes |
| *otc* **Choline Salicylate** | | |
| *Arthropan* | **Liquid:** 870 mg/tsp | No |

| Generic Name<br>*Brand Name Examples* | Supplied As | Generic<br>Available |
|---|---|---|
| **Magnesium Salicylate** | | |
| *otc*   *Backache Maximum Strength Relief, Bayer Select Maximum Strength Backache, Extra Strength Doan's PM, Momentum Muscular Backache Formula, Original Doan's* | **Caplets:** 325 mg, 467 mg, 500 mg, 580 mg | No |
| *Rx*   *Magan, Mobidin* | **Tablets:** 545 mg, 600 mg | No |
| *Rx*   **Salsalate** | | |
| *Amigesic, Disalcid* | **Capsules:** 500 mg | No |
| *Amigesic, Disalcid Amigesic, Argesic-SA, Artha-G, Disalcid, Marthritic, MonoGesic, Salflex, Salsitab* | **Tablets:** 500 mg, 750 mg | Yes |
| *otc*   **Sodium Salicylate** | **Tablets, enteric coated:** 325 mg, 650 mg | Yes |
| *Rx*   **Salicylate Combinations** | | |
| *Trilisate* | **Tablets:** 500 mg salicylate (as 293 mg choline salicylate and 362 mg magnesium salicylate); 750 mg salicylate (as 440 mg choline salicylate and 544 mg magnesium salicylate); 1000 mg salicylate (as 587 mg choline salicylate and 725 mg magnesium salicylate) | No |
| *Trilisate* | **Liquid:** 500 mg salicylate (as 293 mg choline salicylate and 362 mg magnesium salicylate)/tsp | No |

[1] Refrigerate.

## Type of Drug:

Aspirin pain reliever, fever reducer and anti-inflammatory agent. ASA.

## How the Drug Works:

Salicylates relieve pain by inhibiting pain perception by pain receptors and by inhibiting the formation of chemicals called prostaglandins. Prostaglandins cause pain receptors to be more sensitive to pain-producing stimuli.

They reduce fever by direct action on the heat regulating center of the brain (the body's "thermostat"). This increases the removal of heat through increased sweating and dilation (widening) of blood vessels in the skin.

Salicylates also help in preventing blood platelets from clumping together to form clots.

## Uses:

To relieve mild to moderate pain.

To reduce fever.

To reduce inflammation, redness, swelling (eg, in arthritis).

*Aspirin:* To reduce the risk of recurrent transient ischemic attacks (TIAs) or stroke in men.

To reduce risk of death or nonfatal heart attacks (myocardial infarction) in people with previous heart attack or unstable angina.

*Unlabeled Use(s):* Occasionally doctors may prescribe aspirin-like pain relievers for the possible protective effect against cataract formation and to prevent toxemia of pregnancy. It may also be of benefit in pregnant women with inadequate uteroplacental blood flow.

## Precautions:

*Do not use in the following situations:*

| | |
|---|---|
| allergy to salicylates | children younger than 18 with |
| allergy to nonsteroidal anti-inflammatory drugs (NSAIDs) | chicken-pox or flu symptoms |
| | hemophilia |
| bleeding disorder | kidney disease (magnesium |
| bleeding ulcers | salicylate only) |
| | tartrazine sensitivity |

*Use with caution in the following situations:*

| | |
|---|---|
| anemia | kidney disease |
| anticoagulant therapy | liver disease |
| bleeding disorders, history | surgery (within 1 week) |
| diabetes, mild | ulcers |
| gout | vitamin K deficiency |

*Ears:* Discontinue use if dizziness, ringing in the ears, or any hearing difficulty occurs. These symptoms are indications that salicylate blood level may be too high. Temporary hearing loss disappears gradually after the drug is stopped.

*Controlled release aspirin* Because of its relatively long onset of action, controlled-released aspirin is not recommended for fevers or short-term pain relief. It is not recommended in children younger than 12 or children with fever accompanied by dehydration.

*Aspirin intolerance:* Symptoms (spasms in bronchioles, hives, swelling, inflammation of the nose) occur within 3 hours after ingestion. Aspirin intolerance is more common in patients with a history of asthma and nasal polyps.

*Foods* containing salicylate may contribute to a reaction. Some foods with salicylate include curry powder, paprika, licorice, Benedictine liqueur, prunes, raisins, tea, and gherkins. A typical American diet contains 10 to 200 mg/day salicylate.

*Desensitization* has been successful. It should be done in a hospital. It is generally maintained with 1 aspirin/day. Any NSAID can maintain desensitization. However, if maintenance is interrupted, sensitivity will reappear (2 to 5 days).

*Pregnancy:* Salicylates cross the placenta. Avoid use during pregnancy, especially the third trimester. Aspirin studies have shown a potential effect to the fetus. Adequate studies have not been done in pregnant women. Use only if clearly needed and potential benefits outweigh the possible hazards to the fetus.

*Breastfeeding:* Salicylates appear in breast milk. Consult your doctor before you begin breastfeeding.

*Children:* Administration of aspirin to children (including teenagers) with fever-causing illnesses (eg, chickenpox, flu) has been associated with the development of Reye syndrome. Reye is a rare illness characterized by vomiting, lethargy, and belligerence that may progress to delirium and coma. Safety and effectiveness of magnesium salicylate or salsalate in children have not been established.

## Drug Interactions:

Tell your doctor or pharmacist if you are taking or if you are planning to take any over-the-counter or prescription medications or dietary supplements with salicylates. Doses of one or both drugs may need to be modified or a different drug may need to be prescribed. The following drugs and drug classes interact with salicylates.

*Drugs affecting aspirin —*

acetazolamide (eg, *Diamox)*
antacids (eg, *Tums)*
charcoal, activated
contraceptives, oral (eg, *Ortho-Novum)*
corticosteroids (eg, prednisone)
dichlorphenamide (*Daranide)*
methazolamide (eg, *Neptazane)*
nizatidine (eg, *Axid)*
ticlopidine (eg, *Ticlid)*
urinary acidifiers (eg, vitamin C)
urinary alkalinizers (eg, sodium bicarbonate)

*Drugs affected by aspirin —*

ACE inhibitors (eg, captopril)
alcohol
anticoagulants, oral (eg, warfarin)
beta-blockers (eg, propranolol)
heparin
hydantoins (eg, phenytoin)
insulin
loop diuretics (eg, furosemide)
methotrexate (eg, *Rheumatrex*)
nitroglycerin (eg, *Nitrostat)*
nonsteroidal anti-inflammatory agents (eg, ibuprofen)
probenecid
spironolactone (eg, *Aldactone)*
sulfinpyrazone (eg, *Anturane)*
sulfonylureas (eg, chlorpropamide)
valproic acid (eg, *Depakene)*

## Side Effects:

Every drug is capable of producing side effects. Many salicylate users experience no, or minor, side effects. The frequency and severity of side effects depend on many factors including dose, duration of therapy, and individual susceptibility. Possible side effects include:

*Allergic Reactions:* Difficulty breathing and inflammation in nose may occur in people with a history of nasal polyps or asthma.

*Digestive Tract:* Stomach upset; nausea; vomiting; appetite loss; indigestion; heartburn; diarrhea; ulcers; GI bleeding.

*Nervous System:* Dizziness; weakness; confusion; headache.

*Other:* Ringing in the ears; difficulty hearing; thirst; sweating; liver problems; prolonged bleeding; abnormal blood counts; black or bloody stools; rapid breathing; iron deficiency anemia (chronic use); dim vision; rash; fever; hives.

---

### Guidelines for Use:

- Dosage is individualized. Take exactly as prescribed.
- Do not stop taking or change the dose unless directed by your doctor.
- May cause stomach upset. Take with food or after meals.
- Do not crush or chew sustained-release preparations.
- Take with a full glass of water (8 oz) to reduce the risk of medication lodging in the throat.
- Patients allergic to tartrazine dye should avoid aspirin; use caution with asthma or nasal polyps.
- Avoid use during pregnancy.
- Avoid use in children with a fever-causing illness.
- Notify your doctor if ringing in ears or persistent stomach pain occurs.
- Do not use aspirin if it has a strong vinegar-like odor.
- Do not place or dissolve on an oral lesion (eg, canker sore, cold sore) or directly on an aching tooth. A serious local inflammatory reaction could occur.

---

*If you have any questions, consult your doctor, pharmacist, or health care provider.*

| | Brand Name Examples | Aspirin | Buffering Agents |
|---|---|---|---|
| otc | Alka-Seltzer Extra Strength Antacid and Pain Relief Effervescent Tablets[1] | 500 mg | 1000 mg citric acid, 1985 mg sodium bicarbonate |
| otc | Bufferin Arthritis Strength Pain Reliever Caplets, Bufferin Extra Strength Coated Caplets | 500 mg | Calcium carbonate, magnesium carbonate, magnesium oxide |
| otc | Maximum Strength Ascriptin Coated Caplets | 500 mg | Alumina-magnesia, calcium carbonate |
| otc | Alka-Seltzer Original Antacid and Pain Relief Effervescent Tablets[1] | 325 mg | 1000 mg citric acid, 1916 mg sodium bicarbonate |
| otc | Alka-Seltzer Flavored Antacid and Pain Relief Effervescent Tablets[1,2] | 325 mg | 1000 mg citric acid, 1700 mg sodium bicarbonate |
| otc | Magnaprin Film Coated Tablets | 325 mg | 50 mg aluminum hydroxide, 50 mg magnesium hydroxide, calcium carbonate |
| otc | Adprin-B Coated Caplets, Bufferin Coated Tablets | 325 mg | Calcium carbonate, magnesium carbonate, magnesium oxide |
| otc | Arthritis Pain Ascriptin Coated Caplets, Ascriptin Regular Strength Coated Tablets | 325 mg | Alumina-magnesia, calcium carbonate |
| otc | Buffered Aspirin Enteric Coated Tablets | 325 mg | |
| otc | Aspirin Regimen Bayer Adult Low Strength with Calcium Caplets | 81 mg | 250 mg calcium carbonate |

[1] Contains sodium.
[2] Contains phenylalanine.

For more information on aspirin, see the Analgesics-Aspirin and Salicylates monograph in this chapter.

## Type of Drug:

Aspirin pain reliever (analgesic); fever reducer (antipyretic); anti-inflammatory agent.

### Guidelines for Use:

- Dosage is individualized. Take exactly as advised.
- May cause stomach upset. Take with food or after meals.
- Take with a full glass of water (8 oz) to reduce the risk of medication sticking in the throat.
- Do not use for pain for more than 10 days or for fever for more than 3 days unless directed by your health care provider.
- Patients allergic to tartrazine dye (FD&C Yellow No. 5) should avoid aspirin.
- Use with caution if you have asthma or nasal polyps.
- Consult your health care provider if pain or fever persists or gets worse, if new symptoms occur, or if redness or swelling is present. These could be signs of a serious condition.
- Discontinue use and notify your doctor if you experience ringing in ears or persistent stomach pain.
- Limit alcohol intake while taking these products.
- Do not use aspirin if it has a strong vinegar-like odor.
- Avoid use during pregnancy unless advised by your health care provider.
- Avoid use in children with fever-causing illness.
- Store at room temperature (59° to 86°F). Protect from moisture.

*If you have any questions, consult your doctor, pharmacist, or health care provider.*

Content given per capsule, tablet, or powder packet.

| | Brand Name Examples | APAP† | Aspirin | Other Analgesics | Other |
|---|---|---|---|---|---|
| Rx | Axocet Capsules, Bupap Tablets, Phrenilin Forte Capsules, Repan CF Tablets, Sedapap Tablets | 650 mg | | | 50 mg butalbital |
| Rx | Esgic-Plus Tablets | 500 mg | | | 50 mg butalbital, 40 mg caffeine |
| otc | Maximum Strength Midol PMS Caplets and Gelcaps, Maximum Strength Multi-Symptom Pamprin Caplets and Tablets, Premsyn PMS Caplets | 500 mg | | | 25 mg pamabrom, 15 mg pyrilamine maleate |
| otc | Maximum Strength Midol Menstrual Caplets and Gelcaps | 500 mg | | | 60 mg caffeine, 15 mg pyrilamine maleate |
| otc | Vitelle Lurline PMS Tablets | 500 mg | | | 25 mg pamabrom, 50 mg pyridoxine HCl |
| otc | Anacin P.M. Caplets | 500 mg | | | 25 mg diphenhydramine HCl |
| otc | Excedrin PM Tablets | 500 mg | | | 38 mg diphenhydramine citrate |
| Rx | Flextra-DS Tablets | 500 mg | | | 50 mg phenyltoloxamine citrate |
| otc | Aspirin Free Excedrin Caplets | 500 mg | | | 65 mg caffeine |
| otc | Fem-1 Tablets, Maximum Strength Midol Teen Caplets, Women's Tylenol Multi-Symptom Menstrual Relief Caplets | 500 mg | | | 25 mg pamabrom |

**Content given per capsule, tablet, or powder packet.**

| | Brand Name Examples | APAP† | Aspirin | Other Analgesics | Other |
|---|---|---|---|---|---|
| otc | Goody's Body Pain Powder | 325 mg | 500 mg | | |
| otc | Aceta-Gesic Tablets | 325 mg | | | 30 mg phenyltoloxamine citrate |
| c-iii | Fiortal Capsules | 325 mg | | | 50 mg butalbital, 40 mg caffeine |
| Rx | Butalbital, Acetaminophen and Caffeine Tablets, Esgic Tablets, Fioricet Tablets, Margesic Capsules, Medigesic Capsules, Repan Tablets, Triad Capsules | 325 mg | | | 50 mg butalbital, 40 mg caffeine |
| Rx | Phrenilin Tablets | 325 mg | | | 50 mg butalbital |
| otc | Goody's Extra Strength Headache Powder | 260 mg | 520 mg | | 32.5 mg caffeine |
| otc | Excedrin Extra Strength Caplets, Geltabs, and Tablets, Summit Extra Strength Coated Tablets | 250 mg | 250 mg | | 65 mg caffeine |
| otc | Maximum Cramp Relief Pamprin Caplets | 250 mg | | 250 mg magnesium salicylate | 25 mg pamabrom |
| otc | Vanquish Caplets | 194 mg | 227 mg | | 25 mg aluminum hydroxide, 33 mg caffeine, 50 mg magnesium hydroxide |
| otc | Extra Strength Goody's Tablets | 130 mg | 260 mg | | 16.25 mg caffeine |
| otc | Saleto Tablets | 115 mg | 210 mg | 65 mg salicylamide | 16 mg caffeine |
| otc | BC Powder Original Formula | | 650 mg | 195 mg salicylamide | 38 mg caffeine |

**Content given per capsule, tablet, or powder packet.**

| | Brand Name Examples | APAP† | Aspirin | Other Analgesics | Other |
|---|---|---|---|---|---|
| otc | Maximum Strength Anacin Tablets | | 500 mg | | 32 mg caffeine |
| otc | Extra Strength Bayer PM Aspirin Plus Sleep Aid Caplets | | 500 mg | | 25 mg diphen-hydramine HCl |
| otc | Cope Analgesic Tablets | | 421 mg | | 32 mg caffeine |
| otc | Anacin Caplets and Tablets, P-A-C Analgesic Tablets | | 400 mg | | 32 mg caffeine |
| c-III | Butalbital Compound Capsules and Tablets, Fiorinal Capsules | | 325 mg | | 50 mg butalbital, 40 mg caffeine |
| c-IV | Equagesic Tablets, Micrainin Tablets | | 325 mg | | 200 mg meprobamate |
| Rx | Magsal Tablets | | | 600 mg magnesium salicylate tetrahydrate | 25 mg phenyltoloxamine dihydrogen citrate |
| otc | Mobigesic Backache Pain Reliever Tablets | | | 404 mg magnesium salicylate tetrahydrate | 30 mg phenyltoloxamine citrate |
| Rx | Arthrotec Tablets | | | 75 mg diclofenac sodium | 200 mcg misoprostol |
| Rx | Arthrotec Tablets | | | 50 mg diclofenac sodium | 200 mcg misoprostol |

† APAP = Acetaminophen.

## Type of Drug:

Nonnarcotic pain reliever combinations.

## Uses:

Components of these combinations include:

*Nonnarcotic analgesics:* Acetaminophen (APAP); aspirin (ASA) and salicylates (eg, salsalate, salicylamide). For more information, see the individual monographs in this chapter.

*Antacids (eg, magnesium hydroxide, aluminum hydroxide):* Used to minimize gastric upset from salicylates. For more information, see the monograph in the Gastrointestinals chapter.

*Barbiturates (eg, butalbital), meprobamate, and antihistamines (eg, diphenhydramine, pyrilamine, phenyltoloxamine):* Used for their sedative effects. For more information on barbiturates or meprobamate, see the individual monographs in this chapter. For more information on antihistamines, see the monograph in the Respiratory Drugs chapter.

*Caffeine:* A traditional component of many analgesic formulations, may be beneficial in certain vascular headaches. For more information, see the monograph in this chapter.

*Misoprostol:* Prevents nonsteroidal anti-inflammatory-induced gastric ulcers in patients at high risk for complications from a gastric ulcer or at high risk of developing gastric ulceration. For more information, see the Anti-Ulcer-Misoprostol monograph in the Gastrointestinals chapter.

*Pamabrom:* Used as a diuretic.

---

### Guidelines for Use:

- Dosage is individualized. Take exactly as prescribed.
- Do not stop taking or change the dose, unless directed by your doctor.
- May cause stomach upset. Take with food or after meals.
- Do not crush or chew sustained-release preparations.
- Take with a full glass (8 oz) of water or other fluid to reduce the risk of lodging medication in the throat.
- Patients allergic to tartrazine dye should avoid aspirin.
- Notify your doctor if you experience ringing in ears, skin rash, difficulty breathing, easy bruising, or persistent stomach pain.
- Do not use an aspirin-containing product if it has a strong vinegar-like odor.
- Severe or recurrent pain or high or continued fever may indicate serious illness. If pain persists for more than 10 days or if redness is present, consult your doctor immediately.
- Consult your doctor before using in arthritic and rheumatic conditions affecting children less than of age.
- Avoid aspirin-containing products in patients suspected of having chickenpox or the flu because of the risk of Reye syndrome.
- Do not exceed the recommended dosage. Consult your doctor for use in children younger than 3 years of age, or for oral use more than 10 days.
- Poisoning or overdose may cause few early symptoms but requires immediate medical treatment.

---

*If you have any questions, consult your doctor, pharmacist, or health care provider.*

| Generic Name Brand Name Example | Supplied As | Generic Available |
|---|---|---|
| **Diflunisal** | | |
| Rx  *Dolobid* | **Tablets**: 250 mg, 500 mg | Yes |

## Type of Drug:

Anti-inflammatory; analgesic (pain reliever).

## How the Drug Works:

Diflunisal decreases inflammation and relieves pain by inhibiting prosta-glandin synthesis. It is not a steroid or a narcotic.

## Uses:

To relieve mild to moderate pain, inflammation, and rheumatoid arthritis and osteoarthritis pain.

## Precautions:

*Do not use in the following situations:*

allergy to aspirin or nonsteroidal anti-inflammatory drugs
allergy to diflunisal or any of its ingredients

pregnancy, third trimester

*Use with caution in the following situations:*

heart disease
high blood pressure

kidney disease
peptic ulcer

*Pregnancy:* Safety for use during pregnancy has not been established. Use with caution during the first and second trimesters. Do not use during the third trimester.

*Breastfeeding:* Diflunisal appears in breast milk. Consult your doctor before you begin breastfeeding.

*Children:* Safety and effectiveness have not been established. Use in children younger than 12 years of age is not recommended. Acetylsalicylic acid has been associated with Reye syndrome. Since diflunisal is a salicylic acid derivative, the possibility of its association with Reye syndrome cannot be excluded. Consult your doctor.

## Drug Interactions:

Tell your doctor or pharmacist if you are taking or if you are planning to take any over-the-counter or prescription medications or dietary supplements with diflunisal. Doses of one or both drugs may need to be modified or a different drug may need to be prescribed. The following drugs and drug classes interact with diflunisal:

acetaminophen (eg, *Tylenol*)
antacids (eg, *Tums*)
anticoagulants, oral (eg, war-farin)
cyclosporine (eg, *Sandimmune*)

hydrochlorothiazide (eg, *Hydro-DIURIL*)
indomethacin (eg, *Indocin*)
methotrexate (eg, *Rheumatrex*)
sulindac (*Clinoril*)

## Side Effects:

Every drug is capable of producing side effects. Many diflunisal users experience no, or minor, side effects. The frequency and severity of side effects depend on many factors including dose, duration of therapy, and individual susceptibility. Possible side effects include:

*Digestive Tract:* Stomach pain; gas; diarrhea; nausea; constipation; ulcers; indigestion; vomiting.

*Nervous System:* Headache; dizziness; nervousness; sleeplessness; confusion; fatigue or tiredness.

*Skin:* Rash; itching; sweating; sensitivity to light.

*Other:* Ringing in the ears or difficulty hearing; edema (fluid retention); swelling.

---

### Guidelines for Use:

- May cause stomach upset. Take with water, milk, or meals.
- Chronic gastrointestinal upset or any signs of bleeding should be reported to your doctor.
- Swallow tablets whole. Do not crush or chew.
- Do not take aspirin or acetaminophen with diflunisal. Consult your doctor.
- If a dose is missed, take it as soon as possible. If several hours have passed or if it is nearing time for the next dose, do not double the dose to catch up, unless advised by your doctor. If more than 1 dose is missed, contact your doctor or pharmacist.
- May cause sensitivity to sunlight. Avoid prolonged exposure to the sun. Use sunscreens and wear protective clothing until tolerance is determined.

---

*If you have any questions, consult your doctor, pharmacist, or health care provider.*

| Generic Name<br>*Brand Name Examples* | Supplied As | Generic<br>Available |
|---|---|---|
| *C-II* **Codeine** | | |
| *Codeine Sulfate* | **Tablets:** 15 mg, 30 mg, 60 mg | Yes |
| *Codeine Phosphate* | **Solution, oral**: 15 mg/5 mL | Yes |
| *C-II* **Fentanyl** | | |
| *Actiq[1]* | **Lozenge on a stick (transmucosal system)**: 200 mcg, 400 mcg, 600 mcg, 800 mcg, 1200 mcg, 1600 mcg | No |
| *Duragesic* | **Transdermal system**: 2.5 mg/hr, 5 mg/hr[1], 7.5 mg/hr[1], 10 mg/hr[1] | No |
| *C-II* **Hydromorphone** | **Solution, oral**: 1 mg/mL | Yes |
| *Dilaudid* | **Tablets:** 2 mg, 4 mg, 8 mg[2] | Yes |
| *Dilaudid* | **Liquid:** 5 mg/5 mL[2] | Yes |
| *Dilaudid* | **Suppositories:** 3 mg | Yes |
| *C-II* **Levomethadyl Acetate HCl** | | |
| *ORLAAM* | **Solution, oral**: 10 mg/mL | No |
| *C-II* **Levorphanol Tartrate** | | |
| *Levo-Dromoran* | **Tablets:** 2 mg | Yes |
| *C-II* **Meperidine HCl** | | |
| *Demerol* | **Tablets:** 50 mg, 100 mg | Yes |
| *Demerol* | **Syrup:** 50 mg/5 mL | Yes |
| *Demerol* | **Injection**: 10 mg/mL, 25 mg/mL, 50 mg/mL, 75 mg/mL, 100 mg/mL | Yes |
| *C-II* **Methadone HCl** | **Solution, oral**: 5 mg/5 mL, 10 mg/5 mL | Yes |
| *Dolophine HCl, Methadose* | **Tablets:** 5 mg, 10 mg | Yes |
| *Methadone HCl Diskets* | **Tablets, dispersible**: 40 mg | Yes |
| *Methadone HCl Intensol, Methadose* | **Liquid, oral concentrate:** 10 mg/mL | Yes |

| Generic Name<br>*Brand Name Examples* | Supplied As | Generic<br>Available |
|---|---|---|
| *C-II* **Morphine Sulfate** | **Tablets, soluble**: 10 mg, 15 mg, 30 mg | Yes |
| *MSIR* | **Tablets**: 15 mg, 30 mg | No |
| *MS Contin, Oramorph SR* | **Tablets, sustained-release**: 15 mg, 30 mg, 60 mg, 100 mg, 200 mg[1] | Yes |
| *MSIR* | **Capsules**: 15 mg, 30 mg | No |
| *Kadian* | **Capsules, sustained-release**: 20 mg, 50 mg, 100 mg | No |
| *MSIR* | **Solution, oral**: 10 mg/5 mL, 20 mg/5 mL, | Yes |
| *MSIR, OMS Concentrate, Roxanol, Roxanol 100, Roxanol T* | **Solution, oral concentrate**: 20 mg/mL, 100 mg/5 mL | Yes |
| *RMS* | **Suppositories**: 5 mg, 10 mg, 20 mg, 30 mg | Yes |
| *Astramorph PF, Dura-morph, Infumorph* | **Injection**: 0.5 mg/mL, 1 mg/mL, 2 mg/mL, 4 mg/mL, 5 mg/mL, 8 mg/mL, 10 mg/mL, 15 mg/mL, 25 mg/mL, 50 mg/mL | |
| *C-II* **Oxycodone HCl** | | |
| *Percolone, Roxicodone* | **Tablets**: 5 mg | No |
| *OxyContin* | **Tablets, controlled-release**: 10 mg, 20 mg, 40 mg, 80 mg[1], 160 mg[1] | No |
| *OxyIR* | **Capsules**: 5 mg | No |
| *Roxicodone* | **Solution, oral**: 5 mg/5 mL | No |
| *OxyFast, Roxicodone Intensol* | **Solution, oral concentrate**: 20 mg/mL | No |
| *C-II* **Oxymorphone HCl** | | |
| *Numorphan* | **Suppositories**: 5 mg | No |
| *C-IV* **Propoxyphene (Detropropoxyphene)** | | |
| *Darvon-N* | **Tablets**: 100 mg (as napsylate) | No |
| *Darvon Pulvules* | **Capsules**: 65 mg (as HCl) | Yes |

[1] For use only in opioid-tolerant patients.
[2] Contains sulfites.

## Type of Drug:

Narcotic analgesics (pain relievers).

## How the Drug Works:

Narcotic pain relievers relieve pain by dulling the pain perception center of the brain. They may also affect other systems in the body at higher doses. Natural narcotics include opium, codeine, and morphine. Other narcotics are synthetic (opioids) and vary in potency, addictive ability, and side effects.

## Uses:

For relief of mild-to-moderate pain and for coughing induced by viral, bacterial, chemical, or mechanical irritation of the respiratory system (codeine only).

For the management of chronic pain in patients requiring continuous opioid analgesia for pain that cannot be managed by lesser means such as acetaminophen-opioid combinations, nonsteroidal analgesics, or PRN (as-needed) dosing with short-acting opioids (fentanyl only).

For the management of breakthrough cancer pain in patients with malignancies who are already receiving and are tolerant to opioid therapy for their underlying persistent cancer pain (fentanyl lozenge only).

For relief of moderate-to-severe pain (hydromorphone, meperidine, methadone, morphine, oxycodone, and oxymorphone only).

For the management of opiate dependence (levomethadyl acetate only).

For the management of moderate-to-severe pain or as a preoperative medication where an opioid analgesic is appropriate (levorphanol only).

For relief of severe pain, and for detoxification and temporary maintenance treatment of narcotic addiction (methadone only).

For relief of moderate-to-severe acute and chronic pain; for the management of pain not responsive to nonnarcotic analgesics; dyspnea (shortness of breath) associated with acute left ventricle failure and pulmonary edema; used preoperatively for patient sedation; to decrease apprehension; effective in the control of postoperative pain (morphine only).

For relief of pain in patients who require opioid analgesics for more than a few days (morphine sustained-release only).

For relief of mild-to-moderate pain (propoxyphene only).

*Unlabeled Use(s):* Occasionally doctors may prescribe injectable morphine for difficult breathing associated with acute left ventricular failure and pulmonary edema.

## Precautions:

*Do not use in the following situations:*

alcoholism, acute (levorphanol only)

allergy to the narcotic or any of its ingredients

bronchial asthma, acute or severe

diarrhea caused by poisoning until the toxic material has been eliminated (opium only)

hypercarbia (oxycodone only)

MAOI use, concurrent or within the last 14 days (fentanyl and meperidine only)

paralytic ileus (oxycodone and oxymorphone sustained-release only)

respiratory depression

upper airway obstruction

*fentanyl lozenge only —*

management of acute pain

management of postoperative pain

opioid nontolerant patients

*fentanyl transdermal system only —*

allergy to adhesives

management of acute pain

management of mild or intermittent pain responsive to

as-needed narcotics or nonnarcotic analgesics

management of postoperative pain

*hydromorphone only —*

intracranial lesions associated with increased intracranial pressure

parenteral narcotic therapy, concurrent

respiratory depression in the absence of resuscitative equipment

status asthmaticus

ventilatory function, severely depressed (eg, chronic obstructive pulmonary disease, cor pulmonale)

*Use with caution in the following situations:*

abdominal condition, acute

abnormal heart rhythm

Addison's disease

alcoholism, acute

arteriosclerosis (hardening of the arteries)

asthma

brain tumor

bronchitis, chronic

chronic obstructive pulmonary disease

circulatory shock

CNS depressant drug therapy (eg, barbiturates, tranquilizers, narcotics, general anesthetics)

coma

curvature of the spine

debilitation

delirium tremens (DTs)

diarrhea

drug abuse, history

elderly

emphysema

fever (fentanyl transdermal system only)

gallbladder disease

gallstones

gastrointestinal bleeding

gastrointestinal surgery, recent

genitourinary surgery, recent

head injury

heart disease

hypercapnia (excess of carbon dioxide in the blood)

hypoxia (low blood oxygen levels)

inflammatory bowel disease

intracranial pressure, increased

kidney disease

kyphoscoliosis

liver disease

low blood pressure
lung disease
MAOI use, concurrent or within the last 14 days
myxedema
obesity, severe
ocular pressure, increased
prostate, enlarged
respiratory depression, pre-existing
respiratory reserve, decreased
seizure disorder
suicidal or addiction-prone individuals
supraventricular tachycardias
toxic psychosis
underactive thyroid
urethra, narrowing

*Labor and Delivery:* Fentanyl transdermal system is not recommended for use.

*Drug dependence:* Narcotic pain relievers have high abuse potential. Dependence and physical tolerance may develop upon repeated use. However, most patients who receive these agents for medical reasons and do not take more than prescribed do not develop dependence.

*Tolerance:* Some patients may develop tolerance to narcotic pain relievers. This may develop after days or months of continuous therapy. Consult your doctor if tolerance is suspected.

*Withdrawal syndrome:* Severity is related to the degree of dependence, the abruptness of withdrawal and the drug used. Generally, withdrawal symptoms begin to develop at the time the next dose would ordinarily be given. For heroin and morphine, symptoms gradually increase in intensity, reach a maximum in 36 to 72 hours and subside over 5 to 10 days. In contrast, methadone withdrawal is slower in onset and the patient may not recover for 6 to 7 weeks. Meperidine withdrawal often runs its course within 4 to 5 days. Hydrocodone withdrawal symptoms peak at 48 to 72 hours. Withdrawal precipitated by narcotic antagonists (antidotes) is manifested by onset of symptoms within minutes and maximum intensity within 30 minutes. Symptoms of withdrawal include:

*Early* — Yawning; tearing; runny nose; restless sleep; sweating.

*Intermediate* — Flushing; increased heart rate; twitching; tremor; restlessness; anxiety; irritability; goosebumps; appetite loss; dilated pupils.

*Late* — Muscle spasm; fever; nausea; diarrhea; vomiting; spontaneous orgasm; severe backache; stomach and leg pains; stomach and muscle cramps; hot and cold flashes; sleeplessness; intestinal spasm; repetitive sneezing; excessively runny nose; increased body temperature, blood pressure, respiratory rate and heart rate; chills; bone and muscle pain.

*Pregnancy:* There are no adequate and well-controlled studies in pregnant women. Regular narcotic use late in pregnancy may cause withdrawal reactions in newborns. Use only if clearly needed and the potential benefits outweigh the possible risks to the fetus.

*Breastfeeding:* Many of these narcotics appear in breast milk, but the effects on the infant may not be significant. Consult your doctor before you begin or continue breastfeeding if narcotic therapy is required.

*Children:* Safety and effectiveness of fentanyl transmucosal in children younger than 16 years of age are not established. Safety and effectiveness of codeine in children younger than 3 years of age have not been established. Do not administer fentanyl transdermal systems to children younger than 12 years of age or patients less than 18 years of age who weigh less than 50 kg except in an authorized investigational research setting. Use of levomethadyl or levorphanol is not recommended in those less than 18 years of age. Safety and effectiveness of oxymorphone in children younger than 18 years of age have not been established. Methadone is not recommended as an analgesic in children; documented clinical experience is insufficient to establish suitable dosage regimens. Safety of propoxyphene, morphine, opium, oxycodone, and hydromorphone are not established in children.

*Elderly:* Appropriately reduce the initial dose in elderly and debilitated patients. Consider the effect of the initial dose in determining supplemental doses. Use caution because opioids have the ability to depress breathing.

*Sulfites:* Some of these products may contain sulfite preservatives which can cause allergic reactions in certain individuals (eg, asthmatics). Check package label when available or consult your doctor or pharmacist.

## Drug Interactions:

Tell your doctor or pharmacist if you are taking or if you are planning to take any over-the-counter or prescription medications or dietary supplements with narcotic pain relievers. Doses of one or both drugs may need to be modified or a different drug may need to be prescribed. The following drugs and drug classes interact with narcotic pain relievers:

agonist/antagonist analgesics
alcohol
amitriptyline (eg, *Elavil*)
anticoagulants (eg, warfarin)
antihistamines (eg, diphenhydramine)
barbiturate anesthetics (eg, thiopental)
carbamazepine (eg, *Tegretol*)
charcoal
chloral hydrate (eg, *Aquachloral*)
chlorpromazine (eg, *Thorazine*)
clomipramine (eg, *Anafranil*)
desipramine (eg, *Norpramin*)
diazepam (eg, *Valium*)
droperidol (*Inapsine*)
fluvoxamine (*Luvox*)
furazolidone (*Furoxone*)
glutethimide (not available in the US)
hydantoins (eg, phenytoin)
hypnotics (eg, zolpidem)
MAOIs (eg, phenelzine)
methocarbamol (eg, *Robaxin*)
nitrous oxide
nortriptyline (eg, *Pamelor*)
protease inhibitors (eg, saquinavir)
rifampin (eg, *Rifadin*)
thioridazine (eg, *Mellaril*)

## Side Effects:

Every drug is capable of producing side effects. Many narcotic analgesic users experience no, or minor, side effects. The frequency and severity of side effects depend on many factors including dose, duration of therapy, and individual susceptibility. Possible side effects include:

*Most Serious:* Respiratory depression; skeletal muscle rigidity; difficulty breathing; slow heartbeat.

*Most Frequent:* Lightheadedness; dizziness; sedation; nausea; vomiting; sweating.

*Digestive Tract:* Nausea; vomiting; diarrhea; stomach cramps or pain; taste alterations; dry mouth; appetite loss; constipation; biliary tract spasm; ileus (obstruction of the bowels); paralytic ileus; toxic megacolon in patients with inflammatory bowel disease; gas; indigestion; difficulty swallowing.

*Nervous System:* Exaggerated sense of well being; restless mood; delirium; sleeplessness; agitation; anxiety; hallucinations; disorientation; drowsiness; sedation; lethargy; mental and physical impairment; uncoordinated movements; coma; mood changes; weakness; headache; mental cloudiness; blurred vision; double vision; pupil constriction; tremor; convulsions; psychic dependence; toxic psychoses; depression; increased intracranial pressure; headache; abnormal skin sensations; confusion; abnormal dreams; continual rapid eye movement; muscle twitching; amnesia; paranoid reaction; drug withdrawal; suicide attempt; decreased mobility; difficulty moving; excessive movement; speech disorder; abnormal gait; abnormal skin sensations; stupor; apathy.

*Circulatory System:* Flushing; faintness; peripheral circulatory collapse; change in heart rate; abnormal heart rhythm; heart pounding in the chest; chest wall rigidity; change in blood pressure; dizziness or lightheadedness when rising from a seated or lying position; fainting; cardiac arrest; shock.

*Urinary and Reproductive Tract:* Urinary retention or hesitancy; infrequent urination; antidiuretic effect; reduced libido; difficult urination; impotence; difficult ejaculation; urinary incontinence.

*Other:* Depression of cough reflex; chills; asthma exacerbation; vision changes; itching; rash; hives; muscle weakness; sweating; runny nose; tearing; yawning; joint pain; general body discomfort; flu syndrome; hot flashes; hiccups; coughing up blood; sore throat; back pain; runny nose; reversible jaundice, including cholestatic jaundice (propoxyphene).

## Guidelines for Use:

- Dosage is individualized.
- Do not change the dose or stop taking unless advised to do so by your doctor.
- May cause drowsiness, dizziness, or blurred vision. Use caution while driving or performing other tasks requiring alertness, coordination, or physical dexterity.
- May cause dizziness or lightheadedness when rising from a seated or lying position.
- Avoid alcohol and drowsiness-causing drugs while taking a narcotic pain reliever.
- May cause nausea, vomiting, or constipation. Notify your doctor if these occur and become a problem.
- Long-term use may lead to addiction. Early signs include drug ineffectiveness. Dependence is not an issue in terminal illness where patient comfort is more important.
- If stomach upset occurs, take with food.
- May cause constipation (long-term use). Stool softeners or fiber laxatives may be required if use is prolonged.
- These drugs work best if taken on a routine basis. Narcotics are more effective in preventing pain than in treating pain after it occurs.
- Give the drug ample time to work before determining if more is needed (at least 30 minutes to 1 hour for oral agents).
- If a dose is missed, take it as soon as possible. If several hours have passed or if it is nearing time for the next dose, do not double the dose to catch up, unless advised to do so by your doctor. If more than one dose is missed or it is necessary to establish a new dosage schedule, contact your doctor or pharmacist.
- Sometimes these drugs are given in combination with other nonnarcotic pain relievers such as aspirin or acetaminophen (eg, *Tylenol*). Make sure your doctor knows if you have had problems taking aspirin or acetaminophen in the past.
- Notify your doctor if shortness of breath or difficulty breathing occurs.
- Do not crush or chew controlled- or sustained-release medications.
- *Fentanyl transdermal system* — Keep both used and unused systems out of the reach of children. Used systems should be flushed down the toilet immediately upon removal.
  If the application site needs to be cleansed before application, the area should be washed with clear water and allowed to dry. Do not use soaps, alcohol, or other products to cleanse skin.
  Do not cut the patch.
  Remove the old patch before applying a new one.
  Avoid exposing the application site to a direct external heart source, such as an electric blanket.
- *Fentanyl transmucosal system* — This product is extremely toxic to children. Carefully follow the storage, administration, and disposal techniques included in the patient package insert and instructional video.
  Remove from the foil pouch just before use.
  The lozenge should be sucked. Do not chew.
  Store in foil pouch at room temperature (59° to 86°F). Do not freeze. Protect from moisture.
- Refrigerate suppositories.
- It is illegal to share these potent, addictive drugs with others.

*If you have any questions, consult your doctor, pharmacist, or health care provider.*

Content given per capsule, tablet, suppository, or 1 mL or 5 mL liquid.

| Brand Name Examples | Narcotic | APAP† | Aspirin | Other |
|---|---|---|---|---|
| **Codeine Phosphate Containing** | | | | |
| c-v *Acetaminophen w/Codeine Elixir²* | 12 mg codeine phosphate | 120 mg | | |
| *Capital w/Codeine Suspension* | | | | |
| *Tylenol w/Codeine Elixir²* | | | | |
| c-iii *Acetaminophen w/Codeine Tablets* | 15 mg codeine phosphate | 300 mg | | |
| *Tylenol w/Codeine No. 2 Tablets¹* | | | | |
| c-iii *Aspirin w/Codeine Tablets No. 2* | 15 mg codeine phosphate | | 325 mg | |
| c-iii *Acetaminophen w/Codeine Tablets* | 30 mg codeine phosphate | 300 mg | | |
| *Tylenol w/Codeine No. 3 Capsules and Tablets* | | | | |
| c-iii *Phenaphen w/ Codeine No. 3 Capsules* | 30 mg codeine phosphate | 325 mg | | |
| c-iii *Margesic No. 3 Tablets* | 30 mg codeine phosphate | 650 mg | | |
| *Phenaphen-650 w/Codeine Tablets¹* | | | | |
| c-iii *Aspirin w/Codeine Tablets No. 3* | 30 mg codeine phosphate | | 325 mg | |
| *Empirin w/Codeine No. 3 Tablets* | | | | |

| Brand Name Examples | Narcotic | APAP† | Aspirin | Other |
|---|---|---|---|---|
| c-III Amaphen w/Co-deine No. 3 Capsules | 30 mg codeine phosphate | 325 mg | | 40 mg caffeine, 50 mg butal-bital |
| Fioricet w/Codeine Capsules | | | | |
| c-III Fiorinal w/Codeine No. 3 Capsules | 30 mg codeine phosphate | | 325 mg | 40 mg caffeine, 50 mg butal-bital |
| c-III Acetaminophen w/Codeine Tablets | 60 mg codeine phosphate | 300 mg | | |
| Tylenol w/Codeine No. 4 Tablets | | | | |
| c-III Phenaphen w/Co-deine No. 4 Capsules | 60 mg codeine phosphate | 325 mg | | |
| c-III Aspirin w/Codeine Tablets No.4 | 60 mg codeine phosphate | | 325 mg | |
| Empirin w/Co-deine No. 4 Tablets | | | | |
| **Hydrocodone Bitartrate Containing** | | | | |
| c-III Lortab Liquid[2] | 2.5 mg hydro-codone bitartrate | 120 mg | | |
| Lortab Tablets | | 500 mg | | |
| c-III Amacodone Tablets | 5 mg hydro-codone bitartrate | 500 mg | | |
| Anexsia 5/500 Tablets | | | | |
| Anodynos DHC Tablets | | | | |
| Bancap HC Capsules | | | | |
| Dolacet Capsules | | | | |

| Brand Name Examples | Narcotic | APAP† | Aspirin | Other |
|---|---|---|---|---|
| Hydrocet Capsules | 5 mg hydrocodone bitartrate | 500 mg | | |
| Hydrocodone Bitartrate and Acetaminophen Capsules and Tablets | | | | |
| Hy-Phen Tablets | | | | |
| Lorcet-HD Capsules | | | | |
| Lorcet Tablets | | | | |
| Lortab 5/500 Tablets | | | | |
| Margesic H Capsules | | | | |
| Vicodin Tablets | | | | |
| Zydone Capsules | | | | |
| c-III Azdone Tablets | 5 mg hydrocodone bitartrate | | 500 mg | |
| Damason-P Tablets | | | | |
| Lortab ASA Tablets | | | | |
| c-III Lortab 7.5/500 Tablets | 7.5 mg hydrocodone bitartrate | 500 mg | | |
| c-III Vicodin ES Tablets | 7.5 mg hydrocodone bitartrate | 750 mg | | |
| c-III Anexsia 7.5/650 Tablets | 7.5 mg hydrocodone bitartrate | 650 mg | | |
| Lorcet Plus Tablets | | | | |

| | Brand Name Examples | Narcotic | APAP† | Aspirin | Other |
|---|---|---|---|---|---|
| C-III | Lorcet 10/650 Tablets | 10 mg hydro-codone bitartrate | 650 mg | | |

### Dihydrocodeine Bitartrate Containing

| | Brand Name Examples | Narcotic | APAP† | Aspirin | Other |
|---|---|---|---|---|---|
| C-III | Synalgos-DC Capsules | 16 mg dihydroco-deine bitartrate | | 356.4 mg | 30 mg caffeine |

### Opium Containing

| | Brand Name Examples | Narcotic | APAP† | Aspirin | Other |
|---|---|---|---|---|---|
| C-II | B & O Supprettes No. 15A Supposi-tories | 30 mg powdered opium | | | 16.2 mg powdered bella-donna extract |
| C-II | Opium and Bella-donna Supposi-tories | 60 mg powdered opium | | | 15 mg bella-donna extract |
| C-II | B & O Supprettes No. 16A Supposi-tories | | | | 16.2 mg powdered bella-donna extract |

### Oxycodone Containing

| | Brand Name Examples | Narcotic | APAP† | Aspirin | Other |
|---|---|---|---|---|---|
| C-II | Oxycodone HCl and Acetamino-phen Tablets | 5 mg oxy-codone HCl | 325 mg | | |
| | Oxycet Tablets | | | | |
| | Percocet Tablets | | | | |
| | Roxicet Tablets and Solution[1] | | | | |

| | Brand Name Examples | Narcotic | APAP† | Aspirin | Other |
|---|---|---|---|---|---|
| | *Oxycodone with Acetaminophen Capsules* | 5 mg oxy-codone HCl | 500 mg | | |
| | *Roxicet 5/500 Caplets* | | | | |
| | *Roxilox Capsules* | | | | |
| | *Tylox Capsules¹* | | | | |
| C-II | *Oxycodone 2 Aspirin Tablets* | 4.5 mg oxy-codone HCl and 0.38 mg oxy-codone terephtha-late | | 325 mg | |
| | *Percodan Tablets* | | | | |
| | *Roxiprin Tablets* | | | | |
| C-II | *Percodan-Demi Tablets* | 2.25 mg oxy-codone HCl and 0.19 mg oxy-codone terephtha-late | | 325 mg | |

**Meperidine Containing**

| | Brand Name Examples | Narcotic | APAP† | Aspirin | Other |
|---|---|---|---|---|---|
| C-II | *Mepergan Fortis Capsules* | 50 mg meperi-dine HCl | | | 25 mg prome-thazine HCl |

**Propoxyphene Nepsylate Containing**

| | Brand Name Examples | Narcotic | APAP† | Aspirin | Other |
|---|---|---|---|---|---|
| C-IV | *Darvocet-N 50 Tablets* | 50 mg propoxy-phene napsylate | 325 mg | | |
| | *Propoxyphene Napsylate and Acetaminophen Tablets* | | | | |

| Brand Name Examples | Narcotic | APAP† | Aspirin | Other |
|---|---|---|---|---|
| Darvocet-N 100 Tablets | 100 mg propoxy-phene napsylate | 650 mg | | |
| Propacet 100 Tablets | | | | |
| Propoxyphene Napsylate and Acetaminophen Tablets | | | | |
| **Propoxyphene HCl Containing** | | | | |
| c-iv E-LOR Tablets | 65 mg propoxy-phene HCl | 650 mg | | |
| Genagesic Tablets | | | | |
| Propoxyphene HCl w/Acetamino-phen Tablets | | | | |
| Wygesic Tablets | | | | |
| c-iv Propoxyphene HCl Compound Capsules | | | 389 mg | 32.4 mg caffeine |
| Darvon Com-pound-65 Pulvules | | | | |

† APAP = Acetaminophen.
¹ Contains sulfites.
² Contains alcohol.

## Type of Drug:

Narcotic pain reliever combinations.

## Uses:

To relieve moderate to severe pain.

Components of these combinations include:

*Narcotic analgesics:* Codeine, hydrocodone bitartrate, dihydrocodeine bitartrate, opium, oxycodone HCl, oxycodone terephthalate, meperidine HCl, propoxyphene HCl, and propoxyphene napsylate are used as pain relievers.

*Nonnarcotic analgesics:* Acetaminophen, salicylates, and salicylamide are used as pain relievers.

*Caffeine* , a traditional component of many analgesic formulations, may be beneficial in certain vascular headaches and may enhance the analgesic effect of selected narcotics.

*Magnesium-aluminum hydroxides and calcium carbonate* are used as buffers.

*Barbiturates, acetylcarbromal, carbromal and bromisovalum,* are used for their sedative effects.

*Promethazine HCl* (a phenothiazine derivative with antihistaminic properties), is used for its sedative effect. It may enhance the analgesic effect of selected narcotics.

*Belladonna alkaloids,* used as antispasmodics.

## Guidelines for Use:
- May cause drowsiness, dizziness or blurred vision. Use caution while driving or performing other tasks requiring alertness, coordination and/or physical dexterity.
- Avoid alcohol and drowsiness-causing drugs.
- May cause nausea, vomiting or constipation. Notify your doctor if these become prominent.
- Notify your doctor if shortness of breath or difficulty in breathing occurs.
- Long-term use may lead to addiction. The early sign of this is drug ineffectiveness. Dependence is not an issue in terminal illness pain where patient comfort is more important.
- May cause nausea; take with food.
- May cause constipation with long-term use. Stool softeners or fiber laxatives may be required if use is prolonged.
- Narcotics are more effective in preventing pain, than in treating pain after it occurs.
- Sometimes these drugs are given in combination with other nonnarcotic pain relievers. Make sure your doctor knows if you have had problems taking aspirin or acetaminophen (eg, *Tylenol*) in the past.
- It is illegal to share these potent, addictive drugs with others.

*If you have any questions, consult your doctor, pharmacist, or health care provider.*

| Generic Name<br>*Brand Name Example* | Supplied As | Generic<br>Available |
|---|---|---|
| *Rx* **Butorphanol Tartrate**[1]<br>*Stadol NS* | **Nasal Spray:** 10 mg/mL | No |

[1] This product is also available as an injection.

## Type of Drug:
Pain reliever; analgesic.

## How the Drug Works:
Butorphanol is a potent pain reliever similar to the opioid (narcotic) analgesics.

## Uses:
To relieve pain (including postoperative and migraine headache pain).

## Precautions:
*Do not use in the following situations:* Allergy to butorphanol tartrate or benzethonium chloride.

*Use with caution in the following situations:*

| | |
|---|---|
| drug addiction or misuse, history | kidney disease |
| | labor |
| elderly | liver disease |
| emotional instability | lung disease |
| head injury | nervous system diseases |
| heart disease | |

*Drug dependence:* Butorphanol has abuse potential. Dependence may develop upon repeated use. However, most patients who receive these agents for medical reasons do not develop dependence.

*Pregnancy:* Adequate studies have not been done in pregnant women. Use only if clearly needed and potential benefits outweigh the possible hazards to the fetus.

*Breastfeeding:* Butorphanol appears in breast milk. Consult your doctor before you begin breastfeeding.

*Children:* Safety and effectiveness have not been established. Use is not recommended.

*Elderly:* Elderly patients may be more sensitive to side effects.

## Drug Interactions:
Tell your doctor or pharmacist if you are taking or if you are planning to take any over-the-counter or prescription medications or dietary supplements with butorphanol. Doses of one or both drugs may need to be modified or a different drug may need to be prescribed. Barbiturates (eg, phenobarbital) interact with butorphanol.

## Side Effects:

Every drug is capable of producing side effects. Many butorphanol users experience no, or minor, side effects. The frequency and severity of side effects depend on many factors including dose, duration of therapy, and individual susceptibility. Possible side effects include:

*Digestive Tract:* Nausea; vomiting; appetite loss; constipation; stomach pain.

*Nervous System:* Dizziness; drowsiness; sleeplessness; weakness; headache; anxiety; confusion; euphoria (exaggerated sense of well being); floating feeling; nervousness; abnormal sensation; tremor.

*Circulatory System:* Palpitations (pounding in the chest).

*Respiratory System:* Cough; difficulty breathing; nasal congestion/irritation; runny nose; sinus/upper respiratory infection.

*Skin:* Sweating; clamminess; itching.

*Other:* Sensation of heat; dry mouth; sore throat; nosebleed; blurred vision; ear pain; ringing in ears; unpleasant taste.

## Guidelines for Use:

- Patient package insert available with product.
- The pharmacist will assemble product before dispensing to patients.
- May cause drowsiness or dizziness. Use caution while driving or performing other tasks requiring alertness.
- Avoid alcohol and other drowsiness-causing drugs.
- Give the drug ample time to work before determining if more is needed (approximately 1 to 1½ hours).

*If you have any questions, consult your doctor, pharmacist, or health care provider.*

| Generic Name<br>*Brand Name Examples* | Supplied As | Generic<br>Available |
|---|---|---|
| *C-IV* **Pentazocine**[1] | | |
| *Talwin Nx* | **Tablets:** 50 mg with 0.5 mg naloxone HCl | No |
| *C-IV* **Pentazocine Combinations** | | |
| *Talwin Compound Caplets* | **Tablets:** 12.5 mg with 325 mg aspirin | No |
| *Talacen Caplets* | **Tablets:** 25 mg with 650 mg acetaminophen | No |

[1] This product is also available as an injection.

## Type of Drug:

Pain reliever; analgesic.

## How the Drug Works:

Pentazocine is a potent pain reliever similar to selected opioid (narcotic) analgesics.

## Uses:

To relieve moderate to severe pain (oral and injection).

To supplement surgical anesthesia (injection only).

## Precautions:

*Do not use in the following situations:* Allergy to pentazocine, naloxone (in *Talwin Nx*) or any component of the products.

*Use with caution in the following situations:*

| | |
|---|---|
| asthma | kidney disease |
| drug abuse, history | liver disease |
| emotional instability | lung disease |
| head injury | pregnancy, premature delivery |
| heart attack with high blood | seizures, history |
| pressure, nausea and vomiting | ulcers (*Talwin Compound* only) |

*Patients receiving narcotics:* Pentazocine is a mild narcotic antagonist. Some patients previously given narcotics, including drugs for narcotic dependence, have experienced withdrawal symptoms after receiving pentazocine.

*Drug dependence:* Emotionally unstable patients and those with a history of drug abuse must be closely supervised when therapy exceeds 4 or 5 days. Dependence has occurred in such patients. Abrupt discontinuation following extended use of pentazocine has resulted in withdrawal symptoms. Pentazocine must be withdrawn gradually following long-term therapy.

*Talwin Nx* is intended for oral use only. Severe, potentially lethal reactions (eg, clots in the lungs, blood vessel blockage, ulcers and abscesses, withdrawal symptoms in narcotic-dependent individuals) may result from misuse of this drug by injection or in combination with other substances.

*Drug abuse:* Injection of oral preparations of pentazocine (*Talwin*, "Ts") and tripelennamine (PBZ, "Blues") has become a common form of drug abuse. The combination is used as a "substitute" for heroin.

The most frequent and serious complication of "Ts and Blues" addiction is pulmonary (lung) disease, caused by the blocking of arteries and arterioles in the lungs with unsterile particles of cellulose and talc used as tablet binders. Nervous system complications from IV injection of "Ts and Blues" include seizures, strokes, and infections.

*Pregnancy:*

*Pentazocine and pentazocine with acetaminophen* – Adequate studies have not been done in pregnant women, and animal studies may have shown a risk to the fetus. Use only if clearly needed and potential benefits outweigh the possible hazards to the fetus.

*Pentazocine with aspirin* – Safe use of pentazocine during pregnancy has not been established. Studies of aspirin have shown a potential effect to the fetus. Use only if clearly needed and potential benefits outweigh the possible risks.

*Breastfeeding:* It is not known if pentazocine appears in breast milk. Acetaminophen is excreted in breast milk in low concentrations. No side effects in nursing infants were reported. Salicylates (eg, aspirin) are excreted in breast milk in low concentrations. Effects on platelet function in the nursing infant have not been reported, but are a potential risk. Consult your doctor before you begin breastfeeding.

*Children:* Safety and effectiveness have not been established in children younger than 12 years of age.

*Sulfites:* Some of these products may contain sulfite preservatives which can cause allergic reactions in certain individuals. Check package labels when available or consult your doctor or pharmacist.

## Drug Interactions:

Tell your doctor or pharmacist if you are taking or if you are planning to take any over-the-counter or prescription medications or dietary supplements while taking this medicine. Doses of one or both drugs may need to be modified or a different drug may need to be prescribed. Alcohol, barbiturate anesthetics and anticoagulants (*Talwin Compound* only) interact with this medicine. The effect of this medicine may decrease if you are a smoker.

## Side Effects:

Every drug is capable of producing side effects. Many patients experience no, or minor, side effects. The frequency and severity of side effects depend on many factors including dose, duration of therapy and individual susceptibility. Possible side effects include:

*Digestive Tract:* Nausea; vomiting; constipation; cramps; appetite loss; stomach ache; diarrhea.

*Nervous System:* Dizziness; lightheadedness; euphoria (exaggerated sense of well being); sleepiness; sleeplessness; disturbed dreams; depression; irritability; excitement; hallucinations; tremor; headache; weakness; fainting; confusion.

*Circulatory System:* Changes in blood pressure; rapid heart rate; shock.

*Skin:* Swelling of the face; rash; hives; stinging on injection; sweating; hardening of skin, sloughing or small lumps at injection site; flushing; itching; abnormal skin sensations; discoloration.

*Other:* Dry mouth; taste changes; ringing in the ears; blurred vision; difficulty focusing; rapid eye movement; pinpoint pupils; double vision; difficulty breathing; urine retention; temporary absence of breathing in newborns whose mothers took this medicine; chills.

---

### Guidelines for Use:

- Take exactly as prescribed.
- May be taken without regard to food.
- After prolonged use, do not discontinue medication without first checking with your doctor or pharmacist.
- If a dose is missed, take it as soon as possible. If several hours have passed, or if it is nearing time for the next dose, do not double the dose to "catch up" (unless directed to do so by your doctor). If more than one dose is missed, or if it is necessary to establish a new dosing schedule, contact your doctor or pharmacist.
- *Talwin Nx* and combination products are intended for oral use only.
- May cause drowsiness, dizziness, or euphoria. Use caution while driving or performing other tasks requiring alertness, coordination, or physical dexterity.
- Avoid alcohol and other depressants (or drowsiness-causing medications).
- Notify your doctor if skin rash, difficulty breathing, confusion, or disorientation occurs.
- Do not use in anticipation of pain, but only for existing pain.
- Store in tight container at room temperature (59° to 86°F). Protect from light.

---

*If you have any questions, consult your doctor, pharmacist, or health care provider.*

| Generic Name<br>*Brand Name Example* | Supplied As | Generic<br>Available |
|---|---|---|
| *Rx* **Tramadol HCl**<br>*Ultram* | **Tablets:** 50 mg | No |

## Type of Drug:
Pain reliever; analgesic.

## How the Drug Works:
Tramadol is a centrally acting, synthetic analgesic compound that acts in the brain to relieve pain. It is not chemically related to opiates, but its actions are similar to those of opioid (narcotic) analgesics.

## Uses:
To relieve moderate to moderately severe pain in patients older than 16 years of age.

## Precautions:
*Do not use in the following situations:*

alcohol use, acute
allergy to this medicine
centrally acting analgesic use, acute

hypnotics use, acute
opioid use, acute
psychotropic drug use, acute

*Use with caution in the following situations:*

abdominal conditions, acute
CNS depressant use (eg, alcohol, opioids, sedatives, tranquilizers)
drug addiction
epilepsy
head injuries
kidney disease

liver disease
monoamine oxidase inhibitor use
narcotic agonist analgesic use (eg, codeine)
promethazine (eg, *Phenergan*)
seizures, history

*Respiratory depression:* When tramadol is taken with anesthetic medications or alcohol, respiratory depression (slow, shallow, or absent breathing) may occur.

*Pregnancy:* Adequate studies have not been done in pregnant women, or animal studies may have shown a risk to the fetus. Use only if clearly needed and potential benefits outweigh the possible hazards to the fetus.

*Breastfeeding:* Tramadol appears in breast milk. Use in nursing mothers is not recommended. Consult your doctor before you begin breastfeeding.

*Children:* Safety and effectiveness in children younger than 16 years of age have not been established.

*Elderly:* Daily doses of more than 300 mg are not recommended in patients older than 75 years of age.

## Drug Interactions:

Tell your doctor or pharmacist if you are taking or if you are planning to take any over-the-counter or prescription medications or dietary supplements while taking this medicine. Doses of one or both drugs may need to be modified or a different drug may need to be prescribed. The following drugs or drug classes interact with this medicine:

carbamazepine (eg, *Tegretol)*
MAO inhibitors (eg, *phenelzine)*
quinidine (eg, *Quinalan)*

## Side Effects:

Every drug is capable of producing side effects. Many patients experience no, or minor, side effects. The frequency and severity of side effects depend on many factors including dose, duration of therapy, and individual susceptibility. Possible side effects include:

*Digestive Tract:* Nausea; constipation; vomiting; stomach ache; appetite loss; gas; indigestion; diarrhea.

*Nervous System:* Dizziness; feeling of whirling motion; headache; drowsiness; nervousness; confusion; agitation; tremor; exaggerated sense of well-being; unstable emotions; weakness; incoordination; sleep disorders; anxiety; hallucinations; spasticity.

*Skin:* Itching; sweating; rash; flushing; redness; warmness of the skin.

*Urinary and Reproductive Tract:* Urinary frequency; urinary retention; menopausal symptoms.

*Other:* Dry mouth; general body discomfort; muscle stiffness; visual problems.

---

### Guidelines for Use:

- Use exactly as prescribed.
- For the treatment of a painful condition, take 50 to 100 mg every 4 to 6 hours, not exceeding 400 mg per day. In patients older than 75 years of age, no more than 300 mg/day in divided doses (every 4 to 6 hours) is recommended.
- May be taken without regard to food.
- Do not take this medicine more frequently or in larger doses than prescribed. This drug may be addicting and can cause breathing difficulties if taken in large doses.
- Withdrawal symptoms may occur if this medicine is discontinued abruptly. Tapering the medication should relieve symptoms.
- May cause drowsiness, dizziness, or confusion. Use caution while driving or performing other tasks requiring alertness, coordination, or physical dexterity.
- Do not use alcohol or other mental depressants (eg, hypnotics, tranquilizers) as they may cause increased drowsiness, dizziness, confusion, or breathing problems.
- Store at room temperature (from 59° up to 77°F) in a tight container.

---

*If you have any questions, consult your doctor, pharmacist, or health care provider.*

| Generic Name<br>*Brand Name Examples* | Supplied As | Generic<br>Available |
|---|---|---|
| *Rx* **Celecoxib** | | |
| *Celebrex* | **Capsules:** 100 mg, 200 mg | No |
| *Rx* **Diclofenac Potassium** | | |
| *Cataflam* | **Tablets:** 50 mg | Yes |
| *Rx* **Diclofenac Sodium** | | |
| *Voltaren* | **Tablets, delayed release:** 25 mg, 50 mg, 75 mg | Yes |
| *Voltaren-XR* | **Tablets, extended release:** 100 mg | Yes |
| *Rx* **Etodolac** | | |
| *Lodine* | **Capsules:** 200 mg, 300 mg | Yes |
| *Lodine* | **Tablets:** 400 mg, 500 mg | Yes |
| *Lodine XL* | **Tablets, extended release:** 400 mg, 500 mg, 600 mg | Yes |
| *Rx* **Fenoprofen Calcium** | **Tablets:** 600 mg | Yes |
| *Nalfon* | **Capsules:** 200 mg, 300 mg | Yes |
| *Rx* **Flurbiprofen** | | |
| *Ansaid* | **Tablets:** 50 mg, 100 mg | Yes |
| **Ibuprofen** | | |
| *Rx* *Motrin* | **Tablets:** 400 mg, 600 mg, 800 mg | Yes |
| *otc* *Junior Strength Advil, Junior Strength Motrin Caplets* | **Tablets:** 100 mg | Yes |
| *otc* *Advil Tablets and Caplets, Genpril, Haltran, Iprin, Menadol Captabs, Maximum Strength Midol Cramp, Motrin IB, Motrin Migraine Pain Caplets* | **Tablets:** 200 mg | Yes |
| *otc* *Advil Gelcaps and Liqui-Gels, Motrin IB Gelcaps, Advil Migraine* | **Capsules:** 200 mg | No |
| *otc* *Children's Advil[1], Children's Motrin[1]* | **Tablets, chewable:** 50 mg | No |
| *otc* *Junior Strength Motrin[1]* | **Tablets, chewable:** 100 mg | No |
| *otc* *Brite-Life Children's Ibuprofen, Children's Advil, Children's Motrin* | **Suspension, oral:** 100 mg/5 mL | Yes |
| *otc* *Infants' Advil, Infants' Motrin* | **Drops, oral:** 50 mg/1.25 mL | No |

| Generic Name<br>*Brand Name Examples* | Supplied As | Generic<br>Available |
|---|---|---|
| Rx Indomethacin[2] | Capsules, sustained release:<br>75 mg | Yes |
| *Indocin* | Capsules: 25 mg, 50 mg | Yes |
| *Indocin* | Suspension, oral: 25 mg/5 mL | No |
| *Indocin* | Suppositories: 50 mg | No |
| Ketoprofen | | |
| Rx *Orudis* | Capsules: 25 mg, 50 mg,<br>75 mg | Yes |
| Rx *Oruvail* | Capsules, extended release:<br>100 mg, 150 mg | Yes |
| otc *Orudis KT* | Tablets: 12.5 mg | No |
| Rx Ketorolac<br>Tromethamine[2] | | |
| *Toradol* | Tablets: 10 mg | Yes |
| Rx Meclofenamate Sodium | Capsules: 50 mg, 100 mg | Yes |
| Rx Meloxicam | | |
| *Mobic* | Tablets: 7.5 mg, 15 mg | No |
| Rx Mefenamic Acid | | |
| *Ponstel* | Capsules: 250 mg | No |
| Rx Nabumetone | | |
| *Relafen* | Tablets: 500 mg, 750 mg | Yes |
| Rx Naproxen | | |
| *Naprosyn* | Tablets: 250 mg, 375 mg,<br>500 mg | Yes |
| *EC-Naprosyn* | Tablets, delayed release:<br>375 mg, 500 mg | Yes |
| *Naprosyn* | Suspension, oral:<br>125 mg/5 mL | Yes |
| Naproxen Sodium | | |
| otc *Aleve Caplets* | Tablets: 220 mg | Yes |
| Rx *Anaprox* | Tablets: 275 mg | Yes |
| Rx *Anaprox DS* | Tablets: 550 mg | Yes |
| Rx *Naprelan* | Tablets, controlled release:<br>412.5 mg, 550 mg | No |

| Generic Name<br>*Brand Name Examples* | Supplied As | Generic<br>Available |
|---|---|---|
| *Rx* **Oxaprozin** | | |
| *Daypro Caplets* | **Tablets**: 600 mg | Yes |
| *Rx* **Piroxicam** | | |
| *Feldene* | **Capsules:** 10 mg, 20 mg | Yes |
| *Rx* **Rofecoxib** | | |
| *Vioxx* | **Tablets:** 12.5 mg, 25 mg, 50 mg | No |
| *Vioxx* | **Suspension, oral:** 12.5 mg/5 mL, 25 mg/5 mL | No |
| *Rx* **Sulindac** | | |
| *Clinoril* | **Tablets:** 150 mg, 200 mg | Yes |
| *Rx* **Tolmetin Sodium** | | |
| *Tolectin 600* | **Tablets:** 600 mg | Yes |
| *Tolectin DS* | **Capsules:** 400 mg | Yes |
| *Rx* **Valdecoxib** | | |
| *Bextra* | **Tablets**: 10 mg, 20 mg | No |

[1] Contains phenylalanine.
[2] Also available as an injection.

## Type of Drug:

Nonsteroidal anti-inflammatory drugs (NSAIDs); mild to moderate pain relievers (analgesics); fever reducers (antipyretics); anti-inflammatory agents; arthritis (eg, osteoarthritis, rheumatoid arthritis) pain relievers.

## How the Drug Works:

Inflammation (pain, redness, swelling, warmth) occurs when chemicals are released from injured tissues. NSAIDs reduce inflammation by inhibiting chemicals that cause the inflammation. It may take several days before maximum relief is noticed. These agents relieve symptoms but do not alter the course of the underlying disease.

## Uses:

To relieve mild to moderate pain in conditions such as headache, post-extraction dental pain, athletic injury, menstrual cramps, colds, flu, or sore throat.

Some of these drugs may also be used for short and long-term (chronic) treatment of pain of rheumatoid arthritis, ankylosing spondylitis, tendinitis, osteoarthritis, and juvenile rheumatoid arthritis.

Some of these drugs may also be used for short-term (acute) treatment of pain associated with acute gout, acute painful shoulder, burstitis, migraine, and primary dysmenorrhea.

Some of these drugs are used to reduce fever and heavy menstrual blood loss of unknown cause.

*Celecoxib:* To reduce the number of adenomatous colorectal polyps in familial adenomatous polyposis (FAP).

*Unlabeled Use(s):* Occasionally doctors may prescribe certain NSAIDs for juvenile rheumatoid arthritis, sunburn, migraine or cluster headaches, or closure of persistent patent ductus arteriosus.

## Precautions:

*Do not use in the following situations:*

allergy to any NSAID
allergy to aspirin
allergy to sulfonamides (celecoxib only)
aspirin or other NSAID use, current
gastritis, colitis, or ulcer (ketorolac, mefenamic acid only)
gastrointestinal bleeding
gastrointestinal bleeding, history of (ketorolac only)
kidney disease, severe
labor and delivery (ketorolac only)
liver disease, severe
peptic ulcer, active
peptic ulcer, history of (ketorolac only)
porphyria (diclofenac only)
rectal bleeding or inflammation of the rectum (indomethacin suppositories only)
surgery, prior to (ketorolac only)

*Use with caution in the following situations:*

alcoholism
anticoagulant (eg, warfarin) use, current
asthma
bleeding disorders
corticosteriod (eg, prednisone) use, current
dehydration
diuretic use
elderly
epilepsy (indomethacin only)
fluid retention (edema)
gastrointestinal bleeding, history of
gastrointestinal lesions (eg, ulcers), active or history of
heart disease or failure
high blood pressure
infection
kidney disease, mild to moderate
liver disease, mild to moderate
low platelet count (thrombocytopenia)
Parkinson disease (indomethacin only)
peptic ulcer, history of
poor general health (debilitation)
psychiatric disturbances (indomethacin only)
smoking

*Allergy:* Severe allergic reactions can occur, especially in patients with asthma who experience runny nose and nasal polyps. Stop using and immediately inform your doctor if signs or symptoms of an allergic reaction occur (eg, rash, hives, sudden shortness of breath, difficulty breathing).

Severe allergic reactions have also occurred in patients who discontinued tolmetin, then restarted the drug.

*Digestive Tract:* Serious effects such as bleeding, ulceration, and perforation of the stomach or small or large intestine can occur at any time, with or without warning symptoms, in patients treated long term with NSAIDs. Although minor upper GI problems are common, report any signs of ulceration or bleeding (eg, bloody vomit, black or bloody stools, dizziness, frequent indigestion, stomach pain).

*Eyes:* Effects include blurred or diminished vision, spots in vision, changes in color vision, and corneal deposits. Stop taking and notify your doctor if eye side effects are noted.

*Headaches:* Some of these agents may cause headaches (most commonly with fenoprofen, indomethacin, and ketorolac). Dosage reduction or discontinuation may be necessary. Consult your doctor or pharmacist.

*Indomethacin:* May aggravate depression or other psychiatric problems, epilepsy, and Parkinson disease. Use with caution. If severe CNS adverse reactions develop, discontinue use. Consult your doctor or pharmacist if persistent or bothersome headaches occur during therapy.

*Phenylketonuria:* Some of these products contain phenylalanine. Consult your doctor or pharmacist.

*Pregnancy:* There are no adequate and well-controlled studies in pregnant women. Use only if clearly needed and potential benefits outweigh the possible hazards to the fetus. Digestive tract side effects are increased in pregnant women in the third trimester of pregnancy. Some of these agents may prolong pregnancy if given before the onset of labor. Avoid use during pregnancy, especially in the third trimester because some NSAIDs may cause premature closure of the ductus arteriosis.

*Breastfeeding:* Most NSAIDs appear in breast milk. Consult your doctor before you begin breastfeeding.

*Children:* The safety and effectiveness of most NSAIDs in children have not been established. Consult your doctor or pharmacist. Indomethacin, meclofenamate, and mefenamic acid are not recommended in children 14 years of age and younger. OTC ibuprofen suspensions may be used in children 2 to 11 years of age. Carefully follow dosing recommendations provided in package label, or consult your doctor or pharmacist. Etodolac extended-release tablets, naproxen, and tolmetin are the only agents labeled for the treatment of juvenile rheumatoid arthritis. Safety and effectiveness of naproxen and tolmetin in infants younger than 2 years of age and of etodolac extended-release tablets in children younger than 6 years of age have not been established.

*Elderly:* Age appears to increase the possibility of side effects, particularly stomach and intestinal irritation, ulcers, and bleeding. Elderly patients should use NSAIDs with great care, begin with reduced dosages, and use for the shortest period possible.

*Lab tests* and exams may be required during treatment. Tests may include eye exams, hearing exams, liver and kidney function tests, blood chemistry, and complete blood counts.

## Drug Interactions:

Tell your doctor or pharmacist if you are taking or if you are planning to take any over-the-counter or prescription medications or dietary supplements while taking this drug. Doses of one or both drugs may need to be modified or a different drug may need to be prescribed. The following drugs and drug classes interact with this drug:

aminoglycosides (eg, neomycin sulfate)
angiotensin converting enzyme (ACE) inhibitors (eg, capto-pril)
anticoagulants (eg, warfarin)
beta-blockers (eg, propranolol)
bisphosphonates (eg, aledro-nate)
cholestyramine *(Questran)*
colestipol *(Colestid)*
cyclosporine (eg, *Neoral*)
dextromethorphan (eg, *Benylin)*
diflunisal *(Dolobid)* (indo-methacin, sulindac only)
digoxin (eg, *Lanoxin)*
dimethyl sulfoxide (DMSO) (sulindac only)
fluconazole *(Diflucan)* (cele-coxib, valdecoxib only)
hydantoins (eg, phenytoin)

ketoconazole (eg, *Nizoral*)
lithium (eg, *Eskalith)*
loop diuretics (eg, furosemide)
methotrexate (eg, *Rheumatrex)*
phenobarbital (eg, *Solfoton)* (fenoprofen only)
potassium-sparing diuretics (eg, amiloride) (indomethacin, diclofenac only)
probenecid
rifampin (eg, *Rifadin)* (rofecoxib only)
ritonavir (*Norvir*) (piroxicam only)
salicylates (eg, aspirin)
sucralfate *(Carafate)*
theophylline (eg, *Slo-Phyllin)* (rofecoxib only)
thiazide diuretics (eg, hydro-chlorothiazide)

## Side Effects:

Every drug is capable of producing side effects. Many patients experience no, or minor, side effects. The frequency and severity of side effects depend on many factors including dose, duration of therapy, and indi-vidual susceptibility. Possible side effects include:

*Digestive Tract:* Nausea; vomiting; indigestion; stomach upset, cramps, or pain; heartburn; diarrhea; constipation; ulcer; bloating; belching; gas; appetite changes; mouth sores; dry mouth; dark, bloody stools; bloody diarrhea; vomiting of blood; salivation; tongue inflammation; feeling of fullness; difficulty swallowing.

*Nervous System:* Headache; drowsiness; fatigue; dizziness; feeling of whirling motion (vertigo); light-headedness; nervousness; depression; sleeplessness; abnormal dreams; tremor; weakness; confusion; migraine; amnesia; anxiety; aggravation of epilepsy and Parkinson dis-ease; mood changes; convulsions; muscle twitching.

*Circulatory System:* Changes in blood pressure; pounding in the chest (pal-pitations); chest pain; irregular heart rhythm or heart rate; congestive heart failure.

*Urinary and Reproductive Tract:* Blood, glucose, or protein in urine; kidney disease; painful, difficult, or increased urination; urinary tract infection; vaginal bleeding; impotence; menstrual problems.

*Skin:* Rash; hives; itching; redness; irritation; peeling; discoloration; bruising; hair loss; abnormal skin sensations; inflammation; flushing; paleness; increased sweating; acne.

*Senses:* Visual disturbances; swollen, dry, or irritated eyes; blurred, diminished, or double vision; cataracts; reversible loss of color vision; ringing in the ears; hearing disturbances or loss; ear pain; change in taste sensation; blind spot; eye pain.

*Other:* Rectal irritation, swelling, or bleeding (indomethacin suppository only); unexplained bleeding or bruising; general body discomfort; abnormal blood cell and platelet counts; abnormal lab tests; liver disease; yellowing of skin or eyes; difficulty breathing; runny nose; shortness of breath; coughing up blood; fainting; weight changes; fluid retention; fever; chills; thirst; sore throat; back, joint, or muscle pain; swelling of the arms or legs; asthma; injection-site reaction (ketorolac injection only); pneumonia; changes in blood sugar; upper respiratory tract infection; bronchitis; changes in skin sensitivity to touch; flu-like symptoms; sensitivity to sunlight; sinus infection; leg cramps; cough; hot flushes.

## Guidelines for Use:

- Dosage will be individualized. Take exactly as prescribed.
- Do not stop taking or change the dose, unless instructed by your doctor.
- If a dose is missed, take it as soon as possible. If several hours have passed or if it is nearing time for the next dose, do not double the dose to catch up, unless instructed by your doctor.
- Avoid aspirin and alcoholic beverages while taking these drugs.
- Take with food, milk, or antacids if stomach upset occurs. Take tolmetin on an empty stomach or with milk only. For stomach upset with tolmetin, use antacids other than sodium bicarbonate. If symptoms persist, notify your doctor.
- Do not crush, chew, or break extended- or delayed-release products.
- Shake suspensions well before use.
- *Digestive tract* — Long-term treatment with NSAIDs may cause serious effects such as bleeding, ulceration, and perforation. Notify your doctor immediately of signs of ulceration and bleeding (eg, bloody vomit, black or bloody stools, dizziness).
- May cause drowsiness, dizziness, or blurred vision. Use caution while driving or performing other tasks requiring alertness, coordination, or physical dexterity until tolerance is determined.
- May cause sensitivity to sunlight. Avoid prolonged exposure to the sun. Use sunscreens and wear protective clothing until tolerance is determined.
- Stop taking and notify your doctor immediately if you experience skin rash, itching, visual disturbances, unexplained weight gain, swelling, stomach pain, black stools, bloody vomit, fatigue, lethargy, flu-like symptoms, yellowing of the skin or eyes, persistent nausea, decreased urination, or persistent headache.
- Inform your doctor if you are pregnant, become pregnant, plan on becoming pregnant, or are breastfeeding.
- *OTC products* — Read package information before using. Do not take for more than 3 days for fever, or more than 10 days for pain. Contact your doctor if these symptoms persist or worsen, if new symptoms develop, or if pain or redness are noted in the painful area.
- *Diclofenac* — Do not use immediate-, extended-, or delayed-release diclofenac concomitantly with other diclofenac-containing products.
- *Ibuprofen (chewable tablets)* — May cause burning sensation in the mouth or throat. Take with water or food.
- *Ketorolac* — Do not use for more than 5 days.
- *Meclofenamate* — Women taking meclofenamate for heavy menstrual flow should notify their doctor if they have spotting or bleeding between cycles or worsening of their menstrual flow. These symptoms may be signs of the development of a more serious condition.
- *Meclofenamate, mefenamic acid* — Stop taking and notify your doctor if you experience rash, diarrhea, or other digestive system problems.
- *Naproxen* — Do not use naproxen immediate- or delayed-release tablets or suspension with other naproxen-containing products.
- *Sulindac* — If unexplained fever, rash, or other signs of allergic reaction occur, discontinue use and consult your doctor.
- Lab tests and exams may be required to monitor therapy. Be sure to keep appointments.
- Store at room temperature (59° to 86°F).

*If you have any questions, consult your doctor, pharmacist, or health care provider.*

| Generic Name<br>*Brand Name Examples* | Supplied As | Generic<br>Available |
|---|---|---|
| *Rx* **Auranofin** | | |
| *Ridaura* | **Capsules:** 3 mg | No |
| *Rx* **Aurothioglucose** | | |
| *Solganal* | **Injection:** 50 mg/mL<br>suspension | No |
| *Rx* **Gold Sodium Thiomalate** | | |
| *Aurolate* | **Injection:** 50 mg/mL | Yes |

## Type of Drug:

Antirheumatic agents.

## How the Drug Works:

The exact mechanism of action of gold compounds is unknown. They suppress or prevent joint swelling and retard cartilage and bone destruction, but do not cure rheumatoid arthritis.

Therapeutic effects from gold compounds occur slowly. Early improvement, often limited to reduction in morning stiffness, may begin after 6 to 8 weeks of treatment, but other beneficial effects may not be observed until after months of therapy.

## Uses:

To treat early active adult or juvenile rheumatoid arthritis not adequately controlled by other therapies (eg, NSAIDs).

*Unlabeled Use(s):* Occasionally doctors may prescribe gold compounds for pemphigus and psoriatic arthritis.

## Precautions:

*Do not use in the following situations:*

allergy to gold compounds or any of their ingredients
blood/bleeding disorders
bone marrow, lack of development (auranofin only)
colitis
congestive heart failure, uncontrolled
debilitation, severe
diabetes mellitus, uncontrolled
eczema
exfoliative dermatitis (auranofin only)
hematologic disorders, severe (auranofin only)
hepatitis, history of
high blood pressure, severe
hives
kidney disease (injectable gold compounds only)
liver disease (injectable gold compounds only)
necrotizing enterocolitis (auranofin only)
pregnancy
pulmonary fibrosis (auranofin only)
radiation therapy, recent (injectable gold compounds only)
systemic lupus erythematosus
toxicity from previous exposure to gold or other heavy metals, severe

*Use with caution in the following situations:*

blood circulation disorders
blood dyscrasis (eg, granulocytopenia, anemia) caused by drug sensitivity, history of (injectable gold only)
bone marrow depression, history of
congestive heart failure
diabetes mellitus
high blood pressure
inflammatory bowel disease
kidney disease, history of
kidney disease, progressive (auranofin only)
liver disease, active (auranofin only)
liver disease, history of
rash

*Injection reaction:* Increased joint pain may occur for 1 or 2 days after injection. They usually subside after the first few injections. These reactions are usually mild, but occasionally may be so severe that treatment is stopped prematurely.

*Use of other antirheumatic drugs:* Use of salicylates, aspirin, NSAIDs, and systemic corticosteroids may be continued when gold injection therapy is started. After improvement begins, slowly discontinue pain relievers and NSAIDs as symptoms permit. Safety of auranofin with injectable gold or high doses of corticosteroids has not been established. Gold salts should not be used concomitantly with penicillamine or hydroxychloroquine. See Drug Interactions.

*Pregnancy:* There are no adequate and well-controlled studies in pregnant women. Gold therapy is generally contraindicated in pregnant patients. Use only if clearly needed and potential benefits to the mother outweigh the possible hazards to the fetus.

*Breastfeeding:* Gold appears in breast milk. A decision should be made whether to discontinue nursing or discontinue the drug, taking into account the importance of the drug to the mother. Consult your doctor before you begin breastfeeding.

*Children:* Safety and effectiveness of auranofin and gold sodium have not been established. Safety and effectiveness of aurothioglucose in children younger than 6 years of age have not been established.

*Elderly:* Tolerance to gold usually decreases with advancing age.

*Lab tests* will be required during treatment. Tests include complete blood cell and platelet counts, urinalysis, and kidney and liver function tests. All women of child-bearing potential must have a pregnancy test before treatment begins to rule out the possibility of pregnancy.

## Drug Interactions:

Tell your doctor or pharmacist if you are taking or if you are planning to take any over-the-counter or prescription medications or dietary supplements with gold compounds. Doses of one or both drugs may need to be modified or a different drug may need to be prescribed. The following drugs and drug classes interact with gold compounds:

antimalarials (eg, hydroxychloroquine)
immunosuppressive agents (eg, azathioprine, cyclophosphamide, methotrexate)
penicillamine (eg, *Depen)*
phenytoin (eg, *Dilantin)* (auranofin only)

## Side Effects:

Every drug is capable of producing side effects. Many gold compound users experience no, or minor, side effects. The frequency and severity of side effects depend on many factors including dose, duration of therapy, and individual susceptibility. Possible side effects include:

*Digestive Tract:* Indigestion; nausea; vomiting; diarrhea; constipation; stomach cramps; appetite loss; gas; dark or loose stools; mouth inflammation or ulcers.

*Skin:* Rash; itching; hives; redness; unusual bruising.

*Other:* Blood in the urine; skin inflammation; metallic taste; abnormal blood cell counts; abnormal liver or kidney function tests; anemia; yellowing of the skin or eyes.

---

### Guidelines for Use:

- Dosage will be individualized. Do not exceed the recommended dosage.
- *Injectable gold products* — The appropriate dose will be prepared and administered by your health care provider.
- Notify your doctor immediately if any of the following occurs: Rash, mouth inflammation, persistent diarrhea, sore mouth, indigestion, metallic taste, unusual bleeding or bruising, itching, blood in the urine, fainting, slow heartbeat, thickening of the tongue, difficulty swallowing or breathing, yellowing of the skin or eyes.
- Notify your doctor immediately if you suspect you have become pregnant during therapy. All women of child-bearing potential must have a pregnancy test before treatment begins to rule out the possibility of pregnancy.
- Increased joint pain may occur for 1 or 2 days after injection. This usually subsides after the first few injections.
- Observe good oral hygiene during therapy.
- Improvement of symptoms is not immediate. Improvement may be seen after 6 to 8 weeks of treatment, although it has not been seen in some patients for up to several months.
- Lab tests and exams will be required to monitor therapy. Be sure to keep appointments.
- Store at room temperature (59° to 86°F). Protect from light.

---

*If you have any questions, consult your doctor, pharmacist, or health care provider.*

| Generic Name<br>*Brand Name Example* | Supplied As | Generic<br>Available |
|---|---|---|
| *Rx* **Hydroxychloroquine** | | |
| *Plaquenil Sulfate* | **Tablets:** 200 mg | No |

## Type of Drug:

Antirheumatic agent; antimalarial drug.

## How the Drug Works:

Although the mechanism by which hydroxychloroquine works is not completely understood, it is believed that it inhibits the actions of various enzymes and results in the reduction of joint inflammation due to chronic rheumatoid arthritis. There now is evidence that early use of this agent will preserve joint function and may prevent progression of disease.

Full benefit of the drug may not be fully realized for 6 to 12 months. Hydroxychloroquine may have serious side effects and is usually prescribed after other drugs have failed.

## Uses:

To treat acute or chronic rheumatoid arthritis. Hydroxychloroquine also is prescribed for treatment of acute attacks of malaria and lupus erythematosus.

## Precautions:

*Do not use in the following situations:*
> allergy to 4-aminoquinoline compounds
> long-term therapy in children
> retinal or visual field changes due to any 4-aminoquinoline compound

*Use with caution in the following situations:*
> alcoholism
> in conjunction with known hepatotoxic drugs
> liver disease
> porphyria
> psoriasis

*Pregnancy:* Avoid use during pregnancy.

*Breastfeeding:* Hydroxychloroquine appears in breast milk. Consult your doctor before you begin breastfeeding.

*Children:* Do not use as long-term therapy in children. A number of fatalities have been reported following ingestion of hydroxychloroquine in very young children. Safe use in the treatment of juvenile rheumatoid arthritis has not been established.

*Lab tests* may be required during treatment with hydroxychloroquine. Tests may include eye exams, blood counts, and knee and ankle reflex testing.

## Drug Interactions:

Tell your doctor or pharmacist if you are taking or if you are planning to take any over-the-counter or prescription medications or dietary supplements with hydroxychloroquine. Doses of one or both drugs may need to be modified or a different drug may need to be prescribed. The following drugs and drug classes interact with hydroxychloroquine.

digoxin (eg, *Lanoxin*)
hepatotoxic drugs
phenylbutazone, gold compounds

## Side Effects:

Every drug is capable of producing side effects. Many hydroxychloroquine users experience no, or minor, side effects. The frequency and severity of side effects depend on many factors including dose, duration of therapy, and individual susceptibility. Possible side effects include:

*Digestive Tract:* Appetite loss; nausea; vomiting; diarrhea; abdominal cramps.

*Nervous System:* Irritability; nervousness; emotional changes; nightmares; psychosis; headache; weakness; dizziness; vertigo (feeling of whirling motion); convulsions; incoordination.

*Eyes or Ocular:* Visual difficulties/disturbances; blurred vision; missing or blacked-out areas in the central or peripheral visual field; light flashes and streaks; sensitivity to light.

*Skin:* Hives; bleaching of hair; hair loss; itching; changes in pigmentation.

*Other:* Muscle weakness; absent or sluggish deep tendon reflexes; ringing in ears; nerve deafness; blood disorders; weight loss.

---

### Guidelines for Use:

- Do not exceed prescribed dosage. Retinal toxicity may occur if dosage is exceeded.
- May cause stomach upset. Take with food or milk.
- Notify your doctor if any of the following occurs: Vision problems; hearing loss; ringing in ears; fever, sore throat; unusual bleeding or bruising; unusual pigmentation of skin or inside of mouth (blue-black); skin rash; itching; unusual muscle weakness; bleaching/loss of hair; mood/mental changes.
- Periodic blood counts should be taken if therapy is prolonged.
- Avoid long-term therapy in children.
- If favorable results do not occur within 6 months, consult your doctor about discontinuing use.

---

*If you have any questions, consult your doctor, pharmacist, or health care provider.*

| Generic Name Brand Name Examples | Supplied As | Generic Available |
|---|---|---|
| Rx **Methotrexate (MTX)** | | |
| *Rheumatrex Dose Pack*[1] | **Tablets:** 2.5 mg | Yes |

[1] Contains lactose.

## Type of Drug:
Agent for rheumatoid arthritis, psoriasis, and certain types of cancer.

## How the Drug Works:
Methotrexate (MTX) is an antimetabolite which interferes with folic acid production, DNA production, and cellular reproduction.

## Uses:
To treat severe, disabling rheumatoid arthritis when other therapy fails.

To treat severe, disabling psoriasis when other therapy fails (see Agent for Psoriasis - Methotrexate in the Topicals chapter).

To treat certain types of cancer, alone or with other anticancer agents (see Antimetabolites in the Antineoplastics chapter).

*Unlabeled Use(s):* Occasionally doctors may prescribe methotrexate for Reiter's disease.

## Precautions:
*Do not use in the following situations:*

alcoholism
allergy to methotrexate or any of its ingredients
blood disorders before MTX therapy (eg, anemia, bone marrow hypoplasia, low platelet and white-cell count)

breastfeeding
immunodeficiency syndrome
liver disease
pregnancy

*Use with caution in the following situations:*

bone marrow depression
infection, active
kidney disease
liver damage

peptic ulcer, active
poor health and debility
ulcerative colitis
women of childbearing potential

*Liver:* Methotrexate may be highly toxic to the liver, particularly at high doses or with prolonged therapy. Liver atrophy, necrosis, cirrhosis, fatty liver, and liver fibrosis may occur. Liver function should be determined before methotrexate therapy begins and monitored regularly.

*Pregnancy:* Methotrexate has caused fetal death and severe birth defects. Defective egg (ovum) or sperm formation caused by methotrexate has been reported. Do not administer to pregnant women and women of childbearing potential unless the benefits outweigh the risks. Not recommended for pregnant patients with psoriasis or rheumatoid arthritis.

*Breastfeeding:* Methotrexate appears in breast milk. Since the drug may accumulate in newborns and cause serious adverse effects, breastfeeding is not recommended. Decide whether to discontinue nursing or discontinue the drug, taking into account the importance of the drug to the mother.

*Children:* Safety and effectiveness in children have not been established other than in cancer chemotherapy.

*Elderly:* Due to diminished liver and kidney function and folate deficiency, consider low doses for elderly patients and closely monitor for early signs of toxicity.

*Lab tests* will be required before and during treatment with methotrexate. Tests will include: Blood counts; urine tests; kidney, liver, and pulmonary function tests; and chest x-rays. Perform a liver biopsy if there are persistent abnormal liver function tests or a decrease in serum albumin below the normal range in patients with well controlled rheumatoid arthritis.

## Drug Interactions:

Tell your doctor or pharmacist if you are taking or if you are planning to take any over-the-counter or prescription medications or dietary supplements with methotrexate. Doses of one or both drugs may need to be modified or a different drug may need to be prescribed. The following drugs or drug classes interact with methotrexate.

aminoglycosides, oral (eg, neomycin sulfate)
broad-spectrum antibiotics, nonabsorbable (eg, polymyxin B, neomycin)
charcoal
chemotherapeutic agents, nephrotoxic (eg, cisplatin)
chloramphenicol (eg, *Chloromycetin Palmitate*)
folic acid (eg, *Folvite*)
leucovorin calcium (*Wellcovorin*)

nonsteroidal anti-inflammatory agents (eg, indomethacin)
penicillins (eg, penicillin G)
phenylbutazone (eg, *Azolid*)
phenytoin (eg, *Dilantin*)
probenecid
retinoids (eg, etretinate)
salicylates (eg, aspirin)
sulfonamides (eg, trimethoprim, sulfamethoxazole)
tetracycline (eg, *Sumycin*)
theophylline (eg, *Slo-Phyllin*)

## Side Effects:

Every drug is capable of producing side effects. Many methotrexate users experience no, or minor, side effects. The frequency and severity of side effects depend on many factors including dose, duration of therapy, and individual susceptibility. Possible side effects include:

*Digestive Tract:* Nausea; vomiting; appetite loss; diarrhea; mouth sores; sore throat; dark, bloody stools; black vomit; stomach pain; stomach bleeding.

*Hematologic:* Decreased platelet count; decreased white blood cell count; excess urea in blood.

*Nervous System:* Dizziness; headache; general body discomfort; ringing in the ears; unusual tiredness; chills; fever; drowsiness; convulsions; partial or incomplete paralysis; mood changes; strange head sensations; mental disease.

*Respiratory System:* Interstitial pneumonitis; cough; nosebleed; upper respiratory tract infection.

*Skin:* Rash; itching; sensitivity to ultraviolet (UV) light; sweating; boils; toxic epidermal necrolysis (blistering, skin sloughing); Stevens-Johnson syndrome; acne; flushing; redness; pigment changes; dilated vessels.

*Urinary and Reproductive Tract:* Vaginal discharge; painful urination; blood in the urine; menstrual problems; kidney disease; infertility.

*Other:* Fever; joint pain; decreased resistance to infection (eg, *Pneumocystis carinii* pneumonia); liver disease; chest pain; hair loss; blurred vision; unusual bleeding or bruising; abnormal liver function tests; low blood pressure; eye discomfort; blood clots; visual changes; eye infection.

## Guidelines for Use:

- For the treatment of rheumatoid arthritis, the usual starting dose of methotrexate is 7.5 mg once weekly, or a divided dose of 2.5 mg at 12-hour intervals for 3 doses given as a course once weekly.
- Taking methotrexate incorrectly can result in serious side effects. If doses are taken too often, notify your doctor immediately.
- Deaths have been reported from methotrexate use. Patients given methotrexate must receive close medical supervision. Risks of therapy must be fully understood.
- Avoid alcohol, antibiotics, aspirin, other salicylates, and NSAIDs.
- May cause sensitivity to sunlight. Avoid prolonged exposure to the sun or other forms of ultraviolet (UV) light (eg, tanning beds). Use sunscreens and wear protective clothing until tolerance is determined.
- May cause dizziness, drowsiness, or blurred vision. Use caution while driving or performing other tasks requiring mental alertness, coordination, or physical dexterity.
- Contact your doctor immediately if nausea, vomiting, appetite loss, infection, hair loss, skin rash, boils, or acne occurs or persists.
- Discontinue the drug and contact your doctor if any of the following symptoms occur: Diarrhea; abdominal pain; fever; signs of infection; unusual bleeding or bruising; cough; shortness of breath; skin rash. Most adverse reactions are reversible if detected early.
- Do not use methotrexate if you are pregnant.
- Avoid pregnancy if either partner is using methotrexate.
- *Conception* — Men should wait at least 3 months and women should wait at least 1 ovulatory cycle after stopping use of methotrexate before attempting to conceive.
- Unrelated conditions, especially dehydration, can increase the risk of toxicity. Upset stomach, especially when accompanied by significant vomiting, diarrhea, or decreased fluid intake can lead to dehydration. Notify your doctor immediately if these symptoms develop.
- For rheumatoid arthritis treatment, stop methotrexate immediately if there is a significant drop in blood counts or if liver function test abnormalities occur.
- Prior to therapy, a complete blood workup, urinalysis, chest x-ray, and kidney and liver function tests are required. Follow-up tests will also be required.
- Store at 77°F. Excursions are permitted between 59° to 86°F.

*If you have any questions, consult your doctor, pharmacist, or health care provider.*

| Generic Name<br>*Brand Name Examples* | Supplied As | Generic<br>Available |
|---|---|---|
| *Rx* **Allopurinol** | | |
| *Zyloprim* | **Tablets:** 100 mg, 300 mg | Yes |

## Type of Drug:

Agent for gout; xanthine oxidase inhibitor.

## How the Drug Works:

Gout is a hereditary form of arthritis caused by increased uric acid levels in the blood. Allopurinol prevents the formation of uric acid in the body by inhibiting an enzyme (xanthine oxidase) involved in the production of uric acid.

## Uses:

To prevent the signs and symptoms of primary or secondary gout (eg, acute attacks, tophi, joint destruction, uric acid kidney stones, kidney damage).

To manage uric acid elevations in serum (hyperuricemia) and urine (uricosuria) in patients treated for leukemia, lymphoma, and other malignancies.

To manage some types of kidney stones (calcium oxalate).

## Precautions:

*Do not use in the following situations:* Allergy or severe reaction to allopurinol.

*Use with caution in the following situations:*

| | |
|---|---|
| blood or bone marrow disorders | liver disease |
| kidney disease | thiazide diuretic use, concurrent |

*Acute attacks of gout* may increase during the early stages of allopurinol use. The attacks usually become shorter and less severe after several months of therapy. Even with adequate therapy, it may require several months to deplete the uric acid pool sufficiently to control acute episodes.

*Fluid intake:* Drink a sufficient amount of fluid to yield a urinary output of at least 2 quarts a day and to maintain a neutral or slightly alkaline urine. This will help prevent the formation of kidney stones while taking allopurinol.

*Allergy:* Discontinue at the first appearance of rash or other signs of an allergic reaction. In some instances, rash may be followed by more severe reactions such as itching; hives; red lesions; and loss of hair, skin, or fingernails.

*Pregnancy:* There are no adequate and well-controlled studies in pregnant women. Use only if clearly needed and potential benefits to the mother outweigh the possible hazards to the fetus.

*Breastfeeding:* Allopurinol appears in breast milk. Consult your doctor before you begin breastfeeding.

*Children:* Allopurinol is rarely used in children with the exception of those with hyperuricemia secondary to malignancy or to certain rare inborn errors of purine metabolism.

*Lab tests* will be required during treatment with allopurinol. Tests may include uric acid level, blood counts, and kidney and liver function tests.

## Drug Interactions:

Tell your doctor or pharmacist if you are taking or if you are planning to take any over-the-counter or prescription medications or dietary supplements with allopurinol. Doses of one or both drugs may need to be modified or a different drug may need to be prescribed. The following drugs and drug classes interact with allopurinol.

amoxicillin (eg, *Amoxil*)
ampicillin (eg, *Principen*)
anticoagulants (eg, dicumarol)
azathioprine (eg, *Imuran*)
chlorpropamide (eg, *Diabinese*)
cyclosporine (eg, *Sandim-mune*)
cytotoxic agents (eg, cyclophos-phamide)

mercaptopurine (*Purinethol*)
theophylline (eg, *Theo-Dur*)
thiazide diuretics (eg, hydro-chlorothiazide)
tolbutamide (eg, *Orinase*)
uricosuric agents (eg, sulfinpyra-zone)

## Side Effects:

Every drug is capable of producing side effects. Many allopurinol users experience no, or minor, side effects. The frequency and severity of side effects depend on many factors including dose, duration of therapy, and individual susceptibility. Possible side effects include:

*Digestive Tract:* Stomach upset; diarrhea; nausea.

*Skin:* Chills; rash; scaling or sloughing of skin.

*Other:* Acute gout attacks; joint pain; drowsiness.

## Guidelines for Use:

- *Gout and secondary hyperuricemia (maintenance)* — The average dose of allopurinol is 200 to 300 mg/day for patients with mild gout and 400 to 600 mg/day for those with moderate-to-severe gout. The dose may be administered in divided doses or as a single equivalent dose with the 300 mg tablet. Daily doses more than 300 mg should be administered in divided doses. The minimum effective dose is 100 to 200 mg/day, and the maximum recommended dose is 800 mg/day. It is recommended that the patient be started with a low dose (100 mg) and increased at weekly intervals by 100 mg until a serum uric acid level of 6 mg/dL or less is attained, not exceeding the maximum recommended dose.
- *Prevention of uric acid kidney disease during the vigorous chemotherapy of tumors* — 600 to 800 mg/day for 2 or 3 days along with a high fluid intake.
- *Recurrent kidney stones in patients with high levels of uric acid in the urine* — 200 to 300 mg/day in single or divided doses.
- *Secondary hyperuricemia in children* — Children 6 to 10 years of age with secondary hyperuricemia (increased uric acid in the blood) associated with severe diseases may be given 300 mg/day, while those less than 6 years of age are generally given 150 mg/day.
- To minimize stomach upset, take after meals.
- If a dose is missed, simply take your next dose at the regularly scheduled time. Do not attempt to make up for the missed dose.
- May take 2 to 6 weeks to become effective. Do not skip doses or stop taking this drug prematurely.
- Drink plenty of fluids while taking allopurinol, at least 10 to 12 full (8 oz) glasses a day, to prevent kidney stones.
- May cause drowsiness. Use caution while driving or performing other tasks requiring alertness, coordination, or physical dexterity.
- Discontinue allopurinol and notify your doctor immediately at the first sign of appetite loss, weight loss, rash, painful urination, blood in the urine, irritation of the eyes, or swelling of the lips or mouth.
- Avoid large doses of vitamin C as this may increase the possibility of kidney stone formation.
- Allopurinol does not treat acute gout attacks. Other medications (eg, colchicine, indomethacin) are used to treat the acute attack.
- Lab tests will be required to monitor therapy. Be sure to keep appointments.
- Store at 59° to 77°F in a dry place. Protect from light.

*If you have any questions, consult your doctor, pharmacist, or health care provider.*

| Generic Name<br>*Brand Name Examples* | Supplied As | Generic<br>Available |
|---|---|---|
| *Rx* Colchicine | **Tablets:** 0.6 mg | Yes |
| | **Injection:** 0.5 mg/mL | |
| *Rx* **Probenecid**[1] **and**<br>**Colchicine**<br>**Combinations** | | |
| *Col-Probenecid* | **Tablets:** 500 mg probenecid<br>and 0.5 mg colchicine | Yes |

[1] For further information on probenecid, see the Probenecid monograph.

## Type of Drug:

Agent for treating acute gout attacks and preventing or delaying a recurrence of symptoms.

## How the Drug Works:

Gout is a hereditary form of arthritis characterized by increased blood levels of uric acid. Colchicine decreases the inflammatory response to uric acid crystals that occurs in gout. However, it does not lower uric acid levels and thus does not treat the underlying cause of gout. Colchicine relieves pain but it is not an analgesic. Its suppressive effect helps reduce the incidence of gout attacks.

## Uses:

*Colchicine —*

To relieve pain of acute gout attacks. Works most effectively if administered early in the attack.

To prevent or delay acute attacks of gout (prophylaxis).

*Probenecid and colchicine combination —*

For the treatment of chronic gouty arthritis when complicated by frequent, recurrent acute attacks of gout.

*Unlabeled Use(s):* Occasionally doctors may prescribe colchicine for treatment of certain types of cirrhosis, familial Mediterranean fever, primary amyloidosis, Behcet's disease, pseudogout, skin manifestations of scleroderma, refractory idiopathic thrombocytopenic purpura, and chronic progressive multiple sclerosis.

## Precautions:

*Do not use in the following situations:*

allergy to colchicine

allergy to probenecid (probene-cid and colchicine combina-tion only)

blood dyscrasias (probenecid and colchicine combination only)

children younger than 2 years of age (probenecid and col-chicine combination only)

gastrointestinal disorders, severe

heart disease, severe

kidney disease, severe

uric acid kidney stones (pro-benecid and colchicine combi-nation only)

*Use with caution in the following situations:*

elderly (especially those with kidney, gastrointestinal, or heart disease)

gastrointestinal disorders

heart disease

kidney disease

peptic ulcer, history (probenecid and colchicine combination only)

*Men:* May adversely affect spermatogenesis.

*Pregnancy:* Colchicine can cause fetal harm when administered to a preg-nant woman. If this drug is used during pregnancy, or if the patient becomes pregnant while taking it, notify the woman of the potential haz-ard to the fetus.

*Breastfeeding:* It is not known if colchicine appears in breast milk. Consult your doctor before you begin breastfeeding.

*Children:* Safety and effectiveness for use in children have not been estab-lished. Do not use the probenecid and colchicine combination in chil-dren younger than 2 years of age.

*Elderly:* Administer colchicine with great caution to elderly and debilitated patients, especially those with kidney, digestive tract, or heart disease. Reduce dosage if weakness, appetite loss, nausea, vomiting, or diarrhea appears.

*Lab tests* may be required during treatment with colchicine. Tests may include blood counts and uric acid levels.

## Drug Interactions:

Tell your doctor or pharmacist if you are taking or if you are planning to take any over-the-counter or prescription medications or dietary supplements with colchicine or the probenecid and colchicine combina-tion. Doses of one or both drugs may need to be modified or a differ-ent drug may need to be prescribed. The following drugs and drug classes interact with colchicine.

*Colchicine:*

CNS depressants (eg, diazepam)

immunomodulatory agents (eg, cyclosporine)

sympathomimetic agents (eg, ephedrine)

vitamin $B_{12}$

*Probenecid and colchicine combination:*

acetaminophen (eg, *Tylenol*)

barbituate anesthetics (eg, midazolam)

beta-lactams (eg, penicillin)

ketamine (*Ketalar*)

lorazepam (eg, *Ativan*)

methotrexate (eg, *Rheumatrex*)

nonsteroidal anti-inflammatory agents (NSAIDs) (eg, indomethacin, sulindac, ketoprofen, meclofenamate, naproxen)

pyrazinamide

rifampin (eg, *Rifadin*)

salicylates (eg, aspirin)

sulfonamide (eg, sulfamethoxazole)

sulfonylureas, oral (eg, tolbutamide)

theophylline (eg, *Theo-Dur*)

thiopental (eg, *Pentothal*)

zidovudine (*Retrovir*)

## Side Effects:

Every drug is capable of producing side effects. Many colchicine users experience no, or minor, side effects. The frequency and severity of side effects depend on many factors including dose, duration of therapy, and individual susceptibility. Possible side effects include:

*Colchicine:* Vomiting; nausea; diarrhea; stomach pain; muscle weakness; hair loss; sore throat; unusual bleeding or bruising; tingling in hands or feet; abnormal blood counts; bone marrow depression; rash; agranulocytosis; decreased blood platelets; red or purple spots under the skin; aplastic anemia.

*Probenecid and colchicine combination:* Headache; dizziness; hepatic necrosis; vomiting; nausea; appetite loss; sore gums; nephrotic syndrome; uric acid stones with or without blood in the urine; renal colic; rib and vertebra pain; frequent urination; precipitation of acute gouty arthritis; allergic reaction; fever; rash; hives; itching; aplastic anemia; decreased white blood counts; hemolytic anemia; anemia; skin inflammation; hair loss; flushing; diarrhea; stomach pain; muscle weakness; sore throat; unusual bleeding or bruising; tingling in hands or feet; agranulocytosis; red or purple spots under the skin; abnormal blood counts; bone marrow depression.

## Guidelines for Use:

- *Colchicine* — Take medicine at the first warning of an acute gout attack. A delay of a few hours reduces the drug's effectiveness. The usual adult dose is 1 or 2 tablets initially, followed by 1 tablet every 1 or 2 hours until pain is relieved or nausea, vomiting, or diarrhea develops. Some doctors prescribe 2 tablets every 2 hours. Since the number of doses may range from 6 to 16, the total dose is variable. As prophylaxis, 1 tablet may be taken 1 to 4 times a week for mild or moderate cases, and once or twice daily for severe cases.

- The colchicine dose that relieves gout pain is very close to the dose that causes side effects. Stop taking colchicine once your pain is relieved or at the first sign of side effects (eg, stomach pain, nausea, vomiting, diarrhea). Continuing to take colchicine is of no benefit and will only worsen the side effects.

- *Probenecid and colchicine* — Do not start therapy until an acute gout attack has subsided. If an acute attack occurs during therapy, use additional colchicine or other appropriate therapy to control the attack. The recommended adult dose is 1 tablet daily for 1 week, followed by 1 tablet twice daily thereafter. In patients with varying degrees of kidney impairment, a daily dose of 2 tablets may be adequate. However, the daily dose may be increased by 1 tablet every 4 weeks within tolerance (and usually not above 4 tablets per day) if symptoms of gouty arthritis are not controlled.

- To reduce the chance of forming uric acid crystals or stones in the kidney, your doctor may want you to take sodium bicarbonate or potassium citrate as well as have you take extra fluid. Follow instructions carefully.

- Notify your doctor if you experience appetite loss, nausea, vomiting, or diarrhea. Dosage may need to be reduced.

- Discontinue use and notify your doctor if rash, sore throat, fever, unusual bleeding or bruising, tiredness, weakness, numbness, or tingling occurs.

- Colchicine does not relieve pain or inflammation from causes other than gout. It is of no value in other (non-gouty) types of arthritis.

- Lab tests will be required to monitor therapy. Be sure to keep appointments.

- Store at room temperature (59° to 86°F). Protect from light and moisture.

*If you have any questions, consult your doctor, pharmacist, or health care provider.*

| Generic Name Brand Name Examples | Supplied As | Generic Available |
|---|---|---|
| Rx **Probenecid** | **Tablets:** 500 mg | Yes |
| Rx **Probenecid and Colchicine[1] Combinations** | | |
| *Col-Probenecid* | **Tablets:** 500 mg probenecid and 0.5 mg colchicine | Yes |

[1] For further information on colchicine, see the colchicine monograph.

## Type of Drug:

Uricosuric; agent for treating gout.

## How the Drug Works:

Gout is a hereditary form of arthritis characterized by increased blood levels of uric acid. Probenecid decreases the amount of uric acid in the body by increasing the excretion of uric acid into the urine. Probenecid also inhibits secretion of many penicillin and cephalosporin antibiotics by the kidneys. This increases the blood levels of the antibiotics, thereby increasing their effectiveness.

## Uses:

To treat increased uric acid blood levels seen with gout and gouty arthritis.

For use with some antibiotics to make them more effective in treating infections.

## Precautions:

*Do not use in the following situations:*

allergy to probenecid or colchicine or any of their ingredients
blood disorders (eg, acute intermittent porphyria, G-6-PD deficiency)
children younger than 2 years of age
gout attack, acute
salicylates use, concurrent
uric acid kidney stones

*Use with caution in the following situations:*

allergy to sulfa drugs
kidney disease
methotrexate use, concurrent
peptic ulcer, history
pregnancy

*Pregnancy:* Routine use during normal pregnancy is not appropriate. Probenecid crosses the placenta. Use only when clearly needed and when the potential benefits to the mother outweigh the potential hazards to the fetus.

*Breastfeeding:* It is not known if probenecid appears in breast milk. Consult your doctor before you begin breastfeeding.

*Children:* Do not use in children younger than 2 years of age.

## Drug Interactions:

Tell your doctor or pharmacist if you are taking or if you are planning to take any over-the-counter or prescription medications or dietary supplements with probenecid or colchicine. Doses of one or both drugs may need to be modified or a different drug may need to be prescribed. The following drugs and drug classes interact with probenecid.

β-lactam antibiotics (eg, penicillin, cephalosporins)
barbiturate anesthetics (eg, thiopental)
cyclosporine (eg, *Sandimmune*)
diflunisal (eg, *Dolobid*)
dyphylline (eg, *Lufyllin*)
ketamine (*Ketalar*)
ketorolac (*Toradol*)
methotrexate (eg, *Rheumatrex*)
salicylates (eg, aspirin)
zidovudine (AZT; *Retrovir*)

Probenecid may give a false-positive result to copper sulfate tests *(Clinitest)* for urine glucose (sugar) but not to enzyme urine glucose tests *(Clinistix)*.

## Side Effects:

Every drug is capable of producing side effects. Many probenecid and pro- benecid and colchicine users experience no, or minor, side effects. The frequency and severity of side effects depend on many factors including dose, duration of therapy, and individual susceptibility. Possible side effects include:

*Probenecid —*

*Digestive Tract:* Nausea; vomiting; loss of appetite.

*Nervous System:* Headache; dizziness.

*Skin:* Rash; redness of face; itching; hives; skin inflammation.

*Other:* Fever, blood in the urine; increased urination; sore gums; anemia; abnormal blood cell counts; hair loss; precipitation of acute gouty arthritis; liver damage; kidney disease; uric acid kidney stones; colicky pain due to kidney stones; flank pain; allergic reaction.

*Colchicine —*

*Digestive Tract:* Nausea; vomiting; stomach pain; diarrhea.

*Skin:* Rash; hives; skin inflammation.

*Other:* Peripheral neuritis; muscular weakness; abnormal blood counts; hair loss; red or purple spots or patches under the skin.

## Guidelines for Use:

- Do not begin therapy until an acute gout attack has subsided. However, if an acute attack is precipitated during therapy, the medicine may be continued without changing the dosage. Take additional appropriate therapy (eg, colchicine) to control the attack.
- Avoid taking aspirin or aspirin-like products since they can block the effect of probenecid. If you require a mild analgesic agent, the use of acetaminophen (eg, *Tylenol*) rather than salicylates (eg, aspirin) is preferred.
- May cause stomach upset. Take with food or antacids.
- If nausea, vomiting, or loss of appetite persist, call your doctor. Stomach problems may be an indication of overdosage.
- Drink plenty of fluids, at least 6 to 8 full (8 oz) glasses daily, to prevent development of kidney stones.
- Your doctor may also want you to "alkalinize" your urine by taking sodium bicarbonate or potassium citrate. Follow directions carefully.
- A gout attack may occur when you first begin taking probenecid. You may need other medications for the gout attack. Continue taking probenecid.
- Probenecid may not be effective in chronic kidney insufficiency.
- Store at room temperature (59° to 86°F).

*Probenecid —*

- *Gout —* Recommended adult dosage is 250 mg (½ tablet) twice a day for 1 week, followed by 500 mg (1 tablet) twice a day thereafter.
- In children between 2 and 14 years of age, initial dose is 25 mg/kg body weight per day. Maintenance dose is 40 mg/kg, divided into 4 doses. For children weighing more than 110 lbs (50 kg), the adult dosage is recommended.
- *Kidney impairment with gout —* Some degree of kidney impairment may be present in patients with gout and this may decrease the effectiveness of probenecid. A daily dosage of 1000 mg may be adequate. However, if necessary, the daily dosage may be increased by 500 mg increments every 4 weeks within tolerance (and usually not above 2000 mg per day) if symptoms of gouty arthritis are not controlled or the 24-hour uric acid excretion is not more than 700 mg.
- Continue therapy at the dose that will maintain normal serum urate levels. When acute attacks have been absent for 6 months or more and serum urate levels remain within normal limits, decrease the daily dose by 1 tablet every 6 months. Do not reduce the maintenance dose to the point at which serum urate levels tend to rise.
- *Probenecid and penicillin therapy (general) —* Recommended dosage is 2000 mg (4 tablets) in divided doses. Reduce the dose in older patients in whom kidney impairment may be present.
- *Neurosyphilis aqueous procaine —* Administer penicillin G 2.4 million units/day IM plus probenecid 500 mg orally 4 times a day for 10 to 14 days.

## Guidelines for Use (cont.):

*Probenecid and Colchicine —*

- Recommended dosage is 1 tablet daily for 1 week, followed by 1 tablet twice a day thereafter.
- Some degree of kidney impairment may be present in patients with gout. A daily dose of 2 tablets may be adequate. However, if necessary, the daily dosage may be increased by 1 tablet every 4 weeks within tolerance (and usually not above 4 tablets per day) if symptoms of gouty arthritis are not controlled or the 24-hour uric acid excretion is not above 700 mg.
- Continue therapy at the dosage that will maintain normal serum urate levels. When acute attacks have been absent for 6 months or more and serum urate levels remain within normal limits, decrease the daily dose by 1 tablet every 6 months. Do not reduce the maintenance dose to the point at which serum urate levels tend to rise.

*If you have any questions, consult your doctor, pharmacist, or health care provider.*

| Generic Name Brand Name Examples | Supplied As | Generic Available |
|---|---|---|
| Rx **Sulfinpyrazone** | | |
| *Anturane* | **Tablets:** 100 mg | Yes |
| *Anturane* | **Capsules:** 200 mg | Yes |

## Type of Drug:
Uricosuric; agent for treating gout.

## How the Drug Works:
Gout is a metabolic form of arthritis caused by increased blood levels of uric acid. Sulfinpyrazone decreases the amount of uric acid in the body by increasing the elimination of uric acid into the urine.

## Uses:
To treat chronic gouty arthritis and intermittent gouty arthritis. Sulfinpyrazone has a minimal anti-inflammatory effect and is not intended for relief of an acute attack of gout.

*Unlabeled Use(s):* Occasionally doctors may prescribe sulfinpyrazone to decrease the risk of blood clots in some patients with a heart valve disorder.

## Precautions:
*Do not use in the following situations:*

| | |
|---|---|
| allergy to phenylbutazone | peptic ulcer, active |
| allergy to sulfinpyrazone | salicylate use, concomitant |
| blood cell disorders | |
| digestive tract inflammation or ulceration | |

*Use with caution in the following situations:*

| | |
|---|---|
| anticoagulants (eg, warfarin), concurrent use of | peptic ulcer, history |
| hypoglycemic agents (eg, tolbutamide), concurrent use | pregnancy |
| insulin, concurrent use | sulfa drugs (eg, sulfisoxazole), concurrent use |
| kidney disease | urolithiasis |

*Pregnancy:* Adequate studies have not been done in pregnant women. Use only if clearly needed and potential benefits to the mother outweigh the possible hazards to the fetus.

*Breastfeeding:* It is not known if sulfinpyrazone appears in breast milk. Consult your doctor before you begin breastfeeding.

*Children:* Safety and effectiveness in children have not been established.

*Lab tests* may be required to monitor therapy. Tests may include blood uric acid, blood cell counts, kidney function, and urine tests.

## Drug Interactions:

Tell your doctor or pharmacist if you are taking or if you are planning to take any over-the-counter or prescription medications or dietary supplements with sulfinpyrazone. Doses of one or both drugs may need to be modified or a different drug may need to be prescribed. The following drugs and drug classes interact with sulfinpyrazone:

acetaminophen (eg, *Tylenol*)
anticoagulants, oral (eg, warfarin)
insulin
niacin (eg, *Nicobid*)

salicylates (eg, aspirin)
sulfonamides (eg, sulfisoxazole)
sulfonylureas (eg, tolbutamide)
theophylline (eg, *Theo-Dur*)
verapamil (eg, *Isoptin*)

## Side Effects:

Every drug is capable of producing side effects. Many sulfinpyrazone users experience no, or minor, side effects. The frequency and severity of side effects depend on many factors including dose, duration of therapy, and individual susceptibility. Possible side effects include: Stomach upset; nausea; aggravation of peptic ulcers; rash; blood cell disorders.

### Guidelines for Use:

- Initial dosage is 200 to 400 mg daily in 2 divided doses. Maintenance dosage is 400 mg daily given in 2 divided doses. Dose may be increased to 800 mg daily. After blood urate levels are controlled, dose may be reduced to 200 mg daily for long-term control.
- Take sulfinpyrazone regularly as prescribed by your doctor. Do not stop taking or change the dose unless directed by your doctor.
- May cause stomach upset. Take with food, milk, or antacids.
- Initiation of therapy may initially cause acute attacks of gouty arthritis. These initial attacks can be treated with colchicine or other agents used to treat gouty attacks. These attacks subside with continued use of sulfinpyrazone. Do not stop taking sulfinpyrazone during these attacks.
- Continue treatment without interruption, even during acute gouty attacks.
- If a dose is missed, take it as soon as possible. If several hours have passed or if it is nearing time for the next dose, do not double the dose to catch up unless advised to do so by your doctor. If more than 1 dose is missed, or if it is necessary to establish a new dosage schedule, contact your doctor or pharmacist.
- Do not take with aspirin or other products that contain aspirin since they can decrease the effect of sulfinpyrazone.
- Drink plenty of fluids while taking sulfinpyrazone.
- Notify your doctor if you experience nausea, vomiting, severe stomach pain, rash, lethargy, blood in vomit or stool, or unusual bleeding or bruising.
- Inform your doctor if you are pregnant, become pregnant, are planning to become pregnant, or are breastfeeding.
- Lab tests may be required. Be sure to keep appointments.
- Store at room temperature (59° to 86°F). Keep in a tightly closed container.

*If you have any questions, consult your doctor, pharmacist, or health care provider.*

| | Brand Name Examples | Supplied As | Generic Available |
|---|---|---|---|
| Rx | Duradrin, Midrin, Migratine | **Capsules**: 65 mg isomethep-tene mucate/100 mg dichloral-phenazone/325 mg acetaminophen | Yes |
| Rx | Wigraine | **Tablets**: 1 mg ergotamine tar-trate/100 mg caffeine | No |
| Rx | Cafatine-PB | **Tablets**: 1 mg ergotamine tar-trate/100 mg caffeine/30 mg pentobarbital sodium/0.125 mg l-alkaloids of belladonna | No |
| Rx | Cafergot | **Suppositories**: 2 mg ergot-amine tartrate/100 mg caffeine | No |
| otc | Excedrin Migraine | **Tablets, coated**: 250 mg aceta-minophen/250 mg aspirin/ 65 mg caffeine | No |
| otc | Excedrin Migraine | **Caplets**: 250 mg acetamino-phen/250 mg aspirin/65 mg caf-feine | No |
| otc | Excedrin Migraine | **Geltabs**: 250 mg acetamino-phen/250 mg aspirin/65 mg caf-feine | No |

## Type of Drug:

Combinations of drugs used to treat migraine attacks.

## How the Drug Works:

Ergotamine tartrate, caffeine, and isometheptene constrict blood vessels in the brain, an action that may be related to the relief of migraines. For more information on caffeine, see the CNS Stimulants-Caffeine mono-graph in this chapter.

Acetaminophen and aspirin are used for their pain-relieving effect. For more information, see the Analgesics-Acetaminophen and Analgesics-Aspirin and Salicylates monographs in this chapter.

Belladonna alkaloids are used to treat nausea and vomiting during migraine attacks.

Barbiturates and dichloralphenazone are used for sedation to reduce the emotional reaction to migraine pain. For more information on barbitu-rates, see the Sedatives-Barbiturates monograph in this chapter.

## Uses:

To stop or prevent vascular (migraine) headaches.

*Isometheptene:* For relief of tension and vascular (migraine) headaches.

## Precautions:

*Do not use in the following situations:*

allergy to the migraine combination or any of its ingredients

chest pain

coronary artery disease (ergotamine and isometheptene only)

glaucoma (isometheptene only)

high blood pressure, severe (ergotamine and isometheptene only)

kidney disease (ergotamine and isometheptene only)

liver disease (ergotamine and isometheptene only)

MAOI therapy, concurrent (isometheptene only)

peripheral vascular disease (ergotamine only)

pregnancy (ergotamine only)

sepsis (blood poisoning) (ergotamine only)

*Use with caution in the following situations:*

heart attack, recent

high blood pressure

kidney problems

liver problems

peripheral vascular disease

*Pregnancy:* Do not use ergotamine/caffeine products if you are pregnant or planning to become pregnant. Use isometheptene, dichloralphenazone, or acetaminophen products only if clearly needed and the potential benefits to the mother outweigh the possible hazards to the fetus.

*Breastfeeding:* It is not known if ergotamine is excreted in breast milk.

*Children:* Safety and effectiveness of use of ergotamine in children have not been established.

## Drug Interactions:

Tell your doctor or pharmacist if you are taking or if you are planning to take any over-the-counter or prescription medications or dietary supplements while taking a migraine combination. Doses of one or both drugs may need to be modified or a different drug may need to be prescribed. The following drugs and drug classes interact with migraine combinations containing belladonna alkaloids or ergotamine. For more information on other agents, see the individual monographs in this chapter:

beta-blockers (eg, propranolol) (ergotamine only)

haloperidol (eg, *Haldol*) (belladonna only)

macrolide antibiotics (eg, erythromycin) (ergotamine only)

MAOIs (eg, phenelzine) (isometheptene only)

NNRT inhibitors (eg, delavirdine) (ergotamine only)

phenothiazines (eg, perphenazine) (belladonna only)

protease inhibitors (eg, ritonavir) (ergotamine only)

selective 5-HT$_1$ receptor agonists (eg, sumatriptan) (ergotamine only)

sibutramine (*Meridia*) (ergotamine only)

## Side Effects:

Every drug is capable of producing side effects. Many migraine combination users experience no, or minor, side effects. The frequency and severity of side effects depend on many factors including dose, duration of therapy, and individual susceptibility. Possible side effects include:

*Ergotamine* — Chest pain; muscle pain in the arms and legs; numbness and tingling in fingers and toes; cold or pale fingers or toes; abnormal heart rhythm; vomiting; nausea; weakness in the legs; diarrhea; localized swelling and itching; vertigo (feeling of whirling motion); rectal or anal ulcer (due to overuse of suppositories).

*Isometheptene* — Dizziness; rash.

---

### Guidelines for Use:
- Dosage is individualized. Take exactly as prescribed.
- Do not stop taking or change the dose, unless directed by your doctor.
- Take at the first sign or "hint" of a migraine attack.
- Suppositories are used when tablets and capsules cannot be taken because the migraine attack caused nausea or vomiting.
- *Ergotamine products* — Stop taking and notify your doctor if you experience numbness, tingling, coldness, or paleness in fingers or toes; muscle pain in arms or legs; weakness in legs; chest pain; heart rate changes; sudden worsening of headache; swelling; or itching.
- Store tablets and capsules at room temperature. Protect from moisture.
- Store suppositories below 77°F in the foil wrapper. If suppository is soft, chill in the refrigerator before opening.

---

*If you have any questions, consult your doctor, pharmacist, or health care provider.*

| Generic Name<br>*Brand Name Examples* | Supplied As | Generic<br>Available |
|---|---|---|
| *Rx* **Almotriptan Malate** | | |
| *Axert* | **Tablets**: 6.25 mg, 12.5 mg | No |
| *Rx* **Frovatriptan Succinate** | | |
| *Frova* | **Tablets**: 2.5 mg | No |
| *Rx* **Naratriptan HCl** | | |
| *Amerge* | **Tablets**: 1 mg, 2.5 mg | No |
| *Rx* **Rizatriptan Benzoate** | | |
| *Maxalt* | **Tablets**: 5 mg, 10 mg | No |
| *Maxalt-MLT* | **Tablets, orally disintegrating**:<br>5 mg, 10 mg | No |
| *Rx* **Sumatriptan Succinate**[1] | | |
| *Imitrex* | **Tablets**: 25 mg, 50 mg, 100 mg | No |
| *Imitrex* | **Spray, nasal**: 5 mg, 20 mg | |
| *Rx* **Zolmitriptan** | | |
| *Zomig* | **Tablets**: 1 mg, 2 mg, 5 mg | No |
| *Zomig-ZMT* | **Tablets, orally disintegrating**:<br>2.5 mg, 5 mg | No |

[1] Also available as an injection.

## Type of Drug:

Agent for treating migraine headaches.

## How the Drug Works:

Serotonin 5-HT$_1$ receptor antagonists constrict blood vessels in the brain and reduce transmission of trigeminal pain pathways, thus providing relief from migraine headaches.

## Uses:

For the acute management of migraine with or without aura in adults. Not intended for the prevention of migraine or for use in the management of hemiplegic or basilar migraine.

*Sumatriptan succinate injection:* For the acute treatment of cluster headache episodes.

## Precautions:

*Do not use in the following situations:*

5-HT$_1$ agonist (eg, naratriptan) use, within 24 hours

allergy to the drug or any of its ingredients

certain types of migraine (eg, basilar, hemiplegic)

ergot-containing drug (eg, methysergide) use, within 24 hours

heart attack, history of

heart disease or symptoms of heart disease

high blood pressure, uncontrolled

kidney disease, severe

liver disease, severe

MAOI (eg, phenelzine) use, within the last 14 days

peripheral vascular disease

*Use with caution in the following situations:*

coronary artery disease, family history of

kidney disease

liver disease

men older than 40 years of age

menopausal women

risk factors for heart disease (eg, smoking, high cholesterol, diabetes, obesity, high blood pressure)

*Pregnancy:* There are no adequate and well-controlled studies in pregnant women. Use only if clearly needed and the potential benefits outweigh the possible hazards to the fetus.

*Breastfeeding:* It is not known if 5-HT$_1$ agonists appear in breast milk. Consult your doctor before you begin breastfeeding.

*Children:* Safety and effectiveness have not been established. Not recommended in patients younger than 18 years of age.

*Lab tests* may be required prior to or during therapy. Tests include cardiovascular system evaluations.

## Drug Interactions:

Tell your doctor or pharmacist if you are taking or planning to take any over-the-counter or prescription medications or dietary supplements while taking these drugs. Doses of one or both drugs may need to be modified or a different drug may need to be prescribed. The following drugs or drug classes interact with these drugs:

another 5-HT$_1$ agonist

cimetidine (eg, *Tagamet*)

contraceptives, oral (eg, *Ortho-Novum*) (frovatriptan only)

ergot-containing drugs (eg, methysergide)

erythromycin (eg, *E-Mycin*)

itraconazole (*Sporanox*)

ketoconazole (eg, *Nizoral*)

MAOIs (eg, phenelzine)

propranolol (eg, *Inderal*)

ritonavir (*Norvir*)

sibutramine (*Meridia*)

## Side Effects:

Every drug is capable of producing side effects. Many patients experience no, or minor, side effects. The frequency and severity of side effects depend on many factors including dose, duration of therapy, and individual susceptibility. Possible side effects include:

*Digestive Tract:* Stomach pain; nausea; dry mouth; vomiting.

*Nervous System:* Drowsiness; headache; abnormal skin sensations (eg, feeling of warmth, heat, numbness, tingling); dizziness; unusual drowsiness or weakness.

*Circulatory System:* Increased blood pressure; chest pain, tightness, heaviness, or pressure; abnormal heart rhythm; fainting; flushing.

*Other:* Light sensitivity; neck, throat, or jaw pain or tightness; fatigue.

---

### Guidelines for Use:

- 5-HT₁ agonists are only used to treat migraine headaches. They should not be used to prevent a migraine.
- Review patient information leaflet before use.
- Your doctor may want you to take the first dose in the office if you have any risk factors for coronary artery disease.
- Dosage is individualized. Take exactly as prescribed.
- Do not stop taking or change the dose, unless instructed by your doctor.
- If the headache returns after the first dose, you may take a second dose 2 hours or more after the first dose. If pain continues after the first dose, do not take a second dose without first checking with your doctor.
- *Orally-disintegrating tablets* — Make sure your hands are dry before removing the tablet from the package. Remove tablet and immediately place it on the tongue. The tablet dissolves within seconds and is swallowed with the saliva. You do not need to drink water or other liquids to swallow the tablets.
- *Nasal spray* — Clear nasal passages before using. May irritate the nose (eg, burning, soreness, discharge).
- Tablets may be taken without regard to food.
- May cause drowsiness or dizziness. Use caution while driving or performing other tasks requiring alertness, coordination, or physical dexterity.
- Notify your doctor immediately if you experience tightness, pain, pressure, or heaviness in your chest, throat, neck, or jaw.
- The safety of treating more than 4 headaches in a 30-day period is unknown.
- Inform your doctor if you are pregnant, become pregnant, are planning to become pregnant, or are breastfeeding.
- Lab tests may be required prior to or during therapy. Be sure to keep appointments. Long-term users who have or develop risk factors for coronary artery disease will need periodic heart tests.
- Store at controlled room temperature (59° to 86°F). Do not store orally-disintegrating tablets in the bathroom or other damp places. Heat or moisture will destroy the medicine.

---

*If you have any questions, consult your doctor, pharmacist, or health care provider.*

| Generic Name<br>*Brand Name Examples* | Supplied As | Generic<br>Available |
|---|---|---|
| *otc* **Cyclizine HCl** | | |
| *Marezine* | **Tablets:** 50 mg | No |
| **Dimenhydrinate** | | |
| *otc* *Calm-X, Dramamine,<br>Motion Sickness, Triptone* | **Tablets:** 50 mg | Yes |
| *otc* *Dramamine[1]* | **Tablets, chewable:** 50 mg | No |
| *otc* *Children's Dramamine* | **Syrup:** 12.5 mg/5 mL | Yes |
| *Rx* *Hydrate* | **Injection:** 50 mg/mL | Yes |
| **Diphenhydramine HCl** | | |
| *otc* *Banophen, Benadryl<br>Allergy Kapseal, Genahist* | **Capsules:** 25 mg, 50 mg | Yes |
| *otc* *AllerMax[2], Banophen,<br>Benadryl Allergy Ultratabs,<br>Genahist* | **Tablets:** 25 mg, 50 mg | Yes |
| *otc* *Benadryl Allergy Chew-<br>ables* | **Tablets, chewable:** 12.5 mg | No |
| *otc* *Banophen* | **Elixir:** 12.5 mg/5 mL | Yes |
| *otc* *AllerMax, Belix, Benadryl<br>Allergy, Diphen Cough[2],<br>Genahist, Hydramine,<br>Tusstat Cough[2]* | **Liquid:** 12.5 mg/5 mL | Yes |
| *Rx* *Benadryl, Hyrexin-50* | **Injection:** 50 mg/mL | Yes |
| **Meclizine HCl** | | |
| *Rx* *Antivert* | **Tablets:** 12.5 mg | Yes |
| *Rx* *Antivert/25* | **Tablets:** 25 mg | Yes |
| *Rx* *Antivert/50* | **Tablets:** 50 mg | Yes |
| *otc* *Bonine* | **Tablets, chewable:** 25 mg | Yes |
| *Rx* *Meni-D* | **Capsules:** 25 mg | No |
| *Rx* **Scopolamine HBr** | | |
| *Scopace* | **Tablets:** 0.4 mg | No |
| *Transderm Scōp* | **Transdermal system:** 1.5 mg | No |
| *Rx* **Trimethobenzamide HCl** | | |
| *Tigan, Trimazide* | **Capsules:** 100 mg, 250 mg | Yes |
| *Tebamide, Tigan,<br>Trimazide* | **Suppositories, pediatric:**<br>100 mg | Yes |
| *Tebamide, Tigan,<br>Trimazide* | **Suppositories:** 200 mg | Yes |
| *Tigan* | **Injection:** 100 mg/mL | No |

[1] Contains tartrazine dye.
[2] Contains alcohol.

## Type of Drug:

Drugs for prevention and treatment of nausea, vomiting, or dizziness associated with motion sickness and vertigo (feeling of whirling motion).

## How the Drug Works:

Chemical-induced vomiting (including vomiting associated with drugs, radiation, and metabolic disorders) is generally stimulated through the chemoreceptor trigger zone (CTZ), which in turn stimulates the vomiting center (VC) in the brain which controls nausea and vomiting. Nausea due to motion sickness is initiated by stimulation of a mechanism of the middle ear (vestibular system), which sends impulses to the CTZ. These drugs act on the vestibular system, CTZ, VC, nerve pathways, and other centers in the brain to reduce nausea and vomiting.

## Uses:

To prevent and treat nausea, vomiting, or dizziness associated with motion sickness.

*Meclizine:* Possibly effective for the management of vertigo associated with diseases affecting the middle ear (vestibular system).

*Trimethobenzamide:* Indicated only for the treatment of nausea and vomiting.

## Precautions:

*Do not use in the following situations:*

allergy to benzocaine or similar local anesthetics (trimethobenzamide only)
allergy to the medicine or any of its ingredients
glaucoma (scopolamine only)
kidney function, impaired (scopolamine tablets only)
liver function, impaired (scopolamine tablets only)
premature or newborn patients (diphenhydramine injection and trimethobenzamide only)
prostate enlargement (scopolamine tablets only)
pyloric obstruction (scopolamine tablets only)

*Use with caution in the following situations:*

abnormal heart rhythm (dimenhydrinate injection only)
asthma
breathing difficulty
bronchitis, chronic
children
elderly (diphenhydramine and scopolamine only)
emphysema
glaucoma
heart disease (scopolamine only)
kidney disease (scopolamine transdermal system only)
liver disease (scopolamine transdermal system only)
metabolic function, impaired (scopolamine transdermal system only)
obstruction of the digestive tract
peptic ulcer (diphenhydramine only)
prostate enlargement
psychosis (scopolamine transdermal system only)
pulmonary disease, chronic
pyloric obstruction (dimenhydrinate, diphenhydramine, scopolamine only)
seizure disorder (scopolamine transdermal system only)
shortness of breath

urinary bladder neck obstruction (dimenhydrinate, diphenhydramine, scopolamine only)

urination difficulty due to prostate gland enlargement

*Scopolamine drug withdrawal:* Dizziness, nausea, vomiting, headache, and disturbances of equilibrium have been reported in a few patients following discontinuation of the use of the transdermal system. This occurred most often in patients who used the system for more than 3 days.

*Pregnancy: Meclizine* – Studies in pregnant women have not shown a risk to the fetus. However, no drug should be used during pregnancy unless clearly needed.
   *Cyclizine, dimenhydrinate, diphenhydramine, trimethobenzamide, scopolamine* – Adequate studies have not been done in pregnant women. Use only if clearly needed and potential benefits to the mother outweigh the possible hazards to the fetus.

*Breastfeeding:* Diphenhydramine appears in breast milk. It is not known if cyclizine, dimenhydrinate, meclizine, trimethobenzamide, or scopolamine appear in breast milk. Consult your doctor before you begin breastfeeding.

*Children:* Do not use cyclizine or diphenhydramine in children younger than 6 years of age unless directed by a doctor. Do not use diphenhydramine in premature infants or newborns. Do not use dimenhydrinate in children younger than 2 years of age. Do not use meclizine in children younger than 12 years of age. Safety of scopolamine has not been established in children. Do not use trimethobenzamide injection in children; do not use trimethobenzamide suppositories in premature infants or newborns. Anticholinergic antiemetic/antivertigo products are **not** recommended for uncomplicated vomiting in children.

*Tartrazine:* Some of these products may contain tartrazine dye (FD&C Yellow No. 5) which can cause allergic reactions in certain individuals. Check package label when available or consult your doctor or pharmacist.

## Drug Interactions:

Tell your doctor or pharmacist if you are taking or if you are planning to take any over-the-counter or prescription medications while taking an anticholinergic antiemetic/antivertigo product. Doses of one or both drugs may need to be modified or a different drug may need to be prescribed. The following drugs and drug classes interact with anticholinergic antiemetic/antivertigo products.

alcohol
anticholinergics, other (eg, belladonna alkaloids, antihistamines, antidepressants) (scopolamine only)
antidepressants (eg, amitriptyline) (scopolamine only)
CNS depressants (hypnotics, sedatives, tranquilizers (dimenhydrinate, diphenhydramine only)

haloperidol (eg, *Haldol*) (scopolamine only)
monoamine oxidase inhibitors (MAOIs)( eg, phenelzine) (diphenhydramine only)
phenothiazines (eg, acetophenazine, fluphenazine)

## Side Effects:

Every drug is capable of producing side effects. Many anticholinergic antiemetic/antivertigo product users experience no, or minor, side effects. The frequency and severity of side effects depend on many factors including dose, duration of therapy, and individual susceptibility. Possible side effects include:

*Digestive Tract:* Appetite loss; nausea; vomiting; diarrhea; constipation; stomach upset.

*Nervous System:* Drowsiness; restlessness; excitability (especially in children); nervousness; sleeplessness; headache; confusion; disorientation; dizziness; sedation; sleepiness; fatigue; feeling of whirling motion; exaggerated sense of well being; irritability; tremor; memory disturbances; hallucinations; sensitivity to light.

*Circulatory System:* Lowering of blood pressure; pounding in chest; increased heart rate.

*Urinary and Reproductive Tract:* Urinary frequency; difficult or painful urination; urinary retention.

*Allergic Reactions:* Hives; rash; yellowing of skin and eyes (trimethobenzamide only).

*Other:* Blurred vision; double vision; dry, itchy, red eyes; eye pain; enlarged pupils; ringing in the ears; dry mouth, nose, and throat; abnormal blood counts; flushing; dry skin; local necrosis (diphenhydramine injection only); excessive sweating; abnormal skin sensations; convulsions; thickening of mucus; tightness in chest or throat; wheezing; stuffy nose; chills.

## Guidelines for Use:

- Consult your doctor and product labeling for individual dosing instructions. Do not exceed the recommended dosage. Use exactly as prescribed.
- For prevention of nausea and vomiting, take the first dose of oral products 30 to 60 minutes before beginning activity associated with motion sickness.
- Injectable forms are used when the oral dose forms are impractical. Doses will be prepared and administered by your health care provider.
- May cause drowsiness or blurred vision. Use caution while driving or performing other tasks requiring alertness, coordination, or physical dexterity.
- Avoid alcohol and other depressants (eg, sleeping pills, tranquilizers, antianxiety agents, narcotic pain relievers) while you are taking this medicine.
- Do not use any other products containing diphenhydramine (eg, some antihistamines, antiparkinsonians, or antitussives) while taking diphenhydramine.
- Oral agents may be ineffective if consumed after vomiting has already begun. Consider use of injectable products or suppositories under such circumstances.
- Not for frequent or prolonged use unless directed by your doctor.
- *Scopolamine transdermal system* – Patient package insert is available with the transdermal products.
  *Initiation of therapy* – Apply 1 patch on a hairless area behind the ear at least 4 hours before the antiemetic effect is required. Scopolamine will be delivered over 3 days. Wear only 1 patch at a time.
  *Handling* – After applying the patch on dry skin behind the ear, wash hands thoroughly with soap and water, then dry them. When removing the patch, discard the removed patch and wash hands and application site thoroughly with soap and water to prevent any traces of scopolamine from coming into direct contact with the eyes. Temporary dilation of the pupils and blurred vision may occur if scopolamine comes in contact with the eyes. In addition, it is important that used patches be disposed of properly to avoid contact with children or pets.
  *Continuation of therapy* – If the patch is displaced, discard it and place a fresh one behind the other ear. If therapy is required for more than 3 days, discard the first patch and place a fresh one behind the other ear.
  Remove the patch immediately and notify your doctor if you experience pain or reddening of the eyes accompanied by dilated pupils or difficult urination.
- *Trimethobenzamide* – Discontinue use and notify your doctor if blurred vision, convulsions, depression, diarrhea, disorientation, dizziness, drowsiness, headache, yellowing of the skin or eyes, or muscle cramps occur.
- Store at room temperature (59° to 77°F). Protect from light and moisture.

*If you have any questions, consult your doctor, pharmacist, or health care provider.*

| Generic Name<br>*Brand Name Examples* | Supplied As | Generic<br>Available |
|---|---|---|
| *C-II* **Dronabinol** | | |
| *Marinol* | **Capsules, gelatin:** 2.5 mg,<br>5 mg, 10 mg | No |

## Type of Drug:

Marijuana-like agents which reduce nausea and vomiting. Dronabinol also acts to increase appetite in patients with AIDS.

## How the Drug Works:

Dronabinol is the principal substance present in *Cannabis sativa L* (marijuana). Non-therapeutic effects of dronabinol are identical to those of marijuana and other cannabinoids. How the cannabinoids decrease nausea and vomiting and stimulate appetite is unknown.

## Uses:

To treat nausea and vomiting associated with cancer chemotherapy in patients who have failed to respond adequately to conventional antiemetic treatment. Dronabinol also is used in the treatment of anorexia associated with weight loss in patients with AIDS. Because the cannabinoids may alter the mental state, they are intended for use when the patient can be closely supervised.

## Precautions:

*Do not use in the following situations:*
    allergy to marijuana or other cannabinoids
    allergy to sesame oil

*Use with caution in the following situations:*

| | |
|---|---|
| alcoholism, history of | high blood pressure |
| depression | mania |
| elderly | schizophrenia |
| heart disease | |

*Hazardous tasks:* Because of the effects on mental status, do not drive, operate complex machinery or engage in any activity requiring sound judgment and unimpaired coordination while receiving treatment. Effects may persist for an unpredictable period of time. Dronabinol may persist in the body for days.

*Supervision* is required. Patients receiving cannabinoids should be observed in a doctor's office or hospital. This is especially important during treatment of naive patients. Even in patients experienced with marijuana, however, dronabinol may have serious responses not predicted by prior exposures. Any patient who has a psychotic experience with dronabinol must be monitored until the mental state returns to normal. Additional doses should not be given until the patient has been examined and the circumstances evaluated.

*Drug abuse and dependence:* Dronabinol is highly abusable. Prescriptions are limited to the amount necessary for a single cycle of chemotherapy or to the amount necessary for the period between clinic visits. Long-term use of cannabinoids has been associated with disorders of motivation, judgment, and knowledge.

A withdrawal syndrome consisting of irritability, insomnia and restlessness was observed in some subjects within 12 hours following abrupt withdrawal of long-term dronabinol use. The syndrome reached its peak intensity at 24 hours when subjects exhibited hot flashes, sweating, runny nose, loose stools, hiccups, and appetite loss. The syndrome was essentially complete within 48 hours.

Electrocardiogram changes following discontinuation were consistent with a withdrawal syndrome. Several subjects reported disturbed sleep for several weeks after discontinuing high doses.

*Pregnancy:* Adequate studies have not been done in pregnant women. Use these drugs only if clearly needed.

*Breastfeeding:* Dronabinol appears in breast milk and is not recommended for use in nursing mothers.

*Children:* Dronabinol is not recommended for AIDS-related anorexia in children. Caution is recommended in prescribing this drug for children with chemotherapy-induced nausea and vomiting because of its pyschoactive effects.

*Elderly:* Use with caution in the elderly because of enhanced sensitivity to psychoactive effects.

## Drug Interactions:

Tell your doctor or pharmacist if you are taking or planning to take any over-the-counter or prescription medications or dietary supplements with cannabinoids. Doses of one or both drugs may need to be modified or a different drug may need to be prescribed. The following drugs and drug classes interact with cannabinoids.

alcohol
anticholinergic agents (eg, atropine)
barbiturates (eg, phenobarbital)
CNS depressants (benzodiazepines)
disulfiram (eg, *Antabuse)*

fluoxetine *(Prozac)*
sympathomimetic agents (eg, epinephrine)
theophylline (eg, *Theobid)*
tricyclic antidepressants (eg, amitriptyline)

## Side Effects:

Every drug is capable of producing side effects. Many cannabinoid users experience no, or minor, side effects. The frequency and severity of side effects depend on many factors including dose, duration of therapy, and individual susceptibility. Possible side effects include:

*Digestive Tract:* Nausea; vomiting; diarrhea; changes in appetite.

*Nervous System:* Drowsiness; heightened awareness; dizziness; unsteadiness; depression; weakness; hallucinations; memory loss; confusion; nightmares.

*Circulatory System:* Increased heart rate; lowered blood pressure.

*Other:* Dry mouth; vision problems (distortions); flushing.

---

### Guidelines for Use:

- Avoid alcohol and barbiturates. Use other drugs that cause drowsiness (eg, antianxiety agents, narcotic pain relievers) with caution.
- May cause dizziness, drowsiness, and impaired reflexes/judgment. Do not drive or perform hazardous tasks requiring alertness.
- Possible changes in mood and other behavioral effects are possible with these drugs. Do not panic in the event of such manifestations.
- When taking dronabinol to stimulate appetite, take 1 hour before lunch or dinner; do not take before breakfast.
- Remain under supervision of a responsible adult.

---

*If you have any questions, consult your doctor, pharmacist, or health care provider.*

| Generic Name<br>*Brand Name Examples* | Supplied As | Generic<br>Available |
|---|---|---|
| *Rx* **Dolasetron Mesylate** | | |
| *Anzemet* | **Tablets**: 50 mg, 100 mg | No |
| *Anzemet* | **Injection**: 12.5 mg/0.625 mL,<br>20 mg/mL | No |
| *Rx* **Granisetron HCl** | | |
| *Kytril* | **Tablets**: 1 mg | No |
| *Kytril* | **Injection**: 1 mg/mL (base) | No |
| *Rx* **Ondansetron HCl** | | |
| *Zofran* | **Tablets**:<br>4 mg, 8 mg, 24 mg (as HCl<br>dihydrate) | No |
| *Zofran ODT*[1] | **Tablets, orally disintegrating**:<br>4 mg, 8 mg (as base) | No |
| *Zofran* | **Solution, oral**: 4 mg/5 mL<br>(5 mg as HCl dihydrate) | No |
| *Zofran* | **Injection**: 2 mg/mL, 32 mg/<br>50 mL, 40 mg/20 mL (as HCl<br>dihydrate) | No |

[1] Contains phenylalanine.

## Type of Drug:

Antinauseants; antiemetics; drugs used to prevent nausea and vomiting.

## How the Drug Works:

Dolasetron, granisetron, and ondansetron are selective serotonin 5-HT$_3$ receptor antagonists that block serotonin stimulation to prevent nausea and vomiting.

## Uses:

*Oral doseforms* — To prevent nausea and vomiting associated with initial and repeat courses of emetogenic cancer chemotherapy.

*Oral dolasetron and ondansetron* — To prevent postoperative nausea and vomiting.

*Oral granisetron and ondansetron* — To prevent nausea and vomiting associated with radiotherapy in patients receiving either total body irradiation, single high-dose fraction, or daily fractions to the abdomen.

*Intravenous (IV; into a vein) dolasetron* — To prevent and treat postoperative nausea or vomiting.

*Unlabeled Use(s):* Dolasetron has been used to treat radiotherapy-induced nausea and vomiting. Granisetron has been used for acute nausea and vomiting following surgery. Ondansetron has been used in the treatment of nausea and vomiting associated with acetaminophen poisoning, acute levodopa-induced psychosis, and prostacyclin therapy; to reduce bulimic episodes in patients with bulimia nervosa; to treat patients with social anxiety disorder; and as treatment of spinal or epidural morphine-induced pruritis.

## Precautions:

*Do not use in the following situations:* Allergy to the 5-HT₃ receptor antagonist or any of its ingredients.

*Use with caution in the following situations:*

anthracycline therapy, cumulative high dose
antiarrythmic drug therapy, concurrent
atrioventricular block II to III (dolasetron only)
class I or III antiarrythmic agent use, concurrent (dolasetron only)
congenital QT syndrome
diuretic use with potential for inducing electrolyte abnormalities
hypokalemia
hypomagnesemia
prolonged QTc, marked (dolasetron only)

*Benzyl alcohol:* Some of these products contain benzyl alcohol, which has been associated with a fatal "gasping syndrome" in premature infants. Consult your doctor or pharmacist.

*Phenylketonuria:* Ondansetron orally-disintegrating tablets contain phenylalanine. Consult your doctor or pharmacist.

*Pregnancy:* There are no adequate and well-controlled studies in pregnant women. Use only if clearly needed and the potential benefits to the mother outweigh the possible hazards to the fetus.

*Breastfeeding:* Ondansetron appears in breast milk. It is not known if other 5-HT₃ receptor antagonists appear in breast milk. Consult your doctor before you begin breastfeeding.

*Children:* Safety and effectiveness for use of dolasetron and the injection form of granisetron in children younger than 2 years of age have not been established. Safety and effectiveness for use of the oral form of granisetron in children of any age have not been established. Safety and effectiveness for use of ondansetron in children 3 years of age and younger have not been established.

## Drug Interactions:

Tell your doctor or pharmacist if you are taking or if you are planning to take any over-the-counter or prescription medications or dietary supplements while taking a 5-HT₃ receptor antagonist. Doses of one or both drugs may need to be modified or a different drug may need to be prescribed. Rifamycins (eg, rifampin) interact with ondansetron. Antiarrythmic drugs interact with dolasetron.

## Side Effects:

Every drug is capable of producing side effects. Many 5-HT$_3$ receptor antagonist users experience no, or minor, side effects. The frequency and severity of side effects depend on many factors including dose, duration of therapy, and individual susceptibility. Possible side effects include:

*Digestive Tract:* Diarrhea; nausea; constipation; stomach pain; appetite loss; taste disorder; indigestion; dry mouth.

*Nervous System:* Headache; drowsiness; weakness; agitation; fatigue; anxiety; stimulation; sleeplessness; dizziness; flushing; shivers; chills; vertigo (feeling of whirling motion); agitation.

*Other:* Changes in blood pressure; fever; heart rhythm changes; hair loss; abnormal blood counts; muscle, joint, chest, or bone pain; general body discomfort; injection site reaction; cold sensation; rash; tremor; itching; urinary retention; tingling or prickling sensation; deficient oxygenation of the blood.

---

### Guidelines for Use:

- Dosage is individualized. Take exactly as prescribed.
- Do not change the dose or stop taking, unless advised by your doctor.
- *Ondansetron orally-disintegrating tablets* — Remove the tablets from the package just before taking. Peel backing off blister and remove tablet gently. Place tablet on the tongue and swallow with saliva. Tablets disintegrate rapidly on the tongue and do not require water for dissolution or swallowing.
- Contact your doctor immediately if you experience rash, itching, shortness of breath, abnormal heart rhythm, dizziness, fainting, low blood pressure, hives, facial swelling, or difficulty breathing.
- Dolasetron injection can be mixed in apple or apple-grape juice and given orally. The mixed product may be kept up to 2 hours at room temperature (59° to 86°F).
- Store at controlled room temperature (68° to 77°F). Protect from light. Do not freeze injection vials.

---

*If you have any questions, consult your doctor, pharmacist, or health care provider.*

| Generic Name / Brand Name Examples | Supplied As | Generic Available |
|---|---|---|
| Rx **Chlorpromazine**[1] | | |
| *Thorazine* | **Tablets:** 10 mg, 25 mg, 50 mg, 100 mg, 200 mg | Yes |
| *Thorazine Spansules* | **Capsules, sustained release:** 30 mg, 75 mg, 150 mg | No |
| *Thorazine* | **Syrup:** 10 mg/tsp | No |
| *Thorazine* | **Concentrate:** 30 mg/mL, 100 mg/mL | Yes |
| *Thorazine* | **Suppositories (as base):** 25 mg, 100 mg | No |
| Rx **Perphenazine**[1] | | |
| *Trilafon* | **Tablets:** 2 mg, 4 mg, 8 mg, 16 mg | No |
| *Trilafon*[2] | **Concentrate:** 16 mg/tsp | No |
| Rx **Prochlorperazine**[1] | | |
| *Compazine* | **Tablets:** 5 mg, 10 mg | Yes |
| *Compazine Spansules* | **Capsules, sustained release:** 10 mg, 15 mg | No |
| *Compazine* | **Syrup:** 5 mg/tsp | No |
| *Compazine* | **Suppositories:** 2.5 mg, 5 mg, 25 mg | No |
| Rx **Promethazine**[1] | | |
| *Phenergan* | **Tablets:** 12.5 mg, 25 mg, 50 mg | Yes |
| *Phenergan Plain*[2], *Phenergan Fortis*[2] | **Syrup:** 6.25 mg/tsp, 25 mg/tsp | Yes |
| *Phenergan* | **Suppositories:** 12.5 mg, 25 mg, 50 mg | Yes |
| Rx **Thiethylperazine**[1,3,4] | | |
| *Torecan*[3] | **Tablets:** 10 mg | No |
| Rx **Triflupromazine HCl** | | |
| *Vesprin*[2] | **Injection:** 10 mg/mL 20 mg/mL | No |

[1] Some of these products are also available as an injection.
[2] Contains alcohol.
[3] Contains the dye tartrazine.
[4] Contains sulfites.

## Type of Drug:

Drugs for nausea and vomiting.

## How the Drug Works:

Drug-induced vomiting (including drugs, radiation, metabolic disorders) is generally stimulated through the chemoreceptor trigger zone (CTZ), which in turn stimulates the vomiting center (VC) in the brain. Nausea from motion sickness is initiated by stimulation of a mechanism of the ear, which sends impulses to the CTZ. The VC may also be stimulated directly (by stomach irritation, motion sickness, etc).

These drugs act on the CTZ, VC, nerve pathways and other centers of the brain to reduce nausea and vomiting.

## Uses:

To control nausea and vomiting.

*Chlorpromazine, Perphenazine* – To relieve hiccups.

*Promethazine* – To treat and prevent motion sickness.

## Precautions:

*Do not use in the following situations:*

| | |
|---|---|
| allergy to these drugs | depression of CNS |
| blood disorders | liver disease |
| bone marrow depression | pregnancy (thiethylperazine |
| brain damage | only) |
| coma | sedative overdose |

*Use with caution in the following situations:*

| | |
|---|---|
| alcohol withdrawal | heart disease |
| asthma | hot weather |
| bladder obstruction | kidney disease |
| convulsive disorder, history of | liver disease |
| emphysema | respiratory impairment (due to |
| glaucoma | lung infections, acute) |

*Sensitivity to light:* Rare instances of skin pigmentation have occurred, primarily in females on long-term, high dose therapy. These changes, restricted to exposed areas of the skin, range from almost imperceptible darkening to a slate gray color, sometimes with a violet hue. Pigmentation may fade following drug discontinuation. These effects occur most commonly with chlorpromazine.

May cause photosensitivity. Avoid prolonged exposure to the sun and other ultraviolet light. Use sunscreens and wear protective clothing until tolerance is determined.

*Neuroleptic Malignant Syndrome* (NMS) is a potentially fatal syndrome associated with phenothiazines. Symptoms include: Increased body heat; muscle rigidity; altered mental abilities, including catatonia; irregular pulse and blood pressure; increased heart rate; sweating; and irregular heart rhythm.

*Tardive dyskinesia:* Involuntary and uncontrollable movements may develop in patients treated with phenothiazines. Occurrence is highest in the elderly, expecially women. The risk of developing these involuntary movements and the likelihood they will become permanent are increased with long-term use and with high doses. However, it is possible to develop these symptoms after short-term treatment at low doses. The syndrome is characterized by rhythmical involutary movements of tongue, face, mouth, or jaw (eg, protrusion of tongue, puffing of cheeks, puckering of mouth, chewing movements), sometimes accompanied by involuntary movements of the arms and legs. Fine worm-like movement of the tongue may be an early sign of the syndrome. If the medication is stopped at this time, the syndrome may not develop. There is no known treatment for established cases of tardive dyskinesia, although the syndrome may stop, partially or completely, if the drug is withdrawn.

*Pregnancy:* Safety for use during pregnancy has not been established. Use only when clearly needed and potential benefits outweigh the possible hazards to the fetus.

*Thiethylperazine* – Do not use during pregnancy. The risk of use in a pregnant woman clearly outweighs any possible benefit.

*Breastfeeding:* Chlorpromazine appears in breast milk. It is not known if other phenothiazines appear in breast milk. Consult your doctor before you begin breastfeeding.

*Children:* In general, these products are not recommended for children younger than 12 years of age. Children with acute illnesses (eg, chickenpox, CNS infections, stomach or intestinal irritation, measles) or dehydration appear much more susceptible to neuromuscular reactions than adults. Symptoms can occur and may be confused with the signs of an undiagnosed primary disease responsible for vomiting (eg, Reye syndrome). Avoid these agents in children and adolescents whose signs and symptoms suggest Reye syndrome.

*Prochlorperazine, promethazine* – Not recommended for children under 20 pounds or younger than 2 years of age. Not for use in pediatric surgery. Children seem more prone to develop reactions, even on moderate doses. Use the lowest effective dose. Occasionally, the patient may react to the drug with signs of restlessness and excitement; if this occurs, do not administer additional doses. Use with caution in children with acute illnesses or dehydration. Not for use in conditions for which children's dosages are not established.

*Elderly:* Low doses are usually sufficient for elderly patients. These patients are more susceptible to lowered blood pressure and other side effects. Doses should be increased gradually.

*Lab tests* may be required to monitor treatment. Be sure to keep appointments. Tests may include blood counts and kidney and liver function.

*Tartrazine:* Some of these products may contain the dye tartrazine (FD&C Yellow No. 5), which can cause allergic reactions in certain individuals. Check package label when available or consult your doctor or pharmacist.

*Sulfites:* Some of these products may contain sulfite preservatives, which can cause allergic reactions in certain individuals (eg, asthmatics). Check package label when available or consult your doctor or pharmacist.

## Drug Interactions:

Tell your doctor or pharmacist if you are taking or if you are planning to take any over-the-counter or prescription medications or dietary supplements with phenothiazines. Doses of one or both drugs may need to be modified or a different drug may need to be prescribed. The following drugs and drug classes interact with phenothiazines.

ACE inhibitors (eg, lisinopril)
alcohol
anorexiants (eg, methamphetamine)
anticholinergics (eg, benztropine)
anticoagulants, oral (eg, warfarin)
atropine
barbiturates (eg, phenobarbital)
beta-blockers (eg, propranolol)
biperiden (*Akineton*)
carbamazepine (eg, *Tegretol*)
charcoal
clidinium (*Quarzan*)

epinephrine (eg, *Adrenalin*)
guanethidine (eg, *Ismelin*)
levodopa (eg, *Larodopa*)
lithium (eg, *Eskalith*)
meperidine (eg, *Demerol*)
methyldopa (*Aldomet*)
metrizamide (*Amipaque*)
metyrosine *(Demser)*
morphine
orphenadrine (*Norflex*)
phenytoin (eg, *Dilantin*)
propranolol (*Inderal*)
trazodone (*Desyrel*)
tricyclic antidepressants (eg, amitriptyline)

## Side Effects:

Every drug is capable of producing side effects. Many phenothiazine users experience no, or minor, side effects. The frequency and severity of side effects depend on many factors including dose, duration of therapy and individual susceptibility. Possible side effects include:

*Liver:* Yellowing of skin and eyes (jaundice); abnormal liver function tests.

*Parkinson Disease-Like Symptoms:* Tremors; drooling; muscle rigidity/restlessness; unusual eye movements; shuffling walk.

*Muscular System:* Muscle spasms including neck and back muscles; abnormal eye movements; aching and numbness of legs and arms; discoloration; rounding of the tongue; tightness in throat; difficulty swallowing; involuntary movement of tongue, face, mouth or jaw (protrusion of tongue, puffing cheeks, puckering of mouth, chewing movements); weakness; muscular deformation; inability to sit still; fixed eyeballs; exaggerated reflexes; difficulty moving; clumsiness; slurred speech; involuntary movements of arms and legs; agitation; jitteriness.

*Circulatory System:* Changes in blood pressure; postural hypotension (lightheadedness when rising quickly from a sitting or lying position); ECG changes; cardiac arrest; rapid heartbeat; irregular heart rhythm; change in pulse rate.

*Psychiatric:* Catatonia; phobia; tiredness; restlessness; hyperactivity; confusion; nightmares; depression; excitement; bizarre dreams; sleeplessness.

*Nervous System:* Swelling of brain; headache; fatigue; drowsiness; paranoia; lethargy; convulsions; sedation; dizziness; faintness.

*Skin:* Hives; rash; swelling; redness; itching; sensitivity to light; skin pigmentation; pallor; flushing; sweating; oily skin.

*Urinary and Reproductive Tract:* Appearance of milk and breast engorgement and aching in women; breast enlargement in men; menstrual irregularities; changes in sex drive; changes in blood sugar levels; infertility and false pregnancy; inhibition of ejaculation.

*Eyes or Ocular:* Glaucoma; sensitivity to light; blurred vision; changes in pupil size; problems with lens, retina and cornea.

*Respiratory System:* Tightness of throat in muscular system; nasal congestion; difficulty breathing; asthma.

*Digestive Tract:* Changes in appetite; nausea; vomiting; constipation; diarrhea, stomach upset; sore throat.

*Other:* Abnormal blood counts; urinary retention; increased urination; painful erections; impotence (male); swollen glands; thirst; pink or reddish brown urine; dry mouth and nose; ringing in the ears; kidney failure, acute; fever; salivation; sugar in the urine; weight change; swelling of arms, legs and face; urinary retention; inability to control urination; angioneurotic edema; death; swelling of arms, hands and face.

## Guidelines for Use:

- *Brand interchange* — Do not change from one brand of this drug to another without consulting your pharmacist or doctor.
- Do not stop taking this medicine without checking with your doctor.
- Oral agents may be ineffective if expelled after vomiting has already begun. Use of suppositories or injection should be considered under such circumstances.
- Take these drugs routinely as directed. They control illness symptoms. They are not addicting.
- May cause drowsiness. Use caution while driving or performing other tasks requiring alertness, coordination, or dexterity.
- Avoid alcohol or other drugs that cause drowsiness.
- *Sensitivity to sunlight* — May cause photosensitivity (sensitivity to sunlight). Avoid prolonged exposure to the sun and other ultraviolet light. Use sunscreens and wear protective clothing until tolerance is determined.
- May discolor the urine pink or reddish-brown. This is not harmful.
- If dizziness or fainting occurs, avoid sudden changes in posture and use caution when climbing stairs, etc. (more common during first week of therapy).
- Use caution in hot weather. These drugs may increase susceptibility to heat stroke.
- Notify your doctor if sore throat, fever, unusual bleeding or bruising, skin rash, weakness, tremors, impaired vision, dark-colored urine, pale stools, jaundice, or involuntary muscle twitching occurs.
- May cause photosensitivity. Avoid prolonged exposure to the sun or other forms of ultraviolet (UV) light (eg, tanning beds). Use sunscreens and wear protective clothing until tolerance is determined.
- Lab tests may be required to monitor treatment. Be sure to keep appointments. Tests may include blood counts and kidney and liver function.

## Guidelines for Use (cont.):

- *Liquid concentrates* are light sensitive. They are usually dispensed in amber or opaque bottles and protected from light. These solutions are most conveniently administered by dilution in fruit juices or other liquids. Shake well. Use these solutions immediately after dilution.

- *Liquid concentrates* — Avoid contact with skin (contact dermatitis may occur). Store at room temperature (59° to 86°F). Protect from light.

- *Chlorpromazine* —
  *Concentrate:* Add desired dosage to 60 mL (2 oz) or more of liquid just prior to use. Suggested liquids are tomato or fruit juice, milk, sugar water, orange syrup, carbonated beverages, coffee, tea, or water. Semi-solid foods (soups, puddings, etc) may also be used. The concentrate is intended for institutional use only.
  *Sustained release capsules:* Do not crush or chew. Swallow whole.

- *Perphenazine* —*Concentrate:* Dilute only with water, saline, *Seven-Up,* homogenized milk, carbonated orange drink and pineapple, apricot, prune, orange, *V-8,* tomato, and grapefruit juices. Do NOT mix with beverages containing caffeine (coffee, cola), tannins (tea), or pectinates (apple juice). Use approximately 60 mL (2 oz) liquid for each 16 mg (5 mL or 1 tsp) concentrate. Store tablets and concentrate at controlled room temperature.

- All dosage forms should be stored between 59° and 77°F. Refrigerate promethazine suppositories between 36° and 46°F.

*If you have any questions, consult your doctor, pharmacist, or health care provider.*

| Generic Name<br>*Brand Name Examples* | Supplied As | Generic<br>Available |
|---|---|---|
| *otc* **Phosphorated Carbohydrate**<br>*Emetrol, Nausetrol* | **Solution:** Fructose, dextrose, and phosphoric acid | No |

## Type of Drug:

Drugs used for nausea and vomiting.

## How the Drug Works:

Carbohydrate solutions with phosphoric acid relieve nausea and vomiting by a direct local action on the wall of the digestive tract reducing stomach contractions.

## Uses:

For symptomatic relief of nausea and vomiting. Effectiveness has not been proven.

## Precautions:

*Do not use in the following situations:* allergy to the drug

*Use with caution in the following situations:*
 diabetes
 hereditary fructose intolerance

*Pregnancy:* Safety for use during pregnancy has not been established. Phosphorated carbohydrate solution has been used for morning sickness.

*Breastfeeding:* It is not known if these agents appear in breast milk. Consult your doctor before you begin breastfeeding.

## Drug Interactions:

Tell your doctor or pharmacist if you are taking or planning to take any over-the-counter or prescription medications or dietary supplements with phosphorated carbohydrate solution. Doses of one or both drugs may need to be modified or a different drug may need to be prescribed.

## Side Effects:

Every drug is capable of producing side effects. Many antiemetic/antivertigo agent users experience no, or minor, side effects. The frequency and severity of side effects depend on many factors including dose, duration of therapy and individual susceptibility. Possible side effects include stomach pain and diarrhea.

## Guidelines for Use:

- Use exactly as prescribed.
- Do not take for more than 1 hour without consulting your doctor.
- Nausea may signal a serious condition. If symptoms are not relieved or recur often, consult your doctor.
- *Diabetic patients* — Avoid phosphorated carbohydrate solutions because they contain significant amounts of sugar.
- *Phosphorated carbohydrate solutions* — Do not dilute. Do not take oral fluids immediately before the dose, or for at least 15 minutes after the dose.
- Store at room temperature (59° to 86°F).

*If you have any questions, consult your doctor, pharmacist, or health care provider.*

| Generic Name Brand Name Example | Supplied As | Generic Available |
|---|---|---|
| Rx **Midodrine HCl** *ProAmatine* | **Tablets:** 2.5 mg, 5 mg | No |

## Type of Drug:

Drugs used to elevate blood pressure.

## How the Drug Works:

Midodrine causes blood vessels to constrict (become smaller), resulting in an increase in blood pressure.

## Uses:

To treat symptoms of orthostatic hypotension (feeling dizzy or lightheaded when rising from a sitting or standing position, or feelings of dizziness while standing). Use only in patients whose lives are considerably impaired despite standard clinical care, such as support stockings, fluid expansion and lifestyle changes.

*Unlabeled Use(s):* To manage urinary incontinence.

## Precautions:

*Do not use in the following situations:*

heart disease, serious
high blood presure while lying down
hyperthyroidism
kidney disease, acute
pheochromocytoma (tumor of the adrenal gland)
urinary retention

*Use with caution in the following situations:*

diabetes
fludrocortisone acetate (*Florinef*) use
kidney disease
liver disease
vasoconstrive medications, use
visual problems, history

*Supine hypertension* is the most potentially serious side effect of midodrine. Supine (lying) and sitting blood pressures should be monitored. Supine hypertension can often be controlled by not lying totally flat (eg, sleeping with the head of the bed elevated).

*Pregnancy:* Adequate studies have not been done in pregnant women, or animal studies may have shown a risk to the fetus. Use only if clearly needed and potential benefits outweigh the possible hazards to the fetus.

*Breastfeeding:* It is not known if midodrine appears in breast milk. Consult your doctor before you begin breastfeeding.

*Children:* Safety and effectiveness are not established.

*Lab tests* will be required to monitor therapy. Lab tests may include blood pressure tests and kidney and liver function tests.

## Drug Interactions:

Tell your doctor or pharmacist if you are taking or planning to take any over-the-counter or prescription medications or dietary supplements while taking this medicine. Doses of one or both drugs may need to be modified or a different drug may need to be prescribed. The following drugs or drug classes may interact with this medicine.

alpha-adrenergic blockers (eg, doxazoxin)
cardiac glycosides (eg, digoxin)
cimetidine (eg, *Tagamet*)
dihydroergotamine (*D.H.E. 45*)
ephedrine
flecainide (*Tambocor*)
fludrocortisone acetate (*Florinef*)
metformin (*Glucophage*)
phenylephrine
phenylpropanolamine (eg, *Contac*)
procainamide (eg, *Pronestyl*)
pseudoephedrine (eg, *Sudafed*)
quinidine (eg, *Quinora*)
ranitidine (eg, *Zantac*)
triamterene (*Dyrenium*)

## Side Effects:

Every drug is capable of producing side effects. Many patients experience no, or minor, side effects. The frequency or severity of side effects depend on many factors including dose, duration of therapy and individual susceptibility. Possible side effects include:

*Nervous System:* Numbness or tingling in scalp, hands or feet; pain; headache; feeling of pressure/fullness in the head; facial flushing; confusion; abnormal thinking; nervousness; anxiety.

*Skin:* Goosebumps; itching; rash.

*Other:* Painful or difficult urination; high blood pressure while lying or sitting; chills; dry mouth.

## Guidelines for Use:

- Use exactly as prescribed.
- Usual dose is 10 mg, taken three times daily. Take during the daytime hours when you are upright and pursuing daily activities. A suggested dosing schedule of approximately 4 hour intervals is: Shortly before or upon arising in the morning, midday and late afternoon (not later than 6 pm). Doses may be taken in 3 hour intervals if required to control symptoms, but not more frequently. Do not take after the evening meal or less than 4 hours before bedtime.
- If a dose is missed, take it as soon as possible. If several hours have passed or if it is nearing time for the next dose, do not double the dose in order to "catch up" (unless advised to do so by your doctor). If more than one dose is missed or it is necessary to establish a new dosage schedule, contact your doctor or pharmacist.
- Supine (lying down) hypertension can often be controlled by not lying totally flat (eg, sleeping with the head of the bed elevated).
- Tell your doctor or pharmacist about any over-the-counter medications you are taking (eg, cold remedies, diet aids); they can increase the side effects of this medicine.
- Contact your doctor if you experience pounding in the ears, headache, blurred vision, slow pulse, increased dizziness, fainting, cardiac awareness, goosebumps, sensation of coldness or urinary retention.
- Continue taking this medicine, even if your symptoms of low blood pressure are controlled.
- Monitor blood pressure in both the lying and sitting positions.
- Lab tests may be required to monitor therapy. Be sure to keep appointments.
- Store at room temperature (59° to 77°F), out of the reach of children.

*If you have any questions, consult your doctor, pharmacist, or health care provider.*

| Generic Name<br>*Brand Name Examples* | Supplied As | Generic<br>Available |
|---|---|---|
| *C-IV* **Alprazolam** | | |
| *Xanax* | **Tablets:** 0.25 mg, 0.5 mg, 1 mg, 2 mg | No |
| *C-IV* **Chlordiazepoxide**[1] | | |
| *Librium, Mitran, Reposans,* | **Capsules:** 5 mg, 10 mg, 25 mg | Yes |
| *Libritabs* | **Tablets:** 5 mg, 10 mg, 25 mg | No |
| *C-IV* **Clonazepam** | | |
| *Klonopin* | **Tablets:** 0.5 mg, 1 mg, 2 mg | No |
| *C-IV* **Clorazepate Dipotassium** | **Capsules:** 3.75 mg, 7.5 mg, 15 mg | Yes |
| *Gen-Xene, Tranxene* | **Tablets:** 3.75 mg, 7.5 mg, 15 mg | Yes |
| *Tranxene-SD, Tranxene-SD Half Strength* | **Tablets, single dose:** 11.25 mg, 22.5 mg | No |
| *C-IV* **Diazepam**[1] | | |
| *Valium* | **Tablets:** 2 mg, 5 mg, 10 mg | Yes |
| *Valrelease* | **Capsules, sustained release:** 15 mg | No |
| *Diazepam, Diazepam Intensol* | **Oral solution:** 5 mg/tsp, 5 mg/mL | No |
| *C-IV* **Halazepam** | | |
| *Paxipam* | **Tablets:** 20 mg, 40 mg | No |
| *C-IV* **Lorazepam**[1] | | |
| *Ativan* | **Tablets:** 0.5 mg, 1 mg, 2 mg | Yes |
| *Lorazepam Intensol* | **Oral solution:** 2 mg/mL | No |
| *C-IV* **Oxazepam** | | |
| *Serax* | **Capsules:** 10 mg, 15 mg, 30 mg | Yes |
| *Serax*[2] | **Tablets:** 15 mg | Yes |
| *C-IV* **Prazepam** | | |
| *Centrax* | **Capsules:** 5 mg, 10 mg, 20 mg | Yes |
| *Centrax* | **Tablets:** 5 mg, 10 mg | Yes |

[1] Some of these products are also available as an injection.
[2] Contains the dye tartrazine.

## Type of Drug:

Agents to relieve nervousness and tension. Sometimes called "minor tranquilizers."

## How the Drug Works:

Benzodiazepines affect the brain to calm nervous tension while causing little drowsiness.

## Uses:

To treat anxiety disorders and for the short-term relief of the symptoms of anxiety. Anxiety or tension associated with the stress of everyday life does not usually require long-term treatment with an antianxiety agent.

*Alprazolam:* To treat panic disorder, with or without agoraphobia and anxiety associated with depression.

*Chlordiazepoxide:* For symptoms of alcohol withdrawal, preoperative apprehension and anxiety.

*Clorazepate:* For symptomatic relief of alcohol withdrawal. For management of seizures (with other drugs).

*Diazepam:* For symptoms of acute agitation, tremor or delirium tremens (DTs). For relief of muscle spasms. For preoperative anxiety (injection only) and with other drugs to help control convulsions.

*Lorazepam:* To treat anxiety associated with depression. For preoperative anxiety and sedation (injection only).

*Oxazepam:* To manage anxiety, tension, agitation and irritability in older patients. To treat anxiety associated with alcohol withdrawal or depression.

*Unlabeled Use(s):* Occasionally doctors may prescribe chlordiazepoxide, diazepam, clorazepate, lorazepam, oxazepam, prazepam or alprazolam for irritable bowel syndrome. Alprazolam and diazepam are occasionally used to treat panic attacks. Alprazolam is occasionally used to treat agoraphobia with social phobia, depression and premenstrual syndrome. Lorazepam is occasionally used to treat chronic insomnia. Lorazepam injection is occasionally used to treat seizures, chemotherapy-induced nausea and vomiting, acute alcohol withdrawal syndrome and psychogenic catatonia.

## Precautions:

*Do not use in the following situations:*

alcoholism, history
allergy to these drugs
children under 6 months, lactation (diazepam only)
drug addiction, history
glaucoma, narrow-angle

intra-arterial administration (lorazepam injection only)
liver disease, significant (clonazepamonly)
psychoses

*Use with caution in the following situations:*

| | |
|---|---|
| depression or other psychiatric disorders | kidney disease |
| | liver disease |
| elderly and very ill | lung disease (clonazepam only) |

*Dependence:* Prolonged use of benzodiazepines can lead to dependence. A withdrawal syndrome may occur after as little as 4 to 6 weeks of treatment. It is more likely if the drug is short-acting (eg, alprazolam), if it is taken regularly for longer than 3 months, if higher dosages are used and if it is abruptly discontinued.

Onset of withdrawal is within 1 to 10 days; it may last 5 days to a month or more. Symptoms may include: Increased anxiety, sleeplessness, irritability, nausea, headache, muscle tension/cramps, tremor, confusion, abnormal perception of movement, muscle twitching, psychosis and seizures.

Abrupt withdrawal of clonazepam, particularly in patients on long-term, high-dose therapy, may precipitate status epilepticus (a rapid series of convulsions without any periods of consciousness between them). While clonazepam is being gradually withdrawn, the substitution of another anticonvulsant may be indicated. Other symptoms include vomiting, diarrhea and sweating.

When discontinuing therapy, decrease dosage gradually over 4 to 8 weeks to avoid the possibility of withdrawal, especially in patients with a history of seizures, regardless of anticonvulsant drug therapy. Clonidine, propranolol and carbamazepine have been used to treat benzodiazepine withdrawal symptoms.

*Unusual reactions:* Excitement, stimulation and acute rage have been reported in psychiatric patients and hyperactive aggressive children. These reactions may be secondary to relief of anxiety and usually appear in the first 2 weeks of therapy. Acute hyperexcited states, anxiety, hallucinations, increased muscle spasms and sleep disturbances have been reported. Should these occur, consult your doctor. Anger, hostility and episodes of mania have been reported with alprazolam.

*Multiple seizure type:* When used in patients in whom several different types of seizure disorders coexist, clonazepam may increase the frequency or precipitate the onset of generalized tonic-clonic (grand mal) seizures. This may require the addition of other anticonvulsants or an increase in dosage.

*Diazepam:* If an increase in the frequency or severity of grand mal seizures occurs, your doctor may need to increase the dosage of standard anticonvulsant medication.

*Pregnancy:* Benzodiazepines cross the placenta. Studies have shown a potential effect on the fetus. Use only if clearly needed and potential benefits outweigh the possible hazards to the fetus.

*Breastfeeding:* Most benzodiazepines appear in breast milk. It is not known if lorazepam appears in breast milk. Do not use these drugs while breastfeeding.

*Children:* Give the smallest dose possible, as children may be more sensitive to benzodiazepines.

*Alprazolam, halazepam, prazepam* – Safety and effectiveness have not been established in children younger than 18.

*Chlordiazepoxide* – Not recommended for use in children younger than 6 (oral) or 12 (injection).

*Clorazepate* – Not recommended for use in children under 9.

*Diazepam* – Do not use in children younger than 6 months (oral). Safety and effectiveness have not been established in newborns (injection).

*Lorazepam* – Safety and effectiveness have not been established in children younger than 12 (oral). Do not use in children younger than 18 (injection).

*Elderly:* Give the smallest dose possible, as the elderly may be more sensitive to benzodiazepines.

*Lab tests* : Because of reports of abnormal blood counts and yellowing of the skin or eyes, blood counts, and liver function tests should be performed during long-term therapy.

*Tartrazine:* Some of these products may contain the dye tartrazine (FD&C Yellow No. 5) which can cause allergic reactions in certain individuals. Check package label when available and consult your doctor or pharmacist.

## Drug Interactions:

Tell your doctor or pharmacist if you are taking or planning to take any over-the-counter or prescription medications or dietary supplements with benzodiazepines. Doses of one or both drugs may need to be modified or a different drug may need to be prescribed. The following drugs and drug classes interact with benzodiazepines.

alcohol
antacids
barbiturates (eg, phenobarbital)
cimetidine (*Tagamet*)
contraceptives, oral (eg, *Ortho-Novum*)
digoxin (eg, *Lanoxin*)
disulfiram (eg, *Antabuse*)
fluoxetine *(Prozac)*
isoniazid (eg, *Laniazid*)
ketoconazole *(Nizoral)*
levodopa (eg, *Larodopa*)
metoprolol *(Lopressor)*
narcotic pain relievers (eg, codeine)
neuromuscular blocking agents
phenytoin (eg, *Dilantin*)
probenecid (eg, *Benemid*)
propoxyphene (eg, *Darvon*)
propranolol (eg, *Inderal*)
ranitidine *(Zantac)*
rifampin (eg, *Rifadin*)
scopolamine
theophylline (eg, *Theo-Dur*)
valproic acid (eg, *Depakene*)

## Side Effects:

Every drug is capable of producing side effects. Many benzodiazepine users experience no, or minor, side effects. The frequency and severity of side effects depend on many factors including dose, duration of therapy and individual susceptibility. Possible side effects include:

*Digestive Tract:* Stomach upset; constipation; diarrhea; nausea; change in appetite; vomiting.

*Nervous System:* Confusion; depression; nervousness; behavior changes; memory loss; drowsiness; fatigue; decreased activity; dizziness; vertigo (feeling of whirling motion); lethargy; apathy; euphoria (exaggerated sense of well being); restlessness; crying; delirium; disorientation; sleep disturbances; incoordination; vivid dreams; headache; seizures; weakness; unsteadiness.

*Circulatory System:* Changes in heart rate; changes in blood pressure; pounding in the chest (palpitations).

*Skin:* Hives; itching; rash; hair loss; excessive hair growth; yellowing of skin or eyes.

*Senses:* Visual disturbances; double vision; decreased hearing; hearing disturbances; nasal congestion; slurred speech; loss of voice.

*Urinary and Reproductive Tract:* Incontinence; changes in sex drive; urine retention; menstrual problems.

*Other:* Dry mouth; difficulty swallowing; hiccups; fever; balance problems; tremors and uncontrollable muscle movement; breathing problems; ankle and facial swelling; breast enlargement; production of breast milk; movement difficulties; "glassy-eyed" appearance; increased salivation; sore gums; coated tongue; fluid retention (edema); excessive perspiration; abnormal blood counts; abnormal liver function; joint pain; weight gain or loss; dehydration; swollen lymph nodes; fainting.

## Guidelines for Use:

- If a dose is missed, take it as soon as possible. If several hours have passed or if it is nearing time for the next dose, do not double the dose in order to "catch up" (unless advised to do so by your doctor). If more than one dose is missed, or it is necessary to establish a new dosage schedule, contact your doctor or pharmacist. Use exactly as prescribed.
- These drugs can be addictive if used in large doses or for a long time. Do not exceed prescribed dose. Discuss overuse with your doctor.
- Avoid alcohol or other drugs that cause drowsiness while taking these drugs.
- May cause drowsiness. Use caution while driving or performing other tasks requiring alertness.
- May be taken with food or water if stomach upset occurs.
- Patients on long-term or high dosage therapy may experience withdrawal symptoms on abrupt cessation of therapy. Do not discontinue therapy abruptly or change dosage except on advice of your doctor.
- Ingestion of antacids with diazepam and chlordiazepoxide may impair absorption of these drugs.
- *Clonazepam, clorazepate and diazepam*–Carry identification (Medic Alert) if these medications are being used for epilepsy.
- *Intensol solutions*– Mix with liquid or semi-solid food (eg, water, juice, applesauce, pudding).

*If you have any questions, consult your doctor, pharmacist, or health care provider.*

| Generic Name<br>*Brand Name Example* | Supplied As | Generic<br>Available |
|---|---|---|
| *Rx* **Buspirone HCl** | | |
| *BuSpar* | **Tablets:** 5 mg, 10 mg, 15 mg | No |

## Type of Drug:
Antianxiety agent; agent to relieve nervousness.

## How the Drug Works:
It is not known exactly how buspirone works to relieve anxiety. It is believed that it may react with specific chemical receptors in the brain.

## Uses:
For short-term relief of symptoms of anxiety.

To manage anxiety disorders.

*Unlabeled Use(s):* Occasionally doctors may prescribe buspirone for the symptoms of premenstrual syndrome.

## Precautions:
*Do not use in the following situations:*
allergy to buspirone or any of its ingredients
kidney disease, severe
liver disease, severe
MAOI use, concurrent

*Use with caution in the following situations:*
kidney disease
liver disease

*Improvement* in symptoms may occur within 7 to 10 days. Optimum results are generally achieved after 3 to 4 weeks of treatment.

*Withdrawal reactions:* Patients should be withdrawn from benzodiazepines and other sedative/hypnotic drugs gradually before starting buspirone, especially those who have been using these drugs for a long period of time. Withdrawal symptoms, including irritability, anxiety, agitation, sleeplessness, tremor, stomach cramps, muscle cramps, vomiting, sweating, flu-like symptoms without fever, and occasionally seizures, may occur.

*Pregnancy:* There are no adequate and well-controlled studies in pregnant women. Use this drug during pregnancy only if clearly needed and the potential benefits to the mother outweigh the possible risks to the fetus.

*Breastfeeding:* It is not known if buspirone appears in breast milk. Consult your doctor before you begin breastfeeding.

*Children:* Safety and effectiveness in children younger than 18 years of age have not been established.

## Drug Interactions:

Tell your doctor or pharmacist if you are taking or planning to take any over-the-counter or prescription medications or dietary supplements with buspirone. Doses of one or both drugs may need to be modified or a different drug may need to be prescribed. The following drugs and drug classes interact with buspirone:

alcohol
azole antifungals (eg, itracona-zole)
cimetidine (eg, *Tagamet*)
haloperidol (eg, *Haldol*)
MAOIs (eg, isocarboxazid, phenelzine, tranylcypromine)

macrolide antibiotics (eg, clarithromycin, erythro-mycin)
nefazodone (eg, *Serzone*)
rifamycins (eg, *Rifabutin*)
trazodone (eg, *Desyrel*)

## Side Effects:

Every drug is capable of producing side effects. Many buspirone users experience no, or minor, side effects. The frequency and severity of side effects depend on many factors including dose, duration of therapy, and individual susceptibility. Possible side effects include:

*Digestive Tract:* Nausea; stomach upset; diarrhea; constipation; vomiting; dry mouth.

*Nervous System:* Dizziness; headache; nervousness; lightheadedness; excitement; dream disturbances; drowsiness; fatigue; weakness; sleeplessness; decreased concentration; anger; confusion; depression; numbness; incoordination; tremor; hostility; tingling in hands or feet.

*Circulatory System:* Chest pain; increased heart rate; pounding in chest.

*Senses:* Ringing in the ears; sore throat; blurred vision; nasal congestion.

*Other:* Muscle aches or pains; abnormal skin sensations; sweating or clamminess; rash.

## Guidelines for Use:

- Dosage will be individualized according to specific patient needs.
- This medication is designed to be taken every day to prevent anxiety symptoms. It does not work if it is only taken "as needed" or only when anxiety symptoms are present.
- If a dose is missed, take it as soon as possible. If several hours have passed or if it is nearing time for the next dose, do not double the dose in order to catch up, unless advised to do so by your doctor. If more than one dose is missed, or it is necessary to establish a new dosage schedule, contact your doctor or pharmacist. Use exactly as pre-scribed.
- Inform your doctor if any restlessness or abnormal muscle movements occur (eg, motor restlessness, involuntary repetitive movements of facial or neck muscles).
- May cause drowsiness or dizziness. Use caution while driving or per-forming other tasks requiring alertness, coordination, and physical dex-terity.
- Inform your doctor of any prescription or nonprescription medications, alcohol, or drugs that you are taking, or plan to take, during buspirone treatment.
- Avoid alcohol and other depressant drugs while taking buspirone.
- Inform your doctor if you are pregnant, become pregnant, or are plan-ning to become pregnant while taking buspirone, or if you are breast-feeding.
- Some improvement in symptoms may be seen after 7 to 10 days, but optimum results may take 3 to 4 weeks to develop.
- Store at room temperature (below 86°F). Protect from light.

*If you have any questions, consult your doctor, pharmacist, or health care provider.*

| Generic Name<br>*Brand Name Examples* | Supplied As | Generic<br>Available |
|---|---|---|
| *Rx* **Hydroxyzine HCl** | | |
| *Atarax* | **Tablets:** 10 mg, 25 mg, 50 mg | Yes |
| *Atarax 100* | **Tablets:** 100 mg | No |
| *Atarax[1]* | **Syrup:** 10 mg/5 ml | Yes |
| *Hyzine 50* | **Injection:** 25 mg/mL, 50 mg/mL | Yes |
| *Rx* **Hydroxyzine Pamoate** | | |
| *Vistaril* | **Capsules:** 25 mg, 50 mg, 100 mg | Yes |
| *Vistaril* | **Oral suspension:** 25 mg/5 mL | No |
| *Vistaril* | **Injection:** 25 mg/mL, 50 mg/mL | Yes |

[1] Contains alcohol.

## Type of Drug:

Antihistamine and agent to relieve nervousness and anxiety.

## How the Drug Works:

Hydroxyzine decreases anxiety by suppressing activity in the anxiety centers in the brain. Antihistamine (anti-allergy), bronchodilator, analgesic, and antiemetic properties have also been demonstrated.

## Uses:

For short-term (4 months or less) relief of anxiety and tension.

To relieve itching due to allergic conditions (eg, hives, rash, insect bites).

For sedation prior to and following surgery.

*Injection* – To treat hysteria, alcohol withdrawal symptoms, or delirium tremens. To control vomiting and pain (with other drugs) before and after surgery or delivery. To control nausea and vomiting from causes other than pregnancy.

## Precautions:

*Do not use in the following situations:*
>        allergy to hydroxyzine or any of its ingredients
>        breastfeeding
>        pregnancy

*Pregnancy:* Do not use during pregnancy. The risk of use in a pregnant woman clearly outweighs any possible benefit.

*Breastfeeding:* It is not known if hydroxyzine appears in breast milk. Consult your doctor before you begin breastfeeding.

## Drug Interactions:

Tell your doctor or pharmacist if you are taking or planning to take any over-the-counter or prescription medications or dietary supplements with hydroxyzine. Doses of one or both drugs may need to be modified or a different drug may need to be prescribed. The following drugs and drug classes interact with hydroxyzine.

alcohol (eg, ethanol)
antihistamines (eg, diphenhydra-mine)

barbiturates (eg, phenobarbital)
narcotics (eg, morphine)

## Side Effects:

Every drug is capable of producing side effects. Many hydroxyzine users experience no, or minor, side effects. The frequency and severity of side effects depend on many factors including dose, duration of therapy, and individual susceptibility. Possible side effects include:

*Other:* Dry mouth; dizziness; involuntary movements.

### Guidelines for Use:

- Dosage will be adjusted according to individual patient response to therapy. Use exactly as prescribed.
- Shake oral suspension vigorously until product is completely resuspended.
- The injection form is only used when tablets, capsules, suspension, or syrup are unable to be taken by the patient.
- The injection form will be prepared and administered by your health care provider.
- Injection solution should be inspected before use. Injection solution should only be administered intramuscularly (IM).
- The effectiveness of hydroxyzine as an antianxiety agent for more than 4 months has not been assessed by clinical studies. Your doctor will reassess the usefulness of the drug periodically.
- If a dose is missed, take it as soon as possible. If several hours have passed or if it is nearing time for the next dose, do not double the dose to catch up, unless advised to do so by your doctor. If more than one dose is missed, or it is necessary to establish a new dosage schedule, contact your doctor or pharmacist.
- May cause drowsiness. Use caution while driving or performing other tasks requiring alertness, coordination, or physical dexterity.
- Avoid alcohol or other depressant drugs (eg, narcotics, tranquilizers, antihistamines) while taking hydroxyzine.
- Store tablets and capsules at room temperature (59° to 86°F). Keep tightly closed. Protect from moisture.
- Store oral suspension and syrup below 86°F. Keep tightly closed. Protect from freezing and light.
- Store injection solution at room temperature (59° to 86°F). Protect from light. Discard unused portion of single-dose vial.

*If you have any questions, consult your doctor, pharmacist, or health care provider.*

| Generic Name<br>*Brand Name Examples* | Supplied As | Generic<br>Available |
|---|---|---|
| *c-iv* **Meprobamate** | | |
| *Equanil, Miltown* | **Tablets:** 200 mg, 400 mg | Yes |

## Type of Drug:

Agent to relieve nervousness and tension.

## How the Drug Works:

Meprobamate works in the brain to relieve anxiety and tension.

## Uses:

To provide short-term relief of symptoms of anxiety.

To manage anxiety disorders.

Anxiety or tension associated with stress of everyday life usually does not require treatment with an antianxiety agent.

## Precautions:

*Do not use in the following situations:*
>        allergy to carisoprodol or related drugs
>        allergy to meprobamate or any of its ingredients
>        porphyria, acute or intermittent

*Use with caution in the following situations:*

| | |
|---|---|
| addiction, history of | liver disease |
| alcoholism | pregnancy |
| kidney disease | seizure disorder (eg, epilepsy) |
| lactation | suicidal tendencies |

*Drug dependence:* Physical and psychological dependence and abuse may occur. Symptoms of chronic intoxication from prolonged use of greater than recommended doses include incoordination, clumsiness, slurred speech, and veritgo (feeling of whirling motion). Avoid prolonged use. Abrupt discontinuation after prolonged and excessive use may cause a withdrawal syndrome characterized by anxiety, appetite loss, sleeplessness, vomiting, incoordination or clumsiness, tremors, muscle twitching, confusional states, hallucinations, and seizures. Onset of withdrawal symptoms usually begins within 12 to 48 hours after discontinuation of meprobamate and symptoms usually cease within the next 12 to 48 hours.

When excessive dosage has continued for weeks or months the dose should be reduced gradually over a period of 1 or 2 weeks rather than stopping abruptly. Alternatively, a short-acting barbiturate may be substituted, then gradually withdrawn.

*Pregnancy:* Studies have shown a potential effect to the fetus. Meprobamate passes the placental barrier and an increased risk of birth defects is associated with its use during the first trimester. Use during pregnancy should almost always be avoided. Use with extreme caution. Use only if clearly needed and potential benefits to the mother outweigh the possible hazards to the fetus.

*Breastfeeding:* Meprobamate appears in breast milk. Consult your doctor before you begin breastfeeding.

*Children:* Do not use in children younger than 6 years of age.

*Elderly:* To avoid oversedation, use lowest effective dose.

## Drug Interactions:

Tell your doctor or pharmacist if you are taking or planning to take any over-the-counter or prescription medications or dietary supplements with meprobamate. Doses of one or both drugs may need to be modified or a different drug may need to be prescribed. The following drugs and drug classes interact with meprobamate.

| | |
|---|---|
| alcohol | narcotic pain relievers |
| barbiturates (eg, phenobarbital) | (eg, codeine) |

## Side Effects:

Every drug is capable of producing side effects. Many meprobamate users experience no, or minor, side effects. The frequency and severity of side effects depend on many factors including dose, duration of therapy, and individual susceptibility. Possible side effects include:

*Allergic Reactions: Mild* — Rash (over the whole body or only the groin area); abnormal blood counts; purplish or brownish-red discoloration of the skin (either small pin-like or large bruise-like coloring); swelling; swollen glands; fever.
   *Severe (Rare)* — Fever; chills; fluid retention associated with discoloration and rash; difficulty breathing; decreased or lack of urination; skin inflammation; inflammation of the mouth and rectum.

*Digestive Tract:* Nausea; vomiting; diarrhea.

*Nervous System:* Drowsiness; dizziness; feeling of whirling motion; incoordination; headache; weakness; overstimulation; exaggerated sense of well being; paradoxical excitement.

*Circulatory System:* Fast or irregular heartbeat; pounding in chest; low blood pressure; fainting; abnormal heart rhythm.

*Skin:* Abnormal skin sensations (burning, prickling, tingling); itching.

*Other:* Slurred speech; fever; impaired vision or vision changes; shortness of breath.

## Guidelines for Use:

- Usual adult dosage is 1200 mg to 1600 mg/day in 3 or 4 divided doses. Doses greater than 2400 mg/day are not recommended. Usual dosage for children 6 to 12 years of age is 100 mg to 200 mg 2 to 3 times daily.
- Do not crush or chew tablets due to bitter taste.
- Physical and psychological dependence and abuse may occur.
- Do not suddenly stop taking this drug after long-term use. Consult your doctor.
- Long-term effectiveness (more than 4 months) of meprobamate has not been established. Your doctor will periodically reassess the usefulness of the drug.
- If a dose is missed, take it as soon as possible. If several hours have passed or if it is nearing time for the next dose, do not double the dose in order to catch up, unless advised to do so by your doctor. If more than one dose is missed, or it is necessary to establish a new dosage schedule, contact your doctor or pharmacist. Use exactly as pre-scribed.
- Inform your doctor if you are pregnant, become pregnant, are planning to become pregnant, or are breastfeeding.
- May cause drowsiness, dizziness, or blurred vision. Use caution while driving or performing other tasks requiring alertness, coordination, or physical dexterity.
- Discontinue use and notify your doctor immediately at first appearance of fever, sore throat, rash, or other signs of allergic reaction. In some instances, rash may be accompanied by more severe allergic reactions (see Side Effects). You may need to begin appropiate symptomatic therapy (eg, epinephrine, antihistamines, corticosteroids), which will be prescribed or administered by your doctor.
- Avoid alcohol and other mental depressants (eg, narcotics, tranquiliz-ers, antihistamines) while taking this medicine.
- Store at controlled room temperature (68° to 77°F). Keep tightly closed. Protect from moisture.

*If you have any questions, consult your doctor, pharmacist, or health care provider.*

| Generic Name<br>*Brand Name Examples* | Supplied As | Generic<br>Available |
|---|---|---|
| *Rx* **Bupropion HCl** | | |
| *Wellbutrin* | **Tablets:** 75 mg, 100 mg | Yes |
| *Wellbutrin SR* | **Tablets, sustained release:** 100 mg, 150 mg, 200 mg | No |

## Type of Drug:
Antidepressant; nonnicotine smoking deterrent.

## How the Drug Works:
It is not fully understood how bupropion improves depression symptoms (elevates mood). It is thought to increase the activity of certain chemicals in the brain (eg, dopamine, norepinephrine, serotonin) that help elevate mood.

## Uses:
To treat depression. Patients who use this drug for extended periods should be periodically reevaluated by their doctor.

Bupropion is also used as an aid to smoking cessation. See the Smoking Deterrents-Bupropion monograph in the Miscellaneous chapter.

*Unlabeled Use(s):* Occasionally doctors may prescribe bupropion for the treatment of attention deficit hyperactivity disorder and sustained-release bupropion for the treatment of neuropathic pain or to enhance weight loss.

## Precautions:
*Do not use in the following situations:*

abrupt discontinuation of alcohol or sedatives (benzodiazepines)
allergy to the drug or any of its ingredients
anorexia nervosa, active or history of
bulimia, active or history of
bupropion (eg, *Zyban*), current use for smoking cessation
monoamine oxidase inhibitor (MAOI) (eg, phenelzine) use, current or within 14 days
seizure disorders

*Use with caution in the following situations:*

alcohol use, excessive
attempted suicide, history of
bipolar manic depression
brain tumor
diabetes treated with oral hypoglycemics or insulin
drug abuse
head injury, history of
heart attack, recent
heart disease
kidney disease
liver disease
sedative (benzodiazepine) use, current
seizure, history or risk of
therapy that lowers seizure threshold (eg, antipsychotics, antidepressants, theophyllines, systemic steroids)

*Pregnancy:* There are no adequate and well-controlled studies in pregnant women. Use only if clearly needed and the potential benefits outweigh the possible risks to the fetus. Notify your doctor if you are pregnant or intend to become pregnant during therapy.

*Breastfeeding:* Bupropion is excreted in breast milk. Serious side effects could potentially occur in the nursing infant. Decide whether to discontinue the drug or discontinue breastfeeding, taking into account the importance of the drug to the mother. Consult your doctor before you begin breastfeeding.

*Children:* Safety and effectiveness have not been established in children younger than 18 years of age.

*Elderly:* Older patients are known to metabolize drugs more slowly and to be more sensitive to antidepressant drugs. Use the lowest effective dose.

## Drug Interactions:

Tell your doctor or pharmacist if you are taking or planning to take any over-the-counter or prescription medications or dietary supplements with this drug. Drug doses may need to be modified or a different drug prescribed. The following drugs and drug classes interact with this drug:

amantadine (eg, *Symmetrel*)
antidepressants (eg, fluoxetine,
 amitriptyline)
antipsychotics (eg, phenothiazines)
beta blockers (eg, metoprolol)
carbamazepine (eg, *Tegretol*)
cimetidine (eg, *Tagamet*)
corticosteroids, systemic
 (eg, prednisone)
levodopa (eg, *Sinemet*)

MAOIs (eg, phenelzine)
nicotine transdermal system
 (eg, *Nicoderm*)
phenobarbital (eg, *Solfoton*)
phenytoin (eg, *Dilantin*)
ritonavir (*Norvir*)
theophylline (eg, *Slo-Phyllin*)
type 1C antiarrythmics
 (eg, propafenone, flecainide)
warfarin (eg, *Coumadin*)

## Side Effects:

Every drug is capable of producing side effects. Many patients experience no, or minor, side effects. The frequency and severity of side effects depend on many factors including dose, duration of therapy, and individual susceptibility. Possible side effects include:

*Parkinson Disease-Like Symptoms:* Stumbling walk; movement disorders.

*Digestive Tract:* Nausea; vomiting; constipation; indigestion; appetite changes; stomach pain; dry mouth; mouth sores; diarrhea; difficulty swallowing; increased salivation.

*Nervous System:* Seizures; tremor; dizziness; delusions; hallucinations; exaggerated sense of well-being (euphoria); confusion; agitation; hostility; restlessness; anxiety; sedation; sleep disturbances; fatigue; headache; activation of psychosis or mania; sleeplessness; decreased memory; CNS stimulation; disturbed concentration; irritability; nervousness; sensory disturbance; drowsiness; depression; migraine headache; paranoia.

*Circulatory System:* Changes in heart rate and rhythm; changes in blood pressure; pounding in the chest (palpitations); chest pain; fainting.

*Skin:* Rash; itching; excessive sweating; flushing; hives; feeling of hot or cold skin.

*Other:* Taste changes; blurred vision; hearing problems; impotence; frequent urination; menstrual problems; fever; chills; weight changes; changes in sex drive; muscle or joint pain; weakness; abnormal skin sensations; urinary retention; muscle spasms; urinary tract infection; twitch; vaginal bleeding; increased cough; sore throat; upper respiratory complaints; vision problems; ringing in ears; infection; flu-like symptoms; hot flashes; facial swelling; sinus infection.

## Guidelines for Use:

- Read the patient information leaflet before starting therapy and each time you receive a refill.
- May be taken without regard to meals. Take with food if stomach upset occurs.
- This medicine should not be used in combination with *Zyban* or any other medication containing bupropion.
- Avoid or minimize alcohol consumption to reduce the risk of seizures.
- Do not take in combination with MAOIs or within 14 days of discontinuing treatment with an MAOI.
- The full antidepressant effects of bupropion may take 4 weeks or longer.
- May cause drowsiness. Use caution while driving or performing other tasks requiring alertness, coordination, or physical dexterity until tolerance is determined.
- Inform your doctor if you are pregnant, become pregnant, are planning to become pregnant, or are breastfeeding.

*Bupropion Tablets:*
- Do not crush or chew tablets. This can cause numbness of the mouth or throat.
- Do not take more than 450 mg bupropion daily. Single doses should not exceed 150 mg due to the risk of seizures.
- If a dose is missed, take it as soon as possible. If several hours have passed or it is less than 6 hours before your next dose, do not double the dose to catch up, unless instructed by your doctor. Never take more than 150 mg at one time. If more than one dose is missed or it is necessary to establish a new dosage schedule, contact your doctor or pharmacist.
- Store at 59° to 77°F. Protect from light and moisture.

*Bupropion Sustained-Release Tablets:*
- Do not crush, chew, or divide tablets. Tablets are designed to gradually release medication.
- Do not take more than 400 mg daily. Single doses should not exceed 200 mg due to the risk of seizures.
- If a dose is missed, take it as soon as possible. If several hours have passed or it is less than 8 hours before your next dose, do not double the dose to catch up, unless instructed by your doctor. Never take more than 200 mg at one time. If more than one dose is missed or it is necessary to establish a new dosage schedule, contact your doctor or pharmacist.
- Sustained-release bupropion has a characteristic odor; this is normal and no cause for concern.
- Store at 68° to 77°F.

*If you have any questions, consult your doctor, pharmacist, or health care provider.*

| Generic Name Brand Name Example | Supplied As | Generic Available |
|---|---|---|
| Rx **Nefazodone HCl** | | |
| *Serzone* | **Tablets:** 50 mg, 100 mg, 150 mg, 200 mg, 250 mg | No |

## Type of Drug:

Antidepressant; mood elevating agent.

## How the Drug Works:

The exact mechanism is unknown. Nefazodone appears to block the uptake of serotonin and norepinephrine (chemicals found in the brain). The effect may take a few weeks to be noticed.

## Uses:

To treat mental depression in patients 18 years of age and older.

*Unlabeled Use(s):* Occasionally, doctors may prescribe nefazodone for posttraumatic stress disorder (PTSD).

## Precautions:

*Do not use in the following situations:*

allergy to the drug or similar antidepressants (eg, trazodone)

MAOI (eg, phenelzine) use, current or within 14 days

*Use with caution in the following situations:*

alcohol use
benign prostatic hyperplasia (BPH)
bowel obstruction, history of
drug abuse, history of
elderly, especially females
glaucoma, narrow angle
heart attack, recent
heart disease, unstable
kidney disease
liver disease
low blood pressure
mania (psychological disturbance)
myocardial infarction, history of
seizures, history of
stroke, history of
suicide attempts, history of
urinary retention

*Liver abnormalities:* Life-threatening liver failure has been reported in patients taking nefazodone. Notify your doctor if you experience yellowing of the skin or eyes, appetite loss, or tiredness.

*Pregnancy:* There are no adequate and well-controlled studies in pregnant women. Use only if clearly needed and potential benefits outweigh the possible hazards to the fetus.

*Breastfeeding:* It is not known if nefazodone appears in breast milk. Consult your doctor before you begin breastfeeding.

*Children:* Safety and effectiveness in patients younger than 18 years of age have not been established.

*Elderly:* Lower initial doses are recommended for patients older than 65 years of age.

## Drug Interactions:

Tell your doctor or pharmacist if you are taking or planning to take any over-the-counter or prescription medications while taking this drug. Doses of one or both drugs may need to be modified or a different drug may need to be prescribed. The following drugs and drug classes interact with this drug:

alcohol
anesthetics, general
benzodiazepines
 (eg, alprazolam)
buspirone (eg, *BuSpar*)
carbamazepine (eg, *Tegretol*)
cyclosporine (eg, *Sandimmune*)
digoxin (eg, *Lanoxin*)
haloperidol (eg, *Haldol*)

MAOIs (eg, phenelzine)
pimozide (eg, *Orap*)
propranolol (eg, *Inderal*)
serotonin 5-HT$_1$ receptor agonists (eg, sumatriptan)
SSRIs (eg, fluoxetine)
tacrolimus (eg, *Prograf*)
triazolam (eg, *Halcion*)

## Side Effects:

Every drug is capable of producing side effects. Many patients experience no, or minor, side effects. The frequency and severity of side effects depend on many factors including dose, duration of therapy, and individual susceptibility. Possible side effects include:

*Digestive Tract:* Nausea; constipation; indigestion; diarrhea; appetite changes; vomiting; stomach pain; gas; dry mouth.

*Nervous System:* Dizziness; sleeplessness; weakness; drowsiness; light-headedness; confusion; headache; memory loss; incoordination; tremor; anxiety; unstable emotions; depression; abnormal dreams; decreased concentration; migraine; agitation.

*Circulatory System:* Low blood pressure; chest pain; pounding in the chest (palpitations); slow heartbeat.

*Respiratory System:* Cough; runny nose; difficulty breathing; sinus infection; bronchitis; sore throat.

*Skin:* Itching; rash; abnormal skin sensations; flushing; sweating; increased sensitivity to touch.

*Urinary and Reproductive Tract:* Prolonged or inappropriate erections; decreased sexual drive; changes in urinary frequency; breast pain; painful menstruation; impotence; painful urination.

*Other:* Eye pain; flu syndrome; chills; fever; stiff neck; swelling in the arms and legs; joint, muscle, back, or neck pain; ringing in the ears; abnormal taste sensations; weight gain; swelling; cramping; blurred or abnormal vision; thirst.

## Guidelines for Use:

- Dosage is individualized. Take exactly as prescribed.
- Take in 2 divided doses on an empty stomach, or as directed by your doctor.
- Do not stop taking or change the dose unless instructed by your doctor.
- Notify your doctor immediately if you develop a rash, hives, or other type of allergic reaction.
- If a dose is missed, take it as soon as possible. If several hours have passed or it is nearing time for the next dose, do not double the dose to catch up, unless instructed by your doctor. If more than one dose is missed, or it is necessary to establish a new dosage schedule, contact your doctor or pharmacist.
- Do not use in combination with MAOIs (eg, phenelzine) or within 14 days of discontinuing treatment with an MAOI. After stopping this medicine, wait at least 1 week before starting an MAOI.
- May impair judgment, thinking, or motor skills. Use caution while driving or performing other tasks requiring alertness, coordination, or physical dexterity until tolerance is determined.
- Inform your doctor if you are pregnant, become pregnant, are planning to become pregnant, or are breastfeeding.
- Avoid alcohol while using this medicine.
- Improvement may not be seen for several weeks. Exams may be necessary. Be sure to keep appointments.
- Store at room temperature (59° to 86°F) in a dry place.

*If you have any questions, consult your doctor, pharmacist, or health care provider.*

| Generic Name<br>*Brand Name Example* | Supplied As | Generic<br>Available |
|---|---|---|
| *Rx* **Escitalopram Oxalate** | | |
| *Lexapro* | **Tablet**: 5 mg, 10 mg, 20 mg | No |
| *Lexapro* | **Solution, oral**: 5 mg/5 mL | No |

## Type of Drug:
Selective serotonin reuptake inhibitor (SSRI).

## How the Drug Works:
Escitalopram blocks the reuptake of serotonin, a chemical found in the brain, increasing the activity of this chemical and resulting in an improved mood.

## Uses:
To treat major depressive disorder.

## Precautions:
*Do not use in the following situations:*

allergy to the drug, its isomer (citalopram), or any of its ingredients
MAOI (eg, phenelzine) use, current or within 14 days
other SSRI (eg, fluoxetine) use, current

*Use with caution in the following situations:*

heart disease, unstable
kidney disease, history of
liver disease
low sodium ions in the blood
 (hyponatremia)

mania, history of
myocardial infarction, recent
seizure, history of

*Pregnancy:* There are no adequate and well-controlled studies in pregnant women. Use only if clearly needed and potential benefits outweigh the possible risks to the fetus.

*Breastfeeding:* Escitalopram is excreted in breast milk. Consult your doctor before you begin breastfeeding.

*Children:* Safety and effectiveness have not been established.

*Elderly:* Dosage may need to be adjusted because of possible increased sensitivity to the drug.

## Drug Interactions:
Tell your doctor or pharmacist if you are taking or planning to take any over-the-counter or prescription medications or dietary supplements with this drug. Drug doses may need to be modified or a different drug prescribed. The following drugs and drug classes interact with this drug:

alcohol
carbamazepine (eg, *Tegretol*)
cimetidine (eg, *Tagamet*)
CNS drugs (eg, lorazepam,
 codeine)

desipramine (eg, *Norpramin*)
lithium (eg, *Eskalith*)
MAOIs (eg, phenelzine)
other SSRIs (eg, fluoxetine)
sumatriptan (*Imitrex*)

## Side Effects:

Every drug is capable of producing side effects. Many patients experience no, or minor, side effects. The frequency and severity of side effects depend on many factors, including dose, duration of therapy, and individual susceptibility. Possible side effects include:

*Digestive Tract:* Nausea; diarrhea; constipation; dry mouth; upset stomach; stomach pain; decreased appetite.

*Nervous System:* Dizziness; sleeplessness; sleepiness.

*Respiratory System:* Sinus infection; runny nose.

*Urinary and Reproductive Tract:* Impotence; decreased sex drive; inability to achieve orgasm; ejaculation disorder (primarily a delay in ejaculation).

*Other:* Excessive sweating; fatigue; flu-like symptoms.

---

### Guidelines for Use:

- Dosage is individualized. Take exactly as prescribed.
- Do not stop taking or change the dose, unless instructed by your doctor.
- Take once daily, in the morning or evening, with or without food.
- If a dose is missed, take it as soon as possible. If several hours have passed or it is nearing time for the next dose, do not double the dose to catch up, unless instructed by your doctor. If more than one dose is missed or it is necessary to establish a new dosage schedule, contact your doctor or pharmacist.
- It may take 1 to 4 weeks of daily therapy before improvement is noticed.
- Do not use in combination with MAOIs or within 14 days of discontinuing treatment with an MAOI. After stopping this medicine, wait at least 2 weeks before starting an MAOI.
- May impair judgment, thinking, or motor skills. Use caution while driving or performing other tasks requiring alertness, coordination, or physical dexterity until tolerance is determined.
- Inform your doctor if you are pregnant, become pregnant, are planning to become pregnant, or are breastfeeding.
- Avoid alcohol while using this medicine.
- Store at room temperature (77°F).

---

*If you have any questions, consult your doctor, pharmacist, or health care provider.*

| Generic Name<br>*Brand Name Examples* | Supplied As | Generic<br>Available |
|---|---|---|
| *Rx* **Fluoxetine HCl** | | |
| *Prozac* | **Tablets**: 10 mg | No |
| *Prozac* | **Pulvules**: 10 mg, 20 mg, 40 mg | No |
| *Prozac Weekly* | **Capsules, delayed-release**: 90 mg | No |
| *Sarafem* | **Pulvules**: 10 mg, 20 mg | No |
| *Prozac* | **Oral solution**: 20 mg/5 mL[1] | Yes |

[1] Contains alcohol.

## Type of Drug:
Antidepressant; mood elevating agent.

## How the Drug Works:
The exact mechanism is not known. It is believed that fluoxetine adjusts or balances how the brain and nervous system produce and respond to their own natural chemicals (called neurotransmitters). Fluoxetine appears to inhibit CNS neuronal uptake of serotonin by the brain. The effect may take a few weeks to be noticed.

## Uses:
*Prozac:* For the treatment of mental depression, bulimia nervosa, and obsessive-compulsive disorder (OCD) in adults.

*Sarafem:* For the treatment of premenstrual dysphoric disorder (PMDD) in women.

*Unlabeled Use(s):* Occasionally doctors may prescribe fluoxetine to treat alcoholism, anorexia nervosa, attention-deficit hyperactivity disorder (ADHD), and a wide variety of other mental and physical disorders.

## Precautions:
*Do not use in the following situations:*
> allergy to fluoxetine or any of its ingredients
> MAOI use, within 14 days
> thioridazine use, within 5 weeks

*Use with caution in the following situations:*
> anxiety
> diabetes
> drug abuse, history of
> electroshock therapy
> heart attack, recent
> heart disease, unstable
> insomnia
> kidney disease
> liver disease
> mania/hypomania (psychological disturbances)
> seizures, history of
> suicide ideation or attempt, history of
> weight and appetite, changes in

*Diabetes:* Decreased blood sugar (glucose) levels (hypoglycemia) have occurred during therapy, and increased blood sugar levels (hyperglycemia) have developed following discontinuation of the drug. The dosage of insulin or the blood glucose-lowering drug may need to be adjusted when fluoxetine is started or discontinued.

*Rash and Possible Allergic Events:* Approximately 7% of patients have developed a rash or hives. Almost one-third were withdrawn from treatment. Most patients improved promptly with discontinuation of fluoxetine or with treatment with antihistamines or steroids.

*Suicidal Tendencies:* Data from clinical trial studies have failed to show an increased rate or risk of suicide among patients taking fluoxetine. Because suicide may be a complication of unresponsive depression or OCD, any suicidal thoughts or tendencies should be reported to your doctor.

*Pregnancy:* Studies in pregnant women have not shown a risk to the fetus. However, the drug should not be used during pregnancy unless clearly needed and the potential benefits to the mother outweigh the possible hazards to the fetus.

*Breastfeeding:* Fluoxetine appears in breast milk. Use of fluoxetine in nursing mothers is not recommended. Consult your doctor before you begin breastfeeding.

*Children:* Safety and effectiveness in children have not been established.

*Elderly:* Fluoxetine has not been sufficiently evaluated in older patients; however, several hundred elderly patients have participated in clinical studies and no unusual adverse age-related problems have been identified.

## Drug Interactions:
Tell your doctor or pharmacist if you are taking or if you are planning to take any over-the-counter or prescription medications or dietary supplements while taking fluoxetine. Doses of one or both drugs may need to be modified or a different drug may need to be prescribed. The following drugs and drug classes interact with fluoxetine:

antidepressants (eg, doxepin)
benzodiazepines (eg, diazepam)
carbamazepine (eg, *Tegretol*)
clozapine (eg, *Clozaril*)
cyproheptadine (eg, *Periactin*)
dextromethorphan HBr
 (eg, *Drixoral*)
haloperidol (eg, *Haldol*)

hydantoins (eg, phenytoin)
lithium (eg, *Eskalith*)
MAOIs (eg, phenelzine)
sumatriptan (eg, *Imitrex*)
thioridazine (eg, *Mellaril*)
tryptophan
warfarin (eg, *Coumadin)*

## Side Effects:

Every drug is capable of producing side effects. Many fluoxetine users experience no, or minor, side effects. The frequency and severity of side effects depend on many factors including dose, duration of therapy, and individual susceptibility. Possible side effects include:

*Digestive Tract:* Stomach upset; indigestion; vomiting; nausea; appetite changes; diarrhea; constipation; gas; dark, bloody stools or vomit; dry mouth.

*Nervous System:* Tremors; anxiety; nervousness; dizziness; lightheadedness; drowsiness; headache; sleeplessness; fatigue; weakness; decreased concentration; sensation disturbances; abnormal dreams or thinking; memory loss; confusion; psychological disturbances; agitation; twitching.

*Circulatory System:* Palpitations (pounding in the chest); chest pain; hot flashes; flushing.

*Respiratory System:* Flu-like syndrome; nasal congestion; sinus headache; sinus infection; cough; yawn; painful or difficult breathing.

*Skin:* Rash; hives; itching; sweating; acne.

*Urinary and Reproductive Tract:* Painful menstruation; sexual dysfunction; impotence; changes in sex drive; frequent urination; urinary tract infections.

   *Rash and Accompanying Events* – Fever; edema (fluid retention); carpal tunnel syndrome; respiratory distress; joint pain; protein in urine; abnormal blood counts; swollen lymph nodes; abnormal enzyme levels.

*Other:* Fever; back, leg, arm, or muscle pain; vision disturbances; taste changes; ringing in the ears; chills; muscle cramps; viral infections; weight changes; accidental injury.

## Guidelines for Use:

- Dosage is individualized. Take exactly as prescribed.
- Because this medicine may cause sleeplessness when taken in the evening, take doses as early as possible in the day. Single doses should be taken in the morning. Twice daily doses should be taken in the morning and at noon.
- May be taken with or without food.
- Do not crush, chew, or open delayed-release capsules. Swallow whole.
- If a dose is missed, take it as soon as possible. If several hours have passed or if it is nearing time for the next dose, do not double the dose to catch up unless advised by your doctor. If more than one dose is missed, or it is necessary to establish a new dosage schedule, contact your doctor or pharmacist.
- *Diabetes* — Monitor blood glucose levels daily. Notify your doctor if low blood sugar (fatigue, excessive hunger, profuse sweating, numbness of extremities) occurs, or if excessive thirst, excessive urination, or other symptoms of high blood sugar levels occur (glucose or ketones in the urine or blood).
- Do not use in combination with MAOIs or within 14 days of discontinuing treatment with an MAOI. After stopping fluoxetine, wait at least 5 weeks before starting an MAOI.
- Use with caution in individuals with a history of attempted suicide or suicidal thoughts.
- Avoid using alcohol or other depressants (eg, pain relievers, sedatives, antihistamines) that may cause drowsiness or other side effects.
- May cause drowsiness, dizziness, or impaired judgment. Use caution while driving or performing other tasks requiring alertness, coordination, or physical dexterity.
- Consult your doctor or pharmacist before taking nonprescription or prescription drugs or dietary supplements.
- Notify your doctor if you are pregnant or intend to become pregnant, or if you are breastfeeding.
- Notify your doctor if rash or hives develop, if anxiety or nervousness become troublesome, or if extreme appetite loss develops (especially in underweight patients).
- Improvement may not be seen for several days to a few weeks.
- Store at room temperature (59° to 86°F). Protect from light.

*If you have any questions, consult your doctor, pharmacist, or health care provider.*

| Generic Name
Brand Name Example | Supplied As | Generic Available |
|---|---|---|
| Rx **Fluvoxamine Maleate** | | |
| Luvox | **Tablets**: 25 mg, 50 mg, 100 mg | Yes |

## Type of Drug:

Antidepressant; mood elevating agent.

## How the Drug Works:

It is believed that fluvoxamine maleate adjusts or balances how the brain and nervous system produce and respond to their natural chemicals (called neurotransmitters). Fluvoxamine maleate inhibits the reuptake of serotonin by the brain.

## Uses:

For the treatment of obsessions and compulsions in patients with obsessive-compulsive disorder (OCD).

## Precautions:

*Do not use in the following situations:*

allergy to fluvoxamine or any of its ingredients
MAOI use (eg, phenelzine), within 14 days
pimozide use, concurrent
thioridazine use, concurrent

*Use with caution in the following situations:*

attempted suicide, history of
benzodiazepine (eg, alprazolam) use, concurrent
elderly
liver disease
mania/hypomania, history of
seizures, history of

*Smoking:* This medicine may not be as effective if you are a smoker.

*Pregnancy:* There are no adequate and well-controlled studies in pregnant women. Use only if clearly needed and the potential benefits to the mother outweigh the possible hazards to the fetus.

*Breastfeeding:* Fluvoxamine appears in breast milk. Consult your doctor before you begin breastfeeding.

*Children:* Safety and effectiveness are not established in children younger than 8 years of age.

*Elderly:* Use lower initial doses; then increase gradually if necessary.

## Drug Interactions:

Tell your doctor or pharmacist if you are taking or if you are planning to take any over-the-counter or prescription medications or dietary supplements while taking fluvoxamine. Doses of one or both drugs may need to be modified or a different drug may need to be prescribed. The following drugs and drug classes interact with fluvoxamine:

benzodiazepines
 (eg, alprazolam)
carbamazapine (eg, *Tegretol*)
clozapine (eg, *Clozaril*)
diltiazem (eg, *Cardizem*)
lithium (eg, *Lithobid*)
methadone (eg, *Dolophine*)
MAOIs (eg, phenelzine)
phenytoin (eg, *Dilantin*)
pimozide (*Orap*)

propranolol (eg, *Inderal*)
quinidine (eg, *Quinora*)
sumatriptan (*Imitrex*)
tacrine (*Cognex*)
theophylline (eg, *Theo-Dur*)
thioridazine (eg, *Mellaril*)
tricyclic antidepressants
 (eg, amitriptyline)
tryptophan
warfarin (eg, *Coumadin*)

## Side Effects:

Every drug is capable of producing side effects. Many fluvoxamine users experience no, or minor, side effects. The frequency and severity of side effects depend on many factors including dose, duration of therapy, and individual susceptibility. Possible side effects include:

*Digestive Tract:* Nausea; vomiting; constipation; indigestion; diarrhea; stomach pain; appetite loss; gas; dry mouth; difficulty swallowing; tooth disorder; sore throat.

*Nervous System:* Headache; memory loss; apathy; twitching; sleeplessness; nervousness; agitation; anxiety; dizziness; drowsiness; depression; weakness; tremors; mania; unstable emotions; CNS stimulation; abnormal thinking; psychotic reaction.

*Circulatory System:* Rapid heart beat; changes in blood pressure; fainting; flushing; palpitations (pounding in the chest).

*Respiratory System:* Nasal congestion; yawn; difficulty breathing; cough; sinus problems; upper respiratory tract infection.

*Other:* Sweating; taste changes; vision problems; frequent urination; decreased sex drive; inability to achieve orgasm; abnormal ejaculation; painful menstruation; muscular hyperactivity; infection; leg cramps; rash; muscle tension; urinary retention; muscle pain; unusual bruising; nosebleed; abnormal liver enzymes; decreased mobility or movement; general body discomfort; flu-like syndrome; weight changes; chills; swelling of feet, ankles, or hands.

## Guidelines for Use:

- Dosage is individualized. Take exactly as prescribed.
- Usual adult starting dose is 50 mg, taken as a single dose at bedtime. The dosage may be increased by 50 mg/day every 4 to 7 days, if necessary, to achieve maximum benefit. The total dosage should not exceed 300 mg/day. Total doses greater than 100 mg should be taken in 2 divided doses. If the doses are not equal, the larger dose should be taken at bedtime.
- Usual pediatric (8 to 17 years of age) starting dose is 25 mg at bedtime. The dosage may be increased by 25 mg/day every 4 to 7 days, if necessary, to achieve maximum benefit. The total dosage should not exceed 200 mg/day. Total doses greater than 50 mg should be taken in 2 divided doses. If the doses are not equal, the larger dose should be given at bedtime.
- Do not discontinue the medication or change the dose unless directed by your doctor.
- May be taken without regard to food.
- If a dose is missed, take it as soon as possible. If several hours have passed or if it is nearing time for the next dose, do not double the dose to catch up, unless advised by your doctor. If more than one dose is missed or it is necessary to establish a new dosage schedule, contact your doctor or pharmacist.
- Contact your doctor if you develop a rash, hives, other allergic reactions, or seizures. Also contact your doctor if nausea, dry mouth, sleeplessness, or drowsiness become troublesome.
- May cause drowsiness, dizziness, or impaired judgement. Use caution while driving or performing other tasks requiring alertness, coordination, or physical dexterity.
- Do not use in combination with MAOIs or within 14 days of discontinuing treatment with an MAOI. After stopping treatment with this medication, wait at least 2 weeks before starting an MAOI.
- Avoid alcohol and smoking while using this medication. Smoking may reduce the effectiveness of the medication.
- Inform your doctor if you are pregnant, become pregnant, are planning to become pregnant, or if you are breastfeeding.
- Store at controlled room temperature (59° to 86°F) in a tightly closed container. Protect from moisture.

*If you have any questions, consult your doctor, pharmacist, or health care provider.*

| Generic Name<br>*Brand Name Example* | Supplied As | Generic<br>Available |
|---|---|---|
| Rx **Citalopram Hydrobromide** | | |
| *Celexa* | **Tablets:** 20 mg, 40 mg | No |

## Type of Drug:
Antidepressant; mood-elevating agent.

## How the Drug Works:
Citalopram blocks the uptake of a chemical found in the brain (serotonin) which increases the activity of this chemical, resulting in improved mood.

## Uses:
To treat depression.

## Precautions:
*Do not use in the following situations:*
>
> allergy to citalopram or any of its ingredients
> monoamine oxidase inhibitor (MAOI) use, concurrent or within 14 days

*Use with caution in the following situations:*

| | |
|---|---|
| alcohol use | liver disease |
| diseases that produce altered metabolic or hemodynamic responses (eg, congestive heart failure) | mania, history |
| | seizure disorder, history |
| | sodium levels, low |
| kidney disease, severe | suicidal tendencies |

*Pregnancy:* Adequate studies have not been done in pregnant women. Use only if clearly needed and potential benefits outweigh the possible hazards to the fetus.

*Breastfeeding:* Citalopram appears in breast milk. A decision should be made whether to discontinue nursing or discontinue the drug, taking into account the risks to the infant of citalopram exposure (eg, excessive drowsiness, decreased feeding, weight loss) and the importance of the drug to the mother. Consult your doctor before you begin breastfeeding.

*Children:* Safety and effectiveness in children have not been established.

*Elderly:* Older individuals may be more sensitive to the effects of citalopram than younger individuals. The recommended dose for most elderly patients is 20 mg/day with titration to 40 mg/day only for nonresponding patients.

## Drug Interactions:

Tell your doctor if you are taking or are planning to take any over-the-counter or prescription medications while taking citalopram. Doses of one or both drugs may need to be modified or a different drug may need to be prescribed. The following drugs and drug classes interact with citalopram:

alcohol
carbamazepine (eg, *Tegretol*)
cimetidine (eg, *Tagamet*)
CNS drugs (eg, antidepressants)
CYP2C19 inhibitors (eg, omeprazole)
CYP3A4 inhibitors (eg, ketoconazole, erythromycin)

imipramine (eg, *Tofranil*)
lithium (eg, *Lithobid*)
metoprolol (eg, *Lopressor*)
monoamine oxidase inhibitors (MAOIs) (eg, phenelzine)
tricyclic antidepressants (eg, amitriptyline)

## Side Effects:

Every drug is capable of producing side effects. Many citalopram users experience no, or minor, side effects. The frequency and severity of side effects depend on many factors including dose, duration of therapy, and individual susceptibility. Possible side effects include:

*Digestive Tract:* Nausea; dry mouth; vomiting; diarrhea; indigestion; stomach pain; gas; increased salivation; appetite changes.

*Nervous System:* Dizziness; sleeplessness; drowsiness; agitation; tremor; fatigue; weakness; anxiety; impaired concentration; amnesia; apathy; worsening of depression; suicide attempt; confusion; headache.

*Circulatory System:* Decreased heart rate; fast heartbeat; postural (standing) low blood pressure; low blood pressure.

*Respiratory System:* Upper respiratory tract infection; runny nose; sinus infection; coughing.

*Urinary and Reproductive Tract:* Painful menstruation; absence of menstruation; excessive urination; ejaculation disorder; decreased sex drive; impotence.

*Other:* Rash; itching; increased sweating; fever; abnormal skin sensations (eg, burning, prickling, tingling); joint or muscle pain; yawning; weight changes; taste pereception changes.

## Guidelines for Use:

- Dosage is individualized. Take exactly as prescribed.
- Do not stop taking or change the dose unless directed by your doctor.
- Usual adult starting dose is 20 mg/day as a single dose. If necessary, dose may be increased to 40 mg/day after at least 1 week.
- Take once daily, in the morning or evening, with or without food.
- For most elderly patients and patients with liver disease, 20 mg/day is the recommended dose, with titration to 40 mg/day only for nonresponding patients.
- If a dose is missed, inhale it as soon as possible. If several hours have passed or it is nearing time for the next dose, do not double the dose to catch up, unless directed by your doctor. If more than one dose is missed or if it is necessary to establish a new dosage schedule, contact your doctor or pharmacist.
- Contact your doctor if you experience suicidal thoughts, sexual problems, appetite loss, nausea, vomiting, weight gain, restlessness, irritability, confusion, or excessive urination.
- Citalopram should not be used in combination with an MAOI, or within 14 days of discontinuing treatment with an MAOI. At least 14 days should be allowed after stopping citalopram before starting an MAOI.
- May cause drowsiness or dizziness. Use caution while driving or performing other tasks requiring alertness, coordination, or physical dexterity.
- Avoid alcohol while taking citalopram.
- Inform your doctor if you are pregnant, become pregnant, are planning to become pregnant, or are breastfeeding.
- Improvement in depression may be noticed in 1 to 4 weeks. Continue to take citalopram as directed even though your depression has improved.
- Contact your doctor if adverse reactions persist and become bothersome.
- Store at controlled room temperature (59° to 86°F).

*If you have any questions, consult your doctor, pharmacist, or health care provider.*

| Generic Name Brand Name Examples | Supplied As | Generic Available |
|---|---|---|
| Rx **Maprotiline HCl** | **Tablets**: 25 mg, 50 mg, 75 mg | Yes |
| Rx **Mirtazapine** | | |
| *Remeron* | **Tablets**: 15 mg, 30 mg, 45 mg | No |
| *Remeron SolTab* | **Tablets, orally disintegrating**: 15 mg, 30 mg, 45 mg | No |

## Type of Drug:

Antidepressant; mood-elevating agent.

## How the Drug Works:

The exact mechanism of action is not known. It is believed that tetracyclic antidepressants adjust or balance how the brain and nervous system produce and respond to natural chemicals (neurotransmitters) that elevate mood.

## Uses:

*Maprotiline:* To treat depressive illness in patients with depressive neurosis (dysthymic disorder) and manic-depressive illness (major depressive episode).

*Mirtazapine:* To treat depression.

*Unlabeled Use(s):* Maprotiline is also effective for the relief of anxiety associated with depression.

## Precautions:

*Do not use in the following situations:*
>  allergy to the tetracyclic compound or any of its ingredients
>  electroshock therapy, concurrent (maprotiline only)
>  heart attack, acute phase (maprotiline only)
>  MAOI therapy (eg, phenelzine), within 14 days
>  seizure disorders, known or suspected (maprotiline only)

*Use with caution in the following situations:*
>  abnormal blood counts (mirtazapine only)
>  alcohol use
>  anesthetics, general
>  angina (chest pain), history of
>  CNS depressant (eg, barbiturates) use
>  elderly
>  glaucoma, narrow-angle, history of (maprotiline only)
>  heart attack, history of
>  heart disease, significant
>  high blood pressure therapy
>  hyperthyroid, history of (maprotiline only)
>  increased intraocular pressure (maprotiline only)
>  kidney disease (mirtazapine only)
>  liver disease (mirtazapine only)
>  mania or hypomania, history of
>  seizures, history of
>  stroke, history of
>  suicidal tendencies
>  surgery (maprotiline only)
>  urinary retention, history of (maprotiline only)

*Seizures:* Maprotiline use has been associated with seizures. The risk is higher in patients with a history of seizures, in patients taking phenothiazines (eg, promethazine), or when benzodiazepines (eg, alprazolam) are being withdrawn.

*Pregnancy:* There are no adequate or well-controlled studies in pregnant women. Use only if clearly needed and the potential benefits to the mother outweigh the possible hazards to the fetus.

*Breastfeeding:* Maprotiline appears in breast milk. It is not known if mirtazapine appears in breast milk. Consult your doctor before you begin breastfeeding.

*Children:* Safety and effectiveness in children (younger than 18 years of age for maprotiline) have not been established.

*Elderly:* The elimination of mirtazapine is reduced in elderly patients. In general, lower doses of maprotiline are recommended for patients older than 60 years of age. Use with caution in elderly patients.

*Lab tests* may be required periodically during treatment. Lab tests may include blood counts and enzyme levels.

## Drug Interactions:

Tell your doctor or pharmacist if you are taking or are planning to take any over-the-counter or prescription medications or dietary supplements while taking a tetracyclic compound. Doses of one or both drugs may need to be modified or a different drug may need to be prescribed. The following drugs and drug classes interact with tetracyclic compounds:

alcohol
barbiturates (eg, phenobarbital)
benzodiazepines
 (eg, alprazolam)
MAOI antidepressants
 (eg, phenelzine)

phenothiazines (eg, promethazine) (maprotiline only)
thyroid hormones (eg, thyroid desiccated) (maprotiline only)

## Side Effects:

Every drug is capable of producing side effects. Many tetracyclic compound users experience no, or minor, side effects. The frequency and severity of side effects depend on many factors including dose, duration of therapy, and individual susceptibility. Possible side effects include:

*Digestive Tract:* Nausea; vomiting; constipation; dry mouth; thirst; increased appetite; stomach pain; indigestion.

*Nervous System:* Confusion; anxiety; agitation; abnormal thinking; nervousness; tremor; twitching; drowsiness; clumsiness; dizziness; vertigo (feeling of whirling motion); weakness; fatigue; tiredness; sleeplessness; headache; abnormal dreams; increased sensitivity; apathy; depression; memory loss; numbness or tingling in the hands or feet.

*Respiratory System:* Difficulty breathing; cough; sinus problems; wheezing.

*Circulatory System:* Rapid heart rate; irregular heartbeat; increased choles-terol and triglyceride levels; increased blood pressure; low blood pres-sure on arising.

*Skin:* Rash; itching; hives; acne; dry skin; flushing; redness; hair loss.

*Other:* Flu syndrome; general body discomfort; swelling in the hands or feet; blurred vision; muscle, joint, or back pain; frequent urination; uri-nary tract infection.

## Guidelines for Use:

- Dosage is individualized. Take exactly as prescribed.
- Do not stop taking or change the dose unless directed by your doctor.
- *Maprotiline* — May be given as a single daily dose or in divided doses.
- *Mirtazapine* — Take in a single dose, preferably at bedtime. May be taken without regard to food.
- *Remeron SolTabs*— Open tablet blisterpack with dry hands and place the tablet on the tongue. The tablet will disintegrate rapidly and can be swallowed with saliva. No water is needed. Do not chew the tablet, split the tablet, or store the tablet for later use.
- If a dose is missed, take it as soon as possible. If several hours have passed or it is nearing time for the next dose, do not double the dose to catch up, unless advised to do so by your doctor. If more than one dose is missed or it is necessary to establish a new dosage sched-ule, contact your doctor or pharmacist.
- Avoid the use of alcohol, barbiturates, or other CNS depressants (eg, tranquilizers) while taking this medicine.
- Contact your doctor if you experience sore throat, fever, chills, mouth sores, or other signs of infection. Pay particular attention to any flu-like symptoms or other symptoms that might suggest infection.
- May cause drowsiness or dizziness. Alcohol use may increase this effect. Use caution while driving or performing other tasks requiring alertness, coordination, or physical dexterity.
- Allow at least 14 days between discontinuation of an MAO inhibitor anti-depressant (eg, phenelzine) and the start of therapy with this medi-cine. Also, allow at least 14 days after stopping this medicine before starting an MAO inhibitor.
- Maprotiline has been associated with seizures. This risk is higher in patients with a history of seizures, in patients taking phenothiazines (eg, promethazine) or withdrawing from benzodiazepines (eg, alprazolam).
- Inform your doctor if you are pregnant, become pregnant, are plan to become pregnant, or are breastfeeding.
- *Maprotiline* — Beneficial effects are sometimes seen within 3 to 7 days, although 2 to 3 weeks are usually necessary.
- *Mirtazapine* — Beneficial effects may take 1 to 4 weeks to occur.
- Lab tests may be required to monitor therapy. Be sure to keep appoint-ments.
- Store at room temperature (59° to 86°F) in a tightly closed container, away from light and moisture.

*If you have any questions, consult your doctor, pharmacist, or health care provider.*

| Generic Name<br>*Brand Name Examples* | Supplied As | Generic<br>Available |
|---|---|---|
| *Rx* **Isocarboxazid** | | |
| *Marplan* | **Tablets:** 10 mg | No |
| *Rx* **Phenelzine** | | |
| *Nardil* | **Tablets:** 15 mg | No |
| *Rx* **Tranylcypromine Sulfate** | | |
| *Parnate* | **Tablets:** 10 mg | No |

## Type of Drug:

Antidepressants; mood-elevating agents; MAOIs.

## How the Drug Works:

Monoamine oxidase inhibitors (MAOIs) prevent the breakdown of the body's own mood-elevating substances. The effect may take several weeks to be noticed.

## Uses:

To treat chronic (long-term) depression in patients who have not responded satisfactorily to other antidepressants. They are rarely used as first-line antidepressant therapy.

*Unlabeled Use(s):* Occasionally doctors may prescribe MAOIs for bulimia and panic disorder associated with agoraphobia (fear of open or public places) and globus hystericus syndrome (choking sensation associated with hysteria). Phenelzine has been investigated for use as an aid in treating cocaine addiction, night terrors, post-traumatic stress disorder, and migraines resistant to other therapies. Tranylcypromine has been used to treat Binswanger's encephalopathy, seasonal affective disorder, and subjective symptoms of multiple sclerosis.

## Precautions:

*Do not use in the following situations:*

allergy to MAOIs or any of their ingredients
cerebrovascular defect, confirmed or suspected (eg, stroke)
dibenzapine-related agents (eg, tricyclic antidepressants)
headaches, history of severe or frequent
heart disease (eg, congestive heart failure)
high blood pressure
kidney disease, severe
liver disease
liver function tests, abnormal
other MAOIs, concurrent therapy
pheochromocytoma (adrenal gland tumor)
sympathomimetics (eg, amphetamine), concurrent use

*Use with caution in the following situations:*

anesthetic agents, concurrent use
angina, history
antihypertensives, (eg, thiazide diuretics, rauwolfia alkaloids)
bupropion, concurrent use
buspirone, concurrent use
caffeine, concurrent use
CNS depressants (eg, alcohol, narcotics, barbiturates)
debilitated patients
dextromethorphan, concurrent use
diabetes
elderly
kidney disease
low blood pressure
meperidine, concurrent use
overactive thyroid
schizophrenia
seizures, history
SSRIs, concurrent use (eg, fluoxetine, sertraline, paroxetine)
suicidal thoughts
tyramine-containing foods (see Precautions)

*Drug abuse and dependence:* Drug abuse and dependence have been reported in patients using excessive doses of tranylcypromine and isocarboxazid. Some of these patients had a history of substance abuse. The following withdrawal symptoms have been reported: Restlessness; anxiety; depression; confusion; hallucinations; headaches; weakness; diarrhea.

*Hypertensive Crisis:* Hypertensive crisis (extreme elevations in blood pressure) can result from coadministraton of MAOIs and certain drugs and foods.

*Chest pain:* MAOIs may suppress chest pain that would otherwise serve as a warning of myocardial ischemia (inadequate circulation of blood to the heart, usually as a result of heart disease).

*Liver Dysfunction:* Discontinue isocarboxazid use at first sign of liver dysfunction or jaundice (yellowing of skin or eyes).

*Depression:* Tranylcypromine and isocarboxazid may aggravate coexisting symptoms in depression, such as anxiety and agitation.

*Tyramine-containing foods:* Do not eat foods with high tyramine, dopamine, or tryptophan content (see the following listing) during or for 2 weeks after the discontinuation of MAOIs. Any high-protein food that is aged or undergoes breakdown by a putrefaction process to improve flavor is suspected of producing a significant increase in blood pressure in patients taking MAOIs. Do not take any new prescription medication without first reviewing it with your doctor or pharmacist. Do not drink alcoholic beverages or self-medicate with dietary supplements, cold, hay fever, or weight-reducing preparations while undergoing therapy. Do not consume excessive amounts of caffeine in any form, and report headache or other unusual symptoms promptly.

## Tyramine-Containing Foods[1]

*Cheese/Dairy Products:* American, processed; blue; Boursault; brick, natural; Brie; Camembert; cheddar; Emmenthaler; Gruyere; mozzarella; Parmesan; Romano; Roquefort; Stilton; sour cream; yogurt.

*Meat/Fish:* Beef or chicken liver, other meats, fish (unrefrigerated, fermented); meats prepared with tenderizer; fermented sausages (bologna, pepperoni, salami, summer sausage); game meat; caviar; dried fish (especially salted herring); herring (pickled or spoiled).

*Alcoholic Beverages (undistilled):* Beer and ale (imports); red wine (especially Chianti); sherry.

*Fruit/Vegetables:* Avocado (especially overripe); yeast extracts (eg, marmite); bananas; figs, canned (overripe); raisins; soy sauce.

*Other Foods:* Fava beans (overripe); chocolate; caffeine (eg, coffee, tea, colas).

[1] Tyramine contents are not predictable and may vary. The amounts of tyramine are estimated from low to very high.

*Other Problem Foods:* Broad beans (fava beans, overripe); chocolate; caffeine (eg, coffee, tea, colas); ginseng.

*Pregnancy:* Safety for use during pregnancy has not been established. Use during pregnancy or in women of childbearing age only when clearly needed and when the potential benefits outweigh the potential hazards to the fetus.

*Breastfeeding:* Tranylcypromine appears in breast milk. It is not known if the other MAOIs appear in breast milk. Because of the potential for serious adverse effects in the nursing infant, decide whether to discontinue nursing or the drug, taking into account the importance of the drug to the mother. Consult your doctor before you begin breastfeeding.

*Children:* Use in children younger than 16 years of age is not recommended.

*Elderly:* The most serious reactions to MAOI use involve changes in blood pressure. Older patients may suffer more problems than younger patients during and following an episode of increased blood pressure or malignant hyperthermia (extremely high fever). Older patients have less compensatory reserve to cope with any serious adverse reactions. Use with caution in the elderly.

*Lab tests* may be required to monitor therapy. Tests may include periodic liver chemistry (isocarboxazid).

## Drug Interactions:

Tell your doctor or pharmacist if you are taking or if you are planning to take any over-the-counter or prescription medications or dietary supplements with MAOIs. Doses of one or both drugs may need to be modified or a different drug may need to be prescribed. The following drugs and drug classes interact with MAOIs:

anesthetic agents (eg, anesthesia, cocaine)
anorexiants (eg, amphetamine, phentermine)
antidiabetic agents (eg, insulin, sulfonylureas, glyburide, tolbutamide)
antihypertensives (eg, thiazide diuretics, rauwolfia alkaloids)
beta blockers (eg, metoprolol, nadolol)
buproprion HCl (eg, *Zyban*)
buspirone HCl (*BuSpar*)
caffeine
CNS depressants (eg, alcohol, narcotics, barbiturates)
dextromethorphan (eg, *Robitussin DM*)
dibenzapine-related agents (eg, tricyclic antidepressants, carbamazepine, cyclobenzaprine)

disulfiram (eg, *Antabuse*)
guanethidine (eg, *Ismelin*)
levodopa (eg, *Larodopa*)
MAOIs, other
meperidine (eg, *Demerol*)
methyldopa (eg, *Aldomet*)
methylphenidate HCl (eg, *Ritalin*)
metrizamide (*Amipaque*)
phenylpropanolamine (eg, *Propagest*)
pseudoephedrine (eg, *Sudafed*)
selective serotonin reuptake inhibitors (SSRIs) (eg, citalopram, fluoxetine)
sulfonamides (eg, sulfisoxazole, paroxetine)
sumatriptan (*Imitrex*)
sympathomimetics (eg, metaraminol, phenylephrine)
tyramine-containing foods or beverages (see Precautions)

## Side Effects:

Every drug is capable of producing side effects. Many MAOI users experience no, or minor, side effects. The frequency and severity of side effects depend on many factors including dose, duration of therapy, and individual susceptibility. Possible side effects include:

*Digestive Tract:* Nausea; constipation; diarrhea; stomach pain; appetite loss.

*Nervous System:* Hyperactivity; tremor; muscle twitching; unusual muscle movements; headache; dizziness; faintness; anxiety; jitteriness; memory impairment; sleep disturbances (eg, sleeplessness, excessively long sleeping periods); weakness; fatigue; drowsiness; restlessness; agitation; exaggerated reflexes; mania (eg, irritability, euphoria, distractability, excitability); abnormal skin sensations; lethargy; sedation.

*Circulatory System:* Changes in heart rate and rhythm; postural and orthostatic hypotension (dizziness or lightheadedness when rising from a seated or lying position); palpitations (pounding in the chest).

*Skin:* Rash; itching; sweating; jaundice (yellowing of skin or eyes).

*Other:* Dilated (widened) pupils; stiff neck; dry mouth; urinary frequency; edema (fluid retention); blurred vision; weight gain; sexual problems; chills; impotence; abnormal blood cell counts; glaucoma; heavy feeling.

## Guidelines for Use:

- *Phenelzine* — Recommended initial dosage is 15 mg 3 times daily. Increase dose to at least 60 mg/day at a fairly rapid pace consistent with patient tolerance. It may be necessary to increase dose up to 90 mg/day to obtain sufficient MAO inhibition. Many patients do not show clinical response until treatment at 60 mg has been continued for 4 weeks or more. After maximum benefit is achieved, reduce dose slowly over several weeks. Maintenance dosage may be as low as 15 mg/day or 15 mg every other day; continued for as long as required.

- *Tranylcypromine* — The usual effective dose is 30 mg/day in divided doses. Improvement should be seen within 48 hours to 3 weeks after starting therapy. If there is no improvement after 2 weeks, increase dose in 10 mg/day increments at 1- to 3-week intervals. Dosage range may be extended to a maximum of 60 mg/day from the usual 30 mg/day. Gradually withdraw tranylcypromine when discontinuing therapy.

- *Isocarboxazid* — Recommended initial dosage is 10 mg twice daily. If tolerated, increase by 10 mg every 2 to 4 days to achieve a dose of 40 mg by the end of the first week of treatment. Dose can then be increased by increments of up to 20 mg/week, if needed and tolerated, to a maximum recommended dose of 60 mg/day. Daily dose should be divided into 2 to 4 doses. After a maximum clinical response is achieved, attempt to reduce the dose slowly over a period of several weeks without jeopardizing therapeutic response. Beneficial effect may not be seen in some patients for 3 to 6 weeks. If no response is obtained by then, discontinue therapy. Caution is indicated in patients for whom a dose of 40 mg/day is exceeded.

- Do not discontinue this medication or adjust dosage except on the advice of your doctor. Consult your doctor before taking any other medication, including nonprescription items, while taking an MAOI.

- This medicine may take several weeks to become effective. Continue to take as directed.

- If a dose is missed, take it as soon as possible. If several hours have passed or if it is nearing time for the next dose, do not double the dose in order to catch up, unless advised to do so by your doctor. If more than one dose is missed, or it is necessary to establish a new dosage schedule, contact your doctor.

- Avoid tyramine-containing foods, alcohol, caffeine, and tryptophan (see Precautions).

- May cause drowsiness or blurred vision. Use caution while driving or performing other tasks requiring alertness, coordination, or physical dexterity.

- Dizziness, weakness, or fainting may occur when rising from a lying or sitting position. If this occurs, get up slowly.

- At doses over 30 mg/day, postural hypotension (dizziness or lightheadedness when rising from a seated or lying position) is a major side effect and may result in fainting. Dosage increases will be more gradual in patients showing a tendency toward low blood pressure at the beginning of therapy. Postural hypotension may be relieved by lying down until blood pressure returns to normal.

## Guidelines for Use (cont.):

- Hypertensive crises (increase in blood pressure) as a result of concurrent use of MAOI and certain foods or drugs (see Precautions) can occur and are potentially fatal. These crises usually occur within several hours after ingestion of the interacting food or drug. Notify your doctor immediately if you experience a headache that starts in the back of the head and moves forward, pounding in the chest, neck stiffness or soreness, nausea, vomiting, sweating (sometimes with fever or cold, clammy skin), dilated pupils, sensitivity to light, or changes in heart rate with or without chest pain or tightness.
- Notify your doctor if you experience rash or intolerable side effects.
- Use may complicate other medical treatment (eg, general anesthesia, surgery). Inform your doctors and dentist about your use of MAOIs. Wear a *Medic Alert* bracelet or carry a card saying that you are taking an MAOI.
- A waiting period of 10 to 14 days is recommended when switching from one MAOI to another or from a dibenzapine-related agent. Other medications that interact with MAOIs (eg, fluoxetine) have different waiting periods. Discuss appropriate waiting periods for changes in therapy with your doctor or pharmacist.
- Blood pressure will need to be monitored frequently.
- Lab tests may be required to monitor therapy. Be sure to keep appointments.
- Store at room temperature.

*If you have any questions, consult your doctor, pharmacist, or health care provider.*

| Generic Name<br>*Brand Name Examples* | Supplied As | Generic<br>Available |
|---|---|---|
| *Rx* **Paroxetine HCl** | | |
| *Paxil* | **Tablets:** 10 mg, 20 mg, 30 mg, 40 mg | No |
| *Paxil* | **Suspension, oral:** 10 mg/5 mL | No |
| *Paxil CR* | **Tablets, controlled-release:** 12.5 mg, 25 mg, 37.5 mg | No |

## Type of Drug:

Antidepressant (SSRI); mood-elevating agent.

## How the Drug Works:

The actual antidepressant mechanism of paroxetine is not known. It is presumed that it works by blocking the uptake of serotonin, a chemical found in the brain.

## Uses:

*Immediate-release:* To treat obsessions and compulsions in patients with obsessive-compulsive disorder (OCD).

To treat major depressive disorder.

To treat social anxiety disorder, also known as social phobia.

To treat generalized anxiety disorder (GAD).

To treat panic disorder (PD).

To treat post-traumatic stress disorder (PTSD).

*Controlled-release:* To treat major depressive disorder.

To treat panic disorder, with or without agoraphobia.

*Unlabeled Use(s):* Has been used to treat bipolar depression in conjunction with lithium; premenstrual dysphoric disorder, chronic headache, premature ejaculation, fibromyalgia syndrome, and diabetic neuropathy.

## Precautions:

*Do not use in the following situations:*
allergy to paroxetine or any of its ingredients
MAOI therapy, within 2 weeks
thioridazine (eg, *Mellaril*) therapy, concurrent

*Use with caution in the following situations:*

| | |
|---|---|
| alcohol use | kidney disease |
| diuretic therapy, concurrent use | liver disease |
| drug abuse, history of | mania, history of |
| glaucoma, angle-closure | seizures, history of |
| illness affecting metabolism or | suicide, high-risk of |
| hemodynamic responses | |
| (eg, congestive heart failure) | |

*Pregnancy:* There are no adequate and well-controlled studies in pregnant women. Use only if clearly needed and the potential benefits to the mother outweigh the possible hazards to the fetus.

*Breastfeeding:* Paroxetine appears in breast milk. Consult your doctor before breastfeeding.

*Children:* Safety and effectiveness in children have not been established.

*Elderly:* Initial dosage in the elderly should be reduced.

## Drug Interactions:

Tell your doctor or pharmacist if you are taking or if you are planning to take any over-the-counter or prescription medications or dietary supplements while taking paroxetine. Doses of one or both drugs may need to be modified or a different drug may need to be prescribed. The following drugs and drug classes interact with paroxetine:

alcohol
antidepressants (eg, fluoxetine)
cimetidine (eg, *Tagamet*)
cyproheptadine (eg, *Periactin*)
digoxin (eg, *Lanoxin*)
lithium (eg, *Eskalith*)
MAOIs (eg, phenelzine)
phenobarbital (eg, *Solfoton*)
phenothiazines (eg, thioridazine)
phenytoin (eg, *Dilantin*)

procyclidine (*Kemadrin*)
quinidine (eg, *Quinora*)
sumatriptan (*Imitrex*)
theophylline (eg, *Slo-Phyllin*)
tricyclic antidepressants
 (eg, amitriptyline)
L-tryptophan
type 1C antiarrhythmics
 (eg, propafenone)
warfarin (eg, *Coumadin*)

## Side Effects:

Every drug is capable of producing side effects. Many paroxetine users experience no or minor side effects. The frequency and severity of side effects depend on many factors including dose, duration of therapy, and individual susceptibility. Possible side effects include:

*Circulatory System:* Chest pain; palpitations (pounding in the chest); high blood pressure; rapid heart rate.

*Digestive Tract:* Nausea; diarrhea; vomiting; constipation; gas; indigestion; appetite changes; dry mouth.

*Nervous System:* Drowsiness; sleeplessness; agitation; tremor; anxiety; weakness; headache; dizziness; nervousness; confusion; twitching; amnesia; inability to concentrate; abnormal dreams; depression; unstable emotions; vertigo (feeling of whirling motion).

*Skin:* Flushing; sweating; rash; itching.

*Other:* Abnormal ejaculation and other male genital disorders; back pain; joint pain; muscle weakness or pain; tightness in throat; abnormal skin sensations; decreased sex drive; blurred vision; runny nose; taste perversion; urinary frequency; urinary disorder; chills; general body discomfort; weight changes; cough; congestion; ringing in the ears; impotence.

## Guidelines for Use:

- Dosage is individualized. Take exactly as prescribed. Small doses are usually used at first and then gradually increased until the desired benefit is obtained. Dosage changes are usually made at intervals more than 1 week.
- Take once daily, preferably in the morning, without regard to meals. Take with food if stomach upset occurs.
- Do not change the dose or stop taking, unless directed by your doctor.
- Avoid alcohol when using this drug.
- Do not use in combination with MAOIs or within 14 days of discontinuing treatment with an MAOI. Similarly, at least 2 weeks should be allowed after stopping paroxetine before starting an MAOI.
- May cause drowsiness or dizziness. Use caution while driving or performing other tasks requiring alertness, coordination, or physical dexterity.
- Improvement may be noticed in 1 to 4 weeks; continue therapy as directed.
- Shake oral suspension well before using.
- Do not chew or crush controlled-release tablets. Swallow whole.
- Consult your doctor or pharmacist before taking any nonprescription or prescription drugs while using paroxetine.
- Inform your doctor if you are pregnant, become pregnant, are planning to become pregnant, or are breastfeeding.
- Significant weight loss may be an undesirable effect of paroxetine therapy.
- Store tablets at controlled room temperature (59° to 86°F).
- Store controlled-release tablets and suspension at or below 77°F.

*If you have any questions, consult your doctor, pharmacist, or health care provider.*

| Generic Name Brand Name Example | Supplied As | Generic Available |
|---|---|---|
| Rx **Sertraline HCl** | | |
| *Zoloft* | **Tablets**: 25 mg, 50 mg, 100 mg | No |
| *Zoloft* | **Oral concentrate**: 20 mg/mL | No |

## Type of Drug:

Antidepressant; SSRI; mood-elevating agent.

## How the Drug Works:

The actual antidepressant mechanism of sertraline is not known. It is presumed that it works by blocking the uptake of serotonin, a chemical found in the brain.

## Uses:

To treat major depressive disorder, obsessions and compulsions in adult patients with obsessive-compulsive disorder (OCD), panic disorder with or without agoraphobia, posttraumatic stress disorder (PTSD), and premenstrual dysphoric disorder (PMDD).

*Unlabeled Use(s):* Has been used to treat generalized social phobia.

## Precautions:

*Do not use in the following situations:*
>    allergy to sertraline or any of its ingredients
>    disulfiram (*Antabuse*) therapy, concurrent
>    MAOI use, concurrent or within 14 days

*Use with caution in the following situations:*

| | |
|---|---|
| alcohol use | liver disease |
| attempted suicide, history of | mania |
| gout | seizures, history of |
| illness, systemic | |

*Pregnancy:* There are no adequate and well-controlled studies in pregnant women. Use only if clearly needed and the potential benefits to the mother outweigh the possible hazards to the fetus.

*Breastfeeding:* It is not known if sertraline appears in breast milk. Consult your doctor before you begin breastfeeding.

*Children:* Safety and effectiveness have not been established for uses other than OCD in children 6 years of age and older.

## Drug Interactions:

Tell your doctor or pharmacist if you are taking or if you are planning to take any over-the-counter or prescription medications or dietary supplements with sertraline. Doses of one or both drugs may need to be modified or a different drug may need to be prescribed. The following drugs and drug classes interact with sertraline:

| | |
|---|---|
| cimetidine (eg, *Tagamet*) | diazepam (eg, *Valium*) |
| clozapine (eg, *Clozaril*) | digitoxin (*Crystodigin*) |

disulfiram (*Antabuse*)
flecainide (*Tambocor*)
hydantoins (eg, phenytoin)
lithium (eg, *Eskalith*)
MAOIs (eg, phenelzine)
propafenone (*Rythmol*)

sumatriptan (*Imitrex*)
tolbutamide (eg, *Orinase*)
tricyclic antidepressants
 (eg, doxepin)
warfarin (eg, *Coumadin*)

## Side Effects:

Every drug is capable of producing side effects. Many sertraline users experience no, or minor, side effects. The frequency and severity of side effects depend on many factors including dose, duration of therapy, and individual susceptibility. Possible side effects include:

*Digestive Tract:* Nausea; vomiting; diarrhea; indigestion; constipation; gas; appetite changes.

*Nervous System:* Headache; dizziness; tremor; fatigue; nervousness; anxiety; drowsiness; agitation; sleeplessness; decreased or abnormal skin sensations.

*Circulatory System:* Pounding in the chest; chest pain.

*Other:* Dry mouth; vision disturbances; ringing in the ears; back pain; muscle pain; decreased sexual interest or performance; excessive sweating; rash; yawning; fatigue; weakness; general body discomfort; flushing.

## Guidelines for Use:

- Dosage will be individualized. Take exactly as prescribed.
- Do not change the dose or stop taking, unless directed by your doctor.
- Administer once daily, either in the morning or evening.
- Shake oral concentrate well before using.
- Do not use in combination with MAOIs or within 14 days of treatment with an MAOI.
- If a dose is missed, take it as soon as possible. If several hours have passed or it is nearing time for the next dose, do not double the dose to catch up, unless advised to do so by your doctor. If several doses are missed or it is necessary to establish a new dosage schedule, contact your doctor or pharmacist.
- Avoid alcohol when using this drug.
- May cause drowsiness, dizziness, or blurred vision. Use caution while driving or performing other tasks requiring alertness, coordination, or physical dexterity.
- Significant weight loss or gain may be an undesirable effect of sertraline therapy.
- Inform your doctor if you are pregnant, become pregnant, are planning to become pregnant, or are breastfeeding.
- Store at room temperature (59° to 86°F).

*If you have any questions, consult your doctor, pharmacist, or health care provider.*

| Generic Name<br>*Brand Name Examples* | Supplied As | Generic<br>Available |
|---|---|---|
| *Rx* **Trazodone HCl** | | |
| *Desyrel* | **Tablets:** 50 mg, 100 mg | Yes |
| *Desyrel Dividose* | **Tablets:** 150 mg, 300 mg | Yes |

## Type of Drug:

Antidepressant; mood-elevating agent.

## How the Drug Works:

It is not known how trazodone works to relieve depression. It is believed trazodone modifies the chemical balance in the brain, which changes behavior. It does not stimulate the brain.

## Uses:

To relieve mental depression.

*Unlabeled Use(s):* Occasionally doctors may prescribe trazodone for cocaine withdrawal, to manage aggressive behavior when used with other medications, and to treat patients with panic disorder or agoraphobia (fear of open or public places) with panic attacks.

## Precautions:

*Do not use in the following situations:* Allergy to trazodone or any of its ingredients.

*Use with caution in the following situations:*

electroshock therapy, concurrent
heart attack, recent
heart disease, preexisting
heart rhythms, abnormal
high blood pressure
suicide attempts, history of

*Priapism:* If you experience prolonged or painful penile erection, discontinue use immediately and consult your doctor. Permanent damage of normal penis function and impotence have occurred.

*Pregnancy:* There are no adequate and well-controlled studies in pregnant women. Use only if clearly needed and potential benefits to the mother outweigh the possible hazards to the fetus.

*Breastfeeding:* It is not known if trazodone appears in breast milk. Consult your doctor before you begin breastfeeding.

*Children:* Safety and effectiveness in children younger than 18 years of age have not been established.

*Lab tests* may be required to monitor therapy. Tests include blood counts.

## Drug Interactions:

Tell your doctor or pharmacist if you are taking or if you are planning to take any over-the-counter or prescription medications or dietary supplements with trazodone. Doses of one or both drugs may need to be modified or a different drug may need to be prescribed. The following drugs and drug classes interact with trazodone:

anesthetics
CNS depressants (eg, alcohol,
  barbiturates, narcotics)

digoxin (eg, *Lanoxin)*
phenytoin (eg, *Dilantin)*
warfarin (eg, *Coumadin)*

## Side Effects:

Every drug is capable of producing side effects. Many trazodone users experience no, or minor, side effects. The frequency and severity of side effects depend on many factors including dose, duration of therapy, and individual susceptibility. Possible side effects include:

*Digestive Tract:* Upset stomach; nausea; vomiting; diarrhea; constipation; decreased appetite; dry mouth.

*Nervous System:* Anger; hostility; sleeplessness; nightmares or vivid dreams; confusion; disorientation; decreased concentration; dizziness; drowsiness; excitement; fatigue; headache; tremor; impaired memory; nervousness; incoordination; lightheadedness.

*Circulatory System:* Changes in blood pressure; pounding in the chest; fast heartbeat.

*Senses:* Ringing in the ears; blurred vision; red, tired, itching eyes; nasal or sinus congestion.

*Other:* Shortness of breath; weight changes; swelling; aches and pains; fainting; bad taste in the mouth; abnormal skin sensations; general body discomfort; feeling of heaviness or fullness in the head; prolonged painful erection; decreased sex drive; clamminess; sweating; orthostatic hypotension (dizziness or lightheadedness when rising from a sitting or lying position).

## Guidelines for Use:

- Dosage is individualized.
- Dosage will be initiated at a low level and increased gradually by your doctor.
- Take shortly after a meal or snack.
- If a dose is missed, take it as soon as possible. If several hours have passed or if it is nearing time for the next dose, do not double the dose to catch up, unless advised to do so by your doctor. If more than one dose is missed, or it is necessary to establish a new dosage schedule, contact your doctor or pharmacist.
- May cause drowsiness, dizziness, or blurred vision. Use caution while driving or performing other tasks requiring alertness, coordination, or physical dexterity.
- Avoid alcohol or other drowsiness-causing medications (eg, antihistamines, barbiturates, narcotic pain relievers) while taking trazodone.
- Notify your doctor if you experience drowsiness, sore throat, fever, or any signs of infection.
- Male patients with prolonged and painful erections (priapism) should immediately discontinue the drug and consult their doctor.
- Lab tests may be required to monitor therapy. Be sure to keep appointments.
- Store at controlled room temperature (59° to 86°F).

*If you have any questions, consult your doctor, pharmacist, or health care provider.*

| Generic Name<br>Brand Name Examples | Supplied As | Generic<br>Available |
|---|---|---|
| Rx **Venlafaxine HCl** | | |
| Effexor | **Tablets:** 25 mg, 37.5 mg,<br>50 mg, 75 mg, 100 mg | No |
| Effexor XR | **Capsules, extended-release:**<br>37.5 mg, 75 mg, 150 mg | No |

## Type of Drug:
Antidepressant; mood-elevating agent

## How the Drug Works:
Venlafaxine inhibits neuronal uptake of serotonin and norepinephrine in the central nervous system, which is believed to combat depression and other behavioral disorders.

## Uses:
The treatment of depression. The extended-release form is also used to treat generalized anxiety disorder.

## Precautions:
*Do not use in the following situations:*
allergy to venlafaxine
current or recent (within the past 14 days) use of a monoamine oxidase inhibitor (MAOI)

*Use with caution in the following situations:*

| | |
|---|---|
| concomitant systemic illness | mania, history of |
| liver disease | seizures, history of |
| kidney disease | suicide, high-risk of |

*Pregnancy:* Adequate studies have not been done in pregnant women. Use only if clearly needed and potential benefits to the mother outweigh the possible hazards to the fetus.

*Breastfeeding:* Venlafaxine appears in breast milk. A decision should be made to either discontinue nursing or discontinue the drug, taking into account the importance of the drug to the mother.

*Children:* Safety and effectiveness in children younger than 18 years of age have not been established.

## Drug Interactions:
Tell your doctor or pharmacist if you are taking or if you are planning to take any over-the-counter or prescription medications or dietary supplements with venlafaxine HCl. Doses of one or both drugs may need to be modified or a different drug may need to be prescribed. The following drugs and drug classes interact with venlafaxine HCl.

MAOIs (eg, phenelzine)
sibutramine (*Meridia*)

## Side Effects:

Every drug is capable of producing side effects. Many venlafaxine HCl users experience no or minor side effects. The frequency and severity of side effects depend on many factors including dose, duration of therapy, and individual susceptibility. Possible side effects include:

*Circulatory System:* Increased blood pressure; increased heart rate; decreased blood pressure upon rising; flushing.

*Digestive Tract:* Nausea; constipation; appetite loss; diarrhea; vomiting; indigestion; stomach pain; gas; difficulty swallowing; dry mouth; belching.

*Nervous System:* Drowsiness; sleeplessness; dizziness; nervousness; headache; vertigo (feeling of whirling motion); migraine; anxiety; tremor; abnormal dreams; abnormal skin sensations; agitation; confusion; impaired memory; depression; abnormal thinking; unstable emotions; lockjaw; twitching; depersonalization; decreased sex drive; muscle stiffness.

*Respiratory System:* Yawning; bronchitis; difficulty breathing; runny nose; cough.

*Senses:* Blurred vision; taste changes; ringing in the ears; dilated pupils; ear pain; vision changes.

*Skin:* Sweating; rash; itching; flushing.

*Urinary and Reproductive Tract:* Abnormal ejaculation or orgasm; impotence; impaired urination; urinary frequency; menstrual disorders; blood in the urine; painful or difficult urination; irregular bleeding between periods; inflammation of the vagina with itching or abnormal discharge; urinary retention.

*Other:* Weakness; infection; chills; chest pain; weight gain or loss; accidental injury; general body discomfort; neck pain; muscle pain; joint pain; swelling of hands or feet; unusual bruising.

## Guidelines for Use:

- *Tablets* — Usual adult starting dose is 75 mg/day, taken in 2 or 3 divided doses. Dosage may be gradually increased to achieve the desired effect.
- *Extended-release capsules* — Usual adult starting dose is 75 mg/day taken as a single dose.
- Take each dose with food.
- Do not crush, chew, or dissolve extended-release capsules in water. Swallow extended-release capsules whole, with fluid.
- If a dose is missed, take it as soon as possible. If several hours have passed or if it is nearing time for the next dose, do not double the dose to catch up, unless advised to do so by your doctor. If several doses are missed or it is necessary to establish a new dosage schedule, contact your doctor or pharmacist. Use exactly as prescribed.
- Do not change the dose or stop taking venlafaxine unless advised to do so by your doctor.
- If venlafaxine therapy is discontinued, the dose should be gradually reduced over a 2-week period.
- Smaller doses should be used in patients with moderate liver or kidney impairment.
- Venlafaxine should not be used in combination with an MAOI, or within at least 14 days of discontinuing treatment with an MAOI. After stopping venlafaxine, at least 7 days should elapse before starting an MAOI.
- Because any psychoactive drug may impair judgment, thinking, or motor skills, do not operate hazardous machinery, including automobiles, until you are reasonably certain that venlafaxine does not adversely affect your ability to engage in such activities.
- Inform your doctor if you are pregnant, become pregnant, are planning to become pregnant, or if you are breastfeeding during therapy.
- Notify your doctor if rash, hives, or other allergic reactions occur.
- Blood pressure will be monitored during treatment.
- Notify your doctor or pharmacist if you are taking other prescription drugs, over-the-counter drugs, or supplements.
- Avoid alcohol use during venlafaxine therapy.
- Store at room temperature (68° to 77°F). Keep container tightly closed.

*If you have any questions, consult your doctor, pharmacist, or health care provider.*

| Generic Name<br>*Brand Name Examples* | Supplied As | Generic<br>Available |
|---|---|---|
| *Rx* **Amitriptyline HCl** | | |
| *Elavil* | **Tablets:** 10 mg, 25 mg, 50 mg,<br>75 mg, 100 mg, 150 mg | Yes |
| *Elavil* | **Injection:** 10 mg/mL | Yes |
| *Rx* **Amoxapine** | | |
| *Asendin* | **Tablets:** 25 mg, 50 mg,<br>100 mg, 150 mg | Yes |
| *Rx* **Clomipramine HCl** | | |
| *Anafranil* | **Capsules:** 25 mg, 50 mg,<br>75 mg | Yes |
| *Rx* **Desipramine HCl** | | |
| *Norpramin* | **Tablets:** 10 mg, 25 mg, 50 mg,<br>75 mg, 100 mg, 150 mg | Yes |
| *Rx* **Doxepin HCl** | | |
| *Sinequan* | **Capsules:** 10 mg, 25 mg,<br>50 mg, 75 mg, 100 mg,<br>150 mg | Yes |
| *Sinequan* | **Oral concentrate:** 10 mg/mL | Yes |
| *Rx* **Imipramine HCl** | | |
| *Tofranil* | **Tablets:** 10 mg, 25 mg, 50 mg | Yes |
| *Rx* **Imipramine Pamoate** | | |
| *Tofranil-PM* | **Capsules:** 75 mg, 100 mg,<br>125 mg, 150 mg | No |
| *Rx* **Nortriptyline HCl** | | |
| *Aventyl Pulvules* | **Capsules:** 10 mg, 25 mg | No |
| *Pamelor* | **Capsules:** 10 mg, 25 mg,<br>50 mg, 75 mg | Yes |
| *Aventyl, Pamelor[1]* | **Oral solution:** 10 mg/5 mL | No |
| *Rx* **Protriptyline HCl** | | |
| *Vivactil* | **Tablets:** 5 mg, 10 mg | Yes |
| *Rx* **Trimipramine Maleate** | | |
| *Surmontil* | **Capsules:** 25 mg, 50 mg,<br>100 mg | Yes |

[1] Contains alcohol.

## Type of Drug:

Antidepressants; mood-elevating agents.

## How the Drug Works:

Tricyclic antidepressants (TCAs) appear to adjust or rebalance the brain's own natural chemicals (neurotransmitters), which control mood, feelings, and behaviors. The effect may take a few weeks (1 to 4) to be noticed.

## Uses:

For the relief of symptoms of depression (except clomipramine).

*Clomipramine:* Only for the treatment of obsessive-compulsive disorder.

*Doxepin:* To treat anxiety.

*Imipramine:* For the treatment of bedwetting in children 6 years of age and older after possible organic causes have been excluded by appropriate tests.

*Unlabeled Use(s):* Occasionally doctors may prescribe doxepin, clomipramine, imipramine, or amitriptyline to control chronic pain and to treat bulimia. Imipramine, clomipramine, nortriptyline, and other tricyclic antidepressants have also been used to treat panic disorder. Amitriptyline has been used to prevent the onset of cluster and migraine headaches and to treat pathologic weeping and laughing secondary to forebrain disease. Protriptyline has been used in the treatment of obstructive sleep apnea. Trimipramine and doxepin have been studied in the treatment of peptic ulcer disease and to treat skin disorders. Desipramine has been used to facilitate cocaine withdrawal and to treat bulimia. Clomipramine and nortriptyline have been used to treat panic disorder. Nortriptyline has also been used to treat skin disorders and premenstrual depression.

## Precautions:

*Do not use in the following situations:*

| | |
|---|---|
| allergy to TCAs or maprotiline | heart attack, recovery phase |
| glaucoma (doxepin only) | urinary retention (doxepin only) |
| MAOI antidepressant use, concurrent or within 14 days | |

*Use with caution in the following situations:*

| | |
|---|---|
| electroshock therapy | liver disease |
| glaucoma, angle-closure | mental illness (schizophrenia, |
| heart disease (eg, heart failure) | mania, paranoia) |
| hyperthyroid (overactive thyroid) | seizure, history |
| | suicidal tendencies |
| increased intraocular pressure | surgery |
| irregular heartbeat (imipramine only) | stroke |
| | tumor of adrenal medulla |
| kidney disease | urinary retention |

*Tardive Dyskinesia:* Involuntary and uncontrollable movements may develop in patients treated with these drugs. Occurrence is highest among the elderly, especially women. The risk of developing these involuntary movements and the likelihood that they will become permanent are increased as the length of treatment and the total amount of drug given increases. However, it is possible to develop these symptoms after short-term treatment at low doses.

*Neuroleptic Malignant Syndrome (NMS)* is a potentially fatal syndrome associated with use of tricyclic antidepressants. Symptoms include increased body heat, muscle rigidity, altered mental abilities including catatonia, irregular pulse or irregular blood pressure, increased heart rate, sweating, and irregular heart rhythm.

*Withdrawal Symptoms:* Stopping abruptly after prolonged therapy may produce nausea, headache, dizziness, nightmares, and malaise. Clomipramine may also cause vomiting, sleep disturbances, hyperthermia (abnormally high temperature), and irritability. Gradual dose reduction may produce, within 2 weeks, transient symptoms including irritability, restlessness, dreams, and sleep disturbances.

*Sensitivity to sunlight* may occur. Avoid prolonged exposure to the sun. Use sunscreens and wear protective clothing until tolerance is determined. These drugs may reduce tolerance to hot weather.

*Pregnancy:* Adequate studies have not been done in pregnant women. Use only if clearly needed and potential benefits outweigh the possible hazards to the fetus. There have been a few reports of birth defects associated with use of imipramine and amitriptyline. Withdrawal symptoms have been seen in newborns of mothers who have taken clomipramine, desipramine, or imipramine until delivery.

*Breastfeeding:* Tricyclic antidepressants appear in breast milk. Because of the potential for adverse reactions, a decision should be made whether to discontinue nursing or discontinue the drug, taking into account the importance of the drug to the mother. Consult your doctor before you begin breastfeeding.

*Children:* Amitriptyline and doxepin are not recommended for patients younger than 12 years of age. Safety and effectiveness have not been established for amoxapine in children younger than 16 years of age. Imipramine HCl use in bedwetting should be limited to children 6 years of age or older. The safety and effectiveness of imipramine HCl in children with conditions other than bedwetting have not been established. Safety and effectiveness have not been established for clomipramine in children younger than 10 years of age. Trimipramine, nortriptyline, desipramine, imipramine pamoate, and protriptyline are not recommended for use in children.

*Elderly:* Elderly patients are particularly sensitive to the anticholinergic effects (eg, constipation; difficulty urinating; confusion) of tricyclic antidepressants and may be at increased risk for falls. Lower than normal adult doses are generally used when starting therapy.

*Lab tests* may be required during treatment with tricyclic antidepressants. Tests may include blood counts, blood sugar levels, ECG, kidney and liver function tests, and drug blood levels.

## Drug Interactions:

Tell your doctor or pharmacist if you are taking or if you are planning to take any over-the-counter or prescription medications or duetary supplements with tricyclic antidepressants. Doses of one or both drugs may need to be modified or a different drug may need to be prescribed. The following drugs and drug classes interact with tricyclic antidepressants.

alcohol
anorexiants (eg, phentermine)
anticholinergics (eg, dicyclomine)
anticoagulants (eg, warfarin)
azole antifungals (eg, ketoconazole)
barbiturates (eg, phenobarbital)
beta blockers (eg, labetalol)
bupropion (eg, *Zyban*)
carbamazepine (eg, *Tegretol*)
catecholamines (*imipramine HCl only*)
charcoal
cholestyramine (eg, *Questran*)
cimetidine (eg, *Tagamet*)
clonidine (eg, *Catapres)*
diltiazem (eg, *Cardizem*)
disulfiram (eg, *Antabuse)*
ethchlorvynol (*amitriptyline only*)
food (see below)
furazolidone (*Furoxone*)
guanethidine (eg, *Ismelin)*
guanfacine (*Tenex)*
hydantoins (eg, phenytoin)
levodopa (eg, *Larodopa)*

lithium (eg, *Eskalith*)
MAOIs (eg, phenelzine)
methyldopa (eg, *Aldomet*)
methylphenidate (*Ritalin*)
phenothiazines (eg, promethazine)
propafenone (*Rythmol*)
primidone (eg, *Mysoline*)
quinidine (eg, *Quinidex Extentabs*)
quinolones (eg, grepafloxacin, sparfloxacin)
rifamycins (rifabutin, rifampin)
sedatives
SSRI antidepressants (eg, fluoxetine)
sulfonylureas (eg, chloropropamide, tolazamide)
sympathomimetics (eg, phenylephrine, ephedrine)
terbinafine (*Lamisil*)
thyroid hormones (eg, thyroxine)
valproic acid and derivatives (eg, divalproex sodium, valproate sodium)
verapamil (eg, *Calan*)

A high-fiber diet (eg, bran muffins or cereals) may decrease the absorption of TCAs. Patients should avoid consuming excess fiber during drug therapy.

## Side Effects:

Every drug is capable of producing side effects. Many tricyclic antidepressant users experience no, or minor, side effects. The frequency and severity of side effects depend on many factors including dose, duration of therapy, and individual susceptibility. Possible side effects include:

*Enuretic (Bedwetting) Children:* Consider side effects reported with adult use. Most common are nervousness, sleep disorders, tiredness, and mild stomach disturbances. These usually disappear with continued therapy or dosage reduction. Other reported reactions include constipation, convulsions, anxiety, emotional instability, and fainting.

*Clomipramine only:* Tremors; sleeplessness; nervousness; muscle twitches or spasms; memory impairment; anxiety; impaired concentration; breathing problems; abnormal dreams; irritability; emotional lability; depersonalization; hot flashes; menstrual disorder; vaginal irritation; ejaculation disorder; acne; dry skin; abnormal vision; abnormal tears; muscle aches; back pain; joint pain.

*Digestive Tract:* Dry mouth; constipation; decreased bowel movement; nausea; vomiting; loss of appetite; diarrhea; stomach discomfort; peculiar taste in mouth; stomach cramps; black tongue; mouth sores.

*Nervous System:* Confusion with hallucinations (especially in the elderly); disorientation; delusions; anxiety; restlessness; agitation; sleeplessness; tremors; nightmares; hypomania; exacerbation of psychosis; numbness, tingling, and decreased sensations in hands and feet; incoordination; unsteady walking; extrapyramidal symptoms; seizures; ringing in ears; changes in brain wave pattern.

*Circulatory System:* Increased or decreased blood pressure; increased heart rate; pounding in chest (palpitations); heart attack; abnormal heart rhythms; stroke; dizziness when sitting or standing up.

*Skin:* Rash; itching; red spots; flushing; hair loss.

*Urinary and Reproductive Tract:* Urinary retention; decreased urination; dilation of urinary tract.

*Other:* Blurred vision; problems focusing eyes; dilated pupils; increased pressure in eyes; light sensitivity; face and tongue swelling; decreased blood counts; breast enlargement in men; breast enlargement and milk production in women; increased or decreased sex drive; impotence; testicular swelling; increased or decreased blood sugar; weight gain or loss; perspiration; drowsiness; dizziness; weakness; fatigue; headache; changes in liver function; parotid gland swelling; increased appetite.

## Guidelines for Use:

- Use exactly as prescribed.
- Lower dosages are recommended for elderly, adolescent, and outpatients, as compared to hospitalized patients who will be under close supervision. Initiate dosage at a low level and increase gradually, noting carefully the clinical response and any evidence of intolerance. Once depressive symptoms are controlled, maintenance doses will be required for a longer period of time, at the lowest dose that will maintain symptom control.
- For many of these medicines, it is not possible to prescribe a single dosage schedule that is therapeutically effective in all patients. Consequently, the recommended dosage regimens are only a guide, which may be modified by factors such as age, chronic disease, severity of the disease, medical condition of the patient, and degree of psychotherapeutic support.
- If a dose is missed, take it as soon as possible. If several hours have passed or if it is nearing time for the next dose, do not double the dose in order to catch up, unless advised to do so by your doctor. If more than one dose is missed, or it is necessary to establish a new dosage schedule, contact your doctor or pharmacist.

## Guidelines for Use (cont.):

- Once symptoms are controlled, therapy may need to be continued for several months to lessen the chance of relapse.
- Do not change the dose or discontinue therapy unless advised to do so by your doctor.
- These drugs may take 1 to 4 weeks to improve symptoms of depression.
- Do not use in combination with an MAOI or within 14 days of discontinuing treatment with an MAOI. After stopping this medicine, wait at least 2 weeks before starting an MAOI.
- Using these drugs with alcohol or other central nervous system depressants (eg, pain relievers, sedatives, barbiturates) may cause added drowsiness.
- May cause drowsiness or blurred vision. Use caution while driving or performing other tasks requiring alertness, coordination, or physical dexterity.
- Symptoms of nausea, headache, or fatigue may develop after abruptly stopping a tricyclic antidepressant (TCA) after long-term use.
- Notify your doctor if dry mouth, constipation, blurred vision, increased heart rate, impaired coordination, difficult urination, excessive sedation, or seizures occur.
- Notify your doctor if you develop a fever or sore throat.
- Notify your doctor if you experience drowsiness, dizziness, or postural hypotension. Your doctor may need to reduce the dose.
- *Be sure your doctor and pharmacist are aware of the following* —
  Other medical conditions.
  All medications, including nonprescription medicines, that you are taking.
  If you have had an unusual or allergic reaction to any TCA or to maprotiline.
  If you are pregnant or may become pregnant.
  If you are breastfeeding.
- May cause sensitivity to sunlight. Avoid prolonged exposure to the sun and UV light (eg, tanning beds). Use sunscreens and wear protective clothing until tolerance is determined.
- Taking these drugs at bedtime may help reduce side effects (eg, daytime drowsiness). Discuss this possibility with your doctor or pharmacist.
- Lab tests may be required to monitor therapy. Be sure to keep appointments.
- Store at room temperature in a child-resistant container. Patients should supervise this drug carefully in the home.

*Amitriptyline:*
- Usual initial adult dosage for outpatients is 75 mg/day in divided doses. If necessary, this may be increased (preferably at bedtime doses) to a total of 150 mg/day. An alternative method is to begin with 50 to 100 mg at bedtime. This may be increased by 25 or 50 mg as necessary in the bedtime dose to a total of 150 mg/day. Smaller initial doses may be needed if side effects appear with higher doses.

## Guidelines for Use (cont.):

*Amitriptyline:* (cont.)

- Hospitalized patients may require 100 mg/day initially, which can be increased gradually to 200 mg/day. A small number of patients may need up to 300 mg/day.
- Usual dosage for children and elderly patients is 10 mg 3 times a day with 20 mg at bedtime.
- Usual maintenance dosage is 50 to 100 mg given as a single dose at bedtime.
- *Injection Dosage* — Injection should be used for initial therapy in hospitalized patients who are unable or unwilling to take tablets. Tablets should replace the injection as soon as possible. Usual initial dosage by injection is 20 to 30 mg (2 to 3 ml) 4 times a day. Intramuscular doses may cause the effects to appear more rapidly than with tablets.

*Amoxapine:*

- Usual starting dosage is 50 mg 2 or 3 times daily. Dosage may be increased to 100 mg 2 or 3 times daily by the end of the first week.
- Increases above 300 mg/day dose should only be made if 300 mg/day had been ineffective during a trial period of at least 2 weeks.
- Usual effective dose is 200 to 300 mg/day. If no response is seen at 300 mg, dosage may be increased to 400 mg/day. Hospitalized patients who have been refractory to antidepressant therapy and who have no history of convulsive seizures may have dosage raised cautiously up to 600 mg/day in divided doses.
- Once the effective dose is established, the daily maintenance dose, if not more than 300 mg, can be given as a single dose at bedtime. If maintenance dose is more than 300 mg per day, then divided doses should be used.

*Clomipramine:*

- During initial titration, clomipramine should be given in divided doses with meals to reduce stomach upset. Maximum benefit may not be achieved until 2 to 3 weeks after dosage change. Therefore, it may be appropriate to wait 2 to 3 weeks between further dosage adjustments.
- Usual adult initial dose is 25 mg daily, gradually increased to 100 mg during the first 2 weeks. Over the next several weeks, the dose may be increased to a daily maximum of 250 mg.
- Usual initial treatment in children is 25 mg daily given with meals. Dose may be increased during the first 2 weeks to a maximum daily dose of 3 mg/kg or 100 mg, whichever is smaller. Over the next several weeks, the dose may be increased to a maximum daily dose of 200 mg.
- After titration, the total daily dose may be given once daily at bedtime to minimize daytime sedation.
- A high incidence of sexual dysfunction in males has been reported. There is also a significant risk of seizures.
- Notify your doctor if you experience drowsiness, dizziness, or postural hypotension (dizziness or lightheadedness when rising from a seated or lying position). Your doctor may need to reduce dose.

## Guidelines for Use (cont.):

*Desipramine:*

- Usual adult target dose is 100 to 200 mg/day. In some patients, dosage may be increased gradually to 300 mg if necessary. Doses above 300 mg/day are not recommended. Patients needing as much as 300 mg should generally be hospitalized.
- The usual target dose for children and elderly is 25 to 100 mg/day. Usual maximum dosage is 100 mg/day. Doses above 150 mg/day are not recommended.
- Initial therapy may be administered in divided doses or as a single daily dose.
- Maintenance dose may be given on a once-daily schedule.
- Usually start with low doses and gradually increase based on response and tolerance.

*Doxepin:*

- For most patients with mild-to-moderate illness, starting dose is 75 mg/day. Usual optimum dose is 75 to 150 mg/day.
- In patients with mild symptoms, doses may be as low as 25 to 50 mg/day.
- The total daily dose may be taken on a divided or once-a-day dosage schedule. If the once-a-day schedule is employed, the maximum recommended dose is 150 mg/day, which may be given at bedtime.
- The 150 mg capsule strength is intended for maintenance therapy only and is not recommended for initiation of treatment.
- *Oral concentrate* should be diluted just prior to administration with 120 mL (½ cup) of water; whole or skimmed milk; or orange, grapefruit, tomato, prune, or pineapple juice. Doxepin oral concentrate is not compatible with a number of carbonated beverages. For those patients requiring antidepressant therapy who are on methadone maintenance, mix oral concentrate and methadone syrup together with *Gatorade*, lemonade, orange juice, sugar water, *Tang*, or water, but not with grape juice. Preparation and storage of bulk dilution is not recommended.

*Imipramine HCl:*

- Usual initial adult dose for outpatients is 75 mg/day increased to 150 mg/day. Doses over 200 mg/day are not recommended. Maintenance dose is 50 to 150 mg/day.
- For hospitalized patients, usual initial adult dosage is 100 mg/day in divided doses gradually increased to 200 mg/day as required. If no response occurs after 2 weeks, increase dose to 250 to 300 mg/day.
- For adolescents and elderly patients, usual initial dose is 30 to 40 mg/day, not to exceed 100 mg/day.
- *Childhood bedwetting* — An oral dosage of 25 mg/day given 1 hour before bedtime should be tried in children 6 years of age and older.
- If satisfactory response does not occur within 1 week, increase the dose to 50 mg nightly in children younger than 12 years of age; children older than 12 may receive up to 75 mg nightly.
- Doses larger than 75 mg do not work better and tend to increase the side effects.
- In early night bedwetters, the drug is more effective given earlier and in divided amounts (ie, 25 mg in midafternoon, repeated at bedtime).

## Guidelines for Use (cont.):

*Imipramine HCl (cont.):*

- Consider instituting a drug-free period following an adequate therapeutic trial with a favorable response.
- To reduce the tendency to relapse, taper dosage gradually rather than discontinue abruptly.

*Imipramine pamoate:*

- Initiate adult dose for outpatients at 75 mg/day and increase to 150 mg/day, which is the dose level at which optimum response is usually obtained. If necessary, dose may be increased to 200 mg/day. Doses higher than 75 mg/day may also be administered on a once-a-day basis at bedtime after the optimum dosage and tolerance have been determined.
- Maintenance dosage is usually 75 to 150 mg/day administered on a once-a-day basis, preferably at bedtime.

*Nortriptyline:*

- Usual adult dosage is 25 mg 3 to 4 times daily. As an alternative regimen, the total daily dose may be given once a day.
- Doses above 150 mg/day per day are not recommended.
- Usual dosage in elderly patients is 30 to 50 mg/day in divided doses.

*Protriptyline:*

- Usual adult dosage is 15 to 40 mg/day divided into 3 or 4 doses. If necessary, dose may be increased to 60 mg/day. Make dose increases with the morning dose.
- Doses above 60 mg/day are not recommended.
- For elderly patients, the usual dosage is 5 mg 3 times a day initially and is increased gradually. The cardiovascular system must be monitored closely if the daily dose exceeds 20 mg.

*Trimipramine:*

- Usual initial adult dosage for outpatients is 75 mg/day in divided doses. May be increased to 150 mg/day if needed.
- Doses over 200 mg/day are not recommended.
- Hospitalized patients may be given 100 mg/day initially in divided doses, increased gradually in a few days to 200 mg/day. If improvement does not occur in 2 to 3 weeks, the dose may be increased to the maximum recommended dose of 250 to 300 mg/day.
- Usual initial dose for adolescents and elderly patients is 50 mg/day, increasing in gradual increments up to 100 mg/day.

*If you have any questions, consult your doctor, pharmacist, or health care provider.*

| Generic Name<br>*Brand Name Examples* | Supplied As | Generic<br>Available |
|---|---|---|
| Rx **Risperidone** | | |
| *Risperdal* | **Tablets:** 0.25 mg, 0.5 mg,<br>1 mg, 2 mg, 3 mg, 4 mg | No |
| *Risperdal* | **Solution, oral:** 1 mg/mL | No |
| Rx **Ziprasidone HCl**[1] | | |
| *Geodon* | **Capsules:** 20 mg, 40 mg,<br>60 mg, 80 mg | No |

[1] Also available as an injection.

## Type of Drug:

Atypical antipsychotic.

## How the Drug Works:

The exact mechanism of action, like other drugs used to treat schizophrenia, is not known. Benzisoxazole drugs may work by antagonizing dopamine type 2 and serotonin type 2 receptors in the brain.

## Uses:

For treatment of schizophrenia.

## Precautions:

*Do not use in the following situations:*

>abnormal heart rhythm (arrythmia), history of
>acute myocardial infarction, recent
>allergy to the drug or any of its ingredients
>drugs that prolong QT interval (see Drug Interactions)
>QT prolongation, history of
>uncompensated heart failure

*Use with caution in the following situations:*

cardiac conduction abnormalities
cerebrovascular disease
dehydration
dysphagia
heart failure
ischemic heart disease
kidney disease (risperidone, ziprasidone injection only)
liver disease
myocardial infarction, history of
seizures, history of

*Tardive dyskinesia:* Involuntary and uncontrollable movements may develop in patients treated with antipsychotic drugs. Occurrence is highest in the elderly, especially women. However, it is impossible to predict which patients are likely to develop the syndrome. The risk of developing these involuntary movements and the likelihood they will become permanent are increased with long-term use and with high doses. However, it is possible to develop these symptoms after short-term treatment at low doses. The syndrome is characterized by rhythmical, involuntary movements of tongue, face, mouth, or jaw (eg, protrusion of tongue, puffing of cheeks, puckering of mouth, chewing movements), sometimes accompanied by involuntary movements of the arms and legs. Fine worm-like movement of the tongue may be an early sign of the syndrome. If the medication is stopped at this time, the syndrome may not develop further. There is no known treatment for established cases of tardive dyskinesia, although the syndrome may stop, partially or completely, if the drug is withdrawn. Antipsychotic treatment, however, may suppress or partially suppress the signs and symptoms of the syndrome and thereby may possibly mask the underlying disease process. The effect that symptomatic suppression has upon the long-term course of the syndrome is unknown.

*Neuroleptic Malignant Syndrome (NMS)* is a potentially fatal syndrome associated with antipsychotic drugs. Symptoms include fever, muscle rigidity, altered mental abilities, irregular pulse and blood pressure, increased heart rate, sweating, and irregular heart rhythm.

*Pregnancy:* There are no adequate and well-controlled studies in pregnant women. Use only if clearly needed and potential benefits outweigh the possible hazards to the fetus.

*Breastfeeding:* It is not known if benisoxazole derivatives appear in breast milk. It is recommended that women not breastfeed while receiving these drugs.

*Children:* The safety and effectiveness in patients younger than 18 years of age have not been established.

*Elderly:* Dose modifications (ie, lower starting dose) of risperidone may be necessary. Ziprasidone injection has not been evaluated in patients 65 years of age and older.

*Lab tests* may be required to monitor ziprasidone therapy. Tests include serum potassium and magnesium levels.

## Drug Interactions:
Tell your doctor or pharmacist if you are taking or planning to take any over-the-counter or prescription medications or dietary supplements with these drugs. Doses of one or both drugs may need to be modified or a different drug may need to be prescribed. The following drugs and drug classes interact with these drugs:

antihypertensive agents (eg, hydrochlorothiazide)
carbamazepine (eg, *Tegretol*)
centrally acting drugs (eg, guanfacine, tramadol)
clozapine (eg, *Clozaril*)
dopamine agonists (eg, pramipexole)

drugs that prolong the QT interval (eg, chlorpromazine, quinidine, sparfloxacin)
fluoxetine (eg, *Prozac*)
ketoconazole (eg, *Nizoral*)

## Side Effects:

Every drug is capable of producing side effects. Many patients experience no, or minor, side effects. The frequency and severity of side effects depend on many factors including dose, duration of therapy, and individual susceptibility. Possible side effects include:

*Digestive Tract:* Nausea; constipation; indigestion; diarrhea; dry mouth; vomiting; stomach pain; increased or decreased saliva; toothache; appetite loss.

*Respiratory System:* Upper respiratory infection; cough; rhinitis; sinus infection; sore throat; difficulty breathing; runny nose.

*Nervous System:* Sleepiness; dizziness; inability to sit still; muscle tension; headache; anxiety; agitation; increased dream activity; abnormal tongue, face, jaw, or mouth movements; involuntary arm and leg movements; tremor; shuffling; rigidity.

*Circulatory System:* Increased or decreased heart rate; postural hypotension (light-headedness when rising quickly from sitting or lying position); increased blood pressure.

*Skin:* Rash; skin irritation; dry skin; sensitivity to light.

*Other:* Weakness; muscle pain; joint pain; fainting; dizziness; erectile dysfunction; weight gain; decreased sexual desire; abnormal vision.

---

### Guidelines for Use:

- Dosage is individualized. Take exactly as prescribed.
- Do not stop taking or change the dose unless instructed by your doctor.
- Swallow the ziprasidone capsules whole; take with food.
- It is best to take ziprasidone at the same time each day.
- It may take a few weeks for this medicine to start working. Continue taking the medication, even when you feel better.
- Avoid alcohol while taking this medicine.
- Use caution in hot weather; be careful not to become dehydrated.
- Notify your doctor immediately if you experience fever, perspiration, muscle rigidity, involuntary movements, abnormal heart rate or rhythm, or fainting.
- May cause drowsiness. Use caution while driving or performing other tasks requiring alertness, coordination, or physical dexterity.
- This medicine may cause dizziness, light-headedness, or fainting, especially when rising or standing. If these symptoms occur, sit or lie down. Contact your doctor if they continue.
- Inform your doctor if you are pregnant, become pregnant, are planning to become pregnant, or if you are breastfeeding.
- Lab tests may be required to monitor therapy. Be sure to keep appointments.
- Store at controlled room temperature (59° to 86°F). Protect from light and moisture.

---

*If you have any questions, consult your doctor, pharmacist, or health care provider.*

| Generic Name<br>*Brand Name Example* | Supplied As | Generic<br>Available |
|---|---|---|
| *Rx* **Clozapine** | | |
| *Clozaril* | **Tablets**: 25 mg, 100 mg | Yes |
| *Rx* **Loxapine Succinate** | | |
| *Loxitane* | **Capsules**: 5 mg, 10 mg,<br>25 mg, 50 mg | Yes |
| *Rx* **Olanzapine** | | |
| *Zyprexa* | **Tablets**: 2.5 mg, 5 mg, 7.5 mg,<br>10 mg, 15 mg, 20 mg | No |
| *Zyprexa* | **Tablets, orally disintegrating**:<br>5 mg, 10 mg, 15 mg, 20 mg | No |
| *Rx* **Quetiapine Fumarate** | | |
| *Seroquel* | **Tablets**: 25 mg, 100 mg,<br>200 mg, 300 mg | No |

## Type of Drug:
Atypical antipsychotic.

## How the Drug Works:
Atypical antipsychotics act upon several neurotransmitter systems, including antagonism at one or more types of dopamine receptors, antagonism at alpha$_1$–adrenergic receptors, and activity at muscarinic, histamine H$_1$, or nicotinic receptors.

## Uses:
For the treatment of schizophrenia.

*Olanzapine:* For the short-term treatment of acute manic episodes associated with Bipolar I disorder.

## Precautions:
*Do not use in the following situations:*
allergy to the drug or any of its ingredients
epilepsy, uncontrolled
drug-induced agranulocytosis, history of
therapy with drugs that cause agranulocytosis or myelosuppression, current
myeloproliferative disorders
severe granulocytopenia, history of

*Use with caution in the following situations:*
agitated state with depression
aspiration pneumonia, at risk for
alcohol withdrawal
exposure to extreme heat
glaucoma, history of
heart disease
kidney disease
narrow-angle glaucoma
paralytic ileus, history of
phosphorus incesticide exposure
prostatic hypertrophy
seizures, history of or predisposition to

*Tardive dyskinesia:* Involuntary and uncontrollable movements may develop in patients treated with antipsychotic drugs. Occurrence is highest in the elderly, especially women. However, it is impossible to predict which patients are likely to develop the syndrome. The risk of developing these involuntary movements and the likelihood they will become permanent are increased with long-term use and with high doses. However, it is possible to develop these symptoms after short-term treatment at low doses. The syndrome is characterized by rhythmical, involuntary movements of tongue, face, mouth, or jaw (eg, protrusion of tongue, puffing of cheeks, puckering of mouth, chewing movements), sometimes accompanied by involuntary movements of the arms and legs. Fine worm-like movement of the tongue may be an early sign of the syndrome. If the medication is stopped at this time, the syndrome may not develop further. There is no known treatment for established cases of tardive dyskinexia, although the syndrome may stop, partially or completely, if the drug is withdrawn. Antipsychotic treatment, however, may suppress or partially suppress the signs and symptoms of the syndrome and thereby may possibly mask the underlying disease process. The effect that symptomatic suppression has upon the long-term course of the syndrome is unknown.

*Neuroleptic Malignant Syndrome (NMS)* is a potentially fatal syndrome associated with antipsychotic drugs. Symptoms include fever, muscle rigidity, altered mental abilities, irregular pulse and blood pressure, increased heart rate, sweating, and irregular heart rhythm.

*Seizures:* Seizures have occurred during therapy with some antipsychotic agents. The likelihood of seizure becomes greater at higher doses.

*Pregnancy:* There are no adequate and well-controlled studies in pregnant women. Use only if clearly needed and the potential benefits outweigh the possible hazards to the fetus.

*Breastfeeding:* It is not known if these drugs are excreted in breast milk. Do not use breastfeed while taking one of these drugs.

*Children:* Safety and effectiveness of loxapine in patients younger than 16 years of age have not been established. Safety and effectiveness of clozapine, olanzapine, and quetiapine have not been established.

*Lab tests* will be required to monitor therapy. Tests include blood counts and liver function.

## Drug Interactions:
Tell your doctor or pharmacist if you are taking or if you are planning to take any over-the-counter or prescription medications or dietary supplements with these drugs. Doses of one or both drugs may need to be modified or a different drug may need to be prescribed. The following drugs and drug classes interact with these drugs:

anticholinergics (eg, diphenhydramine)
antihypertensives (eg, methyldopa)
carbamazepine (eg, *Tegretol*)
cimetidine (eg, *Tagamet*)

dopamine agonists (eg, bromocriptine)
lorazepam (eg, *Ativan*)
phenytoin (eg, *Dilantin*)
risperidone (*Risperdal*)
thioridazine (eg, *Mellaril*)

## Side Effects:

Every drug is capable of producing side effects. Many patients experience no, or minor, side effects. The frequency and severity of side effects depend on many factors including dose, duration of therapy and individual susceptibility. Possible side effects include:

*Circulatory System:* Increased heart rate; changes in blood pressure; chest pain; abnormal blood counts; increased cholesterol levels.

*Nervous System:* Drowsiness; dizziness; agitation; confusion; seizures; aggressiveness; amnesia; anxiety; disturbed sleep; personality disorder; restlessness; rigidity; slurred speech; stuttering; fainting; tremor.

*Digestive Tract:* Constipation; dry mouth; stomach pain; diarrhea; indigestion; nausea; vomiting; increased appetite.

*Respiratory System:* Coughing; difficulty breathing; runny nose; nasal congestion; upper respiratory tract infection.

*Other:* Rash; orthostatic hypotension (dizziness or light-headedness that occurs when rising quickly from a seated or lying position); prolonged erection; Parkinson-like symptoms; Neuroleptic Malignant Syndrome; tardive dyskinesia; dry skin; toothache; premenstrual syndrome; swelling of the arms or legs; joint, muscle, or back pain; twitching; sore throat; weakness; fever; sweating; visual disturbances; weight gain; false-positive pregnancy tests.

## Guidelines for Use:

- Dosage is individualized. Take exactly as prescribed.
- Do not stop taking or change the dose, unless instructed by your doctor.
- *Orally-disintegrating tablets* — Peel back foil blister; do not push tablet through the foil. Using dry hands, remove and place the entire tablet in your mouth. The tablet will dissolve with or without liquid.
- If a dose is missed, take it as soon as possible. If several hours have passed or it is nearing time for the next dose, do not double the dose to catch up, unless instructed by your doctor. If more than one dose is missed or it is necessary to establish a new dosage schedule, contact your doctor or pharmacist.
- May take several weeks before maximum benefit is obtained.
- May cause drowsiness, dizziness, or seizures. Use caution while driving or performing other tasks requiring alertness, coordination, or physical dexterity.
- Orthostatic hypotension (dizziness or drowsiness when rising quickly from a seated or lying position) may occur. Avoid sudden changes in posture.
- Notify your doctor immediately if you experience abnormal or impaired vision, lethargy, weakness, sore throat, general body discomfort, mucous membrane ulcerations, flu-like symptoms, tremor, muscle twitching or stiffness, or yellowing of the skin or eyes (jaundice).
- Use caution in hot weather. These drugs may increase the possibility of heat stroke. Avoid overheating and dehydration.
- Avoid consuming alcoholic beverages and other mental depressants (eg, narcotics, antihistamines) while taking this medicine.
- Inform your doctor if you are pregnant, become pregnant, plan on becoming pregnant, or are breastfeeding.
- Lab tests will be required to monitor therapy. Be sure to keep appointments.
- Store at controlled room temperature (59° to 86°F). Protect from light and moisture.

*If you have any questions, consult your doctor, pharmacist, or health care provider.*

| Generic Name<br>*Brand Name Example* | Supplied As | Generic<br>Available |
|---|---|---|
| *Rx* **Molindone HCl** | | |
| *Moban* | **Tablets:** 5 mg, 10 mg, 25 mg,<br>50 mg, 100 mg | No |
| *Moban*[1] | **Oral concentrate:** 20 mg/mL | No |

[1] Contains sulfites.

## Type of Drug:
Typical (conventional) antipsychotic.

## How the Drug Works:
The exact mechanism of action, like other drugs used to treat psychotic disorders, is not known.

## Uses:
For the management of manifestation of psychotic disorders (mental illnesses).

## Precautions:
*Do not use in the following situations:*
allergy to molindone or any of its ingredients
central nervous system depression (due to alcohol, barbiturates, or other drugs) or comatose states

*Tardive dyskinesia:* Involuntary and uncontrollable movements may develop in patients treated with antipsychotic drugs. Occurrence is highest in the elderly, especially women. However, it is impossible to predict which patients are likely to develop the syndrome. The risk of developing these involuntary movements and the likelihood they will become permanent are increased with long-term use and with high doses. However, it is possible to develop these symptoms after short-term treatment at low doses. The syndrome is characterized by rhythmical, involuntary movements of tongue, face, mouth, or jaw (eg, protrusion of tongue, puffing of cheeks, puckering of mouth, chewing movements), sometimes accompanied by involuntary movements of the arms and legs. Fine worm-like movement of the tongue may be an early sign of the syndrome. If the medication is stopped at this time, the syndrome may not develop further. There is no known treatment for established cases of tardive dyskinexia, although the syndrome may stop, partially or completely, if the drug is withdrawn. Antipsychotic treatment, however, may suppress or partially suppress the signs and symptoms of the syndrome and thereby may possibly mask the underlying disease process. The effect that symptomatic suppression has upon the long-term course of the syndrome is unknown.

*Neuroleptic Malignant Syndrome (NMS)* is a potentially fatal syndrome associated with antipsychotic drugs. Symptoms include fever, muscle rigidity, altered mental abilities, irregular pulse and blood pressure, increased heart rate, sweating, and irregular heart rhythm.

*Pregnancy:* There are no adequate and well-controlled studies in pregnant women. Use only if clearly needed and the potential benefits outweigh the possible hazards to the fetus.

*Breastfeeding:* It is not known if molindone appears in breast milk. Consult your doctor before you begin breastfeeding.

*Children:* Safety and effectiveness in children younger than 12 years of age have not been established; use is not recommended.

*Sulfites:* Molindone concentrate contains sodium metabisulfite, a sulfite that may cause allergic-type reactions, including anaphylactic symptoms and life-threatening or less severe asthmatic episodes in certain susceptible people. The overall prevalence of sulfite sensitivity in the general population is unknown and probably low. Sulfite sensitivity is seen more frequently in asthmatic than in nonasthmatic people.

## Drug Interactions:

Tell your doctor or pharmacist if you are taking or are planning to take any over-the-counter or prescription medications or dietary supplements while taking this drug. Doses or one or both drugs may need to be modified or a different drug may need to be prescribed. The following drugs and drug classes may interact with this drug:

CNS depressants (eg, antianxiety agents, narcotics, sedatives/hypnotics)

phenytoin (eg, *Dilantin*)
tetracyclines (eg, doxycycline)

## Side Effects:

Every drug is capable of producing side effects. Many patients experience no, or minor, side effects. The frequency and severity of side effects depend on many factors including dose, duration of therapy, and individual susceptibility. Possible side effects include:

*Digestive Tract:* Constipation; dry mouth; increased salivation; nausea.

*Nervous System:* Drowsiness; inability to sit still; euphoria (exaggerated sense of well being); depression; tremor; twitching, abnormal movements; rigidity; immobility; abnormal movement of tongue, face, mouth, or jaw; involuntary arm or leg movement.

*Urinary and Reproductive Tract:* Urinary retention; absence of menstrual bleeding; heavy menstrual bleeding.

*Other:* Rash; weight changes; increased libido; blurred vision, persistent penile erection; impotence; fever; perspiration; rapid heart beat.

## Guidelines for Use:

- Dosage is individualized. Take exactly as prescribed.
- Do not stop taking or change the dose, unless instructed by your doctor.
- A combination of factors, (eg, people older than 65 years of age, females) may require dose adjustment.
- May be taken with or without food.
- If a dose is missed, take it as soon as possible. If several hours have passed or it is nearing time for the next dose, do not double the dose to catch up, unless instructed by your doctor. If more than one dose is missed or if it is necessary to establish a new dosage schedule, contact your doctor or pharmacist.
- Avoid alcohol and other mental depressants (eg, narcotics, tranquilizers, antihistamines) while you are taking this medicine.
- May cause drowsiness. Use caution while driving or performing other tasks requiring alertness, coordination, or physical dexterity.
- Contact your doctor immediately if you experience fever, sweating, muscle rigidity, involuntary movements (of the face, tongue, arms, or legs), menstrual irregularities, rash, or abnormal heart rate or rhythm.
- Inform your doctor if you are pregnant, become pregnant, are planning to become pregnant, or are breastfeeding.
- Store at controlled room temperature (59° to 86°F) away from light and moisture.

*If you have any questions, consult your doctor, pharmacist, or health care provider.*

| Generic Name<br>*Brand Name Examples* | Supplied As | Generic Available |
|---|---|---|
| Rx **Chlorpromazine HCl**[1] | **Concentrate, oral:**[2] 30 mg/mL, 100 mg/mL | Yes |
| *Thorazine* | **Tablets:** 10 mg, 25 mg, 50 mg, 100 mg, 200 mg | Yes |
| *Thorazine* | **Syrup:** 10 mg/5 mL | No |
| *Thorazine* | **Suppositories:** 25 mg, 100 mg | No |
| Rx **Fluphenazine HCl**[1] | **Tablets:** 1 mg, 2.5 mg, 5 mg, 10 mg | Yes |
| Rx **Mesoridazine**[1] | | |
| *Serentil* | **Tablets:** 10 mg, 25 mg, 50 mg, 100 mg | No |
| *Serentil* | **Concentrate, oral:** 25 mg/mL | No |
| Rx **Perphenazine**[1] | | |
| *Trilafon* | **Tablets:** 2 mg, 4 mg, 8 mg, 16 mg | Yes |
| Rx **Prochlorperazine**[1] | | |
| *Compazine* | **Tablets:** 5 mg, 10 mg | Yes |
| *Compazine* | **Capsules, sustained release:** 10 mg, 15 mg | No |
| *Compazine* | **Suppositories:** 2.5 mg, 5 mg | No |
| *Compazine, Compro* | **Suppositories:** 25 mg | Yes |
| *Compazine* | **Syrup:** 5 mg/5 mL | No |
| Rx **Thioridazine HCl** | | |
| *Mellaril* | **Tablets:** 10 mg, 15 mg, 25 mg, 50 mg, 100 mg, 200 mg | Yes |
| *Mellaril* | **Concentrate, oral:** 30 mg/mL, 100 mg/mL | Yes |
| *Mellaril-S* | **Suspension:** 5 mg/5 mL, 20 mg/5 mL | No |
| Rx **Trifluoperazine HCl**[1] | | |
| *Stelazine* | **Tablets:** 1 mg, 2 mg, 5 mg, 10 mg | Yes |
| *Stelazine* | **Concentrate, oral:** 10 mg/mL | No |

[1] Also available as an injection.
[2] Contains sulfites.

## Type of Drug:

Typical (conventional) antipsychotic.

## How the Drug Works:

The exact mechanism of action of antipsychotic agents is not fully understood. It is believed antipsychotic agents reduce nerve sensitivity in different areas of the brain. They are not used to treat anxiety but can improve concentration and self control in severely mentally ill (psychotic or schizophrenic) patients.

## Uses:

*All phenothiazine derivatives:* To reduce symptoms of psychosis (mental illness).

*Chlorpromazine:* To control the manic phase of manic depression.

To relieve restlessness and apprehension prior to surgery.

To treat tetanus when used with other drugs.

To treat acute intermittent porphyria.

To treat severe behavioral problems in children, including combativeness, explosive hyperactivity, and hyperactivity (short-term).

To control nausea and vomiting.

To relieve intractable hiccups.

*Mesoridazine:* To treat schizophrenia.

*Perphenazine:* To treat schizophrenia.

To control nausea and vomiting.

*Prochlorperazine:* For short-term treatment of non-psychotic anxiety. Not the drug of choice.

To control severe nausea and vomiting.

*Thioridazine:* To treat schizophrenia in patients who fail to respond to other antipsychotic drugs.

*Trifluoperazine:* To treat schizophrenia.

For short-term treatment of non-psychotic anxiety. Not the drug of choice.

*Unlabeled Use(s):* Occasionally doctors may prescribe antipsychotic agents to treat migraine headaches (chlorpromazine, prochlorperazine), severe vascular or tension headaches (prochlorperazine), hemiballismus (perphenazine), Huntington chorea (chlorpromazine, fluphenazine), hiccups (perphenazine), or PCP psychosis (chlorpromazine).

## Precautions:

*Do not use in the following situations:*

allergy to the drug or any of its ingredients
blood disorders due to antipsychotics

blood pressure, extremes (thioridazine only)
bone marrow depression
brain damage

CNS depressants (alcohol, barbiturates, narcotics), large
amounts
CNS depression, severe
coma
coronary artery disease
epilepsy
glaucoma
liver disease
overactive thyroid
pediatric surgery (prochlorperazine only)
sedation

*Use with caution in the following situations:*
alcohol withdrawal
angina (trifluoperazine only)
anticholinergics (eg, atropine)
  use
brain damage
breast cancer
bronchitis, chronic
chronic respiratory problems
  (eg, severe asthma, emphysema, acute respiratory infections, especially in children)
circulatory problems
depression
elderly
electroshock therapy, previous
exposure to extreme heat or
  cold
exposure to organophosphorus
  insecticides
glaucoma
heart disease
kidney disease
lithium (eg, *Lithobid*) use, current
liver disease
myelogram testing (within 24
  hours)
Neuroleptic Malignant Syndrome, history of
pheochromocytoma (vascular
  tumor of adrenal medulla)
seizures, history
skin inflammation
surgery
urinary retention, tendency
thyroid, overactive

*Tardive dyskinesia:* Involuntary and uncontrollable movements may
develop in patients treated with antipsychotic drugs. Occurrence is highest in the elderly, especially women. However, it is impossible to predict which patients are likely to develop the syndrome. The risk of
developing these involuntary movements and the likelihood they will
become permanent are increased with long-term use and with high
doses. However, it is possible to develop these symptoms after short-
term treatment at low doses. The syndrome is characterized by rhythmical, involuntary movements of tongue, face, mouth, or jaw (eg, protrusion
of tongue, puffing of cheeks, puckering of mouth, chewing movements),
sometimes accompanied by involuntary movements of the arms and
legs. Fine worm-like movement of the tongue may be an early sign of the
syndrome. If the medication is stopped at this time, the syndrome may
not develop further. There is no known treatment for established cases
of tardive dyskinesia, although the syndrome may stop, partially or completely, if the drug is withdrawn. Antipsychotic treatment, however, may
suppress or partially suppress the signs and symptoms of the syndrome and thereby may possibly mask the underlying disease process.
The effect that symptomatic suppression has upon the long-term course
of the syndrome is unknown.

*Neuroleptic Malignant Syndrome (NMS)* is a potentially fatal syndrome
associated with antipsychotic drugs. Symptoms include fever, muscle
rigidity, altered mental abilities, irregular pulse and blood pressure,
increased heart rate, sweating, and irregular heart rhythm.

*Abrupt withdrawal:* These drugs are not known to cause dependence and do not produce tolerance or addiction. However, following abrupt withdrawal of high dose therapy, symptoms such as nausea, vomiting, dizziness, tremors, headache, upset stomach, and increased heart rate have been reported. Symptoms occurred in 1 to 4 days and subsided in 1 to 2 weeks. These symptoms can be reduced by a gradual decrease in dosage or by continuing antiparkinson agents for several weeks after the antipsychotic agent is withdrawn.

*Skin discoloration:* Rare instances of skin pigmentation have occurred, primarily in females on long-term, high dose therapy. These changes, restricted to exposed areas of the skin, range from a very slight darkening to a slate gray color, sometimes with a violet hue. Pigmentation may fade following drug discontinuation. Use caution against exposure to ultraviolet light (eg, tanning booths) or undue exposure to sunlight. These effects occur most commonly with chlorpromazine.

*Eye changes:* Ocular changes have occasionally occurred in patients receiving long-term, high dose therapy. Eye changes are characterized by deposits of fine particular matter in the lens and cornea. Eye lesions may regress after drug discontinuation. Exposure to light, along with dosage and duration of therapy, seem to be the most significant factor in this reaction.

*PKU tests:* These drugs may produce false-positive phenylketonuria (PKU) test results.

*Pregnancy:* Safety for use during pregnancy is not established. Some newborns of women using these medicines have experienced prolonged jaundice and abnormal movements and reflexes. Use only when clearly needed and the potential benefits outweigh the possible hazards to the fetus.

*Breastfeeding:* Chlorpromazine appears in breast milk. Consult your doctor about this and other antipsychotic agents before you begin breastfeeding.

*Children:* In general, these products are not recommended for children younger than 12 years of age. Phenothiazine use in children younger than 1 year of age may be a factor in sudden infant death syndrome (SIDS). Children with acute illnesses (eg, chickenpox, measles) or dehydration appear much more susceptible to neuromuscular reactions than adults. Symptoms can occur and may be confused with the signs of an undiagnosed primary disease responsible for the vomiting (eg, Reye syndrome). Avoid antipsychotic agents in children and adolescents whose symptoms (eg, vomiting, hyperactivity, confusion) suggest Reye syndrome.

*Mesoridazine* – Safety and effectiveness is not established in children.

*Prochlorperazine* – Contraindicated in children under 20 pounds or younger than 2 years of age. Do not use in pediatric surgery. Children seem more prone to develop Parkinson-like reactions. Use the lowest effective dose. Occasionally, the patient may react to the drug with restlessness and excitement. If this occurs, do not administer additional doses. Use with caution in children with acute illnesses or dehydration. Not for use in conditions for which children's dosages are not established.

*Trifluoperazine* – This drug is for children, aged 6 to 12 years, who are hospitalized or under close supervision. Dosage must be adjusted to the weight of the child and severity of symptoms.

*Elderly:* Low doses are usually sufficient for elderly patients. These patients are more susceptible to lowered blood pressure and other side effects. Doses should be increased gradually.

*Lab tests* may be required during therapy. Tests include eye exams, blood counts, and kidney and liver function tests.

*Sulfites:* Some of these products may contain sulfite preservatives that can cause allergic reactions in certain individuals. Check package label when available or consult your doctor or pharmacist.

## Drug Interactions:

Tell your doctor or pharmacist if you are taking or if you are planning to take any over-the-counter or prescription medications or dietary supplements while taking these drugs. Doses of one or both drugs may need to be modified or a different drug may need to be prescribed. The following drugs and drug classes may interact with these drugs:

ACE inhibitors (eg, captopril)
alcohol
aluminum-containing antacids
 (eg, *Rolaids*)
anticholinergics (eg, atropine)
anticoagulants (eg, warfarin)
antihistamines (eg, diphenhydramine)
appetite suppressants
barbiturate anesthetics
 (eg, methohexital)
beta-blockers (eg, propranolol)
bromocriptine (*Parlodel*)
charcoal
cimetidine (eg, *Tagamet*)
clonidine (eg, *Catapres*)
clozapine (*Clozaril*)
CNS depressants (eg, anesthetics, barbiturates, narcotics)
diazoxide (eg, *Proglycem*)
disulfiram (eg, *Antabuse*)
dopamine (eg, *Intropin*)
epinephrine (eg, *Adrenalin*)

guanethidine (eg, *Ismelin*)
hydantoins (eg, phenytoin)
hydroxyzine (eg, *Atarax*)
levodopa (eg, *Larodopa*)
lithium (eg, *Eskalith*)
meperidine (eg, *Demerol*)
methyldopa (eg, *Aldomet*)
metrizamide (*Amipaque*)
norepinephrine (*Levophed*)
opiates
piperazine (eg, *Antepar*)
polypeptide antibiotics (eg, polymyxin B)
quinidine (eg, *Quinora*)
succinylcholine (eg, *Anectine*)
sympathomimetics
thiazide diuretics (eg, hydro-
 chorothiazides)
trazodone (eg, *Desyrel*)
tricyclic antidepressants
 (eg, amitriptyline)
valproic acid (eg, *Depakene*)
vitamin C

## Side Effects:

Every drug is capable of producing side effects. Many patients experience no, or minor, side effects. The frequency and severity of side effects depend on many factors including dose, duration of therapy, and individual susceptibility. Possible side effects include:

*Hormones:* Appearance of milk and breast engorgement in women; breast enlargement in men; menstrual irregularities; loss of menstruation; changes in sex drive or ability; changes in blood sugar levels; false-positive pregnancy tests; dry vagina.

*Muscular System:* Muscle spasms or aches; aching and numbness of legs and arms; lockjaw; protrusion, discoloration, aching, and rounding of the tongue; tightness in throat; weakness; inability to sit still; exaggeration of reflexes; joint pain or stiffness; difficulty moving.

*Digestive Tract:* Appetite changes; nausea; vomiting; constipation; diarrhea; stomach pain or upset; fecal impaction; dry mouth; excess salivation; reduced salivation; swallowing difficulty; tongue protrusion; swollen tongue; excessive thirst; reduced thirst; sore mouth or gums; excessive eating.

*Circulatory System:* Changes in blood pressure; orthostatic hypotension (dizziness or light-headedness when rising quickly from a sitting or lying position); fainting; changes in heart rate; heart attack; blood cholesterol level changes; abnormal blood counts; anemia.

*Psychiatric:* Hallucinations; catatonia; restlessness; hyperactivity; confusion; depression; agitation; increased dream activity; bizarre dreams; exaggerated sense of well being (euphoria); excitement; lethargy; paranoid reactions; aggressiveness; sedation.

*Nervous System:* Headache; drowsiness (about 1 to 2 weeks); increased sleep duration; dizziness; light-headedness; nervousness; tremors; jitteriness; clumsiness; sleeplessness; anxiety; feeling of whirling motion (vertigo); slurred speech; seizures; fatigue; twitching; tension; numbness.

*Respiratory System:* Spasms of larynx and bronchial tubes (breathing passages); nasal congestion; increased depth of breathing; painful or difficult breathing; asthma; sore throat; cough; sinus problems; upper respiratory infections.

*Skin:* Hives; rash; oily skin; redness; itching; sensitivity to light; hair loss; pallor; flushing; sweating; discoloration; lesions; swelling; dry skin; yellowing of skin.

*Eyes or Ocular:* Glaucoma; sensitivity to light; blurred vision; changes in pupil size; cataracts; problems with cornea, lens, and retina; abnormal vision; drooping eyelid; brownish coloring of vision, abnormal eye movements; impairment of night vision (thioridazine only); yellowing of eyes.

*Urinary and Reproductive Tract:* Urinary retention; increased urination; glucose in urine; lack of bladder control; persistent or painful erections; frequent urination; painful or difficult urination; bedwetting.

*Other:* Toothache; swelling in hands or feet; weight gain; heatstroke; fever; chills; problems with body temperature regulation; back or chest pain; swollen glands; Parkinson-like symptoms; tardive dyskinesia; Neuroleptic Malignant Syndrome.

## Guidelines for Use:

- Dosage is individualized. Use exactly as prescribed.
- Do not stop taking or change the dose, unless instructed by your doctor.
- If a dose is missed, take it as soon as possible. If several hours have passed or it is nearing time for the next dose, do not double the dose to catch up, unless instructed by your doctor. If more than one dose is missed or it is necessary to establish a new dosage schedule, contact your doctor or pharmacist.
- Oral agents may be ineffective if expelled after vomiting has already begun. Consider use of injection or suppositories under such circumstances.
- Take these drugs routinely as directed. They control illness symptoms. They are not addicting.
- Improvement may not be seen for several weeks.
- May cause dizziness, drowsiness, or blurred vision. Use caution while driving or performing other tasks requiring alertness, coordination, or physical dexterity.
- Avoid alcohol or other drugs that cause drowsiness while taking this medicine.
- May cause sensitivity to sunlight. Avoid prolonged exposure to the sun and other sources of ultraviolet (UV) light (eg, tanning beds). Use sunscreens and wear protective clothing until tolerance is determined.
- If dizziness or fainting occurs (more common after first injection), avoid sudden changes in posture.
- May increase susceptibility to heatstroke. Use caution in hot weather.
- Inform your doctor if you are pregnant, become pregnant, are planning to become pregnant, or are breastfeeding.
- Contact your doctor if you experience involuntary muscle twitching, involuntary movements of the tongue, stomach cramping, sore throat, fever, lethargy, decreased sensation of thirst, irregular pulse, excessive sweating, soreness of mouth, gums, or throat, symptoms of upper respiratory infection, unusual bleeding or bruising, weakness, impaired vision, pale stools, skin rash, tremors, or yellowing of skin or eyes.
- *Liquid concentrates* — Liquid concentrates are light sensitive. Keep in amber or opaque bottles and protect from light.
  These solutions are most conveniently used when diluted in fruit juices or other liquids. Use these solutions immediately after dilution.
  Avoid contact with skin (contact dermatitis may occur).
  Shake well before using.
- *Chlorpromazine concentrate*— Add desired dose to 2 oz or more of liquid just prior to use. Suggested liquids are tomato or fruit juice, milk, simple syrup, orange syrup, carbonated beverages, coffee, tea, or water. Semisolid foods (eg, soups, puddings) may also be used.
- *Mesoridazine* — Use the calibrated dropper enclosed with the package to measure the dose.
  Concentrate may be diluted just prior to use with distilled water or orange or grape juice. Do not prepare and store in bulk.
- *Thioridazine* — Add dose to 2 oz or more just prior to use. Liquids suggested are tomato or fruit juices, milk, simple syrup, orange syrup, carbonated beverages, coffee, tea, or water. Semisolid foods (eg, soup, puddings) may also be used.

## Guidelines for Use (cont.):

- *Trifluoperazine* — Concentrate is for institutional use only. Use in severe neuropsychiatric conditions when oral medication is preferred and other oral forms are impractical.
  Add concentrate dose to 2 oz or more just prior to use. Liquids suggested are tomato or fruit juices, milk, simple syrup, orange syrup, carbonated beverages, coffee, tea or water. Semisolid foods (eg, soup, puddings) may also be used.
- Store as directed by package labeling.

*If you have any questions, consult your doctor, pharmacist, or health care provider.*

| Generic Name<br>*Brand Name Example* | Supplied As | Generic<br>Available |
|---|---|---|
| *Rx* **Haloperidol**[1] | | |
| *Haldol* | **Tablet**: 0.5 mg, 1 mg, 2 mg,<br>5 mg, 10 mg, 20 mg | Yes |
| *Haldol* | **Concentrate, oral**: 2 mg/mL | Yes |
| *Rx* **Pimozide** | | |
| *Orap* | **Tablet**: 1 mg, 2 mg | No |

[1] Also available as an injection.

## Type of Drug:

Typical (conventional) antipsychotics.

## How the Drug Works:

The mechanism of action is not well defined, but thought to be related to central dopamine receptor antagonist activity.

## Uses:

Haloperidol is used in the management of manifestations of serious psychotic disorders, including schizophrenia.

Pimozide and haloperidol may be used to suppress motor and phonic tics in patients with Tourette disorder who have failed to respond to standard treatment.

*Unlabeled Use(s):* Bipolar disorder; management of patients with demetia-related psychotic symptoms.

## Precautions:

*Do not use in the following situations:*

| | |
|---|---|
| allergy to the drug or any of its ingredients | comatose states |
| | toxic CNS depression, severe |

*Use with caution in the following situations:*

| | |
|---|---|
| Alzheimer disease | liver disease |
| angina pectoris | low blood pressure |
| elderly | Parkinson disease |
| heart disease | seizures, history of |
| kidney disease | |

*Tardive dyskinesia:* Involuntary and uncontrollable movements may develop in patients treated with antipsychotic drugs. Occurrence is highest in the elderly, especially women. However, it is impossible to predict which patients are likely to develop the syndrome. The risk of developing these involuntary movements and the likelihood they will become permanent are increased with long-term use and with high doses. However, it is possible to develop these symptoms after short-term treatment at low doses. The syndrome is characterized by rhythmical, involuntary movements of tongue, face, mouth, or jaw (eg, protrusion of tongue, puffing of cheeks, puckering of mouth, chewing movements), sometimes accompanied by involuntary movements of the arms and legs. Fine worm-like movement of the tongue may be an early sign of the syndrome. If the medication is stopped at this time, the syndrome may not develop further. There is no known treatment for established cases of tardive dyskinesia, although the syndrome may stop, partially or completely, if the drug is withdrawn. Antipsychotic treatment, however, may suppress or partially suppress the signs and symptoms of the syndrome and thereby may possibly mask the underlying disease process. The effect that symptomatic suppression has upon the long-term course of the syndrome is unknown.

*Neuroleptic Malignant Syndrome (NMS)* is a potentially fatal syndrome associated with antipsychotic drugs. Symptoms include fever, muscle rigidity, altered mental abilities, irregular pulse and blood pressure, increased heart rate, sweating, and irregular heart rhythm.

*Pregnancy:* There are no adequate and well-controlled studies in pregnant women. Use only if clearly needed and the potential benefits outweigh the possible hazards to the fetus.

*Breastfeeding:* It is not known if these drugs appear in breast milk. Consult your doctor before you begin breastfeeding.

*Children:* Safety and effectiveness of haloperidol have not been established. Safety and effectiveness of pimozide in children younger than 12 years of age have not been established.

*Elderly:* A lower starting dose is recommended for elderly patients.

## Drug Interactions:
Tell your doctor or pharmacist if you are taking or planning to take any over-the-counter or prescription medications or dietary supplements with these drugs. Doses of one or both drugs may need to be modified or a different drug may need to be prescribed. The following drugs and drug classes interact with these drugs:

alcohol
amphetamines (eg, dextro-amphetamine) (pimozide only)
antiarrhythmic agents (eg, quinidine) (pimozide only)
azole antifungals (eg, fluconazole) (pimozide only)
blood pressure-lowering medicines (eg, clonidine)
buspirone (eg, *BuSpar*)
carbamazepine (eg, *Tegretol*)
clozapine (*eg, Clozaril*)
dopamine (eg, *Intropin*)
epinephrine (eg, *Adrenalin Chloride*)

fluoxetine (eg, *Prozac*)
levodopa (eg, *Larodopa*)
macrolide antibiotics (eg, clarithromycin) (pimozide only)
methylphenidate (eg, *Ritalin*) (pimozide only)
nefazodone (*Serzone*) (pimozide only)
phenothiazines (eg, promethazine) (pimozide only)
protease inhibitors (eg, saquinavir) (pimozide only)
rifampin (eg, *Rifadin*)
tricyclic antidepressants (eg, amitriptyline)

## Side Effects:

Every drug is capable of producing side effects. Many patients experience no, or minor, side effects. The frequency and severity of side effects depend on many factors including dose, duration of therapy, and individual susceptibility. Possible side effects include:

*Digestive Tract:* Constipation; dry mouth; diarrhea; nausea; indigestion; vomiting; stomach pain; decreased or increased saliva; toothache; appetite changes.

*Nervous System:* Tremor; restlessness; headache; dizziness; sleeplessness; agitation; anxiety; drowsiness; aggressive reaction; increased sleep duration; increased dream activity; nervousness; depression; excitement.

*Respiratory System:* Upper respiratory infection; sinus irritation; congested or runny nose; coughing; sore throat; difficulty breathing.

*Urinary and Reproductive Tract:* Frequent urination; heavy menstrual bleeding; difficulty with orgasm; vaginal dryness; difficulty with erection; decreased sexual desire; impotence; lactation; breast enlargement.

*Skin:* Rash; dry skin; excessively oily skin; dark spots on the skin; sensitivity to sunlight; hair loss.

*Other:* Fast heartbeat; back, chest, or joint pain; muscle stiffness or rigidity; difficult or abnormal movement; clumsiness; difficulty walking; involuntary muscle contractions; fatigue; dizziness or light-headedness upon rising or standing; visual changes; weight gain; fever; sweating.

## Guidelines for Use:

- Dosage is individualized. Take exactly as prescribed.
- Do not stop taking or change the dose, unless instructed by your doctor.
- Can be taken with or without food. Take with food if stomach upset occurs. Avoid grapefruit juice while taking pimozide.
- Generally, low starting doses are used and then the dose is increased to achieve the best effects.
- Contact your doctor immediately if you experience skin rash, sexual dysfunction, difficulty breathing, involuntary muscle movements, muscle rigidity, fever, irregular or fast heartbeat, or profuse sweating.
- May cause dizziness, light-headedness, or fainting when rising or standing, particularly during initial use. Get up slowly and avoid sudden changes in posture.
- May cause drowsiness. Use caution while driving or performing other tasks requiring alertness, coordination, and physical dexterity.
- Avoid alcohol while you are taking this medicine.
- May cause sensitivity to sunlight. Avoid prolonged exposure to the sun or other forms of ultraviolet (UV) light (eg, tanning beds). Use sunscreens and wear protective clothing.
- Consult your doctor or pharmacist before taking prescription or OTC drugs or dietary supplements with phenylbutylpiperadine derivatives.
- Inform your doctor if you are pregnant, become pregnant, are planning to become pregnant, or are breastfeeding.
- Store tablets at controlled room temperature (59° to 86°F) in a tightly closed container and protect from light. Store oral solution at controlled room temperature (59° to 86°F) and protect from light. Do not freeze.

*If you have any questions, consult your doctor, pharmacist, or health care provider.*

| Generic Name<br>*Brand Name Example* | Supplied As | Generic<br>Available |
|---|---|---|
| *Rx* **Aripiprazole** | | |
| *Abilify* | **Tablets**: 10 mg, 15 mg, 20 mg,<br>30 mg | No |

## Type of Drug:
Antipsychotic agent.

## How the Drug Works:
The exact mechanism of action, like other drugs used to treat schizophrenia, is not known.

## Uses:
For treatment of schizophrenia.

## Precautions:
*Do not use in the following situations:* Allergy to the drug of any of its ingredients.

*Use with caution in the following situations:*

| | |
|---|---|
| cerebrovascular disease | heart disease |
| changes (primarily decreases)<br>  in blood pressure | seizures, history of |

*Neuroleptic Malignant Syndrome (NMS):* NMS is a potentially fatal syndrome associated with antipsychotic drugs. Symptoms include fever, muscle rigidity, altered mental abilities, irregular pulse and blood pressure, increased heart rate, sweating, and irregular heart rhythm.

*Tardive dyskinesia:* Involuntary and uncontrollable movements may develop in patients treated with antipsychotic drugs. Occurrence is highest in the elderly, especially women. However, it is impossible to predict which patients are likely to develop the syndrome. The risk of developing these involuntary movements and the likelihood they will become permanent are increased with long-term use and with high doses. However, it is possible to develop these symptoms after short-term treatment at low doses. The syndrome is characterized by rhythmical, involuntary movements of the tongue, face, mouth, or jaw (eg, protrusion of tongue, puffing of cheeks, puckering of mouth, chewing movements), sometimes accompanied by involuntary movements of the arms and legs. Fine worm-like movement of the tongue may be an early sign of the syndrome. If the medication is stopped at this time, the syndrome may not develop further. There is no known treatment for established cases of tardive dyskinesia, although the syndrome may stop partially or completely if the drug is withdrawn. Antipsychotic treatment, however, may suppress or partially suppress the signs and symptoms of the syndrome and thereby may mask the underlying disease process. The effect that symptomatic suppression has upon the long-term course of the syndrome is unknown.

*Pregnancy:* There are no adequate and well-controlled stuides in pregnant women. Use only if clearly needed and the potential benefits outweigh the possible risks to the fetus.

*Breastfeeding:* It is not known if quinolone derivatives appear in breast milk. Consult your doctor before you begin breastfeeding.

*Children:* Safety and effectiveness have not been established.

*Elderly:* Safety and effectiveness in patients with psychosis associated with Alzheimer disease is not known.

## Drug Interactions:

Tell your doctor or pharmacist if you are taking or planning to take any over-the-counter or prescription medications or dietary supplements with this drug. Drug doses may need to be modified or a different drug prescribed. The following drugs and drug classes interact with this drug:

alcohol
carbamazepine (eg, *Tegretol*)
fluoxetine (eg, *Prozac*)

ketoconazole (eg, *Nizoral*)
paroxetine (eg, *Paxil*)
quinidine

## Side Effects:

Every drug is capable of producing side effects. Many patients experience no, or minor, side effects. The frequency and severity of side effects depend on many factors, including dose, duration of therapy, and individual susceptibility. Possible side effects include:

*Digestive Tract:* Nausea; vomiting; constipation.

*Nervous System:* Anxiety; sleeplessness; light-headedness; sleepiness; inability to remain in a sitting position; tremor.

*Respiratory System:* Runny nose; cough.

*Other:* Headache; weakness; fever; rash; weight gain; blurred vision.

## Guidelines for Use:

- Dosage is individualized. Take exactly as prescribed.
- Do not stop taking or change the dose, unless instructed by your doctor.
- May be taken without regard to food.
- Generally, low starting doses are used and then the dose is increased to achieve the best effects.
- Contact your doctor immediately if you experience involuntary movements, muscle rigidity, fever, or rash.
- If a dose is missed, take it as soon as possible, If several hours have passed or it is nearing time for the next dose, do not double the dose to catch up, unless instructed by your doctor. If more than one dose is missed, or it is necessary to establish a new dosage schedule, contact your doctor or pharmacist.
- May impair judgment, thinking, or motor skills. Use caution while driving or performing other tasks requiring alertness, coordination, or physical dexterity until tolerance is determined.
- Inform your doctor if you are pregnant, become pregnant, are planning to become pregnant, or are breastfeeding.
- Avoid alcohol while using this medicine.
- Avoid becoming overheated or dehydrated.
- Store at 77°F.

*If you have any questions, consult your doctor, pharmacist, or health care provider.*

| Generic Name<br>*Brand Name Example* | Supplied As | Generic<br>Available |
|---|---|---|
| Rx **Thiothixene** | | |
| *Navane* | **Capsules:** 1 mg, 2 mg, 5 mg,<br>10 mg, 20 mg | Yes |

## Type of Drug:
Typical (conventional) antipsychotic.

## How the Drug Works:
The exact mechanism is not known. Drugs of this type usually work by altering nerve transmission in the brain.

## Uses:
For the management of the manifestations of psychotic mental disorders.

## Precautions:
*Do not use in the following situations:*

allergy to the drug or any of its ingredients
blood disorders (eg, agranulocytosis)
circulatory collapse
CNS depression
comatose states

*Use with caution in the following situations:*

breast cancer, active or history of
cardiac conduction abnormalities
cerebrovascular disease
dehydration
exposure to extreme heat
heart disease
long-term use (longer than 6 weeks)
seizures, history of
strenuous exercise
suicidal tendency
underactive thyroid (hypothyroidism)

*Neuroleptic Malignant Syndrome (NMS):* NMS is a potentially fatal syndrome associated with antipsychotic drugs. Symptoms include fever, muscle rigidity, altered mental abilities, irregular pulse and blood pressure, increased heart rate, sweating, and irregular heart rhythm.

*Tardive dyskinesia:* Involuntary and uncontrollable movements may develop in patients treated with antipsychotic drugs. Occurrence is highest in the elderly, especially women. However, it is impossible to predict which patients are likely to develop the syndrome. The risk of developing these involuntary movements and the likelihood they will become permanent are increased with long-term use and with high doses. However, it is possible to develop these symptoms after short-term treatment at low doses. The syndrome is characterized by rhythmical, involuntary movements of tongue, face, mouth, or jaw (eg, protrusion of tongue, puffing of cheeks, puckering of mouth, chewing movements), sometimes accompanied by involuntary movements of the arms and legs. Fine worm-like movement of the tongue may be an early sign of the syndrome. If the medication is stopped at this time, the syndrome may not develop further. There is no known treatment for established cases of tardive dyskinexia, although the syndrome may stop, partially or completely, if the drug is withdrawn. Antipsychotic treatment, however, may suppress or partially suppress the signs and symptoms of the syndrome and thereby may possibly mask the underlying disease process. The effect that symptomatic suppression has upon the long-term course of the syndrome is unknown.

*Pregnancy:* There are no adequate and well-controlled studies in pregnant women. Use only if clearly needed and potential benefits outweigh the possible risks to the fetus.

*Breastfeeding:* It is not known if thiothixene appears in breast milk. Consult your doctor before you begin breastfeeding.

*Children:* Safety and effectiveness in children younger than 12 years of age have not been established.

*Lab tests* or exams may be required to monitor treatment. Tests include blood and liver tests and periodic eye exams.

## Drug Interactions:

Tell your doctor or pharmacist if you are taking or planning to take any over-the-counter or prescription medications or dietary supplements with this drug. Doses of one or both drugs may need to be modified or a different drug may need to be prescribed. The following drugs and drug classes interact with this drug:

alcohol
atropine (eg, *Isopto Atropine*)
barbiturates (eg, phenobarbital)
benztropine (eg, *Cogentin*)
bromocriptine (*Parlodel*)
chloroquine (eg, *Aralen*)
guanadrel (eg, *Hylorel*)
guanethidine (eg, *Ismelin*)

levodopa (eg, *Larodopa*)
lithium (eg, *Eskalith*)
phenytoin (eg, *Dilantin*)
propranolol (eg, *Inderal*)
trazodone (eg, *Desyrel*)
tricyclic antidepressants (eg, amitriptyline)

## Side Effects:

Every drug is capable of producing side effects. Many patients experience no, or minor, side effects. The frequency and severity of side effects depend on many factors, including dose, duration of therapy and individual susceptibility. Possible side effects include:

*Digestive Tract:* Indigestion; stomach pain; constipation; appetite changes; diarrhea; nausea; vomiting.

*Nervous System:* Altered mental status; orthostatic hypotension (dizziness or light-headedness when rising quickly from a sitting or lying position); fainting; drowsiness; impaired judgment, thinking or motor skills; headache; restlessness; agitation; light-headedness; sleeplessness; seizures.

*Circulatory System:* Rapid heartbeat; changes in blood pressure; pounding in the chest (palpitations); abnormal blood counts.

*Other:* Rash; fever; muscle rigidity; sweating; acute kidney failure; involuntary and uncontrollable movements (eg, protrusion of tongue, puffing of cheeks; puckering of mouth, chewing movements); lens problems; dry mouth; weakness; weight gain; tight muscles; joint pain; swelling of arms and legs; lactation; moderate breast enlargement (women); absence of menstruation; increased or decreased blood sugar; blurred vision; nasal congestion; increased salivation; impotence; increased thirst; itching; sensitivity to light.

## Guidelines for Use:

- Dosage is individualized. Take exactly as prescribed.
- Do not stop taking or change the dose, unless instructed by your doctor.
- If a dose is missed, take it as soon as possible. If several hours have passed or it is nearing time for the next dose, do not double the dose to catch up, unless instructed by your doctor. If more than one dose is missed or if it is necessary to establish a new dosage schedule, contact your doctor or pharmacist.
- May cause dizziness, light-headedness, or fainting, especially when rising or standing and during the first 3 to 5 days. If these symptoms should occur, sit or lie down and contact your doctor. Use caution while driving or performing hazardous tasks requiring alertness, coordination, or physical dexterity.
- Do not take other medications without your doctor's approval. This includes nonprescription medicines for appetite control, asthma, colds, cough, hay fever, or sinus problems.
- Avoid alcohol and other mental depressants (eg, narcotics, tranquilizers, antihistamines) while you are taking this medicine.
- Inform your doctor if you are pregnant, become pregnant, are planning to become pregnant, or are breastfeeding.
- Avoid overheating and dehydration.
- Lab tests may be required to monitor treatment. Be sure to keep appointments.
- Store at a controlled room temperature (59° to 77°F).

*If you have any questions, consult your doctor, pharmacist, or health care provider.*

| Generic Name<br>*Brand Name Examples* | Supplied As | Generic<br>Available |
|---|---|---|
| *Rx* **Ergoloid Mesylates** | **Tablets, sublingual:** 1 mg | Yes |
| *Hydergine* | **Tablets:** 1 mg | Yes |
| *Hydergine LC* | **Capsules, liquid:** 1 mg | No |
| *Hydergine*[1] | **Liquid:** 1 mg/mL | No |

[1] Contains alcohol.

## Type of Drug:

Dihydrogenated ergot alkaloids. Drugs used to treat age-related decreases in mental ability.

## How the Drug Works:

It is not known how ergoloid mesylates produce beneficial mental effects. It is possible that they may increase brain metabolism, possibly increasing blood flow in the brain.

## Uses:

To treat the signs and symptoms of age-related decreases in mental ability, including decreased alertness, short-term memory loss, decreased self-care, and sociability, or age-related changes in mood in patients older than 60 years of age.

Patients who respond may suffer from an aging disorder or have some underlying condition (eg, primary progressive dementia, Alzheimer disease, senile onset, multi-infarct [stroke] dementia).

## Precautions:

*Do not use in the following situations:*
allergy to ergoloid mesylates or any of their ingredients
psychosis

*Use with caution in the following situations:* Mental decline of unknown origin.

*Before prescribing ergoloid mesylates,* your doctor may need to rule out other conditions that could cause a decrease in mental ability. Periodic doctor visits may be required after beginning therapy.

## Side Effects:

Every drug is capable of producing side effects. Many ergoloid mesylate users experience no, or minor, side effects. The frequency and severity of side effects depend on many factors including dose, duration of therapy, and individual susceptibility. Possible side effects include: Nausea; stomach upset.

## Guidelines for Use:

- Use exactly as prescribed.
- Usual starting dosage is 1 mg 3 times daily.
- Allow sublingual tablets to dissolve under your tongue. Do not crush, chew, or swallow sublingual tablets whole.
- Liquid dose form comes with calibrated dropper to measure dose accurately.
- May cause nausea and stomach upset during start of treatment. Take with food if this occurs.
- If a dose is missed, take it as soon as possible. If several hours have passed or if it is nearing time for the next dose, do not double the dose in order to catch up, unless advised to do so by your doctor. If more than one dose is missed, or it is necessary to establish a new dosage schedule, contact your doctor or pharmacist.
- Improvement of symptoms is gradual and may take 3 to 4 weeks to be noticed.
- Treatment for up to 6 months may be necessary to determine effectiveness.
- Do not stop therapy or change the dose unless advised to do so by your doctor.
- Store tablets below 77°F and protect from light. Store liquid capsules between 59° and 77°F, protect from light, and do not freeze. Store liquid below 86°F.

*If you have any questions, consult your doctor, pharmacist, or health care provider.*

| Generic Name<br>*Brand Name Examples* | Supplied As | Generic<br>Available |
|---|---|---|
| Rx **Lithium Carbonate** | **Tablets:** 300 mg (8.12 mEq lithium) | Yes |
| | **Capsules:** 150 mg (4.06 mEq lithium); 300 mg (8.12 mEq lithium); 600 mg (16.24 mEq lithium) | Yes |
| *Eskalith* | **Capsules:** 300 mg (8.12 mEq lithium) | Yes |
| *Eskalith CR* | **Tablets, controlled release:** 450 mg (12.18 mEq lithium) | No |
| *Lithobid* | **Tablets, slow release:** 300 mg (8.12 mEq lithium) | No |
| Rx **Lithium Citrate** | **Syrup:** 300 mg (8 mEq lithium carbonate)/5 mL | Yes |

## Type of Drug:

Antimanic drug.

## How the Drug Works:

Lithium reduces the extremes of emotional states, behavior, and feelings during periods of mania by stabilizing nerve and muscle cells.

## Uses:

To treat manic episodes of manic-depressive illness (bipolar disorder). Maintenance therapy prevents or decreases the frequency and intensity of subsequent manic episodes.

*Unlabeled Use(s):* Occasionally doctors may prescribe lithium for cluster headaches, premenstrual tension, postpartum psychosis, eating disorders, alcoholism related to depression, psychosis caused by corticosteroid use, certain movement disorders (eg, tardive dyskinesia), and hyperthyroidism (overactive thyroid); and to increase white blood cell counts in individuals undergoing cancer chemotherapy, AIDS patients taking zidovudine, and in childhood disorders in which white blood cell counts are extremely low.

## Precautions:

*Do not use in the following situations:* Allergy to lithium.

*Use with caution in the following situations:*

angiotensin-converting enzyme (ACE) inhibitors use
CNS impairment
debilitation, severe
dehydration (fluid loss), severe
diarrhea, chronic
diuretic use
heart disease, moderate-to-severe
infection with fever
kidney disease, severe
low sodium blood level
neuroleptic drug use
organic brain syndrome
pregnancy
psychiatric condition, life-threatening
sweating, chronic and excessive
thyroid function, low
vomiting

*Decreased thyroid function* (hypothyroidism) may occur with long-term use. Contact your doctor if neck swelling or skin coarsening occurs, or if your activity level decreases. Lithium-induced hypothyroidism may be treated with thyroid hormone therapy.

*Chronic lithium therapy* may be associated with a reduction in the kidney's concentrating ability, occasionally presenting as nephrogenic diabetes insipidus (thirst and frequent urination). This condition is usually reversible when lithium is discontinued.

*Pregnancy:* Studies have shown lithium may cause harm to the fetus. Use only if clearly needed and potential benefits to the mother outweigh the possible risks to the fetus. If possible, lithium should be withdrawn for at least the first trimester.

*Breastfeeding:* Lithium appears in breast milk. Consult your doctor before you begin breastfeeding.

*Children:* Safety and effectiveness in children younger than 12 years of age have not been established.

*Elderly:* Because of an increased risk of toxicity, lower doses and more frequent monitoring are necessary.

*Lab tests* may be required during lithium therapy. Tests may include lithium blood levels, blood counts, urinalysis, electrolytes (eg, sodium, potassium), glucose, electrocardiogram, and thyroid and kidney function tests. Lithium blood levels should be checked twice weekly until dosage is stabilized. When a consistent blood level is reached, testing may be reduced to once weekly. Eventually blood levels will be checked every 2 to 3 months (more frequently in the elderly). See Side Effects.

## Drug Interactions:

Tell your doctor or pharmacist if you are taking or if you are planning to take any over-the-counter or prescription medications with lithium. Doses of one or both drugs may need to be modified or a different drug may need to be prescribed. The following drugs and drug classes interact with lithium.

ACE inhibitors (eg, captopril, lisinopril)
carbamazepine (eg, *Tegretol*)
haloperidol *(Haldol)*
iodide salts (eg, *SSKI*)
nonsteroidal anti-inflammatory agents (NSAIDS) (eg, ibuprofen)

succinylcholine (eg, *Anectine)*
thiazide diuretics (eg, hydrochlorothiazide)
urinary alkalinizers (eg, sodium bicarbonate)

## Side Effects:

Every drug is capable of producing side effects. Many lithium users experience no, or minor, side effects. The frequency and severity of side effects depend on many factors including dose, duration of therapy, and individual susceptibility. Possible side effects include:

*Toxicity:* The likelihood of toxicity increases with increasing serum lithium levels. Lithium blood levels greater than 1.5 mEq/L carry a greater risk than lower levels. Diarrhea, vomiting, drowsiness, muscle weakness, and lack of coordination may be early signs of lithium toxicity, and can occur at lithium levels below 2 mEq/L. At higher levels, giddiness, blurred vision, ringing in the ears, vertigo (feeling of whirling motion), and a large output of urine may be seen. Serum lithium levels should not be permitted to exceed 2 mEq/L during the acute treatment phase.
Fine hand tremor, excessive urination, and mild thirst may occur when starting therapy for the acute manic phase and may persist throughout treatment. Mild nausea and general discomfort may also appear during the first few days of treatment. These side effects are an inconvenience rather than a disabling condition, and usually subside with continued treatment or a temporary dosage reduction.

*Digestive Tract:* Nausea; appetite loss; vomiting; diarrhea; gastritis; salivary gland swelling; stomach pain; excessive salivation; gas; indigestion; dry mouth; metallic taste; salty taste; taste distortion; swollen lips; thirst.

*Nervous System:* Tremor; muscle twitches or jerking movement of whole limbs; hypertonicity; incoordination; clumsiness; uncontrolled muscle movement; hyperactive deep tendon reflex; extrapyramidal symptoms (acute dystonia, cogwheel rigidity); blackout spells; seizures; slurred speech; dizziness; feeling of whirling motion; downbeat nystagmus; drowsiness; psychomotor retardation; restlessness; confusion; stupor; coma; uncontrolled tongue movements; tics; ringing in the ears; hallucinations; poor memory; slowed intellectual function; startled response; worsening of organic brain syndromes; pseudotumor cerebri (increased intracranial pressure and papilledema); lethargy; headache; drowsiness; fatigue; giddiness; blurred vision.

*Circulatory System:* Abnormal heart rhythm; low blood pressure; slow heartbeat; chest tightness.

*Skin:* Drying and thinning of hair; hair loss; numbness of skin; acne; chronic folliculitis; dry skin; itching; rash; skin ulcers; skin inflammation; hives; worsening of psoriasis.

*Urinary and Reproductive Tract:* Urinary problems; inability to urinate; increased or decreased urine output; impotence; sexual dysfunction; incontinence of urine or feces.

*Laboratory changes:* Sugar in urine; decreased kidney function; albumin in urine; increased white blood cell count; increased blood sugar; increased blood calcium.

*Other:* Transient blind spots; bulging of the eyes; ankle or wrist swelling or painful joints; dental cavities; thyroid abnormalities; fever; weight loss or gain.

## Guidelines for Use:

- Use exactly as prescribed.
- Dosage will be individualized according to serum levels and clinical response. Examples of usual doses are as follows:
  *Acute mania* — 600 mg (capsules, tablets, or syrup) 3 times daily; 900 mg (controlled release, slow release) twice daily.
  *Maintenance therapy* — 300 mg (capsules, tablets, or syrup) 3 or 4 times daily; 450 mg (controlled release, slow release) twice daily.
- The syrup and immediate release capsules and tablets are usually given 3 to 4 times daily. Controlled and slow release tablets are usually given 2 times daily (every 12 hours), but can be given 3 times daily (every 8 hours).
- Do not crush or chew slow release or controlled release products.
- Take after meals or with food or milk if stomach upset occurs.
- Maintain a normal diet, including salt and adequate fluid intake (8 to 12 glasses of water) daily.
- Watch for signs of overdose or toxicity, such as diarrhea, vomiting, drowsiness, muscle weakness, lack of coordination, giddiness, blurred vision, ringing in the ears, feeling of whirling motion, or increased urination. Stop the medication and contact your doctor immediately.
- May take 2 to 3 weeks to normalize symptoms when used to treat a manic episode.
- If a dose is missed, take it as soon as possible. If several hours have passed or if it is nearing time for the next dose, do not double the dose in order to catch up, unless advised to do so by your doctor. If more than one dose is missed, or it is necessary to establish a new dosage schedule, contact your doctor or pharmacist.
- May cause drowsiness. Use caution while driving or performing other tasks requiring alertness, coordination, or physical dexterity.
- Notify your doctor if you become pregnant or are planning to become pregnant while taking this medicine. Lithium is a potential hazard to the fetus.
- Notify your doctor if sweating and diarrhea occur since this may decrease your tolerance to lithium. Supplemental fluid and salt should be administered under medical supervision until the condition is resolved.
- Lab tests, including lithium blood levels, may be required periodically during treatment. Be sure to keep appointments.
- Lithium blood levels, to be most accurate, should be drawn just before a scheduled dose.
- *Brand interchange* — Do not change from one brand of this drug to another without consulting your pharmacist or doctor. Products manufactured by different companies may not be equally effective.
- Store between 59° to 86°F in a tight, child-resistant container. Protect from moisture.

*If you have any questions, consult your doctor, pharmacist, or health care provider.*

| Generic Name<br>*Brand Name Examples* | Supplied As | Generic Available |
|---|---|---|
| *Rx* **Donepezil HCl** | | |
| *Aricept* | **Tablets**: 5 mg, 10 mg | No |
| *Rx* **Galantamine HBr** | | |
| *Reminyl* | **Tablets**: 4 mg, 8 mg,<br>12 mg | No |
| *Rx* **Rivastigmine Tartrate** | | |
| *Exelon* | **Capsules**: 1.5 mg, 3 mg,<br>4.5 mg, 6 mg | No |
| *Exelon* | **Solution**: 2 mg/mL | No |
| *Rx* **Tacrine HCl** | | |
| *Cognex* | **Capsules**: 10 mg, 20 mg,<br>30 mg, 40 mg | No |

## Type of Drug:

Reversible cholinesterase inhibitor used in managing mild to moderate Alzheimer disease-associated dementia.

## How the Drug Works:

The exact mechanism is unknown. Cholinesterase inhibitors act by enhancing cholinergic function. Deterioration or loss of cholinergic neurons may be a primary cause of cognitive dysfunction associated with Alzheimer disease. Cholinesterase inhibitors may enhance cholinergic transmission in this setting. If this mechanism of action is correct, the effect of cholinesterase inhibitors may lessen as the disease advances and fewer cholinergic neurons remain functionally intact. There is no evidence that cholinesterase inhibitors alter the course of the underlying dementing process.

## Uses:

To treat mild to moderate dementia of the Alzheimer type.

## Precautions:

*Do not use in the following situations:*

allergy to acridine derivatives (tacrine only)
allergy to carbamate derivatives (rivastigmine only)
allergy to a cholinesterase inhibitor or any of its ingredients
allergy to piperidine derivatives (donepezil only)
treatment-associated jaundice from previous treatments (tacrine only)

*Use with caution in the following situations:*

abnormally slow heart rate
anesthesia (succinylcholine type)
asthma, history of
bladder outflow difficulty
cardiac conduction abnormalities
gastrointestinal disease or dysfunction (eg, peptic ulcer, bleeding disorder)
heart disease
kidney disease (galantamine only)
liver disease, active or history of
NSAID use, concurrent
obstructive lung disease, history of
seizures
sick sinus syndrome
ulcers (gastric, duodenal), history of
urinary obstruction

*Nicotine:* Nicotine use increases the elimination of tacrine from the body.

*Gender:* Tacrine and galantamine are eliminated from the body more slowly in women.

*Pregnancy:* There are no adequate and well-controlled studies in pregnant women. Use only if clearly needed and the potential benefits to the mother outweigh possible hazards to the fetus.

*Breastfeeding:* It is not known if cholinesterase inhibitors are excreted in breast milk. Contact your doctor before you begin breastfeeding.

*Children:* Safety and effectiveness in children have not been established.

*Elderly:* Rivastigmine and galantamine are eliminated from the body more slowly in the elderly.

*Lab tests* will be required to monitor therapy with tacrine. Tests include liver function tests every other week from at least week 4 to week 16, after which monitoring may be decreased to every 3 months, and blood counts.

## Drug Interactions:

Tell your doctor or pharmacist if you are taking or if you are planning to take any over-the-counter or prescription medications or dietary supplements with a cholinesterase inhibitor. Doses of one or both drugs may need to be modified or a different drug may need to be prescribed. The following drugs and drug classes interact with cholinesterase inhibitors:

anticholinergics (eg, atropine, scopolamine)
cholinergic agonists (eg, bethanechol)
cholinesterase inhibitors (eg, neostigmine)
cimetidine (eg, *Tagamet*)
erythromycin (eg, *E-mycin*)
fluvoxamine (eg, *Luvox*) (tacrine only)
food (rivastigmine only)
ketoconazole (eg, *Nizoral*)
NSAIDs (eg, ibuprofen)
paroxetine (*Paxil*)
succinylcholine (eg, *Quelicin*)
theophylline (eg, *Theo-Dur*) (tacrine only)

## Side Effects:

Every drug is capable of producing side effects. Many cholinesterase inhibitor users experience no, or minor, side effects. The frequency and severity of side effects depend on many factors including dose, duration of therapy, and individual susceptibility. Possible side effects include:

*Digestive Tract:* Nausea; vomiting; diarrhea; appetite loss; stomach bleeding; black tarry stools; loss of bowel control; bloating; gas; belching; indigestion; stomach pain; weight loss; constipation.

*Nervous System:* Sleeplessness; fatigue; drowsiness; headache; pain; difficulty moving; dizziness; fainting; depression; abnormal dreams; abnormal thinking; hallucinations; tremors; irritability; numbness or tingling in hands or feet; abnormal skin sensations (eg, burning, prickling, tingling); aggression; feeling of whirling motion; clumsiness; twitching; restlessness; nervousness; anxiety; paranoia; convulsions; weakness; confusion; hostility; difficulty speaking.

*Circulatory System:* Chest pain; abnormal heartbeat; heart pounding; blood pressure changes; flushing; hot flashes.

*Skin:* Itching; hives; rash; excessive sweating; unusual bruising or bleeding.

*Respiratory System:* Difficulty breathing; sore throat; nasal congestion; sinus problems; runny nose; coughing; upper respiratory infection; pulmonary congestion.

*Urinary and Reproductive Tract:* Loss of bladder control; frequent urination; excessive urination at night; urinary tract infection; blood in the urine.

*Other:* Flu-like syndrome; chills; fever; general body discomfort; muscle cramps; muscle or joint pain; muscle tension; back pain; swelling in hands or feet; anemia; dehydration; eye irritation; blurred vision; elevated transaminase; accidental trauma; abnormal gait; ringing in the ears; nosebleed.

## Guidelines for Use:

- Dosage is individualized. Take exactly as prescribed.
- *Donepezil* — Take in the evening just before bedtime with or without food.
- *Galantamine* — Take during morning and evening meal if possible. Follow recommended dosage and administration. If therapy is interrupted for several days or longer, restart treatment at the lowest dose. Nausea may be reduced by administering with food, antiemetic medication, or ensuring adequate fluid intake.
- *Tacrine* — Take between meals if possible; however, it may be taken with meals to avoid stomach upset. The effect of tacrine is thought to depend upon its administration at regular intervals.
- *Rivastigmine capsules*— Take with food in divided doses in the morning or evening.
- *Rivastigmine solution* — Remove the oral dosing syringe provided in its protective case and, using the provided syringe, withdraw the prescribed amount of rivastigmine. Each dose may be swallowed from the syringe or first mixed with a small glass of water, cold fruit juice, or soda. Stir the mixture before drinking.
- If a dose is missed, take it as soon as possible. If several hours have passed or if it is nearing time for the next dose, do not double the dose to catch up, unless advised by your doctor. If more than one dose is missed or it is necessary to establish a new dosage schedule, contact your doctor or pharmacist.
- *Tacrine* — Do not stop taking this medicine suddenly or change the dosage unless instructed to do so by your doctor. Abrupt discontinuation or large reduction in the total daily dose of tacrine may cause a decline in mental function and behavioral disturbances. Unsupervised increases in the dose of tacrine may also have serious consequences.
- Inform your doctor if you are pregnant, become pregnant, planning to become pregnant, or are breastfeeding before beginning therapy.
- Report any new or worsening side effects to your doctor.
- May cause dizziness or blurred vision. Use caution while driving or performing other tasks requiring alertness, coordination, or physical dexterity.
- *Rivastigmine* — There is a high incidence of nausea and vomiting associated with the use of the drug, along with the possibility of anorexia and weight loss. Monitor for these adverse events and inform your doctor if they occur.
- *Tacrine* — Contact you doctor if you experience side effects that occur soon after taking a dose (eg, nausea, vomiting, loose stools) or develop side effects that are delayed (eg, rash, yellowing of the skin, changes in stool color).
- Lab tests will be required to monitor therapy. Be sure to keep appointments.
- Store capsules and tablets at controlled room temperature (59° to 86°F) away from moisture. Store rivastigmine solution below 77°F in an upright position. Protect from freezing.

*If you have any questions, consult your doctor, pharmacist, or health care provider.*

| Generic Name<br>*Brand Name Examples* | Supplied As | Generic<br>Available |
|---|---|---|
| *c-ɪv* **Chlordiazepoxide and Amitriptyline HCl** | **Tablets:** 5 mg chlordiazepoxide and 12.5 mg amitriptyline | Yes |
| *Limbitrol[1], Limbitrol DS[1]* | **Tablets:** 10 mg chlordiaze-poxide and 25 mg amitriptyline | Yes |
| *Rx* **Perphenazine and Amitriptyline HCl** | **Tablets:** 4 mg perphenazine and 10 mg amitriptyline; 4 mg perphenazine and 50 mg ami-triptyline | Yes |
| *Etrafon 2-10* | **Tablets:** 2 mg perphenazine and 10 mg amitriptyline | Yes |
| *Etrafon* | **Tablets:** 2 mg perphenazine and 25 mg amitriptyline | Yes |
| *Etrafon Forte* | **Tablets:** 4 mg perphenazine and 25 mg amitriptyline | Yes |

[1] As hydrochloride salt.

For complete information, see the chlordiazepoxide monograph and the amitriptyline monograph.

## Type of Drug:

Amitriptyline is a tricyclic antidepressant, chlordiazepoxide is a benzodiazepine antianxiety agent, and perphenazine is an antipsychotic agent.

## How the Drug Works:

Amitriptyline acts on the central nervous system (brain) to exert its antidepressant effects. Chlordiazepoxide acts on the central nervous system to effect emotional responses. Perphenazine acts on the central nervous system to exert its antipsychotic effects.

## Uses:

To treat moderate-to-severe depression associated with moderate-to-severe anxiety. Perphenazine and amitriptyline HCl combination is also indicated for anxiety and depression associated with chronic physical disease, depression and anxiety that cannot be clearly differentiated, and schizophrenia with associated symptoms of depression.

## Precautions:

*Do not use in the following situations:*

allergy to these medicines or any of their ingredients

allergy to benzodiazepines or tricyclic antidepressants (chlordiazepoxide and amitriptyline only)

allergy to phenothiazines or tricyclic antidepressants (perphenazine and amitriptyline only)

blood dyscrasias (perphenazine only)

bone marrow depression (perphenazine only)

elective surgery

heart attack, acute recovery phase

liver damage (perphenazine only)

MAOI therapy, concurrent

subcortical brain damage (perphenazine only)

*Use with caution in the following situations:*

asthma, severe (perphenazine only)

drug addiction, history of

electroshock therapy

emphysema (perphenazine only)

glaucoma, closed angle

heart disease

increased eye pressure (perphenazine only)

kidney impairment

liver impairment

lung disease (perphenazine only)

overactive thyroid

seizure, history of

suicidal tendencies

urinary retention, history of

*Neuroleptic Malignant Syndrome (NMS)* is a potentially fatal syndrome associated with perphenazine. Symptoms include increased body heat, muscle rigidity, altered mental abilities including catatonia (eg, confusion, withdrawal, unresponsivness), irregular pulse and blood pressure, increased heart rate, and sweating.

*Tardive dyskinesia:* Involuntary and uncontrollable movements may develop in patients treated with perphenazine. The likelihood that these symptoms will become permanent increases with long-term use and with high doses. However, it is possible to develop these symptoms after short-term treatment at low doses. Occurrence is highest among the elderly. The syndrome is characterized by rhythmical involuntary movements of the tongue, face, mouth, or jaw (eg, protrusion of tongue, puffing of cheeks, puckering of mouth, chewing movements), sometimes accompanied by involuntary movement of the arms and legs. Fine worm-like movements of the tongue may be an early sign of the syndrome. If the medication is stopped at this time, the syndrome may not develop. There is no known treatment for established cases of tardive dyskinesia, although the syndrome may stop, partially or completely, if the drug is withdrawn.

*Pregnancy:* Safety and effectiveness of psychotherapeutic combinations during pregnancy have not been established. Studies suggest an increased risk of congenital malformations associated with use of minor tranquilizers (chlordiazepoxide, diazepam, meprobamate) during the first trimester of pregnancy. Use of these drugs during pregnancy should almost always be avoided. Use only if clearly needed and potential benefits to the mother outweigh the possible risk to the fetus.

*Breastfeeding:* It is not known whether these drugs are excreted in human milk. As a general rule, breastfeeding should not be undertaken while on these drugs, because many drugs are excreted in human milk. Consult your doctor before you begin breastfeeding.

*Children:* Safety and effectiveness of chlordiazepoxide and amitriptyline HCl in children younger than 12 years of age have not been established. Perphenazine and amitriptyline HCl combination is not recommended for use in children.

*Elderly:* Lowest effective dose is recommended to prevent incoordination, oversedation, confusion, or anticholinergic effects (eg, dry mouth, confusion, blurred vision, constipation, urinary retention).

*Lab tests* or exams may be required during treatment with psychotherapeutic combinations. Tests may include periodic kidney and liver function tests and blood counts.

## Drug Interactions:

Tell your doctor or pharmacist if you are taking or if you are planning to take any over-the-counter or prescription medications or dietary supplements with psychotherapeutic combinations. Doses of one or both drugs may need to be modified or a different drug may need to be prescribed. The following drugs and drug classes interact with psychotherapeutic combinations:

alcohol
anticholinergics (eg, scopolamine) (perphenazine only)
anticoagulants (eg, dicumarol)
antifungal agents (eg, ketoconazole)
beta blockers (eg, propranolol) (chlordiazepoxide only)
carbamazepine (eg, *Tegretol*)
cimetidine (eg, *Tagamet*)
clonidine (eg, *Catapres*)
CNS depressants (eg, barbiturates, narcotics)
contraceptves, oral (eg, *Ortho-Novum*) (chlordiazepoxide only)
disulfiram (eg, *Antabuse*)
drugs metabolized by P450 2D6 (eg, fluoxetine)
ethclorvynol (perphenazine only)
guanethidine (eg, *Ismelin*)
histamine $H_2$ antagonists (eg, cimetidine, ranitidine)
MAOIs (eg, phenelzine)
quinolones (eg, ciprofloxacin)
rifampin (eg, *Rifadin*)
SSRIs (eg, fluoxetine)
sympathomimetics (eg, epinephrine)
theophyllines (eg, *TheoDur*) (chlordiazepoxide only)
thyroid medications (eg, *Synthroid*)
valproic acid (eg, *Depakote*)

## Side Effects:

Every drug is capable of producing side effects. Many patients taking psychotherapeutic combinations experience no, or minor, side effects. The frequency and severity of side effects depend on many factors including dose, duration of therapy, and individual susceptibility. Possible side effects include:

*Withdrawal* symptoms include convulsions, tremor, stomach and muscle cramps, vomiting, sweating.

*Chlordiazepoxide/amitriptyline* —

*Digestive Tract:* Constipation; loss of appetite; bloating; nausea; stomach upset; vomiting; peculiar taste; diarrhea.

*Nervous System:* Drowsiness; dizziness; vivid dreams; confusion; tremor; fatigue; weakness; restlessness; lethargy; apprehension; poor concentration; delusions; hallucinations; incoordination; clumsiness; numbness; tingling and abnormal skin sensations of the arms and legs; fainting; headache.

*Other:* Dry mouth; impotence; nasal congestion; fast heartbeat; pounding in the chest; blurred vision; inability to urinate; rash; hives; increased sensitivity to light; itching; excessive or spontaneous flow of breast milk; menstrual irregularities; changes in blood sugar levels; increased sweating; frequent urination; dilated pupils; yellowing of the skin and eyes; hair loss; glandular swelling.

*Perphenazine/amitriptyline* —

*Digestive Tract:* Constipation; appetite loss.

*Nervous System:* Abnormal or involuntary muscle movements; drowsiness; dizziness; vivid dreams; confusion; tremor; fatigue; restlessness; lethargy.

*Other:* Dry mouth; elevated body temperature; urinary retention; blurred vision; changes in blood pressure; abnormal blood counts; abnormal skin pigmentation.

## Guidelines for Use:

- Optimum dosage varies with the severity of the symptoms and the patient response. When satisfactory response is obtained, dosage should be reduced to the smallest amount needed to maintain satisfactory response.
- *Chlordiazepoxide and amitriptyline* — Initial dosage of 3 or 4 tablets daily in divided doses is recommended. The larger portion of the total daily dose may be taken at bedtime. In some patients, a single dose at bedtime may be sufficient.
- *Perphenazine and amitriptyline* — Usual inital dose is 3 to 4 tablets daily in divided doses. Lower inital doses may be used in adolescents and the elderly.
- Take only the amount prescribed by your doctor. Some of these medicines may be habit-forming and may produce dependence. Consult your doctor before increasing the dose or stopping the medicine.
- To avoid withdrawal symptoms after long-term use, a gradual dosage tapering schedule should be followed.
- Do not use in combination with MAOIs or within 14 days of discontinuing treatment with an MAOI. After stopping these medicines, wait at least 14 days before starting an MAOI.
- Avoid alcohol and other mental depressants (eg, narcotics, tranquilizers, antihistamines) while you are taking psychotherapeutic combinations.
- May cause drowsiness. Use caution while driving or performing other tasks requiring alertness, coordination, or physical dexterity.
- Inform your doctor if you are pregnant, become pregnant, are planning to become pregnant, or if you are breastfeeding.
- *Perphenazine and amitriptyline HCl* — Contact your doctor immediately if you notice a rise in body temperature (eg, fever), because this may suggest intolerance to perphenazine. May cause sensitivity to sunlight. Avoid prolonged exposure to the sun or other forms of ultraviolet (UV) light (eg, tanning beds). Use sunscreen and wear protective clothing until tolerance is determined.
- Store at controlled room temperature (36° to 77°F). Keep tightly closed. Protect from light and moisture.

*If you have any questions, consult your doctor, pharmacist, or health care provider.*

| Generic Name<br>*Brand Name Examples* | Supplied As | Generic<br>Available |
|---|---|---|
| *c-II* **Amobarbital Sodium** | | |
| *Amytal Sodium* | **Powder for Injection:** 500 mg/vial | No |
| *c-III* **Butabarbital Sodium** | | |
| *Butisol* | **Tablets:** 15 mg, 30 mg[2], 50 mg[2] | Yes |
| *Butisol[1,2]* | **Elixir**: 30 mg/5 mL | Yes |
| *c-IV* **Mephobarbital** | | |
| *Mebaral* | **Tablets:** 32 mg, 50 mg, 100 mg | Yes |
| **Pentobarbital and Pentobarbital Sodium** | | |
| *c-II Nembutal Sodium* | **Capsules:** 50 mg, 100 mg[2] | No |
| *c-II Nembutal[1]* | **Elixir**: 18.2 mg pentobarbital/5 mL[3] | No |
| *c-II Nembutal[1]* | **Injection**: 50 mg/mL | Yes |
| *c-III Nembutal Sodium* | **Suppositories:** 30 mg, 60 mg, 120 mg, 200 mg | No |
| *c-IV* **Phenobarbital** | **Tablets**: 15 mg, 30 mg, 60 mg, 90 mg, 100 mg | Yes |
| | **Elixir**: 20 mg/5 mL[1] | Yes |
| *c-II* **Secobarbital Sodium** | | |
| *Seconal Sodium* | **Capsules**: 100 mg | Yes |
| **Barbiturate Combinations** | | |
| *c-II Tuinal 100 mg Pulvules* | **Capsules:** 50 mg amobarbital sodium, 50 mg secobarbital sodium | No |
| *c-II Tuinal 200 mg Pulvules* | **Capsules:** 100 mg amobarbital sodium, 100 mg secobarbital sodium | No |

[1] Contains alcohol.
[2] Contains tartrazine dye.
[3] Equivalent to 20 mg pentobarbital sodium/5 mL.

## Type of Drug:

Central nervous system (CNS) depressants; sedatives; antianxiety agents; anticonvulsants; "barbs"; "downers."

## How the Drug Works:

Barbiturates are capable of producing all levels of CNS mood alternation, from excitation to mild sedation, sleep, and deep coma. They also decrease the severity and or frequency of certain types of seizures. Overdose can produce death. In high therapeutic doses, barbiturates induce anesthesia. Barbiturates depress the sensory cortex, decrease motor activity, alter cerebellar function, and produce drowsiness, sedation, and hypnosis (sleep).

## Uses:

To treat sleeplessness by inducing sleep (hypnotic). Do not use for more than 2 weeks. Other drugs have replaced barbiturates as primary sleep aids (all except mephobarbital, phenobarbital).

To calm down (sedate) patients who are agitated (all except pentobarbital injection).

To treat certain seizure disorders. Mephobarbital is indicated for the treatment of grand and petit mal epilepsy. Phenobarbital is indicated for the treatment of generalized and partial seizures. May be used alone or in combination with other medications.

As a preoperative medication (preanesthetic) to lessen anxiety and to assist in induction of anesthesia (amobarbital, secobarbital, and pentobarbital).

## Precautions:

*Do not use in the following situations:*

| | |
|---|---|
| allergy to barbiturates or any of their ingredients | lung disease, severe |
| liver disease, marked | porphyria |

*Use with caution in the following situations:*

| | |
|---|---|
| alcohol use | hypoadrenal function |
| children | kidney disease |
| corticosteroid therapy | liver disease |
| debilated patients | lung disease |
| depression | pain, acute or chronic |
| drug abuse, history of | pregnancy |
| elderly | suicidal tendencies |
| heart disease | |

*Vitamin D requirements* may be increased when taking barbiturates. Long-term barbiturate use may increase the chance for developing rickets or osteoporosis (weakening of bones).

*Vitamin K:* Bleeding in the early neonatal period due to coagulation defects may follow exposure to anticonvulsant drug *in uterto*; therefore, vitamin K should be given to the mother before delivery or to the child at birth.

*Acute or chronic pain:* Caution should be exercised when barbiturates are administered to patients with acute or chronic pain because paradoxical excitement could be induced or symptoms could be masked. However, use of barbiturates as sedatives in postoperative surgical period and as adjunct to cancer chemotherapy is well established.

*Steroid-dependent patients:* Steroids (eg, hydrocortisone, prednisone) may lose some effect when barbiturates are started. Tell your doctor if you take steroid medications regularly.

*Barbiturates may be habit forming.* Tolerance and dependence may occur with continued use, especially following prolonged use of high doses. To minimize the possibility of overdosage or the development of dependence, the prescribing and dispensing of sedative-hypnotic barbiturates should be limited to the amount required for the interval until the next appointment.

*Symptoms of acute intoxication* include unsteady walk, slurred speech, and sustained involuntary eye movements. Mental signs of chronic intoxication include confusion, poor judgment, irritability, sleeplessness, and body aches.

*Symptoms of dependence* are similar to those of chronic alcoholism and include: A strong desire or need to continue taking the drug, tendency to increase the dose, and dependence on the effects of the drug.

*Elderly or debilitated patients* may be more susceptible to side effects. Lower initial doses may be appropriate.

*Pregnancy:* Studies have shown a potential effect on the fetus. Withdrawal symptoms may occur in infants born to women who receive barbituates throughout the last trimester of pregnancy. Use only if clearly needed and potential benefits outweigh the possible risks to the fetus.

*Breastfeeding:* Small amounts of barbiturates appear in breast milk. Drowsiness in the nursing infant has been reported. Consult your doctor before you begin breastfeeding.

*Children:* Safety and effectiveness have not been established for children younger than 6 years of age. Some children may become irritable, excitable, unexpectedly tearful, or aggressive when taking barbiturates.

*Lab tests* may be required during long-term therapy. Tests may include blood counts and kidney and liver function tests.

*Tartrazine:* Some of these products may contain the dye tartrazine (FD&C Yellow No. 5), which can cause allergic reactions in certain individuals. Check package label when available or consult your doctor or pharmacist.

## Drug Interactions:

Tell your doctor or pharmacist if you are taking or if you are planning to take any over-the-counter or prescription medications or dietary supplements with barbiturates. Doses of one or both drugs may need to be modified or a different drug may need to be prescribed. The following drugs and drug classes interact with barbiturates.

alcohol
anesthetics, general
 (eg, methoxyflurane)
anticoagulants (eg, warfarin)
carbamazepine (eg, *Tegretol)*
charcoal
corticosteroids (eg, prednisone)
contraceptives, oral
 (eg, *Ortho-Novum)*
CNS depressant drugs
divalproex sodium (*Depakote)*
doxycycline (eg, *Vibramycin)*
estrogens (eg, estradiol)
felodipine (*Plendil)*
griseofulvin (eg, *Grisactin)*
MAOIs (eg, phenelzine)

methadone (eg, *Dolophine)*
metoprolol (eg, *Lopressor)*
metronidazole (eg, *Flagyl)*
nifedipine (eg, *Procardia)*
phenytoin (eg, *Dilantin)*
propranolol (eg, *Inderal)*
quinidine (eg, *Quinidex-
 Extentabs)*
steroidial hormones (eg, estradiol, estrone, progrestone)
theophyllines (eg, amino-
 phylline)
tricyclic antidepressants
 (eg, amitriptyline)
valproate
valproic acid (eg, *Depakene)*

## Side Effects:

Every drug is capable of producing side effects. Many barbiturate sedative users experience no, or minor, side effects. The frequency and severity of side effects depend on many factors including dose, duration of therapy, and individual susceptibility. Possible side effects include:

*Withdrawal:* Symptoms of withdrawal can be severe and may cause death. Minor symptoms may appear 8 to 12 hours after the last dose of a barbiturate and usually appear in the following order: Anxiety, muscle twitching, tremor of hands and fingers, progressive weakness, dizziness, visual perception problems, nausea, vomiting, sleeplessness, and dizziness or lightheadedness when arising from a seated or lying position. Major symptoms, inclusing convulsions and delirium, may occur within 16 hours and last 5 days or less after abrupt stopping of these drugs. Intensity of withdrawal symptoms gradually declines over a period of approxmately 15 days.

*Digestive Tract:* Nausea; vomiting; constipation.

*Nervous System:* Drowsiness; agitation; confusion; nightmares; hangover feeling; nervousness; hallucinations; sleeplessness; headache; depression; dizziness; stumbling gait.

*Circulatory System:* Slowed heart rate; decreased blood pressure.

*Respiratory System:* Decreased breathing rate; difficulty breathing.

*Other:* Rash; pain; fever; anemia; injection site reactions; fainting.

## Guidelines for Use:

- Doses of barbiturates will be individualized with full knowledge of the patient's particular characteristics, including the patient's age, weight, the condition being treated, and other concurrent medical conditions and medications.
- Take only the amount of drug prescribed by your doctor. Barbiturates may be habit forming both psychologically and physically. Do not change the dose or discontinue therapy unless advised to do so by your doctor.
- *Seizures* — When treating seizures with barbiturates, a barbiturate-induced depression may occur along with a postictal depression once the seizures are controlled; therefore, it is important to use the minimal amount required and to wait for the anticonvulsant effect to develop before administering a second dose.
- Too rapid administration of IV or IM dosing may cause respiratory depression, difficult breathing, larynx spasms, or flushing and redness of the skin with a fall in blood pressure.
- Tell you doctor if you experience pain in the limbs during administration of an injection. This may be a sign of a serious condition. Parenteral solutions of barbiturates are highly alkaline and therefore extreme care should be taken to avoid perivascular extravasation or intra-arterial injection. Results of inappropiate injection may be local tissue damage and pain or gangrene to the limb.
- Tell your doctor if you are pregnant, become pregnant, are planning to become pregnant, or if you are breastfeeding.
- Oral contraceptive effectiveness may be decreased by barbituates. An alternative form of contraceptive (eg, barrier methods) is recommended.
- May decrease alertness or physical ability. Use caution when driving or performing tasks requiring alertness, coordination, or physical dexterity.
- Avoid alcohol and other mental depressants (eg, narcotics, tranquilizers, and antihistamines) while you are taking barbiturates.
- Contact your doctor if you notice fever or excessive sedation.
- Use as an aid to sleep is limited. Do not use for more than 2 weeks.
- *Seizure control* — Do not stop therapy suddenly. Status epilepticus (severe, prolonged seizures) may result from the abrupt discontinuation of mephobarbital or phenobarbital, even when administered in small daily doses for treatment of epilepsy.
- To avoid withdrawal symptoms after long-term use, a gradual dosage tapering schedule should be used.
- Lab tests may be required during prolonged therapy. Be sure to keep appointments.
- Store tablets, capsules, and elixirs at controlled room temperature (68° to 77°F) in a safe place, away from children.

*If you have any questions, consult your doctor, pharmacist, or health care provider.*

| Generic Name<br>*Brand Name Examples* | Supplied As | Generic<br>Available |
|---|---|---|
| *c-iv* **Chloral Hydrate** | **Syrup:** 500 mg/5 mL | Yes |
| *Somnote* | **Capsules:** 500 mg | Yes |
| *Aquachloral Supprettes* | **Suppositories:** 325 mg[1],<br>650 mg | No |
| *c-iv* **Estazolam** | | |
| *ProSom* | **Tablets:** 1 mg, 2 mg | Yes |
| *c-iv* **Ethchlorvynol** | | |
| *Placidyl* | **Capsules:** 200 mg, 500 mg,<br>750 mg[1] | No |
| *c-iv* **Flurazepam HCl** | | |
| *Dalmane* | **Capsules:** 15 mg, 30 mg | Yes |
| *c-iv* **Quazepam** | | |
| *Doral* | **Tablets:** 7.5 mg, 15 mg | No |
| *c-iv* **Temazepam** | | |
| *Restoril* | **Capsules:** 7.5 mg, 15 mg,<br>30 mg | Yes |
| *c-iv* **Triazolam** | | |
| *Halcion* | **Tablets:** 0.125 mg, 0.25 mg | Yes |
| *c-iv* **Zaleplon** | | |
| *Sonata[1]* | **Capsules:** 5 mg, 10 mg | No |
| *c-iv* **Zolpidem Tartrate** | | |
| *Ambien* | **Tablets:** 5 mg, 10 mg | No |

[1] Contains tartrazine.

Estazolam, flurazepam, quazepam, temazepam, and triazolam are benzodiazepines. For more information, see the Antianxiety Agents — Benzodiazepines monograph in this chapter.

## Type of Drug:

Nonbarbiturate sedative/hypnotics. Central nervous system depressant. Short-term sleep aid.

## How the Drug Works:

Nonbarbiturate sedatives and hypnotics act on the central nervous system (brain), causing drowsiness to aid in falling asleep. They are less likely to cause a slower breathing rate than barbiturate-type sedative/hypnotics.

## Uses:

To treat insomnia (sleeplessness) for short (1 to 2 weeks) periods of time. Long-term use is generally not recommended and requires periodic medical evaluation.

Should sleeplessness persist, a drug-free interval of 1 or more weeks should elapse before retreatment is considered. An attempt should be made to find alternative nondrug therapy in chronic sleeplessness.

*Chloral hydrate:* To lessen anxiety and produce sleep before surgery. After surgery, chloral hydrate may be used with other medications to control pain. Also used to prevent or suppress alcohol withdrawal symptoms (suppositories).

*Unlabeled Use(s):* Occasionally doctors may prescribe ethchlorvynol as a sedative at doses of 100 mg to 200 mg 2 or 3 times daily.

## Precautions:

*Do not use in the following situations:*

allergy to the medicine or any of its ingredients
heart disease, severe (chloral hydrate only)
itraconazole use, concurrent (triazolam only)
ketoconazole use, concurrent (triazolam only)
kidney disease, marked (chloral hydrate only)
liver disease, marked (chloral hydrate only)
nefazodone use, concurrent (triazolam only)
porphyria (ethchlorvynol only)
pregnancy (benzodiazepines only)
sleep apnea, established or suspected (quazepam only)

*Use with caution in the following situations:*

depression
disease affecting metabolism or hemodynamic responses (zaleplon, zolpidem only)
drug abuse and dependence
elderly or debilitated patients
esophagitis (chloral hydrate only)
gastritis (chloral hydrate only)
kidney disease
liver disease
lung disease
porphyria (chloral hydrate only)
psychiatric or physical disorder
ulcer, duodenal or gastric (chloral hydrate only)

*Dependence:* Long-term use may result in dependence. Withdrawal symptoms (eg, rebound insomnia) may occur when the drug is stopped abruptly after long-term use.

*Ethchlorvynol:* Patients who exhibit unpredictable behavior, restlessness, or excitement in response to barbiturates or alcohol may react in this manner to ethchlorvynol. This drug should not be used for the management of insomnia in the presence of pain, unless sleep loss persists after pain is controlled with pain relievers.

*Triazolam:* Short-term episodes of significant memory loss have been reported with the use of triazolam. Patients, especially the elderly, may become confused or disoriented and may attempt to wander after taking the drug. Upon waking in the morning, the patient may not remember the episode.

*Pregnancy:* Do not use benzodiazepines during pregnancy. The risk of use in a pregnant woman clearly outweighs any possible benefit. Use of ethchlorvynol is not recommended during the first and second trimesters of pregnancy. Use during the third trimester of pregnancy may produce symptoms in the newborn (eg, jitteriness, hyperactivity, restlessness, irritability, disturbed sleep, hunger). There are no adequate and well-controlled studies for other sedative/hypnotics in pregnant women. Use only if clearly needed and potential benefits outweigh the possible hazards to the fetus.

*Breastfeeding:* Benzodiazepines, chloral hydrate, zaleplon, and zolpidem appear in breast milk. It is not known if the other sedative/hypnotics appear in breast milk. Consult your doctor before you begin breastfeeding.

*Children:* Safety and effectiveness of estazolam, ethchlorvynol, quazepam, temazepam, triazolam, zaleplon, and zolpidem have not been established in patients younger than 18 years of age. Safety and effectiveness of flurazepam have not been established in patients younger than 15 years of age. These drugs are generally not recommended for use in children.

*Elderly:* Use with caution. Elderly patients may be more sensitive to these drugs. There is a risk of oversedation, "morning hangover" (grogginess in the morning), dizziness, and confusion. Smaller doses may be needed. See triazolam precaution.

*Lab tests* may be required to monitor therapy. Tests may include blood counts, urinalysis, blood chemistry, and liver and kidney function tests.

*Tartrazine:* Some of these products may contain tartrazine dye (FD&C Yellow No. 5), which can cause allergic reactions in certain individuals. Check package label when available or consult your doctor or pharmacist.

## Drug Interactions:

Tell your doctor or pharmacist if you are taking or planning to take any over-the-counter or prescription medications with nonbarbiturate sedatives. Doses of one or both drugs may need to be modified or a different drug may need to be prescribed. The following drugs and drug classes interact with nonbarbiturate sedatives:

*All* —

ethanol

*Benzodiazepines only* —

azole antifungal agents (eg, ketoconazole)
cimetidine (eg, *Tagamet*)
contraceptives, oral (eg, *Ortho-Novum*)
disulfiram (eg, *Antabuse*)
grapefruit juice
macrolide antibiotics (eg, erythromycin)
nefazodone (*Serzone*)

NNRT inhibitors (eg, delavirdine)
omeprazole (*Prilosec*)
protease inhibitors (eg, indinavir, ritonavir)
rifamycins (eg, rifampin)
SSRIs (eg, fluvoxamine)
theophyllines (eg, aminophylline)

*Chloral hydrate and ethchlorvynol only —*

anticoagulants (eg, warfarin)

*Zolpidem only —*

azole antifungal agents
(eg, ketocaonzole)
protease inhibitors (eg, indinavir, ritonavir)

rifamycins (eg, rifampin)
SSRIs (eg, fluoxetine)

## Side Effects:

Every drug is capable of producing side effects. Many nonbarbiturate sedative users experience no, or minor, side effects. The frequency and severity of side effects depend on many factors including dose, duration of
therapy, and individual susceptibility. Possible side effects include:

*Digestive Tract:* Stomach pain or upset; vomiting; nausea; diarrhea; constipation; indigestion; appetite loss; gastric irritation; colitis.

*Nervous System:* Confusion; drowsiness; dizziness; hallucinations; headache; anxiety; depression; facial numbness; nervousness; vertigo (feeling of whirling motion); memory loss; drugged feeling; lethargy;
sleeplessness; abnormal thinking; depersonalization; agitation; lightheadedness; abnormal dreams; sleep disorder; euphoria (exaggerated
sense of well being); incoordination; weakness; tremor.

*Circulatory System:* Abnormal blood counts; palpitations (pounding in the
chest).

*Skin:* Jaundice (yellowing of skin or eyes); rash; hives; itching; abnormal
skin sensations.

*Other:* Allergy; back pain; chest pain; fatigue; flu-like symptoms; blurred
vision; mild "hangover"; aftertaste; dry mouth; urinary tract infection;
conjunctivitis; migraine; arthritis; fever; double vision; abnormal vision;
muscle, joint, ear, or eye pain; swelling of the arms or legs; general body
discomfort; photosensitivity; sinus infection; sore throat; runny nose;
bronchitis; distorted sense of smell; nosebleed; painful menstruation;
abnormal acuteness of hearing; muscle tension; muscle pain; falling.

*Benzodiazepines only —*

*Digestive Tract:* Heartburn; appetite loss; nausea; vomiting; diarrhea; constipation; stomach pain; indigestion; taste alterations; dry mouth.

*Nervous System:* Drowsiness; nervousness; talkativeness; apprehension;
irritability; euphoria (exaggerated sense of well being); relaxed feeling;
tremor; memory loss; tiredness; general body discomfort; dreaming or
nightmares; depression; incoordination; confusion; hangover; abnormal
thinking; anxiety; dizziness; disorientation; weakness; agitation; speech
disorder; daytime drowsiness; feeling of whirling motion.

*Circulatory System:* Palpitations (pounding in the chest); chest pain.

*Other:* Abnormal skin sensations; joint or body pain; weakness; headache; genitourinary complaints; falling; staggering; rash; itching; leg or
back pain; stiffness.

## Guidelines for Use:

- Dosage is individualized.
- Do not change the dose or stop taking unless advised by your doctor.
- Take immediately before going to bed.
- May cause dizziness, drowsiness, or blurred vision. Do not drive or perform other tasks requiring alertness, coordination, or physical dexterity.
- Avoid alcohol and other drugs that cause drowsiness (eg, pain relievers, sedatives).
- Contact your doctor if you notice any unusual or disturbing thoughts or behaviors during treatment with any sleep medicine.
- Do not take any sleep medicine unless you are able to get a full night of sleep before you must be active again.
- May cause photosensitivity (sensitivity to light). Avoid prolonged exposure to the sun. Use sunscreens and wear protective clothing until tolerance is determined.
- May be habit forming. Do not discontinue drug abruptly after prolonged use, especially if you have a history of seizures, regardless of other antiseizure medications you may be taking.
- Contact your doctor if visual changes, irregular heartbeats, chest pains, yellowing of skin or eyes, rash, or unusual bleeding or bruising occurs.
- Lab tests may be required to monitor therapy. Be sure to keep appointments.
- *Benzodiazepines* — Nighttime sleep may be disturbed for 1 or 2 nights following stopping of the drug.
  Tell your doctor if you are pregnant, plan to become pregnant, or become pregnant while taking this medicine.
- *Chloral hydrate* — May cause stomach upset. Take capsules with a full glass of water or other liquid.
  Swallow capsules whole. Do not crush or chew.
  Dilute syrup in a half glass of water, ginger ale, or fruit juice.
- *Ethchlorvynol* — Symptoms of giddiness, incoordination, and stomach upset may be reduced if medication is taken with food.
- *Triazolam* — Do not take when a full night's sleep and elimination of the drug from the body are not possible before the need to be active and functional. May cause amnesia.
- *Zaleplon* — Do not take with or immediately following a high-fat or heavy meal.
  May cause sleepiness during the day. Daytime drowsiness can be best avoided by taking the lowest possible dose.
  May cause amnesia. In most cases, memory problems can be avoided if zaleplon is taken only when you are able to get 4 hours or more of sleep before being active.
- *Zolpidem* — For faster sleep onset, do not take with or immediately after a meal.

*If you have any questions, consult your doctor, pharmacist, or health care provider.*

| | Brand Name Examples | Supplied As | Generic Available |
|---|---|---|---|
| otc | Unisom Nighttime Sleep Aid | **Tablets:** 25 mg doxylamine succinate | No |
| otc | Nervine, Nytol QuickCaps, Sominex | **Tablets:** 25 mg diphenhydramine HCl | Yes |
| otc | Sominex Pain Relief | **Tablets:** 25 mg diphenhydramine HCl and 500 mg acetaminophen | No |
| otc | Extra Strength Tylenol PM Geltabs | **Capsules:** 25 mg diphenhydramine HCl and 500 mg acetaminophen | No |
| otc | Maximum Strength Compōz Nighttime Sleep Aid, Maximum Strength Sominex, Twilite | **Tablets:** 50 mg diphenhydramine HCl | No |
| otc | Maximum Strength Compōz Nighttime Sleep Aid, Maximum Strength Nytol QuickGels, Maximum Strength Sleepinal Softgels, Maximum Strength Unisom Sleep-Gels | **Capsules:** 50 mg diphenhydramine HCl | Yes |
| otc | Unisom with Pain Relief | **Tablets:** 50 mg diphenhydramine HCl and 650 mg acetaminophen | No |

## Type of Drug:

Nonprescription (over-the-counter) sleep aids.

## How the Drug Works:

These drugs contain antihistamines (eg, doxylamine, diphenhydramine) which act on the central nervous system to increase feelings of drowsiness or sleepiness which can help induce and maintain sleep. A few products also contain a pain reliever (eg, acetaminophen) for the relief of minor aches and pains.

## Uses:

To treat occasional difficulty in falling asleep.

To relieve sleeplessness with accompanying minor aches, pains, or headache (products containing acetaminophen).

## Precautions:

*Do not use in the following situations:*

alcohol consumption more than 3 drinks a day
allergy to these medicines or any of their ingredients

breastfeeding (doxylamine only)
pregnancy (doxylamine only)

*Use with caution in the following situations:*

| | |
|---|---|
| asthma | glaucoma |
| breathing problems (eg, emphysema, chronic bronchitis) | peptic ulcer, active |
| | prostate gland enlargement |
| difficult urination due to prostate gland enlargement | urinary tract obstruction |

*Pregnancy and breastfeeding:* Pregnant or breastfeeding women should not use products containing doxylamine. Consult your doctor before using any of these products during pregnancy or breastfeeding.

*Long-term insomnia:* Sleep aids should not be used continuously for more than 2 weeks. Contact your doctor if insomnia lasts more than 2 weeks.

Consider all precautions reported for antihistamines when using nonprescription sleep aids. See the Antihistamines monograph in the Respiratory Drugs chapter.

*Children:* Do not use in children younger than 12 years of age unless directed by a doctor.

*Elderly:* The elderly may require lower than usual doses. Antihistamines are more likely to cause dizziness, sedation, confusion, and decrease in blood pressure in elderly people.

## Drug Interactions:

Tell your doctor or pharmacist if you are taking or if you are planning to take any over-the-counter or prescription medications with nonprescription sleep aids. Doses of one or both drugs may need to be modified or a different drug may need to be prescribed. Alcohol interacts with nonprescription sleep aids. The following drugs or drug classes interact with nonprescription sleep aids containing acetaminophen.

| | |
|---|---|
| anticoagulants, oral | hydantoins (eg, phenytoin) |
| ethanol (alcohol) | sulfinpyrazone (eg, *Anturane)* |

## Side Effects:

Every drug is capable of producing side effects. Many nonprescription sleep aid users experience no, or minor, side effects. The frequency and severity of side effects depend on many factors including dose, duration of therapy, and individual susceptibility. For information on possible side effects of antihistamines. See the Antihistamines monograph in the Respiratory Drugs chapter. Possible side effects include:

*Other:* Dry mouth; confusion; blurred vision; urinary retention; constipation; drowsiness.

## Guidelines for Use:

- Consult individual product information for specific dosage instructions. Do not exceed recommended dosage.
- Take 30 minutes before desired sleep time.
- May cause drowsiness. Use caution while driving or performing tasks which require alertness, coordination, or physical dexterity.
- Do not drink alcoholic beverages while taking any sleep aid. Do not take other sedatives or tranquilizers without first consulting your doctor.
- Do not use nonprescription sleep aids containing acetaminophen if you drink 3 or more alcoholic beverages every day, unless directed to do so by your doctor.
- Do not use nonprescription sleep aids containing acetaminophen for pain for more than 10 days or for fever for more than 3 days, unless directed by your doctor.
- Do not use nonprescription sleep aids containing acetaminophen with other products containing acetaminophen (eg, *Tylenol*) unless advised by your doctor.
- Do not give to children younger than 12 years of age unless directed by your doctor.
- Notify your doctor if your symptoms persist or worsen, if new ones occur, or if sleeplessness continues for more than 2 weeks. Sleeplessness may be a symptom of a serious underlying illness.
- Store at room temperature. Avoid excessive heat or humidity.

*If you have any questions, consult your doctor, pharmacist, or health care provider.*

| Generic Name<br>*Brand Name Examples* | Supplied As | Generic<br>Available |
|---|---|---|
| *Rx* **Acetazolamide** | | |
| *Diamox* | **Tablets:** 125 mg, 250 mg | Yes |
| *Diamox* | **Injection:** 500 mg | Yes |
| *Diamox Sequels* | **Capsules, sustained release:** 500 mg | No |

## Type of Drug:

Anticonvulsant; diuretic or "water pill"; antiglaucoma drug; carbonic anhydrase inhibitor.

## How the Drug Works:

*Anticonvulsant:* Prevents or reduces seizures by slowing abnormal nerve impulses in the brain and central nervous system.

*Diuretic:* Reduces amount of fluid in the body by increasing urine formation.

*Antiglaucoma:* Reduces pressure in the eyes by decreasing the formation of fluid inside the eye.

## Uses:

To treat petit mal and unlocalized seizures.

To treat edema (excess fluid in tissues) which may accompany congestive heart failure, other circulatory system disorders, or other drug therapy.

*Sustained-release capsules:* To treat certain types of glaucoma. Usually used in combination with drugs applied directly to the eye.

To prevent or treat the effects of acute mountain sickness.

## Precautions:

*Do not use in the following situations:*

adrenocortical insufficiency (Addison's disease)
allergy to acetazolamide
chronic noncongestive angle-closure glaucoma
cirrhosis
electrolyte imbalance (eg, low potassium or sodium levels)
hyperchloremic acidosis
kidney disease, severe
liver disease, severe
lung obstruction, severe

*Use with caution in the following situations:*

allergy to sulfa drugs (eg, *Bactrim)*
aspirin, high-dose, concurrent
emphysema
lung obstruction

*Blood disorders* can occur while taking this medication. Patients should be routinely monitored to avoid this problem.

*Potassium loss:* By increasing urine formation, acetazolamide may cause loss of potassium from the body. Low potassium levels may be treated by eating foods and drinking fluids high in potassium, such as citrus (orange) juice, bananas, dates, raisins, melons, and tomatoes. If increasing potassium in the diet does not raise potassium levels to normal, a potassium supplement may be necessary to replace lost potassium.

*Pregnancy:* Adequate studies have not been done in pregnant women. Use only if clearly needed and potential benefits outweigh the possible hazards to the fetus.

*Breastfeeding:* Acetazolamide may appear in breast milk. Because of the potential for serious adverse reactions in nursing infants, a decision should be made whether to discontinue nursing or discontinue the drug, taking into account the importance of the drug to the mother. Consult your doctor before you begin breastfeeding.

*Children:* Safety and effectiveness in children have not been established.

*Lab tests* are required during treatment with acetazolamide. Tests may include blood counts, electrolytes (eg, potassium, sodium, chloride), and liver and kidney function tests.

## Drug Interactions:

Tell your doctor or pharmacist if you are taking or if you are planning to take any over-the-counter or prescription medications or dietary supplements with acetazolamide. Doses of one or both drugs may need to be modified or a different drug may need to be prescribed. The following drugs interact with acetazolamide.

cyclosporine (eg, *Sandimmune*)
lithium (eg, *Eskalith*)
primidone (eg, *Mysoline*)
quinidine (eg, *Quinidex*)

salicylates (eg, aspirin, *Arthropan, Doan's, Tusal*)
salsalate (eg, *Disalcid*)
steroid therapy (eg, prednisone)

## Side Effects:

Every drug is capable of producing side effects. Many acetazolamide users experience no, or minor, side effects. The frequency and severity of side effects depend on many factors including dose, duration of therapy, and individual susceptibility. Possible side effects include:

*Digestive Tract:* Nausea; vomiting; loss of appetite; diarrhea.

*Skin:* Unusual bleeding or bruising; rash; red or purple spots under the skin; sensitivity to light.

*Other:* Fever; tingling or numbness in hands or feet; drowsiness; confusion; allergic reaction; taste alterations; ringing in the ears; hearing dysfunction; excessive urination; electrolyte imbalance; metabolic acidosis; crystals in urine; kidney stones; abnormal blood cell counts; transient nearsightedness; sore throat.

## Guidelines for Use:

- *Epilepsy* — Suggested total daily dose is 8 to 30 mg/kg in divided doses. Optimum range appears to be from 375 to 1000 mg daily. When given in combination with other anticonvulsants, the starting dose should be 250 mg once daily in addition to existing medications.
- *Tablets* can be crushed and mixed with sweet foods to mask bitter taste.
- *Capsules* can be opened and contents sprinkled on food, if necessary.
- *Sustained-release capsules* — Do not crush or chew.
- Doses more than 1 g per 24 hours do not produce an increased effect.
- For use of acetazolamide in acute mountain sickness, congestive heart failure, drug-induced edema, and glaucoma, see the Diuretics-Carbonic Anhydrase Inhibitors monograph.
- May cause stomach upset. Take with food.
- May cause drowsiness. Use caution when driving or performing other tasks requiring alertness, coordination, or physical dexterity.
- May cause loss of potassium from the body. Contact your doctor if signs of potassium loss (eg, weakness, muscle cramps, nausea, dizziness) occur.
- Notify your doctor if sore throat, fever, unusual bleeding or bruising, tingling or numbness in the hands or feet, flank or loin pain, or skin rash occurs.
- When using acetazolamide, urination may increase; if possible, take early in the day.
- Temporary nearsightedness (change in vision) has occasionally occurred with this medicine. It subsides when the dose is reduced or the medicine is stopped.
- May cause sensitivity to sunlight. Avoid prolonged exposure to the sun or other forms of ultraviolet (UV) light (eg, tanning beds). Use sunscreens and wear protective clothing until tolerance is determined.
- Store at room temperature (59° to 86°F).

*If you have any questions, consult your doctor, pharmacist, or health care provider.*

| Generic Name<br>*Brand Name Examples* | Supplied As | Generic Available |
|---|---|---|
| *Rx* **Carbamazepine** | | |
| *Epitol, Tegretol* | **Tablets:** 200 mg | Yes |
| *Tegretol* | **Tablets, chewable:** 100 mg | Yes |
| *Tegretol* | **Suspension:** 100 mg/tsp | No |
| *Tegretol-XR* | **Tablets, extended release:**<br>100 mg, 200 mg, 400 mg | No |

## Type of Drug:

Anticonvulsant; drug used to treat a variety of seizure disorders. Analgesic (pain reliever) for certain types of nerve pain (eg, trigeminal neuralgia).

## How the Drug Works:

Carbamazepine appears to prevent or reduce the number of seizures by controlling the activity of nerve impulses in the central nervous system. In trigeminal neuralgia, carbamazepine may reduce the activity of nerve impulses in the trigeminal nerve (nerve to the face), decreasing pain transmission.

## Uses:

To control partial seizures with complex symptoms (eg, psychomotor, temporal lobe), grand mal and mixed seizures, alone or with other anticonvulsant drugs.

To treat trigeminal neuralgia (tic douloureux), a condition causing severe, stabbing pain in the face. Carbamazepine is not a simple pain reliever and should not be used for the relief of minor aches and pains.

*Unlabeled Use(s):* Occasionally doctors may prescribe carbamazepine for neurogenic diabetes insipidus; certain psychiatric disorders; restless leg syndrome; nonneuritic pain syndrome (eg, phantom limb pain); and alcohol, cocaine, and benzodiazepine withdrawal management.

## Precautions:

*Do not use in the following situations:*
>       allergy to carbamazepine
>       allergy to tricyclic antidepressants (eg, amitriptyline)
>       bone marrow depression, history
>       monoamine oxidase inhibitor (eg, phenelzine) use (current or within
>           14 days)

*Use with caution in the following situations:*

anemia or other blood disorders, including drug-induced blood disorders
glaucoma
heart disease
kidney disease
liver disease
lupus erythematosus
mixed seizure disorders with atypical absence (petit mal) seizures

*Potentially fatal blood cell abnormalities* have been reported rarely following treatment with carbamazepine. Early detection of blood changes is important since some abnormalities may be reversible.

*Minor pain:* Do not use carbamazepine to relieve minor aches and pains.

*Pregnancy:* Reports suggest an association between use of anticonvulsant drugs by women with epilepsy and an increased number of birth defects in children born to these women. Other factors (eg, genetics or the epileptic condition) may also contribute to the higher incidence of birth defects. Most mothers receiving anticonvulsant medication during pregnancy deliver normal infants. Tests to detect defects should be considered a part of routine prenatal care in childbearing women receiving carbamazepine. Do not abruptly or suddenly discontinue anticonvulsant drugs used to prevent major seizures. This could result in the occurrence of seizures, oxygen deficiency in body tissues, and an increased risk to both the mother and the unborn child. In cases where seizures do not pose a serious threat, your doctor may recommend gradual discontinuation of anticonvulsants prior to and during pregnancy. It is not known whether even minor seizures constitute some risk to the developing embryo or fetus. Use only when clearly needed and when the potential benefits outweigh the potential hazards to the fetus.

*Breastfeeding:* Carbamazepine appears in breast milk. Consult your doctor before you begin breastfeeding.

*Children:* Use in children under 6 years of age should be directed by clinicians expert in treating seizure disorders (eg, a neurologist).

*Elderly:* Carbamazepine may be more likely to cause confusion or agitation in elderly patients than in younger patients. Use with caution.

*Lab tests* may be required before and during treatment with carbamazepine. Tests may include: Complete blood counts, liver function tests, urinalysis, blood urea nitrogen, eye tests, thyroid tests, and carbamazepine blood levels. Carbamazepine may interfere with thyroid function tests and some pregnancy tests.

## Drug Interactions:
Tell your doctor or pharmacist if you are taking or if you are planning to take any over-the-counter or prescription medications or dietary supplements with carbamazepine. Doses of one or both drugs may need to be modified or a different drug may need to be prescribed. The following drugs and drug classes interact with carbamazepine.

acetaminophen (eg, *Tylenol)*
alprazolam (*Xanax*)
anticoagulants, oral (eg, warfarin)
anticonvulsants (eg, valproic acid, phenytoin, phenobarbital, ethosuximide, primidone, felbamate)
azole antifungals (eg, itraconazole)
bupropion HCl (*Wellbutrin*)

charcoal
cimetidine (*Tagamet*)
cisplatin (*Platinol*)
clomipramine HCl (*Anafranil*)
clozapine (*Clozaril*)
contraceptives, oral (eg, *Ortho-Novum)*
cyclosporine (eg, *Neoral*)
danazol (eg, *Danocrine*)
diltiazem (eg, *Cardizem)*
doxycycline (*Vibramycin*)

doxorubicin (eg, *Rubex*)
felodipine (*Plendil*)
fluoxetine (*Prozac*)
haloperidol (*Haldol)*
isoniazid (*Nydrazid)*
lamotrigine (*Lamictal*)
lithium (eg, *Eskalith)*
loratadine (*Claritin*)
macrolide antibiotics
 (eg, erythromycin)

muscle relaxants (eg, pancuronium)
niacinamide
propoxyphene (eg, *Darvon)*
rifampin (*Rifadin*)
theophylline (eg, *Theo-Dur)*
verapamil (eg, *Calan)*

## Side Effects:

Every drug is capable of producing side effects. Many carbamazepine users experience no, or minor, side effects. The frequency and severity of side effects depend on many factors including dose, duration of therapy, and individual susceptibility. Possible side effects include:

*Digestive Tract:* Nausea; vomiting; stomach upset and pain; diarrhea; constipation; appetite loss; dry mouth or throat; sores on mouth and tongue; sore throat.

*Nervous System:* Drowsiness; dizziness; incoordination; headache; confusion; mood changes; behavior changes (especially in children); unusual body movements; slurred speech; hallucinations; depression; fatigue.

*Circulatory System:* Changes in blood pressure; changes in heart rhythm; blood disorder; decreased blood cell counts (eg, platelets, white blood cells); blood clots.

*Respiratory System:* Difficulty breathing; pneumonia.

*Skin:* Yellowing of skin or eyes; changes in pigmentation; easy bruising or bleeding; rash; hives; skin lesions; peeling; sensitivity to sunlight; sweating; hair loss.

*Eyes or Ocular:* Double vision; unusual eye movements; blurred vision; red, itchy eyes.

*Urinary and Reproductive Tract:* Changes in urinary frequency; urinary retention; kidney failure.

*Other:* Fainting; fever; chills; sore throat; aches in muscles and joints; leg cramps; swelling of legs or ankles; swollen glands; numbness or tingling in hands or feet; ringing in ears; abnormal sensitivity to sounds; altered liver and kidney function tests; altered thyroid function tests; decreased sexual ability; edema (fluid retention); hemorrhaging or bleeding; aggravation of lupus erythematosus; abnormal skin sensations.

## Guidelines for Use:

- Take as directed by your doctor. Daily dose varies depending on individual needs.
- May cause upset stomach. Take with food.
- Shake suspension well before using.
- Suspension should not be administered simultaneously with other liquid medicinal agents or diluents.
- Since the suspension produces higher blood levels than tablets, it is recommended that patients given the suspension be started on lower doses and increased slowly to avoid unwanted side effects.
- Do not use to treat ordinary types of aches or pain. This drug should be used only to treat pain of trigeminal neuralgia.
- *Tegretol-XR* tablets must be swallowed whole and never crushed or chewed. Tablets should be inspected for chips or cracks; damaged tablets should not be consumed. The tablet coating remains in the intestine and is excreted in the stool and may be noticable.
- Carry Medic Alert identification indicating that you are using this drug.
- If you stop taking this drug suddenly, your convulsions may return. Do not stop taking this drug without talking to your doctor.
- If a dose is missed, take it as soon as possible. If several hours have passed or if it is nearing time for the next dose, do not double the dose in order to catch up (unless advised to do so by your doctor). If more than one dose is missed, or it is necessary to establish a new dosage schedule, contact your doctor or pharmacist.
- Stop taking MAO inhibitors at least 14 days before beginning taking carbamazepine.
- Notify your doctor if any of the following occurs: Unusual bleeding or bruising; yellowing of skin or eyes; stomach pain; pale stools; darkened urine; decreased sexual ability; confusion; dizziness; incoordination; hallucinations; excessive sedation; abnormal movements; mood changes; double vision; swelling; fever; chills; sore throat; ulcers in the mouth; rash.
- May cause drowsiness, dizziness, or blurred vision. Use caution when driving or performing other tasks requiring alertness, coordination, or physical dexterity until tolerance is determined.
- Absence (petit mal) seizures do not appear to be controlled by carbamazepine.
- Lab tests will be required before and during treatment, especially during the first 2 months, to make certain the drug is working properly and to screen for possible blood count disorders. Interference with some pregnancy tests had been reported. Be sure to keep appointments.
- Store *Epitol* tablets at room temperature in a tightly sealed, preferably glass container. Protect from moisture. Store *Tegretol* tablets and suspension at room temperature in a tightly sealed, light-resistant container. Protect from moisture.

*If you have any questions, consult your doctor, pharmacist, or health care provider.*

| Generic Name<br>*Brand Name Example* | Supplied As | Generic<br>Available |
|---|---|---|
| c-iv **Clonazepam** | | |
| *Klonopin* | **Tablets:** 0.5 mg, 1 mg, 2 mg | Yes |

## Type of Drug:

Benzodiazepine. Anticonvulsant; drug used to treat epilepsy (seizures) and panic disorder.

## How the Drug Works:

The actual mechanism of clonazepam's action is unknown. However, it is believed that clonazepam prevents or reduces the number of seizures and controls panic attacks by acting on the central nervous system to control the activity of nerve impulses.

## Uses:

To control Lennox-Gastaut syndrome (petit mal variant), akinetic, and myo-clonic seizures either alone or in combination with other anticonvulsant drugs.

To treat absence (petit mal) seizures when succinimides have failed.

To treat panic disorder with or without agoraphobia (fear of crowds, public places, open areas).

## Precautions:

*Do not use in the following situations:*
>>allergy to any other benzodiazepine (eg, alprazolam)
>>allergy to clonazepam or any of its ingredients
>>glaucoma, acute narrow angle
>>liver disease

*Use with caution in the following situations:*
>>alcoholism
>>chronic respiratory disease
>>drug abuse, history of
>>kidney disease
>>multiple seizure disorders

*Multiple seizure type:* When used in patients in whom several different types of seizure disorders coexist, clonazepam may increase the fre-quency or precipitate the onset of generalized tonic-clonic (grand mal) seizures. This may require the addition of other anticonvulsants or an increase in dosage.

*Chronic respiratory disease:* Clonazepam may produce respiratory depres-sion and an increase in salivation. In some patients, increased saliva-tion can cause difficulty breathing. Because of these possibilities, use clonazepam with caution in patients with chronic respiratory disease.

*Withdrawal syndrome:* Withdrawal symptoms (eg, convulsions, psychosis, hallucinations, behavioral disorder, tremor, abdominal and muscle cramps) have occurred following abrupt discontinuation of clonazepam. Severity is related to the degree of dependence and length of time used. The more severe withdrawal symptoms occurred in patients who received excessive doses over an extended period of time. After extended therapy, avoid abrupt discontinuation and follow a gradual dosage tapering schedule.

*Drug dependence:* Addiction prone individuals (ie, alcoholics, drug addicts) must be closely supervised during clonazepam therapy. Dependence has occurred in such patients.

*Pregnancy:* Reports suggest an association between use of anticonvulsant drugs by women with epilepsy and an increased number of birth defects in children born to these women. Other factors (eg, genetics or the epileptic condition) may also contribute to the higher incidence of birth defects. Most mothers receiving anticonvulsant medication deliver normal infants. Do not discontinue anticonvulsant drugs used to prevent major seizures. This could result in the occurrence of seizures, oxygen deficiency in body tissues, and an increased risk to both the mother and the unborn child. In cases where seizures do not pose a serious threat, your doctor may recommend discontinuation of anticonvulsants prior to and during pregnancy. It is not known whether even minor seizures constitute some risk to the developing embryo or fetus. In addition, children born to mothers taking benzodiazepines late in pregnancy may exhibit side effects (eg, flaccid muscles, breathing or feeding difficulties) or withdrawal symptoms. Use this medicine during pregnancy only when benefits to the mother outweigh risks to the fetus.

*Breastfeeding:* Do not breastfeed while receiving clonazepam.

*Children:* Children being treated for seizure disorder may be more sensitive to the effects of this drug. Consult your doctor. Safety and effectiveness for use in children younger than 18 years of age with panic disorder have not been established.

*Lab tests* may be required during treatment with clonazepam. Tests may include blood counts and liver function tests.

## Drug Interactions:
Tell your doctor or pharmacist if you are taking or if you are planning to take any over-the-counter or prescription medications or dietary supplements with clonazepam. Doses of one or both drugs may need to be modified or a different drug may need to be prescribed. The following drugs and drug classes interact with clonazepam:

alcohol
antidepressants (eg, fluvoxamine)
anticonvulsants, other (eg, carbamazepine)
azole antifungal agents (eg, ketoconazole)
cimetidine (eg, *Tagamet*)
contraceptives, oral (eg, *Ortho-Novum*)
disulfiram (eg, *Antabuse*)
indinavir (*Crixivan*)
MAOIs (eg, phenelzine)
omeprazole (*Prilosec*)
rifamycins (eg, rifampin)
ritonavir (*Norvir*)
valproic acid (eg, *Depakene*)

Consider all drug interactions reported for benzodiazepines, in the Antianxiety Agents-Benzodiazepines monograph in this chapter when using this drug.

## Side Effects:

Every drug is capable of producing side effects. Many clonazepam users experience no, or minor, side effects. The frequency and severity of side effects depend on many factors, including dose, duration of therapy, and individual susceptibility. Possible side effects include:

*Digestive Tract:* Constipation; diarrhea; nausea; appetite changes.

*Nervous System:* Drowsiness; incoordination; behavior problems; headache; confusion; depression; memory loss; hysteria; bizarre behavior; mood changes; behavior changes; sleeplessness; tremor; dizziness; vertigo (feeling of whirling motion); partial paralysis; reduced intellectual ability; suicidal thoughts; nightmares; abnormal involuntary body movements; coma; hallucinations.

*Respiratory System:* Difficult breathing; chest congestion; "runny" nose; coughing; sore throat.

*Skin:* Rash; excessive growth or loss of hair.

*Eyes or Ocular:* Blurred vision; double vision; "glassy-eyed" appearance; unusual eye movements.

*Other:* Fever; fatigue; loss of voice; increased salivation or dry mouth; coated tongue; changes in urination; fluid retention; difficulty speaking; sore gums; swollen lymph nodes; weight changes; increased or decreased sex drive; incontinence of urine or feces; muscle pain or weakness; dehydration; menstruation problems; sexual problems; general deterioration; pounding in the chest; slurred speech.

## Guidelines for Use:

- Dosage will be individualized.
- Do not discontinue use or change the dose without first checking with your doctor. If you stop taking this drug suddenly, the frequency of your seizures could increase or you could experience withdrawal symptoms.
- Take with food if stomach upset occurs.
- If a dose is missed, take it as soon as possible. If several hours have passed or if it is nearing time for the next dose, do not double the dose to catch up, unless advised to do so by your doctor. If several doses are missed or it is necessary to establish a new dosage schedule, contact your doctor or pharmacist. Use exactly as prescribed.
- Inform your doctor if you are pregnant, become pregnant, are planning to become pregnant, or if you are breastfeeding.
- May cause drowsiness, dizziness, or blurred vision. Use caution when driving or performing other tasks requiring alertness, coordination, or physical dexterity.
- Using this drug with alcohol or other central nervous system depressants (eg, pain relievers, sedatives) may cause added drowsiness.
- If the drug does not seem to be working as well after taking it for a few weeks, check with your doctor. A dosage adjustment may be needed.
- Carry Medic Alert identification indicating that you are using this drug and have epilepsy.
- Lab tests may be required to monitor therapy. Be sure to keep appointments.
- Store at room temperature (59° to 86°F).

*If you have any questions, consult your doctor, pharmacist, or health care provider.*

| Generic Name<br>*Brand Name Example* | Supplied As | Generic<br>Available |
|---|---|---|
| Rx **Felbamate** | | |
| *Felbatol[1]* | **Tablets:** 400 mg, 600 mg | No |
| *Felbatol[1]* | **Oral suspension:**<br>600 mg/5 mL | |

[1] It has been recommended that use of this drug be discontinued if aplastic anemia or hepatic failure occurs unless, in the judgement of the doctor, continued therapy is warranted. For further information contact Wallace Laboratories at 800-526-3840.

## Type of Drug:
Anticonvulsant; antiepileptic.

## How the Drug Works:
Felbamate acts on the central nervous system to decrease the frequency of seizures.

## Uses:
Felbamate is not indicated as a first-line antiepileptic treatment. Felbamate is recommended for use only in those patients who respond inadequately to alternative treatments and whose epilepsy is so severe that a substantial risk of aplastic anemia or liver failure is deemed acceptable in light of the benefits conferred by its use.

Felbamate is indicated as monotherapy or adjunctive therapy in the treatment of partial seizures with and without generalization in adults with epilepsy.

Also indicated as adjunctive therapy in the treatment of partial or generalized seizures associated with Lennox-Gastaut syndrome in children.

## Precautions:
*Do not use in the following situations:*

allergy to felbamate or any of its ingredients
allergy to other carbamates (eg, meprobamate)

blood disease, history of
liver dysfunction, history of

*Aplastic anemia:* This drug should be used only in cases so severe that the risk of aplastic anemia (bone marrow failure) is deemed acceptable.

*Liver failure:* There have been cases of acute liver failure, some fatal, in association with the use of felbamate.

*Discontinuation:* Antiepileptic drugs should not be suddenly discontinued because of the risk of increasing seizure frequency.

*Sensitivity to light:* May cause photosensitivity (sensitivity to sunlight). Avoid prolonged exposure to the sun and other ultraviolet light. Use sunscreens and wear protective clothing until tolerance is determined.

*Pregnancy:* There are no adequate and well-controlled studies in pregnant women. Use only if clearly needed and potential benefits outweigh the possible hazards to the fetus.

*Breastfeeding:* Felbamate appears in breast milk. Consult your doctor before you begin breastfeeding.

*Children:* Safety and effectiveness in children other than those with Lennox-Gastaut syndrome have not been established.

*Lab tests* may be required to monitor therapy. Tests may include liver function tests (ALT, AST, and bilirubin).

## Drug Interactions:

Tell your doctor or pharmacist if you are taking or if you are planning to take any over-the-counter or prescription medications or dietary supplements while taking felbamate. Doses of one or both drugs may need to be modified or a different drug may need to be prescribed. The following drugs and drug classes interact with felbamate:

carbamazepine (eg, *Tegretol)*  phenobarbital (eg, *Solfoton*)
hydantoins (eg, phenytoin)  valproic acid (eg, *Depakene)*
methsuximide (*Celontin*)

## Side Effects:

Every drug is capable of producing side effects. Many felbamate users experience no, or minor, side effects. The frequency and severity of side effects depend on many factors including dose, duration of therapy, and individual susceptibility. Possible side effects include:

*Digestive Tract:* Upset stomach; vomiting; constipation; indigestion; diarrhea; nausea; appetite loss; stomach pain or bloating; hiccough.

*Nervous System:* Sleeplessness; headache; anxiety; drowsiness; dizziness; nervousness; tremor; depression; abnormal walking; abnormal skin sensations; stupor; confusion; mood changes (especially in children); unstable emotions; abnormal thinking; pinpoint pupils; incoordination; agitation.

*Respiratory System:* Upper respiratory tract (ie, nose, throat) infection; nasal congestion; sinus inflammation; sore throat; coughing.

*Skin:* Acne; rash; itching; yellowing of the skin; unusual bruising; sensitivity to light.

*Urinary and Reproductive Tract:* Urinary incontinence; irregular menstrual bleeding; urinary tract infection.

*Other:* Aplastic anemia (bone marrow failure); acute liver failure; fatigue; fever; chest pain; palpitations (pounding in the chest); weight fluctuation; face edema (fluid retention or swelling); pain; weakness; impaired vision; changes in taste perception; dry mouth; muscle pain; bleeding or bruising; flu symptoms; general body discomfort; fast heartbeat; middle ear infection; abnormal blood counts; abnormal lab tests.

## Guidelines for Use:

- Dosage is individualized. Take exactly as prescribed.
- Do not change the dose or stop taking, unless advised by your doctor.
- May be taken with or without food.
- Shake suspension well before use.
- Do not discontinue use without first checking with your doctor. If you stop taking this drug suddenly, the frequency of your seizures could increase.
- May cause photosensitivity (sensitivity to sunlight). Avoid prolonged exposure to the sun and other ultraviolet (UV) light. Use sunscreens and wear protective clothing until tolerance is determined.
- Notify your doctor immediately if you experience fever, yellowing of the skin or eyes, appetite loss, stomach pain or bloating, weakness, sore throat, unusual bleeding or bruising, rash, or dark urine.
- Lab tests will be required to monitor therapy. Be sure to keep appointments.
- Store at room temperature in a tightly closed container.

*If you have any questions, consult your doctor, pharmacist, or health care provider.*

| Generic Name<br>*Brand Name Example* | Supplied As | Generic<br>Available |
|---|---|---|
| *Rx* **Gabapentin** | | |
| *Neurontin* | **Capsules**: 100 mg, 300 mg, 400 mg | No |
| *Neurontin* | **Tablets, film coated**: 600 mg, 800 mg | No |
| *Neurontin* | **Solution, oral**: 250 mg/mL | No |

## Type of Drug:
Anticonvulsant; drug used to treat epilepsy and seizures.

## How the Drug Works:
It is not known how gabapentin works to prevent seizures.

## Uses:
Used in combination with other anticonvulsant therapy in the treatment of partial seizures with and without secondary generalization in patients older than 12 years of age with epilepsy.

Used in combination with other therapy in the treatment of partial seizures in patients 3 to 12 years of age.

*Unlabeled Use(s):* Occasionally doctors may prescribe gabapentin for neuropathic pain, tremors associated with multiple sclerosis, bipolar disorder, and migraine prophylaxis.

## Precautions:
*Do not use in the following situations:* Allergy to gabapentin or any of its ingredients.

*Use with caution in the following situations:*
kidney disease
pediatric patients (3 to 12 years of age)

*Pregnancy:* There are no adequate and well-controlled studies in pregnant women. Use only if clearly needed and the potential benefits to the mother outweigh the possible hazards to the fetus.

*Breastfeeding:* Gabapentin appears in breast milk. Consult your doctor before you begin breastfeeding.

*Children:* Safety and effectiveness in children younger than 3 years of age have not been established.

*Elderly:* Use with caution. Dosage may need to be adjusted.

## Drug Interactions:
Tell your doctor or pharmacist if you are taking or if you are planning to take any over-the-counter or prescription medications or dietary supplements while taking gabapentin. Doses of one or both drugs may need to be modified or a different drug may need to be prescribed. Antacids (eg, *Maalox*) interact with gabapentin.

## Side Effects:

Every drug is capable of producing side effects. Many gabapentin users experience no, or minor, side effects. The frequency and severity of side effects depend on many factors including dose, duration of therapy, and individual susceptibility. Possible side effects include:

*Digestive Tract:* Appetite changes; gas; indigestion; constipation; gum inflammation; nausea; vomiting.

*Nervous System:* Abnormal skin sensations; hyperactivity; change in reflexes; anxiety; nervousness; tremor; hostility; amnesia; vertigo (feeling of whirling motion); depression; abnormal thinking; twitching; drowsiness; dizziness; incoordination; fatigue; emotional lability; concentration problems; difficulty speaking.

*Respiratory System:* Pneumonia; sore throat; cough; respiratory infection; bronchitis; runny nose.

*Skin:* Abrasion; itching; bruise-like spots under the skin.

*Other:* Abnormal vision; joint, back, or muscle pain; weakness; general body discomfort; impotence; high blood pressure; face edema (fluid retention); dry throat or mouth; rapid eye movement; involuntary muscle movements; weight gain; worsening of seizures; abnormal urine tests; viral infection; fever; swelling of the arms or legs; dental abnormalities; abnormal blood counts; bone fracture.

---

### Guidelines for Use:

- Dosage is individualized. Take exactly as prescribed.
- Do not change the dose or stop taking, unless advised by your doctor.
- Take without regard to food.
- Use a dosing spoon or syringe to measure and administer oral solution.
- Convulsions may return or worsen if gabapentin is stopped suddenly.
- Maximum time between doses should not exceed 12 hours.
- If a dose is missed, take it as soon as possible. If several hours have passed or if it is nearing time for the next dose, do not double the dose to catch up, unless advised by your doctor. If more than one dose is missed or it is necessary to establish a new dosage schedule, contact your doctor or pharmacist.
- Small doses are generally used when starting therapy. The dose is then gradually increased as tolerated until an effective dose level is reached.
- Adjust dosage for patients with kidney disease or those undergoing hemodialysis.
- May cause dizziness, drowsiness, or blurred vision. Use with caution while driving or performing other tasks requiring alertness, coordination, and physical dexterity.
- Do not take gabapentin until at least two hours after taking an antacid.
- Carry *MedicAlert* identification indicating that you have epilepsy and the drugs that you are taking.
- Store tablets and capsules at controlled room temperature (59° to 86°F). Store oral solution under refrigeration (36° to 46°F).

---

*If you have any questions, consult your doctor, pharmacist, or health care provider.*

| Generic Name<br>*Brand Name Examples* | Supplied As | Generic<br>Available |
|---|---|---|
| Rx **Ethotoin** | | |
| *Peganone* | **Tablets:** 250 mg, 500 mg | No |
| Rx **Fosphenytoin** | | |
| *Cerebyx* | **Injection:** 100 mg, 500 mg | No |
| Rx **Mephenytoin** | | |
| *Mesantoin* | **Tablets:** 100 mg | No |
| Rx **Phenytoin** | | |
| *Dilantin Infatab* | **Tablets, chewable:** 50 mg | No |
| *Dilantin-125*[1] | **Oral Suspension:**<br>125 mg/5 mL | No |
| Rx **Phenytoin Sodium,<br>Prompt**[2] | | |
| *Phenytoin Sodium* | **Capsules:** 100 mg | Yes |
| Rx **Phenytoin Sodium,<br>Extended** | | |
| *Dilantin Kapseals* | **Capsules:** 30 mg, 100 mg | Yes |
| Rx **Phenytoin Sodium with<br>Phenobarbital** | | |
| *Dilantin with Phenobarbital<br>Kapseals* | **Capsules:** 100 mg with 16 mg<br>phenobarbital; 100 mg with<br>32 mg phenobarbital | No |

[1] Contains alcohol.
[2] Also available as an injection.

## Type of Drug:

Anticonvulsants; drugs used to treat epilepsy and seizures.

## How the Drug Works:

These agents work in the central nervous system to decrease the frequency of seizures.

## Uses:

To control grand mal and psychomotor seizures.

*Fosphenytoin, Phenytoin:* To prevent and treat seizures during or after neurosurgery.

*Mephenytoin:* To control focal and Jacksonian seizures.

*Unlabeled Use(s):* Occasionally doctors may use phenytoin to control irregular heartbeats (arrhythmia), trigeminal neuralgia (tic douloureux), recessive dystrophic epidermolysis bullosa and junctional epidermolysis bullosa.

## Precautions:

*Do not use in the following situations:*

Adams-Strokes syndrome (fos-phenytoin, phenytoin)
allergy to these medicines
AV block, advanced (phenytoin only)
blood disorders (ethotoin only)

liver disease (ethotoin only)
sino-atrial block (fosphenytoin, phenytoin)
sinus bradycardia (fosphenytoin, phenytoin)

*Use with caution in the following situations:*

AV block, advanced
cardiac insufficiency (fosphe-nytoin, phenytoin)
liver disease

low blood pressure ((fosphe-nytoin, phenytoin)
porphyria, acute, intermittent

*Diabetics* may experience loss of glucose control. Be prepared to monitor blood sugar more often.

*Gum disease* occurs frequently with phenytoin. Incidence may be reduced by good oral hygiene, including gum massage, frequent brushing and flossing and appropriate dental care.

*Pregnancy:* Reports suggest an association between use of anticonvulsant drugs by women with epilepsy and an increased number of birth defects in children born to these women. Other factors (eg, genetics or the epileptic condition) may also contribute to the high incidence of birth defects. Most mothers receiving anticonvulsant medication deliver *normal* infants. Do not discontinue anticonvulsant drugs used to prevent major seizures. This could result in the occurrence of severe seizures and an increased risk to both the mother and the unborn child. In cases where seizures do not pose a serious threat, your doctor may recommend discontinuation of anticonvulsants prior to and during pregnancy. It is not known whether even minor seizures constitute some risk to the developing embryo or fetus. Reports suggest that a mother's use of anticonvulsant drugs, particularly barbiturates, is associated with a blood clotting defect in the newborn that may cause a bleeding problem within 24 hours of birth. It has been suggested that vitamin K be given to the mother one month prior to and during delivery, and to the infant immediately after birth. An increase in seizure frequency often occurs during pregnancy because of altered phenytoin absoption or metabolism. Periodic lab tests will be required to measure phenytoin levels during pregnancy and doses may need to be adjusted. After birth, the dosage will probably go back to what it was before pregnancy.

*Breastfeeding:* Hydantoins appear in breast milk. Because of the potential for serious side effects in breastfed infants, decide whether to discontinue breastfeeding or discontinue the drug. Consult your doctor.

*Lab tests* may be required to monitor therapy. Tests may include blood counts, urinalysis, blood sugar levels (especially in diabetics), liver function tests and phenytoin blood levels.

## Drug Interactions:

Tell your doctor or pharmacist if you are taking or if you are planning to take any over-the-counter or prescription medications or dietary supplements while taking this medicine. Doses of one or both drugs may need to be modified or a different drug may need to be prescribed. The following drugs and drug classes interact with this medicine.

*Increased effects of hydantoins may occur when the following drugs are administered with hydantoins:*

alcohol
allopurinal (eg, *Zyloprim*)
amiodarone (*Cordarone*)
anticoagulants, oral (eg, warfarin)
barbiturates (eg, phenobarbital)
benzodiazepines
  (eg, diazepam)
chloramphenicol (*Chloromycetin*)
chlorpheniramine (eg, *Chlor-Trimeton*)
cimetidine (eg, *Tagamet*)
clonazepam (*Klonopin*)
disulfiram (eg, *Antabuse*)
felbamate (*Felbatol*)
fluconazole (*Diflucan*)
fluoxetine (*Prozac*)
ibuprofen (eg, *Motrin*)
isoniazid (eg, *Nydrazid*)
methylphenidate (eg, *Ritalin*)
metronidazole (eg, *Flagyl*)
miconazole (eg, *Monistat*)
omeprazole (*Prilosec*)
phenacemide (*Phenurone*)
phenothiazines (eg, chlorpromazine)
propoxyphene (eg, *Darvon*)
ranitidine (*Zantac*)
salicylates (eg, aspirin)
sodium valproate
succinimides (eg, ethosuximide)
sulfonamides (eg, sulfamethoxazole/trimethoprim)
trazodone (eg, *Desyrel*)
trimethoprim (eg, *Proloprim*)
tricyclic antidepressants
  (eg, imipramine)
valproic acid (eg, *Depakene*)

*Decreased effects of hydantoins may occur when the following drugs are administered with hydantoins:*

alcohol
antacids containing calcium
  (eg, *Tums*)
antineoplastics (eg, methotrexate)
barbiturates (eg, phenobarbital)
charcoal
carbamazepine (eg, *Tegretol*)
chloral hydrate (eg, *Noctec*)
clonazepam (*Klonopin*)
diazoxide (*Proglycem*)
folic acid (eg, *Folvite*)
influenza vaccine
loxapine (eg, *Loxitane*)
nitrofurantoin (eg, *Furadantin*)
paroxetin (*Paxil*)
pyridoxine (eg, vitamin $B_6$)
quinolones (eg, ciprofloxacin)
rifamycins (eg, rifampin)
sucralfate (*Carafate*)
theophylline (eg, *Theo-Dur*)

*Phenytoin may decrease effects of the following drugs:*

acetaminophen (eg, *Tylenol*)
amiodarone (*Cordarone*)
barbiturates (eg, phenobarbital)
carbamazepine (eg, *Tegretol*)
cardiac glycosides (eg, digitoxin)
clonazepam (*Klonopin*)
contraceptives, oral (eg, *Ortho-Novum*)
corticosteroids (eg, prednisone)
cyclosporine (*Sandimmune*)
dicumarol
disopyramide (eg, *Norpace*)
dopamine (eg, *Dopastat*)
doxycycline (eg, *Vibramycin*)
estrogens (eg, estradiol)
furosemide (eg, *Lasix*)
haloperidol (eg, *Haldol*)
itraconazole (*Sporanox*)
levodopa (eg, *Laradopa*)
levonorgestrel (*Norplant System*)
mebendazole (eg, *Vermox*)
meperidine (eg, Dermerol)
methadone (eg, *Dolophine HCl*)
metyrapone
mexiletine (*Mexitil*)
muscle relaxants, nondepolarizing (eg, pancuronium)
phenothiazines (eg, chlorpromazine)
praziquantel (*Biltricide*)
primidone (eg, *Mysoline*)
quinidine (eg, *Quinora*)
sulfonylureas (eg, tolbutamide)
theophylline (eg, *Theo-Dur*)
thyroid hormones (eg, thyroid)
valproic acid (eg, *Depakene*)
verapamil (eg, *Calan*)
vitamin D
warfarin (*Coumadin*)

*Other:*

enteral nutrition
lithium (eg, *Lithobid*)
warfarin (*Coumadin*)

## Side Effects:

Every drug is capable of producing side effects. Many patients experience no, or minor, side effects. The frequency and severity of side effects depend on many factors including dose, duration of therapy and individual susceptibility. Possible side effects include:

*Digestive Tract:* Nausea; vomiting; diarrhea; constipation.

*Nervous System:* Clumsiness; slurred speech; confusion; dizziness; sleeplessness; nervousness; twitchings; tiredness; irritability; sleepiness; depression; numbness; tremors; headache

*Respiratory System:* Sore throat; sinus inflammation; nasal congestion; asthma; coughing; nosebleed; difficulty breathing; chest pain.

*Urinary and Reproductive Tract:* Difficult, infrequent, painful or excessive urination; loss of bladder control; vaginal infection; genital swelling; kidney failure.

*Skin:* Rash; hives; yellowing of skin or eyes; irritation at injection site.

*Senses:* Rapid eye movement; double or impaired vision; light sensitivity; pupil dilation; eye pain or redness; taste changes or loss; distorted sense of smell; tender, bleeding or swollen gums; ear ache; ringing in the ears.

*Other:* Coarsening of facial features; lip enlargement; hair loss; weight gain; swelling of legs, ankles or hands; joint pain; fever; breast growth in men; swelling of lymph nodes; anemia; high blood sugar levels.

## Guidelines for Use:

- Use exactly as prescribed.
- May cause stomach upset. Taking this medicine with or immediately after meals may help prevent stomach discomfort.
- Do not stop taking this medicine suddenly or change the dosage without checking with your doctor.
- *Brand interchange* — Do not change from one brand of this drug to another without consulting your pharmacist or doctor. Products manufactured by different companies may not be equally effective.
- *Phenytoin* — Do not take at the same time with antacids that contain calcium.
- May cause drowsiness, dizziness or blurred vision; alcohol may intensify these effects. Use caution while driving or performing hazardous tasks requiring mental alertness, coordination or physical dexterity.
- Do not stop taking this medicine or change the dose without checking with your doctor. Abrupt stopping of hydantoins in epileptic patients may precipitate seizures.
- It is important to brush and floss your teeth and to see your dentist regularly, in order to reduce the risk of gum swelling.
- *Diabetics* — Monitor blood sugar regularly and report any abnormalities to your doctor.
- Avoid alcohol, antihistamines and other mental depressants (eg, tranquilizers) while taking this medicine.
- Tell your doctor if you are pregnant, become pregnant, are planning to become pregnant or if you are breastfeeding.
- Contact your doctor immediately if rash appears.
- Contact your doctor if any of the following occurs: Drowsiness; slurred speech; clumsiness; rash; severe nausea or vomiting; swollen glands; bleeding, swollen or tender gums; yellowish discoloration of the skin or eyes; joint pain; unexplained fever; sore throat; nosebleed; unusual bleeding or bruising; persistent headache; general body discomfort; bleeding tendencies; pregnancy or any indication of an infection.
- Inform your doctor of any condition in which it is not possible to take this medicine orally (eg, surgery).
- Carry Medic Alert identification indicating that you are have epilepsy and are taking these drugs.
- Lab tests will be required to monitor treatment. Be sure to keep appointments.
- *Capsules* — Do not use if discolored.
- *Dilantin Suspension* — Shake well before use.
- Store at room temperature below 86°F in a tight-fitting container. Protect from freezing, moisture and light.

*If you have any questions, consult your doctor, pharmacist, or health care provider.*

| Generic Name<br>*Brand Name Example* | Supplied As | Generic<br>Available |
|---|---|---|
| *Rx* **Trimethadione** | | |
| *Tridione* | **Tablets, chewable:** 150 mg | No |
| *Tridione* | **Capsules:** 300 mg | No |
| *Tridione* | **Solution:** 40 mg/mL | No |

Because of the potential of these drugs to cause fetal abnormalities and serious side effects, these drugs are used only when less toxic drugs have been found ineffective in controlling petit mal seizures.

## Type of Drug:

Anticonvulsants; drug used to treat epilepsy and seizures.

## How the Drug Works:

Oxazolidinediones act on the central nervous system to decrease the frequency of seizures.

## Uses:

To control absence (petit mal) seizures that do not respond to other antiseizure medications.

## Precautions:

*Do not use in the following situations:* Allergy to these drugs.

*Use with caution in the following situations:*

| | |
|---|---|
| blood disorders | kidney dysfunction |
| eye diseases (retina, optic nerve) | liver disease |
| | porphyria, acute intermittent |
| kidney disease | rash (after therapy was started) |

*Photosensitivity,* sensitivity to sunlight, may occur. Therefore, use caution and take protective measures (ie, sunscreens, protective clothing) against exposure to ultraviolet light or sunlight until tolerance is determined.

*Pregnancy:* Reports suggest an association between use of anticonvulsant drugs by women with epilepsy and an increased number of birth defects in children born to these women. Other factors (eg, genetics or the epileptic condition) may also contribute to the higher incidence of birth defects. Most mothers receiving anticonvulsant medication deliver normal infants. Do not discontinue anticonvulsant drugs used to prevent major seizures. This could result in the occurrence of seizures and oxygen deficiency in body tissues and an increased risk to both the mother and the unborn child. In cases where seizures do not pose a serious threat, your doctor may recommend discontinuation of anticonvulsants prior to and during pregnancy. It is not known whether even minor seizures constitute some risk to the developing embryo or fetus. Reports suggest that mother's use of anticonvulsant drugs, particularly barbiturates, is associated with a blood clotting defect in the newborn that may cause a bleeding problem within 24 hours of birth. It has been suggested that vitamin K be given to the mother one month prior to and during delivery, and to the infant, immediately after birth.

*Breastfeeding:* It is not known if oxazolidinediones appear in breast milk. Consult your doctor before you begin breastfeeding.

*Children:* Safety and effectiveness in children under 16 years of age have not been established.

*Lab tests* may be required during treatment with oxazolidinediones. Be sure to keep appointments. Tests may include blood counts, liver and kidney function tests, eye exams and urinalysis.

## Side Effects:

Every drug is capable of producing side effects. Many oxazolidinedione users experience no, or minor, side effects. The frequency and severity of side effects depend on many factors including dose, duration of therapy and individual susceptibility. Possible side effects include:

*Digestive Tract:* Nausea; vomiting; abdominal pain; appetite loss; gastric distress.

*Nervous System:* Drowsiness; dizziness; headache; personality changes; irritability; fatigue; sleeplessness; muscle weakness.

*Skin:* Rash; unusual bleeding or bruising; yellowing of eyes or skin; hair loss; itching; peeling skin.

*Other:* Vision changes, double vision; sore throat; fever; muscle weakness (especially eyes, eyelids, face, lips, tongue, throat or neck); sensitivity to sunlight; fatigue; abnormal lab tests (see Precautions); weight loss; hiccoughs; blood pressure changes; protein in urine; day blindness; bleeding gums; nosebleeds; vaginal bleeding; blood disorder; decreased blood platelets; anemia; bleeding.

---

### Guidelines for Use:

- If stomach upset occurs, take with food.
- Do not change the dose or stop taking this medication without consulting your doctor.
- Keep scheduled appointments with your doctor, and carry Medic Alert identification listing your medical condition (epilepsy) and medication.
- May cause drowsiness or blurred vision. Use caution while driving or performing other tasks requiring alertness.
- Notify your doctor if any of the following should occur: Visual disturbances, excessive drowsiness or dizziness, sore throat, fever, unusual bleeding or bruising, skin rash, pregnancy, body discomfort or nosebleed.
- Withdraw drug gradually unless serious adverse effects dictate otherwise.
- May cause sensitivity to sunlight. Avoid prolonged exposure to the sun. Use sunscreens and wear protective clothing until tolerance is determined.
- Store capsules below 77°F. Store tablets in refrigerator and keep container tightly closed. Store solution below 86°F.

---

*If you have any questions, consult your doctor, pharmacist, or health care provider.*

| Generic Name<br>*Brand Name Example* | Supplied As | Generic<br>Available |
|---|---|---|
| Rx **Oxcarbazepine** | | |
| *Trileptal* | **Tablets:** 150 mg, 300 mg,<br>600 mg | No |

## Type of Drug:

Anticonvulsant; drug used to treat a variety of seizure disorders.

## How the Drug Works:

Oxcarbazepine prevents or reduces some types of seizures by controlling abnormal nerve impulses in the brain.

## Uses:

For use alone or in combination therapy for the treatment of partial seizures in adults with epilepsy and as combination therapy for the treatment of partial seizures in children 4 to 16 years of age with epilepsy.

*Unlabeled Use(s):* Oxcarbazepine has been used for atypical panic disorder.

## Precautions:

*Do not use in the following situations:* Allergy to oxcarbazepine or any of its ingredients.

*Use with caution in the following situations:*

| | |
|---|---|
| allergy to carbamazepine (eg, *Tegretol*) | kidney disease |
| blood sodium levels, low | liver disease, severe |

*Pregnancy:* There are no adequate and well-controlled clinical studies in pregnant women; however, it is closely related structurally to carbamazepine, which is considered to be teratogenic in humans. Use during pregnancy only if clearly needed and the potential benefits to the mother outweigh the possible hazards to the fetus.

*Breastfeeding:* Oxcarbazepine and its active metabolite MHD are excreted in human breast milk. Because of the potential for serious adverse reactions, decide whether to discontinue nursing or to discontinue the drug in nursing women, taking into account the importance of the drug to the mother.

*Children:* Oxcarbazepine has been shown to be effective as adjunctive therapy combined with other drugs for partial seizures in patients 4 to 16 years of age.

*Lab tests* will be required to monitor therapy. Tests may include blood sodium levels, liver function, kidney function, and blood tests.

## Drug Interactions:

Tell your doctor or pharmacist if you are taking or if you are planning to take any over-the-counter or prescription medications or dietary supplements with oxcarbazepine. Doses of one or both drugs may need to be modified or a different drug may need to be prescribed. The following drugs and drug classes interact with oxcarbazepine:

calcium channel blockers
 (eg, felodipine)
carbamazepine (eg, *Tegretol*)
phenobarbital (eg, *Solfoton*)

phenytoin (eg, *Dilantin*)
oral contraceptives (eg, *Ortho-Novum*)
valproic acid (eg, *Depakene*)

## Side Effects:

Every drug is capable of producing side effects. Many oxcarbazepine users experience no, or minor, side effects. The frequency and severity of side effects depend on many factors including dose, duration of therapy, and individual susceptibility. Possible side effects include:

*Digestive Tract:* Nausea; vomiting; stomach pain; inflammation of the stomach; appetite changes; dry mouth; toothache; diarrhea; indigestion; constipation; rectal bleeding or pain.

*Nervous System:* Headache; dizziness; drowsiness; anxiety; fatigue; weakness; incoordination; tremors; continual rapid eye movement; abnormal gait; sleeplessness; impaired concentration; amnesia; worsening of seizures; involuntary muscle contractions; unstable emotions; decreased sensation to stimuli; nervousness; agitation; speech disorder; confusion; feeling of whirling motion; abnormal EEG; abnormal thinking.

*Respiratory System:* Sinus congestion; runny nose; upper respiratory infection; cough; breathing difficulties; sore throat; nosebleed; chest infection.

*Skin:* Acne; hot flashes; flushing; rash; unusual bruising; increased sweating; itching.

*Other:* Double vision; abnormal vision; earache; ear infection; fever; allergy; swelling of the legs; chest pain; weight increase; low blood pressure; falling down; swollen lymphnodes; viral infection; urinary tract infection; frequent urination; inflammation or pain of the vagina; low blood sodium levels; thirst.

## Guidelines for Use:

- Dosage is individualized. Take exactly as prescribed.
- Do not stop taking or change the dose unless advised to do so by your doctor.
- May be taken without regard to meals.
- Avoid alcohol and other mental depressants (eg, narcotics, tranquilizers, antihistamines) while you are taking this medicine.
- Treatment should be withdrawn gradually to minimize the potential of increased seizure frequency.
- If a dose is missed, take it as soon as possible. If several hours have passed or if it is nearing time for the next dose, do not double the dose to catch up, unless advised by your doctor. If more than one dose is missed, or it is necessary to establish a new dosage schedule, contact your doctor or pharmacist.
- Additional nonhormonal forms of contraception (eg, latex condoms) are recommended because of a reduction in hormonal contraceptive efficacy during therapy.
- Avoid alcohol during therapy; it may cause drowsiness.
- May cause drowsiness, dizziness, or blurred vision. Use caution while driving or performing hazardous tasks requiring alertness, coordination, or physical dexterity until tolerance is determined.
- Store at controlled room temperature (59° to 86°F). Keep tightly closed.

*If you have any questions, consult your doctor, pharmacist, or health care provider.*

| Generic Name<br>*Brand Name Example* | Supplied As | Generic<br>Available |
|---|---|---|
| *Rx* **Zonisamide** | | |
| *Zonegran* | **Capsules:** 100 mg | No |

## Type of Drug:

Anticonvulsant; sulfonamide used to treat a certain type of seizure disorder.

## How the Drug Works:

Zonisamide works in the brain to prevent seizures. Its mechanism of action is not fully understood.

## Uses:

For adjunctive therapy in the treatment of partial seizures in adults with epilepsy.

## Precautions:

*Do not use in the following situations:*
>allergy to the drug or any of its ingredients
>allergy to sulfonamides

*Use with caution in the following situations:*
>kidney disease
>liver disease

*Pregnancy:* There are no adequate and well-controlled studies in pregnant women. Use only if clearly needed and the potential benefits outweigh the possible hazards to the fetus.

*Breastfeeding:* It is not known whether zonisamide is excreted in breast milk. Because of the potential for serious adverse reactions in nursing infants from zonisamide, decide whether to discontinue breastfeeding or the drug, taking into account the importance of the drug to the mother. Consult your doctor before you begin breastfeeding.

*Children:* Safety and efficacy in patients younger than 16 years of age have not been established. Zonisamide is not approved for pediatric use.

*Elderly:* Older patients may be more sensitive to the effects of zonisamide. Lower starting doses should be considered.

*Lab tests* may be required during treatment. Tests include blood counts and kidney and liver function tests.

## Drug Interactions:

Tell your doctor or pharmacist if you are taking or planning to take any over-the-counter or prescription medications or dietary supplements with this drug. Drug doses may need to be modified or a different drug prescribed. The following drugs and drug classes interact with this drug:

carbamazepine (eg, *Tegretol*)
ketoconazole (eg, *Nizoral*)
phenobarbital (eg, *Solfoton*)

phenytoin (eg, *Dilantin*)
valproate (eg, *Depakene*)

## Side Effects:

Every drug is capable of producing side effects. Many patients experience no, or minor, side effects. The frequency and severity of side effects depend on many factors including dose, duration of therapy, and individual susceptiblity. Possible side effects include:

*Digestive Tract:* Stomach pain; appetite loss; constipation; diarrhea; indigestion; nausea; vomiting.

*Nervous System:* Agitation or irritability; anxiety; incoordination; confusion; depression; difficulty concentrating; difficulty with memory; dizziness; fatigue; headache; sleeplessness; mental slowing; nervousness; continual rapid eye movement; tremor; convulsion; abnormal walking; weakness; unusual thoughts (schizophrenic behavior); drowsiness; tiredness; speech problems.

*Respiratory System:* Sore throat; cough; runny nose.

*Skin:* Itching; rash; abnormal skin sensations (eg, burning, prickling, tingling).

*Other:* Dry mouth; unusual bruising; flu symptoms; weight loss; vision problems; ringing in ear; kidney stones; taste sensation changes.

---

### Guidelines for Use:

- Dosage is individualized. Take exactly as prescribed.
- Do not stop taking or change the dose, unless instructed by your doctor. Abrupt stopping of zonisamide in patients with epilepsy may increase seizure frequency.
- May be taken with or without food.
- Capsules should be swallowed whole.
- Contact your doctor immediately if you experience decreased sweating with or without fever, sore throat, oral ulcers, easy bruising, rash, or worsening seizures.
- Contact your doctor if you experience sudden back pain, stomach pain, or blood in the urine. These could be signs of a kidney stone.
- If dose is missed, take as soon as possible. If several hours have passed or it is nearing time for the next dose, do not double the dose to catch up, unless instructed by your doctor. If more than one dose is missed or it is necessary to establish a new dosage schedule, contact your doctor or pharmacist.
- Drink at least 6 to 8 glasses of fluid per day while taking this drug to decrease the risk of kidney stones.
- Inform your doctor if you are pregnant, become pregnant, plan on becoming pregnant, or are breastfeeding.
- Women of child-bearing potential taking zonisamide should use effective contraception.
- May cause drowsiness, dizziness, or blurred vision. Use caution when driving or performing other tasks requiring alertness, coordination, or physical dexterity until tolerance is determined.
- Store at room temperature (59° to 86°F). Protect from moisture and light.

---

*If you have any questions, consult your doctor, pharmacist, or health care provider.*

| Generic Name *Brand Name Example* | Supplied As | Generic Available |
|---|---|---|
| Rx **Primidone** | | |
| *Mysoline* | **Tablets:** 50 mg, 250 mg | Yes |
| *Mysoline* | **Oral suspension:** 250 mg/tsp | No |

## Type of Drug:

Anticonvulsant; drug used to treat epilepsy and seizures.

## How the Drug Works:

Primidone prevents or reduces the number of seizures by acting on the central nervous system to control the activity of nerve impulses in the brain.

## Uses:

To control grand mal, psychomotor or focal epileptic seizures, alone or in combination with other anticonvulsant drugs.

*Unlabeled Use(s):* Occasionally doctors may prescribe may primidone for benign familial tremor.

## Precautions:

*Do not use in the following situations:*
    allergy to phenobarbital
    porphyria

*Use with caution in the following situations:*
    kidney disease
    liver disease

*Pregnancy:* Reports suggest an association between use of anticonvulsant drugs by women with epilepsy and an increased number of birth defects in children born to these women. Other factors (eg, genetics or the epileptic condition) may also contribute to the higher incidence of birth defects. Most mothers receiving anticonvulsant medication deliver *normal* infants. Do not discontinue anticonvulsant drugs used to prevent major seizures. This could result in the occurrence of seizures and oxygen deficiency in body tissues and an increased risk to both the mother and the unborn child. In cases where seizures do not pose a serious threat, your doctor may recommend discontinuation of anticonvulsants prior to and during pregnancy. It is not known whether even minor seizures constitute some risk to the developing embryo or fetus. Reports suggest that mother's use of anticonvulsant drugs, particularly barbiturates, is associated with a blood clotting defect in the newborn that may cause a bleeding problem within 24 hours of birth. It has been suggested that vitamin K be given to the mother one month prior to and during delivery, and to the infant, immediately after birth.

*Breastfeeding:* Primidone appears in breast milk. It may cause the infant to be unusually drowsy or sleepy. Consult your doctor before you begin breastfeeding.

*Lab tests* may be required during treatment with primidone. Tests may include complete blood counts, liver and kidney function tests and blood levels of primidone.

## Drug Interactions:

Tell your doctor or pharmacist if you are taking or if you are planning to take any over-the-counter or prescription medications or dietary supplements with primidone. Doses of one or both drugs may need to be modified or a different drug may need to be prescribed. The following drugs and drug classes interact with primidone.

acetazolamide (eg, *Diamox*)
alcohol
anticoagulants, oral
(eg, *Coumadin*)
carbamazepine (eg, *Tegretol*)
corticosteroids (eg, prednisone)
contraceptives, oral (eg, *Ortho Novum*)
doxycycline (eg, *Vibramycin*)

griseofulvin (eg, *Grisactin*)
isoniazid (eg, *Laniazid*)
methoxyflurane (*Penthrane*)
metoprolol (*Lopressor*)
phenytoin (eg, *Dilantin*)
propranolol (eg, *Inderal*)
quinidine (eg, *Cin-Quin*)
theophylline (eg, *Theo-Dur*)
valproic acid (eg, *Depakene*)

Consider all drug interactions reported for barbiturates in the Sedatives-Barbiturates monograph in this chapter when using this drug.

## Side Effects:

Every drug is capable of producing side effects. Many primidone users experience no, or minor, side effects. The frequency and severity of side effects depend on many factors including dose, duration of therapy and individual susceptibility. Possible side effects include:

*Digestive Tract:* Nausea; vomiting; loss of appetite.

*Nervous System:* Drowsiness; clumsiness; mood changes; unusual weakness; tiredness; dizziness.

*Other:* Double vision; blurred vision; unusual movements of the eyes; fever; sore throat; decreased sexual ability; rash.

---

### Guidelines for Use:

- May cause drowsiness or sleepiness. Use caution when driving or performing other tasks requiring alertness.
- May cause stomach upset. May be taken with food.
- Do not stop taking this drug or change the dose without talking with your doctor. If you stop taking this drug suddenly, seizures may suddenly return.
- Carry Medic Alert identification listing your medical condition (epilepsy) and medications.
- Using this drug with alcohol or other central nervous system depressants may cause added drowsiness.
- See your doctor regularly when you begin taking this drug to ensure that you are getting the proper dosage. Lab tests will be needed to monitor therapy. Full effect may not be seen for several weeks.
- Contact your doctor if visual disturbance, rash, fever, sore throat, clumsiness or excessive sleepiness occurs.
- *Oral suspension* — Shake well before using.

---

*If you have any questions, consult your doctor, pharmacist, or health care provider.*

| Generic Name<br>*Brand Name Example* | Supplied As | Generic<br>Available |
|---|---|---|
| *Rx* **Topiramate** | | |
| *Topamax* | **Tablets:** 25 mg, 100 mg,<br>200 mg | No |
| *Topamax* | **Capsules, sprinkle:** 15 mg,<br>25 mg | No |

## Type of Drug:

Anticonvulsant; drug used to prevent certain types of seizures.

## How the Drug Works:

Topiramate reduces the incidence of seizures by acting on the central nervous system to alter certain neurological transmissions in the brain.

## Uses:

To treat adults and children older than 2 years of age with partial onset seizures or primary generalized tonic-clonic seizures and seizures associated with Lennox-Gastaut syndrome in combination with other anticonvulsant drugs.

## Precautions:

*Do not use in the following situations:* Allergy to topiramate or any of its ingredients.

*Use with caution in the following situations:*

| | |
|---|---|
| alcohol ingestion | kidney failure |
| glaucoma | kidney stones |
| impaired liver function | |

*Pregnancy:* There are no adequate and well-controlled studies in pregnant women. Use only if clearly needed and the potential benefits to the mother outweigh the possible hazards to the fetus.

*Breastfeeding:* It is not known if topiramate appears in breast milk. Consult your doctor before you begin breastfeeding.

*Children:* Safety and effectiveness in children younger than 2 years of age have not been established.

## Drug Interactions:

Tell your doctor or pharmacist if you are taking or planning to take any over-the-counter or prescription medications or dietary supplements while taking topiramate. Doses of one or both drugs may need to be modified or a different drug may need to be prescribed. The following drugs and drug classes interact with topiramate:

carbamazepine (eg, *Tegretol*)
carbonic anhydrase inhibitors (eg, acetazolamide, dichlorphenamide)
CNS depressants (eg, narcotics, hypnotics)
contraceptives, oral (eg, *Ortho-Novum*)
digoxin (eg, *Lanoxin*)
phenytoin (eg, *Dilantin*)
valproic acid (eg, *Depakene*)

## Side Effects:

Every drug is capable of producing side effects. Many topiramate users experience no, or minor, side effects. The frequency and severity of side effects depend on many factors including dose, duration of therapy, and individual susceptibility. Possible side effects include:

*Digestive Tract:* Nausea; indigestion; stomach pain; constipation; diarrhea; vomiting; dry mouth; gingivitis; stomach or intestinal irritation; hemorrhoids; changes in taste sensation.

*Nervous System:* Dizziness; incoordination; speech disorders; rapid eye movement; abnormal skin sensations; tremor; drowsiness; nervousness; memory difficulty; confusion; depression; appetite loss; agitation; aggressive reaction; hallucination; apathy; slow thinking; difficulty concentrating; anxiety; sleepiness; fatigue; dizziness; mood swings.

*Circulatory System:* Abnormal blood counts; low blood pressure; AV block; heart rhythm changes.

*Respiratory System:* Sore throat; upper respiratory infection; sinus infection; difficulty breathing.

*Urinary and Reproductive Tract:* Breast pain (females); menstrual disorder; blood in urine; urinary tract infection; frequency of urination; urinary incontinence; kidney stones; impotence; difficult or painful urination.

*Skin:* Rash; itching; increased sweating; acne.

*Other:* Influenza-like symptoms; hot flushes; body odor; fluid retention; muscle pain or weakness; weight decrease; nosebleed; dehydration; abnormal vision; double vision; joint, bone, back, chest, or leg pain; increased muscle tone; decreased hearing; fever; ringing in the ears.

## Guidelines for Use:

- Dosage is individualized. Take exactly as prescribed.
- Do not stop taking or change the dose, unless directed by your doctor.
- May be taken without regard to meals.
- If using the sprinkle capsule, sprinkle contents on a small amount (teaspoonful) of soft food (eg, custard, applesauce, yogurt). Swallow without chewing. Do not store any of the sprinkle capsule/food mixture for later use.
- Because of the bitter taste, tablets should not be broken, crushed, or chewed.
- Maintain adequate fluid intake to decrease the risk of kidney stones.
- Inform your doctor immediately of blurred vision or pain around the eye.
- May cause dizziness, confusion, drowsiness, and difficulty concentrating. Use caution when driving or performing tasks requiring alertness, coordination, or physical dexterity.
- Should be withdrawn gradually to minimize potential of increase in seizures.
- Inform your doctor of prolonged periods of dialysis.
- Consider forms of contraception other than estrogen-containing birth control pills.
- See your doctor regularly to ensure correct dosage is being administered. Lab tests will be needed to monitor therapy.
- Store at 59° to 86°F in a tightly sealed container. Protect from moisture.

*If you have any questions, consult your doctor, pharmacist, or health care provider.*

| Generic Name<br>*Brand Name Examples* | Supplied As | Generic<br>Available |
|---|---|---|
| Rx **Ethosuximide** | | |
| *Zarontin* | **Capsules:** 250 mg | No |
| *Zarontin* | **Syrup:** 250 mg/5 mL | Yes |
| Rx **Methsuximide** | | |
| *Celontin Kapseals* | **Capsules:** 150 mg, 300 mg | No |

## Type of Drug:

Anticonvulsants; drugs used to treat childhood absence (petit mal) epilepsy.

## How the Drug Works:

Succinimides act on the central nervous system to decrease the frequency of seizures.

## Uses:

To control absence (petit mal) seizures, particularly when refractory to other drugs.

## Precautions:

*Do not use in the following situations:* Allergy to the drug or any of its ingredients.

*Use with caution in the following situations:*

| | |
|---|---|
| blood diseases | mixed seizures |
| kidney diseases | rash (after therapy was started) |
| liver disease | |

*Lupus:* Cases of systemic lupus erythematosus have occurred during treatment with succinimides. Symptoms include fever, tiredness, skin lesions, pleurisy, joint pain, headaches, and personality changes.

*Pregnancy:* Reports suggest an association between use of anticonvulsant drugs by women with epilepsy and an increased number of birth defects in children born to these women. Other factors (eg, genetics, epileptic condition) may also contribute to the higher incidence of birth defects. Most mothers receiving anticonvulsant medication deliver normal infants. Do not discontinue anticonvulsant drugs used to prevent major seizures. This could result in the occurrence of seizures and oxygen deficiency in body tissues and an increased risk to both the mother and the unborn child. In cases where seizures do not pose a serious threat, your doctor may recommend discontinuation of anticonvulsants prior to and during pregnancy. It is not known whether even minor seizures constitute some risk to the developing embryo or fetus. Reports suggest that a mother's use of anticonvulsant drugs, particularly barbiturates, is associated with a blood clotting defect in the newborn that may cause a bleeding problem within 24 hours of birth. It has been suggested that vitamin K be given to the mother one month prior to and during delivery, and to the infant immediately after birth.

*Breastfeeding:* Consult your doctor before you begin breastfeeding.

*Children:* Safety and effectiveness in children younger than 3 years of age have not been established.

*Lab tests* may be required during treatment. Tests include blood counts, urinalysis, and liver function.

## Drug Interactions:

Tell your doctor or pharmacist if you are taking or planning to take any over-the-counter or prescription medications or dietary supplements with these drugs. Drug doses may need to be modified or a different drug prescribed. The following drugs and drug classes interact with these drugs:

| | |
|---|---|
| hydantoins (eg, phenytoin) | primidone (eg, *Mysoline*) |
| phenobarbital | valproic acid (eg, *Depakene*) |

## Side Effects:

Every drug is capable of producing side effects. Many patients experience no, or minor, side effects. The frequency and severity of side effects depend on many factors including dose, duration of therapy, and individual susceptibility. Possible side effects include:

*Digestive Tract:* Nausea; vomiting; stomach discomfort; appetite loss; diarrhea; constipation; weight loss; cramps.

*Nervous System:* Drowsiness; dizziness; headache; euphoria; dream-like feeling; hyperactivity; confusion; sleep disturbances; night terror; hiccup; fatigue; incoordination; depression; irritability; lethargy; sleeplessness; mental slowness; hypochondriacal behavior; aggressiveness; inability to concentrate.

*Skin:* Rash; unusual bleeding or bruising; hives; increased growth and darkening of fine body hairs; hair loss; itching; skin eruptions.

*Other:* Joint pain; fever; sore throat; blurred vision; abnormal blood counts; eyes sensitive to light; urinary frequency; blood in urine; muscle weakness; swelling of tongue and gums; swelling around eyes; nearsightedness; vaginal bleeding.

## Guidelines for Use:

- Dosage is individualized. Use exactly as prescribed.
- Do not change the dose or stop taking this medication without consulting your doctor. Abrupt withdrawal may cause seizures.
- If stomach upset occurs, take with food or milk.
- If a dose is missed, take it as soon as possible. If several hours have passed or it is nearing time for the next dose, do not double the dose to catch up, unless instructed by your doctor. If more than one dose is missed or it is necessary to establish a new dosage schedule, contact your doctor or pharmacist.
- Avoid alcoholic beverages while taking this medicine.
- May cause drowsiness, dizziness, or blurred vision. Use caution while driving or performing other tasks requiring alertness, coordination, or physical dexterity.
- Notify your doctor if you experience skin rash, joint pain, unexplained fever, sore throat, unusual bleeding or bruising, drowsiness, dizziness, blurred vision, pregnancy, seizures, depression, aggressiveness, or behavioral changes.
- Succinimides, when used alone in mixed types of epilepsy, may increase the frequency of grand mal seizures.
- Keep scheduled appointments with your doctor and carry *Medic-Alert* identification listing your medical condition and medicine.
- Lab tests may be required during treatment. Be sure to keep appointments.
- Store at room temperature (77° to 86°F). Protect from light, moisture, and excessive heat. Do not use *Celontin Kapseals* that are not full or in which contents have melted.

*If you have any questions, consult your doctor, pharmacist, or health care provider.*

| Generic Name Brand Name Example | Supplied As | Generic Available |
|---|---|---|
| Rx **Lamotrigine** | | |
| *Lamictal* | **Tablets:** 25 mg, 100 mg, 150 mg, 200 mg | No |

## Type of Drug:

Anticonvulsant; antiepileptic.

## How the Drug Works:

It is not known exactly how lamotrigine works. It is believed that lamotrigine prevents or reduces the number of seizures by acting on stabilizing the brain to control the activity of nerve impulses.

## Uses:

As an additional therapy in the treatment of partial seizures in patients older than 16 years of age with epilepsy.

*Unlabeled Use(s):* Occasionally, doctors may prescribe lamotrigine to adults with generalized clonic-tonic seizures.

## Precautions:

*Do not use in the following situations:*
    allergy to lamotrigine or its ingredients
    rash in children

*Use with caution in the following situations:*

| | |
|---|---|
| anemia | rash |
| heart disease | valproic acid use |
| kidney disease | visual disorders |
| liver disease | |

*Rash* may occur during treatment with this medicine and may be a symptom of a serious allergic reaction. If a rash should develop, discontinue lamotrigine if the drug is suspected and contact your doctor immediately. The incidence of severe, potentially life-threatening rash in pediatric patients is very much higher than that reported in adults using lamotrigine. Specifically, reports from clinical trials suggest that as many as 1 in 50 to 1 in 100 pediatric patients develop a potentially life-threatening rash. Thus, lamotrigine is not approved for use in patients below the age of 16.

*Pregnancy:* Adequate studies have not been done in pregnant women or animal studies may have shown a risk to the fetus. Use only if clearly needed and potential benefits outweigh the possible hazards to the fetus.

*Breastfeeding:* Lamotrigine appears in breast milk. Breastfeeding while taking lamotrigine is not recommended. Consult your doctor before you begin breastfeeding.

*Children:* Safety and effectiveness in children younger than 16 years of age have not been established.

*Lab tests* to monitor the amount of lamotrigine and other seizure drugs in the blood may be needed. Since it is possible that lamotrigine may collect in the tissues of the eyes, testing may be necessary if visual impairment occurs.

## Drug Interactions:

Tell your doctor or pharmacist if you are taking or if you are planning to take any over-the-counter or prescription medications or dietary supplements while taking lamotrigine. Doses of one or both drugs may need to be modified or a different drug may need to be prescribed. The following drugs and drug classes interact with lamotrigine:

carbamazepine (eg, *Tegretol)*
folate inhibitors (eg, trimetrexate glucuronate)
phenobarbital (eg, *Solfoton)*

phenytoin (eg, *Dilantin)*
primidone (eg, *Mysoline)*
valproic acid (eg, *Depakene)*

## Side Effects:

Every drug is capable of producing side effects. Many lamotrigine users experience no, or minor, side effects. The frequency and severity of side effects depend on many factors including dose, duration of therapy and individual susceptibility. Possible side effects include:

*Circulatory System:* Hot flashes; pounding in the chest (palpitations); chest pain.

*Digestive Tract:* Stomachache; nausea; vomiting; diarrhea; indigestion; constipation; dry mouth; loss of appetite; tooth disorder.

*Nervous System:* Dizziness; incoordination; drowsiness; sleeplessness; tremor; depression; anxiety; nervousness; hostility; convulsions; worsened seizures; irritability; speech disorder; memory loss; confusion; thinking abnormality; unstable emotions; mind racing; rapid eye movement; concentration disturbance; feeling of whirling motion.

*Respiratory System:* Sore throat; increased cough; difficulty breathing; congestion.

*Urinary and Reproductive Tract:* Painful menstruation; inflammation of the vagina; absence of menstrual bleeding;

*Skin:* Rash; itching; hair loss; acne.

*Senses:* Double vision; blurred vision.

*Other:* Headache; flu syndrome; fever; neck, joint or back pain; general body discomfort; chills; weakness; abnormal vision; ear pain; ringing in the ears; muscle spasm; accidental injury; infection; weight gain.

## Guidelines for Use:

- Use exactly as prescribed.
- May be taken without regard to food.
- For long-term therapy, take in two equally divided doses.
- If a rash should develop, it could be a sign of a serious medical condition. Contact your doctor immediately. Also report any fever or gland swelling.
- Notify your doctor if seizures become worse.
- If a dose is missed, take it as soon as possible. If several hours have passed or if it is nearly time for the next dose, do not double the dose to "catch up" (unless advised to do so by your doctor). If more than one dose is missed or it is necessary to establish a new dosage schedule, contact your doctor or pharmacist.
- May cause dizziness and drowsiness. Avoid driving or performing other tasks requiring alertness or coordination until effects are known, then use caution.
- Do not discontinue medication or change the dose without first consulting with your doctor. Seizures could increase. Unless safety concerns require a faster withdrawal, the dose of lamotrigine should be tapered over 2 weeks.
- Inform your doctor if you are pregnant, become pregnant, are planning to become pregnant during therapy, or if you are breastfeeding or intend to breastfeed an infant.
- Lab tests may be required to monitor therapy. Be sure to keep appointments.
- Store in a dry place at room temperature; protect from light.

*If you have any questions, consult your doctor, pharmacist, or health care provider.*

| Generic Name<br>*Brand Name Examples* | Supplied As | Generic<br>Available |
|---|---|---|
| Rx **Tiagabine HCl** | | |
| *Gabitril Filmtab* | **Tablets:** 4 mg, 12 mg, 16 mg,<br>20 mg | No |

## Type of Drug:
Anticonvulsant; drug used to treat seizures.

## How the Drug Works:
It is not known exactly how tiagabine works. It is believed that tiagabine prevents or reduces the number of seizures by altering chemicals in the brain to inhibit nerve impulses which cause certain types of seizures.

## Uses:
As an additional therapy in the treatment of partial seizures in patients older than 12 years of age.

## Precautions:
*Do not use in the following situations:* Allergy to tiagabine or any of its ingredients.

*Use with caution in the following situations:*

| | |
|---|---|
| EEG abnormalities | preexisting cognitive/neuropsy- |
| change of epilepsy drugs | chiatric disorders |
| liver disease | withdrawal, abrupt |
| non-induced patients | |

*Pregnancy:* Adequate studies have not been done in pregnant women. Use only if clearly needed and potential benefits outweigh the possible hazards to the fetus.

*Breastfeeding:* It is not known if tiagabine appears in breast milk. Consult your doctor before you begin breastfeeding.

*Children:* Safety and effectiveness in children younger than 12 years of age have not been established.

*Lab tests* may be required with tiagabine.

## Drug Interactions:
Tell your doctor or pharmacist if you are taking or if you are planning to take any over-the-counter or prescription medications or dietary supplements with tiagabine. Doses of one or both drugs may need to be modified or a different drug may need to be prescribed. The following drugs and drug classes interact with tiagabine.

| | |
|---|---|
| carbamazepine (eg, *Tegretol*) | phenytoin (eg, *Dilantin*) |
| CNS depressants (eg, diaze-<br>  pam, alcohol, tranquilizers,<br>  hypnotics) | primidone (eg, *Mysoline*)<br>triazolam<br>valproate (eg, *Depakote*) |
| ethanol | |
| phenobarbitol (eg, *Solfoton*) | |

## Side Effects:

Every drug is capable of producing side effects. Many tiagabine users experience no, or minor, side effects. The frequency and severity of side effects depend on many factors including dose, duration of therapy and individual susceptibility. Possible side effects include:

*Digestive Tract:* Nausea; stomach pain; diarrhea; vomiting; increased appetite; mouth sores; constipation; appetite loss; dry mouth; gas; indigestion; inflammation of the gums.

*Nervous System:* Dizziness; lightheadedness; drowsiness; nervousness; irritability; tremor; abnormal thinking; difficulty concentrating; depression; confusion; incoordination; sleeplessness; speech disorder; difficulty with memory; abnormal skin sensations; unstable emotions; abnormal walk; hostility; continual rapid eye movement; language problems; agitation; accidental injury; anxiety; depersonalization; slurred speech; headache; fainting; exaggerated sense of well-being; hallucinations; excessive or decreased movement; decreased sensitivity to touch; muscle twitching; migraine; paranoid reaction; personality disorder; decreased reflexes; stupor; feeling of whirling motion.

*Circulatory System:* High blood pressure; pounding in the chest (palpitations); rapid heartbeat.

*Respiratory System:* Bronchitis; difficulty breathing; nosebleed; pneumonia; increased cough.

*Skin:* Flushing; rash; itching; unusual bruising; acne; hair loss; dry skin; sweating.

*Other:* Weakness/lack of energy; pain; muscle weakness; sore throat; chest pain; flu-like syndrome; sinus infection; back pain; fever; vision problems; eye irritation; urinary tract infection; urinary frequency; infection; allergic reaction; chills; cyst; neck pain; general body discomfort; swelling; swelling of arms and legs; weight gain or loss; joint pain; weak or tight muscles; ear pain; ringing in the ears; ear infection; painful menstruation; painful or difficult urination; irregular menstruation; inability to control urination; inflammation of the vagina with itching and vaginal discharge; lymph node disorder.

## Guidelines for Use:

- Usual starting dose is 4 mg once daily.
- Take with food.
- Take as directed by your doctor. The daily dose varies depending on individual needs. Do not adjust the dose or discontinue therapy without consulting your doctor. This could have serious adverse effects.
- If a dose is missed, take it as soon as possible. If several hours have passed or if it is nearing time for the next dose, do not double the dose in order to "catch up" (unless advised by your doctor). If more than one dose is missed or it is necessary to establish a new dosage schedule, contact your doctor or pharmacist. Use exactly as prescribed.
- This medicine may cause drowsiness or dizziness. Use caution while driving or performing other tasks requiring mental alertness, coordination or physical dexterity.
- Avoid alcohol and other mental depressants (eg, narcotics, tranquilizers, antihistamines) while you are taking this medicine.
- Inform your doctor if you are pregnant, become pregnant, are planning to become pregnant or if you are breastfeeding.
- Withdraw tiagabine gradually to minimize the potential of increased seizure frequency, unless safety concerns require a more rapid withdrawal.
- Keep scheduled appointments with your doctor and carry Medic Alert identification listing your medical condition and medicine.
- Lab tests may be required to monitor treatment. Be sure to keep appointments.
- Store at controlled room temperature (68° to 77°F). Protect from light and moisture.

*If you have any questions, consult your doctor, pharmacist, or health care provider.*

| Generic Name<br>*Brand Name Example* | Supplied As | Generic<br>Available |
|---|---|---|
| *Rx* **Levetiracetam** | | |
| *Keppra* | **Tablets**: 250 mg, 500 mg, 750 mg | No |

## Type of Drug:
Anticonvulsant; antiseizure agent.

## How the Drug Works:
Although the precise mechanism of action is not known, it appears that levetiracetam inhibits bursts of neural impulses and propagation of seizure activity.

## Uses:
For adjunctive therapy in the treatment of partial onset seizures in adults with epilepsy.

## Precautions:
*Do not use in the following situations:* Allergy to levetiracetam or any of its ingredients.

*Use with caution in the following situations:* Moderate to severe kidney disease.

*Pregnancy:* There are no adequate and well-controlled studies in pregnant women. Use only if clearly needed and the potential benefits to the mother outweigh the possible risks to the fetus.

*Breastfeeding:* It is not known if levetiracetam appears in breast milk. Consult your doctor before you begin breastfeeding.

*Children:* Safety and effectiveness in patients younger than 16 years of age have not been established.

## Drug Interactions:
Tell your doctor or pharmacist if you are taking or planning to take any over-the-counter or prescription medications or dietary supplements while taking levetiracetam. Doses of one or both drugs may need to be modified or a different drug may need to be prescribed.

## Side Effects:

Every drug is capable of producing side effects. Many patients experience no, or minor, side effects. The frequency and severity of side effects depend upon many factors including dose, duration of therapy, and individual susceptibility. Possible side effects include:

*Nervous System:* Drowsiness; incoordination; dizziness; depression; nervousness; vertigo (feeling of whirling motion); amnesia; anxiety; hostility; emotional lability; hostility; fatigue.

*Respiratory System:* Sore throat; runny nose; increased cough; sinus irritation.

*Other:* Abnormal skin sensations; weakness; headache; infection; pain; appetite loss; double vision

---

### Guidelines for Use:

- Dosage is individualized.
- Do not change the dose or stop taking unless advised to do so by your doctor.
- May be taken without regard to meals or snacks.
- If a dose is missed, take it as soon as possible. If several hours have passed or if it is nearing time for the next dose, do not double the dose in order to catch up, unless advised to do so by your doctor. If several doses are missed, or it is necessary to establish a new dosage schedule, contact your doctor or pharmacist.
- May cause dizziness or drowsiness. Use caution while driving or performing other tasks requiring alertness, coordination, or physical dexterity.
- Notify your doctor if you experience drowsiness, fatigue, coordination difficulties, or behavior abnormalities.
- Notify your doctor if you are pregnant, become pregnant, or are planning to become pregnant while undergoing therapy with levetiracetam.
- Store at controlled room temperature (59° to 86°F).

---

*If you have any questions, consult your doctor, pharmacist, or health care provider.*

| Generic Name<br>*Brand Name Examples* | Supplied As | Generic<br>Available |
|---|---|---|
| *Rx* **Valproic Acid**[1] | | |
| *Depakene* | **Capsules**: 250 mg | Yes |
| *Depakote* | **Capsules, sprinkle**: 125 mg<br>(as divalproex sodium) | No |
| *Depakote* | **Tablets, delayed release**:<br>125 mg, 250 mg, 500 mg (as<br>divalproex sodium) | No |
| *Depakote ER* | **Tablets, extended release**:<br>250 mg, 500 mg (as divalproex<br>sodium) | No |
| *Depakene* | **Syrup**: 250 mg/5 mL | Yes |

[1] Also available as an injection.

## Type of Drug:

Anticonvulsant; drug used to treat epilepsy, seizures, and other conditions.

## How the Drug Works:

Valproic acid prevents or reduces the number of seizures by controlling the abnormal activity of nerve impulses in the brain and central nervous system. Sodium valproate and divalproex sodium are converted to valproic acid in the body.

## Uses:

Used alone or in combination with other anticonvulsants to control simple and complex absence seizures (petit mal).

Used alone or in combination with other anticonvulsants to control isolated complex partial seizures or complex partial seizures associated with other types of seizures.

*Delayed-release tablets:* To treat manic episodes associated with bipolar disorder.

*Delayed-release, extended-release tablets:* For the prevention of migraine headaches.

*Unlabeled Use(s):* May be effective as an adjunct to antipsychotic drugs in the symptomatic management of schizophrenia in patients who fail to respond to an adequate trial of the antipsychotic agent alone. Also may be a useful adjunct in schizophrenic patients with EEG abnormalities suggestive of seizure activity, or in those patients with agitated or violent behavior. May be effective in relieving tardive dyskinesia in patients receiving long-term antipsychotic drug therapy. For the treatment of aggressive outbursts in children with attention deficit hyperactivity disorder. Has been shown to be effective in a limited number of patients with organic brain syndrome.

## Precautions:

*Do not use in the following situations:*
>> allergy to valproic acid, sodium valproate, divalproex, or any of their ingredients
>> liver disease or impairment
>> urea cycle disorders

*Use with caution in the following situations:*

blood or bleeding disorders
children younger than 2 years of age
congenital metabolic disorders
kidney disease
liver disease, history of

organic brain disorder
other anticonvulsant use
pregnancy
severe seizure disorders with mental retardation
suicidal thoughts

*Liver disease:* Liver failure resulting in death has occurred in patients receiving valproic acid and its derivatives. Children younger than 2 years of age are at an increased risk of developing fatal liver toxicity, especially if they are taking several anticonvulsant medications or have birth-related metabolic disorders, severe seizure disorders accompanied by mental retardation, or brain damage. Liver problems usually occur during the first 6 months of treatment. Loss of seizure control, general feeling of ill health, weakness, drowsiness, facial swelling, appetite loss, yellowing of skin and eyes, or persistent or unexplained vomiting may be warning signs of possible liver problems.

*Pancreatitis:* Cases of life-threatening pancreatitis have been reported in children and adults receiving valproate. Pancreatitis can occur at any time while using valproic acid. Abdominal pain, nausea, vomiting, or anorexia can be symptoms of pancreatitis that require prompt medical evaluation.

*Pregnancy:* Studies have shown a potential risk to the fetus. Using these drugs during pregnancy may result in birth defects. If you are pregnant or are planning to become pregnant, discuss with your doctor the possible risks to the unborn infant. Use only if clearly needed and the potential benefits outweigh the possible risks.

*Breastfeeding:* Valproic acid appears in breast milk. Consult your doctor before you begin breastfeeding.

*Children:* Children younger than 2 years of age may be particularly sensitive to the possible liver damage caused by valproic acid, especially if taking other anticonvulsant drugs at the same time. Safety and effectiveness have not been established in children younger than 18 years of age for treatment of acute mania. Safety and efficacy of divalproex sodium for the prevention of migraines has not been established in children younger than 16 years of age. Safety and effectiveness of divalproex sodium extended-release tablets for the prevention of migraine headache and treatment of epilepsy have not been established in children younger than 18 years of age. Sprinkle capsules are for adults and children 10 years of age and older. Consult your doctor. See *Liver disease.*

*Elderly:* Elderly patients may be at an increased risk of drowsiness and tremor. Lower doses are usually used when starting therapy.

*Lab tests* will be required during treatment. Tests may include liver function, blood cell counts, blood-clotting tests, and valproic acid blood levels.

## Drug Interactions:

Tell your doctor or pharmacist if you are taking or planning to take any over-the-counter or prescription medications or dietary supplements with this drug. Drug doses may need to be modified or a different drug prescribed. The following drugs and drug classes interact with this drug:

anticoagulants, oral (eg, warfarin)
carbamazepine (eg, *Tegretol*)
clonazepam (eg, *Klonopin*)
diazepam (eg, *Valium*)
ethanol
ethosuximide (eg, *Zarontin*)
felbamate (*Felbatol*)
hydantoins (eg, phenytoin)

lamotrigine (*Lamictal*)
phenobarbital (eg, *Solfoton*)
primidone (eg, *Mysoline*)
rifampin (eg, *Rifadin*)
salicylates (eg, aspirin)
tricyclic antidepressants
 (eg, amitriptyline)
zidovudine (AZT; *Retrovir*)

## Side Effects:

Every drug is capable of producing side effects. Many patients experience no, or minor, side effects. The frequency and severity of side effects depend on many factors including dose, duration of therapy, and individual susceptibility. Possible side effects include:

*Senses:* Abnormal vision; eye redness or pain; blurred or double vision; spots before the eyes; unusual eye movements; dry eyes; hearing loss; ear pain or disorder; ringing in the ears; taste perversion.

*Digestive Tract:* Appetite changes; nausea; vomiting; stomach cramps or pain; indigestion; diarrhea; fecal incontinence; constipation; gas; tongue inflammation; vomiting of blood; belching; pancreatitis.

*Nervous System:* Weakness; tiredness; nervousness; forgetfulness; clumsiness; drowsiness; behavior changes; depression; headache; tremors; hallucinations; dizziness; slurred speech; abnormal dreams; abnormal thinking; agitation; abnormal gait; twitching; abnormal skin sensations (eg, burning, prickling, tingling); feeling of whirling motion; exaggerated sense of well-being; decreased sense of stimulation; difficulty moving; increased reflexes; confusion; sleeplessness; behavioral deterioration; anxiety.

*Circulatory System:* Changes in blood pressure; pounding in the chest (palpitations); dizziness or light-headedness when rising from a sitting or lying position (postural hypotension); fast heartbeat; flushing; chest pain.

*Skin:* Yellowing of skin or eyes; unusual bleeding or bruising; sensitivity to sunlight; rash; itching; dry or oily skin; skin redness; hair follicle infection; hair loss.

*Other:* Swelling of the face, hands, or feet; weight changes; abscessed teeth; muscle, joint, and back pain; leg cramps; tight muscles; difficulty breathing; increased cough; runny nose; frequent, painful, or difficult urination; loss of bladder control; chills; fever; neck pain or stiffness; changes in menstrual periods; painful menstruation; injection site reactions; sore throat; flu-like syndrome; sweating; general body discomfort; vaginal infection; bronchitis; respiratory infection; muscle weakness; nosebleed; sinus infection; difficulty speaking.

## Guidelines for Use:

- Dosage is individualized. Take exactly as prescribed.
- Do not stop taking or change the dose, unless instructed by your doctor. If you stop taking this medicine suddenly, your seizures may suddenly begin again.
- May cause stomach upset. Take with food.
- *Tablets, capsules* — Swallow whole; do not chew or crush. Chewing or crushing may cause irritation in the mouth or throat.
- *Sprinkle capsules* — May be swallowed whole or taken by opening the capsule and sprinkling the contents on a small amount (teaspoonful) of soft foods such as applesauce or pudding. Swallow quickly without chewing. Do not store drug/food mixture for future use. Some of the specially coated sprinkles may be seen in the stool. This is normal and no cause for concern.
- May cause dizziness, drowsiness, or sleepiness. Use caution when driving or performing other tasks requiring alertness, coordination, or physical dexterity until tolerance is determined. Taking at bedtime may help decrease drowsiness.
- Contact your doctor immediately if you experience loss of seizure control, weakness, swelling of the face, unusual bleeding or bruising, skin reactions, lethargy, general body discomfort, appetite loss, yellowing of skin or eyes, vomiting, nausea, or stomach pain.
- If dose is missed, take as soon as possible. If several hours have passed or it is nearing time for the next dose, do not double the dose to catch up, unless instructed by your doctor. If more than one dose if missed or it is necessary to establish a new dosage schedule, contact your doctor or pharmacist.
- When you first begin taking this medicine, see your doctor regularly. Your doctor may want to adjust the dose you are taking to make sure it is the best dose to control your condition and minimize side effects. Checkups are particularly important if you are taking other anticonvulsant drugs with valproic acid.
- Inform your doctor if you are pregnant, become pregnant, are planning to become pregnant, or are breastfeeding.
- *Diabetes* — These drugs may interfere with urine tests for ketones and may give inaccurate test results.
- Using these drugs with alcohol or other central nervous system depressants (eg, narcotic pain relievers, sedatives) may cause additional drowsiness.

## Guidelines for Use (cont.):

- Carry *MedicAlert* identification indicating that you are taking these drugs and have epilepsy.
- May cause sensitivity to sunlight. Avoid prolonged exposure to the sun and other ultraviolet light. Use sunscreens and wear protective clothing until tolerance is determined.
- Store capsules at 59° to 77°F. Store tablets and syrup below 86°F.

*If you have any questions, consult your doctor, pharmacist, or health care provider.*

| Generic Name<br>*Brand Name Example* | Supplied As | Generic<br>Available |
|---|---|---|
| *Rx* **Baclofen** | | |
| *Lioresal* | **Tablet**: 10 mg, 20 mg | Yes |
| *Lioresal Intrathecal* | **Injection**: 10 mg/20 mL<br>(500 mcg/mL), 10 mg/5 mL<br>(2000 mcg/mL) | No |

## Type of Drug:
Skeletal muscle relaxant.

## How the Drug Works:
Baclofen reduces the frequency and severity of muscle spasms that occur as a result of neurological disorders such as multiple sclerosis.

## Uses:
*Tablets:* To relieve the spasticity, pain, and rigidity from muscle spasms due to multiple sclerosis. May help with spinal cord injuries and other spinal cord diseases.

*Injection:* To manage severe spasticity of spinal cord origin in patients who do not respond to or have side effects from the tablets.

*Unlabeled Use(s):* Occasionally doctors may prescribe oral baclofen for trigeminal neuralgia (tic douloureux), tardive dyskinesia in combination with neuroleptics, and intractable hiccoughs; the injection form may reduce spasticity in cerebral palsy in children.

## Precautions:
*Do not use in the following situations:*

allergy to the drug or any of its ingredients
cerebral palsy (tablets only)
muscle spasms due to rheumatic disorders (tablets only)
Parkinson disease (tablets only)

*Use with caution in the following situations:*

autonomic dysreflexia (lesions on the spinal cord)
epilepsy
infection (injection only)
kidney disease
psychotic disorders
stroke (tablets only)

*Abrupt withdrawal:* Hallucinations and seizures have occurred when treatment with baclofen has been stopped suddenly. Except in cases of serious side effects, the dose must be reduced slowly when the drug is discontinued.

*Epilepsy:* Increased frequency of seizures has occurred in epileptic patients taking baclofen. Frequent physical exams and neurological tests may be required.

*Ovarian cysts:* Ovarian cysts are sometimes found in women who have taken baclofen for up to one year. The cysts often disappear despite continued treatment.

*Pregnancy:* There are no adequate and well-controlled studies in pregnant women. Use only if clearly needed and potential benefits outweigh the possible risks to the fetus.

*Breastfeeding:* Oral baclofen appears in breast milk. It is not known if injectable baclofen appears in breast milk. Consult your doctor before you begin breastfeeding.

*Children:* Safety and effectiveness in children younger than 12 years of age (oral) and in children younger than 4 years of age (injection) have not been established.

## Drug Interactions:

Tell your doctor or pharmacist if you are taking or if you are planning to take any over- the-counter or prescription medications or dietary supplements while taking this medicine. Doses of one or both drugs may need to be modified or a different drug may need to be prescribed. The following drugs and drug classes interact with this medicine.

> alcohol
> morphine
> narcotic pain relievers (eg, *Percodan*)
> sleep aids (eg, flurazepam)
> tricyclic antidepressants (eg, amitriptyline)

## Side Effects:

Every drug is capable of producing side effects. Many patients experience no, or minor, side effects. The frequency and severity of side effects depend on many factors including dose, duration of therapy and individual susceptibility. Possible side effects include:

*Digestive Tract:* Nausea; constipation; vomiting.

*Nervous System:* Drowsiness; dizziness; lightheadedness; weakness; tiredness; headache; seizures; sleeplessness; numbness; tingling; slurred speech.

*Skin:* Rash; itching; excessive sweating.

*Other:* Visual disturbances; ankle swelling (edema); weak muscles; weight gain; nasal congestion; difficulty breathing; frequent urination; low blood pressure.

## Guidelines for Use:

- Use exactly as prescribed.
- If a dose is missed, take it as soon as possible. If several hours have passed or if it is nearing time for the next dose, do not double the dose in order to "catch up" (unless advised to do so by your doctor). If more than one dose is missed or it is necessary to establish a new dosage schedule, contact your doctor or pharmacist.
- May cause drowsiness, dizziness and tiredness. Use caution when driving or performing other tasks requiring alertness. Avoid alcohol and other drugs that cause drowsiness during use of baclofen.
- Sudden discontinuation of baclofen can result in hallucinations. Discontinue only under doctor's supervision.
- Notify your doctor if frequent urges to urinate, painful urination, constipation, nausea, headache, insomnia, confusion, palpitations or chest pain occurs and persists.
- *Injections* — Not for IV, IM, subcutaneous, or epidermal use. Visually inspect solutions for particles or discoloration.
- Store at room temperature. Do not freeze. Do not heat or sterilize solution.

*If you have any questions, consult your doctor, pharmacist, or health care provider.*

| Generic Name<br>*Brand Name Example* | Supplied As | Generic<br>Available |
|---|---|---|
| *Rx* **Dantrolene Sodium** | | |
| *Dantrium* | **Capsules**: 25 mg, 50 mg, 100 mg | No |
| *Dantrium Intravenous* | **Powder for injection**: 20 mg/vial | No |

## Type of Drug:

Skeletal muscle relaxant.

## How the Drug Works:

Dantrolene relaxes skeletal muscle by acting directly on the muscle.

In rare cases, the use of anesthetics in certain individuals can lead to a life-threatening rapid rise in body temperature known as "malignant hyperthermia". It may be due to anesthetics triggering a complex series of events in the muscles that ultimately lead to very high body temperatures. Dantrolene is used to treat or prevent malignant hyperthermia because it is thought that it interferes with the necessary sequence of events which lead to malignant hyperthermia.

## Uses:

To treat muscle spasms (spasticity) due to certain nerve disorders (eg, cerebral palsy, multiple sclerosis, spinal cord injury or stroke). It is best used for individuals with reversible spasms and in whom the spasms interfere with rehabilitation. It may also be used on a long-term basis for some individuals in whom the spasms are painful or disabling. It should not be used in individuals for whom spastic movements are important for gaining or sustaining upright posture or balance or for moving about, or for treatment of spasm resulting from rheumatism.

To treat or prevent malignant hyperthermia (life-threatening rapid rises in body temperature resulting from the use of an anesthetic). These reactions usually occur in the operating room during the course of an operation. Dantrolene is given intravenously in these situations. However, certain individuals considered at risk for malignant hyperthermia from an anesthetic will often be given dantrolene orally prior to an operation. In addition, dantrolene may be given intravenously after malignant hyperthermia has occurred during an operation to prevent a recurrence.

*Unlabeled Use(s):* Occasionally doctors may prescribe dantrolene for exercise-induced muscle pain, neuroleptic malignant syndrome and heat stroke.

## Precautions:

*Do not use in the following situations:*
> allergy to dantrolene
> liver disease (eg, cirrhosis, hepatitis)
> rheumatic disorder

*Use with caution in the following situations:*

| | |
|---|---|
| females | lung disease |
| heart disease | patients older than 35 years of |
| long-term use | age |

*Liver:* Serious liver disorders, including some that were fatal, have occurred as a result of using dantrolene. Risk of hepatitis appears to be greatest in women, in patients older than 35 and in patients taking other drugs in addition to dantrolene. It is important that liver function be checked routinely by physical exam and blood tests.

*Photosensitivity:* May cause photosensitivity (sensitivity to sunlight). Avoid prolonged exposure to the sun or other forms of ultraviolet (UV) light (eg, tanning beds). Use sunscreens and wear protective clothing until tolerance is determined.

*Pregnancy:* Adequate studies have not been done in pregnant women, or animal studies may have shown a risk to the fetus. Use only if clearly needed and potential benefits outweigh the possible hazards to the fetus.

*Breastfeeding:* Do not use dantrolene during breastfeeding.

*Children:* Safety and effectiveness in children under 5 have not been established. Use is not recommended.

## Drug Interactions:

Tell you doctor or pharmacist if you are taking or planning to take any over-the-counter or prescription medications or dietary supplements while taking this medicine. Doses of one or both drugs may need to be modified or a different drug may need to be prescribed. The following drugs and drug classes interact with this medicine.

anticoagulants, oral (eg, warfarin)
clofibrate (eg, *Atromid-S*)
estrogens (eg, *Premarin*)

## Side Effects:

Every drug is capable of producing side effects. Many patients experience no, or minor, side effects. The frequency and severity of side effects depend on many factors including dose, duration of therapy and individual susceptibility. Possible side effects include:

*Urinary and Reproductive Tract:* Change in frequency of urination; blood in urine; loss of urine control (incontinence); difficulty obtaining erection; painful urination; difficulty with urination; frequent urination at night.

*Digestive Tract:* Diarrhea; constipation; black, tarry stools; loss of appetite; difficulty swallowing; upset stomach; abdominal cramps.

*Nervous System:* Drowsiness; dizziness; difficulty with speech; seizures; headache; lightheadedness; sleeplessness; depression; confusion; anxiety (nervousness); weakness; tiredness.

*Circulatory System:* Rapid heart rate; changes in blood pressure; swelling, redness, pain and tenderness over a vein (phlebitis).

*Skin:* Unusual hair growth; rash; itching; hives; redness; sweating; yellowing of skin and eyes.

*Other:* Hepatitis; general feeling of ill health; vision problems; double vision; taste changes; sore muscles; backache; chills and fever; feeling of suffocation; excessive tearing; difficulty breathing; chest pain.

## Guidelines for Use:

- Use exactly as prescribed.
- If a dose is missed, take it as soon as possible. If several hours have passed or if it is nearing time for the next dose, do not double the dose in order to "catch up" (unless advised to do so by your doctor). If more than one dose is missed or it is necessary to establish a new dosage schedule, contact your doctor or pharmacist.
- If no apparent benefit is observed after 45 days of treatment, the drug should be stopped.
- May cause drowsiness, dizziness or lightheadedness. Use caution when driving or performing other tasks requiring alertness, coordination or physical dexterity.
- Avoid alcohol and other drugs that can cause drowsiness, dizziness or lightheadedness.
- May cause weakness, tiredness, nausea, diarrhea and a general feeling of ill health. A decrease in grip strength and weakness of leg muscles (particularly when walking down stairs) may occur after receiving dantrolene intravenously. Notify your doctor if any of these symptoms persist.
- Use caution while eating because choking and difficulty swallowing can occur on the day dantrolene is administered.
- May cause photosensitivity (sensitivity to sunlight). Avoid prolonged exposure to sunlight or other forms of ultraviolet (UV) light (eg, tanning beds). Use sunscreens and wear protective clothing until tolerance is determined.
- Notify your doctor if skin rash, itching, bloody or black tarry stools, or yellowish discoloration of the skin or eyes occurs.
- Store at room temperature. Protect from light.

*If you have any questions, consult your doctor, pharmacist, or health care provider.*

| Generic Name<br>*Brand Name Example* | Supplied As | Generic<br>Available |
|---|---|---|
| *Rx* **Tizanidine HCl** | | |
| *Zanaflex* | **Tablets:** 4 mg | No |

## Type of Drug:
Centrally acting muscle relaxant.

## How the Drug Works:
Tizanidine activates chemical receptors in the brain which inhibit nerve stimulation of muscles.

## Uses:
For acute and intermittent treatment of increased muscle tone associated with spasticity.

## Precautions:
*Do not use in the following situations:* Allergy to tizandine or any of its ingredients.

*Use with caution in the following situations:*

| | |
|---|---|
| antihypertensive drug therapy | kidney disease |
| cardiac rhythm disturbance | liver disease |
| elderly | long-term use |
| females taking oral contra-<br>ceptives | low blood pressure |

*Liver injury:* Tizanidine occasionally causes liver injury which is usually reversible when the medicine is stopped. Liver enzyme testing is used to identify this problem. Report any symptoms of nausea, vomiting, appetitie loss or jaundice (yellowing of skin or eyes) to your doctor.

*Pregnancy:* Adequate studies have not been done in pregnant women. Use only if clearly needed and potential benefits outweigh the possible hazards to the fetus.

*Breastfeeding:* It is not known if tizanidine appears in breast milk.

*Children:* Safety and effectiveness in children have not been established.

*Elderly:* Use with caution in elderly patients.

*Lab tests* may be required to monitor treatment. Be sure to keep appointments. Tests may include: Liver function and kidney function.

## Drug Interactions:

Tell your doctor or pharmacist if you are taking or if you are planning to take any over-the-counter or prescription medications or dietary supplements with tizanidine. Doses of one or both drugs may need to be modified or a different drug may need to be prescribed. The following drugs and drug classes interact with tizanidine.

alcohol
acetaminophen (eg, *Tylenol*)
alpha-adrenergic agonists
 (eg, clonidine)
antihypertensives (eg, prazosin)

baclofen (*Lioresal*)
CNS depressants (eg, benzodi-azepines)
oral contraceptives (eg, *Ortho-Novum 1/35*)

## Side Effects:

Every drug is capable of producing side effects. Many tizanidine users experience no, or minor, side effects. The frequency and severity of side effects depend on many factors including dose, duration of therapy and individual susceptibility. Possible side effects include:

*Digestive Tract:* Dry mouth; constipation; vomiting; stomach pain; diarrhea; indigestion.

*Nervous System:* Sedation; drowsiness; hallucinations; increased spasms; dizziness; nervousness; depression; anxiety; abnormal skin sensations.

*Circulatory System:* Low blood pressure; slow or irregular heartbeat.

*Endocrine:* Rash; sweating; skin ulcer.

*Other:* Abnormal liver function tests; general body weakness; urinary tract infection; infection; speech disorder; blurred vision; urinary frequency; flu-like syndrome; difficulty moving; sore throat; fever; muscle weakness; back pain; nasal congestion; runny nose.

## Guidelines for Use:

- Usual starting dose is 4 mg daily to reduce side effects. Gradual increases in dose will be made to maximize muscle relaxant effect.
- Each dose can be taken as needed every 6 to 8 hours up to three times a day.
- May be taken with or without food.
- If a dose is missed, take it as soon as possible. If several hours have passed or it is nearing time for the next dose, do not double the dose to "catch up" (unless advised by your doctor). If more than one dose is missed or it is necessary to establish a new dosage schedule, contact your doctor or pharmacist.
- If dry mouth, drowsiness or weakness occurs, contact your doctor immediately.
- May cause dizziness, lightheadedness or fainting, especially when rising or standing. If these symptoms should occur, sit or lie down and contact your doctor. Use caution while driving or performing hazardous tasks requiring alertness, coordination or physical dexterity.
- This medicine may cause some other medicines (eg, benzodiazepines, baclofen) and alcohol to have increased sedative or drowsiness effects.
- Inform you doctor if you are pregnant, become pregnant, are planning to become pregnant or if you are breastfeeding.
- Inform your doctor if you are taking oral contraceptives so that necessary dosage adjustments may be made.
- Limited information exists regarding long-term use of this medicine.
- Lab tests or exams may be required to monitor treatment. Be sure to keep appointments. Tests may include: Liver function and kidney function.
- Store at 59° to 86°F.

*If you have any questions, consult your doctor, pharmacist, or health care provider.*

| Generic Name<br>*Brand Name Examples* | Supplied As | Generic<br>Available |
|---|---|---|
| *Rx* **Carisoprodol** | | |
| *Soma* | **Tablets**: 350 mg | Yes |
| *Rx* **Chlorphenesin Carbamate** | | |
| *Maolate*[1] | **Tablets**: 400 mg | No |
| *Rx* **Chlorzoxazone** | | |
| *Paraflex Caplets, Remular-S* | **Tablets**: 250 mg | Yes |
| *Parafon Forte DSC Caplets* | **Tablets**: 500 mg | Yes |
| *Rx* **Cyclobenzaprine** | | |
| *Flexeril* | **Tablets**: 10 mg | Yes |
| *c-iv* **Diazepam**[2] | | |
| *Valium* | **Tablets**: 2 mg, 5 mg, 10 mg | Yes |
| *Diazepam* | **Oral solution**: 5 mg/tsp | Yes |
| *Diazepam Intensol* | **Oral solution, concentrated**: 5 mg/mL | Yes |
| *Rx* **Metaxalone** | | |
| *Skelaxin* | **Tablets**: 400 mg | No |
| *Rx* **Methocarbamol**[2] | | |
| *Robaxin, Robaxin-750* | **Tablets**: 500 mg, 750 mg | Yes |
| *Rx* **Orphenadrine Citrate**[2] | **Tablets**: 100 mg | Yes |
| *Norflex* | **Tablets, sustained release**: 100 mg | No |

[1] Contains the dye tartrazine.
[2] Some of these products are available as an injection.

## Type of Drug:

Skeletal muscle relaxants.

## How the Drug Works:

These drugs indirectly affect nerves that cause muscle tension or spasm. They also have sedative effects on the central nervous system.

## Uses:

To relieve muscle discomfort due to strain, sprain or injury. These agents are not a substitute for rest or physical therapy needed for proper healing. Sometimes given in combination with other pain relieving drugs (such as aspirin or acetaminophen).

*Diazepam* is also used for spasticity caused by upper motor neuron disorders (eg, cerebral palsy, paraplegia); athetosis; stiff-man syndrome.

*Methocarbamol and injectable diazepam* may have a beneficial effect for tetanus.

*Unlabeled Use(s):* Occasionally doctors may prescribe these medicines for other conditions. Cyclobenzaprine may be useful as an adjunct in managing fibrositis syndrome; orphenadrine citrate taken at bedtime may be beneficial in treating leg cramps.

## Precautions:

*Do not use in the following situations:*

abnormal heartbeats
allergy to the drug
allergy to meprobamate (carisoprodol only)
anemia (metaxolone only)
bladder neck obstruction
 (orphenadrine only)
congestive heart failure (CHF)
gastrointestinal obstruction
 (orphenadrine only)

hyperthyroidism (overactive thyroid)
MAOI use
myasthenia gravis (orphenadrine only)
peptic ulcer (orphenadrine only)
porphyria
prostate enlargement (orphenadrine only)

*Use with caution in the following situations:*

addiction-prone individuals
epilepsy
glaucoma (increased intraocular pressure)
kidney disease
liver disease
long-term use
urine retention

*Pregnancy:* Adequate studies have not been done in pregnant women, or animal studies may have shown a risk to the fetus. Use only if clearly needed and potential benefits outweigh the possible hazards to the fetus.

*Diazepam* – Studies have shown a potential adverse effect on the fetus. Use only if clearly needed and potential benefits outweigh the possible risks.

*Breastfeeding:* Carisoprodol appears in breast milk. It is not known if the other skeletal muscle relaxants appear in breast milk. Consult your doctor before you begin breastfeeding.

*Children:* Use in children is generally not recommended. Usage may vary. Consult your doctor.

*Elderly:* In elderly and debilitated patients, it is recommended that dosage of diazepam be limited to the smallest effective amount to guard against development of incoordination and sedation.

*Lab tests* may be required to monitor therapy. Be sure to keep appointments. Tests may include: Urinalysis, blood counts, liver and kidney function tests.

*Tartrazine:* Some of these products may contain the dye tartrazine (FD&C Yellow No. 5) which can cause allergic reactions in certain individuals. Check package label when available or consult your doctor or pharmacist.

*Sulfites:* Some of these products contain sulfite preservatives which can cause allergic reactions in certain individuals (eg, asthmatics). Check package label when available or consult your doctor or pharmacist.

## Drug Interactions:

Tell your doctor or pharmacist if you are taking or if you are planning to take any over-the-counter or prescription medications or dietary supplements while taking this medicine. Doses of one or both drugs may need to be modified or a different drug may need to be prescribed. The following drugs and drug classes interact with this medicine.

> alcohol
> anticholinergic drugs (eg, atropine)
> barbiturates (eg, phenobarbital)
> narcotic analgesics (eg, codeine)
> monoamine oxidase inhibitors (eg, phenylzine)
> phenothiazines (eg, promethazine)
> propoxyphene (eg, *Darvon*)

> *orphenadrine citrate only* –

> amantadine (eg, *Symadine*)
> haloperidol (eg, *Haldol*)

Consider all drug interactions reported for benzodiazepines (see the Antianxiety Agents-Benzodiazepines monograph in this chapter) when using diazepam as a muscle relaxant.

## Side Effects:

Every drug is capable of producing side effects. Many patients experience no, or minor, side effects. The frequency and severity of side effects depend on many factors including dose, duration of therapy and individual susceptibility. Possible side effects include:

Because of cyclobenzaprine's similarity to tricyclic antidepressants (TCAs), consider all side effects for TCAs listed in the monograph in this chapter.

*Allergic Reactions:* Rash; itching; redness; hives; asthma attack; eye discomfort; breathing problems; fever.

*Digestive Tract:* Stomach upset; constipation; indigestion; nausea; vomiting.

*Nervous System:* Tremor; dizziness; drowsiness; headache; nervousness; depression; fatigue; sleeplessness; confusion; weakness; slurred speech; irritability; incoordination; paralysis.

*Circulatory System:* Changes in heartbeat; lightheadedness after standing quickly from a sitting or lying position; fainting; abnormal heartbeat; pounding in the chest; heart attack; low blood pressure.

*Skin:* Yellowing of skin or eyes; unusual bleeding or bruising; flushing; hives; rash.

*Other:* Stuffy nose; sore throat; fever; balance problems; discolored urine; blurred vision; dry mouth; anemia; hiccups; general body discomfort; overstimulation; double vision; rapid eye movement; hallucinations; decreased urination; loss of bladder control; discoloration of urine; temporary vision loss; pupil dilation; increased tension in eyes; sloughing, pain or inflammation at injection site; taste changes.

## Guidelines for Use:

- Use exactly as prescribed.
- May cause stomach upset. Take with food.
- If a dose is missed, take it as soon as possible. If several hours have passed or if it is nearing time for the next dose, do not double the dose in order to "catch up" (unless advised to do so by your doctor). If more than one dose is missed or it is necessary to establish a new dosage schedule, contact your doctor or pharmacist.
- May cause dry mouth, difficult urination, constipation, headache or stomach upset. Notify your doctor if these effects persist, or if skin rash or itching, yellowing of skin or eyes, fever, nasal congestion, rapid heart rate, palpitations or confusion occurs.
- *Orthostatic hypotension* — Dizziness or lightheadedness may occur if you stand up too fast from a lying or sitting position. If this occurs, get up slowly and avoid sudden changes in posture.
- *Chlorzoxazone* may discolor urine orange or purple-red.
- *Methocarbamol* may darken urine to brown, black or green.
- These drugs make an injury temporarily feel better. Do not push your recovery. Lifting or exercising too soon may further damage muscles.
- Muscle relaxants are related to tranquilizers. With the exception of diazepam, they are not considered to be addictive. They should not be used to treat other general body pain.
- May cause drowsiness, dizziness or lightheadedness. Use caution when driving or performing other tasks requiring alertness, coordination or physical dexterity.
- Avoid alcohol or other drugs that cause drowsiness during treatment with skeletal muscle relaxants.
- Do not use a larger dose or use more often than prescribed.
- Store at room temperature.

*If you have any questions, consult your doctor, pharmacist, or health care provider.*

| Generic Name<br>*Brand Name Examples* | Supplied As | Generic<br>Available |
|---|---|---|
| *Rx* **Methocarbamol w/ASA** | | |
| *Robaxisal* | **Tablets**: 400 mg methocarba-mol and 325 mg aspirin | Yes |
| **Carisoprodol Compound** | | |
| *Rx* *Sodol Compound, Soma Compound* | **Tablets**: 200 mg carisoprodol and 325 mg aspirin | Yes |
| *c-III* *Soma Compound w/Codeine* | **Tablets**: 200 mg carisoprodol, 325 mg aspirin and 16 mg codeine phosphate | No |
| *Rx* **Chlorzoxazone w/APAP** | | |
| *Flexaphen* | **Capsules**: 250 mg chlorzoxa-zone and 300 mg aceta-minophen | No |
| *Rx* **Orphenadrine Citrate w/ASA** | | |
| *Norgesic* | **Tablets**: 25 mg orphenadrine citrate, 385 mg aspirin and 30 mg caffeine | No |
| *Norgesic Forte* | **Tablets**: 50 mg orphenadrine citrate, 770 mg aspirin and 60 mg caffeine | No |

## Type of Drug:

Skeletal muscle relaxant combinations.

## Uses:

As adjuncts to rest, physical therapy and other measures for relief of dis-comfort associated with acute, painful musculoskeletal conditions. The other combinations are classified as "probably effective" for this indica-tion. Components of these combinations include:

*Muscle relaxants:* Methocarbamol; chlorzoxazone; carisoprodol; orphena-drine citrate.

*Analgesics:* Acetaminophen; aspirin; codeine.

*Caffeine* used as a CNS stimulant, also has minor analgesic activity. It increases the pain relieving effects and helps the medication begin working faster.

See the corresponding monographs for more information on these components.

## Guidelines for Use:

- Use exactly as prescribed.
- If stomach upset occurs, take with food.
- If a dose is missed, take it as soon as possible. If several hours have passed or if it is nearing time for the next dose, do not double the dose in order to "catch up" (unless advised to do so by your doctor). If more than one dose is missed or it is necessary to establish a new dosage schedule, contact your doctor or pharmacist.
- May cause dry mouth, difficult urination, constipation, headache or stomach upset. Notify your doctor if these effects persist, or if skin rash or itching, yellowing of skin or eyes, fever, nasal congestion, rapid heart rate, pounding in the chest or confusion occurs.
- *Orthostatic hypotension* — Dizziness or lightheadedness may occur if you stand up too fast from a sitting or lying position. If this occurs, get up slowly and avoid sudden changes in posture.
- *Chlorzoxazone* may discolor urine orange or purple-red.
- *Methocarbamol* may darken urine to brown, black or green.
- These drugs make an injury temporarily feel better. Do not push your recovery. Lifting or exercising too soon may further damage muscles.
- Muscle relaxants are related to tranquilizers. They are not considered to be addictive. They should not be used to treat other general body pain.
- May cause drowsiness, dizziness or lightheadedness. Use caution when driving or performing other tasks requiring alertness, coordination or physical dexterity.
- Avoid alcohol or other drugs that cause drowsiness during treatment with these drugs.
- Do not use a larger dose or use more often than prescribed.
- Store at room temperature.

*If you have any questions, consult your doctor, pharmacist, or health care provider.*

| Generic Name<br>*Brand Name Examples* | Supplied As | Generic<br>Available |
|---|---|---|
| *Rx* **Benztropine Mesylate**[1] | | |
| *Cogentin* | **Tablets:** 0.5 mg, 1 mg, 2 mg | No |
| *Rx* **Biperiden**[1] | | |
| *Akineton* | **Tablets:** 2 mg | No |
| **Diphenhydramine**[1] | | |
| *otc* *Banophen, Benadryl,*<br>*Benadryl Allergy*<br>*Kapseals, Benadryl Dye-*<br>*Free Allergy Liqui Gels* | **Capsules:** 25 mg, 50 mg | Yes |
| *Rx* *Banophen, Benadryl,*<br>*Benadryl Kapseals,*<br>*Genahist* | **Capsules:** 25 mg, 50 mg | Yes |
| *otc* *AllerMax, Banophen,*<br>*Benadryl Allergy, Benadryl*<br>*25, Diphenhist Captabs,*<br>*Dormarex 2* | **Tablets:** 25 mg, 50 mg | Yes |
| *Rx* *Genahist* | **Tablets:** 25 mg | Yes |
| *Rx* *Diphenhydramine HCl* | **Tablets:** 50 mg | Yes |
| *otc* *Benadryl Allergy* | **Tablets, chewable:** 12.5 mg | No |
| *otc* *Banophen[2], Belix[2,3],*<br>*Diphenhist, Genahist[2],*<br>*Nidryl[2], Phendry[2],*<br>*Siladryl[2]* | **Elixir:** 12.5 mg/tsp | Yes |
| *Rx* *Benadryl[2]* | **Elixir:** 12.5 mg/tsp | Yes |
| *otc* *Benadryl Allergy, Benadryl*<br>*Dye-Free, Scot-Tussin*<br>*Allergy* | **Liquid:** 6.25 mg/tsp,<br>12.5 mg/tsp | No |
| *otc* *Benylin Cough[2], Diphen*<br>*Cough* | **Syrup:** 12.5 mg/tsp | Yes |
| *Rx* *Hydramyn[2], Tusstat[2]* | **Syrup:** 12.5 mg/tsp | Yes |
| *Rx* **Ethopropazine** | | |
| *Parsidol* | **Tablets:** 10 mg, 50 mg | No |
| *Rx* **Procyclidine** | | |
| *Kemadrin* | **Tablets:** 5 mg | No |

| Generic Name<br>*Brand Name Examples* | Supplied As | Generic<br>Available |
|---|---|---|
| Rx **Trihexyphenidyl HCl** | | |
| *Artane, Trihexy-2,*<br>*Trihexy-4* | **Tablets:** 2 mg, 5 mg | Yes |
| *Artane Sequels* | **Capsules, sustained release:**<br>5 mg | No |
| *Artane*[2] | **Elixir:** 2 mg/tsp | No |

[1] Some of these products are also available as an injection.
[2] Contains alcohol.
[3] Sugar free.

## Type of Drug:

Antiparkinson agents.

## How the Drug Works:

Parkinsonism is a neurological disease with a variety of origins character-ized by tremor, rigidity, and disorders of posture and equilibrium. The onset is slow and progressive with symptoms advancing over months to years.

The group of drugs known as "anticholinergic agents" can reduce the fre-quency and severity of the symptoms of parkinsonism by restoring the chemical imbalance that causes Parkinson disease. The effectiveness of anticholinergics for parkinsonism is not dependent on the origin of the symptoms. These agents are typically used for milder cases of parkin-sonism.

## Uses:

To reduce the frequency and severity of the symptoms of parkinsonism and to control drug-induced parkinsonism-like disorders. Used alone or with other antiparkinson agents. Anticholineric agents do *not* cure the causes of these symptoms.

## Precautions:

*Do not use in the following situations:*

allergy to anticholinergic agents
children younger than 3 years
 of age
glaucoma
myasthenia gravis

prostate enlargement
stomach or intestinal disorders
 (eg, obstruction, ulcers)
urinary bladder obstruction

*Use with caution in the following situations:*

constipation
digestive tract obstruction
elderly (older than 60 years of
 age)
heat intolerance
heart rate, irregular or rapid
high blood pressure

kidney disease
liver disease
low blood pressure
pounding sensation in chest
psychiatric disorder
urinary difficulties

*Pregnancy:* Adequate studies have not been done in pregnant women. Use only if clearly needed and potential benefits outweigh the possible hazards to the fetus.

*Breastfeeding:* Anticholinergic agents appear in breast milk and may reduce milk production. Consult your doctor before you begin breastfeeding.

*Children:* Do not use benztropine in children younger than 3 years old. Safety and effectiveness in older children have not been established.

*Elderly:* Geriatric patients, particularly over 60, frequently develop increased sensitivity to anticholinergic drugs and require strict dosage monitoring. Use with caution. Mental confusion and disorientation, agitation, hallucinations and psychotic-like symptoms may develop. Administer carefully to elderly patients with hardening of the arteries because side effects may be more severe.

## Drug Interactions:

Tell your doctor or pharmacist if you are taking or if you are planning to take any over-the-counter or prescription medications or dietary supplements with anticholinergic agents. Doses of one or both drugs may need to be modified or a different drug may need to be prescribed. The following drugs and drug classes interact with anticholinergic agents.

antihistamines (eg, diphenhydramine)
chlorpromazine (eg, *Thorazine)*
digoxin (eg, *Lanoxin)*
haloperidol (eg, *Haldol)*
levodopa (eg, *Larodopa)*
narcotic pain relievers (eg, *Percodan)*

phenothiazines (eg, promethazine)
quinidine (eg, *Cin-Quin)*
tricyclic antidepressants (eg, amitriptyline)

## Side Effects:

Every drug is capable of producing side effects. Many anticholinergic users experience no, or minor, side effects. The frequency and severity of side effects depend on many factors including dose, duration of therapy and individual susceptibility. Possible side effects include:

*Possible Side Effects Specific to Ethopropazine:* Seizures; brain wave changes, blood disorders; hormone disorders; yellow discoloration of skin and eyes (jaundice); and hallucinations.

*Digestive Tract:* Nausea; vomiting; stomach pain; constipation.

*Nervous System:* Disorientation; confusion; memory loss; hallucinations; lightheadedness; dizziness; weakness; agitation; nervousness; paranoia; delusions; delirium; excessive elation; excitement; depression.

*Circulatory System:* Rapid heart rate; pounding of chest (palpitations); low blood pressure; lightheadedness and dizziness upon rising quickly from a lying position.

*Skin:* Rash; flushing; decreased sweating; hives.

*Eyes or Ocular:* Blurred vision; double vision; widened pupils; visual disturbances; glaucoma.

*Other:* Difficulty urinating; painful urination; muscle weakness; cramping; dry mouth; fever; numbness of fingers; difficulty achieving or maintaining erection; blood disorders (orphenadrine citrate); swollen glands.

---

### Guidelines for Use:

- May cause drowsiness, dizziness, or blurred vision. Use caution when driving or performing other tasks requiring alertness.
- Avoid alcohol and other drugs that cause drowsiness when using anticholinergic agents.
- Stomach upset may occur. Take with food.
- Sucking on hard candy, drinking fluids, or maintaining good dental hygiene can relieve the dry mouth that can result from taking any of the anticholinergic agents.
- Difficult urination and constipation can occur. Use "stool softeners" if necessary. Notify your doctor if either difficult urination or constipation persist.
- Notify your doctor if a rapid heartbeat, pounding sensation in chest, confusion, eye pain, or rash occurs.
- Anticholinergic agents can reduce the ability to sweat, an important function by which overheating is prevented. Avoid excess sun or exercise which may cause excessive sweating.
- Elderly patients may be highly sensitive to anticholinergic drugs. Use with caution. See Precautions.

---

*If you have any questions, consult your doctor, pharmacist, or health care provider.*

| Generic Name<br>*Brand Name Examples* | Supplied As | Generic<br>Available |
|---|---|---|
| *Rx* **Amantadine HCl** | **Capsules:** 100 mg | Yes |
| *Symmetrel* | **Tablets:** 100 mg | No |
| *Symmetrel* | **Syrup:** 50 mg/5 mL | Yes |
| *Rx* **Bromocriptine Mesylate** | | |
| *Parlodel SnapTabs* | **Tablets:** 2.5 mg | No |
| *Parlodel* | **Capsules:** 5 mg | No |
| *Rx* **Carbidopa** | | |
| *Lodosyn* | **Tablets:** 25 mg | No |
| *Rx* **Levodopa** | | |
| *Larodopa* | **Tablets:** 100 mg, 250 mg,<br>500 mg | No |
| *Rx* **Carbidopa/Levodopa** | | |
| *Sinemet 10-100, Sinemet<br>25-100, Sinemet 25-250* | **Tablets:** 10 mg carbidopa,<br>100 mg levodopa; 25 mg carbi-<br>dopa, 100 mg levodopa; 25 mg<br>carbidopa, 250 mg levodopa | Yes |
| *Sinemet CR* | **Tablets, sustained-release:**<br>25 mg carbidopa, 100 mg levo-<br>dopa; 50 mg carbidopa, 200 mg<br>levodopa | No |

For more information, see the amantadine monograph in the Anti-infectives chapter and the bromocriptine monograph in the Miscellaneous chapter.

## Type of Drug:

Antiparkinson agents.

## How the Drug Works:

Parkinsonism is a neurological disease with a variety of causes character-ized by tremor, rigidity, and disorders of posture and balance. The onset is slow and progressive, with symptoms advancing over months to years. Currently, there is no cure for the disease. The goal of therapy is to provide symptomatic relief and attempt to maintain the independence and mobility of the patient.

It is thought that the involuntary muscle movements (shaking) of Parkin-son's disease are due to reduced amounts of the chemical transmitter dopamine in the nervous system. Levodopa is transformed by the body and the nervous system into dopamine. Carbidopa prevents levodopa from being broken down outside the nervous system. Bromocriptine stimulates dopamine receptors. The action of amantadine is not fully understood. It may increase dopamine concentrations in the nervous sys-tem or make the nervous system more sensitive to dopamine.

## Uses:

To treat Parkinson's disease, which may develop spontaneously or follow injury to the nervous system. Amantadine is also used for drug-induced extrapyramidal reactions (symptoms of Parkinson's disease caused by medication).

*Unlabeled Use(s):* Occasionally doctors may prescribe levodopa for herpes zoster (shingles) and restless legs syndrome.

## Precautions:

*Do not use in the following situations:*

> allergy to ergot alkaloids (bromocriptine only)
> allergy to these drugs or any of their ingredients
> angle-closure (narrow angle) glaucoma, untreated (amantadine, levodopa only)
> high blood pressure, uncontrolled (bromocriptine only)
> melanoma, history of (levodopa only)
> monoamine oxidase inhibitor (MAOI) therapy, concurrent or within the previous 14 days (carbidopa/levodopa only)
> skin cancer, possibility of (levodopa only)

*Use with caution in the following situations:*

bronchial asthma (levodopa only)
depression
endocrine gland disease (levodopa only)
glaucoma, chronic wide-angle (levodopa only)
heart attack, history of (bromocriptine, levodopa only)
heart disease, history of
irregular heartbeat (bromocriptine, levodopa only)
kidney disease
liver disease
lung disease, severe (levodopa only)
orthostatic hypotension (drop in blood pressure when standing up)
peptic ulcer, history of (levodopa only)
peripheral edema, history of
postpartum period (bromocriptine only)
psychiatric disorders, history of
psychoses
recurrent eczema, history of (amantadine only)
seizures, history of
substance abuse, history of

*Carbidopa:* Carbidopa had no antiparkinsonian effect when given alone. It is always used in combination with levodopa or carbidopa/levodopa products.

*Neuroleptic malignant-like syndrome (NMS):* NMS, including muscular rigidity, involuntary movements, altered consciousness, elevated body temperature, fast heartbeat, changes in blood pressure, mental changes, and increased serum enzymes, has been reported when antiparkinson agents were stopped suddenly. Do not abruptly reduce the dosage or discontinue use of amantadine or levodopa without consulting your doctor.

*"On-off" phenomenon:* Some patients who initially respond to levodopa therapy may develop the "on-off" phenomenon, a condition in which patients suddenly swing between an improved condition to a worsened condition. This effect may occur within minutes or hours and is associated with long-term levodopa therapy. Other patients may experience a deteriorating response. These conditions can be managed. Contact your doctor.

*Pregnancy:* There are no adequate and well-controlled studies in pregnant women. Use only if clearly needed and potential benefits to the mother outweigh the possible hazards to the fetus.

*Breastfeeding:* Use of amantadine, bromocriptine, and levodopa while breastfeeding is not recommended. It is not known if carbidopa appears in breast milk. Consult your doctor before you begin breastfeeding.

*Children:* Safety and effectiveness of amantadine in children younger than 1 year of age have not been established. Safety and effectiveness of bromocriptine in children younger than 15 years of age have not been established. Safety and effectiveness of carbidopa/levodopa in children younger than 18 years of age have not been established.

*Elderly:* Elderly patients may require less amantadine or carbidopa/levodopa than younger patients.

*Lab tests* will be required to monitor therapy. Tests may include blood counts, eye tests, pituitary tests, blood pressure monitoring, and liver, kidney, and heart function tests.

## Drug Interactions:

Tell your doctor or pharmacist if you are taking or planning to take any over-the-counter or prescription medications or dietary supplements with dopaminergic agents. Doses of one or both drugs may need to be modified or a different drug may need to be prescribed. The following drugs and drug classes interact with dopaminergic agents:

*Amantadine* —

anticholinergics (eg, belladonna)
triamterene/hydrochlorothiazide (eg, *Dyazide*)

*Bromocriptine* —

antihypertensives (eg, diltiazem)
ergot alkaloids (eg, ergotamine)
erythromycin (eg, *Ilosone*)

*Carbidopa/levodopa* —

antihypertensives (eg, diltiazem)
hydantoins (eg, phenytoin)
iron salts (eg, ferrous fumarate)

phenelzine (*Nardil*)
pyridoxine (vitamin $B_6$)
tranylcypromine (*Parnate*)

## Side Effects:

Every drug is capable of producing side effects. Many dopaminergic users experience no, or minor, side effects. The frequency and severity of side effects depend on many factors including dose, duration of therapy, and individual susceptibility. Possible side effects include:

*Digestive Tract:* Nausea; vomiting; diarrhea; constipation; gas; appetite loss; stomach pain or cramps; gastrointestinal bleeding; indigestion; heartburn.

*Nervous System:* Uncontrolled movement (twitching) of face, eyelids, mouth, hands, or legs; abnormally slow movement; mood swings; mental changes; anxiety; fatigue; euphoria (exaggerated sense of well-being); delusions; hallucinations; abnormal dreams; confusion; weakness; agitation; nervousness; dizziness; fainting; orthostatic hypotension (dizziness or lightheadedness when rising quickly from a sitting or lying position); headache; depression; increased tremor; incoordination; sleeplessness; faintness; "on-off" phenomenon; falling; dementia; lightheadedness; irritability; drowsiness; vertigo (feeling of whirling motion).

*Circulatory System:* Palpitations (pounding in the chest); irregular heartbeat; chest pain; changes in blood pressure.

*Skin:* Flushing; rash; increased sweating; hives; itching; hair loss; abnormal skin sensations.

*Other:* Difficult urination; urinary incontinence; difficulty swallowing; numbness; increased salivation; dry mouth or nose; grinding of the teeth; difficulty opening mouth; taste changes; bitter taste; burning tongue; general body discomfort; hot flashes; double vision; blurred vision; dilated pupils; weight changes; dark sweat, saliva, or urine; abnormal blood counts; abnormal liver, kidney, and heart function tests; back, leg, or shoulder pain; abnormal or difficult breathing; suicidal ideation; vein inflammation; visual disturbances; shortness of breath; fluid retention; frequent urination; persistent erection of the penis, accompanied by pain and tenderness; urinary retention; nasal congestion; throat pain; intestinal ulcer; cough; hoarseness; sense of stimulation; hiccups.

## Guidelines for Use:

- Dosage is individualized.
- Be patient. Take this drug routinely as directed. It may take several weeks to a few months to notice benefit from use because the dose is carefully adjusted over time.
- May upset stomach. Take with food at regular intervals.
- Do not change the dose or stop taking unless advised by your doctor. Suddenly stopping treatment may induce neuroleptic malignant-like syndrome (ie, muscle stiffness, involuntary movement, altered consciousness, elevated body temperature, fast heartbeat, changes in blood pressure, mental changes).
- Do not crush or chew sustained-release products.
- *Sustained-release carbidopa/levodopa* — The onset of effect of the first morning dose may be delayed for up to 1 hour. Notify your doctor if this delayed response poses a problem.
- Avoid alcohol during therapy. It may increase the potential for nervous system effects such as dizziness, confusion, lightheadedness, or dizziness when standing up.
- Discontinue MAOIs at least 14 days before starting levodopa or carbidopa/levodopa therapy.
- *Diabetic patients* — Levodopa may interfere with urine tests for sugar or ketones. Report any abnormal results to your doctor before adjusting dosage of antidiabetic medications.
- Gradually increase physical activity as symptoms of Parkinson's disease improve.
- Notify your doctor if you experience uncontrollable movements of the face, eyelids, mouth, tongue, neck, arms, hands, or legs; mood or mental changes; difficult urination; severe or persistent nausea and vomiting; swelling of the arms or legs; or shortness of breath.
- Do not get up quickly after sitting or lying down. Notify your doctor if you experience dizziness or lightheadedness when you rise from a sitting or lying position.
- May cause dizziness, drowsiness, or blurred vision. Use with caution while driving or performing other tasks requiring alertness, coordination, and physical dexterity.
- Levodopa may darken urine, saliva, or sweat. This is not harmful.
- Do not take levodopa along with vitamins containing vitamin $B_6$ (pyridoxine). This vitamin can reduce drug benefits. Carbidopa-containing products may be taken with vitamin $B_6$.
- Using carbidopa together with levodopa may allow a smaller dose of levodopa to be used and reduce its side effects (eg, nausea, vomiting).
- Lab tests will be required to monitor therapy. Be sure to keep appointments.
- Store at controlled room temperature (59° to 86°F). Store bromocriptine below 77°F.

*If you have any questions, consult your doctor, pharmacist, or health care provider.*

| Generic Name<br>*Brand Name Example* | Supplied As | Generic<br>Available |
|---|---|---|
| *Rx* **Pramipexole Dihydrochloride** | | |
| *Mirapex* | **Tablets:** 0.125 mg, 0.25 mg, 1 mg, 1.5 mg | No |

## Type of Drug:

Antiparkinson agent.

## How the Drug Works:

Parkinsonism is a neurological disease with a variety of origins characterized by tremor, rigidity and disorders of posture and balance. The onset is slow and progressive with symptoms advancing over months to years. There is no cure for the disease. The goal of therapy is to provide relief from the symptoms, and to attempt to maintain the independence and mobility of the patient.

It is thought that the involuntary muscle movements (shaking) of Parkinson disease are caused by reduced amounts of dopamine in the nervous system. Pramipexole may exert its effects by stimulating the dopamine receptors in the nervous system.

## Uses:

To manage or treat signs and symptoms of Parkinson disease. May be used with levodopa in the later stages of the disease.

## Precautions:

*Do not use in the following situations:* Allergy to pramipexole

*Use with caution in the following situations:*
      hallucinations
      low blood pressure
      kidney disease
      movement difficulty
      retinal disease (of the eye)

*Pregnancy:* Adequate studies have not been done in pregnant women. Use only if clearly needed and potential benefits outweigh the possible hazards to the fetus.

*Breastfeeding:* It is not known if pramipexole appears in breast milk. Consult your doctor before you begin breastfeeding.

*Children:* Safety and effectiveness have not been established.

*Elderly:* Elderly patients have a greater tendency to develop hallucinations.

## Drug Interactions:

Tell your doctor or pharmacist if you are taking or if you are planning to take any over-the-counter or prescription medications or dietary supplements with pramipexole dihydrochloride. Doses of one or both drugs may need to be modified or a different drug may need to be prescribed. The following drugs and drug classes interact with pramipexole.

butyrophenones (eg, halo-
  peridol)
cimetidine (eg, *Tagamet)*
diltiazem(eg, *Cardizem)*
metoclopramide (eg, *Reglan)*
phenothiazines (eg, chlorpromazine)

quinidine (eg, *Quinora)*
quinine (eg, quinine sulfate)
ranitidine (eg, *Zantac)*
thioxanthenes (eg, chlorprothixene)
triamterene (*Dyrenium)*
verapamil (eg, *Calan)*

## Side Effects:

Every drug is capable of producing side effects. Many pramipexole users experience no, or minor, side effects. The frequency and severity of side effects depend on many factors including dose, duration of therapy and individual susceptibility. Possible side effects include:

*Digestive Tract:* Nausea; constipation; appetite loss; difficulty swallowing; dry mouth; gas; diarrhea; vomiting; indigestion; stomach pain.

*Nervous System:* Dizziness; drowsiness; sleeplessness; hallucinations; confusion; amnesia; reduced skin sensations; muscle tone abnormalities; inability to sit still; thinking abnormalities; decreased sex drive; muscle twitches; movement disorders; dream abnormalities; walking abnormalities; stiffness; paranoid reaction; delusions; sleep disorders; headache; nervousness; leg cramps; tremor.

*Circulatory System:* Low blood pressure.

*Respiratory System:* Difficulty breathing; sinus infection; runny nose/congestion; pneumonia.

*Urinary and Reproductive Tract:* Impotence; increased urination; urinary tract infection; inability to control urination.

*Skin:* Skin disorders; rash.

*Senses:* Vision abnormalities; double vision; abnormal taste.

*Other:* Weakness; swelling; general body discomfort; fever; decreased weight; accidental injury; chest pain; joint pain; muscle weakness; pain; back pain; fainting; depression; sore throat; sweating; flushing; flu syndrome; increased saliva; tooth disease; increased cough; allergic reaction; voice alteration.

## Guidelines for Use:

- Take pramipexole only as directed by your doctor.
- Taking pramipexole with food may reduce nausea.
- Dosage will be started low and gradually increased to achieve maximum effect. Do not change dose sooner than recommended.
- Do not change the dose or discontinue unless advised to do so by your doctor.
- It is recommended that pramipexole be discontinued gradually over a period of a week.
- Hallucinations may occur, especially in the elderly.
- Dizziness or lightheadedness may occur if you stand up too fast from a lying or sitting position. If this occurs, get up slowly and avoid sudden changes in posture.
- Kidney disease patients may need dosage adjustments.
- This medication may cause drowsiness or dizziness. Use caution while driving or performing other tasks requiring mental alertness, coordination or physical dexterity.
- Caution should be used when taking other CNS depressants (eg, alcohol, sedatives) in combination with pramipexole.
- Inform your doctor if you are pregnant, become pregnant, are planning to become pregnant or if you are breastfeeding.
- Store at controlled room temperature (59° to 86° F) and protect from light.

*If you have any questions, consult your doctor, pharmacist, or health care provider.*

| Generic Name<br>*Brand Name Examples* | Supplied As | Generic<br>Available |
|---|---|---|
| *Rx* **Ropinirole HCl** | | |
| *Requip* | **Tablets:** 0.25 mg, 0.5 mg,<br>1 mg, 2 mg, 5 mg | No |

## Type of Drug:
Antiparkinson agent.

## How the Drug Works:
Parkinsonism is a neurological disease with a variety of origins character-ized by tremor, rigidity and disorders of posture and balance. The onset is slow and progressive with symptoms advancing over months to years. There is no cure for the disease. The goal of therapy is to provide relief from the symptoms, and to attempt to maintain the independence and mobility of the patient.

It is thought that the involuntary muscle movements (shaking) of Parkin-son disease are caused by reduced amounts of dopamine in the ner-vous system. Ropinirole may exert its effects by stimulating the dopamine receptors in the nervous system.

## Uses:
To treat signs and symptoms of Parkinson disease. May be used with levo-dopa in the later stages of the disease.

## Precautions:
*Do not use in the following situations:* Allergy to ropinirole.

*Use with caution in the following situations:*

| | |
|---|---|
| fainting | pulmonary (lung) disease |
| hallucinations | movement difficulty |
| kidney impairment, severe | neuroleptic malignant syndrome |
| liver impairment, severe | retinal disease (of the eye) |
| low blood pressure | |

*Pregnancy:* Adequate studies have not been done in pregnant women. Use only if clearly needed and potential benefits outweigh the possible haz-ards to the fetus.

*Breastfeeding:* It is not known if ropinirole appears in breast milk. Consult your doctor before you begin breastfeeding.

*Children:* Safety and effectiveness have not been established.

*Elderly:* Elderly patients have a greater tendency to develop hallucinations.

## Drug Interactions:

Tell your doctor or pharmacist if you are taking or if you are planning to take any over-the-counter or prescription medications or dietary supplements with ropinirole. Doses of one or both drugs may need to be modified or a different drug may need to be prescribed. The following drugs and drug classes interact with ropinirole:

butyrophenones (haloperidol)
cipofloxacin (eg, *Cipro*)
estrogens (eg, *Premarin*)
L-dopa (*Sinemet*)

metoclopramide (eg, *Reglan*)
phenothiazines (eg, chlorpromazine)
thioxanthenes (chlorprothixene)

## Side Effects:

Every drug is capable of producing side effects. Many ropinirole users experience no, or minor, side effects. The frequency and severity of side effects depend on many factors including dose, duration of therapy and individual susceptibility. Possible side effects include:

*Digestive Tract:* Constipation; stomach pain; appetite loss; indigestion; gas; nausea; vomiting.

*Nervous System:* Flushing; dry mouth; increased sweating; dizziness; hyperactivity; decreased sensitivity to touch; whirling feeling; inability to sleep; anxiety; nervousness.

*Circulatory System:* High blood pressure; low blood pressure; orthostatic symptoms (dizziness when rising quickly); fainting; premature heart beat; pounding in the chest; fast heart beat; slow heart beat; high blood sugar.

*Respiratory System:* Bronchitis; difficulty breathing; sore throat; sinus infection; cough.

*Skin:* Abnormal sensations; rash.

*Other:* Weakness; chest pain; fluid accumulation in the lower extremities; fatigue; feeling poorly; pain; headache; increased alkaline phosphatase; amnesia; impaired concentration; confusion; hallucination; drowsiness; yawning; impotence; viral infection; urinary tract infection; cold feet and hands; abnormal vision; double vision; night blindness; joint pain; tremor; back pain; difficulty moving; aggravated Parkinsonism; depression; falls; muscle pain; leg cramps; arthritis; weight loss; muscle spasm; joint degeneration; abnormal dreams; muscular deformation; increased salivation; gout; gum inflammation; blood in the urine; rigidity; inability to control urine; pus in the urine; ringing in the ears.

## Guidelines for Use:

- Take ropinirole only as directed by your doctor (three times daily).
- May be taken with or without food. Taking with food may reduce nausea.
- Dosage will be increased to achieve maximum effect.
- Do not discontinue or change the dose unless advised to do so by your doctor.
- Hallucinations may occur, especially in the elderly.
- Dizziness or lightheadedness may occur if you stand up too fast from a lying or sitting position. If this occurs, get up slowly and avoid sudden changes in posture.
- Caution should be used when taking other CNS depressants (eg, antidepressants) or alcohol.
- This medication may cause drowsiness or dizziness. Use caution while driving or performing other tasks requiring mental alertness, coordination or physical dexterity.
- Inform your doctor if you are pregnant, become pregnant, are planning to become pregnant or if you are breastfeeding.
- Store at controlled room temperature (59° to 77°F) and protect from light.

*If you have any questions, consult your doctor, pharmacist, or health care provider.*

| Generic Name<br>*Brand Name Example* | Supplied As | Generic<br>Available |
|---|---|---|
| Rx **Pergolide Mesylate** | | |
| *Permax* | **Tablets:** 0.05 mg, 0.25 mg,<br>1 mg | No |

## Type of Drug:

Antiparkinson agent.

## How the Drug Works:

Parkinsonism is a neurological disease characterized by tremor, rigidity, and disorders of posture and equilibrium. It has multiple causes. The onset is slow and progressive with symptoms advancing over months to years.

It is thought that the involuntary muscle movements (shaking) of Parkinson disease are due to reduced amounts of the chemical dopamine in the central nervous system (brain). Pergolide may exert its effects by directly stimulating the dopamine receptors in the brain.

## Uses:

To manage the signs and symptoms of Parkinson's disease. Used along with levodopa and carbidopa.

For complete information on levodopa and carbidopa as antiparkinson agents, see the Antiparkinson-Dopaminergic Agents monograph in this chapter.

## Precautions:

*Do not use in the following situations:* Allergy to pergolide or other ergot derivatives.

*Use with caution in the following situations:*
    abnormal heart rhythms
    confusion, recent
    hallucinations, recent
    hypotension (low blood pressure)
    movement disorders

*Neuroleptic Malignant-like Syndrome (NMS):* NMS, including muscular rigidity, elevated body temperature, mental changes, and increased serum enzymes, has been reported when antiparkinson agents were stopped suddenly. Therefore, do not reduce the dosage of pergolide abruptly or discontinue it without consulting your doctor.

*Pregnancy:* There are no adequate and well-controlled studies in pregnant women. Use during pregnancy only if clearly needed.

*Breastfeeding:* It is not known if pergolide appears in breast milk. Consult your doctor before you begin breastfeeding.

*Children:* Safety and effectiveness have not been established.

## Drug Interactions:

Tell your doctor or pharmacist if you are taking or planning to take any over-the-counter or prescription medications or dietary supplements with pergolide mesylate. Doses of one or both drugs may need to be modified or a different drug may need to be prescribed. The following drugs and drug classes interact with pergolide mesylate:

> butyrophenones (eg, haloperidol)
> metoclopramide (eg, *Reglan)*
> phenothiazines (eg, chlorpromazine)
> thioxanthines (eg, thiothixene)

## Side Effects:

Every drug is capable of producing side effects. Many pergolide users experience no, or minor, side effects. The frequency and severity of side effects depend on many factors including dose, duration of therapy, and individual susceptibility. Possible side effects include:

*Digestive Tract:* Nausea; vomiting; constipation; diarrhea; indigestion; stomach pain; appetite loss; difficulty swallowing.

*Nervous System:* Hallucinations; difficult or abnormal movement; restlessness; twitching; confusion; dizziness; drowsiness; fainting; sleeplessness; anxiety; tremor; depression; abnormal dreams; personality changes; headache; weakness; incoordination; difficulty walking.

*Circulatory System:* High or low blood pressure; orthostatic hypotension (dizziness or lightheadedness when arising from a seated or lying position); palpitations (pounding in the chest); irregular heartbeat; heart attack.

*Respiratory System:* Runny nose; difficulty breathing.

*Skin:* Rash; sweating; abnormal skin sensations.

*Other:* Dry mouth; taste changes; general body pain; joint, muscle, or nerve pain; abnormal vision; double vision; frequent urination; urinary tract infections; blood in urine; edema (fluid retention); back, neck, and chest pain; flu-like symptoms; nosebleed; hiccups; weight gain; chills; difficulty speaking; anemia.

## Guidelines for Use:

- Dosage will be individualized.
- Do not change the dose or stop taking this medicine unless advised to do so by your doctor.
- If a dose is missed, take it as soon as possible. If several hours have passed or it is nearing time for the next dose, do not double the dose to catch up, unless advised by your doctor. If more than one dose is missed or it is necessary to establish a new dosage schedule, contact your doctor or pharmacist.
- Notify your doctor if you experience confusion, hallucinations, pounding in the chest, irregular heart rate, or difficulty in movement.
- *Orthostatic hypotension* — Dizziness or lightheadedness may occur when arising quickly from a seated or lying position. Avoid sudden changes in posture while taking pergolide.
- May cause drowsiness. Use caution while driving or performing other tasks requiring alertness, coordination, or physical dexterity.
- Inform your doctor if you are pregnant, become pregnant, are planning to become pregnant, or if you are breastfeeding.
- Store at controlled room temperature (59° to 86°F).

*If you have any questions, consult your doctor, pharmacist, or health care provider.*

| Generic Name<br>*Brand Name Examples* | Supplied As | Generic<br>Available |
|---|---|---|
| *Rx* **Selegiline HCl** | | |
| *Eldepryl* | **Capsules:** 5 mg | No |
| *Carbex* | **Tablets:** 5 mg | Yes |

## Type of Drug:

Monoamine oxidase type B inhibitor, (MAOI); drug used to treat Parkinson's disease.

## How the Drug Works:

Selegiline prolongs the anti-Parkinson activity of levodopa and interferes with normal enzyme activities.

## Uses:

To treat Parkinson disease in conjunction with levodopa/carbidopa in patients whose response to levodopa/carbidopa is deteriorating. There is no evidence that it has any benefit without the concurrent use of levodopa.

*Tyramine-containing foods:* Avoid foods which can interact with monoamine oxidase inhibitors (isocarboxazid, phenelzine, tranylcypromine).

---

### Tyramine-Containing Foods[1]

*Cheese/Dairy Products:* American, processed; blue; Boursault; brick, natural; Brie; Camembert; cheddar; Emmenthaler; Gruyere; mozzarella; Parmesan; Romano; Roquefort; Stilton; sour cream; yogurt.

*Meat/Fish:* Beef or chicken liver, other meats, fish (unrefrigerated, fermented); meats prepared with tenderizer; fermented sausages (bologna, pepperoni, salami, summer sausage); game meat; caviar; dried fish (especially salted herring); herring (pickled or spoiled).

*Alcoholic Beverages (undistilled):* Beer and ale (imports); red wine (especially Chianti); sherry.

*Fruit/Vegetables:* Avocado (especially overripe); yeast extracts (eg, marmite); bananas; figs, canned (overripe); raisins; soy sauce.

*Other Foods:* Fava beans (overripe); chocolate; caffeine (eg, coffee, tea, colas).

---

[1] Tyramine contents are not predictable and may vary. The amounts of tyramine are estimated from low to very high.

## Precautions:

*Do not use in the following situations:*
> allergy to selegiline
> meperidine (eg, *Demerol*) use, concurrent
> tyramine-containing foods

*Use with caution:*
> antidepressant (eg, amitriptyline) use, concurrent or recent
> SSRI (eg, fluxetine) use, concurrent or recent

*Pregnancy:* There are no adequate or well-controlled studies in pregnant women. It is not known if this drug can harm the fetus or interfere with reproduction. Use only if clearly needed and if potential benefit to the mother justifies the potential risk to the fetus.

*Breastfeeding:* It is not known if selegiline appears in breast milk. Consult your doctor before you begin breastfeeding.

*Children:* Safety and effectiveness have not been established.

## Drug Interactions:

Tell your doctor or pharmacist: if you are pregnant, are planning to become pregnant, or are breastfeeding; and if you are taking, will be taking, or stop taking any prescrition or nonprescription medications or dietary supplements. Dosage of levodopa may need to be decreased after you begin taking selegiline.

> contraceptives, oral (eg,*Ortho-Novum*)
> meperidine (eg, *Demerol*)
> SSRIs (eg, fluoxetine)
> sympathomimetics (eg, ephedrine)
> tricyclic antidepressants (eg, amitriptyline)

## Side Effects:

Every drug is capable of producing side effects. Many selegiline users experience no, or minor, side effects. The frequency and severity of side effects depend on many factors including dose, duration of therapy, and individual susceptibility. Possible side effects include:

*Other:* Increased or decreased urination (especially at night); difficult urination.

*Digestive Tract:* Nausea; vomiting; diarrhea; constipation; loss of appetite; stomach pain; heartburn; difficulty swallowing; dry mouth.

*Nervous System:* Weakness; confusion; anxiety; dreams and nightmares; headache; depression; affected speech; tremor; restlessness; sleeplessness; involuntary or abnormal movements; agitation; loss of balance; spasms of eyelid; hallucinations.

*Circulatory System:* Dizziness when arising quickly from a seated or lying position (orthostatic hypotension); changes in blood pressure; pounding of the chest (palpitations); irregular pulse; angina (chest pain); irregular heartbeats; fainting.

*Respiratory System:* Shortness of breath; asthma.

*Skin:* Increased sweating; hair loss; sensitivity to sunlight; facial hair growth; rash; bruising.

---

## Guidelines for Use:

- Dosage is individualized.
- To avoid interference with sleep, take as a single dose with breakfast or in 2 divided doses with breakfast and lunch.
- Do not exceed the recommended daily dose of 10 mg.
- Dosage of levodopa may need to be decreased after the patient begins to take selegiline. Discuss this possibility with your doctor. Do not change the dosage unless advised to do so by your doctor.
- Immediately report any severe headaches or unusual symptoms to your doctor.
- Do not change the dose or stop taking unless advised to do so by your doctor.
- Store at controlled room temperature (59° to 86°F)

---

*If you have any questions, consult your doctor, pharmacist, or health care provider.*

| Generic Name<br>*Brand Name Example* | Supplied As | Generic<br>Available |
|---|---|---|
| *Rx* **Entacapone** | | |
| *Comtan* | **Tablets, film-coated:** 200 mg | No |

## Type of Drug:

Antiparkinson agent; catechol-O-methyltransferase (COMT) inhibitor.

## How the Drug Works:

Entacapone interferes with one of the enzymes (COMT) in the body responsible for eliminating levodopa. It is used in combination with levodopa/carbidopa (eg, *Sinemet*) to prolong the beneficial effects of levodopa in treating symptoms of Parkinson's disease. Entacapone has no antiparkinsonian effects of its own and must always be administered in combination with levodopa/carbidopa.

## Uses:

Entacapone is used in combination with levodopa/carbidopa to treat patients with idiopathic Parkinson's disease who experience the signs and symptoms of end-of-dose "wearing-off" (worsening of Parkinson's symptoms between doses of levodopa/carbidopa). The effectiveness of entacapone has not been evaluated in patients with idiopathic Parkinson's disease who do not experience end-of-dose "wearing-off."

## Precautions:

*Do not use in the following situations:* Allergy to entacapone or any of its ingredients.

*Use with caution in the following situations:*
  dyskinesia, pre-existing
  liver disease
  low blood pressure

*Pregnancy:* There are no adequate and well-controlled studies in pregnant women. Use only if clearly needed and potential benefits outweigh the possible hazards to the fetus.

*Breastfeeding:* It is not known if entacapone appears in breast milk. Consult your doctor before you begin breastfeeding.

*Children:* Safety and effectiveness for use in children have not been established.

## Drug Interactions:

Tell your doctor or pharmacist if you are taking or planning to take any over-the-counter or prescription medications or dietary supplements while taking entacapone. Doses of one or both drugs may need to be modified or a different drug may need to be prescribed. The following drugs and drug classes interact with entacapone:

ampicillin (eg, *Omnipen*)
apomorphine
bitolterol (*Tornalate*)

chloramphenicol (eg, *Chloromycetin*)
cholestyramine (eg, *Questran*)

dobutamine (*Dobutrex*)
dopamine (eg, *Intropin*)
epinephrine (eg, *Epipen*)
erythyromycin (eg, *E-mycin*)
isoetherine
isoproterenol (eg, *Isuprel*)

MAO inhibitors (eg, phenelzine)
methyldopa (eg, *Aldomet*)
norepinephrine (*Levophed*)
probenecid
rifampin (eg, *Rifadin*)

## Side Effects:

Every drug is capable of producing side effects. Many entacapone users experience no, or minor side effects. The frequency and severity of side effects depend on many factors including dose, duration of therapy, and individual susceptibility. Possible side effects include:

*Digestive Tract:* Nausea; diarrhea; stomach pain; constipation; vomiting; dry mouth; indigestion; gas; gastritis.

*Nervous System:* Difficulty moving; abnormal movements; muscular hyperactivity; muscle pain; slow mobility; dizziness; hallucinations; anxiety; agitation; drowsiness.

*Other:* Difficulty breathing; elevated body temperature; increased sweating; unusual bleeding or bruising; little red spots under the skin; brown-orange discoloration of urine; back pain; altered taste; fatigue; weakness; bacterial infection.

---

### Guidelines for Use:

- Dosage is individualized. Use exactly as prescribed.
- Do not change the dose or stop taking this medicine unless advised to do so by your doctor.
- May be taken without regard to meals or snacks.
- Your doctor may reduce your levodopa/carbidopa dose while taking this medicine.
- Each dose is taken at the same time as a dose of levodopa/carbidopa.
- If you experience hallucinations, severe or persistent nausea, or difficult or abnormal movement, contact your doctor immediately.
- May cause dizziness, lightheadedness, or fainting when rising or standing, particularly during initial use. Get up slowly and avoid sudden changes in posture.
- Do not drive a car or operate complex machinery until the effects of entacapone on your mental or motor performance can be gauged.
- Urine color may change to a brownish-orange discoloration. This is normal and of no concern.
- Inform your doctor if you are pregnant, become pregnant, are planning to become pregnant, or are breastfeeding.
- This medicine should not be stopped suddenly. If a decision is made to discontinue this medicine, the dose should be reduced slowly if possible.
- Store at controlled room temperature (59° to 86°F).

---

*If you have any questions, consult your doctor, pharmacist, or health care provider.*

**Antacids**, 903

**Antacid Combinations**, 907

**Anticholinergics/ Antispasmodics**, 916

**Anticholinergic Combinations**, 921

**Mouth and Throat Products**
Doxycycline, 924

**H. Pylori Agents**
Ranitidine Bismuth Citrate, 927
Bismuth Subsalicylate/Metron- idazole/Tetracycline, 929
Lansoprazole/Amoxicillin/ Clarithromycin, 932

**Histamine H$_2$ Antagonists**, 935

**Anti-Ulcer**
Misoprostol, 940
Sucralfate, 942

**Antiflatulents**, 944

**Digestive Aids**
Digestive Enzymes, 946
Metoclopramide, 950

**Proton Pump Inhibitors**, 953

**Gallstone Dissolving Agents**
Oral, 957
Infusion, 959

**Laxatives**
Bulk-Reducing, 961
Glycerin, 965
Lactulose, 967
Mineral Oil, 969
Saline, 971
Stimulant, 973
Stool Softeners, 977
Laxative Combinations, 980

**Bowel Evacuants**
Polyethylene Glycol, 985
Bowel Evacuant Kits, 987

**Antidiarrheals**
Bismuth Subsalicylate, 989
Difenoxin and Diphenoxylate, 992
Lactobacillus, 995
Loperamide, 996
Antidiarrheal Combination Products, 998

**5-Aminosalicylate (5-ASA) Agents**, 1001

**Infliximab**, 1004

**Anti-obesity Agents**
Orlistat, 1006

**Tegaserod Maleate**, 1009

| Generic Name<br>*Brand Name Examples* | Supplied As | Generic<br>Available |
|---|---|---|
| *otc* **Aluminum Carbonate Gel, Basic** | | |
| *Basaljel* | **Capsules:** Equivalent to 608 mg dried aluminum hydroxide gel or 500 mg aluminum hydroxide | No |
| *Basaljel* | **Tablets:** Equivalent to 608 mg dried aluminum hydroxide gel or 500 mg aluminum hydroxide | No |
| *otc* **Aluminum Hydroxide Gel** | | |
| *Alu-Cap* | **Capsules:** 400 mg | No |
| *Amphojel* | **Tablets:** 300 mg, 600 mg | No |
| *Alu-Tab* | **Tablets:** 500 mg | No |
| *ALternaGEL, Amphojel* | **Suspension:** 320 mg/5 mL, 600 mg/5 mL | Yes |
| *otc* **Calcium Carbonate** | **Tablets:** 500 mg, 600 mg, 648 mg, 1250 mg | Yes |
| | **Suspension:** 1250 mg/5 mL | Yes |
| *Gastro-Relief* | **Tablets, chewable:** 250 mg | No |
| *Amitone* | **Tablets, chewable:** 350 mg | No |
| *Mallamint* | **Tablets, chewable:** 420 mg | No |
| *Alkets, Antacid Tablets, Chooz[1], Tums* | **Tablets, chewable:** 500 mg | Yes |
| *Extra Strength Alkets, Extra Strength Antacid Tablets, Tums E-X[2]* | **Tablets, chewable:** 750 mg | Yes |
| *Alka-Mints* | **Tablets, chewable:** 850 mg | No |
| *Tums Ultra[2]* | **Tablets, chewable:** 1000 mg | No |
| *Calcichew* | **Tablets, chewable:** 1250 mg | Yes |
| *otc* **Magaldrate (Aluminum Magnesium Hydroxide Sulfate)** | | |
| *Iosopan, Lowsium* | **Suspension:** 540 mg/5 mL | Yes |

| Generic Name<br>*Brand Name Examples* | Supplied As | Generic<br>Available |
|---|---|---|
| *otc* **Magnesia (Magnesium Hydroxide)** | | |
| *Phillips' Milk of Magnesia* | **Tablets, chewable:** 311 mg | No |
| *Milk of Magnesia, Phillips' Milk of Magnesia* | **Suspension:** 400 mg/5 mL | Yes |
| *Concentrated Phillips' Milk of Magnesia* | **Suspension:** 800 mg/5 mL | No |
| *otc* **Magnesium Oxide** | **Tablets:** 500 mg | Yes |
| *Uro-Mag* | **Capsules:** 140 mg | No |
| *Mag-Ox 400* | **Tablets:** 400 mg | Yes |
| *otc* **Sodium Bicarbonate** | **Tablets:** 325 mg, 650 mg | Yes |
| *Bell/ans* | **Tablets:** 520 mg | No |
| *otc* **Sodium Citrate** | | |
| *Citra pH* | **Solution:** 450 mg/5 mL | No |

[1] Contains phenylalanine.
[2] Contains tartrazine.

## Type of Drug:
Antacids.

## How the Drug Works:
Antacids neutralize stomach acid and increase the pH of the stomach. This action also inhibits activity of pepsin, a digestive enzyme that can be irritating to the stomach lining. They also increase the tone of the muscular valve between the stomach and the esophagus, which helps prevent stomach acids from getting into the esophagus and causing heartburn.

## Uses:
To treat upset stomach due to excessive acid production (including heartburn, acid indigestion, and sour stomach).

To treat excess acid secretion associated with peptic ulcer (ulcers in the stomach or intestine).

*Aluminum carbonate:* To treat or control hyperphosphatemia.

*Calcium carbonate, magnesium oxide:* To treat calcium or magnesium deficiencies, respectively.

*Magnesium hydroxide:* To relieve occasional constipation (irregularity).

*Unlabeled Use(s):* Occasionally doctors may prescribe aluminum hydroxide, aluminum carbonate, and calcium carbonate to reduce phosphorus levels in certain kidney conditions. Aluminum hydroxide or aluminum hydroxide with magnesium hydroxide may be used to prevent stress ulcer bleeding (stress ulcers occur with serious illnesses such as life-threatening infections or blood loss).

## Precautions:

*Use with caution in the following situations:*

kidney disease (magnesium-containing products only)
stomach-emptying disorders (aluminum-containing products only)
upper digestive tract hemorrhage (aluminum hydroxide only)

*Sodium content:* Some antacids have a high sodium content. Select a low-sodium antacid product if you have high blood pressure, heart conditions, kidney disease, fluid retention, or are on a low-sodium diet. Check package label when available or consult your doctor or pharmacist.

*Sodium bicarbonate:* Sodium bicarbonate products can alter normal blood chemistry if used for long periods of time or in excessive doses.

*Phenylketonuria:* Some of these products contain phenylalanine. Check package label when available or consult your doctor or pharmacist.

*Pregnancy:* There are no adequate and well-controlled studies in pregnant women. Use only if clearly needed and the potential benefits to the mother outweigh the possible risks to the fetus.

*Breastfeeding:* It is not known if antacids appear in breast milk. Consult your doctor before you begin breastfeeding.

*Tartrazine:* Some of these products may contain the dye tartrazine (FD&C Yellow No. 5), which can cause allergic reactions in certain individuals. Check package label when available or consult your doctor or pharmacist.

## Drug Interactions:

Tell your doctor or pharmacist if you are taking or if you are planning to take any over-the-counter or prescription medications or dietary supplements with antacids. Doses of one or both drugs may need to be modified or a different drug may need to be prescribed. The following drugs and drug classes interact with antacids:

allopurinol (eg, *Zyloprim*) (aluminum products only)
chloroquine (eg, *Aralen*) (aluminum products only)
digoxin (eg, *Lanoxin*) (aluminum products only)
ethambutol (*Myambutol*) (aluminum products only)
hydantoins (eg, phenytoin)
iron salts (eg, ferrous fumarate)
isoniazid (eg, *Nydrazid*) (aluminum products only)
ketoconazole *(Nizoral)*
levothyroxine (eg, *Synthroid*)
penicillamine (eg, *Cuprimine*) (aluminum products only)
quinidine (eg, *Cin-Quin*)
quinolone antibiotics (eg, ciprofloxacin)
salicylates (eg, aspirin)
sodium polystyrene sulfonate (eg, *Kayexalate)*
tetracyclines (eg, doxycycline) (aluminum products only)
valproic acid (eg, *Depakote*)

## Side Effects:

Every drug is capable of producing side effects. Many antacid users experience no, or minor, side effects. The frequency and severity of side effects depend on many factors including dose, duration of therapy, and individual susceptibility. Possible side effects include:

*Aluminum-containing antacids:* Constipation; high aluminum blood levels; low phosphorus levels.

*Calcium-containing antacids:* Appetite loss; nausea; vomiting; dry mouth; increased urination; constipation; stomach pain; thirst; confusion; high blood calcium levels.

*Magnesium-containing antacids:* Diarrhea; high magnesium blood levels; muscle weakness; slow reflexes.

---

### Guidelines for Use:

- Consult individual product labeling for dosage. Antacids contain a variety of different ingredients. Do not exceed the maximum recommended dosage.
- *Chewable tablets* — Chew thoroughly before swallowing. May be followed with a glass of water.
- *Suspensions* — Shake well before using.
- *Product choice* — Liquid products work faster and have greater activity than other forms. Tablets and capsules may be more acceptable and convenient, particularly when you are away from home or when the liquid would be inconvenient to carry.
- Antacids reduce acidity for about 30 to 60 minutes when taken on an empty stomach. Acidity is reduced for about 2 to 3 hours when antacids are taken 1 hour after meals.
- Antacids can interfere with the absorption of some drugs. Do not take medication within 2 hours of taking the antacid.
- Notify your doctor if "coffee-ground" vomiting or black, tarry stools occur.
- Taking too much of these products can cause the stomach to secrete excess stomach acid. Consult your doctor or pharmacist about the appropriate dose.
- *Long-term use* — Do not take for longer than 2 weeks for the relief of indigestion, unless advised to do so by your doctor. If discomfort continues, consult your doctor.
- Store at room temperature (59° to 86°F) in a dry place. Refrigeration of liquid antacids may improve the flavor. Avoid freezing. If the taste of one antacid product is not satisfactory, talk to your doctor or pharmacist about switching to another product.

---

*If you have any questions, consult your doctor, pharmacist, or health care provider.*

| | Brand Name Examples | Aluminum Hydroxide | Magnesium Hydroxide | Calcium Carbonate | Other Content | Sodium (mg)[2] |
|---|---|---|---|---|---|---|
| otc | Tempo | 133 | 81 | 414 | 20 mg simethi-cone | 3 |
| otc | Maalox | 200 | 200 | | | |
| otc | Mintox | | | | | |
| otc | Rulox #1 | | | | | |
| otc | Almacone | | | | 20 mg simethi-cone | |
| otc | Mylanta | | | | | 0.77 |
| otc | Gelusil | | | | 25 mg simethi-cone | < 5 |
| otc | Maalox Plus | | | | | |
| | Magalox Plus | | | | | |
| otc | Mintox Plus | | | | | |
| otc | RuLox | | | | | |
| otc | Entra Strength Maalox | 350 | 350 | | 30 mg simethi-cone | |
| otc | Extra Strength Maalox Plus | | | | | |
| otc | Rulox #2 | 400 | 400 | | | |
| otc | Mylanta Double Strength | | | | 40 mg simethi-cone | |
| otc | Calcium Rich Rolaids | | 80 | 412 | | 0.4 |
| otc | Advanced Formula Di-Gel | | 128 | 280 | 20 mg simethi-cone | |
| otc | Foamicon | 80 | | | 20 mg magnesium trisili-cate, sodium bicarbonate | 18.4 |
| otc | Genaton | | | | | |
| otc | Gaviscon | | | | | |
| otc | Double Strength Gaviscon-2 | 160 | | | Alginic acid, sodium bicarbonate, 40 mg magnesium trisilicate | 36.8 |

| | Brand Name Examples | Aluminum Hydroxide | Magnesium Hydroxide | Calcium Carbonate | Other Content | Sodium (mg)[2] |
|---|---|---|---|---|---|---|
| otc | Extra Strength Genaton | 160 | | | 105 mg magnesium carbonate, alginic acid, sodium bicarbonate | 29.9 |
| otc | Gaviscon Extra Strength Relief Formula | | | | | |
| otc | Gas-Ban | | | 300 | 40 mg simethicone | |
| otc | Mylanta Gelcaps | | | 311 | 232 mg magnesium carbonate | |
| otc | Mylagen Gelcaps | | | | | |
| otc | Calglycine[2] | | | 420 | 150 mg glycine | |
| otc | Titralac[2] | | | | | 0.3 |
| otc | Titralac Plus | | | | 21 mg simethicone | 1.1 |
| otc | Alkets | | | 500 | | ≤ 2 |
| otc | Marblen | | | 520 | 400 mg magnesium carbonate | |
| otc | Titralac Extra Strength[2] | | | 750 | | 0.6 |
| otc | Riopan Plus | † | | | 480 mg magaldrate, 20 mg simethicone | |
| otc | Riopan Plus Double Strength | | | | 1080 mg magaldrate, 20 mg simethicone | |

† See Other Content column.
[1] Content given in mg per capsule, tablet or wafer.
[2] Sugar free.

## Type of Drug:
Antacid combinations.

## Uses:

To treat upset stomach due to too much acid secretion (including heartburn, gastroesophageal reflux, acid indigestion and sour stomach).

To treat excess acid secretion associated with peptic ulcer, irritation of the stomach, irritation of the esophagus or hiatal hernia.

*Unlabeled Use(s):* To prevent significant stress ulcer bleeding. To treat duodenal and gastric ulcers.

---

### Guidelines for Use:

- *Chewable tablets* — Chew before swallowing. Follow with a glass of water.
- If you are currently taking a prescription drug or other medications, do not take an antacid without checking with your doctor or pharmacist.
- Magnesium-containing products may cause diarrhea; aluminum and calcium-containing products may cause constipation.
- Antacids reduce acidity for about 30 minutes when taken on an empty stomach and for about 3 hours when taken 1 hour after meals.
- Notify your doctor if "coffee-ground" vomiting or black, tar-like stools occur.
- Taking too much of these products can cause the stomach to secrete excess stomach acid. Consult your doctor or pharmacist about the appropriate dose.
- *Long-term use* — Do not take for longer than 2 weeks for the relief of indigestion. If discomfort continues, consult your doctor.

---

*If you have any questions, consult your doctor, pharmacist, or health care provider.*

| Brand Name Examples | Aluminum Hydroxide | Magnesium Hydroxide | Calcium Carbonate | Other Content | Sodium (mg)[2] |
|---|---|---|---|---|---|
| otc  Almacone | 200 | 200 | | 20 mg simethicone | |
| otc  Di-Gel | | | | | |
| otc  Gelusil | | | | 25 mg simethicone | |
| otc  Mi-Acid | | | | 20 mg simethicone | |
| otc  Mygel Suspension | | | | | |
| otc  Mylagen | | | | | < 1.25 |
| otc  Mylanta | | | | | 0.68 |
| otc  Alumina, Magnesia, and Simethicone Suspension | 213 | 200 | | 20 mg simethicone | |
| otc  Alamag Suspension | 225 | 220 | | | < 1.25 |
| otc  Alamag Plus Suspension | | | | 25 mg simethicone | |
| otc  Antacid Suspension | | | | | |
| otc  Maalox Suspension | | | | | |
| otc  Magnalox | | | | | |
| otc  Magnox Suspension | | | | | |
| otc  Rulox Suspension | | | | | |
| otc  Aludrox Suspension | 307 | 103 | | simethicone | |
| otc  Almacone II Double Strength Suspension | 400 | 400 | | 40 mg simethicone | |
| otc  Gas-Ban DS | | | | | |
| otc  Mygel II Suspension | | | | | |
| otc  Mylagen II | | | | | < 1.25 |

| | Brand Name Examples | Aluminum Hydroxide | Magnesium Hydroxide | Calcium Carbonate | Other Content | Sodium (mg)[2] |
|---|---|---|---|---|---|---|
| otc | Mylanta Double Strength | 400 | 400 | | 40 mg simethicone | |
| otc | Extra Strength Maalox Suspension | 500 | 450 | | | |
| otc | Extra Strength Maalox Plus Suspension | | | | | |
| otc | Extra Strength Mintox Plus | | | | | |
| otc | Kudrox Double Strength Suspension | | | | | |
| otc | Rulox Plus Suspension | | | | | |
| otc | Maalox Therapeutic Concentrate Suspension | 600 | 300 | | | |
| otc | Genaton | 31.7 | | | 137.3 mg magnesium carbonate, sodium alginate, EDTA | 13 |
| otc | Gaviscon | | | | 119.3 mg magnesium carbonate, sodium alginate, EDTA | 13 |
| otc | Gaviscon Extra Strength Relief Formula | 254 | | | 237.5 mg magnesium carbonate, simethicone | |
| otc | Nephrox | 320 | | | 10% mineral oil | |
| otc | Titralac Plus[2] | | | 500 | 20 mg simethicone | 0.15 |

| Brand Name Examples | Aluminum Hydroxide | Magnesium Hydroxide | Calcium Carbonate | Other Content | Sodium (mg)[2] |
|---|---|---|---|---|---|
| otc Marblen | | | 520 | 400 mg magnesium carbonate | |
| otc Lowsium Plus Suspension | †† | | | 540 mg magaldrate, 40 mg simethicone | |
| otc Magaldrate Plus Suspension | | | | | |
| otc Riopan Plus Suspension | | | | | |
| otc Riopan Plus Double Strength Suspension | | | | 1080 mg magaldrate and 40 mg simethicone | |
| otc Maalox Heartburn Relief | | | | 140 mg aluminum hydroxide magnesium carbonate, 175 mg magnesium carbonate | |

† See Other Content column.
[1] Content given in mg per 5 mL.
[2] Sugar free.

## Type of Drug:

Antacid combinations.

## Uses:

To treat upset stomach due to too much acid secretion (including heartburn, gastroesophageal reflux, acid indigestion and sour stomach).

To treat excess acid secretion associated with peptic ulcer, irritation of the stomach, irritation of the esophagus or hiatal hernia.

Unlabeled Use(s): To prevent significant stress ulcer bleeding. To treat duodenal and gastric ulcers.

## Guidelines for Use:

- *Suspension* — Shake well before using.
- If you are currently taking a prescription drug or other medications, do not take an antacid without checking with your doctor or pharmacist.
- Magnesium-containing products may cause diarrhea; aluminum and calcium-containing products may cause constipation.
- *Refrigeration* of liquid antacids may improve the flavor (avoid freezing). Talk to your doctor or pharmacist about switching to another product if the taste is not satisfactory.
- Antacids reduce acidity for about 30 minutes when taken on an empty stomach and for about 3 hours when taken 1 hour after meals.
- Notify your doctor if "coffee-ground" vomiting or black, tar-like stools occur.
- Taking too much of these products can cause the stomach to secrete excess stomach acid. Consult your doctor or pharmacist about the appropriate dose.
- *Long-term use* — Do not take for longer than 2 weeks for the relief of indigestion. If discomfort continues, consult your doctor.

*If you have any questions, consult your doctor, pharmacist, or health care provider.*

| | Brand Name Examples | Supplied As |
|---|---|---|
| otc | Citrocarbonate[1] | **Effervescent granules:** 780 mg sodium bicarbonate, 1820 mg sodium citrate and 700.6 mg sodium per dose |
| otc | Bromo Seltzer | **Effervescent granules:** 2781 mg sodium bicarbonate, 325 mg acetaminophen, 2224 mg citric acid and 761 mg sodium per dose |
| otc | Gold Alka-Seltzer | **Effervescent tablets:** 958 mg sodium bicarbonate, 832 mg citric acid, 312 mg potassium bicarbonate and 311 mg sodium |
| otc | Alka-Seltzer | **Effervescent tablets:** 1700 mg sodium bicarbonate, 1000 mg citric acid, 9 mg phenylalanine, 325 mg aspirin and 506 mg sodium |
| otc | Original Alka-Seltzer | **Effervescent tablets:** 1916 mg sodium bicarbonate (heat treated), 1000 mg citric acid, 325 mg aspirin and 567 mg sodium |
| otc | Extra Strength Alka-Seltzer | **Effervescent tablets:** 1985 mg sodium bicarbonate (heat treated), 1000 mg citric acid, 500 mg aspirin and 588 mg sodium |

[1] Sugar free.

## Type of Drug:

Antacid combinations.

## Uses:

To treat upset stomach due to too much acid secretion (including heartburn, gastroesophageal reflux, acid indigestion and sour stomach).

To treat excess acid secretion associated with peptic ulcer, irritation of the stomach, irritation of the esophagus or hiatal hernia.

Unlabeled Use(s): To prevent significant stress ulcer bleeding. To treat duodenal and gastric ulcers.

## Guidelines for Use:

- *Effervescent tablets* — Allow to completely dissolve in water. Allow most of the bubbling to stop before drinking.
- If you are currently taking a prescription drug or other medications, do not take an antacid without checking with your doctor or pharmacist.
- Magnesium-containing products may cause diarrhea; aluminum and calcium-containing products may cause constipation.
- Antacids reduce acidity for about 30 minutes when taken on an empty stomach and for about 3 hours when taken 1 hour after meals.
- Notify your doctor if "coffee-ground" vomiting or black, tar-like stools occur.
- Taking too much of these products can cause the stomach to secrete excess stomach acid. Consult your doctor or pharmacist about the appropriate dose.
- *Long-term use* — Do not take for longer than 2 weeks for the relief of indigestion. If discomfort continues, consult your doctor.

*If you have any questions, consult your doctor, pharmacist, or health care provider.*

| Generic Name Brand Name Examples | Supplied As | Generic Available |
|---|---|---|
| Rx **Dicyclomine**[1] | | |
| *Bentyl*[1,2] | **Capsules:** 10 mg | Yes |
| *Bentyl*[1,2] | **Tablets:** 20 mg | Yes |
| *Bentyl*[1,3] | **Syrup:** 10 mg/5 mL | Yes |
| Rx **Hyoscyamine Sulfate** | | |
| *Anaspaz*[4], *Cystospaz*[2], *Levsin*[1,5], *Donnamar* | **Tablets:** 0.125 mg, 0.15 mg | No |
| *Cystospaz-M, Levsinex Timecaps* | **Capsules, timed release:** 0.375 mg | No |
| *Levsin Drops*[6] | **Solution:** 0.125 mg/mL | No |
| *Levsin*[6] | **Elixir:** 0.125 mg/5 mL | No |
| Rx **Glycopyrrolate** | | |
| *Robinul* | **Tablets:** 1 mg | Yes |
| *Robinul Forte* | **Tablets:** 2 mg | Yes |
| Rx **Mepenzolate Bromide** | | |
| *Cantil*[2,7] | **Tablets:** 25 mg | No |
| Rx **Methscopolamine Bromide** | | |
| *Pamine*[2] | **Tablets:** 2.5 mg | No |
| Rx **Propantheline Bromide** | | |
| *Pro-Banthine*[2] | **Tablets:** 7.5 mg, 15 mg | Yes |

[1] This product also available as an injection.
[2] Contains lactose.
[3] Contains parabens.
[4] Contains lactose, mannitol.
[5] Contains sugar, lactose.
[6] Contains alcohol.
[7] Contains the dye tartrazine.

## Type of Drug:

Drugs used to treat stomach and intestinal disorders; anticholinergic; anti-spasmodic.

## How the Drug Works:

These drugs inhibit actions of nerves in smooth muscle, secretory glands and the central nervous system. They slow certain activity of the stomach and intestines and reduce cramping, reduce secretions (acids, enzymes, etc) of the stomach and intestines, relax the urinary bladder (reduce spasm) and promote closure of the sphincter valve (these actions tend to cause urinary retention). They also slow or increase the heart rate, block sweating (causing the body temperature to rise), reduce salivary gland secretions (causing dry mouth), widen the pupils of the eyes and reduce the ability of the eyes to focus.

## Uses:

To treat peptic ulcers.

To treat diarrhea.

To treat irritable bowel syndrome (spastic colon).

To treat irritation or inflammation of the stomach and intestines (eg, colitis).

To treat infant colic.

To treat spasms of the bile and urinary tracts.

To treat frequent urination problems and bedwetting.

To reduce symptoms of runny or congested nose.

## Precautions:

*Do not use in the following situations:*

allergy to these drugs or any of their ingredients
diarrhea
enlarged colon
enlarged prostate
glaucoma (narrow-angle)
heart problems (eg, ischemia, rapid or irregular heart rate)
infants less than 6 months of age (dicyclomine only)
intestinal obstructions
lack of intestinal muscle tone in elderly or debilitated patients
myasthenia gravis
nursing mothers (dicyclomine)
ulcerative colitis, severe
urinary obstruction

*Use with caution in the following situations:*

abnormal heart rhythm
asthma
bile duct disorders
congestive heart failure
colon problems (eg, ulcerative colitis)
coronary artery disease
dementia, elderly
drowsiness, blurred vision
elderly
esophagitis, reflux
gastric or duodenal ulcers
heart disease
hiatal hernia with gastric reflux
high blood pressure
hot weather
hyperthyroidism (overactive thyroid)
kidney disease
liver disease
nerve disorder
prostate gland problems
psychosis

*Exposure to heat:* These drugs can reduce sweating if you are exposed to hot weather. This can cause heat prostration, fever and heatstroke.

*Diarrhea* can be an early symptom of incomplete intestinal obstruction. Check with your doctor or pharmacist before self-medicating diarrhea with these drugs.

*Contact lens use:* These products can cause drying of the eyes. Contact lens wearers should use an appropriate lubricating solution while taking these products.

*Anticholinergic psychosis* has been reported in sensitive individuals given anticholinergic drugs. CNS signs and symptoms include confusion, disorientation, short-term memory loss, hallucinations, slurred speech, incoordination, coma, exaggerated sense of well-being, decreased anxiety, fatigue, sleeplessness, agitation and inappropriate affect. These CNS signs and symptoms usually resolve within 12 to 24 hours after discontinuation of the drug.

*Pregnancy:* Studies in pregnant women or in animals have been judged not to show a risk to the fetus in patients taking dicyclomine and mepenzolate bromide. Adequate studies have not been done in pregnant women in association with the other listed drugs. Use only if clearly needed and potential benefits outweigh the possible hazards to the fetus.

*Breastfeeding:* These drugs appear in breast milk. They may reduce milk production and cause side effects in the infant. Breastfeeding is contraindicated in patients taking dicyclomine. Consult your doctor before you begin breastfeeding.

*Children:* Safety and effectiveness in children have not been established. Hyoscyamine has been used in infant colic. Some infant deaths have been associated with the use of dicyclomine. Dicyclomine is not recommended for use in children under 6 months of age.

*Elderly:* These drugs can cause agitation and mental confusion in older patients.

*Lab tests* may be required during therapy including upper gastrointestinal contrast radiology or endoscopy, as well as tests for blood in the stool. Be sure to keep appointments.

*Tartrazine:* Some of these products may contain the dye tartrazine (FD&C Yellow No. 5) which can cause allergic reactions in certain individuals. Check package label when available or consult your doctor or pharmacist.

## Drug Interactions:

Tell your doctor or pharmacist if you are taking or if you are planning to take any over-the-counter or prescription medications or dietary supplements with gastrointestinal anticholinergics or antispasmodics. Doses of one or both drugs may need to be modified or a different drug may need to be prescribed. The following drugs and drug classes interact with gastrointestinal anticholinergics or antispasmodics.

amantadine (eg, *Symmetrel*)
antacids (eg, *Maalox)*
anticholinergics, other (eg, belladonna alkaloids)
benzodiazepines (eg, diazepam)
beta blockers (eg, atenolol)
cholinergics (eg, pilocarpine)
cholinesterase inhibitors (eg, physostigmine)
corticosteroids (eg, prednisone)
digoxin (eg, *Lanoxin)*
haloperidol (eg, *Haldol)*
isocarboxazid *(Marplan)*
levodopa (eg, *Dopar*)

MAO inhibitors (eg, phenelzine)
meperidine (eg, *Demerol)*
metoclopramide (eg, *Reglan)*
nitrates (eg, nitroglycerin)
phenothiazines (eg, promethazine)
selegiline *(Eldepryl)*
sympathomimetics (eg, epinephrine)
thioxanthenes (eg, thiothixene)
tranylcypromine *(Parnate)*
tricyclic antidepressants (eg, amitriptyline)

## Side Effects:

Every drug is capable of producing side effects. Many anticholinergic or antispasmodic users experience no, or minor, side effects. The frequency and severity of side effects depend on many factors including dose, duration of therapy and individual susceptibility. Possible side effects include:

*Digestive Tract:* Nausea; vomiting; bloating; constipation; abdominal pain; appetite loss; difficulty swallowing.

*Nervous System:* Confusion; excitement; restlessness; hallucinations; headache; nervousness; drowsiness; dizziness; lightheadedness; tingling; numbness; difficulty moving; fainting; disorientation; short-term memory loss; slurred speech; incoordination; coma; exaggerated sense of well-being; decreased anxiety; tiredness; speech disturbance; weakness; sleeplessness; fever; tremor.

*Circulatory System:* Pounding in the chest (palpitations); fast or irregular heartbeat.

*Respiratory System:* Difficulty breathing; nasal stuffiness; nasal congestion.

*Skin:* Rash; itching; flushing; decreased sweating; hives; skin disorder.

*Other:* Difficult urination; muscle weakness; visual problems; blurred vision; dry mouth; taste changes; urinary retention; impotence; reduced breast milk production and flow; enlarged pupils; eye sensitivity to light; increased eye pressure.

## Guidelines for Use:

- Take exactly as prescribed.
- Take 30 minutes before meals. Take mepenzolate with meals and at bedtime.
- If a dose is missed, take it as soon as possible. If several hours have passed or if it is nearing time for the next dose, do not double the dose to "catch up" (unless advised by your doctor). If more than one dose is missed or it is necessary to establish a new dosage schedule, contact your doctor or pharmacist.
- May cause drowsiness, dizziness or blurred vision. Use caution when driving or performing other tasks requiring mental alertness, coordination or physical dexterity.
- Notify your doctor if skin rash, flushing, rapid heartbeat, urinary retention, blurred vision or eye problems occur.
- May cause dry mouth, difficulty in urination or constipation, or increased sensitivity to light. Notify your doctor if these effects persist or become severe.
- If symptoms of fever, heatstroke and decreased sweating occur, discontinue the drug and contact a doctor immediately.
- Signs of overdosage with these drugs include: Headache, nausea, vomiting, dizziness, dry mouth, blurred vision, rapid heartbeat or loss of heart rhythm, dry skin, fever, difficulty in swallowing, excitation, tiredness, stupor, coma, respiratory depression and paralysis. Contact your doctor if these instances occur.
- Avoid alcohol and medicines (eg, tranquilizers, sedating antihistamines) that cause drowsiness.
- Sucking on hard sugarless candy, drinking fluids and maintaining good oral hygiene can relieve dry mouth.
- Inform your doctor if you are pregnant, become pregnant, are planning to become pregnant or are breastfeeding.
- Store at room temperature.

*If you have any questions, consult your doctor, pharmacist, or health care provider.*

| Generic Name<br>*Brand Name*<br>*Examples* | Anticholinergic | Sedative |
|---|---|---|
| *Rx* **Atropine-<br>containing<br>Combinations** | | |
| *Barbidonna No. 2*[1] | **Tablets:** 0.025 mg atropine sulfate, 0.0074 mg scopolamine HBr, 0.1286 mg hyoscyamine HBr or $SO_4$ | 32 mg pheno-barbital |
| *Barbidonna*[1] | | 16 mg pheno-barbital |
| *Donnatal* | **Tablets:** 0.0194 mg atropine sulfate, 0.0065 mg scopolamine HBr, 0.1037 mg hyoscyamine HBr or $SO_4$ | 16.2 mg phenobarbital |
| *Donnatal Extentabs* | **Tablets, sustained release:** 0.0582 mg atropine sulfate, 0.0195 mg scopolamine HBr, 0.3111 mg hyoscyamine sulfate | 48.6 mg phenobarbital |
| *Donnatal* | **Capsules:** 0.0194 mg atropine sulfate, 0.0065 mg scopolamine HBr, 0.1037 mg hyoscyamine HBr or $SO_4$ | 16.2 mg phenobarbital |
| *Donnatal*[2], *Hyosophen*[2], *Belladonna Alkaloids with Phenobarbital*[2] | **Elixir:** 0.0194 mg atropine sulfate, 0.0065 mg scopolamine HBr, 0.1037 mg hyoscyamine HBr or $SO_4$/5 mL | 16.2 mg phenobarbital/5 mL |

| | Generic Name<br>*Brand Name*<br>*Examples* | Anticholinergic | Sedative |
|---|---|---|---|
| *Rx* | **Belladonna-<br>containing<br>Combinations** | | |
| | *Butibel* | **Tablets:** 15 mg bella-<br>donna extract | 15 mg buta-<br>barbital<br>sodium |
| | *Chardonna-2* | **Tablets:** 15 mg bella-<br>donna extract | 15 mg pheno-<br>barbital |
| | *Bellergal-S*[3] | **Tablets, sustained<br>release:** 0.2 mg<br>l-alkaloids of bella-<br>donna | 40 mg pheno-<br>barbital |
| | *Butibel*[2] | **Elixir:** 15 mg bella-<br>donna extract/5 mL | 15 mg buta-<br>barbital<br>sodium/5 mL |
| *Rx* | **L-hyoscyamine-<br>containing<br>Combinations** | | |
| | *Levsin w/Pheno-<br>barbital* | **Tablets:** 0.125 mg<br>hyoscyamine sulfate | 15 mg pheno-<br>barbital |
| | *Levsin-PB Drops*[2] | **Elixir:** 0.125 mg hyo-<br>scyamine sulfate/mL | 15 mg pheno-<br>barbital/mL |
| *Rx* | **Clidinium<br>Bromide-<br>containing<br>Combinations** | | |
| | *Librax, Chlordiaze-<br>poxide and Clidin-<br>ium Bromide* | **Capsules:** 2.5 mg<br>clidinium bromide | 5 mg chlor-<br>diazepoxide<br>HCl |

[1] Contains lactose.
[2] Contains alcohol.
[3] Contains 0.6 mg ergotamine tartrate.

## Type of Drug:

Gastrointestinal anticholinergic combinations.

## Uses:

Combination anticholinergic preparations may include the following components:

*Antihistamines:* May be included for antihistaminic effects, sedative or anti-cholinergic side effects. For more information, see the Antihistamines monograph in the Respiratory Drugs chapter.

*Ergotamine tartrate:* Provides inhibition of the nervous system. For more information, see the Agents for Migraine-Migraine Combinations monograph in the CNS Drugs chapter.

*Kaolin:* Used for its adsorbent properties.

*Sedatives and antianxiety agents:* For more information, see the individual monographs in the CNS Drugs chapter.

---

### Guidelines for Use:

- Dosage is individualized. Take exactly as prescribed.
- Do not stop taking or change the dose unless directed by your doctor.
- Some agents must be taken 30 minutes before meals. Consult your doctor or pharmacist.
- May cause drowsiness. Use caution when driving or performing other tasks requiring alertness, coordination, or physical dexterity.
- Notify your doctor if you experience skin rash, flushing, or eye pain.
- May cause dry mouth, difficult urination, constipation, blurring of vision, headache, nausea, vomiting, dilated pupils, dry skin, dizziness, difficulty swallowing, or increased sensitivity to light. Notify your doctor if these effects persist or become severe.
- Barbiturates may be habit-forming; tolerance, psychological dependence, and physical dependence may occur following prolonged use of high doses.

---

*If you have any questions, consult your doctor, pharmacist, or health care provider.*

| Generic Name *Brand Name Example* | Supplied As | Generic Available |
|---|---|---|
| Rx **Doxycycline** | | |
| *Periostat* | **Tablets**: 20 mg (as hyclate) | No |

## Type of Drug:
Antibiotic; tetracycline.

## How the Drug Works:
Doxycycline reduced elevated collagenase activity in the gingival crevicular fluid of adult patients with periodontitis.

## Uses:
As an adjunct to tooth scaling and root planing to promote attachment level gain and to reduce pocket depth in patients with adult periodontitis.

## Precautions:
*Do not use in the following situations:*
   acutely abscessed periodontal pocket
   allergy to doxycycline or any of its ingredients
   breastfeeding
   infancy and childhood (up to 8 years of age)
   pregnancy

*Use with caution in the following situations:*
   esophageal or peptic ulcer disease, preexisting
   oral candidiasis, history of or predisposition to

*Tooth discoloration:* Use of a tetracycline during tooth development (last half of pregnancy, infancy, and childhood up to 8 years of age) may cause permanent discoloration of the teeth (yellow-gray-brown). This is more common during long-term use but has been observed following repeated short-term courses. Enamel hypoplasia has also been reported. Do not use a tetracycline in this age group or in pregnant or nursing mothers unless the potential benefits outweigh the possible risks.

*Superinfection:* Use of broad spectrum antibiotics (especially prolonged or repeated therapy) may result in bacterial or fungal overgrowth. Such overgrowth may lead to a second infection. The tetracycline may need to be stopped and another antibiotic may need to be prescribed for the second infection.

*Pseudotumor cerebri:* Tetracyclines have been associated with pseudotumor cerebri (benign intracranial hypertension). Early signs and symptoms include headache, nausea, vomiting, and blurred vision. If these symptoms develop, stop the drug immediately and contact your doctor.

*Cross resistance:* Antimicrobial activity of the tetracyclines is similar. Resistance to one tetracycline may mean resistance to most or all of the others.

*Pregnancy:* May cause harm when administered to a pregnant woman. Do not use during pregnancy. The risk of use in a pregnant woman clearly outweighs any possible benefit.

*Breastfeeding:* Tetracyclines are excreted in breast milk. Do not use while breastfeeding because of the potential for serious adverse effects in nursing infants.

*Children:* Tetracyclines should not be used in children under 8 years of age, unless other drugs are not likely to be effective or are not advised.

*Lab tests* may be required during long-term treatment with tetracyclines. Tests may include blood counts and liver and kidney function tests.

## Drug Interactions:

Tell your doctor or pharmacist if you are taking or if you are planning to take any over-the-counter or prescription medications or dietary supplements with doxycycline. Doses of one or both drugs may need to be modified or a different drug may need to be prescribed. The following drugs and drug classes interact with tetracyclines:

aluminum salts (eg, aluminum hydroxide)
anticoagulants (eg, warfarin)
barbiturates (eg, phenobarbital)
bismuth salts (eg, bismuth subsalicylate)
calcium salts (eg, calcium citrate)
carbamazepine (eg, *Tegretol*)
charcoal
contraceptives, oral (eg, *Ortho-Novum*)
digoxin (eg, *Lanoxin*)
iron salts (eg, ferrous fumarate)
magnesium salts (eg, magnesium hydroxide)
methoxyflurane (*Penthrane*)
penicillins (eg, amoxicillin)
phenytoin (eg, *Dilantin*)
rifampin (eg, *Rifadin*)
sodium bicarbonate
tricalcium phosphate (eg, *Posture*)
urinary alkalinizers (eg, sodium bicarbonate)
zinc salts (eg, zinc gluconate)

## Side Effects:

Every drug is capable of producing side effects. Many doxycycline users experience no, or minor, side effects. The frequency and severity of side effects depend on many factors including dose, duration of therapy, and individual susceptibility. Possible side effects include:

*Digestive Tract:* Acid indigestion; appetite loss; vomiting; diarrhea; nausea; mouth sores; sore throat; toothache; tooth disorder; swollen gums.

*Respiratory System:* Bronchitis; cough; sinus congestion; sinus headache; runny nose.

*Other:* Backache; common cold; flu-like symptoms; headache; infection; injury; joint or muscle pain; menstrual cramps; vaginal candidiasis; pain; rash; hives; sensitivity to light; anemia.

## Guidelines for Use:

- Dosage will be individualized. Take exactly as prescribed.
- Do not stop taking or change the dose unless directed by your doctor.
- Take 1 tablet 2 times daily at 12 hour intervals, preferably 1 hour before or 2 hours after a meal. Therapy lasts for up to 9 months.
- If a dose is missed, take it as soon as possible. If several hours have passed or it is nearing time for the next dose, do not double the dose to catch up, unless advised to do so by your doctor. If more than one dose is missed, or it is necessary to establish a new dosage schedule, contact your doctor or pharmacist.
- To prevent irritation or ulceration of the esophagus (food pipe), take with a full glass of water or other nondairy liquid. Do not lie down for at least 30 minutes after a dose.
- Do not use during pregnancy or breastfeeding.
- Do not use in children under 8 years of age unless other drugs are not likely to be effective or are inadvisable. Use during tooth development may cause permanent discoloration and inadequate hardening of baby and permanent teeth.
- Avoid use of tetracyclines with antacids, laxatives, alcohol, dairy products (eg, milk, cheese), or iron-containing products. If any of these products must be taken, take at least 2 hours before or after tetracyclines.
- May cause photosensitivity (sensitivity to sunlight). Avoid prolonged exposure to the sun and other sources of ultraviolet (UV) light (eg, tanning beds). Use sunscreens and wear protective clothing until tolerance is determined.
- Concurrent use of tetracyclines with oral contraceptives (eg, *Ortho-Novum*) may cause the oral contraceptives to be less effective. Discuss alternative contraceptive methods with your doctor.
- Notify your doctor if you experience skin redness, flushing, itching, or hives.
- *Do not use outdated tetracyclines.* Outdated tetracyclines may be highly toxic to the kidneys.
- Lab tests may be required to monitor therapy. Be sure to keep appointments.
- Store at controlled room temperature (59° to 86°F).

*If you have any questions, consult your doctor, pharmacist, or health care provider.*

| Generic Name<br>*Brand Name Examples* | Supplied As | Generic<br>Available |
|---|---|---|
| *Rx* **Ranitidine Bismuth Citrate** | | |
| *Tritec* | **Tablets:** 400 mg | No |

## Type of Drug:

*H. pylori* agent; anti-ulcer drug.

## How the Drug Works:

This drug, when combined with other drugs, acts as an anti-infective to help eliminate the bacteria that is responsible for many cases of peptic ulcer disease.

## Uses:

Used in combination with clarithromycin to treat active duodenal ulcers caused by *H. pylori* infection. Do not use ranitidine bismuth citrate alone.

## Precautions:

*Do not use in the following situations:*
  allergy to this medicine or its ingredients
  hangover

*Use with caution in the following situations:*
  kidney disease
  porphyria
  urine tests (may give false results)

*Clarithromycin therapy:* If *H. pylori* infection is not eradicated after ranitidine bismuth citrate and clarithromycin treatment, the infection may be resistant to clarithromycin. Any patients who do not respond to this therapy should not be retreated with a regimen containing clarithromycin.

*Darkening of the tongue:* The bismuth may cause a temporary and harmless darkening of the tongue or stool. Stool darkening should not be confused with blood in the stool.

*Pregnancy:* Adequate studies have not been done in pregnant women, or animal studies may have shown a risk to the fetus. Use only if clearly needed and potential benefits outweigh possible risks to the fetus.

*Breastfeeding:* It is not known if ranitidine bismuth citrate appears in breast milk. Consult your doctor before you begin breastfeeding.

*Children:* Safety and effectiveness in children have not been established.

## Drug Interactions:

Tell your doctor or pharmacist if you are taking or planning to take any over-the-counter or prescription medications or dietary supplements while taking this medicine. Doses of one or both drugs may need to be modified or a different drug may need to be prescribed. The following drugs and drug classes interact with this medicine:

> antacids
> aspirin

## Side Effects:

Every drug is capable of producing side effects. Many patients experience no, or minor, side effects. The frequency and severity of side effects depend on many factors including dose, duration of therapy and individual susceptibility. Possible side effects include:

*Digestive Tract:* Diarrhea; nausea; vomiting; constipation.

*Nervous System:* Headache; dizziness.

*Other:* Itching; gynecological problems; taste changes; sleep problems; chest pain.

---

### Guidelines for Use:

- The usual dose of ranitidine bismuth citrate is 400 mg twice a day for 4 weeks in conjunction with clarithromycin 500 mg three times a day for the first 2 weeks.
- Both ranitidine bismuth citrate and clarithromycin may be taken without regard to food.
- If a dose is missed, take it as soon as possible. If several hours have passed or if it is nearing time for the next dose, do not double the dose in order to "catch up" (unless advised to do so by your doctor). If more than one dose is missed or it is necessary to establish a new dosage schedule, contact your doctor or pharmacist. Use exactly as prescribed.
- The bismuth may cause a temporary and harmLess darkening of the tongue or stool. Stool darkening should not be confused with blood in the stool.
- May cause dizziness. Use caution while driving or performing other tasks which require alertness, coordination or physical dexterity.
- Avoid alcohol, aspirin and NSAIDS (eg, ibuprofen) while taking this medicine.
- Store at room temperature or in the refrigerator (36° to 86°F). Protect from moisture and light.

---

*If you have any questions, consult your doctor, pharmacist, or health care provider.*

| Generic Name Brand Name Examples | Supplied As | Generic Available |
|---|---|---|
| Rx **Bismuth Subsalicylate/ Metronidazole/Tetra- cycline HCl** | | |
| *Helidac* | **Tablets:** 262.4 mg bismuth subsalicylate | No |
| | **Tablets:** 250 mg metronidazole | |
| | **Capsules:** 500 mg tetracycline HCl | |

## Type of Drug:
*H. pylori* agents; anti-ulcer drug.

## How the Drug Works:
The three drugs used in this combination treatment are used to eliminate the *H. pylori* bacteria known to cause certain kinds of ulcers.

## Uses:
Used in combination with an $H_2$ antagonist to treat active duodenal ulcers cause by *H. pylori* infection.

## Precautions:
*Do not use in the following situations:*

allergy to bismuth subsalicylate, metronidizole or other nitroim- idazole derivatives, any of the tetracyclines, aspirin or salicy- lates

breastfeeding
children
kidney disease
liver disease
pregnancy

*Use with caution in the following situations:*

blood disorders
blurred vision
candidiasis infection

headache
nervous system diseases

*Dark tongue/stools:* The bismuth may cause a temporary and harmLess darkening of the tongue and stool. Stool darkening should not be con- fused with blood in the stool.

*Children (over 8) and teenagers* who have or who are recovering from chicken pox or flu should not use this medicine to treat nausea and vomiting. If nausea and vomiting are present, contact your doctor because this could be an early sign of Reye syndrome.

*Superinfection:* Use of antibiotics (especially prolonged or repeated therapy) may result in bacterial or fungal overgrowth. Such overgrowth may lead to a second infection. This medicine may need to be stopped and another antibiotic may need to be prescribed for the second infection.

*Photosensitivity:* May cause photosensitivity (risk of sunburn). Avoid prolonged exposure to the sun or other forms of ultraviolet (UV) light (eg, tanning beds). Use sunscreens and wear protective clothing until tolerance is determined.

*Pregnancy:* Do not use this combination during pregnancy.

*Breastfeeding:* Metronidazole and tetracycline appear in breast milk. Do not breastfeed while taking this medicine. Consult your doctor.

*Children:* Do not use this medicine in children under 8 years of age. Tetracycline may cause discoloration and damage to developing teeth. Safety and effectiveness in children with *H. Pylori* have not been established.

*Elderly:* Use with caution in elderly patients because of potential kidney and liver dysfunction.

## Drug Interactions:

Tell your doctor or pharmacist if you are taking or planning to take any over-the-counter or prescription medications or dietary supplements while taking this medicine. Doses of one or both may need to be modified or another drug may need to be prescribed. See the individual Bismuth Subsalicylate monograph in this chapter, and the Metronidazole and Tetracyclines monographs in the Anti-Infectives chapter for further information.

## Side Effects:

Every drug is capable of producing side effects. Many patients experience no, or minor, side effects. The frequency and severity of side effects depend on many factors including dose, duration of therapy and individual susceptibility. Possible side effects include:

*Digestive Tract:* Diarrhea; nausea; vomiting; stomach pain; dark bloody stools; anal discomfort; appetite loss; constipation.

*Nervous System:* Dizziness; abnormal skin sensations; weakness; sleeplessness; pain.

## Guidelines for Use:

- Use exactly as prescribed.
- Each dose contains four pills: two pink round chewable tablets (bismuth subsalicylate), one white tablet (metronidazole) and one pale orange and white capsule (tetracycline). Take each dose four times a day with meals and at bedtime. Chew and swallow the bismuth subsalicylate (pink) tablets, and swallow the metronidazole (white) tablets and tetracycline (pale orange and white) capsules whole with a full glass of water (8 ounces). Do not take with milk or other dairy products.
- Drink adequate amounts of fluid, especially with the bedtime tetracycline dose to reduce the risk of irritation and ulceration of the esophagus.
- If a dose is missed, continue the normal dosing schedule until the medication is gone. Do not double the dose in order to "catch up." If more than four doses are missed, contact your doctor or pharmacist.
- This treatment includes salicylates. If ringing in the ears occurs while taking with aspirin, consult your doctor about stopping the aspirin therapy until treatment is completed.
- Using tetracyclines may render oral contraceptives less effective. Use a different or additional form of contraception. Breakthrough bleeding has been reported.
- Inform your doctor if you are pregnant, become pregnant, are planning to become pregnant or if you are breastfeeding.
- Avoid alcohol while taking metronidazole and for one day afterward.
- This medication may cause dizziness. Use caution while driving or performing other tasks requiring alertness, coordination or physical dexterity.
- May cause photosensitivity (sensitivity to sunlight). Avoid prolonged exposure to the sun or other forms of ultraviolet light (eg, tanning beds). Use sunscreens and wear protective clothing until tolerance is determined.
- Bismuth subsalicylate may cause temporary and harmLess darkening of the tongue and stool. Stool darkening should not be confused with blood in the stool.
- Store at room temperature.

*If you have any questions, consult your doctor, pharmacist, or health care provider.*

| Generic Name Brand Name Examples | Supplied As | Generic Available |
|---|---|---|
| Rx **Lansoprazole/Amoxicillin/ Clarithromycin** | | |
| *Prevpac* | **Capsules and Tablets**: 30 mg[1]/500 mg[2]/500 mg[3] | No |

[1] Lansoprazole (contains sucrose).
[2] Amoxicillin.
[3] Clarithromycin (contains povidone).

## Type of Drug:

A combination of drugs used to reduce the risk of duodenal (stomach/ intestinal) ulcer recurrence caused by infection with *H. pylori*.

## How the Drug Works:

Lansoprazole reduces gastric (stomach) acid secretion by blocking the final step of gastric acid production. Amoxicillin kills bacteria by preventing the production of the bacterial cell wall. Clarithromycin suppresses the formation of vital proteins by bacteria, slowing bacterial growth.

## Uses:

For the treatment of *H. pylori* infection and duodenal (stomach/intestinal) ulcers (active or 1-year history of a duodenal ulcer) to eradicate *H. pylori* and prevent ulcer recurrence.

## Precautions:

*Do not use in the following situations:*

allergy to any ingredients
astemizole (*Hismanal* therapy)
cisapride (*Propulsid* therapy)
macrolide antibiotic allergy
 (eg, erythromycin)
penicillin allergy (eg, ampicillin)
pimozide (*Orap* therapy)

*Use with caution in the following situations:*

kidney impairment, severe
pregnancy (clarithromycin)

*Diarrhea:* If diarrhea develops during lansoprazole/amoxicillin/clarithro-mycin use, pseudomembranous colitis must be considered. This inflammatory condition of the colon is due to overgrowth of bacteria that are not killed by lansoprazole/amoxicillin/clarithromycin. The primary cause is a toxin produced by a bacteria known as *Clostridia difficile*. Coli-tis symptoms may range in severity from mild to life-threatening. Mild cases usually respond by stopping the antibiotic. In more severe cases, other antibiotics may need to be used.

*Pregnancy:* Adequate studies have not been done in pregnant women. Use only if clearly needed and potential benefits outweigh the possible haz-ards to the fetus.

*Breastfeeding:* Amoxicillin appears in breast milk. Because of the poten-tial for serious adverse effects, decide whether to discontinue nursing or discontinue the drug. Consult your doctor.

*Children:* Safety and effectiveness in children have not been established.

## Drug Interactions:

Tell your doctor or pharmacist if you are taking or if you are planning to take any over-the-counter or prescription medications or dietary supplements while taking this medicine. Doses of one or both drugs may need to be modified or a different drug may need to be prescribed. The following drugs and drug classes interact with this medicine.

*amoxicillin only –*

allopurinol (eg, *Zyloprim*)
contraceptives, oral (eg, *Ortho-Novum, Ovral*)
probenecid (*Benemid*)
tetracyclines (eg, tetracycline HCl)

*clarithromycin only –*

anticoagulants, oral (eg, warfarin)
astemizole (*Hismanal*)
benzodiazepines (eg, alprazolam, diazepam, midazolam, triazolam)
buspirone (*Buspar*)
cisapride (*Propulsid*)
cyclosporine (eg, *Neoral, Sandimmune*)
dihydroergotamine or ergotamine (eg, *Ergomar*)
disopyramide (*Norpace*)
fluconazole (*Diflucan*)
HMG-CoA reductase inhibitors (eg, atorvastatin, fluvastatin, simvastatin)
pimozide (*Orap*)
rifabutin (*Mycobutin*)
rifampin (*Rifadin, Rimactane*)
tacrolimus (*Prograf*)

*lansoprazole only –*

ampicillin (eg, *Omnipen*)
cyanocobalamin (eg, *Crystamine*)
drugs metabolized by the cytochrome P 450 system
    (eg, diazepam, ibuprofen, indomethacin, phenytoin, prednisone, propanolol)
iron salts
ketoconazole (*Nizoral*)
sucralfate (*Carafate*)

*lansoprazole and clarithromycin only –*

carbamazepine (eg, *Tegretol*)
digoxin (eg, *Lanoxin*)
theophylline (eg, *Theo-Dur*)

## Side Effects:

Every drug is capable of producing side effects. Many patients experience no, or minor, side effects. The frequency and severity of side effects depend on many factors including dose, duration of therapy, and individual susceptibility. Possible side effects include:

*Digestive Tract:* Diarrhea; taste changes; nausea; dark stools; sore tongue; mouth sores; tongue discoloration; dry mouth; thirst; indigestion; stomach pain or irritation; vomiting; rectal itching.

*Urinary and Reproductive Tract:* Vaginal inflammation; vaginal infection.

*Nervous System:* Headache; confusion; dizziness.

*Other:* Muscle pain; itching; rash; hives.

---

## Guidelines for Use:

- Take exactly as prescribed.
- Each medication packet contains enough medication for 2 doses.
- Usual adult dose is 30 mg lansoprazole (1 pink and black capsule), 1 g amoxicillin (2 maroon and light pink capsules), and 500 mg clarithromycin (1 yellow tablet) taken together twice daily before eating (morning and evening) for 14 days. Swallow each pill whole.
- Failure to complete full course of therapy may allow the infection to return.
- If a dose is missed, take it as soon as possible. If several hours have passed or if it is nearing time for the next dose, do not double the dose in order to catch up unless advised to do so by your doctor. If more than 1 dose is missed, or if it is necessary to establish a new dosage schedule, contact your doctor or pharmacist.
- Discontinue therapy immediately and contact your doctor if any of the following occurs: Rash; hives; difficulty breathing; swelling of the eyelids, face, tongue, or lips.
- Notify your doctor if diarrhea develops while taking this medicine or shortly after completing therapy.
- This product contains a penicillin. Tell your doctor if you have a penicillin allergy.
- Decreased dosage or dosing intervals of clarithromycin may be necessary for patients with severe kidney impairment and will be determined by your doctor.
- Store at controlled room temperature (59° to 86°F). Protect from light and moisture.

---

*If you have any questions, consult your doctor, pharmacist, or health care provider.*

| Generic Name<br>*Brand Name Examples* | Supplied As | Generic<br>Available |
|---|---|---|
| **Cimetidine**[1] | | |
| *otc Tagamet HB 200* | **Tablets**: 200 mg | Yes |
| *Rx Tagamet* | **Tablets**: 200 mg, 300 mg,<br>400 mg, 800 mg | Yes |
| *otc Tagamet HB 200* | **Suspension**: 200 mg/20 mL | No |
| *Rx Tagamet* | **Liquid**: 300 mg/5 mL | Yes |
| **Famotidine**[1] | | |
| *otc Pepcid AC* | **Tablets**: 10 mg | Yes |
| *Rx Pepcid* | **Tablets**: 20 mg, 40 mg | Yes |
| *otc Pepcid AC*[2] | **Tablets, chewable**: 10 mg | No |
| *Rx Pepcid RPD*[2] | **Tablets, orally disintegrating**:<br>20 mg, 40 mg | No |
| *otc Pepcid AC* | **Gelcaps**: 10 mg | Yes |
| *Rx Pepcid* | **Powder for oral suspension**:<br>40 mg/5 mL | No |
| **Nizatidine** | | |
| *Rx Axid Pulvules* | **Capsules**: 150 mg, 300 mg | No |
| *otc Axid AR* | **Tablets**: 75 mg | No |
| **Ranitidine**[1] | **Capsules**: 150 mg, 300 mg | Yes |
| *otc Zantac 75* | **Tablets**: 75 mg | Yes |
| *Rx Zantac 150* | **Tablets**: 150 mg | Yes |
| *Rx Zantac 300* | **Tablets**: 300 mg | Yes |
| *Rx Zantac 150 EFFERdose*[2] | **Tablets, effervescent**: 150 mg | No |
| *Rx Zantac 150 EFFERdose*[2] | **Granules, effervescent**:<br>150 mg | No |
| *Rx Zantac* | **Syrup**: 15 mg/mL | Yes |
| *otc* **Famotidine/Calcium<br>Carbonate/Magnesium<br>Hydroxide** | | |
| *Pepcid Complete* | **Tablets, chewable**: 10 mg<br>famotidine/800 mg calcium<br>carbonate/165 mg magnesium<br>hydroxide | No |

[1] This product is also available as an injection.
[2] Contains phenylalanine.

## Type of Drug:

Anti-ulcer drugs.

## How the Drug Works:

Histamine H$_2$ antagonists reduce acid in the stomach by blocking one of the chemical transmitters (histamine) that is responsible for stimulating the production of stomach acid.

## Uses:

To treat and prevent recurrence of duodenal (first part of small intestine) ulcers.

To treat gastric (stomach) ulcers.

To prevent recurrence of gastric (stomach) ulcers (ranitidine only).

To treat hypersecretory (increased acid secretion) conditions (eg, Zollinger-Ellison syndrome).

To treat erosive gastroesophageal reflux disease (GERD) (reflux of stomach acid into the food pipe, which causes heartburn).

To treat (over-the-counter cimetidine, famotidine, and nizatidine only) or prevent (over-the-counter cimetidine, famotidine, and nizatidine only) heartburn, acid indigestion, or sour stomach.

*Unlabeled Use(s):* Occasionally doctors may prescribe:

*Cimetidine* – To prevent stress-induced or peptic ulcers and certain types of respiratory complications (aspiration pneumonia) during anesthesia. It may be used to treat hyperparathyroidism (overactive parathyroid gland), indigestion, ringworm, herpes virus infections, chronic warts, chronic hives, allergic skin reactions, acetaminophen overdose, colorectal cancer, and abnormal hair growth in women.

*Famotidine* – To prevent stress-induced or peptic ulcers and certain types of respiratory conditions (aspiration pneumonia) during anesthesia. It may also be used to treat bleeding of the stomach or intestines.

*Nizatidine* – To treat peptic ulcers.

*Ranitidine* – To prevent stomach and intestinal damage associated with long-term nonsteroidal anti-inflammatory drug therapy (eg, ibuprofen), stress-induced or peptic ulcers, certain types of respiratory complications (aspiration pneumonia) during anesthesia, and to treat bleeding of the stomach or intestines.

## Precautions:

*Do not use in the following situations:* Allergy to the histamine H$_2$ antagonist or any of its ingredients.

*Use with caution in the following situations:*

| | |
|---|---|
| immunocompromised patients | liver disease |
| kidney disease | porphyria, acute (ranitidine only) |

*Phenylketonuric patients:* Some of these products contain phenylalanine. Consult your doctor or pharmacist.

*Pregnancy:* There are no adequate and well-controlled studies in pregnant women. Use only if clearly needed and the potential benefits to the mother outweigh the possible hazards to the fetus.

*Breastfeeding:* Cimetidine, famotidine, nizatidine, and ranitidine appear in breast milk. Consult your doctor before you begin breastfeeding.

*Children:* Safety and effectiveness of nizatidine in children have not been established. Safety and effectiveness of famotidine in children under 1 year of age and of ranitidine in children under 1 month of age have not been established. Cimetidine use is not usually recommended in children less than 16 years of age. Over-the-counter cimetidine, famotidine, nizatidine, or ranitidine use is not recommended in children under 12 years of age.

*Elderly:* Safety and effectiveness are similar to younger patients. Elderly patients may have reduced kidney function. Smaller cimetidine doses may be prescribed.

*Lab tests* may be required to monitor therapy. Tests may include liver function tests.

## Drug Interactions:

Tell your doctor or pharmacist if you are taking or if you are planning to take any over-the-counter or prescription medications or dietary supplements while taking histamine H$_2$ antagonists. Doses of one or both drugs may need to be modified or a different drug may need to be prescribed. The following drugs and drug classes interact with histamine H$_2$ antagonists:

*cimetidine only –*

aminoquinolones (eg, chloroquine)
anticoagulants, oral (eg, warfarin)
beta-blockers (eg, propranolol)
benzodiazepines (except lorazepam, oxazepam, temazepam)
carbamazepine (eg, *Tegretol*)
carmustine (*BiCNU*)
dofetilide (*Tikosyn*)
hydantoins (eg, phenytoin)
ketoconazole (eg, *Nizoral*)
lidocaine (eg, *Xylocaine*)
metformin (eg, *Glucophage*)
moricizine (*Ethmozine*)
nifedipine (eg, *Procardia*)
pentoxifylline (*Trental*)
praziquantel (*Biltricide*)
procainamide (eg, *Pronestyl*)
quinidine (eg, *Quinora*)
theophylllines (eg, aminophylline)
tricyclic antidepressants (eg, amitriptyline)

*famotidine and ranitidine only –*

ketoconazole (eg, *Nizoral*)

*nizatidine only –*

charcoal
ketoconazole (eg, *Nizoral*)
ketoprofen (eg, *Orudis*)

## Side Effects:

Every drug is capable of producing side effects. Many histamine H$_2$ antagonist users experience no, or minor, side effects. The frequency and severity of side effects depend on many factors including dose, duration of therapy, and individual susceptibility. Possible side effects include:

*Digestive Tract:* Diarrhea; constipation; stomach pain.

*Nervous System:* Confusion; hallucinations; fatigue; dizziness; sleepiness; headache.

*Other:* Impotence; breast enlargement (males).

## Guidelines for Use:

- Dosage is individualized. Take exactly as prescribed or as directed by the package label.
- Do not stop taking or change the dose, unless directed by your doctor.
- May be taken without regard to meals.
- If a dose is missed, take it as soon as possible. If several hours have passed or it is nearing time for the next dose, do not double the dose to catch up, unless advised to do so by your doctor. If more than one dose is missed or it is necessary to establish a new dosage schedule, contact your doctor or pharmacist.
- It may be necessary to make lifestyle changes to assist in the treatment and prevention of ulcers and other digestive problems. These changes may include stress-reduction programs, exercise, and dietary changes.
- Notify your doctor if you experience diarrhea, dizziness, confusion, anxiety, depression, disorientation, agitation, or hallucinations.
- Notify your doctor if you experience any symptoms that suggest a bleeding ulcer, such as black, tarry stools or "coffee-ground" vomit.
- Antacids can be used at the same time to help control acid symptoms. Stagger doses of antacids and cimetidine or ranitidine.
- May cause dizziness or drowsiness. Use caution while driving or performing other tasks requiring alertness, coordination, or physical dexterity.
- *Over-the-counter products* — Contact your doctor if you have trouble swallowing or persistent stomach pain. Do not take maximum daily dosage for more than 2 weeks continuously except under the advice and supervision of your doctor.
- *Famotidine suspension* — Shake well before using. Do not freeze. Discard unused suspension after 30 days.
- *Famotidine orally disintegrating tablets* — Keep tablets in unopened package until time of use. Open tablet blister pack with dry hands and place tablet on tongue to dissolve and be swallowed with saliva. No water is needed for taking the tablet.
- *Pepcid Complete* — Do not swallow tablets whole; chew completely before swallowing.
- *Ranitidine effervescent tablets or granules* — Dissolve in 6 to 8 oz of water before drinking.
- Inform your doctor if you are pregnant, become pregnant, are planning to become pregnant, or are breastfeeding.
- Lab tests or exams may be required to monitor therapy. Be sure to keep appointments.
- Store at room temperature in a tight container away from light.

*If you have any questions, consult your doctor, pharmacist, or health care provider.*

| Generic Name<br>*Brand Name Example* | Supplied As | Generic<br>Available |
|---|---|---|
| *Rx* **Misoprostol** | | |
| *Cytotec* | **Tablets**: 100 mcg, 200 mcg | No |

## Type of Drug:

Anti-ulcer drug; prostaglandin.

## How the Drug Works:

Misoprostol reduces the amount of acid secreted by the stomach. It also helps to protect the stomach lining.

## Uses:

To prevent formation of stomach ulcers in patients who are taking nonsteroidal anti-inflammatory drugs (NSAIDs), including aspirin. For high-risk individuals taking NSAIDs who are at greater risk for developing ulcers or who are at greater risk for complications from ulcers (eg, elderly, patients with a history of ulcers, patients with other debilitating diseases).

*Unlabeled Use(s):* Occasionally doctors may prescribe misoprostol to treat duodenal ulcers or to reduce the risk of organ rejection in kidney transplants.

## Precautions:

*Do not use in the following situations:*
     allergy to misoprostol or any of its ingredients
     allergy to prostaglandins
     pregnancy

*Use with caution in the following situations:*
     kidney disease
     women of childbearing age

*Diarrhea:* Usually develops early in the course of therapy and resolves after approximately 8 days. Discontinuation may be required.

*Pregnancy:* Do not use during pregnancy. The risk of use in a pregnant woman clearly outweighs any possible benefit. Women of childbearing potential should not receive the drug unless the patient requires NSAIDs and is at high risk of complications from stomach ulcers associated with the use of NSAIDs, or is at high risk of developing stomach ulceration. Such patients may use misoprostol if the following criteria are met:

- The patient is capable of complying with effective contraceptive measures.
- The patient has received both oral and written warnings of the hazards of misoprostol, the risk of possible contraception failure, and the danger to other women of childbearing potential should the drug be taken by mistake.
- The patient has a negative serum pregnancy test within 2 weeks prior to beginning therapy.
- The patient will begin therapy only on the second or third day of the next normal menstrual period.

*Breastfeeding:* It is unlikely that misoprostol is excreted in breast milk. It is not known if active metabolites are excreted in breast milk. Do not use while breastfeeding; the drug may cause significant diarrhea in nursing infants.

*Children:* Safety and effectiveness in children under 18 years of age have not been established.

## Drug Interactions:

Tell your doctor or pharmacist if you are taking or if you are planning to take any over-the-counter or prescription medications or dietary supplements with misoprostol. Doses of one or both drugs may need to be modified or a different drug may need to be prescribed. Antacids interact with misoprostol.

## Side Effects:

Every drug is capable of producing side effects. Many misoprostol users experience no, or minor, side effects. The frequency and severity of side effects depend on many factors including dose, duration of therapy and individual susceptibility. Possible side effects include:

*Digestive Tract:* Diarrhea; nausea; vomiting; constipation; abdominal pain; gas; indigestion.

*Other:* Menstrual irregularities; painful menstruation; vaginal bleeding or spotting; headache.

---

### Guidelines for Use:

- Take misoprostol for the duration of NSAID therapy.
- Contraceptive measures (birth control) are recommended during therapy.
- If a dose is missed, take it as soon as possible. If several hours have passed or if it is nearing time for the next dose, do not double the dose in order to "catch up" (unless advised to do so by your doctor). If more than one dose is missed, or it is necessary to establish a new dosage schedule, contact your doctor or pharmacist. Use exactly as prescribed.
- Diarrhea may occur early in the course of therapy. It may be minimized by taking after meals and at bedtime.
- Discontinue the drug and notify your doctor immediately if pregnancy is suspected. Misoprostol produces contractions of the uterus that may cause a miscarriage (see Precautions).
- Avoid magnesium-containing antacids.
- Never give your misoprostol tablets to anyone else.

---

*If you have any questions, consult your doctor, pharmacist, or health care provider.*

| Generic Name<br>*Brand Name Example* | Supplied As | Generic<br>Available |
|---|---|---|
| *Rx* **Sucralfate** | | |
| *Carafate* | **Tablets:** 1 g | No |
| *Carafate* | **Suspension:** 1 g/10 mL | No |

## Type of Drug:

Anti-ulcer drug.

## How the Drug Works:

Sucralfate helps ulcers heal by forming a protective layer on the ulcer to serve as a barrier against acid, bile salts and enzymes present in the stomach and duodenum.

## Uses:

For short-term treatment (up to 8 weeks) of duodenal ulcers.

For maintenance therapy for duodenal ulcer patients at reduced dosage after healing of acute ulcers.

*Unlabeled Use(s):* Occasionally doctors may prescribe sucralfate for oral and esophageal ulcers caused by chemotherapy or radiation, drug-induced digestive tract irritation, prevention of stress ulcers, long-term treatment of gastric (stomach) ulcers or inflammation of the esophagus. Sucralfate has also been shown to speed the healing of gastric ulcers.

## Precautions:

*Use with caution in the following situations:*
> dialysis
> kidney disease

*Pregnancy:* Adequate studies have not been done in pregnant women. Use only if clearly needed and potential benefits outweigh the possible hazards to the fetus.

*Breastfeeding:* It is not known if sucralfate appears in breast milk. Consult your doctor before you begin breastfeeding.

*Children:* Safety and effectiveness in children have not been established.

## Drug Interactions:

Tell your doctor or pharmacist if you are taking or if you are planning to take any over-the-counter or prescription medications or dietary supplements with sucralfate. Doses of one or both drugs may need to be modified or a different drug may need to be prescribed. The following drugs and drug classes interact with sucralfate.

antacids (aluminum-containing)
cimetidine (eg, *Tagamet*)
ciprofloxacin (eg, *Cipro*)
digoxin (eg, *Lanoxin*)
ketoconazole (eg, *Nizoral*)
norfloxacin (eg, *Noroxin*)

penicillamine (eg, *Cuprimine)*
phenytoin (eg, *Dilantin*)
rantidine (eg, *Zantac)*
tetracycline (eg, *Sumycin*)
theophylline (eg, *Theolair*)
warfarin (eg, *Coumadin*)

## Side Effects:

Every drug is capable of producing side effects. Many sucralfate users experience no, or minor, side effects. The frequency and severity of side effects depend on many factors including dose, duration of therapy and individual susceptibility. Possible side effects include:

*Other:* Red or black stools; coughing up or vomiting bright red or "coffee ground-like" material.

*Digestive Tract:* Constipation; diarrhea; nausea; stomach discomfort; indigestion.

*Skin:* Rash; itching; hives.

*Other:* Dry mouth; back pain; dizziness; sleepiness; facial swelling; difficulty breathing.

---

## Guidelines for Use:

- Take on an empty stomach at least 1 hour before meals and at bedtime.
- Do not take antacids 30 minutes before or after taking sucralfate.
- If a dose is missed, take it as soon as possible. If several hours have passed or if it is nearing time for the next dose, do not double the dose in order to "catch up" (unless advised to do so by your doctor). If more than one dose is missed, or it is necessary to establish a new dosage schedule, contact your doctor or pharmacist. Use exactly as prescribed.
- If red or black stools, coughing up or vomiting bright red or "coffee ground-like" material occur, contact your doctor.
- Duodenal ulcer is a chronic recurrent disease. While a single course of therapy of 4 to 8 weeks may completely heal the ulcer, ulcers may occur again and may be more severe.
- *Suspension* — Shake well before using.

---

*If you have any questions, consult your doctor, pharmacist, or health care provider.*

| Generic Name<br>*Brand Name Examples* | Supplied As | Generic<br>Available |
|---|---|---|
| *otc* **Charcoal** | | |
| *Charcoal* | **Tablets:** 325 mg | No |
| *Charcoal* | **Capsules:** 260 mg | No |
| *CharcoCaps* | **Capsules:** 260 mg activated charcoal | No |
| *otc* **Simethicone** | | |
| *Phazyme, Phazyme 95* | **Tablets:** 60 mg, 95 mg | No |
| *Extra Strength Gas-X, Gas-X, Mylicon, Mylicon-125* | **Tablets, chewable:** 40 mg, 80 mg, 125 mg | No |
| *Phazyme 125* | **Capsules:** 125 mg | No |
| *Flatulex, Mylicon, Phazyme* | **Drops:** 40 mg/0.6 mL | Yes |

## Type of Drug:

Anti-gas agents.

## How the Drug Works:

"Flatulence" refers to excessive amounts of air or gases in the stomach or intestines that result in abdominal discomfort (eg, pain, fullness, bloating). The air or gases are trapped in small bubbles. Simethicone relieves discomfort due to flatulence by helping the formation of larger gas bubbles which are easier to eliminate by belching or passing rectally.

Excessive air and gases that can accumulate in the stomach or intestines will bind to charcoal. As the charcoal is eliminated from the body, the air and gases are also eliminated, resulting in relief.

Other substances that bind to charcoal include certain poisons, drugs and naturally occurring substances. By binding to charcoal, absorption of these substances into the bloodstream is reduced. This can be an advantage in the treatment of poisonings but a disadvantage when it interferes with the effects of a drug.

## Uses:

*Charcoal:* For relief of intestinal gas, diarrhea and intestinal distress associated with indigestion.

For prevention of itching associated with kidney dialysis treatment and intestinal motility testing.

To treat certain poisonings and drug overdoses by decreasing absorption into the bloodstream and speeding up removal of the poisons and drugs from the body.

*Simethicone:* To relieve abdominal discomfort due to excess air or gases in the stomach, intestines or both. Conditions where antiflatulents may be helpful include: Surgery, peptic ulcer, air swallowing, spastic or irritable bowel, acid indigestion and diverticulitis.

## Precautions:

*Children:* Do not use charcoal in children under 3 years of age.

## Drug Interactions:

Tell your doctor or pharmacist if you are taking or if you are planning to take any over-the-counter or prescription medications or dietary supplements with charcoal. Doses of one or both drugs may need to be modified or a different drug may need to be prescribed. The following drugs and drug classes interact with charcoal.

acetaminophen (eg, *Tylenol)*
barbiturates (eg, phenobarbital)
carbamazepine (eg, *Tegretol)*
digitoxin (eg, *Crystodigin)*
digoxin (eg, *Lanoxin)*
furosemide (eg, *Lasix)*
glutethimide
hydantoins (eg, phenytoin)
methotrexate (eg, *Rheumatrex)*
nizatidine (*Axid)*
phenothiazines (eg, chlorpromazine)

propoxyphene (eg, *Darvon)*
salicylates (eg, aspirin)
sulfonamides (eg, sulfisoxazole)
sulfones
sulfonylureas (eg, glipizide)
tetracyclines (eg, doxycycline)
theophyllines (eg, aminophylline)
tricyclic antidepressants
(eg, amitriptyline)
valproic acid (eg, *Depakene)*

## Guidelines for Use:

*Charcoal:*

- Take either 2 hours before or 1 hour after taking other oral drugs, because many drugs bind to charcoal in the stomach or intestines and never reach the bloodstream.
- Swallow 2 tablets whole after eating, as needed. Do not chew. Do not exceed 20 tablets per day.
- Stool will turn black. This is normal.

*Simethicone:*

- Take 1 to 2 tablets as needed after each meal and at bedtime. Do not exceed 4 tablets in 24 hours unless directed by your doctor.
- *Gas-X* — Do not exceed 6 tablets in 24 hours.
- *Phazyme* — Do not exceed 3 softgels per day.
- Swallow softgels whole with water.
- Drops — Shake well before using.
- Chewable tablets — Chew thoroughly before swallowing.
- Store at room temperature. Protect from moisture. Keep out of reach of children.

*If you have any questions, consult your doctor, pharmacist, or health care provider.*

| | Generic Name<br>*Brand Name Examples* | Lipase<br>(units) | Protease<br>(units) | Amylase<br>(units) |
|---|---|---|---|---|
| *Rx* | *Ku-Zyme Capsules[1]* | 1200 | 15,000 | 15,000 |
| *Rx* | *Kutrase Capsules[1]* | 2400 | 30,000 | 30,000 |
| *Rx* | *Pancrease MT 4 Capsules[1]* | 4000 | 12,000 | 12,000 |
| *Rx* | *Pancrecarb MS-4 Delayed-Release Capsules[1]* | 4000 | 25,000 | 25,000 |
| *Rx* | *Lipram 4500 Delayed-Release Capsules,[1] Pancrease Capsules,[1] Pangestyme EC Capsules,[1] Ultrase Capsules[1]* | 4500 | 25,000 | 20,000 |
| *otc* | *Hi-Vegi-Lip Tablets* | 4800 | 60,000 | 60,000 |
| *Rx* | *Creon 5 Delayed-Release Capsules[1]* | 5000 | 18,750 | 16,600 |
| *Rx* | *Lipram-CR5 Delayed-Release Capsules[1]* | 5000 | 18,750 | 16,600 |
| *Rx* | *Ku-Zyme HP Capsules,[1] Plaretase 8000 Tablets,[1] Viokase 8 Tablets[1]* | 8000 | 30,000 | 30,000 |
| *Rx* | *Pancrecarb MS-8 Delayed-Release Capsules[1]* | 8000 | 45,000 | 40,000 |
| *Rx* | *Lipram-PN10 Delayed-Release Capsules,[1] Pancrease MT 10 Capsules[1]* | 10,000 | 30,000 | 30,000 |
| *Rx* | *Creon 10 Delayed-Release Capsules,[1] Lipram-CR10 Delayed-Release Capsules,[1] Pangestyme CN-10 Delayed-Release Capsules[1]* | 10,000 | 37,500 | 33,200 |
| *Rx* | *Lipram-UL12 Delayed-Release Capsules,[1] Pangestyme UL12 Capsules,[1] Ultrase MT12 Capsules[1]* | 12,000 | 39,000 | 39,000 |
| *Rx* | *Lipram-PN16 Delayed-Release Capsules,[1] Pancrease MT 16 Capsules,[1] Pangestyme MT16 Capsules[1]* | 16,000 | 48,000 | 48,000 |

| Generic Name<br>*Brand Name Examples* | Lipase<br>(units) | Protease<br>(units) | Amylase<br>(units) |
|---|---|---|---|
| *Rx*   *Panokase 16 Tablets,[1]*<br>*Viokase 16 Tablets[1]* | 16,000 | 60,000 | 60,000 |
| *Rx*   *Viokase Powder[1,2]* | 16,8000 | 70,000 | 70,000 |
| *Rx*   *Lipram-UL18 Delayed-*<br>*Release Capsules,[1]*<br>*Pangestyme UL18*<br>*Capsules,[1] Ultrase MT18*<br>*Capsules[1]* | 18,000 | 58,500 | 58,500 |
| *Rx*   *Lipram-PN20 Delayed-*<br>*Release Capsules,[1]*<br>*Pancrease MT 20 Capsules[1]* | 20,000 | 44,000 | 56,000 |
| *Rx*   *Lipram-UL20 Delayed-*<br>*Release Capsules,[1]*<br>*Pangestyme UL20*<br>*Capsules,[1] Ultrase MT20*<br>*Capsules[1]* | 20,000 | 65,000 | 65,000 |
| *Rx*   *Creon 20 Delayed-Release*<br>*Capsules,[1] Lipram-CR20*<br>*Delayed-Release Capsules,[1]*<br>*Pangestyme CN-20 Delayed-*<br>*Release Capsules[1]* | 20,000 | 75,000 | 66,400 |

[1] Pork source product.
[2] Amount in 1/4 teaspoon.

## Type of Drug:

Digestive enzymes.

## How the Drug Works:

Pancreatic enzymes (lipase, protease, and amylase) help digest and absorb the fats, proteins, and carbohydrates (starches and sugars) from food. Lipase accelerates the breakdown of fat, protease accelerates the breakdown of protein, and amylase accelerates the breakdown of starch.

## Uses:

To replace pancreatic enzymes in patients who do not produce normal amounts (eg, patients with cystic fibrosis, chronic pancreatitis, removal of the pancreas, obstruction of the pancreatic duct, and pancreatic insufficiency).

To treat excess fat in a bowel movement due to malabsorption syndrome or stomach bypass surgery.

To test pancreatic function.

## Precautions:

*Do not use in the following situations:*

> allergy to pork (pork source products only)
> allergy to the drugs or any of their ingredients
> chronic pancreatic disease, acute exacerbation of
> pancreatitis, acute

*Powder:* Do not inhale or spill powder on skin because it may irritate skin or mucous membranes. Inhalation can precipitate an allergic reaction, coughing spell, bronchospasm, nasal irritation, watery eyes, or asthma attack. If it is necessary to open the capsules, wear a mask and gloves.

*Pregnancy:* There are no adequate and well-controlled studies in pregnant women. Use only if clearly needed and potential benefits outweigh the possible hazards to the fetus.

*Breastfeeding:* It is not known if these drugs are excreted in breast milk. Consult your doctor before you begin breastfeeding.

*Lab tests* may be required during treatment. Tests include stool fat content monitoring, blood albumin levels, and blood-clotting tests.

## Drug Interactions:

Tell your doctor or pharmacist if you are taking or planning to take any over-the-counter or prescription medications or dietary supplements with these drugs. Drug doses may need to be modified or a different drug prescribed. The following drugs and drug classes interact with these drugs:

> calcium carbonate (eg, *Tums)*
> folic acid
> iron supplements (eg, *Feosol* )
> magnesium hydroxide (eg, *Milk of Magnesia)*

## Side Effects:

Every drug is capable of producing side effects. Many patients experience no, or minor, side effects. The frequency and severity of side effects depend on many factors including dose, duration of therapy, and individual susceptibility. Possible side effects include:

*Digestive Tract:* Nausea; stomach cramps; diarrhea; constipation; vomiting; stomach pain or burning; belching; gas; intestinal obstruction; anal irritation; stool abnormalities (eg, greasy stool); bloating; loose stools; diarrhea.

*Other:* Skin irritation.

## Guidelines for Use:

- Consult your doctor and product labeling for individual dosing instructions. Do not exceed the recommended dosage.
- Do not change the dose or stop taking unless advised to do so by your doctor.
- Take with meals and snacks. Do not take on an empty stomach.
- Do not inhale or spill powder on skin. Inhaling may cause an allergic reaction, coughing spell, bronchospasm, nasal irritation, or asthma attack.
- Do not crush or chew coated tablets or capsules. If an intact capsule cannot be swallowed whole, it may be opened and the contents taken with a small amount of food that does not require chewing and has a pH less than 5.5 (eg, applesauce, apricot, banana, and sweet potato baby foods, gelatin snacks). Do not mix with dairy products. Consume immediately after mixing. Wear a mask and gloves while handling open capsules containing powder.
- Drink a full glass of water or juice with medicine to insure swallowing.
- Avoid using antacids or supplements containing calcium carbonate or magnesium hydroxide while taking digestive enzymes. Antacids may negate the beneficial effect of the enzymes.
- Maintain an adequate fluid intake (at least 64 oz per day) while taking this medicine.
- May interfere with the absorption of folic acid. Women who are pregnant or planning to become pregnant during treatment with this medicine should take folic acid supplements.
- Do not change brands without consulting with your pharmacist or doctor.
- Stop taking and notify your doctor if you experience allergy symptoms (eg, rash, wheezing, shortness of breath), bloody diarrhea, or stomach pain with ongoing diarrhea and poor weight gain.
- Vegetarians or patients with allergies to pork can use *Hi-Vegi-Lip* tablets, which are of vegetable origin.
- Lab tests may be required to monitor therapy. Be sure to keep appointments.
- Store at room temperature (below 77°F) in a cool, dry place.

*If you have any questions, consult your doctor, pharmacist, or health care provider.*

| Generic Name<br>*Brand Name Examples* | Supplied As | Generic<br>Available |
|---|---|---|
| *Rx* **Metoclopramide**[1] | | |
| *Clopra, Maxolon,*<br>*Octamide,*<br>*Reclomide, Reglan* | **Tablets:** 10 mg | Yes |
| *Reglan*[2] | **Syrup:** 5 mg/tsp | No |
| *Metoclopramide Intensol* | **Concentrated solution:**<br>10 mg/mL | No |

[1] Some of these products may be available as an injection.
[2] Sugar free.

## Type of Drug:

Digestive tract (gastrointestinal) stimulant.

## How the Drug Works:

These drugs stimulate the contractions/movements of the stomach and small intestine.

## Uses:

To treat symptoms of diabetic gastroparesis (eg, nausea, vomiting, heartburn, persistent fullness after meals and appetite loss).

To treat the nausea and vomiting associated with cancer chemotherapy.

To treat gastroesophageal reflux (reflux of stomach contents into the throat).

*Unlabeled Use(s):* Occasionally doctors may prescribe metoclopramide to improve breast milk secretion, to improve response to migraine medications, for nausea and vomiting, to treat anorexia nervosa, to treat gastric ulcers, for intestinal blockage after operations, diabetic cystoparesis (weak bladder), and bleeding from the esophagus.

## Precautions:

*Do not use in the following situations:*
allergy to metoclopramide
epilepsy or seizure conditions
intestinal obstruction or perforation
pheochromocytoma (adrenal tumor)
stomach or intestinal bleeding

*Use with caution in the following situations:*
breast cancer, history
diabetes

*Diabetics:* Metoclopramide affects the movement of food from the stomach to the intestines and also the absorption of food. Insulin dose may need to be adjusted.

*Pregnancy:* Metoclopramide crosses the placenta. Studies in pregnant women have not shown a risk to the fetus. However, no drug should be used during pregnancy unless clearly needed.

*Breastfeeding:* Metoclopramide appears in breast milk. Consult your doctor before you begin breastfeeding.

*Children:* Metoclopramide has been used in children. However, muscle spasms of the neck, face and jaw, and involuntary movement of the eyes have been reported more commonly in children.

## Drug Interactions:

Tell your doctor or pharmacist if you are taking or if you are planning to take any over-the-counter or prescription medications or dietary supplements with metoclopramide. Doses of one or both drugs may need to be modified or a different drug may need to be prescribed The following drugs and drug classes interact with metoclopramide.

acetaminophen (eg, *Tylenol)*
alcohol
anticholinergics (eg, atropine)
butyrophenone (eg, *Haldol)*
cimetidine (*Tagamet)*
cyclosporine (eg, *Sandimmune)*
digoxin (eg, *Lanoxin)*
hypnotics (eg, phenobarbital)
insulin
levodopa (eg, *Larodopa)*

narcotic pain relievers
 (eg, codeine)
phenothiazines (eg, promethazine)
sedatives (eg, flurazepam)
succinylcholine (eg, *Anectine)*
tetracycline (eg, *Sumycin)*
thioxanthene(eg, *Navane)*
tranquilizers (eg, *Valium)*

## Side Effects:

Every drug is capable of producing side effects. Many metoclopramide users experience no, or minor, side effects. The frequency and severity of side effects depend on many factors including dose, duration of therapy and individual susceptibility. Possible side effects include:

*Digestive Tract:* Nausea; diarrhea.

*Nervous System:* Restlessness; drowsiness; fatigue; weakness; involuntary trembling, jerky movements; shaking muscle spasms; dizziness; anxiety; sleeplessness; headache; depression; hallucinations; facial grimacing; slurred speech; teeth grinding.

*Other:* Increased blood pressure; excessive or spontaneous flow of breast milk; stopping of menstrual period; nipple tenderness; breast enlargement in males; impotence in males; rash; asthma-like symptoms; impaired vision; uncontrolled urination or bowel movements; difficult breathing; decreased blood pressure; neuroleptic malignant syndrome (NMS).

**Guidelines for Use:**

- May cause drowsiness. Use caution when driving or performing other tasks requiring alertness.
- Take 30 minutes before each meal.
- Notify your doctor if involuntary movement of the eyes, face or limbs occurs.

*If you have any questions, consult your doctor, pharmacist, or health care provider.*

| Generic Name<br>*Brand Name Examples* | Supplied As | Generic<br>Available |
|---|---|---|
| *Rx* **Esomeprazole Magnesium** | | |
| *Nexium* | **Capsules, delayed release**: 20 mg, 40 mg | No |
| *Rx* **Lansoprazole** | | |
| *Prevacid* | **Capsules, delayed release**: 15 mg, 30 mg | No |
| *Prevacid* | **Enteric-coated granules for oral suspension, delayed release**: 15 mg, 30 mg | No |
| *Prevacid SoluTab*[1] | **Orally-disintegrating tablets, delayed release**: 15 mg, 30 mg | No |
| *Rx* **Omeprazole** | | |
| *Prilosec* | **Capsules, delayed release**: 10 mg, 20 mg, 40 mg | Yes |
| *Rx* **Pantoprazole Sodium**[2] | | |
| *Protonix* | **Tablets, delayed release**: 20 mg, 40 mg | No |
| *Rx* **Rabeprazole Sodium** | | |
| *Aciphex* | **Tablets, delayed release**: 20 mg | No |

[1] Contains phenylalanine.
[2] Also available as an injection.

## Type of Drug:

Proton pump inhibitors (PPIs); gastric (stomach) acid secretion inhibitors.

## How the Drug Works:

PPIs reduce gastric acid secretion significantly and for a prolonged period by blocking the final step of acid production by the stomach lining.

## Uses:

For short-term treatment (8 weeks or less) of gastroesophageal reflux disease (GERD, the reflux of stomach contents into the food pipe, which can cause heartburn), and to maintain healing and reduce relapse rates of heartburn symptoms in patients with erosive or ulcerative GERD.

*Esomeprazole, lansoprazole, omeprazole:* For short-term treatment (4 to 8 weeks for esomeprazole and omeprazole; 8 weeks or less for lansoprazole) or to maintain healing of inflammation and erosion of the food pipe (erosive esophagitis).

*Esomeprazole, lansoprazole, omeprazole, rabeprazole:* In combination therapy with antibiotics for treatment and elimination of *Helicobacter pylori* infection and associated active duodenal ulcer and to reduce the risk of ulcer recurrence.

*Lansoprazole:* For short-term treatment (up to 12 weeks) to reduce the risk of NSAID-associated gastric ulcers.

*Lansoprazole, omeprazole:* For short-term treatment (4 to 8 weeks for omeprazole; 8 weeks or less for lansoprazole) of active benign gastric ulcers; to treat and reduce the risk of gastric ulcers associated with the use of nonsteroidal anti-inflammatory drugs (NSAIDs) (lansoprazole only).

*Lansoprazole, omeprazole, pantoprazole, rabeprazole:* For long-term treatment of hypersecretory (increased acid secretion) conditions (eg, Zollinger-Ellison syndrome).

*Lansoprazole, omeprazole, rabeprazole:* For short-term treatment (4 to 8 weeks for omeprazole; 4 weeks or less for lansoprazole, rabeprazole) of active duodenal ulcers; to maintain healing of duodenal ulcers (lansoprazole only).

*Unlabeled Use(s):* These agents may increase the effectiveness of pancreatic enzyme replacements used to treat the "fatty stools" of patients with cystic fibrosis. Omeprazole has been prescribed to treat laryngitis.

## Precautions:

*Do not use in the following situations:* Allergy to the drug or any of its ingredients.

*Use with caution in the following situations:*
    Asian patients (omeprazole only)
    liver disease, severe

*Pregnancy:* There are no adequate and well-controlled studies in pregnant women. Use only if clearly needed and the potential benefits outweigh the possible risks to the fetus.

*Breastfeeding:* It is not known if proton pump inhibitors are excreted in breast milk. Because of the potential for serious adverse reactions in nursing infants from PPI, decide whether to discontinue nursing or the drug, taking into account the importance of the drug to the mother. Consult your doctor before you begin breastfeeding.

*Children:* Omeprazole can be used in children 2 years of age and older. Safety and effectiveness of other agents have not been established.

## Drug Interactions:

Tell your doctor or pharmacist if you are taking or planning to take any over-the-counter or prescription medications or dietary supplements with these drugs. Drug doses may need to be modified or a different drug prescribed. The following drugs and drug classes interact with these drugs:

ampicillin (eg, *Principen*)
benzodiazepines (eg, diazepam)
    (omeprazole only)

clarithromycin (eg, *Biaxin*)
cyclosporine (eg, *Neoral*)
disulfiram (eg, *Antabuse*)

iron salts (eg, ferrous sulfate)
phenytoin (eg, *Dilantin*) (omeprazole only
sucralfate (eg, *Carafate*)

theophylline (eg, *Theo-Dur*)
   (lansoprazole only)
warfarin (eg, *Coumadin*)

## Side Effects:

Every drug is capable of producing side effects. Many patients experience no, or minor, side effects. The frequency and severity of side effects depend on many factors including dose, duration of therapy, and individual susceptibility. Possible side effects include:

*Digestive Tract:* Diarrhea; nausea; vomiting; stomach pain; constipation; gas; belching.

*Nervous System:* Dizziness; headache; weakness.

*Other:* Rash; back pain; upper respiratory tract infection; cough; high blood sugar.

## Guidelines for Use:

- Dosage is individualized. Take exactly as prescribed.
- Do not stop taking or change the dose, unless instructed by your doctor.
- Usually taken once daily, at least 1 hour before a meal. Dosages and dosing regimens may vary depending on condition being treated.
- Take rabeprazole after the morning meal when treating duodenal ulcers.
- Take pantoprazole with or without regard to food.
- These medicines must be taken daily to be effective in treating and preventing acid-related gastrointestinal diseases. Do not take on an "as needed" basis.
- Antacids may be used as needed with these medicines.
- Do not chew, crush, or split capsules or tablets. Swallow whole. If you have difficulty swallowing esomeprazole, omeprazole, or lansoprazole capsules, they may be opened, sprinkled on 1 tablespoon of applesauce, *Ensure* pudding, cottage cheese, yogurt, or strained pears, and swallowed immediately without chewing the granules. Lansoprazole capsules can also be emptied into a small glass of either orange or tomato juice (60 mL; approximately 2 oz), mixed briefly, and swallowed immediately. To ensure complete ingestion, rinse the glass with 4 or more oz of juice and swallow the contents immediately.
- *Orally-disintegrating tablets* — Place tablet on the tongue. Allow to melt with or without water until particles can be swallowed.
- *Lansoprazole suspension* — Empty the packet contents into a container with 2 tablespoons (30 mL) of water. Do not use other liquids or foods. Stir well and drink immediately. More water can be added if material remains in the container; drink immediately.
- If a dose is missed, take it as soon as possible. If several hours have passed or it is nearing time for the next dose, do not double the dose to catch up, unless instructed by your doctor. If more than one dose is missed, or it is necessary to establish a new dosage schedule, contact your doctor or pharmacist.
- Inform your doctor if you are pregnant, become pregnant, plan on becoming pregnant, or are breastfeeding.
- PPIs should be taken at least 30 minutes prior to taking sucralfate.
- Store at controlled room temperature (59° to 86°F) in a tightly closed container. Protect from light and moisture.

*If you have any questions, consult your doctor, pharmacist, or health care provider.*

| Generic Name<br>*Brand Name Example* | Supplied As | Generic<br>Available |
|---|---|---|
| *Rx* **Ursodiol**<br>**(Ursodeoxycholic Acid)** | | |
| *Actigall* | **Capsules**: 300 mg | Yes |

## Type of Drug:

Gallstone dissolving agent.

## How the Drug Works:

Ursodiol helps dissolve cholesterol gallstones. It is most effective if the gallstones are small or "floatable." Patients must have a working gallbladder.

## Uses:

To dissolve cholesterol gallstones smaller than 20 mm in diameter in patients who are not good candidates for surgery because of systemic disease, advanced age, or reaction to general anesthesia.

For the prevention of gallstones in obese patients experiencing rapid weight loss.

## Precautions:

*Do not use in the following situations:*

allergy to bile acids
allergy to the drug or any of its ingredients
biliary-gastrointestinal fistula
biliary obstruction
calcified cholesterol gallstones
cholangitis
cholecystitis, acute and unremitting
gallstone pancreatitis
liver disease, chronic
radiolucent bile pigment stones
radiopaque stones

*Use with caution in the following situations:* Liver disease.

*Gallstone recurrence:* Treatment requires months of therapy. Complete dissolution does not always occur and recurrence within 5 years has been observed in 50% or fewer patients. Consider alternative therapy if possible.

*Pregnancy:* There are no adequate and well-controlled studies in pregnant women. Use only if clearly needed and the potential benefits outweigh the possible hazards to the fetus.

*Breastfeeding:* It is not known if ursodiol appears in breast milk. Consult your doctor before you begin breastfeeding.

*Children:* Safety and effectiveness have not been established.

*Lab tests* will be required during treatment. Tests include liver function analysis.

## Drug Interactions:

Tell your doctor or pharmacist if you are taking or planning to take any over-the-counter or prescription medications or dietary supplements with this drug. Drug doses may need to be modified or a different drug prescribed. The following drugs and drug classes interact with this drug:

antacids, aluminum-based (eg, aluminum hydroxide)
bile acid sequestrants (eg, cholestyramine)

clofibrate (eg, *Atromid-S*)
contraceptives, oral (eg, *Ortho-Novum*)
estrogens (eg, ethinyl estradiol)

## Side Effects:

Every drug is capable of producing side effects. Many patients experience no, or minor, side effects. The frequency and severity of side effects depend on many factors including dose, duration of therapy and individual susceptibility. Possible side effects include.

*Digestive Tract:* Nausea; vomiting; diarrhea; severe abdominal pain (especially in upper right side); indigestion; constipation; gas; gallbladder inflammation; inflammation of the mouth.

*Nervous System:* Headache; fatigue; anxiety; depression; sleep problems.

*Skin:* Rash; itching; hives; dry skin; sweating; hair thinning.

*Other:* Metallic taste; joint and muscle pain; cough; runny nose; back pain; mouth sores.

---

### Guidelines for Use:

- Use exactly as prescribed. Otherwise, the gallstones may dissolve very slowly or not at all.
- If a dose is missed, take it as soon as possible. If several hours have passed or if it is nearing time for the next dose, do not double the dose in order to "catch up" (unless advised to do so by your doctor). If more than one dose is missed or it is necessary to establish a new dosage schedule, contact your doctor or pharmacist.
- Carefully follow the diet your doctor has prescribed.
- Contact your doctor if diarrhea, stomach pain, severe sudden pain in upper right side, nausea or vomiting occurs.
- Therapy usually takes months. Complete dissolving of gallstones does not occur in all patients, and recurrence within 5 years occurs in up to 50% of patients.
- The long-term effects (more than 24 months) of this medicine are not known.
- Lab tests will be required to monitor therapy. Be sure to keep appointments.
- Store below 86°F.

---

*If you have any questions, consult your doctor, pharmacist, or health care provider.*

| Generic Name Brand Name Examples | Supplied As | Generic Available |
|---|---|---|
| **Monoctanoin** | | |
| Rx  Moctanin | **Infusion** | No |

## Type of Drug:

Gallstone dissolving agent.

## How the Drug Works:

Monoctanoin is a liquid given through a catheter into the bile duct. Gallstones (found in the gallbladder or bile duct) may remain in the bile duct after surgical removal of the gallbladder. If these stones are made of cholesterol and are too large to pass out of the body on their own, monoctanoin may help dissolve them. Complete dissolution is more likely when there is a single stone than when there are multiple stones.

## Uses:

To dissolve cholesterol gallstones that remain in the bile duct after the gallbladder has been removed. Used when other means of removing the stones have failed, or in patients who are not good candidates for surgery.

## Precautions:

*Do not use in the following situations:*

biliary tract infection, significant
duodenal ulcer, recent
jejunitis, history
liver disease
pancreatitis, acute
porto-systemic shunting

*Use with caution in the following situations:* Obstructive jaundice.

*Pregnancy:* Adequate studies have not been done in pregnant women, or animal studies may have shown a risk to the fetus. Use only if clearly needed and potential benefits outweigh the possible hazards to the fetus.

*Breastfeeding:* It is not known if monoctanoin appears in breastmilk. Consult your doctor before you begin breastfeeding.

*Children:* Safety and effectiveness have not been established.

*Lab tests* may be required to monitor therapy. Lab tests include liver function tests.

## Side Effects:

Every drug is capable of producing side effects. Many patients experience no, or minor, side effects. The frequency and severity of side effects depend on many factors including dose, duration of therapy and individual susceptibility. Possible side effects include: Stomach pain; nausea; vomiting; diarrhea; appetite loss; loose stools; indigestion; fever.

## Guidelines for Use:

- This agent must be given by your doctor through a catheter or tube into the bile duct. It is given continuously for 2 to 10 days.
- Tell your doctor immediately if stomach pain, nausea, diarrhea, vomiting, fever, appetite loss, chills, severe pain in the upper right side, or yellowing or skin or eyes occurs.

*If you have any questions, consult your doctor, pharmacist, or health care provider.*

| Generic Name<br>*Brand Name Examples* | Supplied As | Generic<br>Available |
|---|---|---|
| *otc* **Methylcellulose** | | |
| *Citrucel* | **Powder:** 2 g/heaping tbsp | No |
| *Citrucel Sugar Free*[1] | **Powder:** 2 g, 52 mg phenylala-<br>nine/heaping tbsp | No |
| *Unifiber* | **Powder** | No |
| *otc* **Barley Malt Extract** | | |
| *Maltsupex* | **Tablets:** 750 mg | No |
| *Maltsupex* | **Powder:** 8 g/tbsp | No |
| *Maltsupex* | **Liquid:** 16 g/tbsp | No |
| *otc* **Polycarbophil** | | |
| *Equalactin, Fiberall,*<br>*Mitrolan* | **Tablets, chewable:** 500 mg,<br>1250 mg | No |
| *FiberCon*[2]*, Fiber-Lax,*<br>*FiberNorm, Konsyl Fiber* | **Tablets:** 500 mg, 625 mg | No |
| *otc* **Psyllium** | | |
| *Fiberall Natural Flavor*[1]*,*<br>*Fiberall Orange Flavor*[1] | **Powder:** 3.4 g with wheat bran,<br>< 10 mg sodium, < 60 mg<br>potassium, < 6 calories/dose | No |
| *Hydrocil Instant*[1] | **Powder:** 3.5 g | No |
| *Konsyl*[1] | **Powder:** 100% psyllium | No |
| *Konsyl-Orange* | **Powder:** 3.4 g/tbsp | No |
| *Maalox Daily Fiber*<br>*Therapy* | **Powder:** ≈ 3.4 g, sucrose,<br>35 calories/12 g | No |
| *Metamucil* | **Powder:** ≈ 3.4 g, 3.5 g car-<br>bohy-drates, < 10 mg sodium,<br>31 mg potassium, 14 calories/<br>dose | No |
| *Metamucil Orange Flavor* | **Powder:** ≈ 3.4 g, 7.1 g carbo-<br>hydrates, < 10 mg sodium,<br>31 mg potassium, 30 calories/<br>dose | No |
| *Metamucil Sugar Free*[1] | **Powder:** ≈ 3.4 g, 0.3 g carbo-<br>hydrates, < 10 mg sodium,<br>31 mg potassium, 1 calorie/<br>dose | No |
| *Mylanta Natural Fiber*<br>*Supplement* | **Powder:** 3.4 g | No |
| *Restore*[4] | **Powder:** 3.4 g/dose, orange<br>flavor, saccharine, sucrose | |

| Generic Name<br>*Brand Name Examples* | Supplied As | Generic<br>Available |
|---|---|---|
| *Metamucil* | **Wafers:** ≈ 1.7 g, 18 g carbohy-drate, 18 mg sodium, 4.5 g fat, 96 calories/dose | No |
| *Fiberall* | **Wafers:** 3.4 g, 0.03 g sodium, 78 calories/wafer | No |
| *Alramucil* [3] | **Effervescent powder:** 3.6 g, citric acid, sucrose, saccharin, potassium bicarbonate, sodium bicarbonate, 4 calories, < 0.01 g sodium/packet | No |
| *Effer-syllium* | **Effervescent powder:** 3 g/rounded tsp | No |
| *Metamucil Lemon-Lime Flavor* | **Effervescent powder:** ≈ 3.4 g, sodium and potassium bicarbo-nate, < 10 mg sodium, calcium carbonate, 290 mg potassium, 1 calorie/dose | No |
| *Metamucil Orange Flavor* | **Effervescent powder:** ≈ 3.4 g, sodium and potassium bicarbonate, < 10 mg sodium, 310 mg potassium, 1 calorie/dose | No |
| *Perdiem Fiber* [5] | **Granules:** 4.03 g 1.8 mg sodium, 36.1 mg potassium, 4 calories/rounded tsp | No |
| *Serutan* | **Granules:** 2.5 g, < 0.03 g sodium/heaping tsp | No |
| *Siblin* | **Granules:** 2.5 g/rounded tsp | No |

[1] Sugar free.
[2] Sodium free.
[3] Also available in orange flavor.
[4] Also available sugar free.
[5] Dye free.

Laxatives promote bowel emptying. Nonprescription laxatives are frequently misued due to lack of understanding of normal bowel function. Restrict self-medication to short-term therapy of constipation. Chronic use of laxatives (particularly stimulants) may lead to dependence. Prior to laxative use, consider living habits affecting bowel function including disease state and drug history. Rational therapy and prevention of constipation include: Adequate fluid intake (4 to 6 glasses of water daily), proper dietary habits including sufficient bulk or roughage, responding to the urge to defecate and daily exercise.

## Type of Drug:

Bulk laxative.

## How the Drug Works:
Bulk laxatives hold water in the stool and dissolve and swell in the intestinal fluids to stimulate intestinal activity. They are considered to be the safest laxative products for the treatment of constipation and to help maintain normal bowel function in some digestive disorders.

## Uses:
For short-term treatment of constipation.

*Psyllium:* To treat irritable bowel syndrome, diverticular disease, spastic colon and hemorrhoids.

*Polycarbophil:* To treat acute nonspecific diarrhea or diarrhea associated with conditions such as diverticulitis or irritable bowel syndrome.

*Unlabeled Use(s):* Occasionally doctors may prescribe psyllium in combination with a dietary program for the reduction of cholesterol levels.

## Precautions:
*Do not use in the following situations:*
>   allergy to any ingredients of these products
>   abdominal pain, undiagnosed
>   abdominal surgery
>   appendicitis symptoms (nausea, vomiting, stomach pain)
>   intestinal obstruction
>   intestinal ulcers, stenosis or adhesions
>   stool impaction

*Use with caution in the following situations:*
>   kidney stones

*Rectal bleeding or failure of the laxative* to produce a bowel movement can indicate a more serious condition which requires medical attention.

*Laxatives that contain sodium* should be used with caution by patients with heart disease, high blood pressure, conditions in which swelling occurs, or patients who are on low-sodium diets.

*Long-term use:* These products should not be used over one week except by the advice of your doctor.

*Failure to drink adequate fluids* with these products can result in intestinal obstruction or fecal impaction.

*Pregnancy:* Bulk laxatives may be used during pregnancy, but only under the direction of a doctor.

## Drug Interactions:
Tell your doctor or pharmacist if you are taking or if you are planning to take any over-the-counter or prescription medications or dietary supplements with this medicine. Doses of one or both drugs may need to be modified or a different drug may need to be prescribed. Tetracycline (eg, *Achromycin V*) interacts with polycarbophil.

## Side Effects:

Every drug is capable of producing side effects. Many patients experience no, or minor, side effects. The frequency and severity of side effects depends on many factors including dose, duration of therapy and individual susceptibility. Possible side effects include:

*Digestive Tract:* Diarrhea; nausea; vomiting; rectal irritation; bloating; gas; stomach pain; intestinal or rectal obstruction.

*Other:* Dizziness; weakness; fainting; sweating; pounding in the chest.

---

### Guidelines for Use:

- Use exactly as prescribed.
- Take with a full glass of water or juice.
- Do not use if abdominal pain, nausea or vomiting occurs.
- Contact your doctor if unrelieved constipation, rectal bleeding, muscle cramps or pain, weakness, or dizziness occurs.
- Bulk laxatives are the safest laxatives. However, laxative use is only a temporary measure. When normal bowel habits return, stop use of these products unless instructed otherwise by your doctor. Prolonged, frequent or excessive use may result in dependence or electrolyte imbalance.

---

*If you have any questions, consult your doctor, pharmacist, or health care provider.*

| Generic Name<br>*Brand Name Examples* | Supplied As | Generic<br>Available |
|---|---|---|
| **Glycerin, USP** | | |
| *otc Sani-Supp* | **Suppositories:** Glycerin and sodium stearate | Yes |
| **Glycerin Rectal Liquid** | | |
| *otc Fleet Babylax* | **Liquid:** 4 mL glycerin applicators | No |

Laxatives promote bowel emptying. Nonprescription laxatives are frequently misued due to lack of understanding of normal bowel function. Restrict self-medication to short-term therapy of constipation. Chronic use of laxatives (particularly stimulants) may lead to dependence. Prior to laxative use, consider living habits affecting bowel function including disease state and drug history. Rational therapy and prevention of constipation include: Adequate fluid intake (4 to 6 glasses of water daily), proper dietary habits including sufficient bulk or roughage, responding to the urge to defecate and daily exercise.

## Type of Drug:

Hyperosmolar laxatives.

## How the Drug Works:

Glycerin irritates the colon and draws water into the colon, stimulating bowel movements.

## Uses:

For short-term treatment of constipation.

To treat constipation in infants and children.

## Precautions:

*Do not use in the following situations:*

abdominal surgery
allergy to any ingredient of these
  products
appendicitis symptoms (nausea,
  vomiting, abdominal pain)

intestinal obstruction
stool impaction

*Frequent use of laxatives and inadequate fluid* can cause an imbalance in fluid and electrolyte levels. Symptoms may include muscle cramps, muscle weakness or dizziness.

*Rectal bleeding or failure of the laxative* to produce a bowel movement can indicate a more serious condition which requires medical attention.

*Children:* Physical manipulation of a glycerin suppository in infants will usually promote bowel movements. Because of this, side effects are usually minimal.

## Side Effects:

Every drug is capable of producing side effects. Many patients experience no, or minor, side effects. The frequency and severity of side effects depends on many factors including dose, duration of therapy and individual susceptibility. Possible side effects include:

*Circulatory System:* Pounding of the chest (palpitations).

*Other:* Bowel cramping; stomach cramps; irritation of the rectal area; diarrhea; nausea; vomiting; weakness; dizziness; fainting; sweating; bloating; gas; excessive bowel activity.

---

### Guidelines for Use:

- Laxative use is only a temporary measure. Do not use longer than one week. Stop use of these products when normal bowel habits return. Prolonged, frequent or excessive use may result in dependence or electrolyte imbalance.
- *Suppositories* — Insert one suppository high in the rectum and retain 15 minutes. It does not need to melt to produce laxative action.
- *Rectal liquid* — With gentle, steady pressure, insert stem with tip pointing towards naval. Squeeze unit until nearly all the liquid is expelled. Remove. A small amount of liquid will remain in unit.
- Do not use if abdominal pain, nausea or vomiting occurs.
- Contact your doctor if unrelieved constipation, rectal bleeding, muscle cramps or pain, weakness or dizziness occurs.
- Effects usually occur within 30 minutes.

---

*If you have any questions, consult your doctor, pharmacist, or health care provider.*

| Generic Name<br>*Brand Name Examples* | Supplied As | Generic<br>Available |
|---|---|---|
| **Lactulose**<br>*Cephulac, Cholac,*<br>*Chronulac, Constilac,*<br>*Constulose, Duphalac,*<br>*Enulose* | **Syrup:** 10 g/tbsp | Yes |

Laxatives promote bowel emptying. Nonprescription laxatives are frequently misued due to lack of understanding of normal bowel function. Restrict self-medication to short-term therapy of constipation. Chronic use of laxatives (particularly stimulants) may lead to dependence. Prior to laxative use, consider living habits affecting bowel function including disease state and drug history. Rational therapy and prevention of constipation include: Adequate fluid intake (4 to 6 glasses of water daily), proper dietary habits including sufficient bulk or roughage, responding to the urge to defecate and daily exercise.

## Type of Drug:

Laxative.

## How the Drug Works:

Lactulose draws water into the colon to create bulk and stimulate bowel movements.

## Uses:

*Chronulac, Constilac, Duphalac* — For the treatment of constipation.

*Cephulac, Cholac, Enulose* — To prevent and treat portal-systemic encephalopathy (liver disease), including the stages of hepatic pre-coma and coma.

## Precautions:

*Do not use in the following situations:*
> allergy to any ingredient in these products
> low galactose-sugar diet

*Use with caution in the following situations:*
> diabetes
> electrocautery procedures
> other laxatives, use

*Lab tests:* Elderly or debilitated patients who receive lactulose for more than 6 months should have electrolyte levels (eg, potassium chloride, carbon dioxide) done
periodically.

*Diabetes:* This product contains sugar. Use with caution.

*Pregnancy:* Studies in pregnant women or in animals have been judged not to show a risk to the fetus. However, no drug should be used during pregnancy unless clearly needed.

*Breastfeeding:* It is not known if lactulose appears in breastmilk. Consult your doctor before you begin breastfeeding.

*Children:* Safety and effectiveness have not been established.

## Drug Interactions:

Tell your doctor or pharmacist if you are taking or if you are planning to take any over-the-counter or prescription medications or dietary supplements while taking this medicine. Doses of one or both drugs may need to be modified or a different drug may need to be prescribed. The following drugs and drug classes interact with this medicine.

antacids
neomycin (eg, *Mycifradin*)

## Side Effects:

Every drug is capable of producing side effects. Many patients experience no, or minor, side effects. The frequency and severity of side effects depends on many factors including dose, duration of therapy and individual susceptibility. Possible side effects include: Gas and belching; stomach pain; bowel cramping; diarrhea; nausea; vomiting.

---

### Guidelines for Use:

- *Chronulac, Constilac, Duphalac* — Usual adult dose is 1 to 2 table-spoonfuls (15 to 30 mL) daily. Do not take more than 4 tablespoon-fuls (60 mL) daily.
- *Cephulac, Cholac, Enulose* — Usual adult dose is 2 to 3 tablespoon-fuls (30 to 45 mL) three to four times daily. Adjust dosage every day or two to produce 2 or 3 soft stools daily.
- May be mixed with fruit juice, water or milk to improve taste.
- May cause belching, gas or cramps. Notify your doctor if these effects become bothersome or if unusual diarrhea occurs.
- Do not take other laxatives while on lactulose therapy.
- Prevention of constipation includes: Adequate fluid intake (4 to 6 glasses of water daily), proper dietary habits including sufficient bulk or rough-age, responding to the urge to defecate and daily exercise.
- Effects may not be seen for 24 to 48 hours.
- *Duphalac* — Darkening of syrup may occur. This is not significant.
- Store below 86°F. Do not freeze.

---

*If you have any questions, consult your doctor, pharmacist, or health care provider.*

| Generic Name<br>*Brand Name Examples* | Supplied As | Generic<br>Available |
|---|---|---|
| *otc* **Mineral Oil** | **Liquid, heavy** | Yes |
| *Neo-Cultol* | **Jelly**: Refined mineral oil | No |
| *Milkinol* | **Emulsion**: Mineral oil in an emulsifying base | No |
| *Kondremul Plain*[1] | **Emulsion**: Mineral oil with Irish moss, acacia, glycerin | No |

Laxatives promote bowel emptying. Nonprescription laxatives are frequently misused due to lack of understanding of normal bowel function. Restrict self-medication to short-term therapy of constipation. Chronic use of laxatives (particularly stimulants) may lead to dependence. Prior to laxative use, consider living habits affecting bowel function including disease state and drug history. Rational therapy and prevention of constipation include: adequate fluid intake (4 to 6 glasses of water daily), proper dietary habits, including sufficient bulk or roughage, responding to the urge to defecate, and daily exercise.

## Type of Drug:
Lubricant or emollient laxative; liquid petrolatum.

## How the Drug Works:
Mineral oil lubricates the colon and softens feces by coating it and holding water in the fecal mass.

## Uses:
For the short-term treatment of constipation, or relief of fecal impaction.

To prevent straining at the stool in patients who have heart conditions or who have had recent rectal surgery.

## Precautions:
*Do not use in the following situations:*
>   abdominal surgery
>   allergy to the drug or any of its ingredients
>   appendicitis symptoms (eg, nausea, vomiting, abdominal pain)
>   intestinal obstruction
>   surfactant laxative (eg, docusate) use, current

*Anal/rectal surgery:* Mineral oil can leak from the rectum and cause itching, hemorrhoids, irritation, and discomfort.

*Frequent use/inadequate fluid:* Frequent use of laxatives and inadequate fluid can cause an imbalance in fluid and electrolyte levels. Symptoms may include muscle cramps, muscle weakness, or dizziness.

*Lipid pneumonia:* Lipid pneumonia can occur if mineral oil is accidentally inhaled into the lungs, especially when the patient is lying down. Patients who are young, elderly, or have difficulty swallowing are at greater risk for this problem.

*Rectal bleeding/failure of the laxative:* Rectal bleeding or failure of the laxative to produce a bowel movement can indicate a more serious condition which requires medical attention.

*Pregnancy:* Mineral oil can decrease absorption of fat-soluble vitamins (A, D, E, K) from the diet or from vitamin tablets. Consult your doctor before using these products.

## Drug Interactions:

Tell your doctor or pharmacist if you are taking or if you are planning to take any over-the-counter or prescription medications or dietary supplements while taking this medicine. Doses of one or both drugs may need to be modified or a different drug may need to be prescribed. The following drugs and drug classes interact with this medicine:

| | |
|---|---|
| surfactant laxatives | vitamin D |
| (eg, docusate) | vitamin E |
| vitamin A | vitamin K |

## Side Effects:

Every drug is capable of producing side effects. Many patients experience no, or minor, side effects. The frequency and severity of side effects depends on many factors including dose, duration of therapy, and individual susceptibility. Possible side effects include:

*Digestive Tract:* Nausea; vomiting; diarrhea; stomach pain; bloating; gas; bowel cramping.

*Nervous System:* Weakness; dizziness; fainting.

*Other:* Irritation, itching, or bleeding of the rectal area; hemorrhoids; anal seepage; sweating; pounding of the chest (palpitations); muscle cramps or pain.

---

### Guidelines for Use:

- The usual adult dose is 5 to 45 mL.
- Take with a full glass of water or juice.
- Most effective when taken on an empty stomach.
- Although the usual directions are to give the dose at bedtime, caution is advised because of lipid pneumonia (see Precautions).
- Laxative use is only a temporary measure. Do not use longer than one week.
- Do not use if you experience stomach pain, nausea, or vomiting.
- Contact your doctor if you experience unrelieved constipation, rectal bleeding, muscle cramps or pain, weakness, or dizziness.
- Mineral oil may seep from the rectum, soiling clothing and causing itching, irritation, hemorrhoids, and rectal discomfort. This is less likely to happen with the emulsion.
- Prevention of constipation includes: adequate fluid intake (4 to 6 glasses of water daily), proper dietary habits, including sufficient bulk or roughage, responding to the urge to defecate, and daily exercise.
- Effects usually occur in 6 to 8 hours. Plan accordingly.

---

*If you have any questions, consult your doctor, pharmacist, or health care provider.*

| Brand Name Examples | Supplied As |
| --- | --- |
| otc Citrate of Magnesia | **Solution**: Magnesium citrate |
| otc Epsom Salt | **Granules**: Magnesium sulfate |
| otc Fleet Phospho-soda[1], Sodium Phosphates[1] | **Solution**: 18 g sodium phosphate and 48 g sodium biphosphate/100 mL |
| otc Milk of Magnesia, Concentrated, Phillips' Milk of Magnesia, Concentrated | **Liquid**: Magnesium hydroxide |
| otc Milk of Magnesia, Phillips' Milk of Magnesia | **Liquid**: Magnesium hydroxide, 7% to 8.5 % aqueous suspension |

[1] Sugar free.

Laxatives promote bowel emptying. Nonprescription laxatives are frequently misused due to lack of understanding of normal bowel function. Restrict self-medication to short-term therapy of constipation. Chronic use of laxatives (particularly stimulants) may lead to dependence. Prior to laxative use, consider living habits affecting bowel function including disease state and drug history. Rational therapy and prevention of constipation include: adequate fluid intake (4 to 6 glasses of water daily), proper dietary habits, including sufficient bulk or roughage, responding to the urge to defecate, and daily exercise.

## Type of Drug:

Saline laxatives.

## How the Drug Works:

Saline laxatives cause water to accumulate in the intestine, thereby increasing pressure in the intestine and causing bowel movements.

## Uses:

For the short-term treatment of constipation.

To clean out the bowel before bowel examinations or bowel surgery.

## Precautions:

*Do not use in the following situations:*
abdominal surgery
allergy to the drug or any of its ingredients
appendicitis symptoms (eg, nausea, vomiting, abdominal pain)
intestinal obstruction
stool impaction

*Use with caution in the following situations:*
congestive heart failure
high blood pressure
kidney disease
sodium-restricted diet
swelling or water retention

*Frequent use/inadequate fluid:* Frequent use of laxatives and inadequate fluid can cause an imbalance in fluid and electrolyte levels. Symptoms may include muscle cramps, muscle weakness, or dizziness.

*Rectal bleeding/failure of the laxative:* Rectal bleeding or failure of the laxative to produce a bowel movement can indicate a more serious condition which requires medical attention.

*Pregnancy:* Saline laxatives can cause an electrolyte imbalance (eg, potassium). Use of a bulk or stool-softening laxative is preferred. Consult your doctor.

## Drug Interactions:

Tell your doctor or pharmacist if you are taking or if you are planning to take any over-the-counter or prescription medications or dietary supplements while taking this medicine. Doses of one or both drugs may need to be modified or a different drug may need to be prescribed. Tetracyclines interact with magnesium-containing products.

## Side Effects:

Every drug is capable of producing side effects. Many patients experience no, or minor, side effects. The frequency and severity of side effects depends on many factors including dose, duration of therapy, and individual susceptibility. Possible side effects include:

*Digestive Tract:* Nausea; vomiting; diarrhea; stomach pain; bloating; gas; bowel cramping; griping.

*Nervous System:* Weakness; dizziness; fainting.

*Other:* Irritation of the rectal area; sweating; pounding of the chest (palpitations); rectal bleeding; muscle cramps or pain; electrolyte imbalance (eg, potassium).

---

### Guidelines for Use:

- Take with a full glass of water or juice.
- Laxative use is only a temporary measure. Do not use longer than one week. Stop use of these products when normal bowel habits return. Prolonged, frequent, or excessive use may result in dependence or electrolyte imbalance.
- Do not use if you experience stomach pain, nausea, or vomiting.
- Contact your doctor if you experience unrelieved constipation, rectal bleeding, muscle cramps or pain, weakness, or dizziness.
- Prevention of constipation includes: adequate fluid intake (4 to 6 glasses of water daily), proper dietary habits, including sufficient bulk or roughage, responding to the urge to defecate, and daily exercise.
- Although the usual directions are to give the dose at bedtime, caution is advised because of lipid pneumonia (see Precautions).
- Effects usually occur in 30 minutes to 3 hours. Plan accordingly.
- Store magnesium citrate solutions in the refrigerator to retain potency and to improve taste.

---

*If you have any questions, consult your doctor, pharmacist, or health care provider.*

| Generic Name<br>*Brand Name Examples* | How Supplied | Generic<br>Available |
|---|---|---|
| *otc* **Bisacodyl** | | |
| *Feen-a-mint* | **Tablets:** 5 mg | No |
| *Dulcagen, Dulcolax, Fleet* | **Tablets, enteric coated:** 5 mg | Yes |
| *Bisacodyl Uniserts, Bisco-Lax, Dulcagen, Dulcolax, Fleet* | **Suppositories:** 10 mg | Yes |
| *otc* **Calcium Salts of Sennosides<br>A & B** | | |
| *Ex-Lax Gentle Nature, Senexon* | **Tablets:** 5.6 mg, 20 mg | No |
| *otc* **Cascara Sagrada** | **Tablets:** 325 mg | Yes |
| *Cascara Sagrada Aromatic Fluid Extract*[1] | **Liquid** | Yes |
| *otc* **Castor Oil** | **Liquid** | Yes |
| *Purge* | **Liquid:** 95% | Yes |
| *Emulsoil*[2] | **Emulsion:** 95% | No |
| *Fleet Flavored Castor Oil* | **Emulsion:** 67% | No |
| *Neoloid*[2] | **Oil:** 36.4% | No |
| *otc* **Phenolphthalein** | | |
| *Alophen Pills, Espotabs, Ex-Lax Maximum Relief, Ex-Lax Unflavored, Feen-a-mint, Lax Pills, Laxative Pills, Modane, Prulet* | **Tablets:** 60 mg, 90 mg, 97.2 mg, 130 mg, 135 mg | No |
| *Evac-U-Gen, Ex-Lax Chocolated, Feen-a-mint, Feen-a-mint Chocolated, Medilax* | **Tablets, chewable:** 65 mg, 90 mg, 97.2 mg, 120 mg | No |
| *Evac-U-Lax Tablets* | **Wafers, chewable:** 80 mg | No |
| *Feen-a-mint* | **Gum:** 97.2 mg | No |

*otc* **Senna**

| | | |
|---|---|---|
| *Black-Draught, Senexon, Senna-Gen, Senolax, Senokot, SenokotXTRA* | **Tablets:** 8.6 mg, 217 mg, 374 mg, 600 mg | No |
| *Black-Draught[3], Gentlax, Senokot* | **Granules:** 15 mg/tsp, 1.65 g/ ½ tsp | No |
| *Senokot* | **Suppositories:** 652 mg | No |
| *Dosalax[1], Senokot[1]* | **Syrup:** 8.8 mg/tsp | No |
| *Dr. Caldwell Senna[1], Fletcher's Castoria[1]* | **Liquid:** 33.3 mg/mL | No |

[1] Contains alcohol.
[2] Sugar free.
[3] Contains the dye tartrazine.

Laxatives promote bowel emptying. Nonprescription laxatives are frequently misued due to lack of understanding of normal bowel function. Restrict self-medication to short-term therapy of constipation. Chronic use of laxatives (particularly stimulants) may lead to dependence. Prior to laxative use, consider living habits affecting bowel function including disease state and drug history. Rational therapy and prevention of constipation include: Adequate fluid intake (4 to 6 glasses of water daily), proper dietary habits including sufficient bulk or roughage, responding to the urge to defecate and daily exercise.

## Type of Drug:
Irritant or stimulant laxatives.

## How the Drug Works:
Stimulant laxatives act directly on the intestines, irritating the digestive tract lining and stimulating intestinal activity.

## Uses:
For short-term treatment of constipation.

To clean out the bowel before bowel examinations or bowel surgery.

## Precautions:
*Do not use in the following situations:*
abdominal pain, undiagnosed
abdominal surgery
allergy to any ingredient of these
 products
appendicitis symptoms (nausea,
 vomiting, abdominal pain)
children under 10 years of age
 (bisacodyl only)
intestinal obstruction
stool impaction
ulcerative lesions of colon (bisacodyl only)

*Use with caution in the following situations:*
multiple enemas (bisacodyl only)

*Frequent use of laxatives and inadequate fluid* can cause an imbalance in fluid and electrolyte levels. Symptoms may include muscle cramps, muscle weakness or dizziness.

*Rectal bleeding or failure of the laxative* to produce a bowel movement can indicate a more serious condition which requires medical attention.

*Discoloration* of the urine (yellow-brown, pink-red, red-violet or red-brown) may occur with phenolphthalein, cascara sagrada or senna.

*Tartrazine:* Some of these products may contain the dye tartrazine (FD&C Yellow No. 5) which can cause allergic reactions in certain individuals. Check package label when available or consult your doctor or pharmacist.

*Pregnancy:* Adequate studies have not been done in pregnant women, or animal studies may have shown a risk to the fetus. Use only if clearly needed and potential benefits outweigh the possible hazards to the fetus. Improper use of these products can cause a dangerous electrolyte imbalance. Use of a bulk or stool-softening laxative is preferred.

   *Castor oil* — Do not use during pregnancy. It can produce premature labor.

*Breastfeeding:* Cascara sagrada appears in breast milk. Use can result in diarrhea in the infant. Consult your doctor before you begin breast-feeding.

*Children:* Do not use bisacodyl tannex in children under 10 years of age.

## Drug Interactions:

Tell your doctor or pharmacist if you are taking or if you are planning to take any over-the-counter or prescription medications or dietary supplements while taking these products. Doses of one or both drugs may need to be modified or a different drug may need to be prescribed. Antacids and milk interact with bisacodyl.

## Side Effects:

Every drug is capable of producing side effects. Many patients experience no, or minor, side effects. The frequency and severity of side effects depends on many factors including dose, duration of therapy and individual susceptibility. Possible side effects include:

*Digestive Tract:* Nausea; vomiting; stomach pain; bowel cramping; diarrhea; bloating; gas.

*Nervous System:* Weakness; dizziness; fainting.

*Other:* Irritation of the rectal area; sweating; pounding of the chest (palpitations).

## Guidelines for Use:

- Use exactly as prescribed.
- Laxative use is only a temporary measure. Do not use longer than one week. Stop use of these products when normal bowel habits return. Prolonged, frequent or excessive use may result in dependence or electrolyte imbalance.
- Take with a full glass of water or juice.
- *Bisacodyl* — Swallow tablets whole (do not crush). Do not take within 1 hours of antacids or milk.
- *Suspensions and emulsions* — Shake well before use.
- Do not use if abdominal pain, nausea or vomiting occurs.
- Contact your doctor if unrelieved constipation, rectal bleeding, muscle cramps or pain, weakness or dizziness occurs.
- *Phenolphthalein* may cause a skin reaction. Stop using if this occurs.
- *Biscodyl suppositories* may cause proctitis and inflammation. Do not take these for long-term use.
- Pink-red, red-violet, yellow-brown or red-brown discoloration of the urine may occur, particularly with phenophthalein, senna or cascara sagrada.
- Some of these products may contain the dye tartrazine (FD&C Yellow No. 5) which can cause allergic reactions in certain individuals. Check package label when available or consult your doctor or pharmacist.
- Prevention of constipation includes: Adequate fluid intake (4 to 6 glasses of water daily), proper dietary habits including sufficient bulk or roughage, responding to the urge to defecate and daily exercise.
- Effects usually occur in 6 to 10 hours with most of these products, except castor oil (2 to 4 hours) and bisacodyl suppositories (15 to 60 minutes). Plan accordingly.
- Store at room temperature.

*If you have any questions, consult your doctor, pharmacist, or health care provider.*

| Generic Name Brand Name Examples | How Supplied | Generic Available |
|---|---|---|
| otc **Docusate Calcium** | | |
| *Correctol, Correctol Extra Gentle* | **Tablets:** 5 mg | No |
| *Correctol, DC Softgels, Pro-Cal-Sof, Surfak Liqui-gels[1], Sulfalax Calcium* | **Capsules:** 5 mg, 50 mg, 240 mg | Yes |
| *Correctol* | **Capsules, soft gel:** 100 mg | No |
| otc **Docusate Potassium** | | |
| *Diocto-K, Kasof* | **Capsules:** 100 mg, 240 mg | No |
| otc **Docusate Sodium** | | |
| *Dialose* | **Tablets:** 100 mg | No |
| *Colace, Colace-T, Disonate, Dioeze, DOK, DOS Softgel, D-S-S, Modane Soft, Pro-Sof Capsules, Regulax SS* | **Capsules:** 50 mg, 100 mg, 240 mg, 250 mg | Yes |
| *Colace[1], Diocto, Disonate, DOK, Silace* | **Syrup:** 50 mg/15 mL, 60 mg/15 mL | Yes |
| *Colace, Diocto, Disonate, DOK* | **Liquid:** 150 mg/15 mL | Yes |
| *Doxinate[1]* | **Solution:** 50 mg/mL | No |

[1] Contains alcohol.

Laxatives promote bowel emptying. Nonprescription laxatives are frequently misued due to lack of understanding of normal bowel function. Restrict self-medication to short-term therapy of constipation. Chronic use of laxatives (particularly stimulants) may lead to dependence. Prior to laxative use, consider living habits affecting bowel function including disease state and drug history. Rational therapy and prevention of constipation include: Adequate fluid intake (4 to 6 glasses of water daily), proper dietary habits including sufficient bulk or roughage, responding to the urge to defecate and daily exercise.

## Type of Drug:
Surfactant laxatives; fecal softeners.

## How the Drug Works:
Fecal softeners soften the stool by mixing fat and water into fecal matter. They are helpful when feces are hard or dry, or in conditions where passage of a firm stool is painful.

## Uses:

For short-term treatment of constipation.

To soften the stool in patients who should not strain at the stool (eg, patients who have had a heart attack or recent rectal surgery).

## Precautions:

*Do not use in the following situations:*

abdominal pain, undiagnosed
abdominal surgery
allergy to any ingredient of these
 products
appendicitis symptoms (nausea,
 vomiting, abdominal pain)
intestinal obstruction
mineral oil use (docusate
 sodium only)
stool impaction

*Frequent use of laxatives and inadequate fluid* can cause an imbalance in fluid and electrolyte levels. Symptoms may include muscle cramps, muscle weakness or dizziness.

*Rectal bleeding or failure of the laxative* to produce a bowel movement can indicate a more serious condition which requires medical attention.

*Pregnancy:* Adequate studies have not been done in pregnant women, or animal studies may have shown a risk to the fetus. Use only if clearly needed and potential benefits outweigh the possible hazards to the fetus.

*Breastfeeding:* It is not known if docusate sodium appears in breast milk. Consult your doctor before you begin breastfeeding.

## Drug Interactions:

Tell your doctor or pharmacist if you are taking or if you are planning to take any over-the-counter or prescription medications or dietary supplements while taking these products. Doses of one or both drugs may need to be modified or a different drug may need to be prescribed. Mineral oil interacts with docusate.

## Side Effects:

Every drug is capable of producing side effects. Many patients experience no, or minor, side effects. The frequency and severity of side effects depends on many factors including dose, duration of therapy and individual susceptibility. Possible side effects include:

*Digestive Tract:* Nausea; vomiting; stomach pain; bowel cramping; diarrhea; bloating; gas.

*Other:* Weakness; dizziness; fainting; irritation of the rectal area; sweating; pounding of the chest (palpitations).

## Guidelines for Use:

- Use exactly as prescribed.
- Laxative use is only a temporary measure. Do not use longer than one week. Stop use of these products when normal bowel habits return. Prolonged, frequent or excessive use may result in dependence or electrolyte imbalance.
- Take with a full glass of water or juice.
- Do not use if abdominal pain, nausea or vomiting occurs.
- Contact your doctor if unrelieved constipation, rectal bleeding, muscle cramps or pain, weakness or dizziness occurs.
- *Liquid* — Give in milk, fruit juice or infant formula to mask taste.
- *Enemas* — Add 1 or 2 tsp liquid to a retention or flushing enema.
- Prevention of constipation includes: Adequate fluid intake (4 to 6 glasses of water daily), proper dietary habits including sufficient bulk or roughage, responding to the urge to defecate and daily exercise.
- Effects usually occur in 24 to 72 hours with most of these products. Plan accordingly.
- Store at room temperature.

*If you have any questions, consult your doctor, pharmacist, or health care provider.*

| | Brand Name Examples | Docusate (mg) | Senna Combinations (mg) | Phenophthalein (mg) | Casanthranol (mg) | Cascara Sagrada (mg) | Sodium Carboxy-methylcellulose (mg) | Generic Available |
|---|---|---|---|---|---|---|---|---|
| otc | Gentlax S Tablets | 50[1] | 8.6[2] | | | | | No |
| otc | Senokot-S Tablets | 50[1] | 187 | | | | | No |
| otc | Doxidan Capsules, Docucal-P Softgels | 60[3] | | 65 | | | | No |
| otc | Ex-Lax Extra Gentle Pills | 75[1] | | 65 | | | | No |
| otc | Phillips' LaxCaps, Phillips' Laxative Gelcaps | 83[1] | | 90 | | | | No |
| otc | Colax Tablets, Correctol Tablets, Dialose Plus Capsules and Tablets, Disolan Capsules, Feen-a-mint Pills, Femilax Tablets, Modane Plus Tablets | 100[1] | | 65 | | | | No |
| otc | Unilax Capsules | 230[1] | | 130 | | | | No |
| otc | Disanthrol Capsules, Doxidan LiquiGels, Genasoft Plus Softgels, Peri-Colace Capsules, Peri-Dos Softgels, Pro-Sof Plus Capsules, Regulace Capsules | 100[1] | | | 30 | | | Yes |
| otc | Dialose Plus Capsules, Diocto-K Plus Capsules, Dioctolose Plus Capsules, DSMC Plus Capsules | 100[4] | | | 30 | | | Yes |
| otc | Disoplex Capsules | 100[1] | | | | | 400 | No |
| otc | Disolan Forte Capsules | 100[1] | | | 30 | | 400 | No |
| otc | Herbal Laxative Tablets[8] | | 125[5] | | | 20[6] | | No |

| | Brand Name Examples | Docusate (mg) | Senna Combinations (mg) | Phenophthalein (mg) | Casanthranol (mg) | Cascara Sagrada (mg) | Sodium Carboxy-methylcellulose (mg) | Generic Available |
|---|---|---|---|---|---|---|---|---|
| otc | Veracolate Tablets | | | 32.4 | | 75[7] | | No |
| otc | Nature's Remedy Tablets | | | | | 150 | | No |

[1] As sodium.
[2] As sennosides.
[3] As calcium.
[4] As potassium.

[5] As senna leaves.
[6] As cascara sagada bark.
[7] As extract.
[8] Sugar free.

Laxatives promote bowel emptying. Nonprescription laxatives are frequently misued due to lack of understanding of normal bowel function. Restrict self-medication to short-term therapy of constipation. Chronic use of laxatives (particularly stimulants) may lead to dependence. Prior to laxative use, consider living habits affecting bowel function including disease state and drug history. Rational therapy and prevention of constipation include: Adequate fluid intake (4 to 6 glasses of water daily), proper dietary habits including sufficient bulk or roughage, responding to the urge to defecate and daily exercise.

## Type of Drug:

Laxative combinations.

## Uses:

To treat constipation.

For more information on laxative ingredients, see the Laxatives – Stimulant and Laxatives – Stool Softeners monographs in this chapter. Casanthranol is a stimulant laxative used in laxative combinations.

## Guidelines for Use:

- Use exactly as prescribed.
- Take 1 or 2 at bedtime with a full glass of water.
- Do not use in the presense of abdominal pain, nausea or vomiting.
- Laxative use if only a tempeorary measure; do not use longer than 1 week. When regularity returns, discontiue use. Prolonged, frequent or excessive use may result in dependence or electrolyte imbalance.
- Contact your doctor if unrelieved constipation rectal bleeding or symptoms of electrolyte imbalance (eg, muscle cramps or pain, weakness, dizziness) occurs.
- Pink-red, red-violet or red-brown discoloration of alkaline urine may occur with cascara sagrada, phenolphthalein or senna.
- Prevention of constipation includes: Adequate fluid intake (4 to 6 glasses of water daily), proper dietary habits including sufficient bulk or roughage, responding to the urge to defecate and daily exercise.

*If you have any questions, consult your doctor, pharmacist, or health care provider.*

| | Brand Name Examples | Supplied As | Generic Available |
|---|---|---|---|
| otc | Agoral[1] | **Emulsion:** 4.2 m mineral oil and 0.2 g phenolphthalein per 15 mL in an emlulsion with agar, traga-canth, egg albumin, acacia and glycerin | No |
| otc | Haley's M-O[1] | **Emulsion:** 900 magnesium hydroxide and 3.75 mL mineral oil/15 mL | No |
| otc | Kondremul w/Phenolphtha-lein | **Emulsion:** 55% mineral oil and 150 mg phenolphthalein per 15 mL with Irish moss as an emul-sifier | No |
| otc | Liqui-Doss[1,2] | **Emulsion:** Mineral oil in an emulsifying base | No |
| otc | Black-Draught[3,4] | **Syrup:** 90 mg per 15 mL casanthranol with senna extract, fluid rhubarb aromatic, methyl salicylate and menthol | No |
| otc | Diocto C[3], Peri-Colace[3] | **Syrup:** 60 mg docusate sodium and 30 mL casanthranol/15 mL | Yes |
| otc | Silace-C[3] | **Syrup:** 30 mg casanthranol and 60 mL docusate sodium per 15 mL | No |

[1] Sugar free.
[2] Alcohol free.
[3] Contains alcohol.
[4] Contains the dye tartrazine.

Laxatives promote bowel emptying. Nonprescription laxatives are frequently misued due to lack of understanding of normal bowel function. Restrict self-medication to short-term therapy of constipation. Chronic use of laxatives (particularly stimulants) may lead to dependence. Prior to laxative use, con-sider living habits affecting bowel function including disease state and drug history. Rational therapy and prevention of constipation include: Adequate fluid intake (4 to 6 glasses of water daily), proper dietary habits including suf-ficient bulk or roughage, responding to the urge to defecate and daily exer-cise.

## Type of Drug:
Laxative combinations.

## Uses:
To treat constipation.

For more information on laxative ingredients, see the Laxatives – Stimulant and Laxatives – Stool Softeners monographs in this chapter. Casanthranol is a stimulant laxative used in laxative combinations.

## Guidelines for Use:

- Use exactly as prescribed.
- Take 5 to 45 mL at bedtime with a full glass of water.
- Do not use in the presence of abdominal pain, nausea or vomiting.
- Laxative use if only a temporary measure; do not use longer than 1 week. When regularity returns, discontinue use. Prolonged, frequent or excessive use may result in dependence or electrolyte imbalance.
- Contact your doctor if unrelieved constipation rectal bleeding or symptoms of electrolyte imbalance (eg, muscle cramps or pain, weakness, dizziness) occurs.
- Pink-red, red-violet or red-brown discoloration of alkaline urine may occur with cascara sagrada, phenolphthalein or senna.
- Some of these products may contain the dye tartrazine (FD&C Yellow No. 5) which can cause allergic reactions in certain individuals. Check package label when available or consult your doctor or pharmacist.
- Prevention of constipation includes: Adequate fluid intake (4 to 6 glasses of water daily), proper dietary habits including sufficient bulk or roughage, responding to the urge to defecate and daily exercise.
- Store at room temperature.

*If you have any questions, consult your doctor, pharmacist, or health care provider.*

| Generic Name<br>*Brand Name Examples* | Supplied As | Generic<br>Available |
|---|---|---|
| *Rx* **Polyethylene Glycol** | | |
| *Colyte, Colyte Flavored* | **Powder for oral solution:**<br>**1 gal:** 227.1 g polyethylene glycol 3350<br>**4 L:** 240 g polyethylene glycol 3350 | No |
| *GoLYTELY* | **Powder for oral solution:**<br>236 g polyethylene glycol 3350/4 L jug | No |
| *OCL* | **Oral solution:** 6 g polyethylene glycol 3350/100 mL | No |

## Type of Drug:

Bowel-cleansing agent administered prior to a diagnostic procedure on the lower portion of the colon.

## How the Drug Works:

Oral polyethylene glycol induces a diarrhea (onset, 30 to 60 minutes) that rapidly cleanses the bowel, usually within 4 hours. The electrolytes contained in the solution allow for the use of large volumes of this solution without significant changes in water or electrolyte balance.

## Uses:

For bowel cleansing prior to diagnostic examination of the lower portion of the colon.

## Precautions:

*Do not use in the following situations:*

allergy to polyethylene glycol or any of its ingredients
bowel perforation
ileus
obstruction of digestive tract
retention of stomach contents
toxic colitis
toxic megacolon

*Use with caution in the following situations:*

impaired gag reflex
regurgitation- or aspiration-prone
ulcerative colitis, severe
unconscious or semiconscious patients

*Pregnancy:* Safety for use during pregnancy has not been established. Use only if clearly needed and the potential benefits outweigh the possible hazards to the fetus.

*Children:* Safety and effectiveness in children have not been established.

## Drug Interactions:

Tell your doctor or pharmacist if you are taking or if you are planning to take any over-the-counter or prescription medications or dietary supplements while using polyethylene glycol. Doses of one or both drugs may need to be modified or a different drug may need to be prescribed. Do not take oral medications within 1 hour of starting polyethylene glycol solution.

## Side Effects:

Every drug is capable of producing side effects. Many polyethylene glycol users experience no, or minor, side effects. Possible side effects include: Nausea; stomach fullness; bloating; stomach cramps; vomiting; anal irritation.

## Guidelines for Use:

- Recommended adult dosage is 4 liters of solution prior to the exam. Drink 8 oz every 10 minutes until the watery stool is clear and free of solid matter or until the 4 liters are consumed. Rapid drinking of each portion is preferred to drinking small amounts continuously. The first bowel movement should occur in about 1 hour.
- *Preparation of solution from powder* — Lukewarm tap water may be used. Shake container vigorously several times to ensure that the powder is completely dissolved. Prepare solution ahead of time and store in refrigerator since solution is more palatable if chilled.
- Do not add additional ingredients (eg, flavorings) to the solution before use.
- Polyethylene glycol is usually administered orally but may be given via nasogastric tube to patients who are unwilling or unable to drink the solution. Nasogastric tube administration is at the rate of 20 to 30 mL/minute. The first bowel movement should occur approximately 1 hour after the start of administration.
- Fasting 3 to 4 hours before drinking the solution produces the best results. However, do not eat solid foods less than 2 hours before solution is administered.
- For midmorning examination, allow 3 hours for drinking and 1 hour to complete bowel evacuation, or drink the solution the evening before the examination, particularly if you are to have a barium enema.
- No foods except clear liquids are permitted after administration of the solution.
- You may experience some stomach bloating and discomfort before the bowels start to move. If severe discomfort or distention occur, stop drinking temporarily or drink each portion at longer intervals until these symptoms disappear.
- Oral medication administered within 1 hour of the start of administration of the solution may be flushed from the gastrointestinal tract and not absorbed.
- Store powder at controlled room temperature (59° to 86°F). Refrigerate the reconstituted solution. Use within 48 hours. Discard unused portion. Store *OCL* solution at room temperature (59° to 86°F). Protect from excessive heat and freezing.

*If you have any questions, consult your doctor, pharmacist, or health care provider.*

|  | Brand Name Examples | Supplied As |
|---|---|---|
| otc | Evac-Q-Kwik | 300 mL magnesium citrate |
|  |  | 3 bisacodyl tablets (5 mg/tablet)[1,2] |
|  |  | 1 bisacodyl suppository (10 mg) |
| otc | Fleet Prep Kit # 1 | 45 mL phospho-soda (21.6 g monobasic sodium phosphate, 8.1 g dibasic sodium phosphate) |
|  |  | 4 bisacodyl tablets (5 mg/tablet) |
|  |  | 1 bisacodyl suppository (10 mg) |
| otc | Fleet Prep Kit # 2 | 45 mL phospho-soda (21.6 g monobasic sodium phosphate, 8.1 g dibasic sodium phosphate) |
|  |  | 4 bisacodyl tablets (5 mg/tablet) |
|  |  | 1 bagenema |
| otc | Fleet Prep Kit # 3 | 45 mL phospho-soda (21.6 g monobasic sodium phosphate, 8.1 g dibasic sodium phosphate) |
|  |  | 4 bisacodyl tablets (5 mg/tablet) |
|  |  | 30 ml bisacodyl enema (10 mg) |
| otc | Tridrate Dry Bowel Cleansing System | 19 g magnesium citrate powder |
|  |  | 3 bisacodyl tablets (5 mg/tablet) |
|  |  | 1 bisacodyl suppository (10 mg) |
| otc | X-Prep Bowel Evacuant Kit-1 | 74 mL extract of senna concentrate (130 mg sennosides)[3,4] |
|  |  | 2 tablets (8.6 mg sennosides, 50 mg docusate sodium per tablet)[1] |
|  |  | 1 bisacodyl suppository (10 mg) |
| otc | X-Prep Bowel Evacuant Kit-2 | 74 mL extract of senna concentrate (130 mg sennosides)[3,4,5] |
|  |  | 30 g granules (8 g magnesium citrate, 5.3 g magnesium sulfate)[4,6] |
|  |  | 1 bisacodyl suppository (10 mg) |
| otc | X-Prep Senna Liquid Bowel Evacuant | 74 mL extract of senna concentrate (130 mg sennosides, 50 g sugar)[3,4] |

[1] Contains lactose.
[2] Contains sugar.
[3] Contains parabens.
[4] Contains sucrose.
[5] Contains alcohol.
[6] Contains saccharin.

## Type of Drug:
Bowel-cleansing drugs.

## Uses:

For bowel cleansing prior to examination or surgery of the digestive tract.

## Precautions:

*Do not use in the following situations:*

kidney disease (*Fleet Prep Kits # 1, 2, and 3; Evac-Q-Kwik; Tridrate; X-Prep Bowel Evacuant Kit-2*)

magnesium-restricted diet (*Evac-Q-Kwik, X-Prep Bowel Evacuant Kit-2; Tridrate*)

megacolon

sodium-restricted diet (*Fleet Prep Kits # 1, 2, and 3*)

*Children:* Safety and effectiveness in children under 5 years of age have not been established.

## Side Effects:

Every drug is capable of producing side effects. Many bowel evacuant kit users experience no, or minor, side effects. The frequency and severity of side effects depend on many factors including dose, duration of therapy, and individual susceptibility, Possible side effects include:

*Other:* Stomach discomfort; faintness; rectal burning; stomach cramps.

---

### Guidelines for Use:

- Review kit insert for complete instructions. Instructions include eating guidelines, minimum fluid requirements, and timing of use of bowel evacuant kit components. Follow directions exactly to ensure best results and to avoid the need for repeat examination.
- Take with a glass of water.
- Do not use for longer than 1 week unless directed by your doctor.
- Consult a doctor before use if you notice a sudden change in bowel habits that persists more than 2 weeks.
- Consult your doctor if you are pregnant, planning to become pregnant, or are breastfeeding.
- Do not use when abdominal pain, nausea, or vomiting are present unless directed to do so by your doctor.
- Notify your doctor immediately if you experience rectal bleeding or a failure to respond to the bowel evacuant.
- Continue to take prescription medications as scheduled, unless advised differently by your doctor.

---

*If you have any questions, consult your doctor, pharmacist, or health care provider.*

| Generic Name<br>*Brand Name Examples* | Supplied As | Generic<br>Available |
|---|---|---|
| *otc* **Bismuth Subsalicylate** | | |
| *Pepto-Bismol*[1,2] | **Tablets:** 262 mg | No |
| *Pepto-Bismol*[1,2] | **Tablets, chewable:** 262 mg | Yes |
| *Pepto-Bismol*[1,2] | **Suspension:** 262 mg/15 mL | Yes |
| *Pepto-Bismol,*<br>*Maximum Strength*[1,2] | **Suspension:** 525 mg/15 mL | No |

[1] Low sodium.
[2] Sugar free.

## Type of Drug:

Antidiarrheal; drug for indigestion.

## How the Drug Works:

The exact mechanism of action of bismuth subsalicylate is not known; however, it appears to reduce stomach secretions, reduce inflammation, and inhibit some bacterial and viral organisms capable of producing intestinal tract diseases.

## Uses:

To control diarrhea, including traveler's diarrhea (generally within 24 hours).

To treat indigestion (eg, upset stomach, heartburn) without causing constipation.

To treat nausea.

To relieve stomach cramps.

*Unlabeled Use(s):* Occasionally doctors and pharmacist may recommend bismuth subsalicylate to prevent traveler's diarrhea and to treat infantile diarrhea.

## Precautions:

*Do not use in the following situations:*
allergy to bismuth subsalicylate
allergy to salicylates (aspirin)

*Use with caution in the following situations:*
chickenpox (children)     radiologic (x-ray) examinations
flu (children)     of GI tract

*Pregnancy:* This product contains salicylates. Do not take bismuth subsalicylate during pregnancy, especially during the third trimester.

*Breastfeeding:* Salicylates appear in breast milk. If bismuth subsalicylate is needed, the patient should stop breastfeeding.

*Children:* Impaction (severe constipation) may occur in infants. Consult your doctor before using in children under 3 years of age.

## Drug Interactions:

Tell your doctor or pharmacist if you are taking or if you are planning to take any over-the-counter or prescription medications or dietary supplements with bismuth subsalicylate. Doses of one or both drugs may need to be modified or a different drug may need to be prescribed. The following drugs and drug classes interact with bismuth subsalicylate.

anticoagulants, oral (eg, warfarin)
corticosteroids (eg, hydrocortisone)
insulin (*Humulin*, *Iletin*)
methotrexate (eg, *Rheumatrex*)

salicylates (eg, aspirin)
spironolactone (eg, *Aldactone)*
sulfinpyrazone (eg, *Anturane)*
tetracyclines (eg, doxycycline)
valproic acid (eg, *Depakene)*

## Side Effects:

Every drug is capable of producing side effects. Many bismuth subsalicylate users experience no, or minor, side effects. Possible side effects include severe constipation, darkening of tongue, and darkening of stools.

Consider all side effects and drug interactions reported for salicylates when using bismuth subsalicylate. See Analgesics – Aspirin and Salicylates monograph in the CNS drugs chapter.

## Guidelines for Use:

- Dosage for tablets and chewable tablets for adults is 2 tablets. For children ages 9 to 12 years old, 1 tablet; children 6 to 9 years old, 2/3 of a tablet; and children 3 to 6 years old 1/3 of a tablet.
- Dosing for suspension for adults is 2 tbsp (30 mL). For children ages 9 to 12, 1 tbsp (15 mL); children 6 to 9 years old, 2 tsp (10 mL); and children 3 to 6, 1 tsp (5 mL).
- Dose may be repeated every 30 to 60 minutes if needed. Do not take more than 8 doses in 24 hours (regular strength) or 4 doses in 24 hours (maximum strength).
- Shake suspension well before using.
- Chewable tablets may be chewed or allowed to dissolve in mouth. Do not swallow whole.
- Swallow regular tablets whole with a glass of water. Do not chew regular tablets.
- Drink plenty of fluids to prevent dehydration which may accompany diarrhea.
- May cause temporary and harmLess darkening of the tongue or stool.
- If taken with other salicylate-containing products (eg, aspirin), and ringing in the ears occurs, discontinue use.
- Contact your doctor if diarrhea is accompanied by high fever or if diarrhea continues for more than 2 days.
- Do not use to treat nausea or vomiting in children or teenagers with the flu or chickenpox without consulting a doctor. If nausea or vomiting is present, consult a doctor because this could be an early sign of Reye syndrome, a rare but serious illness.
- *Suspension:* Store at room temperature. Refrigeration may improve taste. Avoid excessive heat and protect from freezing.
- *Tablets:* Avoid excessive heat.

*If you have any questions, consult your doctor, pharmacist, or health care provider.*

| Generic Name<br>*Brand Name Examples* | Supplied As | Generic<br>Available |
|---|---|---|
| c-iv **Difenoxin with Atropine Sulfate** | | |
| *Motofen* | **Tablets:** 1 mg difenoxin, 0.025 mg atropine sulfate | No |
| c-v **Diphenoxylate with Atropine Sulfate** | | |
| *Lomotil, Lonox* | **Tablets:** 2.5 mg diphenoxylate, 0.025 mg atropine sulfate | Yes |
| *Lomotil* | **Liquid:** 2.5 mg diphenoxylate, 0.025 mg atropine sulfate/5 mL | Yes |

## Type of Drug:

Antidiarrheal.

## How the Drug Works:

Difenoxin and diphenoxylate, related to the narcotic pain reliever meperidine, act on intestinal tract muscles and slow intestinal motility. Atropine is present to discourage deliberate misuse of these drugs.

## Uses:

To relieve diarrhea.

## Precautions:

*Do not use in the following situations:*
>   allergy to the drug or any of its ingredients
>   children under 2 years of age
>   diarrhea associated with antibiotic therapy (eg, pseudomembranous colitis)
>   diarrhea associated with enterotoxin-producing bacteria (eg, toxigenic *E. coli*, *Salmonella*, *Shigella*)
>   jaundice (yellowing of skin or eyes)

*Use with caution in the following situations:*

children (diphenoxylate only)
dehydration
Down syndrome (diphenoxylate only)
drug addiction, history
kidney disease
liver disease
MAOI use, concurrent
patients receiving addictive drugs
ulcerative colitis, acute

*Diphenoxylate can be habit forming.* If you have been taking large doses and suddenly stop taking the medication, symptoms of withdrawal may occur. These symptoms include muscle cramps, stomach cramps, "goose bumps," unusual sweating, nausea, vomiting, and shaking or trembling. Recommended doses used to treat diarrhea do not cause addiction.

*Pregnancy:* Adequate studies have not been done in pregnant women. Use only if clearly needed and potential benefits outweigh the possible hazards to the fetus.

*Breastfeeding:* Difenoxin and diphenoxylate may appear in breast milk. Atropine appears in breast milk. Because of the potential for serious side effects in nursing infants, a decision should be made whether to discontinue nursing or to discontinue the drug, taking into account the importance of the drug to the mother.

*Children:* Do not use difenoxin tablets or diphenoxylate liquid in children under 2 years of age. Do not use diphenoxylate tablets in children under 13 years of age. Safety and effectiveness of difenoxin tablets have not been established in children under 12 years of age. Use with caution in children with Down syndrome due to presence of atropine.

## Drug Interactions:
Tell your doctor or pharmacist if you are taking or if you are planning to take any over-the-counter or prescription medications or dietary supplements with antidiarrheals containing difenoxin, diphenoxylate, or atropine sulfate. Doses of one or both drugs may need to be modified or a different drug may need to be prescribed. The following drugs and drug classes interact with antidiarrheals containing difenoxin, diphenoxylate, or atropine sulfate.

alcohol
barbiturates (eg, phenobarbital)
MAOIs (eg, isocarboxazid, phenelzine, tranylcypromine, selegiline)

narcotic pain relievers (eg, meperidine)
tranquilizers (eg, benzodiazepines)

## Side Effects:
Every drug is capable of producing side effects. Many antidiarrheal users experience no, or minor, side effects. The frequency and severity of side effects depend on many factors including dose, duration of therapy, and individual susceptibility. Possible side effects include:

*Both:* Nausea; vomiting; dizziness; drowsiness; headache.

*Difenoxin only:* Constipation; lightheadedness; dry mouth; stomach pain.

*Diphenoxylate only:* Stomach ache; appetite loss; toxic megacolon; paralytic ileus; pancreatitis; restlessness; confusion; depression; exaggerated sense of well-being; itching; hives; swelling of gums; numbness of arms or legs; general body discomfort; allergic reaction.

*Atropine only:* Dry skin; flushing; fever; fast heartbeat; urinary retention.

## Guidelines for Use:

- *Difenoxin* — Starting dose in adults is 2 mg by mouth, then 1 mg after each loose stool or 1 mg every 3 to 4 hours as needed. Total dose in any 24-hour period should not exceed 8 mg.
- *Diphenoxylate* — Initial dosage in adults is 2 tablets by mouth 4 times daily or 10 mL (2 tsp) of liquid 4 times daily (20 mg/day). Once control of diarrhea is achieved, reduce the dose to the lowest possible level (eg, 2 tablets daily) to maintain control.
  Do not use tablets for children under 13 years of age. Only use the plastic dropper included with the liquid to measure doses for children. Doses for children must be carefully determined. Talk to your doctor or pharmacist about the correct dose for your child.
- If clinical improvement of acute diarrhea is not observed within 48 hours, do not continue the medication. If improvement of chronic diarrhea is not seen within 10 days of using diphenoxylate (with a maximum daily dose of 20 mg), symptoms are unlikely to be controlled by further administration.
- Do not take more than the prescribed dose.
- Appropriate fluid and electrolyte therapy should be used in conjunction with diphenoxylate therapy in the treatment of diarrhea in children.
- Avoid alcohol and other sedatives that may cause drowsiness.
- May cause drowsiness or dizziness. Use caution when performing tasks requiring alertness, coordination, or physical dexterity.
- May cause dry mouth. Chew sugarless gum or suck sugarless hard candies if desired.
- Keep out of reach of children because accidental overdose may result in severe, even fatal, breathing problems.
- Notify your doctor if diarrhea persists or if fever, rapid heart rate, or stomach swelling occur.
- Store at room temperature (59° to 86°F) in a child resistant container. Protect diphenoxylate from light.

*If you have any questions, consult your doctor, pharmacist, or health care provider.*

| Generic Name<br>*Brand Name Examples* | Supplied As | Generic<br>Available |
|---|---|---|
| *otc* **Lactobacillus** | | |
| *Bacid* | **Capsules:** Cultured strain of not less than 500 million viable L acidophilus with 100 mg sodium carboxymethylcellulose | No |
| *Lactinex* | **Granules** | No |
| *Lactinex* | **Chewable tablets** | No |
| *More-Dophilus[1]* | **Powder:** 4 billion units of acidophilus-carrot derivative/g | No |

[1] Sugar free.

## Type of Drug:
Antidiarrheal.

## How the Drug Works:
Lactobacillus creates a more normal bacterial environment in the digestive tract and prevents the growth of unfavorable bacteria that may contribute to diarrhea.

## Uses:
To treat uncomplicated diarrhea, including diarrhea due to long-term antibiotic therapy.

To treat fever blisters (cold sores).

## Precautions:
*Do not use in the following situations:*
allergy to milk or lactose

*Use with caution in the following situations:*
children under 3 years of age
presence of high fever

---

## Guidelines for Use:
- Some of the available products need to be refrigerated. Check package label.
- Do not use for more than 2 days unless directed by your doctor.
- If high fever is present, do not use unless directed by your doctor.

---

*If you have any questions, consult your doctor, pharmacist, or health care provider.*

| Generic Name<br>Brand Name Examples | Supplied As | Generic<br>Available |
|---|---|---|
| **Loperamide HCl** | | |
| Rx  Imodium | **Capsules:** 2 mg | No |
| otc  Imodium A-D Caplets,<br>Kaopectate II Caplets,<br>Maalox Anti-Diarrheal<br>Caplets | **Tablets:** 2 mg | No |
| otc  Imodium A-D[1],<br>Pepto Diarrhea Control | **Liquid:** 1 mg/tsp | Yes |

[1] Contains alcohol.

## Type of Drug:

Antidiarrheal.

## How the Drug Works:

Loperamide decreases movement of the digestive tract. This allows more time for reabsorption of water and electrolytes from the stool.

## Uses:

For relief of nonspecific acute diarrhea, chronic diarrhea associated with inflammatory bowel disease and for Traveler's diarrhea.

To deacrease the volume of discharge from ileostomies.

## Precautions:

*Do not use in the following situations:*
     allergy to loperamide
     blood in the stools
     high fever

*Use with caution in the following situations:*
     diarrhea associated with antibiotic therapy
     liver disease
     ulcerative colitis

*Pregnancy:* There are no adequate and well-controlled studies in pregnant women. Safety for use during pregnancy has not been established. Use only when clearly needed and when the potential benefits outweigh the potential hazards to the fetus.

*Breastfeeding:* It is not known if loperamide appears in breast milk. Consult your doctor before you begin breastfeeding.

*Children:* Not recommended in children under 6. Use with caution and consult your doctor.

## Drug Interactions:

Tell your doctor or pharmacist if you are taking of if you are planning to take any over-the-counter or prescription medications or dietary supplements with loperamide. Doses of one or both drugs may need to be modified or a different drug may need to be prescribed. Cholestyramine (*Questran*) interacts with loperamide.

## Side Effects:

Every drug is capable of producing side effects. Many loperamide users experience no, or minor, side effects. The frequency and severity of side effects depend on many factors including dose, duration of therapy and individual susceptibility. Possible side effects include:

*Digestive Tract:* Constipation; nausea; vomiting; appetite loss; stomach ache; abdominal distention or bloating.

*Other:* Dry mouth; fever; rash; drowsiness; dizziness.

---

### Guidelines for Use:

- Do not take more than the prescribed dose.
- May cause drowsiness or dizziness. Use caution when driving or performing other tasks requiring alertness, coordination or physical dexterity.
- Drink plenty of clear fluids to help prevent dehydration, which may accompany diarrhea.
- May cause dry mouth. Chew sugarless gum or suck sugarless hard candies if desired.
- Notify your doctor if diarrhea does not stop after a few days or if abdominal pain, distention or fever occurs.

---

*If you have any questions, consult your doctor, pharmacist, or health care provider.*

| Generic Name *Brand Name Examples* | Supped As | Generic Available |
|---|---|---|
| **Opiate-containing combinations** | | |
| c-ii *Opium Tincture*[1] | **Solution:** 10 mg opium/2 tsp | |
| c-iii *Paregoric*[1] | **Solution:** 2 mg morphine/1 tsp | Yes |
| c-ii *B&O Suprettes* | **Suppositories:** 30 mg opium, 16.2 mg belladonna | Yes |
| c-ii *B&O Suprettes* | **Suppositories:** 60 mg opium, 16.2 mg belladonna | Yes |
| otc **Opiate-free combinations** | | |
| *Rheaban* | **Tablets:** 750 mg activated attapulgite. Pectin. | No |
| *Kaopectate* | **Tablets:** 750 mg attapulgite | No |
| *Donnagel* | **Tablets, chewable:** 600 mg activated attapulgite | No |
| *Devrom* | **Tablets, chewable:** 200 mg bismuth subgallate | No |
| *Kaopectate* | **Liquid:** 750 mg attapulgite/tbsp | No |
| *Kao-Tin* | **Liquid:** 750 mg attapulgite/tbsp | Yes |
| *Diasorb*[2] | **Liquid:** 750 mg activated attapulgite/tsp | No |
| *Children's Kaopectate* | **Liquid:** 300 mg attapulgite/ ½ tbsp | No |
| *K-Pek* | **Suspension:** 750 mg attapulgite/tbsp | Yes |
| *Donnagel*[1] | **Suspension:** 600 mg activated attapulgite/2 tbsp | Yes |
| *Kaolin w/Pectin, Kapectolin* | **Suspension:** 5.85 g kaolin and 130 mg pectin/2 tbsp | Yes |
| *Kao-Spen* | **Suspension:** 5.2 g kaolin and 260 mg pectin/2 tbsp | No |
| *K-C* | **Suspension:** 5.2 g kaolin, 260 mg pectin, and 260 mg bismuth subcarbonate/2 tbsp | No |
| *Kaodene Non-Narcotic* | **Suspension:** 3.9 g kaolin, 194.4 mg pectin, and bismuth subsalicylate/2 tbsp | No |

[1] Contains alcohol.
[2] Sugar free.

## Type of Drug:

Antidiarrheal combination products.

## How the Drug Works:

These drugs reduce intestinal movement, absorb fluid, reduce the severity of intestinal inflammation and modify intestinal bacteria.

## Uses:

To treat diarrhea and the cramps and pain that accompany it. Adequate controlled studies demonstrating the effectiveness of these antidiarrheal combinations are lacking.

*Opium (tincture, powder, or paregoric)* is used to reduce the intestinal activity, to relieve the urge to have a bowel movement without success and to relieve the pain associated with diarrhea.

*Belladonna alkaloids* are used to control hyperactivity and increased secretion in the digestive tract.

*Activated attapulgite, kaolin and pectin* are used for their absorbent actions to bind up and remove digestive tract irritants.

*Bismuth salts (see Antidiarrheals – Bismuth Subsalicylate in this chapter)* have antacid and absorbent properties.

## Precautions:

*Do not use opium-containing products in the following situations:*

| | |
|---|---|
| glaucoma | convulsive disorders |
| hepatic disease, severe | acute alcoholism |
| renal disease, severe | delirium tremens |
| bronchial asthma | premature labor |
| narcotic idiosyncrasies | diarrhea caused by poisoning |
| respiratory depression | |

*Use opium-containing products with caution in the following situations:*

| | |
|---|---|
| idiosyncrasy to atropine or atropine-like compounds | cerebral arteriosclerosis |
| | hepatic cirrhosis |
| addiction to morphine or morphine-like products | liver insufficiency |
| | gastrointestinal hemorrhage |
| cardiac disease | myxedema |
| glaucoma, incipient | emphysema |
| prostatic hypertrophy | bronchial asthma |
| debilitated patients | toxic psychosis |
| increased intracranial pressure | |

Addiction may result from opium usage.

*Pregnancy:* Adequate studies have not been done in pregnant women. Use only if clearly needed and potential benefits to the mother outweigh the possible hazards to the fetus.

*Breastfeeding:* It is not known if opium appears in breast milk. Consult your doctor before you begin breastfeeding.

*Children:* Not for use in children younger than 13 years of age.

*Elderly:* Use with caution in the elderly.

## Drug Interactions:

Tell your doctor or pharmacist if you are taking of if you are planning to take any over-the-counter or prescription medications or dietary supplements with this drug. Doses of one or both drugs may need to be modified or a different drug may need to be prescribed. CNS depressants interact with this drug.

## Side Effects:

Every drug is capable of producing side effects. Many ptients experience no, or minor, side effects. The frequency and severity of side effects depend on many factors including dose, duration of therapy, and individual susceptibility. Possible side effects include: blurred vision; constipation; dizziness; drowsiness; dry mouth; hives, rash; itching; nausea; photophobia; rapid pulse; urinary retention; vomiting.

---

### Guidelines for Use:

- Follow individual product instructions.
- Do not use if diarrhea is accompanied by a fever or if blood or mucus is present in stool.
- If severe diarrhea, stomach pain/cramps, or bloody stools occur, contact your doctor immediately. This could be a symptom of a serious side effect requiring immediate medical attention. Do not treat diarrhea without first consulting your doctor.
- If you are taking a prescription medicine, consult your doctor before taking these products.
- Inform your doctor if you are pregnant or nursing a baby.
- Drink clear fluids to prevent dehydration.
- Do not use agents that slow digestive tract motility for diarrhea associated with antibiotic-caused colitis or in diarrhea caused by bacteria.
- Do not use these preparations for more than 2 days, in the presence of high fever or in infants and children under 3, except under a doctor's direction.
- Salicylate absorption may occur from bismuth sabsalicylate. Observe caution in patients with bleeding disorders or aspirin sensitivity and in children.
- *Liquids* — Shake well before using.
- Store at room temperature (68° to 77°F).

---

*If you have any questions, consult your doctor, pharmacist, or health care provider.*

| Generic Name<br>*Brand Name Examples* | Supplied As | Generic<br>Available |
|---|---|---|
| *Rx* **Balsalazide Disodium** | | |
| *Colazal* | **Capsules**: 750 mg | No |
| *Rx* **Mesalamine (5-ASA)** | | |
| *Asacol* | **Tablets, delayed-release**: 400 mg | No |
| *Rowasa* | **Suppositories**: 500 mg | Yes |
| *Rowasa*[1] | **Suspension, rectal**: 4 g/60 mL | No |
| *Rx* **Olsalazine Sodium** | | |
| *Dipentum* | **Capsules**: 250 mg | No |

[1] Contains sulfites.

## Type of Drug:

Intestinal anti-inflammatory agents.

## How the Drug Works:

The exact mechanism of action of the 5-aminosalicylic acid (5-ASA) agents is unknown. They appear to work topically, reducing inflammation of the colon by preventing the production of substances involved in the inflammatory process.

## Uses:

*Balsalazide Disodium:* To treat mild to moderate active ulcerative colitis (inflammation of the colon or rectum).

*Mesalamine:* To treat mild to moderate inflammation of the colon or rectum (eg, ulcerative colitis) and to reduce chances of reoccurance (delayed-release tablets).

To treat active mild to moderate distal ulcerative colitis, proctosigmoiditis, or proctitis (rectal suppositories and suspension).

*Olsalazine Sodium:* To reduce the chances that ulcerative colitis will reoccur in patients who cannot take sulfasalazine.

## Precautions:

*Do not use in the following situations:*
allergy to the 5-ASA agent or any of its ingredients
allergy to salicylates (eg, aspirin)

*Use with caution in the following situations:*
allergy to sulfasalazine, history of
kidney disease
pyloric stenosis (tablets and capsules only)
sulfite sensitivity (rectal suspension only)

*Intolerance:* Mesalamine can cause an intolerance syndrome characterized by cramping, acute stomach pain, bloody diarrhea, fever, headache, and rash. Prompt withdrawal is required. Consult your doctor.

*Worsening of symptoms:* Worsening of symptoms of colitis (thought to have been caused by mesalamine or sulfasalazine) has occurred.

*Pregnancy:* There are no adequate and well-controlled studies in pregnant women. Use during pregnancy only if clearly needed and the potential benefits to the mother outweigh the possible hazards to the fetus.

*Breastfeeding:* Oral mesalamine appears in breast milk. It is not known if rectal mesalamine, balsalazide, or olsalazine appear in breast milk. Consult your doctor before you begin breastfeeding.

*Children:* Safety and effectiveness in children have not been established.

*Sulfites:* Some of these products contain sulfite preservatives that can cause allergic reactions in certain individuals. Check package label when available or consult your doctor or pharmacist.

## Drug Interactions:

Tell your doctor or pharmacist if you are taking or if you are planning to take any over-the-counter or prescription medications or dietary supplements with 5-ASA. Doses of one or both drugs may need to be modified or a different drug may need to be prescribed. Thiopurines (eg, mercaptopurine) and anticoagulants (eg, warfarin) interact with olsalazine.

## Side Effects:

Every drug is capable of producing side effects. Many 5-ASA users experience no, or minor, side effects. The frequency and severity of side effects depend on many factors including dose, duration of therapy, and individual susceptibility. Possible side effects include:

*Digestive Tract:* Diarrhea; constipation; frequent stools; indigestion; heartburn; bloating; gas; stomach pain or cramps; nausea; vomiting; belching; worsening of colitis; appetitie loss; rectal bleeding; mouth inflammation.

*Nervous System:* Dizziness; headache; tiredness; weakness; disorientation; sleeplessness; fatigue; drowsiness; depression; vertigo (feeling of whirling motion); lightheadedness.

*Other:* Sweating; chills; hair loss; fever; flu-like symptoms; cough; muscle pain, cramps, or tension; general pain; painful urination; fever; leg, back, chest, joint, or rectal pain; hemorrhoids; sore throat; edema (fluid retention); general body discomfort; dry mouth; sore throat; congestion; runny nose; sinus inflammation; upper respiratory infection; painful menstruation; eye inflammation; hives; rash; itching; acne; increased bowel swelling; urinary tract infection.

## Guidelines for Use:

- Dosage is individualized. Take exactly as prescribed.
- If a dose is missed, take it as soon as possible. If several hours have passed or if it is nearing time for the next dose, do not double the dose to catch up, unless advised by your doctor. If more than one dose is missed, or it is necessary to establish a new dosage schedule, contact your doctor or pharmacist.
- Inform your doctor if you are pregnant, become pregnant, planning to become pregnant, or are breastfeeding.

*Mesalamine:*
- Tablets — Swallow whole. Do not break outer coating. Intact or partially intact tablets may appear in stool. Contact your doctor if this occurs repeatedly.
- Rectal suspension — For rectal use only. Review the patient instructions included. Shake bottle well. Remove protective sheath from the applicator tip. Holding the bottle at the neck will not allow medication to be discharged. The position most often used is to lie on the left side (to help flow into the sigmoid colon), with the lower leg extended and the upper right leg bent forward for balance. An alternative is the knee-chest position. Gently insert the applicator tip in the rectum pointing toward the navel. A steady squeezing of the bottle will discharge most of the preparation. After administering, withdraw and discard the bottle. Remain in position for at least 30 minutes.
- Suspension should be given once daily, preferably at bedtime. The drug should be retained in the rectum all night if possible.
- Suppositories — Usual dosage is twice daily. The drug should be retained in the rectum for 1 to 3 hours or longer. Review the patient instructions included for the proper insertion technique.
- Improvement may not be seen for up to 3 weeks. Usual treatment is one enema or 2 suppositories daily for 3 to 6 weeks.
- Contents of suspension and suppositories can cause staining of clothes, sheets, or flooring. Choose a location where this will not be a problem.
- Store tablets at controlled room temperature (68° to 77°F); store suspension at room temperature (59° to 86°F); store suppositories at a temperature of 66° to 79°F.

*Olsalazine sodium:*
- Take with food. Take in evenly divided doses.
- May cause diarrhea in some patients. Contact your doctor if diarrhea occurs.
- Contact your doctor before stopping treatment. Abrupt withdrawal may cause adverse effects.
- Store at room temperature (59° to 86°F).

*Balsalazide disodium:*
- Store at room temperature (59° to 86°F).

*If you have any questions, consult your doctor, pharmacist, or health care provider.*

| Generic Name *Brand Name Example* | Supplied As | Generic Available |
|---|---|---|
| Rx **Infliximab** | | |
| *Remicade* | **Powder for injection**: 100 mg/20 mL vial | No |

## Type of Drug:

Immunomodulator; monoclonal antibody.

## How the Drug Works:

Infliximab inhibits certain proteins (tissue necrosis factor) responsible for the inflammation and immune responses that may cause Crohn disease and rheumatoid arthritis.

## Uses:

For reducing the signs and symptoms of moderately to severely active Crohn disease in patients who have had an inadequate response to conventional therapy.

For reducing the number of draining abdominal fistulas in fistulizing Crohn disease.

For use in combination with methotrexate to reduce signs and symptoms of rheumatoid arthritis in patients who have had an inadequate response to methotrexate alone.

## Precautions:

*Do not use in the following situations:*
allergy to the drug or any of its ingredients (eg, mice proteins)
congestive heart failure, moderate to severe
live vaccinations, concurrent

*Use with caution in the following situations:*
CNS demyelinating disease, current or history of
congestive heart failure, mild
immunosuppression
infection, chronic or recurrent
seizure disorder

*Autoimmune antibodies:* Auto antibodies may develop and, rarely, a lupus-like syndrome (eg, difficulty breathing, chest pain, joint pain) may occur.

*Tuberculosis:* A TB skin test should be administered before starting therapy to check for latent tuberculosis. Treatment of latent TB should be started before beginning therapy with infliximab.

*Pregnancy:* It is not known whether infliximab can cause fetal harm when administered to a pregnant woman. Use only if clearly needed and the potential benefits outweigh the possible hazards to the fetus.

*Breastfeeding:* It is not known if infliximab appears in breast milk. Consult your doctor before you begin breastfeeding.

*Children:* Safety and effectiveness have not been established.

*Elderly:* There is a higher incidence of infections in the elderly population in general. Use caution when administering infliximab to elderly patients.

## Drug Interactions:

Tell your doctor or pharmacist if you are taking or planning to take any over-the-counter or prescription medications or dietary supplements with this drug. Doses of one or both drugs may need to be modified or a different drug may need to be prescribed. Specific studies on drug interactions have not been conducted; however, immunosuppressants and live vaccines may interact with this drug.

## Side Effects:

Every drug is capable of producing side effects. Many patients experience no, or minor, side effects. The frequency and severity of side effects depend on many factors including dose, duration of therapy, and individual susceptibility. Possible side effects include:

*Digestive Tract:* Diarrhea; nausea; stomach pain or swelling; vomiting; indigestion; difficulty swallowing.

*Nervous System:* Headache; fatigue; dizziness; depression; sleeplessness.

*Respiratory System:* Difficulty breathing; upper or lower respiratory tract infection; sinus infection; cough; sore throat; throat inflammation.

*Skin:* Itching; fungal skin infection; hot flushes.

*Other:* Infections; muscle, joint, or back pain; swelling; abscess; fluid retention (edema); urinary tract infection; heart failure; high blood pressure.

*Infusion Reactions:* Fever; chills; itching; rash; hives; chest pain; low blood pressure; high blood pressure; difficulty breathing; flushing.

---

### Guidelines for Use:

- This medicine will be prepared and administered by your health care provider in a medical setting.
- Dosage is individualized.
- Inform your doctor if you are pregnant, become pregnant, planning to become prenant, or are breastfeeding before beginning therapy.
- Notify your health care provider if you experience severe rash, hives, difficulty breathing, low blood pressure, swelling of the eyes, mouth, or throat, or other signs of an allergic reaction.
- Notify your health care provider of you experience new or worsening joint or msucle pain, fever or other signs of an infection, sore throat, difficulty swallowing, swelling of the hands, feet, or face, or headache.

---

*If you have any questions, consult your doctor, pharmacist, or health care provider.*

| Generic Name<br>*Brand Name Examples* | Supplied As | Generic<br>Available |
|---|---|---|
| *Rx*  **Orlistat** | | |
| *Xenical* | **Capsules**: 120 mg | No |

## Type of Drug:

Lipase inhibitor.

## How the Drug Works:

Inhibits enzyme in intestine (lipase) which breaks down dietary fats into small absorbable particles. By preventing breakdown and absorption of fat in the intestine and increasing its subsequent loss in the stool, fewer calories are absorbed, which may result in weight loss.

## Uses:

For obesity management including weight loss and weight maintenance when used in conjunction with a reduced-calorie diet. Orlistat is indicated for obese patients with an initial body mass index (BMI) of at least 30 kg/m$^2$ (27 kg/m$^2$ in the presence of other risk factors [eg, high blood pressure, diabetes, dyslipidemia]).

To reduce the risk of weight regain after prior loss.

## Precautions:

*Do not use in the following situations:*

allergy to orlistat or any of its ingredients
cholestasis
chronic malabsorption syndrome

*Use with caution in the following situations:*

| | |
|---|---|
| anorexia nervosa | hyperoxaluria, history |
| bulimia | hypothyroidism |
| cyclosporine therapy, | kidney stones |
|  concomitant | warfarin therapy, concomitant |
| high fat diet | |

*Diabetes:* Weight loss induction by orlistat may be accompanied by improved metabolic control in diabetic patients, which might require a reduction in dose of oral hypoglycemic medication (eg, sulfonylureas, metformin) or insulin.

*Organic causes of obesity* (eg, hypothyroidism) should be excluded before orlistat is prescribed.

*Pregnancy:* There are no adequate and well-controlled studies in pregnant women. Orlistat is not recommended for use during pregnancy.

*Breastfeeding:* It is not known if orlistat appears in breast milk. Therefore, orlistat should not be taken by nursing women. Consult your doctor before you begin breastfeeding.

*Children:* Safety and effectiveness of orlistat in children have not been established.

## Drug Interactions:

Tell your doctor or pharmacist if you are taking or plan to take any over-the-counter or prescription medications or dietary supplements while taking orlistat. Doses of one or both drugs may need to be modified or a different drug may need to be prescribed. The following drugs and drug classes interact with orlistat:

| | |
|---|---|
| beta-carotene | vitamin E acetate |
| cyclosporine (eg, *Sandimmune*) | warfarin (eg, *Coumadin*) |
| pravastatin (*Pravachol*) | |

## Side Effects:

Every drug is capable of producing side effects. Many orlistat users experience no, or minor, side effects. The frequency and severity of side effects depend on many factors including dose, duration of therapy, and individual susceptibility. Possible side effects include:

*Digestive Tract:* Oily spotting; gas with discharge; fecal urgency; fatty or oily stool; oily evacuation; stomach pain or discomfort; nausea; infectious diarrhea; rectal pain or discomfort; tooth disorder; gum disorder; nausea; vomiting; inability to control bowel movements; increased frequency of bowel movements.

*Nervous System:* Headache; dizziness; fatigue; sleep disorder; anxiety; depression.

*Respiratory System:* Flu; upper or lower respiratory tract infection; ear, nose, and throat symptoms.

*Skin:* Rash; dry skin.

*Other:* Back pain; pain in legs or feet; swollen feet; joint pain; muscle pain; joint disorder; tendonitis; menstrual irregularity; inflammation of the vagina with itching or abnormal discharge; urinary tract infection; ear infection.

## Guidelines for Use:

- The recommended dose of orlistat is 120 mg (1 capsule) 3 times daily with each main meal containing fat (during or up to 1 hour after the meal). Doses over 120 mg 3 times daily have not been shown to provide additional benefit.

- If a meal is occasionally missed or contains no fat, the dose of orlistat can be omitted.

- Eat a nutritionally balanced, reduced-calorie diet that contains about 30% of calories from fat. Gastrointestinal events may increase when orlistat is taken with a diet high in fat (greater than 30% total daily calories from fat). The daily intake of fat, carbohydrate, and protein should be distributed over 3 main meals. If orlistat is taken with any one meal very high in fat, the possibility of gastrointestinal adverse effects increases.

- Take a multivitamin supplement that contains fat-soluble vitamins (A, D, E, and K) to ensure adequate nutrition, because orlistat has been shown to reduce the absorption of some fat-soluble vitamins. Take the multivitamin supplement (with food to reduce gastrointestinal discomfort) once a day at least 2 hours before or after the administration of orlistat, such as at bedtime.

- Based on fecal fat measurements, the effect of orlistat is seen as soon as 24 to 48 hours after dosing. Upon discontinuation of therapy, fecal fat content usually returns to pretreatment levels within 48 to 72 hours.

- Safety and effectiveness of orlistat beyond 2 years have not been established.

- Store between 59° to 86°F in a tightly closed container. Do not use after expiration date.

*If you have any questions, consult your doctor, pharmacist, or health care provider.*

| Generic Name<br>*Brand Name Example* | Supplied As | Generic<br>Available |
|---|---|---|
| *Rx* **Tegaserod Maleate** | | |
| *Zelnorm* | **Tablets:** 2 mg, 6 mg | No |

## Type of Drug:

Serotonin-receptor agonist.

## How the Drug Works:

Increases the movement of stool through the bowels by activating serotonin type-4 receptors.

## Uses:

For short-term treatment of women with irritable bowel syndrome (IBS) whose primary bowel symptom is constipation.

## Precautions:

*Do not use in the following situations:*

abdominal adhesions
allergy to the drug or any of its ingredients
bowel obstruction, history of
kidney impairment, severe
liver impairment, moderate or severe
suspected sphincter of Oddi dysfunction
symptomatic gallbladder disease

*Use with caution in the following situations:*

diarrhea
stomach pain, new or suddenly worsening

*Pregnancy:* There are no adequate and well-controlled studies in pregnant women. Use only if clearly needed and the potential benefits outweigh the possible risks to the fetus.

*Breastfeeding:* It is not known if tegaserod maleate appears in breast milk. Consult your doctor before you begin breastfeeding.

*Children:* Safety and effectiveness in patients younger than 18 years of age have not been established.

## Drug Interactions:

Tell your doctor or pharmacist if you are taking or planning to take any over-the-counter or prescription medications or dietary supplements with this drug. Drug doses may need to be modified or a different drug prescribed.

## Side Effects:

Every drug is capable of producing side effects. Many patients experience no, or minor, side effects. The frequency and severity of side effects depend on many factors including dose, duration of therapy, and individual susceptibility. Possible side effects include:

*Digestive Tract:* Stomach pain or cramping; diarrhea; nausea; gas; increased appetite; irritable colon.

*Nervous System:* Headache; fainting; impaired concentration; dizziness; migraine; feeling of whirling motion (vertigo); depression; sleeplessness.

*Circulatory System:* Low blood pressure; irregular heartbeat; rapid heartbeat; chest pain.

*Other:* Back, joint, or leg pain; flushing; facial swelling; sweating; itching.

---

### Guidelines for Use:

- Dosage is individualized. Take exactly as prescribed.
- Do not stop taking or change the dose, unless instructed by your doctor.
- Take before a meal on an empty stomach.
- If a dose is missed, skip that dose. If several hours have passed or it is nearing time for the next dose, do not double the dose to catch up, unless instructed by your doctor. If more than one dose is missed or if it is necessary to establish a new dosage schedule, contact your doctor or pharmicist.
- Contact your doctor if you experience severe diarrhea, or if diarrhea is accompanied by severe cramping, stomach pain, or dizziness.
- Contact your doctor if you experience new or worsening abdominal pain.
- Inform your doctor if you are pregnant, become pregnant, plan to become pregnant, or if you are breastfeeding.
- Store at controlled room temperature (59° to 86°F).

---

*If you have any questions, consult your doctor, pharmacist, or health care provider.*

## Antibiotics
Aminoglycosides, Oral, 1013
Aztreonam, 1016
Cephalosporins, 1019
Chloramphenicol, 1027
Lincosamides, 1030
Macrolides, 1034
Spectinomycin, 1039
Erythromycin, Topical, 1041
Vancomycin, 1043
Oxalodinones, 1046
Fluoroquinolones, 1049
Carbapenem Antibiotics
   Meropenem, 1055
   Ertrapenem, 1057
   Imipenem-Cilastatin, 1059
Metronidazole, 1062
Mupirocin, 1065
Penicillins, Oral, 1067
Tetracyclines, 1072
Tetracyclines, Topical, 1077
Trimethoprim (TMP), 1079
Topical, Miscellaneous, 1081

## Sulfonamides, 1084
Erythromycin Ethylsuccinate/
   Sulfisoxazole, 1087
Trimethoprim/Sulfamethoxazole
   (TMP-SMZ), 1090

## Vaginal Anti-infectives, 1093

## Antifungals
Clotrimazole, 1096
Fluconazole, 1098
Griseofulvin, 1100
Itraconazole, 1102
Ketoconazole, 1105
Nystatin, 1109
Voriconazole, 1111
Topical Preparations, 1113
Topical Combinations, 1118
Vaginal Preparations, 1121

## Antimalarials
Aminoquinolines, 1124
Mefloquine, 1127
Pyrimethamine, 1129
Sulfadoxine/Pyrimethamine, 1131
Halofantrine, 1134
Atovaquone/Proguanil, 1136
Quinine Sulfate, 1138

## Antiviral Agents
Foscarnet, 1140
Ganciclovir, 1143
Valganciclovir, 1146
Adefovir, 1149
Antiherpes Virus Agents, 1151
Amantadine, 1154
Cidofovir, 1157
Ribavirin, 1160
Rimantadine, 1163
Zanamivir, 1165
Oseltamivir Phosphate, 1167

## Antiretroviral Agents
Protease Inhibitors, 1169
Nucleotide Analog Reverse
   Transcriptase Inhibitors, 1173
Nucleoside Reverse
   Transcriptase Inhibitors, 1176
Non-Nucleoside Reverse
   Transcriptase Inhibitors, 1181

## Antiparasitics
Albendazole, 1185
Mebendazole, 1187
Pyrantel, 1189
Thiabendazole, 1191
Ivermectin, 1193

## Urinary Anti-infectives
Methenamine/Methenamine
   Salts, 1195
Fosfomycin Tromethamine, 1197
Nalidixic Acid, 1199
Nitrofurantoin, 1201
Combinations, 1204

**Miscellaneous Anti-infectives**
Antituberculosis Drugs, 1207
Atovaquone, 1217
Pentamidine Isethionate, 1219
Interferon Alfa-n3, 1222
Interferon Alfacon-1, 1224
Interferon Gamma-1b, 1227
Scabicides/Pediculicides, 1229

| Generic Name<br>*Brand Name Examples* | Supplied As | Generic<br>Available |
|---|---|---|
| *Rx* **Kanamycin Sulfate** | | |
| *Kantrex* | **Capsules:** 500 mg | No |
| *Rx* **Neomycin Sulfate** | **Tablets:** 500 mg | Yes |
| *Neo-fradin* | **Solution, oral:** 125 mg/5 mL | No |
| *Rx* **Paromomycin Sulfate** | | |
| *Humatin* | **Capsules:** 250 mg | No |

The aminoglycosides are antibiotics with a broad spectrum of activity and effectiveness. The oral aminoglycosides are not significantly absorbed and are used primarily to suppress bacteria within the digestive tract. The injectable aminoglycosides (eg, neomycin, streptomycin, kanamycin, gentamicin, tobramycin, amikacin, netilmicin) are used in the treatment of serious infections. The following monograph discusses only the oral aminoglycosides.

For detailed information regarding injectable aminoglycosides and their uses, contact your pharmacist or doctor.

## Type of Drug:

Anti-infective; antibiotic used to suppress the growth of bacteria normally found in the digestive tract.

## How the Drug Works:

Aminoglycosides inhibit production of essential proteins in bacteria, causing bacterial cell death.

## Uses:

*Capsules and tablets:* To suppress growth of intestinal bacteria.

In combination with other therapies to manage hepatic coma.

*Neomycin oral solution:* Used in hepatic coma to reduce ammonia-formulating bacteria in the intestinal tract. This reduction in blood ammonia has resulted in neurological improvement.

*Paromomycin:* To treat intestinal amebiasis (parasites).

## Precautions:

*Do not use in the following situations:*
allergy to these drugs or any of their ingredients
inflammation or ulceration of digestive tract
obstruction of digestive tract

*Use with caution in the following situations:*

hearing loss
kidney disease
liver disease
myasthenia gravis

parkinsonism
ulcerative lesions, bowel (paromomycin only)

*Hearing and kidney toxicity:* Aminoglycosides (particularly the injectable products) can cause significant hearing and kidney damage. Toxicity may develop with routine doses, particularly in people with preexisting kidney disease and preexisting hearing loss. Evidence of toxicity requires discontinuation of the drug.

*Superinfection:* Use of antibiotics (especially prolonged or repeated therapy) may result in bacterial or fungal overgrowth of nonsusceptible organisms (secondary infection). The aminoglycoside may need to be stopped and another antibiotic may need to be prescribed.

*Pregnancy:* Safety for use during pregnancy has not been established. Some aminoglycosides (eg, neomycin) can cause fetal harm. Use only when clearly needed and when potential benefits outweigh the possible hazards to the fetus.

*Breastfeeding:* Most aminoglycosides appear in breast milk. It is not known if neomycin appears in human breast milk. Because of the potential for serious adverse reactions from the aminoglycosides in nursing infants, a decision should be made whether to discontinue nursing or to discontinue the drug, taking into account the importance of the drug to the mother.

*Children:* Safety and efficacy in patients under 18 years of age have not been established. If treatment is necessary, use with caution. Do not exceed a treatment period of 3 weeks because of absorption from the gastrointestinal tract.

*Elderly:* Patients may have reduced kidney function that is not evident in the results of routine screening tests. Monitoring of kidney function and hearing during treatment is very important if oral therapy is prolonged.

*Lab tests* may be required during treatment with aminoglycosides. Tests may include blood counts, hearing tests, kidney function tests, and urine tests.

## Drug Interactions:

Tell your doctor or pharmacist if you are taking or if you are planning to take any over-the-counter or prescription medications with aminoglycosides. Doses of one or both drugs may need to be modified or a different drug may need to be prescribed. The following drugs and drug classes interact with aminoglycosides.

| | |
|---|---|
| 5-fluorouracil (eg, *Adrucil)* | methotrexate (eg, *Rheumatrex*) |
| aminoglycosides, other | neuromuscular blocking agents |
| anticoagulants, oral (eg, warfarin) | (eg, tubocurarine) |
| | penicillin V potassium |
| antimicrobial drugs, ototoxic or | (eg, *Veetids*) |
| nephrotoxic (eg, gentamicin) | polypeptide antibiotics (eg, polymyxin B) |
| digitalis (eg, digoxin) | |
| diuretics (eg, furosemide) | vitamin A |
| mannitol (eg, *Osmitrol*) | vitamin $B_{12}$, oral |

## Side Effects:

Every drug is capable of producing side effects. Many aminoglycoside users experience no, or minor, side effects. The frequency and severity of side effects depend on many factors including dose, route of administration, duration of therapy, and individual susceptibility. Possible side effects include:

*Kidney problems:* Blood and protein in urine; increased urination; problems urinating; abnormal kidney function tests; destruction of kidney cells.

*Hearing loss (may be no warning):* Ringing in the ears; hearing impairment; ear problems; dizziness.

*Other:* Rash; itching; nausea; vomiting; diarrhea; fatty stools; abdominal cramps; malaborption syndrome (increased fecal fat, decreased serum carotene, fall in xylose absorption).

---

## Guidelines for Use:

- Complete full course of therapy.
- *Kanamycin sulfate* – As an adjunct to mechanical cleansing of the large bowel in short-term therapy, usual dosage is 1 g (2 capsules) every hour for 4 hours followed by 1 g (2 capsules) every 6 hours for 36 to 72 hours. As an adjunct in extended therapy of hepatic coma, usual dosage is 8 g to 12 g (16 to 24 capsules) per day in divided doses.
- *Neomycin sulfate* – As an adjunct to mechanical cleansing of the bowel before bowel surgery, usual dosage is 1 g (2 tablets) with 1 g erythromycin at 19 hours, 18 hours, and again at 11 hours before surgery. As an adjunct in extended therapy of hepatic coma, usual dosage is 4 g (8 tablets) per day in divided doses.
  For oral solution management of hepatic coma, withdraw protein from diet, avoid the use of diuretic agents, and give supportive therapy (eg, blood products). Recommended dosage is 4 g to 12 g/day in divided doses over 5 to 6 days, during which protein should be returned incrementally to the diet.
- *Paromomycin sulfate* – For intestinal amebiasis in adults and children, usual dosage is 25 mg to 35 mg/kg body weight daily, administered in 3 doses with meals, for 5 to 10 days.
  For management of hepatic coma in adults, usual dosage is 4 g daily in divided doses, given at regular intervals for 5 to 6 days.
- If a dose is missed, take it as soon as possible. If several hours have passed or if it is nearing time for the next dose, do not double the dose in order to catch up (unless advised to do so by your doctor). If more than one dose is missed or it is necessary to establish a new dosage schedule, contact your doctor or pharmacist.
- May cause nausea, vomiting, or diarrhea.
- Notify your doctor if ringing in the ears, hearing impairment, rash, problems urinating, or dizziness occurs.
- Drink plenty of fluids.
- Lab tests may be required. Be sure to keep appointments.
- Store at room temperature (59° to 86°F) and protect from moisture.

*If you have any questions, consult your doctor, pharmacist, or health care provider.*

| Generic Name<br>*Brand Name Examples* | Supplied As | Generic<br>Available |
|---|---|---|
| *Rx* **Aztreonam** | | |
| *Azactam* | **Powder for Injection:** 500 mg,<br>1 g, 2 g | No |

## Type of Drug:
Synthetic anti-infective, antibiotic.

## How the Drug Works:
Aztreonam kills susceptible bacteria by interfering with formation of the bacterial cell wall. This increases the likelihood that the cell wall will rupture and result in cell death. Aztreonam is a particularly effective antibiotic against susceptible gram-negative bacteria.

## Uses:
To treat serious infections caused by susceptible bacteria. Aztreonam may be particularly useful in treating urinary tract infections (eg, bladder infections), lower respiratory tract infections (eg, pneumonia), septicemia (blood poisoning), skin infections, abdominal infections, and gynecologic infections caused by gram-negative bacteria.

*Unlabeled Use(s):* Occasionally doctors may prescribe aztreonam to treat gonorrhea.

## Precautions:
*Do not use in the following situations:*
> allergy to aztreonam or any of its ingredients

*Use with caution in the following situations:*
> allergy to beta-lactam antibiotics (eg, cephalosporins, penicillins)
> aminoglycoside use, concurrent (eg, gentamicin)
> kidney disease
> liver disease

*Elderly patients and patients with decreased kidney function:* Drug may not be eliminated as rapidly in these patients. Dosage of the drug may be decreased or dosage interval altered in some instances.

*Superinfection:* Use of antibiotics (especially prolonged or repeated therapy) may result in bacterial or fungal overgrowth of organisms (secondary infection). Aztreonam may need to be stopped and another antibiotic prescribed for the second infection.

*Diarrhea:* If diarrhea develops during aztreonam use, pseudomembranous colitis must be considered. This inflammatory condition of the colon is due to overgrowth of bacteria that are not killed by aztreonam. The primary cause is a toxin produced by a bacteria known as *Clostridia difficile*. Colitis symptoms may range in severity from mild to life-threatening. Mild cases usually respond by stopping the antibiotic. In more severe cases, other antibiotics may need to be used.

*Pregnancy:* Adequate studies have not been done in pregnant women. Use only if clearly needed and potential benefits outweigh the possible hazards to the fetus.

*Breastfeeding:* Aztreonam appears in breast milk. Consult your doctor before you begin breastfeeding.

*Children:* The safety and effectiveness of aztreonam have been established in children 9 months to 16 years of age. It is not known whether aztreonam is safe and effective in children less than 9 months of age or in any child with septicemia (blood poisoning) or skin infections due to some types of organisms.

*Lab tests* may be required. Be sure to keep appointments.

## Drug Interactions:

Tell your doctor or pharmacist if you are taking or if you are planning to take any over-the-counter or prescription medications with aztreonam. Doses of one or both drugs may need to be modified or a different drug may need to be prescribed. Beta-lactamase-inducing antibiotics (eg, cefoxitin) interact with aztreonam.

## Side Effects:

Every drug is capable of producing side effects. Many aztreonam users experience no, or minor, side effects. The frequency and severity of side effects depend on many factors including dose, duration of therapy, and individual susceptibility. Possible side effects include:

*Local:* Inflammation of the vein (IV); discomfort, pain, redness, or swelling at injection site (IM).

*Digestive Tract:* Nausea; vomiting; diarrhea.

*Other:* Rash; fever; hives; itching; difficulty breathing; wheezing; dizziness; vaginal itching; headache.

## Guidelines for Use:

- Aztreonam is usually administered by health care professionals in a health care setting.
- Aztreonam may occasionally be prescribed for home therapy. If so, carefully follow the storage, preparation, administration, and disposal directions given to you by your doctor.
- Given intramuscularly (IM) or intravenously (IV) only.
- The IV route of administration is preferred in patients requiring single doses greater than 1 g or in bacterial septicemia (blood poisoning), localized abscess, peritonitis (inflammation of the lining of the abdomen), and other severe or life-threatening infections.
- Duration of therapy depends on severity of infection. Usually continued for 48 hours after symptoms disappear or evidence of bacterial absence is confirmed. Persistent infections may require therapy for several days to several weeks.
- If diarrhea occurs, notify your doctor immediately. This could be a symptom of a severe side effect (pseudomembranous colitis) requiring immediate medical attention. Mild cases of colitis usually respond by stopping the drug. In more severe cases, other antibiotics may need to be used.
- Aztreonam may cause abnormal liver, kidney, and blood tests.
- Lab tests may be required. Be sure to keep appointments.
- Store at room temperature. Avoid excessive heat.

*If you have any questions, consult your doctor, pharmacist, or health care provider.*

| Generic Name<br>*Brand Name Examples* | Supplied As | Generic<br>Available |
|---|---|---|
| **Rx Cefaclor** | | |
| *Ceclor* | **Capsules:** 250 mg, 500 mg | Yes |
| *Ceclor* | **Oral suspension:**<br>125 mg/5 mL, 187 mg/5 mL,<br>250 mg/5 mL, 375 mg/5 mL | Yes |
| *Ceclor CD* | **Tablets, extended release:**<br>375 mg, 500 mg | No |
| **Rx Cefadroxil** | | |
| *Duricef* | **Capsules:** 500 mg | Yes |
| *Duricef* | **Tablets:** 1 g | Yes |
| *Duricef* | **Oral suspension:**<br>125 mg/5 mL, 250 mg/5 mL,<br>500 mg/5 mL | No |
| **Rx Cefazolin Sodium** | | |
| *Ancef, Kefzol* | **Injection:** 500 mg, 1 g, 5 g,<br>10 g | Yes |
| *Ancef*[1] | **Injection, (frozen):** 500 mg,<br>1 g | No |
| **Rx Cefdinir** | | |
| *Omnicef* | **Capsules:** 300 mg | No |
| *Omnicef*[2] | **Oral suspension:**<br>125 mg/5 mL | No |
| **Rx Cefepime Hydrochloride** | | |
| *Maxipime* | **Injection:** 500 mg, 1 g, 2 g | No |
| **Rx Cefixime** | | |
| *Suprax* | **Tablets:** 200 mg, 400 mg | No |
| *Suprax* | **Oral suspension:**<br>100 mg/5 mL | No |
| **Rx Cefmetazole Sodium** | | |
| *Zefazone* | **Injection:** 1 g, 2 g | No |
| *Zefazone* | **Injection (frozen):** 1g/50 mL,<br>2 g/50 mL | No |
| **Rx Cefonicid Sodium** | | |
| *Monocid* | **Powder for Injection, lyophi-<br>lized:** 500 mg, 1 g, 10 g | No |

| Generic Name<br>*Brand Name Examples* | Supplied As | Generic<br>Available |
|---|---|---|
| *Rx* **Cefoperazone Sodium** | | |
| *Cefobid* | **Injection:** 1 g, 2 g, 10 g | No |
| *Cefobid* | **Injection (frozen):** 1 g/50 mL,<br>2 g/50 mL | No |
| *Rx* **Cefotaxime Sodium** | | |
| *Claforan* | **Injection:** 500 mg, 1 g, 2 g,<br>10 g | No |
| *Claforan* | **Injection (frozen):** 1 g/50 mL,<br>2 g/50 mL | No |
| *Rx* **Cefotetan Disodium** | | |
| *Cefotan* | **Injection:** 1 g, 2 g, 10 g | No |
| *Cefotan* | **Injection (frozen):** 1 g/50 mL,<br>2 g/50 mL | No |
| *Rx* **Cefoxitin Sodium** | | |
| *Mefoxin* | **Injection:** 1 g, 2 g, 10 g | No |
| *Mefoxin* | **Injection (frozen):** 1 g, 2 g | No |
| *Rx* | | |
| *Vantin* | **Tablets:** 100 mg, 200 mg | No |
| *Vantin* | **Oral suspension:** 50 mg/5 mL,<br>100 mg/5 mL | No |
| *Rx* **Cefprozil** | | |
| *Cefzil* | **Tablets:** 250 mg, 500 mg | No |
| *Cefzil*[β] | **Oral suspension:** 125<br>mg/5 mL, 250 mg/5 mL | No |
| *Rx* **Ceftazidime** | | |
| *Ceptaz, Fortaz, Tazicef,*<br>*Tazidime* | **Injection:** 500 mg, 1 g, 2 g,<br>6 g, 10 g | No |
| *Fortaz, Tazicef* | **Injection (frozen):** 1 g, 2 g | No |
| *Rx* **Ceftibuten** | | |
| *Cedax* | **Capsules:** 400 mg | No |
| *Cedax* | **Oral suspension:** 90 mg/5 mL,<br>180 mg/5 mL | No |
| *Rx* **Ceftizoxime Sodium** | | |
| *Cefizox* | **Injection:** 500 mg, 1 g, 2 g,<br>10 g | No |
| *Cefizox* | **Injection (frozen):** 1 g | No |

| Generic Name<br>*Brand Name Examples* | Supplied As | Generic<br>Available |
|---|---|---|
| *Rx* **Ceftriaxone Sodium** | | |
| *Rocephin* | **Injection:** 250 mg, 500 mg, 1 g, 2 g, 10 g | No |
| *Rocephin* | **Injection (frozen):** 1 g, 2 g | No |
| *Rx* **Cefuroxime** | | |
| *Ceftin* | **Tablets:** 125 mg, 250 mg, 500 mg | No |
| *Ceftin* | **Oral suspension:** 125 mg/5 mL, 250 mg/5 mL | No |
| *Kefurox, Zinacef* | **Injection:** 750 mg, 1.5 g, 7.5 g | Yes |
| *Zinacef* | **Injection (frozen):** 750 mg, 1.5 g | No |
| *Rx* **Cephalexin HCl Monohydrate** | | |
| *Keftab* | **Tablets:** 500 mg | No |
| *Rx* **Cephalexin Monohydrate** | | |
| *Keflex* | **Capsules:** 250 mg, 500 mg | Yes |
| | **Tablets:** 250 mg, 500 mg, 1 g | Yes |
| | **Oral suspension:** 125 mg/5 mL, 250 mg/5 mL | Yes |
| *Rx* **Cephapirin Sodium** | | |
| *Cefadyl* | **Injection:** 500 mg, 1 g, 2 g, 4 g, 20 g | No |
| *Rx* **Cephradine** | | |
| *Velosef* | **Capsules:** 250 mg, 500 mg | Yes |
| *Velosef* | **Oral suspension:** 125 mg/5 mL, 250 mg/5 mL | Yes |
| *Velosef* | **Injection:** 250 mg, 500 mg, 1 g, 2 g | No |
| *Rx* **Loracarbef** | | |
| *Lorabid* | **Capsules:** 200 mg, 400 mg | No |
| *Lorabid* | **Oral suspension:** 100 mg/5 mL, 200 mg/5 mL | No |

[1] Contains dextrose.
[2] Contains sucrose (2.86 g/5 mL).
[3] Contains sucrose, aspartame, and phenylalanine (28 mg/5 mL).

## Type of Drug:

Anti-infective; antibiotic.

## How the Drug Works:

Cephalosporins kill susceptible bacteria by preventing the formation and maintenance of the normal bacterial cell wall. This increases the likelihood that the cell wall will rupture. Effectiveness of the cephalosporins depends on factors such as dose, concentration of drug in blood, other body fluids and tissue, and the susceptibility of the organism. They are most effective when organisms are growing rapidly.

## Uses:

To treat infections caused by various susceptible bacteria. Cephalosporins are particularly useful in treating respiratory tract infections (eg, bronchitis, pneumonia, otitis media), middle ear infections, skin and skin structure infections, urinary tract infections, bone and joint infections, blood poisoning, inflammation of the heart, sore throat (pharyngitis and tonsillitis), central nervous system infections (eg, meningitis), gynecologic infections, genital infections, abdominal infections, early Lyme disease, and sexually transmitted diseases.

Some cephalosporins are used before, during, and after surgery to reduce the risk of developing an infection. Certain injectable cephalosporins may be used in combination with other antibiotics to treat serious infections, but careful monitoring of kidney function is required.

*Unlabeled Use(s):* Ceftriaxone may be used to treat nervous system complications, joint pain, or inflammation of the heart associated with Lyme disease in patients who cannot use penicillin G.

## Precautions:

*Do not use in the following situations:*
allergy to cephalosporins or any of their ingredients
hemolytic anemia, cephalosporin-associated

*Use with caution in the following situations:*

| | |
|---|---|
| allergy to penicillins | liver disease |
| bleeding disorders | malnourished |
| breastfeeding | prolonged or repeated cephalo- |
| elderly | sporin therapy |
| gallbladder disease, symptoms | stomach or intestinal disease, |
| kidney disease (especially in | history (eg, colitis) |
| conjunction with dialysis) | |

*Superinfection:* Use of antibiotics (especially prolonged or repeated therapy) may result in bacterial or fungal overgrowth (secondary infection). The cephalosporin may need to be stopped and another antibiotic prescribed for the second infection.

*Bleeding complications:* Bleeding complications seen with use of certain injectable cephalosporins (eg, cefmetazole, cefoperazone, cefotetan, ceftriaxone) are not generally a problem with oral therapy. Factors which may increase risk of bleeding complications are liver and kidney disease, low blood platelet count, poor nutrition, concurrent cancer, use of anticoagulants or aspirin, and use in elderly or debilitated patients.

*Penicillin allergy:* Penicillin-allergic patients should use cephalosporins cautiously. If a patient is allergic to penicillins, he or she may also be allergic to cephalosporins and vice versa. Cephalosporins are not an absolutely safe alternative to penicillins in the penicillin-allergic patient. Consult your doctor or pharmacist.

*Serum sickness-like reactions:* Serum sickness-like reactions (skin rashes with inflammation, joint pain, and fever) have been reported, usually following a second course of therapy and usually occur more frequently in children than adults. Symptoms usually occur a few days after beginning therapy and resolve after the drug is discontinued. Antihistamines and corticosteroids may be helpful in managing symptoms.

*Coomb's test:* Positive direct Coomb's tests may be caused by cephalosporins.

*Immune mediated hemolytic anemia:* Immune mediated hemolytic anemia has been observed in patients receiving cephalosporins. Rare cases of severe hemolytic anemia, including fatalities, have been reported. If a patient develops anemia any time within 2 to 3 weeks after the administration of a cephalosporin, consider the diagnosis of a cephalosporin-associated anemia and stop the drug until the cause is determined. Periodically monitor patients receiving prolonged courses of a cephalosporin for treatment of infections for signs and symptoms of hemolytic anemia.

*Disulfiram-like reactions:* Disulfiram-like reactions such as flushing, sweating, headache, and fast heartbeat may occur when alcoholic beverages are ingested within 72 hours after the use of certain cephalosporins (cefazolin, cefmetazole, cefoperazone, cefotetan).

*Diarrhea:* If diarrhea develops during cephalosporin use, pseudomembranous colitis must be considered. This inflammatory condition of the colon is due to overgrowth of bacteria that are not killed by cephalosporins. The primary cause is a toxin produced by a bacteria known as *Clostridia difficile*. Colitis symptoms may range in severity from mild to life-threatening. Mild cases usually respond to stopping the antibiotic. In more severe cases, other antibiotics may need to be used.

*Seizures:* Certain cephalosporins (usually injectables) may cause convulsions (seizures) in patients with decreased kidney function if the dose is not reduced. If seizures occur, the drug should be discontinued.

*Pregnancy:* There are no adequate and well controlled studies in pregnant women. Use only if clearly needed and the possible benefits outweigh the possible risks to the fetus.

*Breastfeeding:* Cephalosporins appear in breast milk. The nursing infant is at risk for certain cephalosporin-induced side effects. Caution should be exercised when administered to a nursing woman. Consult your doctor before you begin breastfeeding.

*Children:* Cephalosporins have been used in children. However, safety and effectiveness of the various cephalosporins are dependent on the age of the child and the organism being treated. Refer to individual package labeling and consult your doctor.

*Lab tests* may be needed to monitor therapy. Tests may include kidney and liver function tests, blood cell counts, and prothrombin time or International Normalized Ratio (INR) (blood-clotting tests).

## Drug Interactions:

Tell your doctor or pharmacist if you are taking or if you are planning to take any over-the-counter or prescription medications while taking cephalosporins. Doses of one or both drugs may need to be modified or a different drug may need to be prescribed. The following drugs and drug classes interact with cephalosporins.

alcohol
aminoglycosides (eg, neomycin)
antacids, aluminum- or magnesium-containing
anticoagulants, oral (eg, warfarin)
carbamazepine (eg, *Tegretol*)
chloramphenicol (eg, *Chloromycetin*)

diuretics (eg, furosemide)
H₂-receptor antagonists (eg, cimetidine) (cefpodoxime and ceftibuten only)
iron supplements (eg, ferrous sulfate)
nephrotoxic drugs (eg, gentamicin)
probenecid

## Side Effects:

Every drug is capable of producing side effects. Many cephalosporin users experience no, or minor, side effects. The frequency and severity of side effects depend on many factors including dose, duration of therapy, and individual susceptibility. Possible side effects include:

*Allergic Reactions:* Rash; hives; itching; fever; joint pain; edema (fluid retention); difficulty breathing; Stevens-Johnson syndrome; toxic epidermal necrolysis; low blood pressure; skin inflammation; weakness; abnormal skin sensations; fainting; flushing; skin redness.

*Serum sickness-like reactions:* Rash; joint pain; fever.

*Local:* Pain, hardness, burning, tenderness, swelling, bleeding, or bruising at injection site; phlebitis (vein inflammation).

*Digestive Tract:* Nausea; vomiting; diarrhea; stomach pain; appetite loss; gas; indigestion; loose, reddish, or frequent stools; oral thrush; swollen tongue; excessive salivation; stomach inflammation.

*Nervous System:* Headache; dizziness; hot flashes; hallucinations; confusion; drowsiness; fatigue; agitation; nervousness; sleeplessness; seizures; irritability; chills; hyperactivity.

*Other:* Fever; nosebleed; low blood pressure; secondary fungal infection, particularly in the mouth, rectal, vaginal, and intestinal areas; taste changes; changes in color perception; abnormal lab tests including liver and kidney function tests, blood counts, urine and blood glucose, urine protein, bilirubin, and creatinine levels; itching in genital, vaginal, and anal areas; anemia; aggravation of myasthenia gravis; chest tightness or pain; yellowing of skin and eyes; difficulty breathing; joint pain and swelling; decreased platelets; transient hepatitis; back pain; kidney dysfunction; bleeding; runny nose; liver dysfunction; thirst; cough; swelling around the eyes; positive Coomb's tests; decreased phosphorus levels; painful or difficult urination; symptoms of gallbladder disease; lockjaw; neck muscle spasm; kidney pain; vaginal discharge; viral illness; arthritis; painful menstruation; flu syndrome.

## Guidelines for Use:

- Use exactly as prescribed by your doctor.
- May be taken with food or milk if stomach upset occurs.
- *Ceftin* oral suspension, *Ceclor CD* tablets, and *Vantin* tablets should be administered with meals. Tablets should not be cut, crushed, or chewed.
- *Cefpodoxime* — Take with food to enhance absorption
- *Ceftibuten and loracarbef* — Take ceftibuten at least 2 hours before or 1 hour after a meal. Take loracarbef on an empty stomach, at least 1 hour before or 2 hours after a meal.
- *Cefuroxime tablets* — Swallow whole; do not crush or chew. Children who cannot swallow the tablet whole should receive the oral suspension.
- Take at prescribed intervals. Do not skip doses.
- Continue use until all of the prescribed drug has been taken. Failure to take a full course of therapy may prevent complete elimination of bacteria, allowing the infection to return. Continue the antibiotic even after a fever or other symptoms disappear.
- Iron supplements, including multivitamins that contain iron, interfere with the absorption of cefdinir. If iron supplements are required during cefdinir therapy, cefdinir should be taken at least 2 hours before or after the iron supplement.
- If a dose is missed, take or inject it as soon as possible. If several hours have passed or if it is nearing time for the next dose, do not double the dose in order to catch up (unless advised to do so by your doctor). If more than one dose is missed, or it is necessary to establish a new dosage schedule, contact your doctor or pharmacist.
- If diarrhea occurs, contact your doctor immediately. This could be a symptom of a severe side effect (pseudomembranous colitis) requiring immediate medical attention. Mild cases of colitis usually respond to stopping the drug. In more severe cases, other antibiotics may need to be used.
- Cephalosporins may cause allergic reactions. These may vary from mild itching and rash to a life-threatening reaction. Report prior allergic reactions to cephalosporins, penicillins, and any other drugs to your doctor. If you experience rash, hives, nausea, severe diarrhea, itching, fever, joint or muscle pain, chest tightness, fluid retention, urinary problems, chills, unusual bleeding or bruising, or difficulty breathing, contact your doctor immediately.

## Guidelines for Use (cont.):

- May trigger seizures, especially in patients with kidney disease. Discontinue use and notify your doctor if seizures occur.
- Notify your doctor if you are breastfeeding. Cephalosporins appear in breast milk.
- May interact with other drugs. Consult your pharmacist or doctor before taking another drug while taking a cephalosporin.
- *Diabetes* — May interfere with urine tests for glucose and may give false test results. Notify your doctor before changing diet or dosage of diabetes medication.
- Some cephalosporins interact adversely with recent alcohol use (before or up to 72 hours after administration).
- A minimum of 10 days of treatment is recommended for any infection caused by group A beta-hemolytic streptococci. This is the bacteria that causes strep throat. This treatment period is necessary to prevent rheumatic fever (and possible heart damage) or kidney inflammation and damage.
- Ceftriaxone is indicated in the treatment of chancroid; uncomplicated gonococcal infections of the cervix, urethra, throat, rectum, and conjunctiva; bacteremia; gonococcal meningitis and endocarditis; ophthalmic neonatorum caused by *N. gonorrheae*; prophylactic treatment of infants whose mothers have a gonococcal infection; arthritis; epididymitis; pelvic inflammatory disease; proctitis; proctocolitis; and enteritis.
- Cefoxitin and cefotan are indicated in the treatment of pelvic inflammatory disease (PID).
- Cefixime, cefotetan, cefoxitin, and cefotaxime are indicated in the treatment of gonococcal infections.
- Ceftriaxone is indicated in the treatment of gonococcal meningitis and endocarditis.
- Cefotetan and cefoxitin are indicated for the treatment of pelvic inflammatory disease.
- Refer to product labeling for specific storage information.
- *Injections* — Carefully follow preparation, administration, and storage instructions provided by your health care provider regarding injections. Do not use injectable solutions if they are discolored or contain particles.
- *Oral suspensions* — Store in refrigerator (except cefixime and loracarbef). Do not freeze. Shake well before using. Check expiration date. May be kept for 14 days without significant loss of potency. Cefixime and loracarbef may be kept at room temperature. Cefuroxime may be kept for 10 days, either in the refrigerator or at room temperature.

*If you have any questions, consult your doctor, pharmacist, or health care provider.*

| Generic Name<br>*Brand Name Examples* | Supplied As | Generic<br>Available |
|---|---|---|
| Rx **Chloramphenicol** | **Capsules:** 250 mg | Yes |
| *Chloromycetin Sodium*<br>*Succinate* | **Powder for Injection:**<br>100 mg/mL | Yes |

## Type of Drug:
Anti-infective; antibiotic.

## How the Drug Works:
Chloramphenicol interferes with or prevents protein production in susceptible bacteria, slowing their growth.

## Uses:
To treat serious infections in children and adults for which potentially less-harmful drugs are ineffective or not recommended.

To treat acute infections of typhoid fever. Not recommended for the routine treatment of the typhoid "carrier state."

To treat certain infections in patients with cystic fibrosis.

## Precautions:
*Do not use in the following situations:*
>       allergy to chloramphenicol or any of its ingredients
>       bacterial infections, prophlaxis
>       minor infections (eg, colds, influenza, throat infections)
>       premature or newborn infants

*Use with caution in the following situations:*
>       bone marrow depression, drugs causing
>       glucose-6-phosphate dehydrogenase (G-6-PD, an enzyme)
>           deficiency
>       kidney disease
>       liver disease
>       porphyria (high concentrations of iron-free pigment)

*Blood disorders:* Serious and even fatal blood disorders have occurred after chloramphenicol use. There have been reports of aplastic anemia (severe form of anemia), granulocytopenia (decreased white blood count, causing increased risk of infections), and thrombocytopenia (decreased platelet count, causing bleeding or bruising). Blood disorders have occurred after short-term as well as long-term use. Monitoring of blood counts will be required frequently during treatment.

*Superinfection:* Use of antibiotics (especially prolonged or repeated therapy) may result in bacterial or fungal overgrowth. Such overgrowth of nonsusceptible organisms may lead to a secondary infection. Chloramphenicol may need to be stopped and another antibiotic prescribed for the second infection.

*Pregnancy:* There are no studies to establish the safety of this drug in pregnancy. Because chloramphenicol readily crosses the placental barrier, cautious use is particularly important during pregnancy at term or during labor because of potential toxic effects on the fetus (gray syndrome). Use only if clearly needed and potential benefits outweigh the possible hazards to the fetus.

*Breastfeeding:* Chloramphenicol appears in breast milk. Use with caution, if at all, while breastfeeding, because of the possibility of toxic effects on the nursing infant. Consult your doctor before you begin breastfeeding.

*Children:* Use with caution and in smaller doses in premature and full-term infants to avoid gray syndrome toxicity.

*Lab tests* are required to monitor treatment. Tests include bacterial cultures, blood counts, and chloramphenicol blood levels.

## Drug Interactions:

Tell your doctor or pharmacist if you are taking or if you are planning to take any over-the-counter or prescription medications while taking chloramphenicol. Doses of one or both drugs may need to be modified or a different drug may need to be prescribed. The following drugs and drug classes interact with chloramphenicol.

anticoagulants, oral (eg, warfarin)
barbiturates (eg, phenobarbital)
cyclophosphamide (eg, *Cytoxan)*
hydantoins (eg, phenytoin)
iron salts (eg, ferrous sulfate)
penicillins (eg, amoxicillin)
rifampin (eg, *Rifadin)*
sulfonylureas (eg, glipizide)
vitamin $B_{12}$

## Side Effects:

Every drug is capable of producing side effects. Many chloramphenicol users experience no, or minor, side effects. The frequency and severity of side effects depend on many factors including dose, duration of therapy, and individual susceptibility. Possible side effects include:

*Gray syndrome* is a potentially life-threatening condition that can occur in premature infants and newborns given high doses of chloramphenicol during the first 48 hours of life. Symptoms include: Swelling of abdomen; ashen (pale) color; vomiting; shock; difficulty breathing; refusal to suck; loose green stools; limp muscles; decreased temperature.

*Hematologic:* Blood disorders (eg, bone marrow suppression, anemia) are the most serious side effects associated with chloramphenicol. Potentially fatal blood disorders may occur. Symptoms include: Fever, difficulty breathing; rash; numb or tingling hands or feet.

*Digestive Tract:* Nausea; vomiting; diarrhea; inflammation of the mouth or tongue.

*Skin:* Rash; hives; itching; unusual bleeding or bruising.

*Other:* Bone marrow depression; fever; confusion; depression; delirium; headache; fatigue; changes in vision; difficulty breathing.

## Guidelines for Use:

- Dosage is individualized. Use exactly as prescribed.
- Usually taken every 6 hours around the clock.
- The injectable intravenous (IV; into a vein) form will usually be pre-pared and administered by a health care provider in a medical set-ting. It may occasionally be prescribed for home therapy.
- An oral dosage form of chloramphenicol will be substituted for the IV form as soon as possible by your health care provider.
- Take the oral dose on an empty stomach (at least 1 hour before or 2 hours after a meal). It may be taken with food if stomach upset occurs.
- Continue use until all of the prescribed medicine has been taken. Fail-ure to take all of the medicine may prevent complete elimination of bac-teria, allowing the infection to return.
- If a dose is missed, take it as soon as possible. If several hours have passed or it is nearing time for the next dose, do not double the dose to catch up unless advised to do so by your doctor. If more than one dose is missed or it is necessary to establish a new dosage sched-ule, contact your doctor or pharmacist.
- The use of this antibiotic, as with other antibiotics, may result in an over-growth of nonsusceptible organisms, including fungi (secondary infec-tion). If infections caused by nonsusceptible organisms appear during therapy, the chloramphenicol may need to be stopped and another anti-biotic prescribed for the second infection.
- Doses are variable and depend on factors such as type of infection, age, liver function, and kidney function.
- Contact your doctor immediately if you experience fever, sore throat, mouth sores, tiredness, unusual bleeding or bruising, visual distur-bances, diarrhea, or unusual sensations in hands or feet.
- Gray Syndrome may occur in premature infants and newborns, particu-larly if chloramphenicol is given during the first 48 hours of life. Symp-toms appear after 3 to 4 days of continual higher-dose treatment and may include swelling of the abdomen, ashen (pale) color, vomiting, shock, difficulty breathing, refusal to suck, loose green stools, limp muscles, and decreased temperature. Death may occur within hours of onset of the symptoms. Death occurs in approximately 40% of patients. Stopping therapy when symptoms first appear increases the chance for complete recovery.
- Do not continue treatment with chloramphenicol longer than necessary. Avoid repeating a course of therapy with chloramphenicol, if possible.
- Do not use to treat minor infections such as colds, flu, or throat infections.
- Do not use to prevent an infection.
- Lab tests are required to monitor treatment. Be sure to keep appointments.
- Store capsules below 86°F. Protect from moisture and excessive heat. Store injection below 104°F, preferably at room temperature (59° to 86°F).

*If you have any questions, consult your doctor, pharmacist, or health care provider.*

| Generic Name<br>*Brand Name Examples* | Supplied As | Generic<br>Available |
|---|---|---|
| *Rx* **Clindamycin HCl** | | |
| *Cleocin HCl* | **Capsules:** 75 mg[1], 150 mg[1], 300 mg | Yes |
| *Cleocin Pediatric* | **Granules, flavored:** 75 mg/5 mL | No |
| *Cleocin Phosphate* | **Injection:** 150 mg/mL | Yes |
| *Rx* **Clindamycin, Topical** | | |
| *Cleocin T* | **Gel:** 10 mg/g (1%) | Yes |
| *Cleocin T* | **Lotion:** 10 mg/mL | Yes |
| *Cleocin T, Clinda-Derm* | **Solution, topical:** 10 mg/mL (1%) | Yes |
| *Rx* **Lincomycin** | | |
| *Lincocin* | **Capsules:** 500 mg | No |
| *Lincocin[2], Lincorex[2]* | **Injection:** 300 mg/mL | Yes |

[1] Contains tartrazine dye.
[2] Contains benzyl alcohol.

## Type of Drug:

Anti-infective; antibiotic.

## How the Drug Works:

Systemic clindamycin and lincomycin cause bacterial cell death by suppressing protein production in susceptible bacteria.

Topical clindamycin treats acne by reducing the skin bacterial count and reducing the presence of free fatty acids that irritate the skin surface.

## Uses:

*Oral or injectable:* To treat serious infections caused by susceptible bacteria. Use should be reserved for those allergic to penicillin or for use when penicillin or erythromycin is not appropriate. Less toxic agents should be used first whenever possible.

*Topical:* To treat acne.

*Unlabeled Use(s):* Occasionally doctors may prescribe topical clindamycin for rosacea. Clindamycin has been used to treat bacterial vaginosis due to *Gardenella vaginalis* and pelvic inflammatory disease.

## Precautions:

*Do not use in the following situations:*
allergy to lincosamides or any of their ingredients
infections, minor bacterial or viral

meningitis (clindamycin only)

*Use with caution in the following situations:*

| | |
|---|---|
| asthma or significant allergies, history of | diarrhea |
| colitis or other digestive tract diseases, history of | kidney disease |
| | liver disease, moderate to severe |

*Benzyl alcohol:* Some of these injectable products contain benzyl alcohol, which has been associated with fatal "gasping syndrome" in premature infants.

*Superinfection:* Use of antibiotics (especially prolonged or repeated therapy) may result in bacterial or fungal overgrowth (secondary infection) of nonsusceptible organisms. Clindamycin or lincomycin may need to be stopped and another antibiotic may need to be prescribed for the second infection.

*Diarrhea:* If diarrhea develops during lincosamide use, consider pseudomembranous colitis. This inflammatory condition of the colon is due to overgrowth of bacteria that are not killed by lincosamides. The primary cause is a toxin produced by a bacteria known as *Clostridia difficile.* Colitis symptoms may range from mild to life-threatening. Mild cases usually respond by stopping the antibiotic. In more serious cases, another antibiotic may need to be used.

*Pregnancy:* Clindamycin and lincomycin cross the placenta. There are no adequate and well-controlled studies in pregnant women. Use only if clearly needed and the potential benefits outweigh the possible hazards to the fetus.

*Breastfeeding:* Oral and injectable clindamycin and lincomycin appear in breast milk. It is not known if topical clindamycin appears in breast milk. Consult your doctor before you begin breastfeeding.

*Children:*

   *Oral and injectable lincosamides* – Use of lincomycin in newborns is not recommended. Use caution when administering clindamycin to newborns and infants and carefully monitor when administering to children under 16 years of age.

   *Topical clindamycin* – Safety and effectiveness in children under 12 years of age have not been determined.

*Elderly:* Use with caution. Older patients with severe illness may not tolerate drug-associated diarrhea well. Watch for changes in frequency of bowel movements.

*Lab tests* may be required during long-term treatment with lincosamides. Tests may include liver and kidney function tests, blood counts, and bacterial cultures.

*Tartrazine:* Some of these products may contain tartrazine dye (FD&C Yellow No. 5), which can cause allergic reactions in certain individuals. Check package label when available or consult your doctor or pharmacist.

## Drug Interactions:

Tell your doctor or pharmacist if you are taking or planning to take any over-the-counter or prescription medications or dietary supplements while taking lincosamides. Doses of one or both drugs may need to be modified or a different drug may need to be prescribed. The following drugs and drug classes interact with lincosamides:

erythromycin (eg, *E-Mycin)*

kaolin-pectin (eg, *Kaopectate)*

neuromuscular blocking agents (eg, pancuronium bromide)

## Side Effects:

Every drug is capable of producing side effects. Many lincosamide users experience no, or minor, side effects. The frequency and severity of side effects depend on many factors including dose, duration of therapy, and individual susceptibility. Possible side effects include:

*Digestive Tract:* Nausea; vomiting; diarrhea; bloody stools; anal itching; stomach pain or cramps; mouth or tongue sores; sore throat; unpleasant taste; heartburn.

*Skin:* Rash; hives; itching; red, dry, flaking, peeling, burning, or oily skin (topical clindamycin only).

*Other:* Ringing in the ears; feeling of whirling motion; vaginal infection; yellowing of skin or eyes; pain or irritation at injection site; abnormal liver function tests; abnormal blood cell counts; difficulty breathing; joint pain; kidney dysfunction including infrequent urination; low blood pressure.

## Guidelines for Use:

- Dosage is individualized. Use exactly as prescribed.
- *Oral —*
  *Lincomycin* — Take on an empty stomach (except for water) at least 1 to 2 hours before or after meals. Take each dose with a full glass of water (6 to 8 oz).
  *Clindamycin* — Take without regard to food. Take each dose with a full glass of water (6 to 8 oz).
  Store at room temperature (59° to 86°F). Do not refrigerate the pediatric solution. Discard after 2 weeks.
- *Topical clindamycin* — For external use only. Shake lotion well immediately before use.
  If using solution with pledget applicator, remove pledget from foil just before use. Discard after single use.
  Apply a thin layer of the gel, lotion, or solution to the affected area twice daily.
  Make sure the area is clean and dry before application.
  Avoid contact with the eyes, nose, mouth, or other mucous membranes and damaged skin. Burning or irritation may occur.
  In case of contact with the eye, damaged skin, or mucous membranes, bathe the area with large amounts of cool tap water for several minutes.
  Store at room temperature (59° to 86°F). Protect from freezing. Keep container tightly closed.
- *Injections —*
  This medication will usually be prepared and administered by your health care provider in a medical setting. This medicine may occasionally be prescribed for home therapy. If so, carefully follow the storage, preparation, administration, and disposal techniques taught to you by your health care provider. Do not use if solution is discolored or contains particles.
- If a dose is missed, apply, take, or inject it as soon as possible. If several hours have passed or it is nearing time for the next dose, do not double the dose to catch up, unless directed by your doctor. If more than one dose is missed or it is necessary to establish a new dosage schedule, contact your doctor or pharmacist.
- Discontinue use and contact your doctor immediately if you experience severe diarrhea, stomach pain or cramps, bloody stools, unusual bleeding, bruising, joint pain, itching, hives, rash, or difficulty breathing. These could be symptoms of severe side effects requiring immediate medical attention. Do not treat diarrhea without consulting your doctor.
- Continue use until all of the prescribed medicine has been taken. Failure to take all of the medicine may prevent complete elimination of bacteria, allowing the infection to return.
- Lab tests may be required during long-term treatment. Be sure to keep appointments.

*If you have any questions, consult your doctor, pharmacist, or health care provider.*

| Generic Name<br>*Brand Name Examples* | Supplied As | Generic<br>Available |
|---|---|---|
| Rx **Azithromycin**[1] | | |
| *Zithromax* | **Tablets:** 250 mg, 500 mg, 600 mg | No |
| *Zithromax* | **Capsules**: 250 mg | No |
| *Zithromax* | **Powder for oral suspension (when reconstituted)**: 100 mg/5 mL, 200 mg/5 mL | No |
| Rx **Clarithromycin** | | |
| *Biaxin* | **Tablets:** 250 mg, 500 mg | No |
| *Biaxin* | **Granules for oral suspension (when reconstituted)**: 125 mg/5 mL, 250 mg/5 mL | No |
| *Biaxin XL* | **Tablets, extended release**: 500 mg | No |
| Rx **Dirithromycin** | | |
| *Dynabac* | **Tablets, enteric coated**: 250 mg | No |
| Rx **Erythromycin Base** | | |
| *E-Mycin, Ery-Tab* | **Tablets, enteric coated:** 250 mg, 333 mg | No |
| *Ery-Tab* | **Tablets, enteric coated**: 500 mg | No |
| *PCE Dispertab* | **Tablets with polymer-coated particles:** 333 mg, 500 mg | No |
| *Eryc* | **Capsules, delayed release:** 250 mg | Yes |
| Rx **Erythromycin Estolate** | **Suspension, oral**: 125 mg/5 mL, 250 mg/5 mL | Yes |
| Rx **Erythromycin Ethylsuccinate** | | |
| *EryPed* | **Tablets, chewable:** 200 mg | No |
| *E.E.S. 400* | **Tablets**: 400 mg | Yes |
| *E.E.S. 200, Ery-Ped 200* | **Suspension:** 200 mg/5 mL | Yes |
| *E.E.S. 400, Ery-Ped 400* | **Suspension:** 400 mg/5 mL | Yes |
| *E.E.S. Granules* | **Powder for oral suspension (when reconstituted):** 200 mg/5 mL | No |
| *EryPed Drops* | **Suspension**: 100 mg/2.5 mL | No |

| Generic Name<br>*Brand Name Examples* | Supplied As | Generic<br>Available |
|---|---|---|
| Rx **Erythromycin Stearate** | **Tablets, film coated:** 250 mg,<br>500 mg | Yes |

[1] Also available as an injection.

## Type of Drug:

Antibiotic; anti-infective.

## How the Drug Works:

Macrolide antibiotics suppress the formation of protein by bacteria, slowing bacterial growth or causing bacterial cell death.

## Uses:

To treat mild to moderate infections (eg, pharyngitis, tonsillitis, chronic bronchitis, pneumonia, skin infections) caused by susceptible bacteria.

*Azithromycin:* To treat lower and upper respiratory tract infections, pharyngitis or tonsillitis, skin infections, middle ear infections (children only), and certain sexually transmitted diseases caused by susceptible organisms.

*Clarithromycin:* To treat lower and upper respiratory tract infections, pharyngitis or tonsillitis, skin infections, sinusitis, middle ear infections (children only); to prevent spread of *Mycobacterium avium* complex (MAC) in patients with advanced HIV infection; and to treat stomach and intestinal ulcers caused by *Helicobacter pylori*.

*Dirithromycin:* To treat acute bacterial exacerbations of chronic bronchitis, secondary bacterial infections of acute bronchitis, community-acquired pneumonia, pharyngitis, tonsilitis, and skin infections.

*Erythromycin:* To treat *Mycoplasma pneumoniae* (respiratory tract infection), Legionnaire disease, intestinal dysenteric amebiasis, pelvic inflammatory disease, whooping cough, diphtheria, erythrasma, and certain sexually transmitted diseases (eg, syphilis, gonorrhea). Also used to prevent recurrent attacks of rheumatic fever and to prevent bacterial endocarditis. As an alternative drug in penicillin or tetracycline allergy or when penicillin or tetracycline is not recommended or not tolerated to treat susceptible organisms.

## Precautions:

*Do not use in the following situations:*
   allergy to the drug or any of its ingredients
   pimozide (*Orap*) therapy, current

*Use with caution in the following situations:*
   bacteremias (blood infections) (dirithromycin only)
   kidney disease, severe (azithromycin, clarithromycin only)
   liver disease (dirithromycin, erythromycin only)
   liver disease, severe (azithromycin only)
   myasthenia gravis (erythromycin only)

*Diarrhea/Pseudomembranous colitis:* If diarrhea develops during use, pseudomembranous colitis must be considered. This inflammatory condition of the colon is due to overgrowth of bacteria that are not killed by macrolide antibiotics. The primary cause is a toxin produced by the bacteria *Clostridia difficile.* Mild cases usually respond to stopping the antibiotic. Severe cases may require treatment with a different antibiotic.

*Superinfection:* Use of antibiotics (especially prolonged and repeated therapy) may result in bacterial or fungal overgrowth (secondary infection). Macrolide antibiotics may need to be stopped and another antibiotic may need to be prescribed for the second infection.

*Pregnancy:* Safety for use during pregnancy has not been established for many of these medications. There are no adequate and well-controlled studies of azithromycin, clarithromycin, dirithromycin, or erythromycin in pregnant women. Use only if clearly needed and the potential benefits outweigh the possible risks to the fetus.

*Breastfeeding:* Erythromycin appears in breast milk. It is not known if other macrolide antibiotics appear in breast milk. Consult your doctor before you begin breastfeeding.

*Children:* Azithromycin is not recommended for middle ear infections in children younger than 6 months of age and is not recommended for pharyngitis or tonsillitis in children younger than 2 years of age. Clarithromycin is not recommended in children younger than 6 months of age for treatment of mycobacterial infections. Dirithromycin is not recommended in children younger than 12 years of age. Safety and effectiveness of erythromycin in children have been established.

*Lab tests* may be required to monitor therapy. Tests may include cultures, blood cell counts, and kidney or liver tests.

## Drug Interactions:

Tell your doctor or pharmacist if you are taking or planning to take any over-the-counter or prescription medications or dietary supplements with these drugs. Drug doses may need to be modified or a different drug prescribed. The following drugs and drug classes interact with these drugs:

alfentanil (*Alfenta*) (azithromycin, dirithromycin, erythromycin only)

antacids, aluminum- or magnesium-containing (eg, *Rolaids*) (azithromycin, dirithromycin only)

anticoagulants, oral (eg, warfarin) (azithromycin, dirithromycin, erythromycin only)

bromocriptine (*Parlodel*)

carbamazepine (eg, *Tegretol*)

cimetidine (eg, *Tagamet*) (dirithromycin only)

corticosteroids (eg, methylprednisolone) (dirithromycin, erythromycin only)

cyclosporine (eg, *Sandimmune)*

digoxin (eg, *Lanoxin)*

disopyramide (eg, *Norpace)*

ergot-containing drugs (eg, *Ergomar)*

felodipine (*Plendil*) (erythromycin only)

fluconazole (*Diflucan*) (clarithromycin only)

HMG-CoA reductase inhibitors (eg, lovastatin) (clarithromycin, erythromycin only)

omeprazole (eg, *Prilosec*) (clarithromycin only)

phenytoin (eg, *Dilantin*)

pimozide (*Orap*)

protease inhibitors (eg, ritonavir) (azithromycin only)
rifamycins (eg, rifampin)
(azithromycin only)
tacrolimus (*Prograf*) (azithromycin, clarithromycin only)
theophyllines (eg, amino-
phylline)

triazolam (eg, *Halcion*)
valproic acid (eg, valproate
sodium) (clarithromycin only)
vinblastine (eg, *Velban*) (erythromycin only)

## Side Effects:

Every drug is capable of producing side effects. Many patients experience no, or minor, side effects. The frequency and severity of side effects depend on many factors including dose, duration of therapy, and individual susceptibility. Possible side effects include:

*Digestive Tract:* Nausea; diarrhea; vomiting; stomach pain; upset stomach.

*Other:* Hives; rash; itching; difficulty breathing; headache.

*Azithromycin:* Vaginal itching or inflammation; dizziness; injection site pain and inflammation.

*Clarithromycin:* Taste changes.

*Dirithromycin:* Gas; weakness; dizziness; feeling of a whirling motion (vertigo); sleeplessness; cough; vaginal inflammation.

*Erythromycin:* Stomach cramps or discomfort; yellowing of eyes or skin; abnormal liver function tests.

---

## Guidelines for Use:

- Dosage is individualized. Take exactly as prescribed.
- Do not stop taking or change the dose, unless instructed by your doctor.
- Take tablets or capsules with a full glass of water (6 to 8 oz).
- Contact your doctor immediately if you experience nausea, vomiting, diarrhea, stomach cramps, unusual tiredness, severe stomach pain, yellow discoloration of skin or eyes, rash, dark urine, pale stools, chest pain, difficulty breathing, mouth sores, rash, hives, itching, or sensitivity to light. These may be signs of a serious allergic reaction. The medicine should be discontinued and appropriate therapy instituted.
- If diarrhea occurs, contact your doctor immediately. This could be a symptom of a severe side effect requiring immediate medical attention. Do not treat diarrhea without consulting your doctor.
- If a dose is missed, take it as soon as possible. If several hours have passed or it is nearing time for the next dose, do not double the dose to catch up, unless instructed by your doctor. If more than one dose is missed or it is necessary to establish a new dosage schedule, contact your doctor or pharmacist.

## Guidelines for Use (cont.):

- Continue use until all of the prescribed medicine has been taken, even if fever or other symptoms have disappeared. Failure to take all of the medicine may prevent complete elimination of bacteria, allowing the infection to return.
- *Azithromycin* – Take capsules and suspension at least 1 hour before or 2 hours after a meal. Tablets can be taken without regard to meals; take with food if stomach upset occurs.
  Do not take aluminum- or magnesium-containing antacids 1 hour before or 2 hours after taking this medicine.
  Store capsules and tablets at 59° to 86°F. Store powder packets at 41° to 86°F.
- *Clarithromycin* – Tablets and suspension may be taken without regard to food; take with food if stomach upset occurs. Take extended-release tablets with food.
  Follow each dose of the suspension with 6 to 8 oz of fluid.
  Take at evenly spaced intervals throughout the day, preferably every 12 hours.
  Adequate birth control is necessary with this product. If pregnancy occurs while taking this medication, there is a potential hazard to the fetus.
  Store tablets at room temperature (59° to 86°F); protect from light in a tightly closed container. Shake suspension well before each use. Do not refrigerate. After mixing suspension, store at room temperature (59° to 86°F) away from light. Use within 14 days. Discard any unused medication.
- *Dirithromycin* – Take with food or within 1 hour of eating. Do not cut, chew, or crush the tablets. Store at room temperature (59° to 86°F).
- *Erythromycin* – Take on an empty stomach, 1 hour before or 2 hours after meals. If stomach upset occurs, take with food. The estolate, ethylsuccinate, and enteric-coated forms of erythromycin are not significantly affected by food.
  Take at evenly spaced intervals throughout the day, preferably around the clock.
  After reconstitution of drops, liquid, and suspension, store at or below 77°F. Shake suspension well before using. Use within 14 days. Refrigerate to maintain the best taste.

*If you have any questions, consult your doctor, pharmacist, or health care provider.*

| Generic Name<br>*Brand Name Example* | Supplied As | Generic<br>Available |
|---|---|---|
| *Rx* **Spectinomycin HCl** | | |
| *Trobicin*[1] | **Powder for injection**<br>**(reconstituted)**: 200 mg/mL | No |

[1] Contains benzyl alcohol.

## Type of Drug:
Anti-infective.

## How the Drug Works:
Spectinomycin inhibits protein synthesis in bacterial cells, resulting in the death of the bacteria.

## Uses:
To treat acute gonorrheal urethritis and proctitis in men and acute gonorrheal cervicitis and proctitis in women due to susceptible strains of *Neisseria gonorrhoeae*, the bacteria that causes gonorrhea. Also used to treat men and women recently exposed to gonorrhea.

## Precautions:
*Do not use in the following situations:* Allergy to the drug or any of its ingredients.

*Use with caution in the following situations:* Patients with a history of atopy.

*Syphilis:* Spectinomycin is not effective in the treatment of syphilis. Antibiotics used in high doses for short periods of time to treat gonorrhea may mask or delay the symptoms of incubating syphilis. All patients with gonorrhea should have a serologic test for syphilis at the time of diagnosis and a follow up test after 3 months.

*Benzyl alcohol:* Spectinomycin contains benzyl alcohol, which has been associated with fatal "gasping syndrome" in premature infants and an increased incidence of neurologic and other complications.

*Pregnancy:* There are no adequate and well-controlled studies in pregnant women. Use only if clearly needed and the potential benefits outweigh the possible risk to the fetus.

*Breastfeeding:* It is not known if spectinomycin appears in breast milk. Consult your doctor before you begin breastfeeding.

*Children:* Safety and effectiveness have not been established.

## Drug Interactions:
Tell your doctor or pharmacist if you are taking or planning to take any over-the-counter or prescription medications or dietary supplements while taking this drug. Drug doses may need to be modified or a different drug prescribed.

## Side Effects:

Every drug is capable of producing side effects. Many patients experience no, or minor, side effects. The frequency and severity of side effects depend on many factors including dose, duration of therapy, and individual susceptibility. Possible side effects include: Soreness at injection site; nausea; dizziness; decreased urination; itching; hives; rash; chills; fever; sleeplessness.

---

### Guidelines for Use:

- This medication will be prepared and administered by your health care provider in a medical setting.
- To alleviate pain or soreness at injection site, apply warm compresses and take over-the-counter analgesics (eg, acetaminophen, ibuprofen).
- Patients treated with spectinomycin should have a follow-up blood test for syphilis after 3 months.

---

*If you have any questions, consult your doctor, pharmacist, or health care provider.*

| Generic Name<br>*Brand Name Examples* | Supplied As | Generic<br>Available |
|---|---|---|
| Rx **Erythromycin, Topical**[1] | | |
| *Staticin* | **Solution:** 1.5% | No |
| *A/T/S, Del-Mycin,*<br>*Erycette, Eryderm 2%,*<br>*Erymax, Erythra-Derm,*<br>*Theramycin Z, T-Stat* | **Solution:** 2% | Yes |
| *A/T/S, Emgel, Erygel* | **Gel:** 2% | Yes |

[1] Contains ethyl alcohol.

## Type of Drug:

Topical antibiotic; acne medicine applied to the skin.

## How the Drug Works:

The mechanism by which topical erythromycin treats acne is not known. Reduction of inflammatory lesions is presumably related to its antibiotic action.

## Uses:

For the topical treatment of acne vulgaris.

## Precautions:

*Do not use in the following situations:*

allergy to erythromycin or any of its ingredients
ophthalmic (eye) use

*Superinfection:* Use of antibiotics (especially long-term or repeated therapy) may result in bacterial or fungal overgrowth of nonsusceptible organisms (secondary infection). Contact your doctor if you suspect an infection unrelated to acne vulgaris.

*Diarrhea:* If diarrhea develops during topical erythromycin use, pseudomembranous colitis must be considered. This inflammatory condition of the colon is due to overgrowth of bacteria that are not killed by topical erythromycin. The primary cause is a toxin produced by a bacteria known as *Clostridia difficile.* Mild cases usually respond to stopping the antibiotic.

*Pregnancy:* There are no adeqate and well controlled studies in pregnant women. Use only when clearly needed and when the potential benefits outweigh the possible hazards to the fetus.

*Breastfeeding:* It is not known if erythromycin appears in breast milk after topical administration. Consult your doctor before you begin breastfeeding.

*Children:* Safety and efficacy in children have not been established.

## Drug Interactions:

Tell your doctor or pharmacist if you are taking or if you are planning to take any over-the-counter or prescription medications while using topical erythromycin. Doses of one or both drugs may need to be modified or a different drug may need to be prescribed.The following drugs and drug classes interact with topical erythromycin.

> acne therapy, topical (eg, abrasive, desquamating, or peeling agents)
> clindamycin (eg, *Cleocin T*)

## Side Effects:

Every drug is capable of causing side effects. Many patients experience no, or minor, side effects. The frequency and severity of side effects depend on many factors including dose, duration of therapy, and individual susceptibility. Possible side effects include:

*Skin:* Flushing, redness, peeling, burning, or tenderness in treated area; dryness; itching; oily skin; eye irritation; skin discoloration; inflammation of the face, eyes, or nose; hives.

---

### Guidelines for Use:

- For topical use only. Do not use in the eyes.
- Keep away from eyes, nose, mouth, and other mucous membranes. If contact occurs, flush with water.
- Apply topical erythromycin to the affected areas in the morning and evening. Wash affected areas with soap and water, rinse well, and pat dry before applying the drug.
- Reduce frequency of application to once a day if excessive drying and peeling occur.
- Apply gels with fingertips. Spread medication lightly. Do not rub into skin.
- Apply solutions with applicator pad or fingertips. Wash hands after application.
- If excessive skin irritation or diarrhea occurs, discontinue use and consult your doctor.
- If there has been no improvement after 6 to 8 weeks, or if condition worsens, discontinue treatment and contact your doctor.
- Use additional topical acne therapy with caution because a cumulative irritant effect may occur.
- Store at room temperature (59° to 77°F). Keep tightly closed.

---

*If you have any questions, consult your doctor, pharmacist, or health care provider.*

| Generic Name
Brand Name Examples | Supplied As | Generic Available |
| --- | --- | --- |
| Rx **Vancomycin HCl** | | |
| Vancocin | **Pulvules:** 125 mg, 250 mg | Yes |
| Vancocin | **Solution, oral:** 1 g, 10 g | Yes |
| Vancocin, Vancoled | **Powder for injection:** 500 mg, 1 g, 5 g, 10 g | Yes |

## Type of Drug:
Anti-infective; antibiotic.

## How the Drug Works:
Vancomycin inhibits RNA production and interferes with the formation of the bacterial cell wall in susceptible bacteria.

## Uses:
To treat staphylococcal enterocolitis and antibiotic-associated pseudomembranous colitis caused by *Clostridia difficile* (oral use only). The injection solution may also be given orally for this use. Oral use of vancomycin is not effective for other types of infection.

To treat serious, resistant, or severe infections (particularly staphylococcal infections) not treatable with other antimicrobials, including penicillins and cephalosporins (injection only).

To prevent bacterial inflammation of the heart (endocarditis) in penicillin-allergic patients who have congenital heart disease or rheumatic or other acquired or valvular heart disease when these patients undergo dental procedures or surgery of the upper respiratory tract (injection only).

## Precautions:
*Do not use in the following situations:* Allergy to vancomycin or any of its ingredients.

*Use with caution in the following situations:*

excessive dose requirements
hearing loss
intestinal lining inflammation
kidney disease
low blood pressure

nephrotoxic agent therapy, concurrent (eg, aminoglycosides)
ototoxic agent therapy, concurrent (eg, aminoglycosides)

*Superinfection:* Use of antibiotics (especially prolonged or repeated therapy) may result in bacterial or fungal overgrowth (secondary infection). Vancomycin may need to be stopped and another antibiotic may need to be prescribed for the second infection.

*Pseudomembranous colitis/diarrhea:* If diarrhea develops during IV use of vancomycin injection, pseudomembranous colitis must be considered. This inflammatory condition of the colon is due to overgrowth of bacteria that are not killed by vancomycin. Mild cases usually respond to stopping the antibiotic.

*Pregnancy:* There are no adequate and well-controlled studies in pregnant women. Use only if clearly needed and the potential benefits to the mother outweigh the possible hazards to the fetus.

*Breastfeeding:* Vancomycin appears in breast milk. A decision should be made whether to discontinue nursing or discontinue the drug, taking into account the importance of the drug to the mother.

*Children:* Dosage may need to be adjusted, especially in premature neonates and young infants.

*Elderly:* Dosage may need to be adjusted, especially when kidney disease is also present.

*Lab tests* may be required to monitor therapy. Tests include hearing tests, kidney function, vancomycin blood levels, and blood count tests.

## Drug Interactions:

Tell your doctor or pharmacist if you are taking or planning to take any over-the-counter or prescription medications or dietary supplements while taking vancomycin. Doses of one or both drugs may need to be modified or a different drug may need to be prescribed. The following drugs and drug classes interact with vancomycin:

> anesthetics (especially in children)
> nephrotoxic agents (eg, aminoglycosides, amphotericin B, cisplatin, bacitracin, polymyxin B)
> nondepolarizing muscle relaxants (eg, tubocurarine)
> ototoxic agents (eg, aminoglycosides)

## Side Effects:

Every drug is capable of producing side effects. Many vancomycin users experience no, or minor, side effects. The frequency and severity of side effects depend upon many factors including dose, duration of therapy, and individual susceptibility. Possible side effects include:

*Injection and oral:* Kidney dysfunction or failure; hearing loss; abnormal blood cell counts; hives; itching; diarrhea; nausea; chills; rash; fever; ringing in the ears; dizziness; feeling of a whirling sensation.

*Injection only:* Pain, tenderness, or inflammation at the injection site; low blood pressure; difficulty breathing; wheezing; pain and muscle spasm of chest and back; flushing of upper body; blood vessel inflammation.

## Guidelines for Use:

- Dosage is individualized. Take exactly as prescribed.
- Do not change the dose or stop taking, unless directed by your doctor.
- *Oral Solution* — Mix thoroughly to dissolve the dose. May be further diluted with 1 oz of water. Common flavoring syrups may be added to the solution to improve the taste. The diluted solution may be administered via nasogastric tube.
- *Injection* — For intravenous (IV; into a vein) use only. Visually inspect solutions for particles or discoloration before use. Follow the injection procedure taught to you by your health care provider. Administer dose over no less than 60 minutes to avoid rapid-infusion-related reactions.
- If a dose is missed, take or inject it as soon as possible. If several hours have passed or it is nearing time for the next dose, do not double the dose to catch up, unless advised by your doctor. If more than one dose is missed or it is necessary to establish a new dosage schedule, contact your doctor or pharmacist.
- Continue use until all of the prescribed medicine has been taken, even if fever or other symptoms have disappeared. Failure to use all of the medicine may prevent complete elimination of bacteria, allowing the infection to return.
- Dosage reduction may be necessary in patients with kidney function impairment and in premature neonates and young infants.
- If diarrhea develops during intravenous vancomycin use, pseudomembranous colitis must be considered. Contact your doctor immediately.
- Contact your doctor immediately if you experience sudden dizziness or lightheadedness with or without rash over the face and body, or hearing loss.
- Lab tests may be required to monitor therapy. Be sure to keep appointments.
- *Pulvules* — Store at controlled room temperature (59° to 86°F).
- *Oral Solution* — Store in the refrigerator. May be refrigerated for up to 2 weeks.
- *Injection* — Prior to reconstitution, store at room temperature (59° to 86°F). After reconstitution, store in the refrigerator. When reconstituted with 5% Dextrose Injection or 0.9% Sodium Chloride Injection, the injection may be kept for 14 days. When reconstituted with any other solution, the injection may stored for 96 hours (4 days).

*If you have any questions, consult your doctor, pharmacist, or health care provider.*

| Generic Name<br>*Brand Name Example* | Supplied As | Generic<br>Available |
|---|---|---|
| Rx **Linezolid**[1] | | |
| *Zyvox*[2] | **Tablets**: 400 mg, 600 mg | No |
| *Zyvox*[2,3] | **Suspension, oral**:<br>100 mg/5 mL | No |

[1] Also available as an intravenous injection
[2] Contains sodium.
[3] Contains phenylalanine.

## Type of Drug:
Anti-infective; antibiotic.

## How the Drug Works:
This drug inhibits bacterial protein synthesis, preventing bacterial reproduction.

## Uses:
For the treatment of vancomycin-resistant *Enterococcus faecium* infections, nosocomial pneumonia, complicated and uncomplicated skin and skin structure infections, and community-acquired pneumonia caused by susceptible bacteria.

## Precautions:
*Do not use in the following situations:* Allergy to linezolid or any of its ingredients.

*Use with caution in the following situations:* History of high blood pressure.

*Phenylketonuria:* Each 5 mL of linezolid oral suspension contains 20 mg phenylalanine. Consult your doctor or pharmacist.

*Myelosuppression:* Myelosuppression has been reported in patients receiving linezolid. Monitor blood counts weekly, particularly in those who receive linezolid for longer than 2 weeks, those with preexisting myelosuppression, those receiving drugs that produce bone marrow suppression, or those with a chronic infection who have received previous or concomitant antibiotic therapy. Consider stopping linezolid therapy in patients who develop or have worsening myelosuppression.

*Pseudomembranous colitis/diarrhea:* If diarrhea develops during linezolid use, pseudomembranous colitis must be considered. This inflammatory condition of the colon is due to overgrowth of bacteria that are not killed by linezolid. Mild cases usually respond when drug use is discontinued.

*Tyramine-containing foods:* Avoid large quantities of food or beverages with high tyramine content while taking linezolid. Quantities of tyramine consumed should be less than 100 mg/meal. Foods high in tyramine content include those that may have undergone protein changes by aging, fermentation, pickling, or smoking to improve flavor, such as aged cheeses (0 to 15 mg tyramine/oz), fermented or air-dried meats (0.1 to 8 mg tyramine/oz), sauerkraut (8 mg tyramine/8 oz), soy sauce (5 mg tyramine/1 tsp), tap beers (4 mg tyramine/12 oz), and red wines (0 to 6 mg tyramine/8 oz). The tyramine content of any protein-rich food may be increased if stored for long periods or improperly refrigerated.

*Pregnancy:* There are no adequate and well-controlled studies in pregnant women. Use only if clearly needed and the potential benefits to the mother outweigh the possible hazards to the fetus.

*Breastfeeding:* It is not known if linezolid appears in breast milk. Consult your doctor before you begin breastfeeding.

*Children:* Safety and effectiveness have not been established.

*Lab tests* may be required to monitor therapy. Tests include weekly blood counts.

## Drug Interactions:

Tell your doctor or pharmacist if you are taking or planning to take any over-the-counter or prescription medications or dietary supplements while taking linezolid. Doses of one or both drugs may need to be modified or a different drug may need to be prescribed. The following drugs or drug classes interact with linezolid:

> adrenergic agents (eg, epinephrine, pseudoephedrine)
> selective serotonin reuptake inhibitors (eg, fluoxetine)
> MAOIs (eg, phenelzine)

## Side Effects:

Every drug is capable of producing side effects. Many linezolid users experience no, or minor, side effects. The frequency and severity of side effects depend on many factors including dose, duration of therapy, and individual susceptibility. Possible side effects include:

*Digestive Tract:* Diarrhea; nausea; vomiting; taste sensation altered; tongue discoloration; constipation.

*Other:* Abnormal blood counts; headache; dizziness; rash; fever; changes in blood pressure; vaginal infection; fungal infection; abnormal lab tests; sleeplessness; itching.

## Guidelines for Use:

- Dosage is individualized. Take exactly as prescribed.
- Do not change or stop taking the dose, unless directed by your doctor.
- May be taken without regard to meals.
- Notify your doctor if you experience frequent and persistent diarrhea.
- Do not vigorously shake the oral suspension before use. Gently invert the bottle a few times to mix.
- Inform your doctor if you are taking medications containing pseudo-ephedrine, such as cold remedies and decongestants.
- Inform your doctor if you are taking selective serotonin reuptake inhibitors or other antidepressants.
- Avoid eating large quantities of food or beverages with a high tyramine content.
- Lab tests may be required to monitor therapy. Be sure to keep appointments.
- Store at room temperature (59° to 86°F) in a tightly-closed container. Protect from light. Use oral suspension within 21 days.

*If you have any questions, consult your doctor, pharmacist, or health care provider.*

| Generic Name<br>*Brand Name Examples* | Supplied As | Generic<br>Available |
|---|---|---|
| *Rx* **Ciprofloxacin**[1] | | |
| *Cipro* | **Suspension, oral:** 5 g/100 mL,<br>10 g/100 mL | No |
| *Cipro* | **Tablets:** 100 mg, 250 mg,<br>500 mg, 750 mg | No |
| *Rx* **Gatifloxacin**[1] | | |
| *Tequin* | **Tablets**: 200 mg, 400 mg | No |
| *Rx* **Levofloxacin**[1] | | |
| *Levaquin* | **Tablets:** 250 mg, 500 mg,<br>750 mg | No |
| *Rx* **Lomefloxacin HCl** | | |
| *Maxaquin* | **Tablets, film-coated:** 400 mg | No |
| *Rx* **Moxifloxacin HCl**[1] | | |
| *Avelox* | **Tablets**: 400 mg | No |
| *Rx* **Norfloxacin** | | |
| *Noroxin* | **Tablets:** 400 mg | No |
| *Rx* **Ofloxacin**[1] | | |
| *Floxin* | **Tablets:** 200 mg, 300 mg,<br>400 mg | No |
| *Rx* **Sparfloxacin** | | |
| *Zagam* | **Tablets:** 200 mg | No |
| *Rx* **Trovafloxacin Mesylate**[2] | | |
| *Trovan* | **Tablets:** 100 mg, 200 mg | No |

[1] Also available as an injection.
[2] Alatrofloxacin mesylate is available as an injection.

## Type of Drug:

Anti-infectives; antibiotics.

## How the Drug Works:

Fluoroquinolones cause an inhibition of DNA production of susceptible bacteria, resulting in inability to reproduce and bacterial cell death.

## Uses:

*Ciprofloxacin:* To treat acute sinusitis, lower respiratory tract infections (eg, bronchitis), nosocomial pneumonia, skin and skin structure infections, bone and joint infections, urinary tract infections, infectious diarrhea, typhoid fever, acute uncomplicated cystitis in women, chronic prostate infection, complicated intra-abdominal infections (in combination therapy), inhalation anthrax (postexposure), and uncomplicated cervical, rectal, and urethral gonorrhea caused by susceptible bacteria. Also used as empirical therapy for febrile neutropenic patients.

*Gatifloxacin:* To treat chronic bronchitis, acute sinusitis, community-acquired pneumonia, complicated and uncomplicated urinary tract infections, pyelonephritis, uncomplicated urethral and cervical gonorrhea, and acute, uncomplicated rectal infections in women.

*Levofloxacin:* To treat sinus infections, lower respiratory system infections (eg, chronic bronchitis, community-acquired pneumonia), complicated and uncomplicated skin and skin structure infections, complicated and uncomplicated urinary tract infections, and acute pyelonephritis.

*Lomefloxacin:* To treat lower respiratory infections (except chronic bronchitis caused by *Streptococcus pneumoniae*) and urinary tract infections. Also used for preoperative prevention of infection in certain types of surgery.

*Moxifloxacin:* To treat acute bacterial sinusitis, acute bacterial exacerbation of chronic bronchitis, community-acquired pneumonia, and uncomplicated skin structure infections.

*Norfloxacin:* To treat sexually transmitted diseases (eg, uncomplicated gonorrhea), urinary tract infections, and prostate infections.

*Ofloxacin:* To treat lower respiratory infections (eg, chronic bronchitis, community-acquired pneumonia), sexually transmitted diseases (eg, uncomplicated gonorrhea, nongonococcal urethritis and cervicitis, acute pelvic inflammatory disease), skin and skin structure infections, uncomplicated cystitis, complicated urinary tract infections, and prostate infections.

*Sparfloxacin:* To treat community-acquired pneumonia and acute bacterial exacerbations of chronic bronchitis.

*Trovafloxacin/alatrofloxacin:* For use as initiating therapy in in-patient health care facilities to treat serious life- or limb-threatening infections such as community-acquired pneumonia, nosocomial pneumonia, complicated intra-abdominal infections, gynecologic and pelvic infections, and skin and skin structure infections.

*Unlabeled Use(s):* Occasionally doctors may prescribe fluoroquinolones for traveler's diarrhea, gonorrheal complications, ear infections, joint infections, bacterial meningitis, blood infections, bronchitis, pneumonia, prostate infections, osteomyelitis, prevention in urological surgery, pelvic inflammatory disease (PID), sinus infections, and endocarditis (inflammation of the lining of the heart).

## Precautions:
*Do not use in the following situations:*
> allergy to any fluoroquinolone antibiotic or any of its ingredients
> allergy to quinolones
> low blood potassium
> tendon rupture associated with quinolone use, history of tendonitis
> $QT_C$ prolongation (abnormal heartbeat, electrocardiogram abnormality) (gatifloxacin, moxifloxacin only)
> $QT_C$ prolonging antiarrythmic drug (eg, disopyramide, amiodarone) therapy, concurrent

*Use with caution in the following situations:*

| | |
|---|---|
| kidney disease | nervous system disorders, |
| liver disease | known or suspected (eg, epi- |
| myasthenia gravis | lepsy) |

*CNS stimulant toxicity:* May produce seizures, psychosis, tremors, restlessness, light-headedness, confusion, hallucinations, paranoia, depression, nightmares, and sleeplessness.

*Pseudomembranous colitis/diarrhea:* If diarrhea develops during fluoroquinolone use, pseudomembranous colitis must be considered. This inflammatory condition of the colon is due to overgrowth of bacteria that are not killed by fluoroquinolones. Mild cases usually respond to stopping the antibiotic.

*Sensitivity to light:* May cause photosensitivity (sensitivity to sunlight), especially in patients using ciprofloxacin, lomefloxacin, ofloxacin, sparfloxacin, or trovafloxacin. Avoid prolonged exposure to the sun and other ultraviolet (UV) light sources (eg, tanning beds). Use sunscreens and wear protective clothing until tolerance is determined.

*Superinfection:* Use of antibiotics (especially prolonged or repeated therapy) may result in bacterial or fungal overgrowth. Such overgrowth may lead to a second infection. Fluoroquinolones may need to be stopped and another antibiotic may need to be prescribed for the second infection.

*Syphilis testing:* These medicines may mask or delay symptoms of syphilis during treatment for gonorrhea. At the time of gonorrhea diagnosis, patients should also be tested for syphilis. Patients should also have a follow-up test for syphilis after 3 months.

*Tendonitis:* Discontinue taking medicine, notify your doctor, rest, and refrain from exercise if you experience joint or muscle pain, inflammation, or rupture of a tendon.

*Pregnancy:* There are no adequate and well-controlled studies in pregnant women. Use only if clearly needed and the potential benefits to the mother outweigh the possible hazards to the fetus.

*Breastfeeding:* Ciprofloxacin, ofloxacin, sparfloxacin, and trovafloxacin appear in breast milk. It is not known if other fluoroquinolones appear in breast milk. Because of the potential for serious adverse reactions, decide whether to discontinue nursing or discontinue the drug, taking into account the importance of the drug to the mother. Consult your doctor before you begin breastfeeding.

*Children:* Safety and effectiveness in children have not been established. Use in patients under 18 years of age is not recommended.

*Elderly:* Elderly patients may require adjusted dosages, particularly if moderate to severe kidney impairment exists.

*Lab tests* may be required to monitor therapy. Tests include blood counts, liver, pancreas, and kidney function tests, blood glucose monitoring, and blood pressure monitoring.

## Drug Interactions:

Tell your doctor or pharmacist if you are taking or if you are planning to take any over-the-counter or prescription medications or dietary supplements while taking a fluoroquinolone. Doses of one or both drugs may need to be modified or a different drug may need to be prescribed. The following drugs and drug classes interact with fluoroquinolones although not every fluoroquinolone may interact similarly:

antacids with aluminum, calcium, or magnesium (eg, *Amphojel, Tums, Milk of Magnesia*)
antiarrythmic agents (eg, amiodarone, quinidine)
anticoagulants (eg, warfarin)
caffeine
cyclosporine (eg, *Neoral*)
didanosine (*Videx*)
disopyramide (eg, *Norpace*)
glyburide (eg, *Micronase*)
iron salts (eg, ferrous fumarate)
macrolide antibiotics (eg, erythromycin)
nitrofurantoin (*Furadantin*)
NSAIDs (eg, ibuprofen)
phenothiazines (eg, promethazine)
phenytoin (eg, *Dilantin*)
procainamide (eg, *Pronestyl*)
sotalol (eg, *Betapace*)
sucralfate (eg, *Carafate*)
theophyllines (eg, aminophylline)
tricyclic antidepressants (eg, amitriptyline)
warfarin (eg, *Coumadin*)
zinc salts

## Side Effects:

Every drug is capable of producing side effects. Many fluoroquinolone users experience no, or minor, side effects. The frequency and severity of side effects depend on many factors including dose, duration of therapy, and individual susceptibility. Possible side effects include:

*Digestive Tract:* Nausea; vomiting; diarrhea; stomach pain; appetite loss; constipation; heartburn; gas; dry or painful mouth; indigestion; taste sensation changes; pseudomembranous colitis; oral fungal infection; mouth sores.

*Nervous System:* Dizziness; drowsiness; headache; sleeplessness; sleep disturbances; vertigo (feeling of whirling motion); nervousness; weakness; fatigue; psychotic reactions; hallucinations; seizures; confusion; depression; anxiety; light-headedness; paranoia; agitation; abnormal dreams; tremor.

*Circulatory System:* Abnormal heart rhythm; fast heartbeat; heart murmur; blood sugar changes; changes in blood pressure; palpitations (pounding in the chest).

*Skin:* Rash; hives; itching; photosensitivity; external vaginal itching; dry skin; sweating; pain and redness at injection site.

*Other:* Restlessness; vaginal irritation or discharge; lack of energy; general body discomfort; fever; vision disturbances; hearing loss; fainting; chills; swelling; abnormal lab tests; ringing in the ears; painful or difficult urination; blood in the urine; sore throat; exacerbated signs of myasthenia gravis; joint pain or stiffness; jaw, arm, back, neck, or chest pain; gout flare up; tingling of the fingers; difficulty breathing; tremor; sweating; runny nose; facial swelling; thirst; leg cramps; fainting; liver damage (trovafloxacin, alatrofloxacin only).

## Guidelines for Use:

- Dosage is individualized. Take exactly as prescribed.
- Do not change the dose or stop taking, unless directed by your doctor.
- Take norfloxacin on an empty stomach, 1 hour before or 2 hours after meals. All other fluoroquinolones may be taken without regard to meals.
- Drink plenty of liquids while taking this medicine.
- Do not consume caffeine-containing products (eg, certain drugs, coffee, tea, certain carbonated beverages) during therapy with fluorquinolones (other than sparfloxacin).
- Do not take antacids containing magnesium, calcium, or aluminum or products containing citric acid buffered with sodium citrate, iron, magnesium, zinc, or didanosine chewable/buffered tablets or buffered solution, or the pediatric powder for oral solution simultaneously or within 6 hours before or 2 hours (8 hours for moxifloxacin) after taking a fluoroquinolone.
- If a dose is missed, take it as soon as possible. If several hours have passed or it is nearing time for the next dose, do not double dose to catch up, unless advised to do so by your doctor. If more than one dose is missed, or it is necessary to establish a new dosage schedule, contact your doctor or pharmacist.
- May cause dizziness or light-headedness. Use caution when driving or performing other tasks requiring alertness, coordination, or physical dexterity until tolerance is determined.
- Stop taking at first appearance of rash, facial swelling, rapid heartbeat, difficulty breathing, or other allergic signs. Report nausea, vomiting, or diarrhea to your doctor.
- Continue use until all of the prescribed drug has been taken, even if fever or other symptoms of infection have disappeared. Failure to take a full course of therapy may prevent complete elimination of bacteria, causing a relapse of infection.
- Discontinue medication and notify your doctor if you experience tremors; light-headedness; appetite loss; yellowing of the skin or eyes; dark urine; pale stools; confusion; hallucinations; palpitations (pounding in the chest); fainting spells; paranoia; depression; nightmares; insomnia; or pain, inflammation, or rupture of a tendon.
- Patients with a history of seizures or other nervous system disorders should consult their doctor before use.
- Diabetic patients should monitor blood sugar regularly while taking a fluoroquinolone. Notify your doctor immediately if you experience a hypoglycemic or hyperglycemic reaction.
- May cause sensitivity to sunlight. Avoid prolonged exposure to sun or other ultraviolet (UV) light (eg, tanning beds). Use sunscreens and wear protective clothing. Discontinue use if you experience burning sensation, redness, swelling, blisters, rash, or itching.
- Lab tests may be required to monitor therapy. Be sure to keep appointments.
- Store as directed by the package labeling.

*If you have any questions, consult your doctor, pharmacist, or health care provider.*

| Generic Name | | Generic |
| Brand Name Example | Supplied As | Available |
| --- | --- | --- |
| Rx **Meropenem** | | |
| *Merrem I.V.* | **Powder for injection:** 500 mg, 1 g | No |

## Type of Drug:
Carbapenem antibiotic.

## How the Drug Works:
Meropenem kills certain bacteria by interfering with formation of the bacterial cell wall.

## Uses:
To treat serious infections caused by susceptible bacteria that produce complicated intra-abdominal infections and bacterial meningitis (in children 3 months of age and older).

## Precautions:
*Do not use in the following situations:*
allergy to meropenem or any of its ingredients
allergy to other carbapenem antibiotics
anaphylactic reaction to β-lactams (eg, penicillin)

*Use with caution in the following situations:*
allergy to cephalosporins
bacterial meningitis
brain lesions
colitis, active
compromised kidney function
diarrhea, active
multiple allergies, history of
seizures, history of

*Kidney function impairment:* A dosage adjustment is required in patients with kidney function impairment.

*Pseudomembranous colitis/diarrhea:* If diarrhea develops during meropenem use, pseudomembranous colitis must be considered. This inflammatory condition of the colon is due to overgrowth of bacteria not killed by meropenem. Mild cases usually respond to stopping the antibiotic.

*Superinfection:* Use of antibiotics (especially prolonged or repeated therapy) may result in bacterial or fungal overgrowth. Such overgrowth may lead to a secondary infection. Meropenem may need to be stopped and another antibiotic prescribed for the secondary infection.

*Pregnancy:* There are no adequate and well-controlled studies in pregnant women. Use only if clearly needed and the potential benefits to the mother outweigh the possible hazards to the fetus.

*Breastfeeding:* It is not known if meropenem appears in breast milk. Consult your doctor before you begin breastfeeding.

*Children:* The safety and effectiveness of meropenem have been established in patients 3 months of age and older. Use of meropenem in pediatric patients with bacterial meningitis or intra-abdominal infections is supported by evidence from adequate and well-controlled studies.

*Elderly:* A dosage adjustment is recommended in elderly patients with diminished kidney function.

*Lab tests* may be required to monitor therapy. Tests may include periodic assessment of organ function, including kidney, liver, and blood function.

## Drug Interactions:

Tell your doctor or pharmacist if you are taking or planning to take any over-the-counter or prescription medications or dietary supplements with this drug. Drug doses may need to be modified or a different drug prescribed. Probenecid interacts with meropenem.

## Side Effects:

Every drug is capable of producing side effects. Many patients experience side effects. The frequency and severity of side effects depend on many factors including dose, duration of therapy, and individual susceptibility. Possible side effects include:

*Digestive Tract:* Diarrhea; nausea; vomiting; constipation; bloody stools; mouth infection; inflammation of the tongue.

*Skin:* Hives; rash; itching.

*Other:* Headache; nosebleed; difficulty breathing; inflammation at injection site; vein inflammation; abnormal lab tests.

---

### Guidelines for Use:

- Dosage is individualized. Use exactly as prescribed.
- Do not stop taking or change the dose, unless instructed by your doctor.
- If a dose is missed, inject it as soon as possible. If several hours have passed or it is nearing time for the next dose, do not double the dose to catch up, unless instructed by your doctor. If more than one dose is missed or it is necessary to establish a new dosage schedule, contact your doctor or pharmacist.
- Notify your doctor if you experience rash, itching, shortness of breath, dizziness, diarrhea or disorientation.
- The dose and duration of therapy is based on location and severity of infection, age, and kidney function.
- This drug is given by injection. Solutions for injection must be prepared using appropriate aseptic techniques.
- This drug should not be added to solutions containing other drugs.
- Lab tests may be required to monitor treatment. Be sure to keep appointments.
- It is best to administer freshly prepared solution; however, solutions remain stable for 1 to 4 hours at room temperature (59° to 86°F) or for 2 to 24 hours if refrigerated, depending on the solution in which it is mixed. Check product literature for specific storage guidelines.

---

*If you have any questions, consult your doctor, pharmacist, or health care provider.*

| Generic Name<br>*Brand Name Example* | Supplied As | Generic<br>Available |
|---|---|---|
| *Rx* **Ertapenem**<br>*Invanz* | **Injection:** 1 g | No |

## Type of Drug:
Anti-infective; antibiotic.

## How the Drug Works:
Ertapenem kills certain bacteria by interfering with the formation of the bacterial cell wall.

## Uses:
To treat serious infections caused by susceptible bacteria that produce complicated intra-abdominal infections, complicated skin and skin structure infections, community-acquired pneumonia, complicated urinary tract infections, and acute pelvic infections.

## Precautions:
*Do not use in the following situations:*

allergy to local anesthetics of the amide type (intramuscular [IM] administration only)

allergy to the drug or any of its ingredients

*Use with caution in the following situations:*

allergy to penicillins, cephalosporins, or other beta-lactams
brain injury or disease

kidney disease
nervous system disorder (eg, seizures)

*Superinfection:* Use of antibiotics (especially prolonged or repeated therapy) may result in bacterial or fungal overgrowth. Such overgrowth may lead to a secondary infection. Ertapenem may need to be stopped and another antibiotic prescribed for the secondary infection.

*Diarrhea/Pseudomembranous colitis:* If diarrhea develops during ertapenem use, pseudomembranous colitis must be considered. This inflammatory condition of the colon is due to overgrowth of bacteria that are not killed by ertapenem. The primary cause is a toxin produced by the bacteria *Clostridia difficile*. Mild cases usually respond to stopping the antibiotic.

*Pregnancy:* There are no adequate and well-controlled studies in pregnant women. Use only if clearly needed and the potential benefits outweigh the possible risks to the fetus.

*Breastfeeding:* Ertapenem appears in breast milk. Consult your doctor before you begin breastfeeding.

*Children:* Safety and effectiveness in pediatric patients have not been established. Therefore, use in patients under 18 years of age is not recommended.

*Lab tests* may be required to monitor treatment. Tests include blood counts and liver and kidney function tests.

## Drug Interactions:

Tell your doctor or pharmacist if you are taking or planning to take any over-the-counter or prescription medications or dietary supplements while taking this drug. Drug doses may need to be modified or a different drug prescribed. Probenecid interacts with ertapenem.

## Side Effects:

Every drug is capable of producing side effects. Many patients experience no, or minor, side effects. The frequency and severity of side effects depend on many factors including dose, duration of therapy, and individual susceptibility. Possible side effects include:

*Digestive Tract:* Upset stomach; diarrhea; constipation; stomach pain; nausea; vomiting; stomach acid regurgitation.

*Nervous System:* Fatigue; anxiety; dizziness; headache; confusion; disorientation; sleeplessness; stupor; sleepiness.

*Circulatory System:* Changes in blood pressure; rapid heartbeat; vein inflammation; chest pain.

*Other:* Death; swelling; fever; cough; difficulty breathing; sore throat; itching; rash; flushing; vaginal inflammation.

---

### Guidelines for Use:

- Dosage is individualized. Take exactly as prescribed.
- Duration of therapy depends on the condition being treated and its severity. Therapy should not be stopped without consulting your doctor.
- If a dose is missed, inject it as soon as possible. If several hours have passed or it is nearing time for the next dose, do not double the dose to catch up, unless instructed by your doctor. If more than one dose is missed, contact your doctor or pharmacist.
- Contact your doctor immediately if you experience rash or other signs of allergic reaction (eg, difficulty breathing).
- Inform your doctor if you are pregnant, become pregnant, plan to become pregnant, or are breastfeeding.
- Lab tests may be required to monitor treatment. Be sure to keep appointments.
- The reconstituted solution may be stored at room temperature (77°F) and used within 6 hours or stored for 24 hours under refrigeration (41°F) and used within 4 hours after removal from refrigeration. Do not freeze.

---

*If you have any questions, consult your doctor, pharmacist, or health care provider.*

| Generic Name<br>*Brand Name Example* | Supplied As | Generic<br>Available |
|---|---|---|
| *Rx* **Imipenem-Cilastatin** | | |
| *Primaxin I.V.*[1] | **Injection:** 250 mg imipenem/<br>250 mg cilastatin, 500 mg imipenem/500 mg cilastatin | No |
| *Primaxin I.M.*[2] | **Injection:** 500 mg imipenem/<br>500 mg cilastatin, 750 mg imipenem/750 mg cilastatin | No |

[1] Contains 75 mg sodium.
[2] Contains 64 mg sodium.

## Type of Drug:
Anti-infection drug; antibiotic.

## How the Drug Works:
Imipenem-cilastatin kills certain susceptible bacteria by interfering with formation of the bacterial cell wall.

## Uses:
*Primaxin I.M.:* To treat serious infections caused by susceptible bacteria that produce lower respiratory tract, intra-abdominal, gynecological, and skin infections.

*Primaxin I.V.:* To treat serious infections caused by susceptible bacteria that produce lower respiratory tract, intra-abdominal, gynecological, skin, urinary tract, bone and joint, and polymicrobic infections (infections due to several species of organisms), bacterial septicemia (blood poisoning), endocarditis (bacterial infection of the heart valves and tissues), and infections resistant to other antibiotics (eg, cephalosporins, penicillins, aminoglycosides).

## Precautions:
*Do not use in the following situations:*
   allergy to local anesthetics of the amide type (IM [intramuscular; into a muscle] only)
   allergy to the drug or any of its ingredients
   severe shock or heart block due to use of lidocaine HCl diluent (IM only)

*Use with caution in the following situations:*
   allergy to penicillins, cephalosporins, or other beta-lactams
   brain injury or disease (IV [intravenous; into a vein] only)
   hemodialysis patients (IV only)
   kidney disease, severe (IV only)
   nervous system disorder (eg, seizures) (IV only)

*Superinfection:* Use of antibiotics (especially prolonged or repeated therapy) may result in bacterial or fungal overgrowth. Such overgrowth may lead to a secondary infection. Imipenem-cilastatin may need to be stopped and another antibiotic prescribed for the secondary infection.

*Diarrhea/Pseudomembranous Colitis:* If diarrhea develops during imipenem-cilastatin use, consider pseudomembranous colitis. This inflammatory condition of the colon is due to overgrowth of bacteria that are not killed by imipenem-cilastatin. The primary cause is a toxin produced by the bacteria *Clostridia difficile*. Mild cases usually respond after stopping the antibiotic.

*Pregnancy:* There are no adequate and well-controlled studies in pregnant women. Use only if clearly needed and the potential benefits outweigh the possible risks to the fetus.

*Breastfeeding:* It is not known if imipenem-cilastatin appears in breast milk. Consult your doctor before you begin breastfeeding.

*Children:* Safety and effectiveness of IM administration in children younger than 12 years of age have not been established. Safety and effectiveness of IV administration have been established in children.

*Lab tests* may be required to monitor treatment. Tests include blood counts and liver and kidney function tests.

## Drug Interactions:
Tell your doctor or pharmacist if you are taking or planning to take any over-the-counter or prescription medications or dietary supplements while taking this drug. Drug doses may need to be modified or a different drug prescribed. The following drugs and drug classes interact with this drug:

> cyclosporine (eg, *Sandimmune*)
> ganciclovir (eg, *Cytovene*) (IV only)

## Side Effects:
Every drug is capable of producing side effects. Many patients experience no, or minor, side effects. The frequency and severity of side effects depend on many factors including dose, duration of therapy, and individual susceptibility. Possible side effects include:

*Local:* Vein and injection site inflammation; pain or redness at injection site.

*Other:* Fever; itching; rash; seizures; drowsiness; dizziness; low blood pressure; nausea; vomiting; diarrhea.

## Guidelines for Use:

- The initial dose is based on location and severity of infection, susceptibility of bacteria to the drug, and patient characteristics (eg, age, weight, kidney function). Duration of therapy depends on the condition being treated and its severity. Take exactly as prescribed.
- Do not stop taking or change the dose, unless instructed by your doctor.
- If a dose is missed, inject it as soon as possible. If several hours have passed or it is nearing time for the next dose, do not double the dose to catch up, unless instructed by your doctor. If more than one dose is missed, contact your doctor or pharmacist.
- Notify your doctor if you experience itching, rash, shortness of breath, difficulty breathing, dizziness, or disorientation.
- Inform your doctor if you are pregnant, become pregnant, plan to become pregnant, or are breastfeeding.
- Lab tests may be required to monitor treatment. Be sure to keep appointments.
- *Primaxin I.M.* — Administer IM injection in the thigh or buttocks only. Use within 1 hour after preparation. Keep refrigerated; do not freeze reconstituted solution.
- *Primaxin I.V.* — Reconstituted solution maintains potency for 4 hours at room temperature (59° to 86°F) and for 24 hours when refrigerated. Do not freeze.

*If you have any questions, consult your doctor, pharmacist, or health care provider.*

| Generic Name Brand Name Examples | Supplied As | Generic Available |
|---|---|---|
| Rx **Metronidazole**[1] | | |
| *Flagyl* | **Tablets:** 250 mg, 500 mg | Yes |
| *Flagyl ER* | **Tablets, extended release:** 750 mg | No |
| *Flagyl 375* | **Capsules:** 375 mg | No |
| *MetroCream* | **Cream:** 0.75% | No |
| *Noritate* | **Cream:** 1% | No |
| *MetroGel* | **Gel:** 0.75% | No |
| *MetroGel Vaginal* | **Gel, vaginal:** 0.75% | No |
| *MetroLotion* | **Lotion:** 0.75% | No |

[1] Some of these products are also available as an injection.

## Type of Drug:

Antibiotic; anti-infection drug active against various bacteria and protozoa.

## How the Drug Works:

Metronidazole enters the bacterial or protozoal cell, impairing production of essential chemicals and leading to cell death.

## Uses:

*Oral:* To treat infections caused by susceptible bacteria, including abdominal infections (peritonitis, abscess), skin infections, gynecologic infections (eg, endometritis), infections of the blood, bone and joint infections, meningitis and brain abscess, lower respiratory infections (eg, pneumonia), and endocarditis.

To treat amebiasis and trichomoniasis (protozoal infections).

*Topical:* To treat inflammatory papules and pustules of rosacea (acne).

*Vaginal:* To treat bacterial vaginal disease.

*Unlabeled Use(s):* Occasionally doctors may prescribe metronidazole to reduce infection rates in gynecologic and abdominal surgery and to treat hepatic encephalopathy, Crohn disease, antibiotic-associated colitis, giardia infections, and stomach ulcers caused by certain bacteria.

## Precautions:

*Do not use in the following situations:*

allergy to the drug, any of its ingredients, or similar drugs
pregnancy, first trimester in patients with trichomoniasis

*Use with caution in the following situations:*

blood disorders
central nervous system disorders (eg, seizures)

liver disease, severe
peripheral neuropathy

*Nervous system effects:* Seizures and numbness or tingling of the hands and feet have been reported. Stop taking this medicine if such symptoms occur. In some cases, the symptoms are not reversible.

*Pregnancy:* There are no adequate and well-controlled studies in pregnant women. Use only during the second and third trimesters if alternative treatment has been inadequate and only if clearly needed and potential benefits outweigh the possible hazards to the fetus.

*Breastfeeding:* Metronidazole appears in breast milk. A nursing mother should express and discard any breast milk produced while on the drug and resume breastfeeding 24 to 48 hours after the drug is stopped.

*Children:* Except for amebiasis treatment, safety and effectiveness have not been established.

*Lab tests* may be required to monitor treatment. Tests include white blood cell counts, prothrombin tests for patients taking oral anticoagulants, and lithium level tests for patients taking lithium.

## Drug Interactions:
Tell your doctor or pharmacist if you are taking or planning to take any over-the-counter or prescription medications or dietary supplements with this drug. Drug doses may need to be modified or a different drug prescribed. The following drugs and drug classes interact with this drug:

alcohol
anticoagulants, oral
 (eg, *Coumadin*)
cimetidine (eg, *Tagamet*)

disulfiram (eg, *Antabuse*)
lithium (eg, *Eskalith*)
phenobarbital (eg, *Bellatal*)
phenytoin (eg, *Dilantin*)

## Side Effects:
Every drug is capable of producing side effects. Many patients experience no, or minor, side effects. The frequency and severity of side effects depend on many factors including dose, duration of therapy, and individual susceptibility. Possible side effects include:

*Oral –*

*Digestive Tract:* Nausea; vomiting; diarrhea; appetite loss; stomachache or cramping; constipation; dry mouth; furry tongue; inflammation of the mouth or tongue.

*Nervous System:* Seizures; feeling of whirling motion (vertigo); depression; lack of coordination; confusion; irritability; weakness; sleeplessness; headache; dizziness.

*Skin:* Rash; hives; flushing; itching.

*Urinary and Reproductive Tract:* Sense of pelvic pressure; pain during sex; decreased sex drive; dryness of vagina or vulva; prostate inflammation; difficult urination; painful or increased urination; incontinence; dark urine.

*Other:* Joint pain; metallic taste; nasal congestion; abnormal blood counts; overgrowth of *Candida* (yeast); tingling in hands and feet; numbness; abnormal skin sensations; fever.

*Topical:* Tearing of eyes (if drug is applied too close to the eye); redness; mild dryness, burning, and irritation of the skin; stinging; metallic taste; tingling or numbness of the arms and legs; nausea.

*Topical vaginal:* Vaginal discharge; cramping; vulva or vaginal irritation or burning sensation; pelvic discomfort; stomach discomfort; nausea; vomiting; metallic taste; diarrhea; decreased appetite; headache; dizziness; abnormal blood counts.

## Guidelines for Use:

*Oral:*
- Dosage is individualized. Take exactly as prescribed.
- Do not stop taking or change the dose, unless instructed by your doctor.
- Take extended-release tablets at least 1 hour before or 2 hours after meals.
- Take the full course of therapy to produce the best response.
- Avoid alcoholic beverages. Concurrent use of alcohol and metronidazole may produce stomach pain, nausea, vomiting, headache, and flushing. Do not consume alcohol until at least 1 full day after therapy with tablets is stopped and until at least 3 days after therapy with capsules and extended-release tablets is stopped.
- Inform your doctor if you are pregnant, become pregnant, are planning to become pregnant, or are breastfeeding.
- May cause a darkening of the urine or a metallic taste sensation. This is no cause for concern.
- Sexual partners of patients with trichomoniasis should be treated simultaneously, whether they have symptoms or not.
- Stop taking this medication and notify your doctor if you experience seizures, numbness, or tingling in arms or legs.

*Topical:*
- Wash area before application. Rub in a thin film twice daily.
- For external use only. Avoid contact with the eyes.
- Store at controlled room temperature (68° to 77°F).

*Vaginal:*
- Usual dosage is one application of gel intravaginally once or twice a day for 5 days. For once-a-day dosing, administer at bedtime.
- Store at controlled room temperature (59° to 86°F).

*Injection:*
- This medicine will be prepared and administered by your health care provider in a medical setting.

*If you have any questions, consult your doctor, pharmacist, or health care provider.*

| Generic Name<br>*Brand Name Example* | Supplied As | Generic<br>Available |
|---|---|---|
| *Rx* **Mupirocin** | | |
| *Bactroban,*<br>*Bactroban Nasal* | **Ointment:** 2% | No |

## Type of Drug:
Topical anti-infective; externally used antibiotic.

## How the Drug Works:
Mupirocin inhibits bacterial protein production by interfering with formation of RNA, causing bacterial cell death in susceptible organisms.

## Uses:
*Topical:* To treat impetigo.

*Nasal:* To eradicate nasal colonization with methicillin-resistant *Staphylococcus aureus* in adult patients and healthcare workers as part of a comprehensive infection control program to reduce the risk of infection among high-risk patients during institutional outbreaks of infections with this pathogen.

## Precautions:
*Do not use in the following situations:*
> allergy to any component of the ointment
> in the eyes

*Superinfection:* Use of antibiotics (especially prolonged or repeated therapy) may result in bacterial or fungal overgrowth. Such overgrowth may lead to a secondary infection. Mupirocin may need to be stopped and another antibiotic prescribed for the secondary infection.

*Pregnancy:* Studies in pregnant women have not shown a risk to the fetus. However, no drug should be used during pregnancy unless clearly needed.

*Breastfeeding:* It is not known if mupirocin appears in breast milk. Consult your doctor before you begin breastfeeding.

*Children:*

> *Nasal* – Safety in children under 12 years of age has not been established.

## Drug Interactions:
Tell your doctor or pharmacist if you are taking or planning to take any over-the-counter or prescription medication while taking mupirocin. Doses of one or both drugs may need to be modified or a different drug may need to be prescribed.

## Side Effects:

Every drug is capable of producing side effects. Many mupirocin users experience no, or minor, side effects. The frequency and severity of side effects depend on many factors including dose, duration of therapy and individual susceptibility. Possible side effects include:

*Skin:* Burning; stinging; pain; itching.

*Other:* Sinus infection, congestion; headache; respiratory disorder; sore throat; throat inflammation; taste perversion; cough.

---

## Guidelines for Use:

*Topical:*

- Apply a small amount of ointment to the affected area 3 times daily. A loose gauze dressing may be used to cover the area, if desired.
- If improvement of impetigo is not seen in 3 to 5 days, contact the doctor.
- Do not use in or near the eyes.
- If an inflammatory reaction persists, it may be due to a chemical irritation or an allergic reaction to the drug. Stop using mupirocin and consult your doctor.

*Nasal:*

- Application should be made in the morning and evening for 5 days.
- Apply half of the ointment into one nostril and the other half into the other nostril.
- Discard the tube. Do not re-use.
- Press the sides of the nose together and gently massage for about 1 minute to spread the ointment throughout the insides of the nostrils.
- Do not use in or near the eyes.
- Do not use any other nasal products at the same time.
- If an inflammatory reaction persists, it may be due to a chemical irritation or an allergic reaction to the drug. Stop using mupirocin and consult your doctor.

---

*If you have any questions, consult your doctor, pharmacist, or health care provider.*

| Generic Name<br>*Brand Name Examples* | Supplied As | Generic<br>Available |
|---|---|---|
| *Rx* **Amoxicillin** | | |
| *Amoxil* | **Tablets:** 500 mg, 875 mg | No |
| *Amoxil, Trimox* | **Tablets, chewable:** 125 mg, 200 mg, 250 mg, 400 mg | Yes |
| *Amoxil, Trimox* | **Capsules:** 125 mg, 250 mg, 500 mg | Yes |
| *Amoxil, Trimox* | **Oral suspension:** 125 mg/5 mL, 200 mg/5 mL, 250 mg/5 mL, 400 mg/5 mL | Yes |
| *Amoxil Pediatric Drops, Trimox Pediatric Drops* | **Oral suspension:** 50 mg/mL | No |
| *Rx* **Amoxicillin and Potassium Clavulanate** | | |
| *Augmentin* | **Tablets:** 250 mg amoxicillin, 125 mg clavulanic acid; 500 mg amoxicillin, 125 mg clavulanic acid; 875 mg amoxicillin, 125 mg clavulanic acid | No |
| *Augmentin* | **Tablets, chewable:** 125 mg amoxicillin, 31.25 mg clavulanic acid; 200 mg amoxicillin, 28.5 mg clavulanic acid; 250 mg amoxicillin, 62.5 mg clavulanic acid; 400 mg amoxicillin, 57 mg clavulanic acid | No |
| *Augmentin* | **Oral suspension:** 125 mg amoxicillin, 31.25 mg clavulanic acid/5 mL; 200 mg amoxicillin, 28.5 mg clavulanic acid/5 mL; 250 mg amoxicillin, 62.5 mg clavulanic acid/5 mL; 400 mg amoxicillin, 57 mg clavulanic acid/5 mL | No |
| *Rx* **Ampicillin** | | |
| *Principen, Totacillin* | **Capsules:** 250 mg; 500 mg | Yes |
| *Principen, Totacillin* | **Oral suspension:** 125 mg/5 mL; 250 mg/5 mL | Yes |
| *Rx* **Bacampicillin HCl** | | |
| *Spectrobid* | **Tablets:** 400 mg | No |
| *Rx* **Carbenicillin Indanyl Sodium** | | |
| *Geocillin* | **Tablets, film coated:** 382 mg | No |

| Rx  **Cloxacillin Sodium** | **Capsules:** 250 mg, 500 mg | Yes |
|---|---|---|
| | **Oral solution:** 125 mg/5 mL | Yes |
| Rx  **Dicloxacillin Sodium** | | |
| *Dycill, Dynapen* | **Capsules:** 125 mg, 250 mg, 500 mg | Yes |
| *Dynapen* | **Oral suspension:** 62.5 mg/5 mL | No |
| Rx  **Oxacillin Sodium** | **Capsules:** 250 mg, 500 mg | Yes |
| | **Oral solution:** 250 mg/5 mL | Yes |
| Rx  **Penicillin V Potassium** | | |
| *Beepen-VK, Veetids* | **Tablets:** 250 mg, 500 mg | Yes |
| *Beepen-VK, Veetids* | **Oral solution:** 125 mg/5 mL, 250 mg/5 mL | Yes |

Penicillins are antibiotics with a broad spectrum of activity and effectiveness. The injectable penicillins (eg, penicillin G, penicillin G procaine, penicillin G benzathine, methicillin sodium, nafcillin sodium, oxacillin sodium, ampicillin sodium, carbenicillin disodium, ticarcillin disodium) are used in the treatment of serious infections. The following monograph discusses only oral penicillins.

For detailed information regarding injectable penicillins and their use, contact your pharmacist or doctor.

## Type of Drug:
Antibiotics; anti-infection drugs; penicillins.

## How the Drug Works:
Penicillins kill susceptible bacteria by preventing the production of the bacterial cell wall. They are most effective in killing bacteria when bacteria are rapidly multiplying.

## Uses:
To treat mild-to-moderate infections caused by penicillin-sensitive bacteria.

## Precautions:
*Do not use in the following situations:*
allergy to any penicillin or any of its ingredients
cholestatic jaundice, drug-induced, history of (amoxicillin and clavulanate potassium only)
infection caused by penicillinase-producing organisms (amoxicillin, ampicillin, bacampicillin, penicillin V only)
liver dysfunction, drug-induced, history of (amoxicillin and clavulanate potassium only)
mononucleosis (amoxicillin, ampicillin, bacampicillin only)

*Use with caution in the following situations:*

| | |
|---|---|
| allergies, history of | kidney impairment |
| allergy to cephalosporins | liver disease (amoxicillin and |
| asthma, history of | clavulanate potassium only) |
| cardiospasm | nausea |
| gastric dilation | rash, history of |
| hay fever, history of | severe illness |
| intestinal hypermotility | vomiting |

*Superinfection:* Use of antibiotics (especially for prolonged or repeated therapy) may result in bacterial or fungal overgrowth. Such overgrowth may lead to a second infection. The penicillin may need to be stopped and another antibiotic prescribed to treat the second infection.

*Diarrhea:* If diarrhea develops during penicillin use, pseudomembranous colitis must be considered. This inflammatory condition of the colon is due to overgrowth of bacteria that are not killed by penicillins. The primary cause is a toxin produced by a bacteria known as *Clostridia difficile*. Mild cases usually respond to stopping the antibiotic.

*Penicillin V:* Penicillin V is preferred over penicillin G for oral therapy. Penicillin V achieves blood levels 2 to 5 times higher than the same dose of penicillin G. Penicillin V is also stable in stomach acid, while penicillin G is not.

*Clavulanic acid:* Oral penicillins may be combined with clavulanic acid, a drug that inactivates enzymes produced by bacteria that destroy the penicillin. Clavulanic acid extends the effectiveness of penicillins.

*Allergy:* A person allergic to one penicillin may be allergic to other penicillins. Reactions to penicillin vary from mild itching and rashes to life-threatening reactions. All allergic reactions to any drug or food should be reported to your doctor.

Cephalosporins are a distinct group of antibiotics closely related to the penicillins. Due to the similarity, people allergic to penicillins may also be allergic to cephalosporins, and people allergic to cephalosporins may also be allergic to penicillins.

*Cross resistance:* Bacteria may become resistant to penicillin. If resistance develops to one of these drugs, it may result in resistance to most, if not all, penicillins.

*Pregnancy:* There are no adequate and well-controlled studies in pregnant women. Use only if clearly needed and the potential benefits to the mother outweigh the possible risks to the fetus.

*Breastfeeding:* Penicillins appear in breast milk. Consult your doctor before you begin breastfeeding.

*Children:* Use with caution in patients under 3 months of age. Safety and effectiveness of carbenicillin in children have not been established.

*Lab tests* may be required to monitor therapy. Tests may include blood counts, kidney and liver function tests, and bacteriologic studies.

## Drug Interactions:

Tell your doctor or pharmacist if you are taking or if you are planning to take any over-the-counter or prescription medications with penicillins. Doses of one or both drugs may need to be modified or a different drug may need to be prescribed. The following drugs and drug classes interact with penicillins:

allopurinol (eg, *Zyloprim*)
amiloride (*Midamor*) (amoxicillin only)
aminoglycosides (eg, amikacin)
anticoagulants (eg, warfarin)
beta blockers (eg, atenolol)
chloramphenicol (eg, *Chloromycetin*)
contraceptives, oral (eg, *Ortho-Novum*)

disulfiram (eg, *Antabuse*)
food
macrolides (eg, erythromycin)
methotrexate (eg, *Rheumatrex*)
probenecid (eg, *Benemid*)
sulfonamides (eg, sulfisoxazole)
tetracyclines (eg, doxycycline)

## Side Effects:

Every drug is capable of producing side effects. Many penicillin users experience no, or minor, side effects. The frequency and severity of side effects depend on many factors including dose, duration of therapy, and individual susceptibility. Possible side effects include:

*Allergy:* Side effects are more likely to occur in individuals with a history of previous allergic reactions. In penicillin-sensitive individuals with a history of allergy, asthma, hay fever, or hives, the reactions may be immediate and severe.

Allergic symptoms include nausea, vomiting, low blood pressure, shortness of breath, swollen joints, flushing, redness, wheezing, hives, itching, spasms in throat and breathing tubes, joint and muscle pain, difficulty breathing, chills, fever, fluid retention, skin rashes, and exhaustion.

*Digestive Tract:* Nausea; vomiting; diarrhea; stomach upset; gas; stomach pain or cramps; inflammation of the tongue or mouth; black, hairy tongue; loose stools.

*Skin:* Hives; itching; rash.

*Other:* Taste changes; abnormal liver function tests and blood counts; vaginal infection.

## Guidelines for Use:

- Use exactly as prescribed. Dosage and duration of therapy will take into account severity of infection, susceptibility of bacteria to the drug, and general health of the patient.
- Take at even intervals, preferably around the clock.
- Absorption of most oral penicillins is decreased by food. These drugs are best taken on an empty stomach (1 hour before or 2 hours after a meal) with a full glass of water. Penicillin V, amoxicillin, and bacampicillin are exceptions and may be taken with food.
- Continue until all the prescribed drug has been taken even if symptoms of infection have disappeared. Failure to take a full course of therapy may prevent complete elimination of bacteria, causing a relapse of the infection.
- A minimum of 10 days of treatment is recommended for any infection caused by group A beta-hemolytic streptococci. This treatment period is necessary to prevent rheumatic fever or kidney inflammation and damage.
- If a dose is missed, take it as soon as possible. If several hours have passed or if it is nearing time for the next dose, do not double the dose to catch up, unless advised to do so by your doctor. If more than one dose is missed or it is necessary to establish a new dosage schedule, contact your doctor or pharmacist.
- Notify your doctor immediately if shortness of breath, wheezing, skin rash, mouth irritation, black tongue, sore throat, itching, nausea, vomiting, severe diarrhea, fever, swollen joints, unusual bleeding or bruising, flushing, redness, hives, or skin inflammation occurs.
- Contact your doctor immediately if severe diarrhea, stomach pain or cramps, or bloody stools occur. These could be symptoms of a serious side effect requiring immediate medical attention. Do not treat diarrhea without consulting your doctor.
- Use of antibiotics (especially prolonged or repeated therapy) may result in bacterial or fungal overgrowth. Such overgrowth may lead to a second infection. The penicillin may need to be stopped and another antibiotic prescribed for the second infection.
- Do not take any additional medications while taking a penicillin without your doctor's approval, including nonprescription drugs such as antacids, laxatives, and vitamins.
- If you have previously experienced an allergic reaction to penicillin, consider wearing a medical identification tag or bracelet documenting this reaction.
- Lab tests may be required to monitor therapy. Be sure to keep appointments.
- *Oral suspensions and solutions* — Do not freeze. Shake well before using. Check expiration date. Discard any liquid forms of penicillin after 7 days if stored at room temperature, or after 14 days if refrigerated.
- *Tablets and capsules* — Store at controlled room temperature (59° to 86°F) in a tightly closed container.

*If you have any questions, consult your doctor, pharmacist, or health care provider.*

| Generic Name<br>*Brand Name Examples* | Supplied As | Generic<br>Available |
|---|---|---|
| *Rx* **Demeclocycline HCl** | | |
| *Declomycin* | **Tablets:** 150 mg, 300 mg | No |
| *Rx* **Doxycycline** | | |
| *Ed-DOXY Caps, Periostat, Vibramycin* | **Capsules (as hyclate):** 20 mg, 50 mg, 100 mg | Yes |
| *Monodox* | **Capsules (as monohydrate):** 50 mg, 100 mg | No |
| *Vibra-Tabs* | **Tablets (as hyclate):** 100 mg | Yes |
| *Doryx* | **Capsules, coated pellets (as hyclate):** 100 mg | No |
| *Vibramycin[1]* | **Oral suspension (as mono-hydrate):** 25 mg/5 mL | No |
| *Vibramycin* | **Syrup (as calcium):** 50 mg/5 mL | No |
| *Vibramycin* | **Injection (as hyclate):** 100 mg/vial | Yes |
| *Rx* **Minocycline HCl** | | |
| *Dynacin, Minocin, Vectrin* | **Capsules:** 50 mg, 75 mg, 100 mg | Yes |
| *Minocin[1]* | **Oral suspension:** 50 mg/5 mL | No |
| *Minocin* | **Injection:** 100 mg/vial | No |
| *Rx* **Oxytetracycline HCl** | | |
| *Terramycin* | **Capsules:** 250 mg | Yes |
| *Terramycin* | **Injection:** 50 mg/mL, 100 mg/2 mL, 250 mg/2 mL | No |
| *Rx* **Tetracycline HCl** | | |
| *Sumycin 250, Sumycin 500* | **Capsules:** 250 mg, 500 mg | Yes |
| *Sumycin 250, Sumycin 500* | **Tablets:** 250 mg, 500 mg | Yes |
| *Sumycin Syrup[1]* | **Oral suspension:** 125 mg/5 mL | Yes |

[1] Contains sulfites (metabisulfites).

## Type of Drug:

Antibiotics; anti-infection drugs; antibacterial drugs.

## How the Drug Works:

Tetracyclines inhibit susceptible bacteria's production of proteins necessary for their growth. This slows and prevents the bacteria's growth and reproduction while body defense mechanisms (eg, white blood cells) destroy them.

## Uses:

To treat a wide variety of infections caused by susceptible bacteria.

As alternative drugs for certain types of infection when penicillin cannot be used (eg, penicillin allergy).

For treatment of uncomplicated urethral, endocervical, or rectal infections caused by *Chlamydia trachomatis.*

To treat severe acne and inclusion conjunctivitis.

Used with amebicides (antiparasitic drugs) to treat acute intestinal amebiasis (parasites).

*Doxycycline:* For use as a preventative against certain types of malaria in short-term (less than 4 months) travelers.

Also used as an adjunct to scaling and root planing to promote attachment level gain and to reduce pocket depth in patients with adult periodontitis (*Periostat* only). See the Mouth and Throat Products – Doxycyclinie monograph in the Gastrointestinals chapter.

*Minocycline:* To treat uncomplicated infections of the rectal and genitourinary tract caused by *Ureaplasma urealyticum.*

*Unlabeled Use(s):* Occasionally doctors may prescribe tetracyclines for other uses.

*Demeclocycline* – Used in patients with decreased blood sodium associated with the syndrome of inappropriate antidiuretic hormone (SIADH) secretion.

*Doxycycline* – To prevent "traveler's diarrhea."

*Minocycline* – Used as an alternative to sulfonamides in nocardiosis.

*Tetracycline* – Used in specialized procedures for certain types of lung cancer. Tetracycline used with gentamicin has been recommended for wound infections or infections caused by eating contaminated seafood. Tetracycline suspension has been used as a mouthwash in the treatment of mouth ulcers and canker sores.

*Tetracycline and doxycycline* – Recommended for early Lyme disease.

## Precautions:

*Do not use in the following situations:* Allergy to any tetracycline or any of its ingredients

*Use with caution in the following situations:*
children under 8 years of age
kidney disease
liver disease (injectable forms only)
oral candidiasis, predisposition or history of (*Periostat* only)
pregnancy

*Bone:* Tetracycline binds to calcium in bone. A decrease in growth rate has been observed in premature infants given oral tetracycline. This effect was reversible when the drug was discontinued.

*Teeth:* Use during tooth development (last half of pregnancy, infancy, and childhood to 8 years of age) may cause permanent discoloration (yellow-gray-brown) and inadequate calcification (hardening) of baby and permanent teeth. This reaction is more common if use is long term or repeated. Doxycycline and oxytetracycline may be less likely to affect teeth than other tetracyclines.

*Pseudotumor cerebri:* Tetracyclines have been associated with pseudotumor cerebri (benign intracranial hypertension). Early signs and symptoms include headache, nausea, vomiting, and blurred vision. Bulging fontanels ("soft spots") have been associated with tetracycline use in infants. If these symptoms develop, stop the drug immediately and contact your doctor.

*Demeclocycline:* Demeclocycline has resulted in the appearance of diabetes insipidus syndrome (eg, increased urination, increased thirst, and craving for ice water) in some patients on long-term therapy. The syndrome is reversible when therapy is discontinued.

*Superinfection:* Use of broad spectrum antibiotics (especially prolonged or repeated therapy) may result in bacterial or fungal overgrowth. Such overgrowth may lead to a second infection. The tetracycline may need to be stopped and another antibiotic may need to be prescribed for the second infection.

*Cross resistance:* Antimicrobial activity of the tetracyclines is similar. Resistance to one tetracycline may mean resistance to most or all of the others.

*Pregnancy:* Do not use during pregnancy. The risk of use in a pregnant woman clearly outweighs any possible benefit (see Children).

*Breastfeeding:* Tetracyclines appear in breast milk. Consult your doctor before you begin breastfeeding.

*Children:* Tetracyclines should not be used in children under 8 years of age, unless other drugs are not likely to be effective or are not advised.

*Lab tests* may be required during long-term treatment with tetracyclines. Tests may include blood counts and liver and kidney function tests.

*Sulfites:* Some of these products may contain sulfite preservatives that can cause allergic reactions in certain individuals. (eg, asthmatics). Check package label when available or consult your doctor or pharmacist.

## Drug Interactions:

Tell your doctor or pharmacist if you are taking or if you are planning to take any over-the-counter or prescription medications with tetracyclines. Doses of one or both drugs may need to be modified or a different drug may need to be prescribed. The following drugs and drug classes interact with tetracyclines:

aluminum salts (eg, aluminum carbonate)
anticoagulants (eg, warfarin)
bismuth salts (eg, bismuth sub-salicylate)
calcium salts (eg, calcium citrate)
charcoal
colestipol (*Colestid*)
contraceptives, oral (eg, *Ortho-Novum*)
digoxin (eg, *Lanoxin)*
food
insulin
iron salts (eg, ferrous sulfate)
lithium (eg, *Eskalith*)
magnesium salts (eg, magnesium sulfate)
penicillins (eg, penicillin V)
urinary alkalinizers (eg, sodium bicarbonate)
zinc salts (eg, zinc gluconate)

## Side Effects:

Every drug is capable of producing side effects. Many tetracycline users experience no, or minor, side effects. The frequency and severity of side effects depend on many factors including dose, duration of therapy, and individual susceptibility. Possible side effects include:

*Diabetes Insipidus Syndrome (demeclocycline):* Weakness; excessive urination; excessive thirst.

*Digestive Tract:* Nausea; vomiting; appetite loss; diarrhea; indigestion; tongue inflammation; difficulty swallowing; indigestion; black, hairy tongue.

*Skin:* Rash; hives; sensitivity to sunlight; red or purple spots under the skin.

*Other:* Joint pain; anemia; decreased platelets; abnormal liver or kidney function tests and blood counts; mouth sores; teeth staining (in children); headache; lightheadedness (minocycline); pancreatic inflammation; exacerbation of lupus; pseudotumor cerebri; dizziness; common cold; sinus congestion; sinus headache; menstrual cramps; pain; decreased hearing; skin inflammation in the anal and genital region; feeling of whirling motion (minocycline); blurred vision.

## Guidelines for Use:

- Dosage will be individualized. Use exactly as prescribed. Do not change the dose or stop taking unless advised to do so by your doctor.
- Injectable tetracyclines are used when oral dosage forms are not suitable.
- If a dose is missed, take it as soon as possible. If several hours have passed or if it is nearing time for the next dose, do not double the dose in order to catch up, unless advised to do so by your doctor. If more than one dose is missed, or it is necessary to establish a new dosage schedule, contact your doctor or pharmacist.
- Continue use until all the prescribed drug has been taken, even if symptoms of infection are gone. Failure to take a full course of therapy may prevent complete elimination of bacteria, causing a relapse of the infection.
- Do not use during pregnancy.
- Do not use in children younger than 8 years of age unless other drugs are not likely to be effective or are inadvisable. Use during tooth development may cause permanent discoloration and inadequate hardening of baby and permanent teeth.
- Take oral doseforms on an empty stomach at least 1 hour before or 2 hours after a meal. Exceptions are doxycycline and minocycline, which are not affected by food or milk.
- *Periostat* — Take at least 1 hour before the morning and evening meals.
- To prevent irritation of the esophagus (food pipe), take capsules or tablets with a full glass of water or other non-dairy liquid. Do not lie down for at least 30 minutes after a dose.
- Shake oral suspensions and syrups well before using.
- Avoid use of tetracyclines with antacids, laxatives, alcohol, dairy products (eg, milk, cheese) or iron-containing products. If any of these products must be taken, take at least 2 hours before or after tetracyclines.
- May cause photosensitivity (sensitivity to sunlight). Avoid prolonged exposure to the sun and other ultraviolet light. Use sunscreens and wear protective clothing until tolerance is determined.
- Concurrent use of tetracyclines with oral contraceptives (eg, *Ortho-Novum*) may cause the oral contraceptives to be less effective. Discuss alternative contraceptive methods with your doctor.
- Notify your doctor if you experience skin redness or flushing.
- *Do not use outdated tetracyclines.* Outdated tetracyclines may be highly toxic to the kidneys.
- *Minocycline* — Minocycline may cause lightheadedness, dizziness and vertigo (feeling of whirling motion). Use caution while driving or performing other tasks requiring alertness.
- Lab tests may be required to monitor therapy. Be sure to keep appointments.
- Store at controlled room temperature (59° to 86°F). Do not freeze oral suspensions or syrups. Check expiration date.

*If you have any questions, consult your doctor, pharmacist, or health care provider.*

| Generic Name<br>*Brand Name Examples* | Supplied As | Generic<br>Available |
|---|---|---|
| *Rx* **Meclocycline Sulfosalicylate** | | |
| *Meclan* | **Cream:** 1% | No |
| **Tetracycline** | | |
| *Rx* *Topicycline* | **Topical solution:** 2.2 mg/mL | No |
| *otc* *Achromycin* | **Ointment:** 3% | No |

## Type of Drug:

Externally applied antibiotic.

## How the Drug Works:

The mechanism by which topical tetracycline treats acne is not well defined. It is probably related, in large part, to its antibacterial activity.

## Uses:

To treat acne vulgaris.

To prevent infection in minor skin abrasions and to treat superficial infections of the skin.

## Precautions:

*Do not use in the following situations:* Allergy to tetracyclines or other ingredients in the formulation

*Use with caution in the following situations:*
    kidney disease
    liver disease

*Pregnancy:* Safety for use during pregnancy has not been established. Use only when clearly needed and when the potential benefits outweight the potential hazards to the fetus.

*Breastfeeding:* Safety for use while breastfeeding has not been established. Consult your doctor.

*Children:* Safety and effectiveness in children under 11 have not been established.

*Sulfites:* Some of these products may contain sulfite preservatives, which can cause allergic reactions in certain individuals. Check package label when available or consult your doctor or pharmacist.

## Side Effects:

Every drug is capable of producing side effects. Many topical tetracycline users experience no, or minor, side effects. The frequency and severity of side effects depend on many factors including dose, duration of therapy and individual susceptibility. Possible side effects include: Irritation of skin; burning after application; rash; itching; slight yellow staining of skin or hair follicles.

## Guidelines for Use:

- For external use only.
- Avoid contact with the eyes and lining of the nose and mouth.
- Apply to the affected area 2 times daily (morning and evening) for best results. Less frequent applications may be used if the response is good.
- Apply generously until the affected skin is thoroughly wet or covered.
- Stinging or burning may occur but should only last for a few minutes. If stinging or burning persists, contact your doctor.
- Excessive use of the cream may stain some fabrics.
- A slight yellowing of the skin may occur. This is not harmful and may be removed by washing.
- Normal use of cosmetics is permissible.

*If you have any questions, consult your doctor, pharmacist, or health care provider.*

| Generic Name<br>*Brand Name Examples* | Supplied As | Generic<br>Available |
|---|---|---|
| *Rx* **Trimethoprim** | | |
| *Proloprim* | **Tablets:** 100 mg, 200 mg | Yes |

## Type of Drug:
Anti-infective agent.

## How the Drug Works:
Trimethoprim (TMP) blocks production of folic acid which is needed by bacteria. Decreased folic acid interferes with the production of protein by the bacterial cell resulting in slowed bacterial growth or cell death.

## Uses:
To treat urinary tract infections caused by susceptible bacteria.

## Precautions:
*Do not use in the following situations:*
>    allergy to trimethoprim
>    anemia due to folic acid deficiency

*Use with caution in the following situations:*

| | |
|---|---|
| folic acid deficiency | kidney disease |
| infants under 2 months | liver disease |

*Pregnancy:* Adequate studies have not been done in pregnant women. Use only if clearly needed and potential benefits outweigh the possible hazards to the fetus.

*Breastfeeding:* Trimethoprim appears in breast milk. Consult your doctor before you begin breastfeeding.

*Children:* Safety in infants under 2 months has not been established. Effectiveness when taken alone in children under 12 has not been established.

## Drug Interactions:
Tell your doctor or pharmacist if you are taking or if you are planning to take any over-the-counter or prescription medications with trimethoprim. Doses of one or both drugs may need to be modified or a different drug may need to be prescribed. Phenytoin (eg, *Dilantin*) interacts with trimethoprim.

## Side Effects:

Every drug is capable of producing side effects. Many trimethoprim users experience no, or minor, side effects. The frequency and severity of side effects depend on many factors including dose, duration of therapy and individual susceptibility. Possible side effects include:

*Digestive Tract:* Stomach upset; nausea; vomiting.

*Skin:* Rash; inflammation; itching; swelling; redness; peeling skin.

*Other:* Inflammation of the tongue; fever; yellowing of skin or eyes; anemia; abnormal liver or kidney function tests.

---

## Guidelines for Use:

- Take medication until it is gone. Do not stop without consulting your doctor.
- Do not use if you have anemia due to folic acid deficiency.
- Notify your doctor immediately if you develop any unusual bleeding or bruising, sore throat, fever, fatigue or skin reactions.
- May cause photosensitivity (sensitivity to sunlight). Avoid prolonged exposure to the sun or other forms of ultraviolet (UV) light (eg, tanning beds). Use sunscreens and wear protective clothing until tolerance is determined.

---

*If you have any questions, consult your doctor, pharmacist, or health care provider.*

| Generic Name Brand Name Examples | Supplied As | Generic Available |
|---|---|---|
| *otc* **Bacitracin** | | |
| *Baciguent* | **Ointment:** 500 units/g | Yes |
| *Rx* **Chloramphenicol** | | |
| *Chloromycetin* | **Cream:** 1% in a water miscible ointment base | No |
| *Rx* **Erythromycin** | | |
| *Akne-mycin* | **Ointment:** 2% | No |
| *Rx* **Gentamicin** | **Ointment:** 0.1% (as 1.7 mg sulfate/g) | Yes |
| | **Cream:** 0.1% (as 1.7 mg sulfate/g) | Yes |
| *otc* **Neomycin Sulfate** | | |
| *Myciguent* | **Ointment:** 0.5% (5 mg neomycin sulfate/g, equal to 3.5 mg neomycin/g) | Yes |
| *Myciguent* | **Cream:** 0.5% (5 mg neomycin sulfate/g, equal to 3.5 mg neomycin/g) | No |
| *otc* **Multiple Antibiotics** | | |
| *Neosporin* | **Cream:** 10,000 units polymyxin B sulfate and 3.5 mg neomycin base/g | No |
| *Polysporin* | **Ointment:** 10,000 units polymyxin B sulfate and 500 units zinc bacitracin/g | No |
| *Polysporin* | **Aerosol:** 200,000 units polymyxin B sulfate and 10,000 units zinc bacitracin/90 g | No |
| *Spectrocin* | **Ointment:** 2.5 mg neomycin base (as sulfate) and 0.25 mg gramicidin/g | No |
| *Terramycin w/Polymyxin B Sulfate* | **Powder:** 30 mg oxytetracycline and 10,000 units polymyxin B sulfate/g | No |
| *Terramycin w/Polymyxin B Sulfate* | **Ointment:** 30 mg oxytetracycline and 10,000 units polymyxin B sulfate/g | No |

| Generic Name<br>*Brand Name Examples* | Supplied As | Generic<br>Available |
|---|---|---|
| **Triple Antibiotic** | | |
| *otc N.B.P., Neomac, Septa* | **Ointment:** 5000 units poly-myxin B sulfate, 3.5 mg neo-mycin base and 400 units bacitracin/g | Yes |
| *otc Lanabiotic* | **Ointment:** 5000 units poly-myxin B, 3.5 mg neomycin base, 500 units bacitracin and 40 mg lidocaine/g | No |
| *otc Mycitracin Triple Antibiotic* | **Ointment:** 5000 units poly-myxin B, 3.5 mg neomycin base and 400 units zinc baci-tracin/g | No |
| *otc Neomixin, Neosporin* | **Ointment:** 5000 units poly-myxin B sulfate, 3.5 mg neo-mycin base and 400 units zinc acitracin/g | No |
| *otc Polysporin* | **Powder:** 10,000 units poly-myxin B sulfate and 500 units zinc bacitracin/g | No |

## Type of Drug:
Externally applied antibiotics.

## How the Drug Works:
Topical antibiotics exert their antibacterial action by different mechanisms with the same effect. The choice of antibiotic(s) depends on the nature of the wound and the suspected bacterial infection.

## Uses:
To prevent infections after minor skin lacerations (cuts) or abrasions (scrapes).

To treat superficial infections of the skin caused by susceptible bacteria.

## Precautions:
*Do not use in the following situations:*
> allergy to any component of the formulation
> in the eyes
> in the outer ear canal (if eardrum is perforated)

*Use with caution in the following situations:*
> deep skin infections
> if redness, swelling, inflammation or pain worsens while using the drug

*Neomycin sensitivity:* Frequent application of neomycin sulfate to inflamed skin increases the chance of sensitivity developing. Reddening, swelling, dry scaling and itching may occur. Consult your doctor.

*Superinfection:* Use of antibiotics (especially prolonged or repeated therapy) may result in bacterial or fungal overgrowth. Such overgrowth may lead to a second infection. The topical antibiotic may need to be stopped and another antibiotic prescribed for the second infection.

## Side Effects:

Every drug is capable of producing side effects. Many miscellaneous topical antibiotic users experience no, or minor, side effects. The frequency and severity of side effects depend on many factors including dose, duration of therapy and individual susceptibility. Possible side effects include:

*Skin:* Rash; itching; burning; redness; swelling; sensitivity to sunlight (gentamicin).

*Other:* Hearing loss (neomycin); kidney damage (neomycin); sensitivity to neomycin (see Precautions).

---

### Guidelines for Use:

- Apply a small amount of drug in a thin layer on the affected area 1 to 5 times daily. Cover the area with a loose gauze dressing, if desired.
- Clean the affected area prior to applying the drug.
- Deeper skin infections may require oral or injectable antibiotic therapy in addition to topical treatment.
- Do not use in or near the eyes.
- If rash or irritation develops or worsens where the antibiotic is applied, contact your doctor.

---

*If you have any questions, consult your doctor, pharmacist, or health care provider.*

| Generic Name<br>*Brand Name Examples* | Supplied As | Generic<br>Available |
|---|---|---|
| *Rx* **Sulfadiazine** | **Tablets:** 500 mg | Yes |
| *Rx* **Sulfamethizole** | | |
| *Thiosulfil Forte* | **Tablets:** 500 mg | No |
| *Rx* **Sulfamethoxazole** | | |
| *Gantanol, Gantanol DS, Urobak* | **Tablets:** 500 mg, 1 g | Yes |
| *Gantanol* | **Oral suspension:** 500 mg/tsp | No |
| *Rx* **Sulfasalazine** | | |
| *Azulfidine* | **Tablets:** 500 mg | Yes |
| *Azulfidine EN-tabs* | **Tablets, enteric coated:** 500 mg | Yes |
| *Azulfidine* | **Oral suspension:** 250 mg/tsp | No |
| *Rx* **Sulfisoxazole** | | |
| *Gantrisin* | **Tablets:** 500 mg | Yes |
| *Gantrisin* | **Syrup:** 500 mg acetyl sulfisoxazole/tsp | No |
| *Gantrisin* | **Pediatric suspension:** 500 mg acetyl sulfisoxazole/tsp | No |
| *Rx* **Multiple Sulfonamides** | | |
| *Triple Sulfa* | **Tablets:** 167 mg sulfadiazine, 167 mg sulfamerazine and 167 mg sulfamethazine | Yes |
| *Triple Sulfa No. 2* | **Tablets:** 162 mg sulfadiazine, 162 mg sulfamerazine and 162 mg sulfamethazine | Yes |
| *Triple Sulfa* | **Suspension:** 167 mg sulfadiazine, 167 mg sulfamerazine and 167 mg sulfamethazine/tsp | Yes |

## Type of Drug:

Anti-infection drugs; sulfa drugs.

## How the Drug Works:

Sulfonamides inhibit the use of Para-aminobenzoic acid (PABA) by the bacterial cell. PABA is an essential component in folic acid production and bacterial cell function.

## Uses:

To treat infections caused by susceptible bacteria. Infections may include: Urinary tract infections (pyelonephritis, pyelitis, cystitis), chancroid, inclusion conjunctivitis, trachoma, nocardiosis, toxoplasmosis, malaria, middle ear infections, meningitis, rheumatic fever and dermatitis herpetiformis.

*Sulfasalazine* is prescribed for treatment of ulcerative colitis.

*Unlabeled Use(s):* Occasionally doctors may prescribe sulfasalazine for rheumatoid arthritis, collagenous colitis, and Crohn's disease. Sulfisoxazole has been used to prevent recurrences of middle ear infections.

## Precautions:

*Do not use in the following situations:*

allergy to salicylates or aspirin (sulfasalazine only)
allergy to sulfonamides or related drugs (oral antidiabetic drugs or thiazide diuretics)
breastfeeding
infants under age 2 (sulfasalazine only)

infants under 2 months (except pyrimethamine to treat toxoplasmosis)
intestinal or urinary obstruction (sulfasalazine only)
porphyria
pregnancy at term

*Use with caution in the following situations:*

acid urine
blood disorders
bronchial asthma
glucose-6-phosphate dehydrogenase (G-6-PD) deficiency

kidney disease
liver disease
pregnancy prior to term
streptococcus infections (eg, strep throat)

*Sensitivity to light:* Sulfonamides may cause sensitivity to light. Avoid prolonged exposure to the sun. Use sunscreens and wear protective clothing until tolerance is determined.

*Avoid drugs which may acidify the urine* in large doses (such as vitamin C, ammonium chloride). Sulfonamides crystallize in an acid urine. This may cause serious complications in the kidneys. Adequate fluid (eg, water) intake is recommended to increase urine flow.

*Pregnancy:* Safety for use during pregnancy has not been established. Sulfonamides cross the placenta and studies have shown a potential effect to the fetus. Consult your doctor if pregnancy is suspected.

*Breastfeeding:* Sulfonamides appear in breast milk. Although the actual amount of drug that a breastfed infant would receive appears to be low, sulfonamides are not recommended while breastfeeding. Consult your doctor.

*Children:* Do not use sulfasalazine in children under 2.

*Tartrazine:* Some of these products may contain the dye tartrazine (FD&C Yellow No. 5) which can cause allergic reactions in certain individuals. Check package label when available or consult your doctor or pharmacist.

## Drug Interactions:

Tell your doctor or pharmacist if you are taking or if you are planning to take any over-the-counter or prescription medications with sulfonamides. Doses of one or both drugs may need to be modified or a different drug may need to be prescribed. The following drugs and drug classes interact with sulfonamides.

chlorpropamide (eg, *Diabinese)*
contraceptives, oral
 (eg, *Ortho-Novum)*
digoxin (eg, *Lanoxin)*
folic acid
iron
local anesthetics (eg, benzocaine)
methotrexate (eg, *Mexate)*
nonsteroidal anti-inflammatory
 agents (eg, ibuprofen)

PABA (eg, *Potaba)*
phenylbutazone
 (eg, *Butazolidin)*
phenytoin (eg, *Dilantin)*
probenecid (eg, *Benemid)*
salicylates (eg, aspirin)
thiazide diuretics (eg, hydrochlorothiazide)
tolbutamide (eg, *Orinase)*
warfarin (eg, *Coumadin)*

## Side Effects:

Every drug is capable of producing side effects. Many sulfonamide users experience no, or minor, side effects. The frequency and severity of side effects depend on many factors including dose, duration of therapy and individual susceptibility. Possible side effects include:

*Digestive Tract:* Nausea; vomiting; diarrhea; appetite loss; stomach ache.

*Nervous System:* Headache; vertigo (feeling of whirling motion); depression; seizures; sleeplessness; drowsiness.

*Skin:* Rash; itching; hives; chills; unusual bleeding or bruising; yellowing of skin or eyes.

*Other:* Blood disorders, abnormal blood counts; abnormal urine tests; numbness or tingling in hands or feet; ringing in the ears; liver damage; hepatitis; sensitivity to light; kidney damage; fever; joint pain; difficult breathing.

---

### Guidelines for Use:

- Complete full course of therapy for the best response.
- Take on an empty stomach. Take with a full glass of water.
- *Sulfasalazine—* Take at evenly spaced intervals after meals.
- *Sulfasalazine* may cause an orange-yellow discoloration of the urine.
- Sensitivity to light — Avoid prolonged exposure to the sun. Use sunscreens and wear protective clothing until tolerance is determined.
- *Oral suspensions—* Shake well before using. Keep bottle tightly closed. Refrigerate after opening. Discard unused portion after 14 days.
- Notify your doctor if any of the following occurs: Blood in urine, yellowing of skin or eyes, easy bruising, rash, ringing in ears, difficulty in breathing, fever, sore throat or chills.

---

*If you have any questions, consult your doctor, pharmacist, or health care provider.*

| Generic Name Brand Name Example | Supplied As | Generic Available |
|---|---|---|
| Rx **Erythromycin Ethylsuc-cinate/Sulfisoxazole** | | |
| *Eryzole* | **Oral suspension:** Erythromycin ethylsuccinate (equivalent to 200 mg erythromycin) and sulfisoxazole acetyl (equivalent to 600 mg sulfisoxazole)/5 mL | Yes |

## Type of Drug:

Antibiotic combination; combination sulfonamide - erythromycin anti-infective.

## Uses:

To treat acute middle ear infections (acute otitis media) in children older than 2 months of age caused by susceptible strains of *Haemophilus influenzae.*

## Precautions:

*Do not use in the following situations:*

allergy to erythromycin
allergy to sulfonamides or related drugs (oral anti-diabetic drugs or thiazide diuretics)
breastfeeding of infants under 2 months of age
infants under 2 months of age
pregnancy at term (after 36 weeks)

*Use with caution in the following situations:*

glucose-6-phosphate dehydro-genase (G6PD) deficiency
kidney disease
liver disease
myasthenia gravis
severe allergies or bronchial asthma

*Avoid the following:* Drugs or vitamins that may acidify the urine in large doses (eg, vitamin C, ammonium chloride). Sulfonamides crystallize in an acid urine. This may cause serious complications in the kidneys. Adequate fluid (eg, water) intake is strongly recommended to increase urine flow.

*Diarrhea:* If diarrhea develops during erythromycin ethylsuccinate/sulfixoxa-zole use, pseuodomembranous colitis must be considered. This inflam-matory condition of the colon is due to overgrowth of bacteria that are not killed by erythromycin ethylsuccinate/sulfisoxazole. The primary cause is a toxin produced by a bacteria known as *Clostridium difficile.* Mild cases usually respond to stopping the antibiotic. More severe cases may need to be treated with another antibiotic.

*Superinfection:* Use of antibiotics (especially for prolonged or repeated therapy) may result in bacterial or fungal overgrowth. Such overgrowth may lead to a second infection. Erythromycin ethylsuccinate/sulfisoxa-zole may need to be stopped and another antibiotic may need to be prescribed for the second infection.

*Pregnancy:* Adequate studies have not been done in pregnant women. Use only if clearly needed and potential benefits to the mother outweigh the possible hazards to the fetus.

*Breastfeeding:* These drugs appear in breast milk. Consult your doctor before you begin breastfeeding. A decision should be made whether to discontinue nursing or discontinue the drug, taking into account the importance of the drug to the mother.

*Children:* Do not give to infants under 2 months of age. Sulfonamides are not recommended for this age group.

*Lab tests* may be required during treatment. Tests may include complete blood counts, urinalysis, and kidney function tests.

## Drug Interactions:

Tell your doctor or pharmacist if you are taking or if you are planning to take any over-the-counter or prescription medications with erythromycin ethylsuccinate/sulfisoxazole. Doses of one or both drugs may need to be modified or a different drug may need to be prescribed. The following drugs and drug classes interact with erythromycin ethylsuccinate/sulfisoxazole:

alfentanil (*Alfenta*)
anticoagulants, oral (eg, warfarin)
benzodiazepines (eg, midazolam, triazolam)
bromocriptine (*Parlodel*)
carbamazepine (eg, *Tegretol*)
cyclosporine (eg, *Neoral*)
digoxin (eg, *Lanoxin*)
dihydroergotamine (*D.H.E. 45*)

disopyramide (eg, *Norpace*)
ergotamine (eg, *Ergomar*)
lovastatin (*Mevacor*)
methotrexate (eg, *Rheumatrex*)
phenytoin (eg, *Dilantin*)
sulfonylureas (eg, chlorpropamide)
theophylline (eg, *Theo-Dur*)
thiopental (eg, *Pentothal*)

## Side Effects:

Every drug is capable of producing side effects. Many erythromycin ethylsuccinate/sulfisoxazole users experience no, or minor, side effects. The frequency and severity of side effects depend on many factors including dose, duration of therapy, and individual susceptibility. Possible side effects include:

*Digestive Tract:* Nausea; vomiting; stomach pain; diarrhea; appetite loss; inflammation of the liver; intestinal bleeding; dark, bloody stools; gas; inflammation and redness of the mouth and tongue.

*Nervous System:* Headache; dizziness; abnormal skin sensations; convulsions; ringing in the ears; vertigo (feeling of whirling motion); incoordination.

*Circulatory System:* Fast heartbeat; pounding in the chest; fainting; bluish discoloration of skin; irregular heart rhythm; inflammation of blood vessels or heart tissue.

*Urinary and Reproductive Tract:* Blood in the urine; infrequent or frequent urination; inability to urinate.

*Skin:* Serious immediate allergic reaction; delayed allergic reaction (days or weeks); giant hives or skin inflammation; rash; itching; mild skin eruption; sensitivity to light.

*Other:* Reversible hearing loss; low blood sugar levels; abnormal blood counts; red or purple spots/patches under the skin; low iron or blood counts sometimes resulting in fatigue; clotting disorders; mental disorder; hallucinations; disorientation; anxiety; depression; inflammation of the eye; cough; shortness of breath; fluid retention; fever; drowsiness; weakness; fatigue; yellowing of the skin or eyes; inflammation of lung tissue; rigidity; chills; flushing; sleeplessness.

---

## Guidelines for Use:

- Dosage will be individualized.
- Doses should be equally divided into 3 or 4 daily doses and administered for 10 days. Continue therapy for entire 10 days even if symptoms of infection have disappeared.
- Shake well before using.
- May be administered without regard to meals.
- Maintain an adequate fluid intake to prevent formation of crystals in the urine and kidney stones.
- Do not stop taking the drug or change the dose unless advised to do so by your doctor.
- *Superinfection* — Use of antibiotics (especially for prolonged or repeated therapy) may result in bacterial or fungal overgrowth. Such overgrowth may lead to a second infection. Erythromycin ethylsuccinate/sulfisoxazole may need to be stopped and another antibiotic may need to be prescribed for the second infection.
- Discontinue use and contact your doctor immediately at first appearance of a rash.
- Contact your doctor immediately if severe diarrhea, stomach pain/cramps, or bloody stools occur. This could be a symptom of a serious side effect requiring medical attention. Do not treat diarrhea without first consulting your doctor.
- May cause sensitivity to ultraviolet (UV) light. Avoid prolonged exposure to the sun. Use sunscreens and wear protective clothing until tolerance is determined.
- May cause nausea, vomiting, diarrhea, unusual tiredness, or stomach pain. Contact your doctor if effects persist and are bothersome.
- Contact your doctor immediately if sore throat, fever, pallor, rash, darkened urine, unusual bleeding or bruising, yellowing of eyes or skin, or difficulty breathing occurs.
- Lab tests or exams may be required to monitor treatment. Be sure to keep appointments.

---

*If you have any questions, consult your doctor, pharmacist, or health care provider.*

| Generic Name<br>*Brand Name Examples* | Supplied As | Generic Available |
|---|---|---|
| *Rx* **Trimethoprim/Sulfa-<br>methoxazole, TMP-SMZ**[1] | | |
| *Bactrim, Bethaprim SS,<br>Cotrim, Septra, Sulfatrim,<br>Uroplus SS* | **Tablets:** 80 mg trimethoprim<br>and 400 mg sulfamethoxazole | Yes |
| *Bactrim DS, Bethaprim<br>DS, Cotrim DS, Septra<br>DS, Sulfatrim DS, Uroplus<br>DS* | **Tablets, double strength:**<br>160 mg trimethoprim and<br>800 mg sulfamethoxazole | Yes |
| *Bactrim*[2] *Bethaprim*[2]*,<br>Cotrim Pediatric,<br>Septra*[2]*, Sulfatrim,<br>Sulmeprim* | **Oral suspension:** 40 mg<br>trimethoprim and 200 mg<br>sulfamethoxazole/tsp | Yes |

[1] Also available as an injection.
[2] Contains alcohol.

For more information, see the Sulfonamides and Antibiotics – Trimethoprim monographs in this chapter.

## Type of Drug:

Combination sulfonamide-trimethoprim anti-infective; TMP-SMZ, Co-tri-moxazole.

## How the Drug Works:

Trimethoprim (TMP) and sulfamethoxazole (SMZ) block the production of folic acid. Decreased folic acid interferes with the production of critical nucleic acids and proteins of bacteria.

## Uses:

To treat certain urinary tract infections; intestinal infections caused by *Shigella; Pneumocystis carinii* pneumonia; middle ear infections; chronic bronchitis.

*Unlabeled Use(s):* Occasionally doctors may prescribe TMP-SMZ for cholera, salmonella-type infections, to prevent urinary tract infections (women), nocardiosis and "traveler's diarrhea," and to prevent infections in patients with a compromised immune system with *Pneumocystis carinii* infections or leukemia.

## Precautions:

*Do not use in the following situations:*
allergy to sulfonamides or
related drugs (oral antidiabetic
drugs or thiazide diuretics)
allergy to trimethoprim
anemia due to folic acid
deficiency
breastfeeding
infants less than 2 months of
age
pregnancy at term

*Use with caution in the following situations:*

- AIDS patients with *carinii* pneumonitis
- alcoholism
- allergy, severe
- anticonvulsant therapy
- asthma
- folic acid deficiency
- glucose-6-phosphate dehydrogenase (G-6-PD) deficiency
- kidney disease
- liver disease
- malnutrition
- strep throat

*Avoid drugs that may acidify the urine* in large doses (such as vitamin C, ammonium chloride) when taking sulfonamides. Sulfonamides crystallize in an acid urine. This may cause serious complications in the kidneys. Adequate fluid intake (eg, water) is recommended to increase urine flow.

*AIDS patients* may not tolerate or respond to TMP-SMZ because of their abnormally functioning immune systems.

*Superinfection:* Use of antibiotics (especially prolonged or repeated therapy) may result in bacterial or fungal overgrowth. Such overgrowth may lead to a second infection. TMP-SMZ may need to be stopped and another antibiotic prescribed for the second infection.

*Pregnancy:* Do not use at term (after 36 weeks). Adequate studies have not been done in pregnant women. Use only if clearly needed and potential benefits outweigh the possible hazards to the fetus.

*Breastfeeding:* TMP-SMZ appears in breast milk. Do not use TMP-SMZ during breastfeeding. Consult your doctor.

*Children:* Use in children less than 2 months is not recommended.

*Elderly:* Patients may be at an increased risk for side effects, particularly when complicating conditions exist (such as kidney or liver disease). Dosage must be adjusted accordingly.

*Sulfites:* Some of these products may contain sulfite preservatives which can cause allergic reactions in certain individuals. Check package label when available or consult your doctor or pharmacist.

## Drug Interactions:

Tell your doctor or pharmacist if you are taking or if you are planning to take any over-the-counter or prescription medications with TMP-SMZ. Doses of one or both drugs may need to be modified or a different drug may need to be prescribed. The following drugs and drug classes interact with TMP-SMZ.

- acetohexamide (eg, *Dymelor*)
- anticoagulants, oral (eg, *Coumadin*)
- chlorpropamide (eg, *Diabinese*)
- cyclosporine *(Sandimmune)*
- methotrexate (eg, *Mexate*)
- phenytoin (eg, *Dilantin)*
- thiazide diuretics (eg, hydrochlorothiazide)
- tolazamide (eg, *Tolinase)*
- tolbutamide (eg, *Orinase)*

Consider all drug interactions reported for sulfamethoxazole when using this drug.

## Side Effects:

Every drug is capable of producing side effects. Many TMP-SMZ users experience no, or minor, side effects. The frequency and severity of side effects depend on many factors including dose, duration of therapy and individual susceptibility. Possible side effects include:

*Digestive Tract:* Nausea; vomiting; appetite loss; stomach pain; diarrhea.

*Nervous System:* Headache; depression; seizures; hallucinations; weakness; nervousness; meningitis; insomnia; vertigo (feeling of whirling motion); sleeplessness.

*Skin:* Rash; peeling of skin; yellowing of the skin or eyes; sensitivity to light; hives; itching.

*Other:* Inflammation of the tongue and mouth; fever; chills; inflammation of the eyes; ringing in the ears; abnormal liver and kidney function tests; joint or muscle pain.

---

### Guidelines for Use:

- Take on an empty stomach. If upset stomach occurs, take with food.
- Take with a full glass of water.
- Treat initial, uncomplicated urinary tract infections with a single antibacterial. Use this combination for more complicated infections resistant to more traditional therapy.
- Complete the full course of therapy for best results and to decrease the risk of a relapse.
- Consult your doctor immediately if sore throat, fever, chills, pale skin, yellowing of skin or eyes, rash or unusual bleeding or bruising occurs.

---

*If you have any questions, consult your doctor, pharmacist, or health care provider.*

| Generic Name<br>*Brand Name Examples* | Supplied As | Generic<br>Available |
|---|---|---|
| *Rx* **Sulfanilamide** | | |
| *AVC* | **Vaginal cream:** 15% | Yes |
| *AVC* | **Vaginal suppositories:** 1.05 g | No |
| *Rx* **Triple Sulfa** | | |
| *Sultrin Triple Sulfa* | **Vaginal tablets:** 172.5 mg sulfathiazole, 143.75 mg sulfacetamide, 184 mg sulfabenzamide and urea | No |
| *Dayto Sulf, Gyne-Sulf, Sulfa-Trip, Sultrin Triple Sulfa, Trysul, V.V.S.* | **Vaginal cream:** 3.42% sulfathiazole, 2.86% sulfacetamide, 3.7% sulfabenzamide and 0.64% urea | Yes |
| *Rx* **Vaginal Anti-infective Combinations** | | |
| *Terramycin w/Polymyxin B Sulfate* | **Vaginal tablets:** 100 mg oxytetracycline and 100,000 units polymyxin B sulfate | Yes |
| *Vagisec Plus* | **Vaginal suppositories:** 6 mg aminacrine HCl, 5.25 mg polyoxyethylene nonyl phenol, 0.66 mg EDTA and 0.07 mg docusate sodium | No |
| *Cantri* | **Vaginal cream:** 10% sulfisoxazole, 0.2% aminacrine HCl and 2% allantoin | No |
| *Nil* | **Vaginal cream:** 15% sulfanilamide, 0.2% aminacrine HCl and 1.5% allantoin | No |
| *Alasulf, Benegyn, Deltavac, D.I.T.1-2* | **Vaginal cream:** 15% sulfanilamide, 0.2% aminacrine HCl and 2% allantoin | No |
| *Cleocin*[1] | **Vaginal cream:** 2% clindamycin phosphate | No |
| *MetroGel* | **Vaginal gel:** 0.75% metronidazole | No |

[1] Contains mineral oil.

## Type of Drug:

Vaginal anti-infection products.

## Uses:

In these combinations:

*Antibiotics:* For infections due to susceptible organisms. Consult mono-graphs on individual agents.

*Triple Sulfa:* For treatment of bacterial vaginosis.

*Sulfanilamide:* For the treatment of *Candida albicans* vulvovaginitis (monilia, yeast) only.

*Sulfonamides:* For infections due to susceptible organisms.

*Estrogens:* To aid in the return of the vaginal mucosa to normal.

*Metronidazole:* For the treatment of bacterial vaginosis.

*Oxyquinoline benzoate and aminacrine:* For use as antiseptics.

*Allantoin:* Aids in the surgical removal of dead tissue and in tissue regeneration.

*Polyoxyethylene nonyl phenol, alkyl aryl sulfonate, sodium lauryl sulfate, and docusate sodium:* Used as wetting agents.

## Precautions:

*Do not use in the following situations:*
>       alcohol use (metronidazole only)
>       allergy to lincomycin (clindamycin only)
>       allergy to the vaginal anti-infective or any of its ingredients
>       colitis, antibiotic-associated (clindamycin only)
>       disulfiram therapy, within 2 weeks (metronidazole only)
>       inflammation of the intestine, history of (clindamycin only)
>       kidney disease (sulfonamides only)
>       ulcerative colitis (clindamycin only)

*Use with caution in the following situations:*
>       CNS diseases (metronidazole only)
>       impaired liver function (metronidazole only)
>       pregnancy

## Drug Interactions:

Tell your doctor or pharmacist if you are taking or if you are planning to take any over-the-counter or prescription medications or dietary supplements with vaginal anti-infectives. Doses of one or both drugs may need to be modified or a different drug may need to be prescribed. Anti-coagulants (eg, warfarin) and disulfiram (eg, *Antabuse)* interact with metronidazole.

## Side Effects:

Every drug is capable of producing side effects. Many vaginal anti-infective users experience no, or minor, side effects. The frequency and severity of side effects depend on many factors including dose, duration of therapy, and individual susceptibility. If local irritation, rash, or itching develops, discontinue treatment and contact your doctor. Cramps, stomach pain, and a change in white blood cell count may occur with metronidazole use.

---

## Guidelines for Use:

- Patient instructions are included with product.
- Dosage is individualized. Use exactly as prescribed.
- Do not stop taking or change the dose unless directed by your doctor. Complete full course of therapy.
- Use the applicator provided to insert high into the vagina. An applicator may not be recommended during pregnancy. Use only on the advice of your doctor.
- Notify your doctor if burning, itching, irritation, or an allergic reaction occurs.
- Mineral oil may weaken latex or rubber products such as condoms or diaphragms. Do not use such products within 72 hours following treatment with mineral oil-containing products.
- Do not engage in vaginal sexual intercourse during treatment.
- Avoid contact with the eyes.

---

*If you have any questions, consult your doctor, pharmacist, or health care provider.*

| Generic Name Brand Name Examples | Supplied As | Generic Available |
|---|---|---|
| **Clotrimazole** | | |
| Rx  Lotrimin | **Cream**: 1% | Yes |
| otc  Cruex, Lotrimin AF | **Cream**: 1% | Yes |
| Rx  Lotrimin | **Lotion**: 1% | No |
| otc  Lotrimin AF | **Lotion**: 1% | No |
| Rx  Fungoid, Lotrimin | **Solution**: 1% | Yes |
| otc  Lotrimin AF | **Solution**: 1% | No |
| Rx  Mycelex | **Troches**: 10 mg | No |

## Type of Drug:
Topical antifungal.

## How the Drug Works:
Fungi apparently bind to the drug. The cell membrane of fungi is altered, allowing fungal cell contents to leak out, resulting in cell death. The troche binds to the oral mucosa (lining of the mouth) and provides a long-term concentration in saliva.

## Uses:
*Solutions, creams, and lotions:* To treat tinea pedis (athlete's foot), tinea cruris (jock itch), and tinea corporis (ringworm).

*Troche (hard lozenge):* To treat thrush (oral candidiasis) or reduce the incidence of thrush in immuncompromised patients.

*Rx products:* To treat tinea versicolor (pityriasis) and candidiasis (yeast).

## Precautions:
*Do not use in the following situations:* Allergy to clotrimazole or any of its ingredients.

*Use with caution in the following situations:* Liver disease.

*Pregnancy:* There are no adequate and well-controlled studies in pregnant women. Use only if clearly needed and the potential benefits to the mother outweigh the possible hazards to the fetus.

*Breastfeeding:* It is not known if clotrimazole appears in breast milk. Consult your doctor before you begin breastfeeding.

*Children:* Do not use in children under 2 years of age, unless directed by your doctor. Supervise use in children under 12 years of age.

## Side Effects:

Every drug is capable of producing side effects. Many clotrimazole users experience no, or minor, side effects. The frequency and severity of side effects depend on many factors including dose, duration of therapy, and individual susceptibility. Possible side effects include:

*Troche:* Nausea; vomiting; abnormal liver function tests; unpleasant mouth sensations; itching.

*Topical:* Redness; stinging; burning; blistering; peeling; swelling; itching; hives; general skin irritation.

### Guidelines for Use:

- Dosage is individualized. Use exactly as prescribed.
- Do not stop taking or change the dose, unless directed by your doctor.
- Avoid contact with eyes. Do not use on scalp or nails.
- Avoid use of occlusive wrappings or dressings.
- If condition persists or worsens, or if irritation, redness, burning, blistering, swelling, oozing, or itching occurs, discontinue use and notify your doctor.
- If a dose is missed, take it as soon as possible. If several hours have passed or it is nearing time for the next dose, do not double the dose in order to catch up, unless advised to do so by your doctor. If more than one dose is missed or it is necessary to establish a new dosage schedule, contact your doctor or pharmacist.
- Continue use until a full course of therapy is completed. Failure to use all of the medicine may prevent complete elimination of the fungi, causing the infection to return.
- Contact your doctor or pharmacist if symptoms persist after a course of treatment is completed.
- Do not use for treating fungal infection other than in the mouth (troches only) or on the skin (creams, lotions, solutions).
- *Troches* — Slowly dissolve in the mouth for maximum effect.
- *Lotions, creams, and solutions* — Apply after cleansing the affected area, unless directed otherwise by your doctor. Apply twice daily, morning and evening. Improvement should be seen within 1 week.
- Avoid sources of infection or reinfection.
- Avoid contact with eyes.

*If you have any questions, consult your doctor, pharmacist, or health care provider.*

| Generic Name<br>*Brand Name Example* | Supplied As | Generic<br>Available |
|---|---|---|
| *Rx* **Fluconazole**[1] | | |
| *Diflucan* | **Tablets:** 50 mg, 100 mg,<br>150 mg, 200 mg | No |
| *Diflucan* | **Oral Suspension:** 50 mg/5 mL,<br>200 mg/5 mL | No |

[1] Also available as an injection.

## Type of Drug:
Antifungal agent.

## How the Drug Works:
Fluconazole interferes with the formation of the cell membrane of fungi. This causes leakage of cellular contents, resulting in fungal cell death.

## Uses:
To treat candidiasis (yeast) infections of the mouth, throat, and vagina.

To treat other serious candidal infections such as urinary tract infection, peritonitis (inflammation of the lining of the abdomen and pelvis), and pneumonia.

To treat cryptococcal meningitis (caused by yeast-like organisms affecting the brain).

To decrease the incidence of candidiasis (yeast) infections in patients undergoing bone marrow transplants who receive chemotherapy or radiation therapy.

## Precautions:
*Do not use in the following situations:* Allergy to fluconazole or any of its ingredients.

*Use with caution in the following situations:*
> allergy to other azole antifungals (eg, ketoconazole)
> kidney disease
> liver disease
> weakened immune system or other serious underlying conditions (eg, AIDS, cancer)

*Pregnancy:* There are no adequate and well-controlled studies in pregnant women. Use only if clearly needed and the potential benefits to the mother outweigh the possible hazards to the fetus.

*Breastfeeding:* Fluconazole appears in breast milk. Consult your doctor before you begin breastfeeding.

*Children:* Safety and effectiveness have not been established in infants under 6 months of age.

## Drug Interactions:

Tell your doctor or pharmacist if you are taking or if you are planning to take any over-the-counter or prescription medications while taking this medicine. Doses of one or both drugs may need to be modified or a different drug may need to be prescribed.The following drugs and drug classes interact with this medicine.

anticoagulants, oral
 (eg, warfarin)
cimetidine (eg, *Tagamet*)
cyclosporine (eg, *Sandimmune*)
hydrochlorothiazide
 (eg, *Esidrix*)
oral contraceptives (eg, *Ortho-Novum*)

phenytoin (eg, *Dilantin)*
rifampin (eg, *Rifadin)*
sulfonylureas (eg, glipizide)
tacrolimus *(Prograf)*
theophylline (eg, *Theo-Dur)*
zidovudine *(Retrovir)*

## Side Effects:

Every drug is capable of producing side effects. Many patients experience no, or minor, side effects. The frequency and severity of side effects depend on many factors including dose, duration of therapy, and individual susceptibility. Possible side effects include:

*Digestive Tract:* Nausea; vomiting; diarrhea; indigestion; stomach ache; changes in taste.

*Other:* Headache; dizziness; rash.

### Guidelines for Use:

- Use exactly as prescribed.
- Continue use until all of the prescribed medicine has been taken. Failure to take or use all of the medicine may prevent complete elimination of the fungi, causing the infection to return.
- If a dose is missed, take or inject it as soon as possible. If several hours have passed or if it is nearing time for the next dose, do not double the dose in order to "catch up" (unless advised to do so by your doctor). If more than one dose is missed or it is necessary to establish a new dosage schedule, contact your doctor or pharmacist.
- Contact your doctor if rash, yellowing of skin or eyes, nausea, weakness, difficulty breathing or facial swelling develops.
- *Intravenous solution* — Do not use if solution is cloudy or contains particles. Follow the administration procedure taught to you by your healthcare provider. Do not remove unit from overwrap until ready for use. Store at room temperature (bottles, 41° to 86°F; bags, 41° to 77°F).
- *Oral suspension* — Shake well before use. Store at room temperature (41°to 86°F) and discard unused portion after 2 weeks. Protect from freezing.
- *Tablets* — Store at room temperature (below 86°F).

*If you have any questions, consult your doctor, pharmacist, or health care provider.*

| Generic Name Brand Name Examples | Supplied As | Generic Available |
|---|---|---|
| Rx **Griseofulvin Ultramicrosize** | | |
| *Fulvicin P/G, Grisactin Ultra, Gris-PEG* | **Tablets:** 125 mg, 165 mg, 250 mg, 330 mg | Yes |

## Type of Drug:
Antifungal agent.

## How the Drug Works:
Griseofulvin is deposited into the skin. Diseased skin tissue gradually flakes off and is replaced by noninfected tissue which contains griseofulvin. The new skin cells become highly resistant to further fungal infections.

## Uses:
To treat ringworm (fungal) infections of the hair, skin and nails.

To treat athlete's foot.

## Precautions:
*Do not use in the following situations:*

allergy to griseofulvin
liver failure
porphyria (high concentrations
 of iron-free pigments)

pregnancy
to treat minor infections which
 will respond to skin-applied
 agents alone

*Use with caution in the following situations:*
allergy to penicillin
long-term therapy
lupus erythematosus

*Sensitivity to light:* May cause photosensitivity (sensitivity to sunlight). Avoid prolonged exposure to the sun and other ultraviolet light. Use sunscreens and wear protective clothing until tolerance is determined.

*Males:* Males should wait at least 6 months after therapy before trying to father a child.

*Lab Tests:* Patients on long-term griseofulvin therapy may be required to have complete blood counts and liver and kidney function tests done periodically. Be sure to keep appointments.

*Pregnancy:* Do not use during pregnancy. The risk of use in pregnant women clearly outweighs any possible benefit.

*Children:* Safety and effectiveness have not been established in children under 2 years of age.

## Drug Interactions:
Tell your doctor or pharmacist if you are taking or if you are planning to take any over-the-counter or prescription medications while taking this

medicine. Doses of one or both drugs may need to be modified or a different drug may need to be prescribed.The following drugs and drug classes interact with this medicine.

alcohol
anticoagulants, oral (eg, warfarin)
barbiturates (eg, phenobarbital)
contraceptives, oral (eg, Ortho-Novum)

cyclosporine (eg, *Sandimmune)*
estrogens (eg, *Premarin)*
salicylates (eg, aspirin)

## Side Effects:

Every drug is capable of producing side effects. Many patients experience no, or minor, side effects. The frequency and severity of side effects depend on many factors including dose, duration of therapy and individual susceptibility. Possible side effects include:

*Digestive Tract:* Nausea; vomiting; diarrhea; stomach ache; whiteness in mouth.

*Other:* Headache; fatigue; dizziness; confusion; sleeplessness; impaired coordination; rash; hives; itching.

---

### Guidelines for Use:

- Use exactly as prescribed.
- Take with food high in fat content (eg, peanut butter).
- If a dose is missed, take it as soon as possible. If several hours have passed or if it is nearing time for the next dose, do not double the dose in order to "catch up" (unless advised to do so by your doctor). If more than one dose is missed or it is necessary to establish a new dosage schedule, contact your doctor or pharmacist.
- Beneficial effects may not be apparent for several weeks. Continue use until all of the prescribed medicine has been taken, even if symptoms have disappeared. Failure to take all of the medicine may prevent complete elimination of fungi, causing the infection to return.
- Observe good hygiene during treatment to help control infection and prevent reinfection.
- Contact your doctor if any of the following occurs: Sore throat, skin rash, facial swelling, yellowing of skin/eyes, difficulty breathing, fatigue, fever or weight loss.
- Inform your doctor if you are pregnant, become pregnant or are planning to become pregnant. Males should wait at least 6 months after therapy before trying to father a child.
- Topical antifungal therapy may accompany oral therapy. Topical therapy is especially useful in athlete's foot (tinea pedis) and jock itch (tinea cruris).
- May cause photosensitivity (sensitivity to sunlight). Avoid prolonged exposure to the sun and other ultraviolet light. Use sunscreens and wear protective clothing until tolerance is determined.
- Lab tests may be necessary to monitor therapy. Be sure to keep appointments.
- Store at room temperature (59° to 86°F) in a tightly closed container.

---

*If you have any questions, consult your doctor, pharmacist, or health care provider.*

| Generic Name *Brand Name Examples* | Supplied As | Generic Available |
|---|---|---|
| Rx **Itraconazole** | | |
| *Sporanox* | **Capsules:** 100 mg | No |

## Type of Drug:
Antifungal agent.

## How the Drug Works:
Itraconazole inhibits the formation of the cell membrane of fungi. This causes leakage of cellular contents, resulting in fungal cell death.

## Uses:
For treatment of fungal infections due to blastomycosis, histoplasmosis, aspergillosis (in patients intolerant of or who do not respond to amphotericin B) and onychomycosis (when due to dermatophytes of the toenail). Occasionally doctors may prescribe this medicine for other fungal infections.

## Precautions:
*Do not use in the following situations:*
>   allergy to itraconazole
>   midazolam (oral) use
>   pregnant woman with onychomycosis (fungal nail disease), treatment of
>   triazolam (*Halcion*) use

*Use with caution in the following situations:*
>   allergy to similar antifungals
>   liver disease

*Lab Tests:* Liver enzyme test values should be monitored in patients with pre-existing liver function abnormalities and in patients receiving itraconazole treatment for over 1 month. Be sure to keep appointments.

*Pregnancy:* Adequate studies have not been done in pregnant women, or animal studies may have shown a risk to the fetus. Use only if clearly needed and the potential benefits outweigh the possible hazards to the fetus. Effective contraception (birth control) must be used throughout itraconazole therapy and for 2 months following treatment.

>   *Onychomycosis (fungal nail disease) treatment* – Do not use itraconazole during pregnancy. The risk of use in a pregnant woman clearly outweighs any possible benefit.

*Breastfeeding:* Itraconazole appears in breast milk. Do not use while breastfeeding.

*Children:* Safety and effectiveness in children have not been established.

## Drug Interactions:

Tell your doctor or pharmacist if you are taking or if you are planning to take any over-the-counter or prescription medications while taking this medicine. Doses of one or both drugs may need to be modified or a different drug may need to be prescribed. The following drugs and drug classes interact with this medicine.

anticoagulants (eg, warfarin)
antidiabetic drugs, oral (eg, glipizide)
calcium channel blockers (dihydropyridine class eg, nifedipine)
carbamazepine (eg, *Tegretol*)
cyclosporine (eg, *Sandimmune*)
didanosine (*Videx*)
digoxin (eg, *Lanoxin*)
HMG-CoA reductase inhibitors (eg, lovastatin)

$H_2$ antagonists (eg, cimetidine)
isoniazid (eg, *Laniazid*)
midazolam, oral
phenytoin (eg, *Dilantin*)
quinidine (eg, *Quinora*)
rifampin (eg, *Rifadin*)
tacrolimus (*Prograf*)
triazolam (*Halcion*)
vincristine (eg, *Oncovin*)

## Side Effects:

Every drug is capable of producing side effects. Many patients experience no, or minor, side effects. The frequency and severity of side effects depend on many factors including dose, duration of therapy, and individual susceptibility. Possible side effects include:

*Digestive Tract:* Nausea; vomiting; stomach pain; diarrhea; appetite loss.

*Nervous System:* Headache; dizziness; fatigue; sleepiness; drowsiness; feeling of whirling motion.

*Skin:* Rash; hives; itching.

*Other:* Fever; general body discomfort; muscle pain; decreased sexual drive; impotence; edema (fluid retention); difficulty breathing; high blood pressure; dizziness or lightheadedness when rising quickly from a sitting or lying position; abnormal lab values; dark urine; pale stools; yellowing of the skin or eyes.

## Guidelines for Use:

- Use exactly as prescribed.
- Usual dose is 200 mg once daily, taken after a full meal.
- Continue use until all of the prescribed drug has been taken, even if symptoms have disappeared. Failure to take a full course of therapy may prevent complete elimination of fungi, causing the infection to return.
- If a dose is missed, take it as soon as possible. If several hours have passed or if it is nearing time for the next dose, do not double the dose in order to "catch up" (unless advised to do so by your doctor). If more than one dose is missed, contact your doctor or pharmacist.
- Contraceptive measures (birth control) are recommended during treatment and for 2 months following treatment. Inform your doctor if you are pregnant, become pregnant, are planning to become pregnant, or if you are breastfeeding.
- Lab tests may be required to monitor therapy. Be sure to keep appointments.
- Contact your doctor if any of the following occurs: Unusual fatigue, appetite loss, nausea, vomiting, yellowing of skin or eyes, dark urine, pale stools, rash, itching, hives or difficulty breathing.
- Store at room temperature (59° to 86°F) away from moisture and light.

*If you have any questions, consult your doctor, pharmacist, or health care provider.*

| Generic Name<br>*Brand Name Examples* | Supplied As | Generic<br>Available |
|---|---|---|
| *Rx* **Ketoconazole** | | |
| *Nizoral*[1] | **Cream:** 2% | No |
| *Nizoral* | **Shampoo:** 2% | No |
| *Nizoral* | **Tablets:** 200 mg | No |

[1] Contains sulfites.

## Type of Drug:
Antifungal agent.

## How the Drug Works:
Ketoconazole interferes with the formation of the cell membrane of fungi. This causes leakage of cellular contents, resulting in fungal cell death.

## Uses:
*Cream:* For topical treatment of ringworm, jock itch, athlete's foot, tinea versicolor (pityriasis), candidiasis (yeast) infections of the skin and seborrheic dermatitis (inflamed scaling skin).

*Shampoo:* To reduce scaling due to dandruff.

*Tablets:* To treat systemic (internal) fungal infections. Also used to treat severe fungal infections of the skin or mouth that have not responded to topical therapy or oral griseofulvin, or in patients who are unable to take griseofulvin.

## Precautions:
*Do not use in the following situations:*
        allergy to ketoconazole
        fungal meningitis (tablets only)
        triazolam (*Halicon*) use, current (tablets only)

*Use with caution in the following situations:*
        lack of adequate stomach acid (tablets only)
        liver disease (tablets only)
        prostatic cancer (tablets only)

*Liver disease:* This medication has caused liver disease in some patients. The injury is usually reversible if treatment is discontinued as soon as symptoms occur. Stop taking this medicine and contact your doctor immediately if any of the following occurs: Fatigue, appetite loss, nausea, vomiting, yellowing of skin or eyes, dark urine or pale stools.

*Pregnancy:* Adequate studies have not been done in pregnant women, or animal studies may have shown a risk to the fetus. Use only if clearly needed and potential benefits outweigh the possible hazards to the fetus.

*Breastfeeding:* Oral ketoconazole probably appears in breast milk. Do not breastfeed during oral ketoconazole treatment. It is not known if ketoconazole cream appears in breast milk. The shampoo does not appear in breast milk. Exercise caution when applying topical ketoconazole to a nursing woman.

*Children:* Safety and effectiveness of topical and oral ketoconazole have not been established in children under 2 years of age. Do not use in children unless the potential benefits outweigh the risks.

*Lab tests* may be required to monitor therapy with oral ketoconazole. Be sure to keep appointments. Lab tests may include liver function tests.

*Sulfites:* Some of these products may contain sulfite preservatives which can cause allergic reactions in certain individuals (eg, asthmatics). Check package label when available or consult your doctor or pharmacist.

## Drug Interactions:
Tell your doctor or pharmacist if you are taking or if you are planning to take any over-the-counter or prescription medications while taking this medicine. Doses of one or both drugs may need to be modified or a different drug may need to be prescribed.The following drugs and drug classes interact with this medicine.

*All doseforms:*

| | |
|---|---|
| alcohol | digoxin (eg, *Lanoxin)* |
| antacids | $H_2$ antagonists (eg, cimetidine) |
| anticholinergics (eg, atropine) | isoniazid (eg, *Laniazid)* |
| didanosine *(Videx)* | theophylline (eg, *Theo-Dur)* |

*Tablets only:*

| | |
|---|---|
| anticoagulants, oral (eg, warfarin) | cyclosporine (eg, *Sandimmune)* |
| | midazolam *(Versed)* |
| antidiabetic agents, oral (eg, sulfonylureas) | phenytoin (eg, *Dilantin)* |
| | rifampin (eg, *Rifadin)* |
| corticosteroids (eg, methylprednisolone) | tacrolimus *(Prograf)* |
| | triazolam *(Halcion)* |

## Side Effects:
Every drug is capable of producing side effects. Many patients experience no, or minor, side effects. The frequency and severity of side effects depend on many factors including dose, duration of therapy and individual susceptibility. Possible side effects include:

*Topical cream:* Skin irritation; itching; stinging.

*Tablets:* Nausea; vomiting; stomach ache; itching; skin reactions.

*Shampoo:* Hair loss; loss of curl in hair; skin irritation or dryness.

## Guidelines for Use:

- Use exactly as prescribed.
- If a dose is missed, take or apply it as soon as possible. If several hours have passed or if it is nearing time for the next dose, do not double the dose in order to "catch up" (unless advised to do so by your doctor). If more than one dose is missed or it is necessary to establish a new dosage schedule, contact your doctor or pharmacist.
- Continue use until all of the prescribed medicine has been taken or used. Failure to use all of the medicine may prevent complete elimination of the fungi, causing the infection to return.
- *Cream—*
  For external use only.
  Apply once daily, covering the affected and surrounding area. (For seborrheic dermatitis, apply twice daily for 4 weeks or until clearing has occurred.)
  Avoid contact with the eyes.
  Discontinue use and contact your doctor if irritation occurs.
  Improvement may be seen soon after treatment is begun. Jock itch, yeast infections and ringworm should be treated for 2 weeks to reduce the possibility of recurrence. Patients with tinea versicolor usually require 2 weeks of treatment; patients with athlete's foot usually require 6 weeks.
  If no clinical improvement is seen after the treatment period, consult your doctor.
  Store at room temperature. Do not freeze.
- *Shampoo—*
  For external use only.
  Moisten hair and scalp thoroughly with water. Apply enough shampoo to produce enough lather to wash the scalp and hair, and gently massage it over entire scalp area for 1 minute. Rinse hair thoroughly with warm water. Repeat, leaving shampoo on scalp for an additional 3 minutes. After the second thorough rinse, dry hair with towel or hair dryer.
  Shampoo twice a week for 4 weeks with at least 3 days between each shampooing and then intermittently as needed to maintain control.
  Avoid contact with the eyes.
  Discontinue use and contact your doctor if irritation occurs.
  Occasionally the use of the shampoo has resulted in removal of curl from permanently waved hair.
  Store below 77°F away from light.
- *Tablets—*
  Usual dose is 200 mg once daily.
  If stomach upset occurs, take with food.
  In cases of achlorhydria (low stomach acidity), dissolve tablets in a 4 mL (approximately 1 teaspoon) solution of 0.2 N HCl. Use a glass or plastic straw to avoid contact with the teeth. Follow with a glass of water.
  Do not take with antacids, anticholinergics or $H_2$-blockers (eg, *Tagamet*). Wait at least 2 hours after having taken the ketoconazole before taking these products.

## Guidelines for Use (cont.):

- *Tablets* (cont.) –
  Contact your doctor if any of the following occurs: Fatigue, appetite loss, nausea, vomiting, yellowing of skin or eyes, dark urine, pale stools, rash or difficulty breathing.

  May cause dizziness, drowsiness or headache. Use caution while driving or performing other tasks requiring alertness, coordination or physical dexterity.

  Lab tests may be required to monitor treatment. Be sure to keep appointments.

  Store at room temperature (59° to 86°F) away from moisture.

*If you have any questions, consult your doctor, pharmacist, or health care provider.*

| Generic Name<br>*Brand Name Examples* | Supplied As | Generic<br>Available |
|---|---|---|
| *Rx* **Nystatin** | | |
| *Mycostatin,, Nilstat* | **Tablets:** 500,000 units | Yes |
| *Mycostatin[1], Nilstat, Nystex[1]* | **Oral suspension:** 100,000 units/mL | Yes |
| *Mycostatin Pastilles* | **Troches (Lozenges):** 200,000 units | No |
| *Mycostatin, Nilstat, Nystex* | **Cream:** 100,000 units/g | Yes |
| *Mycostatin, Nilstat, Nystex* | **Ointment:** 100,000 units/g | Yes |
| *Mycostatin, Pedi-Dri* | **Powder:** 100,000 units/g | Yes |
| *Nilstat* | **Powder:** 50 million units, 150 million units, 500 million units, 1 billion units, 2 billion units, 5 billion units | Yes |

[1] Contains alcohol.

## Type of Drug:
Antifungal agent.

## How the Drug Works:
Nystatin interferes with the formation of the cell membrane of fungi. This causes leakage of cellular contents, resulting in fungal cell death.

## Uses:
To treat oral (thrush), intestinal, skin or mucous membrane fungal infections due to *Candida* species (yeast).

## Precautions:
*Do not use in the following situations:* Allergy to this medicine

*Pregnancy:* Adequate studies have not been done in pregnant women, or animal studies may have shown a risk to the fetus. Use only if clearly needed and potential benefits outweigh the possible hazards to the fetus.

*Breastfeeding:* Since it is not known whether nystatin appears in breast milk, it should be used with caution. Contact your doctor before you begin breastfeeding.

*Children:* Safety and effectiveness have not been established.

## Side Effects:
Every drug is capable of producing side effects. Many patients experience no, or minor, side effects. The frequency and severity of side effects depend on many factors including dose, duration of therapy and individual susceptibility. Possible side effects include: Nausea; vomiting; diarrhea; stomach ache.

## Guidelines for Use:

- Use exactly as prescribed.
- Avoid contact with the eyes.
- If a dose is missed, take or apply it as soon as possible. If several hours have passed or if it is nearing time for the next dose, do not double the dose in order to "catch up" (unless advised to do so by your doctor). If more than one dose is missed or it is necessary to establish a new dosage schedule, contact your doctor or pharmacist.
- Continue use until all of the prescribed medicine has been taken. Failure to use all of the medicine may prevent complete elimination of the fungi, causing the infection to return.
- Discontinue use and contact your doctor if mouth or skin irritation occurs.
- *Tablets*— Usually taken 3 times a day. Store at room temperature protected from light and moisture.
- *Oral Suspension*— Shake well before using. Swish thoroughly (as long as possible) in mouth before swallowing. Store at room temperature protected from light. Avoid freezing. Doses vary depending upon age. Keep out of the reach of children.
- *Troches (Lozenges/Pastilles)*— Dissolve slowly in the mouth. Do not chew or swallow whole. Good oral hygiene, including proper care of dentures, is of the utmost importance. Store refrigerated (36° to 46°F).
- *Cream and Ointment*— Apply liberally after cleansing the affected area (unless otherwise directed) until healing is complete. These medications do not stain skin or mucous membranes. Store at room temperature. Do not freeze.
- *Children*— Nystatin has been specially compounded by pharmacists and administered in the form of flavored frozen popsicles to improve oral retention. Consult your doctor or pharmacist.

*If you have any questions, consult your doctor, pharmacist, or health care provider.*

| Generic Name<br>*Brand Name Example* | Supplied As | Generic<br>Available |
|---|---|---|
| Rx **Voriconazole**[1] | | |
| *Vfend* | **Tablets:** 50 mg, 200 mg | No |

[1] Also available as an injection.

## Type of Drug:

Anti-infective; azole antifungal.

## How the Drug Works:

Voriconazole kills fungal organisms by interfering with the formation of the fungus.

## Uses:

To treat invasive aspergillosis (invasion of blood vessels and tissue infarction by *Aspergillus fumigatus*).

To treat serious fungal infections caused by *Scedosporium apiospermum* and *Fusarium* species in patients intolerant of, or refactory to, other therapy.

## Precautions:

*Do not use in the following situations:*

allergy to the drug or any of its ingredients
galactose intolerance
hepatic cirrhosis, severe
lactase deficiency

*Use with caution in the following situations:*

allergy to other azole antifungals
hepatic cirrhosis, moderate to severe
kidney insufficiency, moderate to severe

*Visual disturbances:* Visual distrubances are common. Approximately one third of patients experience altered or enhanced visual perception, blurred vision, color vision changes, or photophobia. Most visual changes are mild.

*Pregnancy:* Studies have shown a potential harmful effect on the fetus. Use only when clearly needed and the potential benefits outweigh the possible risks to the fetus.

*Breastfeeding:* It is not known if voriconazole appears in breast milk. Consult your doctor before you begin breastfeeding.

*Children:* Safety and effectiveness in children younger than 12 years of age have not been established.

*Lab tests* may be required during treatment. Tests include visual acuity, visual field, color perception, and renal and hepatic function.

## Drug Interactions:

Tell your doctor or pharmacist if you are taking or planning to take any over-the-counter or prescription medications or dietary supplements while taking this drug. Drug doses may need to be modified or a different drug prescribed. The following drugs and drug classes interact with this drug:

barbiturates (eg, phenobarbital)
benzodiazepines (eg, midazolam, triazolam)
calcium channel blockers (eg, diltiazem)
carbamazepine (eg, *Tegretol*)
cimetidine (eg, *Tagament*)
cyclosporine (eg, *Neoral*)
ergot alkaloids (eg, ergotamine)
HMG-CoA reductase inhibitors (eg, lovastatin)
NNRTIs (eg, delavirdine)
phenytoin (eg, *Dilantin*)
pimozide (*Orap*)

prednisolone (eg, *Prelone*)
protease inhibitors (eg, ritonavir, saquinavir)
proton pump inhibitors (eg, omeprazole)
quinidine (eg, *Quinora*)
rifamycins (eg, rifampin)
sirolimus (eg, *Rapamune*)
sulfonylureas (eg, glyburide)
tacrolimus (eg, *Prograf*)
vinca alkaloids (eg, vincristine, vinblastine)
warfarin (eg, *Coumadin*)

## Side Effects:

Every drug is capable of producing side effects. Many patients experience no, or minor, side effects. The frequency and severity of side effects depend on many factors including dose, duration of therapy, and individual susceptibility. Possible side effects include:

*Digestive Tract:* Vomiting; nausea; diarrhea; stomach pain.

*Other:* Visual disturbances; fever; rash; headache; infection of blood or tissues; swelling; breathing disorder; elevated liver function tests; chills; fast heartbeat; hallucinations; sensitivity to light.

---

### Guidelines for Use:

- Dosage is individualized. Take exactly as prescribed.
- Do not stop taking or change the dose, unless directed by your doctor.
- Take at least one hour before or after a meal.
- If a dose is missed, take it as soon as possible. If several hours have passed or it is nearing time for the next dose, do not double the dose to catch up, unless instructed by your doctor. If more than one dose is missed or it is necessary to establish a new dosage schedule, contact your doctor or pharmacist.
- Do not drive at night while taking voriconazole. It may cause blurred vision and sensitivity to light (photophobia). Do not operate machinery or drive if you experience vision changes.
- Avoid direct sunlight during therapy.
- Lab tests may be required to monitor therapy. Be sure to keep appointments.
- Store at controlled room temperature (59° to 86°F).

---

*If you have any questions, consult your doctor, pharmacist, or health care provider.*

| Generic Name<br>*Brand Name Examples* | Supplied As | Generic<br>Available |
|---|---|---|
| *Rx* **Amphotericin B** | | |
| *Fungizone* | **Cream**: 3% | No |
| *Fungizone* | **Lotion**: 3% | No |
| *Rx* **Ciclopirox Olamine** | | |
| *Loprox* | **Cream**: 0.77% | No |
| *Loprox* | **Lotion**: 0.77% | No |
| *Loprox* | **Gel**: 0.77% | No |
| *Penlac Nail Lacquer* | **Solution**: 8% | No |
| **Clotrimazole** | | |
| *otc* *Cruex, Desenex, Lotrimin AF* | **Cream**: 1% | Yes |
| *otc* *Lotrimin AF* | **Lotion**: 1% | No |
| *Rx* *Fungoid* | **Solution**: 1% | Yes |
| *otc* *Lotrimin AF* | **Solution**: 1% | No |
| *Rx* **Econazole Nitrate** | | |
| *Spectazole* | **Cream**: 1% | No |
| *otc* **Gentian Violet** | **Solution**: 1% | Yes |
| **Miconazole Nitrate** | | |
| *otc* *Micatin* | **Cream**: 2% | Yes |
| *Rx* *Monistat-Derm* | **Cream**: 2% | No |
| *otc* *Lotrimin AF, Micatin, Zeasorb-AF* | **Powder**: 2% | No |
| *otc* *Fungoid Tincture* | **Solution**: 2% | No |
| *otc* *Lotrimin AF, Micatin* | **Spray**: 2% | No |
| *otc* *Cruex, Desenex, Lotrimin AF, Micatin, Ting* | **Spray powder**: 2% | No |
| *Rx* **Naftifine Hydrochloride** | | |
| *Naftin* | **Cream**: 1% | No |
| *Naftin* | **Gel**: 1% | No |
| *Rx* **Nystatin** | | |
| *Pedi-Dri* | **Powder**: 100,000 U/g | No |
| *Rx* **Oxiconazole Nitrate** | | |
| *Oxistat* | **Cream**: 1% | No |
| *Oxistat* | **Lotion**: 1% | No |

| Generic Name<br>*Brand Name Examples* | Supplied As | Generic<br>Available |
|---|---|---|
| *Rx* **Sulconazole Nitrate** | | |
| *Exelderm* | **Cream:** 1% | No |
| *Exelderm* | **Solution:** 1% | No |
| *otc* **Terbinafine Hydrochloride** | | |
| *Lamisil AT* | **Cream:** 1% | No |
| *otc* **Tolnaftate** | | |
| *NP•27, Tinactin* | **Cream:** 1% | Yes |
| *Odor-Eaters, Quinsana Plus, Tinactin* | **Powder**: 1% | Yes |
| *Aftate for Athlete's Foot, Aftate for Jock Itch, Tinactin, Tinactin for Jock Itch* | **Spray powder**: 1% | Yes |
| *Absorbine Jr., Aftate for Athlete's Foot, Odor-Eaters, Tinactin, Ting* | **Spray liquid**: 1% | No |
| *Absorbine Jr., Dr. Scholl's Fungi Solution, Tinactin* | **Solution**: 1% | Yes |
| *Absorbine Jr.* | **Gel**: 1% | No |
| *Tinactin* | **Wipes**: 1% | |
| *otc* **Undecylenic Acid and Derivatives** | | |
| *Breezee Mist* | **Powder**: Undecylenic acid | No |
| *FungiCure* | **Liquid**: 10% undecylenic acid | No |

## Type of Drug:

Topical antifungals; drugs used to treat fungal infections of the skin or nails.

## How the Drug Works:

Topical antifungals exert their action by different mechanisms and treat a wide variety of fungi. The choice of topical antifungal depends on the nature of the infection.

## Uses:

Products and their uses are listed in the following table:

| | Uses | | | | |
|---|---|---|---|---|---|
| Generic Name | Athlete's Foot | Jock Itch | Ring-worm | Tinea versicolor (pityriasis) | Other |
| Amphotericin B | | | | | Candidiasis[1] |
| Ciclopirox | ✔ | ✔ | ✔ | ✔ | Candidiasis[1] infections on skin |
| Clotrimazole | ✔ | ✔ | ✔ | ✔ | Candidiasis,[1] seborrheic dermatitis of scalp; see clotrimazole monograph in this chapter |
| Econazole | ✔ | ✔ | ✔ | ✔ | Candidiasis[1] infections on skin |
| Gentian Violet | | | | | Anti-infective and antifungal dye |
| Miconazole | ✔ | ✔ | ✔ | ✔ | Candidiasis[1] infections on skin |
| Naftifine | ✔ | | ✔ | ✔ | |
| Nystatin | | | | | Candidiasis[1]; see nystatin monograph in this chapter |
| Oxiconazole | ✔ | ✔ | ✔ | ✔ | |
| Sulconazole | ✔ | ✔ | ✔ | ✔ | |
| Terbinafine | ✔ | ✔ | ✔ | ✔[2] | Candidiasis[1] infections on skin[2] |
| Tolnaftate | ✔ | ✔ | ✔ | ✔ | Adjunctive therapy in other fungal infections |
| Undecylenic Acid | ✔ | ✔ | | | Prickly heat, diaper rash, itching, burning and chafing, excessive perspiration and irritation in the groin area, foul-smelling perspiration |

[1] Also called canida, moniliasis, albicans, or yeast.
[2] Unlabeled use.

## Precautions:

*Do not use in the following situations:* Allergy to the topical antifungal or any of its ingredients.

*Use with caution in the following situations:*
blistered, raw, or oozing areas of skin
worsening skin irritation during drug therapy

*Pregnancy:* There are no adequate and well-controlled studies in pregnant women. Use only if clearly needed and the potential benefits to the mother outweigh the possible hazards to the fetus.

*Breastfeeding:* Some topical antifungals may appear in breast milk. Consult your doctor before you begin breastfeeding. Avoid direct application of terbinafine to the breast.

*Children:* Do not use undecylenic acid, clotrimazole, miconazole, or tolnaftate on children under 2 years of age. Amphotericin B and nystatin can be used in infants. Safety and effectiveness for use of the other topical antifungals in children under 10 years of age have not been established.

## Side Effects:

Every drug is capable of producing side effects. Many topical antifungal users experience no, or minor, side effects. The frequency and severity of side effects depend on many factors including dose, duration of therapy, and individual susceptibility. Possible side effects include: Allergic contact dermatitis; burning; hives; blistering; peeling; itching; stinging; redness; swelling; dryness.

## Guidelines for Use:

- Use exactly as directed.
- For external use only. Avoid contact with the eyes, nose, or mouth or other mucous membranes.
- Cleanse and dry the area to be treated before application.
- Avoid inhalation of spray products.
- Apply with caution to blistered or raw skin, oozing skin, or skin over a deep puncture wound.
- Wash hands before and after applying.
- Avoid the use of occlusive wraps or dressings unless directed by your health care provider.
- Patients with decreased circulation, including diabetic patients, should consult their doctor or pharmacist before using undecylenic acid.
- Allergic reactions may occur. If the condition being treated worsens or irritation, burning, redness, swelling, or stinging persists, discontinue use and inform your health care provider.
- Frequency of application and duration of therapy is dependent on the condition being treated, its location, the drug, the strength of the drug, and the doseform used. For assistance in drug selection and dosage guidelines, consult your pharmacist or doctor.
- Amphotericin B and gentian violet may stain fabric, skin, or hair.
- For athlete's foot, wear well-fitting and ventilated shoes. Change socks at least once a day.
- Use these medications for the full treatment time, even after the symptoms improve.
- Notify your physician if there is no improvement after 4 weeks.
- Shake ciclopirox lotion well before each use.
- Spray powders and liquids and tolnaftate solution and gel are flammable. Do not use near heat or open flame.
- *Penlac Nail Lacquer* — Do not shower or bathe for at least 8 hours after applying the solution. Do not use polish or other nail cosmetic products on treated nails. Product is flammable. Do not use near heat or open flame. Must be used as part of a comprehensive management program including the removal of the unattached, infected nails. Store in the original carton after each use to protect from light.
- Store at room temperature (68° to 77°F). Avoid freezing.

*If you have any questions, consult your doctor, pharmacist, or health care provider.*

| | Brand Name Examples | Supplied As |
|---|---|---|
| otc | Blis-To-Sol | **Liquid:** Undecylenic acid and salicylic acid |
| | | **Powder:** Benzoic acid and salicylic acid |
| otc | Castaderm | **Liquid:** Resorcinol, boric acid, acetone, basic fuchsin, phenol and 9% alcohol |
| Rx | Castellani Paint | **Solution:** Basic fuchsin, phenol, resorcinol, acetone and alcohol. Also available as a colorless solution without basic fuchsin |
| otc | Castel Minus | **Liquid:** 10% resorcinol, acetone, basic fuchsin, hydroxyethylcelluose and 11.5% alcohol |
| otc | Castel Plus | **Liquid:** 10% resorcinol, acetone, basic fuchsin, hydroxyethylcellulose and 11.5% alcohol |
| otc | Dermasept Antifungal | **Liquid:** 6.098% tannic acid, 5.081% zinc chloride, 2.032% benzocaine, 3.049% methylbenzethonium HCl, 1.017% tolnaftate, 5.081% undecylenic acid, 58.539% ethanol 38B, phenyl, benzyl alcohol, benzoic acid, coal tar, camphor, menthol |
| otc | Fungi•Nail | **Liquid:** 10% undecylenic acid, 5% salicylic acid, 70% isopropyl alcohol |
| Rx | Gordochom | **Liquid:** 25% undecylenic acid and 3% chloroxylenol in an oil base |
| Rx | Mycolog-II | **Cream:** 100,000 units nystatin and 1 mg triamcinolone acetonide per gram |
| | | **Ointment:** 100,000 units nystatin and 1 mg triamcinolone acetonide per gram |
| otc | Neo-Castaderm | **Liquid:** Resorcinol, boric acid, acetone, sodium bisulfite, phenol and 9% alcohol |
| otc | Prophyllin | **Ointment:** 5% sodium propionate and 0.0125% chlorophyll derivatives |
| | | **Powder:** Makes a solution containing 1% sodium propionate and 0.0025% water soluble chlorophyllin |

| | Brand Name Examples | Supplied As |
|---|---|---|
| otc | SteriNail | **Solution:** Undecylenic acid, tolnaftate, propylene glycol, acetone, acetic acid, propionic acid, benzyl alcohol, eucalyptol and benzyl acetate, *Steri-Scrub* and *Steri-Brush* included |
| otc | Ting | **Powder:** Benzoic acid, boric acid, zinc oxide, zinc stearate and propylene glycol |
| | | **Cream:** Benzoic acid, boric acid, zinc oxide, zinc stearate, sodium stearate, titanium dioxide and 19% alcohol |
| Rx | Tinver | **Lotion:** 25% sodium thiosulfate, 1% salicylic acid, 10% isopropyl alcohol, menthol, propylene glycol, EDTA and colloidal alumina |
| otc | Whitfield's | **Ointment:** 6% benzoic acid and 3% salicylic acid |

## Type of Drug:

Antifungal agents. Drugs used to treat fungal infections.

## How the Drug Works:

Topical antifungals exert their action by different mechanisms and treat a wide variety of fungi. The choice of topical antifungal depends on the nature of the infection.

## Uses:

The principal active components of these formulations include:

Antifungal agents—

> Undecylenic acid
> Nystatin
> Iodochlorhydroxyquin
> Parachlorometaxylenol
> Sodium propionate, sodium caprylate, zinc caprylate, zinc propionate, zinc stearate, benzoic acid, sodium thiosulfate, phenol and resorcinol
> Tolnaftate
> Triamcinolone acetonide

See individual monographs for more information.

Other components include:

*Salicylic acid* for its topical keratolytic (softening or peeling).

*Tannic acid* as an astringent (agent that causes shrinking or puckering of tissue, eg, styptic pencil).

*Boric acid* as an astringent and antiseptic.

*Zinc oxide* for its astringent, antiseptic and protective properties.

*Chloroxylenol* as an antiseptic.

*Benzocaine* as an anesthetic.

*Menthol* for its anti-itch, anesthetic and antiseptic effects.

*Chlorophyll derivatives* to promote healing, relieve pain and inflammation and reduce smell in wounds, burns, surface ulcers, cuts, scrapes and skin irritations.

*Basic fuchsin* for its antifungal and antibacterial activity.

In general, powders are used with other products. Ointments, creams and liquids are used as primary therapy in very mild conditions or as preventative agents, especially in moist areas. In addition, powders with a cornstarch base may be preferred over those with a talc base.

---

### Guidelines for Use:

- For external use only. Avoid contact with the eyes, nose, mouth or other mucous membranes.
- Cleanse and dry the area to be treated before application.
- Avoid the use of occlusive dressings, unless directed by the doctor.
- Allergic reactions may occur. If the condition being treated worsens or irritation, burning, redness, swelling or stinging persists, do not reapply the drug and contact your doctor.
- *Undecylenic acid* - Patients with decreased circulation, including diabetics, should consult their doctor before use.
- Frequency of application and duration of therapy is dependent on the condition being treated, its location, the drug, the strength of the drug and the dosage form used. For assistance in drug selection and dosage guidelines, consult your pharmacist or doctor.

---

*If you have any questions, consult your doctor, pharmacist, or health care provider.*

| Generic Name<br>*Brand Name Examples* | Supplied As | Generic<br>Available |
|---|---|---|
| *Rx* **Butoconazole Nitrate** | | |
| *Femstat* | **Vaginal cream:** 2% | No |
| **Clotrimazole** | | |
| *otc Femcare, Gyne-Lotrimin, Mycelex-7, Sweent'n fresh clotrimazole-7* | **Vaginal tablets:** 100 mg | Yes |
| *Rx Mycelex-G* | **Vaginal tablets:** 500 mg | No |
| *otc Gyne-Lotrimin Combination Pack* | **Cream:** 1% **Tablets:** 500 mg | No |
| *Rx Mycelex Twin Pack* | **Cream:** 1% **Tablets:** 500 mg | No |
| *otc Femcare, Gyne-Lotrimin, Mycelex-7, Sweent'n fresh clotrimazole-7* | **Vaginal cream:** 1% | Yes |
| *Rx* **Gentian Violet** | | |
| *Genapax* | **Tampons:** 5 mg | No |
| **Miconazole Nitrate** | | |
| *otc Monistat 7* | **Vaginal suppositories:** 100 mg | No |
| *Rx Monistat 3* | **Vaginal suppositories:** 200 mg | No |
| *otc Monistat 7* | **Vaginal cream:** 2% | Yes |
| *otc Monistat 7 Combination Pack* | **Cream:** 2%<br>**Vaginal suppositories:** 100 mg | No |
| *Rx Monistat-Derm* | **Topical Cream;** 2% | No |
| *Rx Monistat Dual-Pak* | **Cream:** 2%<br>**Vaginal suppositories:** 200 mg | No |
| *Rx* **Nystatin** | | |
| *Mycostatin* | **Vaginal tablets:** 100,000 units | Yes |
| *Rx* **Terconazole** | | |
| *Terazol 3* | **Vaginal suppositories:** 80 mg | No |
| *Terazol 3, Terazol 7* | **Vaginal cream:** 0.4%, 0.8% | No |
| *Rx* **Tioconazole** | | |
| *Vagistat-1* | **Vaginal ointment:** 6.5% | No |

## Type of Drug:
Vaginal antifungal agents.

## How the Drug Works:
These drugs apparently weaken the cell membrane and allow leakage of cellular contents, producing cell death.

## Uses:

To treat vaginal candidiasis (monilia or "yeast") infections.

## Precautions:

*Do not use in the following situations:* Allergy to the drug or any of its ingredients.

*Pregnancy:* Adverse effects or complications have not been reported in infants born to women treated with these agents. Avoid use of a vaginal applicator during pregnancy. Insertion of tablets by hand is preferred. Use only on advice of your doctor. Because small amounts of these drugs may be absorbed from the vagina, use during the first trimester only when essential. Use butoconazole during the second and third trimesters only. Possible exposure of the fetus through direct transfer of terconazole from an irritated vagina may occur.

*Breastfeeding:* It is not known if vaginal antifungals appear in breast milk. Consult your doctor before you begin breastfeeding.

*Children:* Safety and effectiveness of terconazole and tioconazole have not been established.

## Side Effects:

Every drug is capable of producing side effects. Many vaginal antifungal users experience no, or minor, side effects. The frequency and severity of side effects depend on many factors including dose, duration of therapy, and individual susceptibility. Possible side effects include:

*General:* Vaginal irritation; burning; itching.

*Clotrimazole:* Stomach cramps; bloating; vaginal rash; painful intercourse.

*Miconazole:* Pelvic cramps; headache; hives; skin rash.

*Butoconazole:* Vaginal swelling, discharge, or soreness.

*Terconazole:* Headache; body aches; local irritation; sensitivity to light; painful menstruation; stomach pain; fever; genital pain.

*Tioconazole:* Vaginal discharge, pain, dryness, or scaling; vulvar edema and swelling; excessive urination at night; difficult urination; painful intercourse.

## Guidelines for Use:

- Patient instructions for proper use are enclosed in each package and should be strictly followed.
- *Vaginal tablets, creams, and suppositories* — Insert high into the vagina, except during pregnancy.
- Complete a full course of therapy. Use continuously, even during the menstrual period.
- If the vaginal medication causes burning or irritation, or if symptoms worsen, contact your doctor.
- Refrain from sexual intercourse during treatment or use condoms to avoid the risk of reinfection.
- A sanitary napkin or minipad may be used to prevent staining of clothing due to seepage or leakage. Do not use a tampon.
- Concurrent use (up to 72 hours) with certain latex products (eg, condoms, diaphragms) is not recommended.
- If candidiasis is chronic and recurrent, other factors may be involved. Factors that increase the risk of candidiasis include diabetes, chronic antibiotic therapy, pregnancy, steroid use, and oral contraceptive use.

*If you have any questions, consult your doctor, pharmacist, or health care provider.*

| Generic Name<br>*Brand Name Examples* | Supplied As | Generic<br>Available |
|---|---|---|
| Rx **Chloroquine Hydrochloride** | | |
| *Aralen HCl* | **Injection**: 50 mg/mL | No |
| Rx **Chloroquine Phosphate** | | |
| *Aralen* | **Tablets**: 250 mg, 500 mg | Yes |
| Rx **Hydroxychloroquine Sulfate** | | |
| *Plaquenil* | **Tablets**: 200 mg | Yes |
| Rx **Primaquine Phosphate** | **Tablets**: 26.3 mg | Yes |

## Type of Drug:

Antimalarial anti-infectives.

## How the Drug Works:

The actual mechanism of action of aminoquinoline antimalarial drugs is unknown. They may destroy malaria parasites by inhibiting normal metabolism inside the parasite.

These drugs can treat and cure malarial infections caused by susceptible strains of *Plasmodium falciparum* but do not cure infections caused by *P. vivax* or *P. malariae*. Their use may lengthen the time period between treatment and relapse in cases that are not cured.

## Uses:

To prevent and treat acute attacks of malaria caused by *Plasmodium vivax, P. malariae, P. ovale*, and susceptible strains of *P. falciparum*.

Chloroquine is also used as an amebicide.

Chloroquine HCl injection is used to treat acute attacks caused by *P. vivax, P. malariae, P. ovale*, and susceptible strains of *P. falciparum*.

Hydroxychloroquine is also used to treat acute or chronic rheumatoid arthritis and chronic discoid and systemic lupus erythematosus.

Primaquine is used only for the prevention of relapse of *P. vivax*, or following termination of chloroquine suppressive therapy in an area where *P. vivax* is endemic.

*Unlabeled Use(s):* Occasionally doctors may prescribe chloroquine to suppress rheumatoid arthritis, or to treat discoid and systemic lupus erythematosus, scleroderma, pemphigus, lichen planus, polymyositis, sarcoidosis, and porphyria cutanea tarda.

## Precautions:

*Do not use in the following situations:*
> allergy to aminoquinolines or any of their ingredients
> retinal or visual field changes (eg, dark holes in vision)

> *Primaquine only —*
> bone marrow depressants, concurrent use
> granulocytopenia tendency
> hemolytic drugs, concurrent use
> quinacrine, recent or concurrent use

*Use with caution in the following situations:*
> alcohol abuse
> children
> favism, history of or family history of (primaquine only)
> glucose-6 phosphate dehydrogenase (G-6-PD) deficiency
> liver disease
> nicotinamide adenine dinucleotide (NADH) methemoglobin reductase deficiency (primaquine only)
> porphyria
> psoriasis
> hepatoxic (toxic to the liver) drugs, concurrent use

*Pregnancy:* Use only if clearly needed and the potential benefits to the mother outweigh the possible hazards to the fetus.

*Breastfeeding:* Aminoquinolines appear in breast milk. Safety for use during breastfeeding has not been established. Consult your doctor before you begin breastfeeding.

*Children:* Children are especially sensitive to aminoquinoline compounds. Deaths following accidental ingestion of relatively small doses and sudden deaths from injections of chloroquine have been reported. Hydroxychloroquine is not for long-term therapy in children.

*Lab tests* will be required to monitor therapy. Tests including reflex and vision assessments and blood counts may be required.

## Drug Interactions:

Tell your doctor or pharmacist if you are taking or planning to take any over-the-counter or prescription medications with aminoquinolines. Doses of one or both drugs may need to be modified or a different drug may need to be prescribed. The following drugs and drug classes interact with aminoquinolines:

> cimetidine (eg, *Tagamet*)
> magnesium salts (eg, magnesium carbonate)

## Side Effects:

Every drug is capable of producing side effects. Many aminoquinoline users experience no, or minor, side effects. The frequency and severity of side effects depend on many factors including dose, duration of therapy, and individual susceptibility. Possible side effects include:

*Eyes or Ocular:* Visual disturbances; blurred vision; difficulty focusing; "foggy" vision; night blindness; abnormal retina found during eye examinations.

*Digestive Tract:* Nausea; vomiting; diarrhea; stomach upset or cramps; appetite loss.

*Skin:* Rash; itching; pigment changes; hair loss.

*Other:* Ringing in the ears; hearing loss; dizziness; seizures; headache; abnormal blood counts; low blood pressure; darkening of the urine.

---

### Guidelines for Use:

- Dosage is individualized. Take exactly as prescribed for the full course of therapy.
- Do not change the dose or stop taking unless advised by your doctor.
- May cause stomach upset. Take with food.
- Notify your doctor if you experience any change in vision, ringing in the ears, rash, muscle weakness, or hearing impairment.
- *Primaquine* — Notify your doctor immediately if you experience darkening of the urine.
- Overdosage can be especially severe and is extremely dangerous in children. Keep this medication in a childproof container and out of the reach of children.
- May cause nausea, vomiting, stomach pain, diarrhea, appetite loss, irregular heartbeat, or low blood pressure. Notify your doctor if these persist or become bothersome.
- Irreversible damage to the retina of the eye, usually with long-term, high-dose use, has been reported. When long-term use is expected, periodic eye exams should be performed. Retinal changes and visual disturbances may continue even after stopping therapy.
- Chloroquine HCl injection is used when oral therapy is not possible. It will be prepared and administered by your health care provider.
- Lab tests will be required to monitor therapy. Be sure to keep appointments.
- Store at controlled room temperature (59° to 86°F). Protect from light.

---

*If you have any questions, consult your doctor, pharmacist, or health care provider.*

| Generic Name<br>*Brand Name Example* | Supplied As | Generic<br>Available |
|---|---|---|
| *Rx* **Mefloquine Hydrochloride** | | |
| *Lariam* | **Tablets:** 250 mg | No |

## Type of Drug:

Antimalarial anti-infective.

## How the Drug Works:

It is not known exactly how mefloquine acts to inhibit malaria-causing organisms (*Plasmodium falciparum*, *P. vivax*) in the blood. This drug does not eliminate the liver phase of *P. vivax* parasite growth. To prevent relapses in this situation, aminoquinoline drugs (eg, primaquine) must be used.

## Uses:

To prevent (prophylax) and malaria caused by susceptible strains of *Plasmodium falciparum* or by *P. vivax*. Also used to treat mild to moderate malarial infections caused by susceptible strains of *P. falciparum* or *P. ovale*.

## Precautions:

*Do not use in the following situations:*

allergy to mefloquine or related drugs (eg, quinine, quinidine)
depression
epilepsy, history of
halofantrine, concurrent with or after mefloquine
psychosis, history of

*Use with caution in the following situations:*

heart disease
liver disease

*Discontinue use:* Discontinue use if unexplained anxiety, depression, restlessness, or confusion appears during use. These symptoms may signal a more serious problem. Contact your doctor immediately.

*Pregnancy:* Adequate studies have not been done in pregnant women. Use only if clearly needed and potential benefits to the mother outweigh the possible hazards to the fetus. Women of childbearing age who travel to areas of the world where malaria exists should avoid becoming pregnant and use reliable contraception for 2 months after the last dose.

*Breastfeeding:* Mefloquine appears in breast milk. Consult your doctor before you begin breastfeeding.

*Children:* Safety and effectiveness in children under 6 months of age have not been established.

*Lab tests* and periodic doctor visits will be required during long-term treatment with mefloquine. Liver function tests, blood counts (platelets and white blood cells), and eye examinations may be required.

## Drug Interactions:

Tell your doctor or pharmacist if you are taking or planning to take any over-the-counter or prescription medications with mefloquine. Doses of one or both drugs may need to be modified or a different drug may need to be prescribed. The following drugs and drug classes interact with mefloquine:

anticonvulsants (eg, valproic acid)

beta-blockers (eg, propranolol)

chloroquine (eg, *Aralen*)

halofantrine (*Halfan*)

quinidine (eg, *Quinora*)

quinine

typhoid vaccine, live attenuated oral

## Side Effects:

Every drug is capable of producing side effects. Many mefloquine users experience no, or minor, side effects. The frequency and severity of side effects depend on many factors including dose, duration of therapy, and individual susceptibility. Possible side effects include:

*Digestive Tract:* Nausea; vomiting; diarrhea; stomach pain; appetite loss.

*Nervous System:* Dizziness; headache; fatigue; seizures; vertigo (feeling of whirling motion); confusion; anxiety; depression; fainting; loss of balance; drowsiness; sleeplessness; abnormal dreams.

*Other:* Ringing in the ears; chills; rash; fever; muscle aches; visual disturbances; abnormal blood tests; changes in blood pressure.

---

### Guidelines for Use:

- Dose and duration of therapy depend on the drug, patient's age, and situation being treated. Take specifically as prescribed for the full course of therapy. Contact your doctor if you are not able to take as prescribed or cannot complete the full course of therapy.
- Take with food to prevent stomach upset.
- Take with at least 8 oz. of water.
- May cause dizziness. Use caution when driving or performing other tasks requiring alertness, coordination, or physical dexterity.
- Side effects of mefloquine may decrease with prolonged therapy. However, if side effects do occur and do not decrease, they may persist up to several weeks after the last dose.
- If a dose is missed, take it as soon as possible. If several hours have passed or if it is nearing time for the next dose, do not double the dose to catch up. If more than one dose is missed or it is necessary to establish a new dosage schedule, contact your doctor or pharmacist.
- Discontinue use and contact your doctor if you experience unexplained anxiety, depression, restlessness, or confusion.
- If you are a woman of childbearing age who travels to areas where malaria exists, avoid becoming pregnant.
- Lab tests may be required to monitor therapy. Be sure to keep appointments.
- Store at controlled room temperature (59° to 86°F).

---

*If you have any questions, consult your doctor, pharmacist, or health care provider.*

| Generic Name<br>*Brand Name Example* | Supplied As | Generic<br>Available |
|---|---|---|
| *Rx* **Pyrimethamine** | | |
| *Daraprim* | **Tablets:** 25 mg | No |

## Type of Drug:

Antimalarial anti-infective.

## How the Drug Works:

This drug works primarily by inhibiting key enzymes critical to the life of susceptible strains of the organisms causing malaria.

## Uses:

In susceptible strains of plasmodia only. It is not suitable as a preventative agent for travelers to most areas because of prevalent resistance worldwide.

Used with a sulfonamide (eg, sulfadoxine) to treat toxoplasmosis.

In conjunction with a sulfonamide to initiate transmission control and suppression for susceptible strains of plasmodia. Fast-acting antimalarial drugs (eg, chloroquine, quinine) are preferable for the treatment of acute malaria attacks.

## Precautions:

*Do not use in the following situations:*
 allergy to pyrimethamine or any of its ingredients
 megaloblastic anemia due to folate deficiency

*Use with caution in the following situations:*

| | |
|---|---|
| alcohol abuse | G-6-PD deficiency |
| convulsive disorders | kidney disease |
| folate deficiency | liver disease |
| folate-reducing therapies (eg, methotrexate, phenytoin) | malabsorption syndrome |

*Pregnancy:* There are no adequate and well-controlled studies in pregnant women. Use only if clearly needed and potential benefits to the mother outweigh the possible hazards to the fetus.

*Breastfeeding:* Pyrimethamine is excreted in breast milk. Consult your doctor before you begin breastfeeding.

*Lab tests* may be required during treatment. Tests may include blood and platelet counts.

## Drug Interactions:

Tell your doctor or pharmacist if you are taking or if you are planning to take any over-the-counter or prescription medications or dietary supplements while taking pyrimethamine. Doses of one or both drugs may need to be modified or a different drug may need to be prescribed. The following drugs and drug classes interact with pyrimethamine:

antifolic drugs (eg, methotrexate, sulfonamides, trimethoprim-sulfamethoxazole)
lorazepam (eg, *Ativan*)

## Side Effects:

Every drug is capable of producing side effects. Many pyrimethamine users experience no, or minor, side effects. The frequency and severity of side effects depend on many factors including dose, duration of therapy, and individual susceptibility. Possible side effects include:

*Digestive Tract:* Appetite loss; vomiting; inflammation and redness of the tongue.

*Circulatory System:* Irregular heart rhythm; abnormal blood counts; blood in the urine.

*Other:* Rash; redness.

---

### Guidelines for Use:

- Dosage is individualized. Take exactly as prescribed.
- Do not exceed the recommended dose.
- Taking with meals may minimize appetite loss and vomiting.
- Discontinue use and notify your doctor immediately at the first appearance of a rash.
- Sore throat, lethargy, pale skin, unusual bruising, or inflamed or reddened tongue may be early signs of a serious disorder. Contact your doctor immediately to determine whether you should discontinue taking the drug and seek medical treatment.
- Contraceptive measures (birth control) are recommended during treatment.
- Inform your doctor if you are pregnant, become pregnant, are planning to become pregnant, or are breastfeeding.
- Lab tests may be required to monitor treatment. Be sure to keep appointments.
- Store in a dry place at room temperature (59° to 77°F). Protect from light.

---

*If you have any questions, consult your doctor, pharmacist, or health care provider.*

| Generic Name *Brand Name Example* | Supplied As | Generic Available |
|---|---|---|
| *Rx* **Sulfadoxine/ Pyrimethamine** | | |
| *Fansidar* | **Tablets:** 500 mg sulfadoxine and 25 mg pyrimethamine | No |

## Type of Drug:

Antimalarial anti-infective.

## How the Drug Works:

The combination of these drugs inhibits the normal enzymatic metabolism within a parasite causing malaria.

## Uses:

For the treatment of *Plasmodium falciparum* malaria for patients in whom chloroquine resistance is suspected.

For prevention of *P. falciparum* malaria for travelers to areas where chloro-quine-resistant malaria is endemic.

## Precautions:

*Do not use in the following situations:*

allergy to pyrimethanmine or sulfonamides
blood dyscrasias
infants under 2 months of age
kidney disease, severe
liver disease, severe (for preven-tion only)
megalobastic anemia due to folate deficiency
nursing mothers
pregnancy (at term)

*Use with caution in the following situations:*

allergy, severe
bronchial asthma
folate deficiency
kidney disease
liver disease

*Stevens-Johnson Syndrome and Toxic Epidermal Necrolysis:* Fatalities, though rare, have been associated with the administration of this medi-cine. Discontinue this medicine and consult your doctor immediately at the first appearance of skin rash, reduction in the count of any formed blood elements, or occurrence of bacterial or fungal infections.

*Pregnancy:* There are no adequate and well-controlled studies in preg-nant women, but women should be cautioned against becoming preg-nant during use. Use only if clearly needed and potential benefits to the mother outweigh the possible hazards to the fetus.

*Breastfeeding:* Sulfonamides appear in breast milk. Women should not breastfeed during therapy.

*Children:* This medicine should not be given to infants under 2 months of age.

*Lab tests* may be required during treatment. Tests may include periodic blood counts, analysis of urine, and organ function (eg, liver, kidney) tests.

## Drug Interactions:

Tell your doctor or pharmacist if you are taking or planning to take an over-the-counter or prescription medications or dietary supplements with sulfadoxine and pyrimethamine. Doses of one or both drugs may need to be modified or a different drug may need to be prescribed. The following drugs and drug classes interact with sulfadoxine and pyrimethamine:

> antifolic drugs (eg, sulfonamides, trimethoprim-sulfamethoxazole)
> chloroquine (eg, *Aralen*)

## Side Effects:

Every drug is capable of producing side effects. Many sulfadoxine and pyrimethamine users experience no, or minor, side effects. The frequency and severity of side effects depend on many factors including dose, duration of therapy, and individual susceptibility. Possible side effects include:

*Digestive Tract:* Inflammation and redness of the tongue or mouth; nausea; vomiting; stomach pain; hepatitis; liver damage; diarrhea; pancreatitis.

*Nervous System:* Headache; inflammation of peripheral nerves; tingling sensation; depression; convulsions; incoordination or clumsiness; hallucinations; ringing in the ears; dizziness; insomnia; apathy; fatigue; muscle weakness; nervousness.

*Hematologic:* Abnormal blood counts; anemia; decreased blood platelets; red or purple spots or patches under the skin; easy bruising or bleeding.

*Respiratory System:* Cough; shortness of breath; difficulty breathing.

*Allergic Reactions:* Flushing or redness of skin; skin eruptions; hives; rash; redness; itching; flaking and sloughing of skin; pale or yellowing of skin; swelling; sensitivity to light.

*Other:* Joint pain; fever; chills; abnormal kidney function.

## Guidelines for Use:

- Dosage is individualized.
- Keep out of reach of children.
- Discontinue this medicine and seek medical attention immediately at the first appearance of a skin rash.
- Notify your doctor immediately if you experience sore throat, fever, joint pain, cough, shortness of breath, pale or yellow skin, unusual bruising, or inflammation or redness of the tongue or mouth. These symptoms may be early indications of a serious disorder that requires immediate treatment.
- Adequate fluid intake must be maintained in order to prevent crystal formation in the urine and stone formation in the kidneys.
- Contraceptive measures (birth control) are recommended during treatment to avoid birth defects should pregnancy occur. Contact your doctor if you suspect you are pregnant.
- Nursing mothers should not breastfeed their infants during treatment with this medicine.
- Lab tests may be required to monitor treatment. Be sure to keep appointments.

*If you have any questions, consult your doctor, pharmacist, or health care provider.*

| Generic Name<br>*Brand Name Example* | Supplied As | Generic<br>Available |
|---|---|---|
| Rx **Halofantrine HCl** | | |
| *Halfan* | **Tablets:** 250 mg | No |

## Type of Drug:

Antimalarial anti-infective.

## How the Drug Works:

The mechanism of antimalarial activity of halofantrine is not known. This drug does not eliminate the liver phase of *Plasmodium vivax* parasite growth. To prevent relapses after initial treatment, aminoquinoline drugs (eg, primaquine) must be used to eradicate hepatic phase parasites.

## Uses:

For the treatment of adults who can tolerate oral medication and who have mild to moderate malaria caused by *P. falciparum* or *P. vivax*.

## Precautions:

*Do not use in the following situations:*

> allergy to halofantrine or any of its ingredients
> AV conduction disorders
> fainting, unexplained
> family history of congenital $QT_c$ prolongation
> heart disease, known or suspected
> mefloquine, used concurrently or after halofantrine

*Pregnancy:* There are no adequate and well-controlled studies in pregnant women. Use only if clearly needed and potential benefits to the mother outweigh the possible hazards to the fetus.

*Breastfeeding:* It is not known if halofantrine appears in breast milk. Consult your doctor before you begin breastfeeding.

*Children:* Safety and effectiveness in children have not been established.

## Drug Interactions:

Tell your doctor or pharmacist if you are taking or if you are planning to take any over-the-counter or prescription medications or dietary supplements while taking halofantrine. Doses of one or both drugs may need to be modified or a different drug may need to be prescribed. The following drugs, drug classes, and foods interact with halofantrine:

> high-fat foods
> mefloquine (*Lariam*)

## Side Effects:

Every drug is capable of producing side effects. Many halofantrine users experience no, or minor, side effects. The frequency and severity of side effects depend on many factors including dose, duration of therapy, and individual susceptibility. Possible side effects include:

*Digestive Tract:* Stomach pain; appetite loss; diarrhea; nausea; vomiting.

*Other:* Dizziness; headache; coughing; itching; shakiness; chills; muscle pain.

---

### Guidelines for Use:

- Dosage is individualized. Take exactly as prescribed.
- Take on an empty stomach at least 1 hour before or 2 hours after food.
- May cause dizziness. Use caution while driving or performing other tasks requiring alertness, coordination, or physical dexterity.
- Inform your doctor if you are pregnant, become pregnant, are planning to become pregnant, or are breastfeeding
- If you are a woman of childbearing age who travels to areas where malaria exists, avoid becoming pregnant.
- May cause photosensitivity (sensitivity to sunlight). Avoid prolonged exposure to the sun or other forms of ultraviolet (UV) light (eg, tanning beds). Use sunscreens and wear protective clothing until tolerance is determined.
- Store at room temperature (68° to 77°F). Protect from light.

---

*If you have any questions, consult your doctor, pharmacist, or health care provider.*

| Generic Name<br>*Brand Name Examples* | Supplied As | Generic<br>Available |
|---|---|---|
| *Rx* **Atovaquone/Proguanil** | | |
| *Malarone* | **Tablets:** 250 mg atovaquone and 100 mg proguanil HCl | No |
| *Malarone Pediatric* | **Tablets:** 62.5 mg atovaquone and 25 mg proguanil HCl | No |

## Type of Drug:

Antimalarial anti-infective.

## How the Drug Works:

Atovaquone and proguanil alter the biochemistry of *Plasmodium falciparum*, causing death of the malaria-producing organism.

## Uses:

For the prevention and treatment of *P. falciparum* malaria, including areas where chloroquine, halofantrine, mefloquine, and amodioquine resistance has been reported.

## Precautions:

*Do not use in the following situations:* Allergy to atovaquone, proguanil HCl, or any of the ingredients in this medicine.

*Use with caution in the following situations:* Kidney failure.

*Pregnancy:* There are no adequate and well-controlled studies in pregnant women. Use only if clearly needed and potential benefits to the mother outweigh the possible hazards to the fetus.

*Breastfeeding:* Proguanil appears in breast milk. It is not known if atovaquone appears in breast milk. Consult your doctor before you begin breastfeeding.

*Children:* Safety and effectiveness for use in children who weigh less than 24 pounds (11 kilograms) have not been established.

*Elderly:* Cautious dose selection for elderly patients is recommended.

*Lab tests* may be required during treatment.

## Drug Interactions:

Tell your doctor or pharmacist if you are taking or if you are planning to take any over-the-counter or prescription medications or dietary supplements while taking atovaquone or proguanil. Doses of one or both drugs may need to be modified or a different drug may need to be prescribed. The following drugs, foods, and drug classes interact with atovaquone or proguanil:

high-fat foods
metoclopramide (eg, *Reglan*)

rifampin (eg, *Rifadin*)
tetracycline (eg, *Sumycin*)

## Side Effects:

Every drug is capable of producing side effects. Many atovaquone or pro-guanil users experience no, or minor, side effects. The frequency and severity of side effects depend on many factors including dose, dura-tion of therapy, and individual susceptibility. Possible side effects include:

*Digestive Tract:* Stomach pain; inflamed stomach; nausea; vomiting; appe-tite loss; indigestion; diarrhea.

*Nervous System:* Headache; dizziness; weakness.

*Other:* Itching; fever; muscle pain; cough; abnormal liver tests.

---

### Guidelines for Use:

- Dosage is individualized. Take exactly as prescribed.
- Do not change the dose or stop taking this medicine unless advised by your doctor.
- Take this medicine at the same time each day with food or a milk drink.
- Take a repeat dose if vomiting occurs within 1 hour of taking the medicine.
- Talk to your doctor about other forms of malaria prevention if this medi-cine is prematurely discontinued.
- Use of protective clothing, insect repellents, and bednets are important in preventing malaria.
- Preventative treatment should be started 1 or 2 days before entering a malaria-endemic area and continued daily during the stay and for 7 days after returning.
- Because medicines are not always 100% effective, seek medical atten-tion for illnesses that occur during or after return from a malaria-en-demic area.
- Inform your doctor if you are pregnant, become pregnant, are planning to become pregnant, or are breastfeeding.
- Pregnant women should talk with their doctors prior to traveling to malaria-endemic areas.
- Store at controlled room temperature (59° to 86°F).

---

*If you have any questions, consult your doctor, pharmacist, or health care provider.*

| Generic Name | Supplied As | Generic Available |
|---|---|---|
| Rx **Quinine Sulfate** | **Capsules:** 200 mg, 325 mg | Yes |
| | **Tablets:** 260 mg | Yes |

## Type of Drug:
Antimalarial anti-infective.

## How the Drug Works:
The antimalarial activity of quinine is unclear. It appears to kill the malaria-causing parasite by disrupting its metabolism.

## Uses:
To treat chloroquine-resistant *Plasmodiurn falciparum* malaria. Used either alone, with pyrimethamine and a sulfonamide, or with a tetracycline. It is also considered alternative therapy for chloroquine-sensitive strains of *P. falciparum, P. malariae, P. ovale*, and *P. vivax.* Mefloquine and clindamycin may also be used with quinine, depending on where the malaria was acquired (eg, Southeast Asia, Bangladesh, East Africa).

*Unlabeled Use(s):* Doctors may occasionally prescribe quinine sulfate for the prevention and treatment of nocturnal recumbency (nighttime) leg cramps.

## Precautions:
*Do not use in the following situations:*

allergy to quinine sulfate or any of its ingredients
blackwater fever, history of glucose-6-phosphate dehydrogenase (G-6-PD) deficiency
inflammation of optic nerve
pregnancy
ringing in the ears
thrombocytopenic purpura with previous quinine use

*Use with caution in the following situations:* Irregular heartbeat.

*Allergy:* Discontinue quinine if there is any evidence of allergy. Flushing, itching, rash, fever, stomach pain, difficulty breathing, ringing in the ears, and vision problems may occur, even with only small doses of quinine. Extreme flushing of the skin with intense itching over most of the body is most common.

*Pregnancy:* Do not use during pregnancy. The risk of use in a pregnant woman clearly outweighs any possible benefit. Birth defects have been reported with large doses.

*Breastfeeding:* Quinine appears in breast milk. Consult your doctor before you begin breastfeeding.

## Drug Interactions:

Tell your doctor or pharmacist if you are taking or planning to take any over-the-counter or prescription medications with quinine sulfate. Doses of one or both drugs may need to be modified or a different drug may need to be prescribed. The following drugs and drug classes interact with quinine sulfate:

anticoagulants, oral (eg, warfarin)
antihistamines, nonsedating (eg, loratadine)
digoxin (eg, *Lanoxin)*

nondepolarizing muscle relaxants (eg, pancuronium)
rifamycins (eg, rifampin)
succinylcholine (eg, *Anectine)*

## Side Effects:

Every drug is capable of producing side effects. Many quinine sulfate users experience no, or minor, side effects. The frequency and severity of side effects depend on many factors including dose, duration of therapy, and individual susceptibility. Possible side effects include:

*Cinchonism:* Ringing in the ears; headache; diarrhea; nausea; disturbed vision.

*Eyes or Ocular:* Disturbed color vision and perception; sensitivity to light; blurred vision; night blindness; double vision; dilated pupil; optic nerve damage.

*Digestive Tract:* Nausea; vomiting; stomach ache.

*Nervous System:* Headache; vertigo (feeling of whirling motion); restlessness; confusion; excitement; apprehension; delirium; dizziness; convulsions.

*Other:* Ringing in the ears; fever; hepatitis; blood cell disorders; lowered body temperature; chest pain; thrombocytopenia purpura; deafness; fainting; rash; itching; flushing.

---

### Guidelines for Use:

- Dosage is individualized.
- Do not change the dose or stop taking unless advised by your doctor.
- May cause stomach upset. Take with food or after meals.
- May cause nausea, vomiting, diarrhea, stomach cramps or pain, or ringing in the ears. Contact your doctor if these symptoms persist.
- May cause blurred vision or dizziness. Use caution when driving or performing other tasks requiring alertness, coordination, and physical dexterity.
- Notify your doctor immediately if you experience any evidence of allergy such as flushing, itching, rash, fever, stomach pain, difficulty breathing, ringing in the ears, or vision problems.
- Store at controlled room temperature (59° to 86°F). Protect from light and moisture.

---

*If you have any questions, consult your doctor, pharmacist, or health care provider.*

| Generic Name Brand Name Examples | Supplied As | Generic Available |
|---|---|---|
| Rx **Foscarnet Sodium (Phosphonoformic acid; PFA)** | | |
| *Foscavir* | **Injection:** 24 mg/ml | No |

## Type of Drug:
Antiviral drug.

## How the Drug Works:
Foscarnet exerts its antiviral activity by selective inhibition of virus-specific DNA. Foscarnet is not necessarily a cure for cytomegalovirus (CMV) retinitis or herpes simplex virus (HSV) infections.

## Uses:
To treat CMV retinitis (infection in lining of eyeball) in patients with acquired immunodeficiency syndrome (AIDS) and acyclovir-resistant mucocutaneous HSV infections in immunocompromised patients only. Safety and effectiveness have not been established for treatment of other CMV infections (eg, pneumonitis, gastroenteritis), other HSV infections (eg, retinitis, encephalitis), congenital or neonatal CMV or HSV disease, or nonimmunocompromised individuals. Also used as combination therapy with ganciclovir for patients who have relapsed after monotherapy with either drug.

## Precautions:
*Do not use in the following situations:* Allergy to foscarnet sodium or any of its ingredients.

*Use with caution in the following situations:*

| | |
|---|---|
| anemia | mineral and electrolyte levels, |
| drugs affecting serum calcium | abnormal (eg, low blood |
| levels, concurrent use of | calcium) |
| heart disease | seizures |
| kidney disease | |

*Pregnancy:* There are no adequate and well-controlled studies in pregnant women. Use only if clearly needed and the potential benefits to the mother outweigh the possible hazards to the fetus.

*Breastfeeding:* The Centers for Disease Control and Prevention (CDC) recommends that HIV-infected mothers not breastfeed their infants to avoid risking postnatal transmission of HIV. It is not known if foscarnet is excreted in breast milk. Consult your doctor before you begin breastfeeding.

*Children:* Safety and effectiveness have not been established. Foscarnet may affect the development of teeth and bones. Use only after careful evaluation and if the potential benefits outweigh the possible risks.

*Elderly:* Monitor kidney function carefully before and during treatment with foscarnet and adjust dosage as necessary.

*Lab tests* will be required to monitor treatment. Tests include kidney function, plasma minerals and electrolytes, serum creatinine, and eye examinations.

## Drug Interactions:

Tell your doctor or pharmacist if you are taking or planning to take any over-the-counter or prescription medications or dietary supplements while taking foscarnet. Doses of one or both drugs may need to be modified, or a different drug may need to be prescribed. The following drugs and drug classes interact with foscarnet:

aminoglycosides
  (eg, gentamycin)
amphotericin B (eg, *Fungizone)*
didanosine (*Videx)*
pentamidine isethionate
  (*Pentam 300*)

ritonavir (*Norvir*)
saquinavir *(Invirase)*
zidovudine (*Retrovir*)

Foscarnet decreases serum levels of ionized calcium. Use caution when other drugs known to influence serum calcium levels are used.

## Side Effects:

Every drug is capable of producing side effects. Many foscarnet users experience side effects. The frequency and severity of side effects depend on many factors including dose, duration of therapy, and individual susceptibility. Possible side effects include:

*Digestive Tract:* Nausea; vomiting; diarrhea; stomach pain; appetite loss; taste sensation changes; constipation; indigestion; gas; dark or bloody stool; inflammation of pancreas; mouth infection; dry mouth; rectal bleeding.

*Nervous System:* Headache; dizziness; abnormal skin sensations; tremor; muscle spasms; seizures; decreased sensitivity to touch; dementia; clumsiness; stupor; sense disturbances; confusion; drowsiness; depression; anxiety; sleeplessness; fatigue; weakness; nervousness; agitation; memory loss; aggressive behavior; hallucinations; abnormal speech; incoordination.

*Circulatory System:* Blood pressure changes; chest pain; palpitations (pounding in the chest); rapid heartbeat; cerebrovascular disorder; blood clots; abnormal heart rhythm.

*Respiratory System:* Cough; difficult breathing; pneumonia; sinus inflammation; sore throat; nasal congestion; wheezing; bronchospasm; spitting up blood.

*Skin:* Rash; sweating; itching; flushing; ulcers; discoloration; redness; seborrhea.

*Urinary and Reproductive Tract:* Protein in urine; decreased urination; painful or difficult urination; urinary tract infections.

*Other:* Fever; general body discomfort; back pain; bacterial or fungal infections; chills; pain or inflammation at injection site; general ill health; flu-like symptoms; abscess; edema (fluid retention); facial swelling; abnormal vision; eye pain; inflammation of eye; abnormal levels of minerals and electrolytes; weight loss; thirst; joint and muscle pain; leg cramps; difficulty swallowing; bone marrow suppression; anemia; abnormal blood counts; abnormal kidney function; death.

## Guidelines for Use:

- Dosage is individualized according to kidney function. Take exactly as prescribed.
- Usual dose is injected intravenously (IV; into a vein) 2 to 3 times daily for 2 to 3 weeks. Take in evenly spaced intervals throughout the day.
- Do not exceed recommended dosage, frequency, or rate of infusion.
- Follow the injection procedure taught to you by your health care provider.
- If a dose is missed, inject it as soon as possible. If several hours have passed or if it is nearing time for the next dose, do not double the dose to catch up, unless advised to do so by your doctor. If more than one dose is missed or it is necessary to establish a new dosage schedule, contact your doctor or pharmacist.
- Drink plenty of fluids.
- Foscarnet is not a cure for CMV retinitis or HSV. You may continue to experience effects of retinitis during or following treatment. While complete healing of HSV may occur, relapse occurs in most patients. Patients should remain under the care of a doctor.
- Foscarnet does not reduce the risk of transmitting HIV to others through sexual contact or blood contamination.
- HIV-infected mothers should not breastfeed because of the risk of transmitting the HIV infection to the infant.
- Kidney function may be impaired during foscarnet therapy. Patients with abnormal kidney function should use with caution. Dose modifications and possible discontinuation may be required.
- Discontinue immediately and contact your doctor if tingling around the mouth, urination problems, numbness in the extremities, or abnormal sensations such as burning or prickling occurs during or after infusion.
- Lab tests and eye exams are required to monitor therapy. Be sure to keep appointments.
- Store at room temperature (59° to 86°F). Do not freeze.

*If you have any questions, consult your doctor, pharmacist, or health care provider.*

| Generic Name *Brand Name Example* | Supplied As | Generic Available |
|---|---|---|
| Rx **Ganciclovir Sodium**[1] | | |
| *Cytovene* | **Capsules:** 250 mg, 500 mg | No |

[1] Also available as an intravenous injection.

## Type of Drug:

Antiviral drug to treat and prevent cytomegalovirus (CMV) infections.

## How the Drug Works:

It is believed that ganciclovir interferes with the ability of cytomegalovirus (CMV) to reproduce by stopping the production of important proteins needed by the virus to grow.

## Uses:

*Ganciclovir capsules* are used as an alternative to intravenous ganciclovir for maintenance treatment of CMV retinitis in immunocompromised patients, including patients with AIDS, in whom retinitis is stable following treatment with intravenous ganciclovir and for whom the risk of more rapid progression is balanced by the benefit associated with avoiding daily IV infusions. Ganciclovir capsules are also used to prevent CMV disease in transplant recipients.

*Intravenous ganciclovir* is used for the treatment of CMV retinitis (inflammation of the retina) in patients with immunocompromised (weakened) immune systems, including patients with acquired immunodeficiency syndrome (AIDS). It is also used to prevent CMV disease in transplant patients at risk for CMV disease.

*Unlabeled Use(s):* Occasionally doctors may prescribe ganciclovir for CMV pneumonia in transplant patients, CMV gastroenteritis in patients with irritable bowel disease, and for CMV pneumonitis.

## Precautions:

*Do not use in the following situations:*

allergy to acyclovir or ganciclovir, or any of its ingredients
nonimmunocomromised patients
treatment of congenital or newborn CMV disease
treatment of other CMV infections

*Use with caution in the following situations:*

cytopenias (low blood cell counts), preexisting cytopenic reactions to other drugs, chemicals, or radiation therapy, history of
kidney disease
transplant recipients

*Pregnancy:* There are no adequate and well-controlled studies in pregnant women. Use only if clearly needed and the potential benefits to the mother outweigh the possible hazards to the fetus. Women of childbearing potential should avoid becoming pregnant during ganciclovir therapy.

*Breastfeeding:* The Centers for Disease Control and Prevention (CDC) recommends that HIV-infected mothers not breastfeed their infants to avoid risking postnatal transmission of HIV. It is not known if ganciclovir is excreted in breast milk. Do not breastfeed while taking ganciclovir. Consult your doctor before you begin breastfeeding.

*Children:* Safety and effectiveness have not been established. Use only after careful evaluation and if the potential benefits outweigh the possible risks.

*Elderly:* Monitor kidney function carefully before and during treatment with ganciclovir and adjust dosage as necessary.

*Lab tests* will be required to monitor treatment. Tests may include blood cell counts, eye exams, and kidney function tests.

## Drug Interactions:

Tell your doctor or pharmacist if you are taking or if you are planning to take any over-the-counter or prescription medications or dietary supplements while taking ganciclovir. Doses of one or both drugs may need to be modified or a different drug may need to be prescribed. The following drugs and drug classes interact with ganciclovir:

cell growth inhibitors (eg, dapsone, pentamidine, flucytosine, vincristine, vinblastine, adriamycin, amphotericin B, trimethoprim/sulfamethoxazole)

didanosine (*Videx)*
imipenem-cilastatin (*Primaxin)*
nephrotoxic drugs (eg, aminoglycosides)
probenecid
zidovudine (*Retrovir)*

## Side Effects:

Every drug is capable of producing side effects. Many ganciclovir users experience no, or minor, side effects. The frequency and severity of side effects depend on many factors including dose, duration of therapy, and individual susceptibility. Possible side effects include:

*Hematologic:* Granulocytopenia (neutropenia), usually within first or second week of therapy; thrombocytopenia.

*Digestive Tract:* Nausea; vomiting; diarrhea; appetite loss.

*Nervous System:* Headache; abnormal sensations in arms or legs.

*Skin:* Itching; sweating.

*Other:* Infections; fever; chills; general body pain; inflammation at injection site; fertility problems; impaired kidney function; abnormal liver function tests; retinal detachment; vision changes; phlebitis; abnormal blood cell counts.

## Guidelines for Use:

- Dosage is individualized. Take exactly as prescribed.
- Do not change the dose or stop taking, unless directed by your doctor.
- The injectable form of ganciclovir is prepared and administered intravenously (IV; into vein) by your health care provider in a medical setting.
- Take capsules with food to maximize effectiveness. Do not open, crush, or chew capsules.
- *Capsules* — If a dose is missed, take it as soon as possible. If several hours have passed or it is nearing time for the next dose, do not double the dose to catch up, unless advised to do so by your doctor. If more than one dose is missed or it is necessary to establish a new dosage schedule, contact your doctor or pharmacist.
- Avoid contact of broken or crushed capsules with skin, mouth or nasal tissues, or eyes. If contact occurs, wash skin thoroughly with soap and water and rinse eyes thoroughly with plain water.
- Notify your doctor immediately if you experience fever or other signs of infection, sore throat, or unusual bleeding or bruising.
- Ganciclovir is not a cure for CMV retinitis. You may continue to experience effects of retinitis during or following treatment. Patients should remain under the care of a doctor.
- Contraceptive (birth control) measures are recommended for men and women during therapy. Men should use barrier contraception during and for at least 90 days following ganciclovir treatment.
- HIV-infected mothers should not breastfeed because of the risk of transmitting the infection to the infant.
- Lab tests and eye exams will be required to monitor therapy. Be sure to keep appointments.
- Store capsules between 41°F and 77°F.

*If you have any questions, consult your doctor, pharmacist, or health care provider.*

| Generic Name Brand Name Example | Supplied As | Generic Available |
|---|---|---|
| Rx **Valganciclovir HCl** | | |
| *Valcyte* | **Tablets**: 450 mg | No |

## Type of Drug:

Antiviral drug used to treat cytomegalovirus (CMV) infections.

## How the Drug Works:

It is believed that valganciclovir, which is converted into ganciclovir in the body, interferes with the ability of CMV to reproduce by stopping the production of important proteins the virus needs to grow.

## Uses:

Used for the treatment of CMV retinitis (infection in lining of eyeball) in patients with acquired immunodeficiency syndrome (AIDS).

## Precautions:

*Do not use in the following situations:*

allergy to valganciclovir, ganciclovir, or any of their ingredients
hemodialysis

*Use with caution in the following situations:*

cytopenias (low blood cell counts), preexisting myelosuppressive (bone marrow depressing) drugs

kidney impairment
radiation therapy

*Pregnancy:* There are no adequate and well-controlled studies in pregnant women. Use only if clearly needed and the potential benefits to the mother outweigh the possible hazards to the fetus.

*Breastfeeding:* The Centers for Disease Control and Prevention (CDC) recommends that HIV-infected mothers not breastfeed their infants to avoid risking postnatal transmission of HIV. It is not known if valganciclovir is excreted in breast milk. Do not breastfeed while taking valganciclovir. Consult your doctor before you begin breastfeeding.

*Children:* Safety and effectiveness have not been established. Use only after careful evaluation and if the potential benefits outweigh the possible risks.

*Elderly:* Monitor kidney function carefully before and during treatment with valcanciclovir and adjust dosage as necessary.

*Lab tests* will be required to monitor treatment. Tests may include blood cell counts, eye exams, and kidney function tests.

## Drug Interactions:

Tell your doctor or pharmacist if you are taking or planning to take any over-the-counter or prescription medications or dietary supplements while taking valganciclovir. Doses of one or both drugs may need to be modified, or a different drug may need to be prescribed. The following drugs and drug classes may interact with valganciclovir:

ganciclovir (eg, Vitrasert)
imipenem-cilastatin
 (eg, *Primaxin*)
nephrotoxic drugs
 (eg, aminoglycosides)

probenecid
didanosine (*Videx*)
zidovudine (*Retrovir*)

## Side Effects:

Every drug is capable of producing side effects. Many valganciclovir users experience no, or minor, side effects. The frequency and severity of side effects depends on many factors including dose, duration of therapy, and individual susceptibility. Possible side effects include:

*Nervous System:* Headache; sleeplessness; abnormal sensations in the arms or legs; abnormal skin sensations; convulsion; psychosis; hallucinations; confusion; agitation; sedation; dizziness; incoordination.

*Digestive Tract:* Diarrhea; nausea; vomiting; stomach pain.

*Hematologic/Lymphatic:* Neutropenia; anemia; thrombocytopenia; pancytopenia; bone marrow depression; aplastic anemia.

*Other:* Fever; retinal detachment; local and systemic infections and sepsis.

## Guidelines for Use:

- Review the patient package insert provided with this medicine before taking.
- Dosage is individualized. Take exactly as prescribed.
- Do not change the dose or stop taking, unless directed by your doctor.
- Valganciclovir tablets cannot be substitiuted for ganciclovir capsules on a one-to-one basis. Patients switching from ganciclovir capsules to valganciclovir capsules risk overdosage if they take more than the pre-scribed number of valganciclovir tablets.
- Take with food to maximize effectiveness. Do not open, crush, or chew tablets.
- Avoid direct contact of broken or crushed tablets with skin or mucous membranes. If contact occurs, wash skin thoroughly with soap and water, and rinse eyes thoroughly with plain water.
- Notify your doctor immediately if you experience fever or other signs of infection, sore throat, or unusual bleeding or bruising.
- Contraceptive (birth control) measures are recommended for men and women during therapy. Men should use barrier contraception during and at least 90 days following treatment.
- May cause sedation, dizziness, incoordination, seizures, or confusion. Use caution while driving or performing other tasks that require alert-ness, coordination, or physical dexterity.
- Valganciclovir is not a cure for CMV retinitis. You may continue to expe-rience effects of retinitis during or following treatment. Patients should remain under the care of a doctor.
- HIV-infected mothers should not breastfeed because of the risk of trans-mitting the infection to the infant.
- Lab tests and eye exams will be required to monitor therapy. Be sure to keep appointments.
- Store at room temperature (59° to 86° F).

*If you have any questions, consult your doctor, pharmacist, or health care provider.*

| Generic Name<br>*Brand Name Example* | Supplied As | Generic<br>Available |
|---|---|---|
| *Rx* **Adefovir Dipivoxil** | | |
| *Hepsera* | **Tablets**: 10 mg | No |

## Type of Drug:
Acyclic nucleotide analog of adenosine monophosphate.

## How the Drug Works:
Adefovir dipivoxil is a prodrug (inactive form) of adefovir. Adefovir stops hepatitis B virus (HBV) replication by inhibiting viral DNA.

## Uses:
For the treatment of chronic hepatitis B in adults with evidence of active viral replication and evidence of either persistent elevations in serum aminotransferases (ALT or AST) or histologically active disease.

## Precautions:
*Do not use in the following situations:* Allergy to the drug or any of its ingredients.

*Use with caution in the following situations:*
lactic acidosis
liver disease
kidney disease

*HIV infection:* Patients with unrecognized or untreated HIV infection may develop HIV-resistant infection if treated with adefovir. HIV antibody testing should be done before starting adefovir therapy.

*Pregnancy:* There are no adequate and well-controlled studies in pregnant women. Use only if clearly needed and the potential benefits outweigh the possible risks to the fetus.

*Breastfeeding:* It is not known if adefovir appears in breast milk. Consult your doctor before you begin breastfeeding.

*Children:* Safety and effectiveness have not been established.

*Elderly:* Use with caution because of greater frequency of decreased heart or kidney function. Safety and effectiveness in patients 65 years of age have not been established.

*Lab tests* may be required during treatment. Tests include blood cell counts, kidney or liver tests, and HIV screening.

## Drug Interactions:
Tell your doctor or pharmacist if you are taking or planning to take any over-the-counter or prescription medications or dietary supplements with this drug. Drug doses may need to be modified or a different drug prescribed.

## Side Effects:

Every drug is capable of producing side effects. Many patients experience no, or minor, side effects. The frequency and severity of side effects depend on many factors, including dose, duration of therapy, and individual susceptibility. Possible side effects include:

*Digestive Tract:* Nausea; stomach pain; gas; diarrhea; upset stomach; vomiting.

*Nervous System:* Headache; weakness; fever.

*Other:* Increased cough; sore throat; sinus infection; rash; itching; weakness; muscle pain; light-headedness; dizziness; yellowing of skin; dark urine; rapid heart rate; liver failure.

---

### Guidelines for Use:

- Dosage is individualized. Take exactly as prescribed.
- Do not stop taking or change the dose, unless instructed by your doctor.
- May be taken without regard to food. Take with food if upset stomach occurs.
- If a dose is missed, take it as soon as possible. If several hours have passed or it is nearing time for the next dose, do not double the dose to catch up, unless instructed by your doctor. If more than one dose is missed or it is necessary to establish a new dosage schedule, contact your doctor or pharmacist.
- Contact your doctor immediately if you experience weakness, muscle pain, difficulty breathing, stomach pain, vomiting, light-headedness, dizziness, fast heartbeat, yellowing of the skin, dark urine, appetite loss, or nausea.
- Inform your doctor if you are pregnant, become pregnant, plan on becoming pregnant, or are breastfeeding.
- Severe exacerbations of hepatitis may occur when anti-hepatitis B therapy is stopped. Patients who stop therapy should be monitored at repeated intervals over a period of time. Anti-hepatitis therapy may need to be restored.
- Lab tests may be required to monitor treatment. Be sure to keep appointments.
- Store at room temperature (59° to 86°F).

---

*If you have any questions, consult your doctor, pharmacist, or health care provider.*

| Generic Name<br>*Brand Name Examples* | Supplied As | Generic<br>Available |
|---|---|---|
| *Rx* **Acyclovir**[1] | | |
| *Zovirax* | **Tablets:** 400 mg, 800 mg | Yes |
| *Zovirax* | **Capsules:** 200 mg | Yes |
| *Zovirax* | **Oral suspension:**<br>200 mg/5 mL | Yes |
| *Zovirax* | **Ointment:** 5% | No |
| *Rx* **Famciclovir** | | |
| *Famvir* | **Tablets**: 125 mg, 250 mg,<br>500 mg | No |
| *Rx* **Valacyclovir** | | |
| *Valtrex* | **Tablets**: 500 mg, 1 g | No |

[1] Also available as an intravenous injection.

## Type of Drug:

Antiviral drug used to treat herpes zoster infections (shingles), genital herpes, and chickenpox.

## How the Drug Works:

Acyclovir prevents the herpes virus from reproducing, reducing the time needed to recover from the infection and the time for the lesion to heal. Acyclovir does not eliminate the virus and is not a cure. It does not prevent transmission of the virus to others.

## Uses:

*Oral:* To treat initial episodes and manage recurrent episodes of genital herpes infections. Also for acute treatment of herpes zoster (shingles) and treatment of chickenpox.

*Topical:* To treat initial episodes of genital herpes infections and limited non-life-threatening HSV skin infections in immunocompromised patients.

*Unlabeled Use(s):* Occasionally doctors may prescribe acyclovir for cytomegalovirus and herpes simplex infections following bone marrow or kidney transplants, disseminated primary eczema herpeticum, herpes infections other than those affecting the genitals (eg, infection of the brain, eye, rectum, finger), infectious mononucleosis and chickenpox-related pneumonia. Valacyclovir has also been used as prophylactic treatment for prevention of cytomegalovirus (CMV) disease in patients with advanced HIV and in patients postrenal transplant.

## Precautions:

*Do not use in the following situations:* Allergy to the antiherpes virus agent or any of its ingredients.

*Use with caution in the following situations:*
    drugs potentially toxic to the kidneys
    kidney disease

*Pregnancy:* There are no adequate and well-controlled studies in pregnant women. Use only if clearly needed and the potential benefits to the mother outweigh the possible hazards to the fetus.

*Breastfeeding:* Acyclovir appears in breast milk. Consult your doctor before you begin breastfeeding.

*Children:* Safety and effectiveness of acyclovir in children younger than 2 years of age have not been established. Saftey and effectiveness of famciclovir have not been established in children younger than 18 years of age. Safety and effectiveness of valcyclovir in children have not been established.

## Drug Interactions:

Tell your doctor or pharmacist if you are taking or if you are planning to take any over-the-counter or prescription medications or dietary supplements with an antiherpes virus agent. Doses of one or both drugs may need to be modified or a different drug may need to be prescribed. The following drugs and drug classes interact with antiherpes virus agents:

cimetidine (eg, *Tagamet*)
digoxin (eg, *Lanoxin*)
interferon (*Roferon*)
methotrexate (eg, *Mexate*)

probenecid
theophylline (eg, *Theo-Dur*)
zidovudine (*Retrovir*)

## Side Effects:

Every drug is capable of producing side effects. Many antiherpes virus agent users experience no, or minor, side effects. The frequency and severity of side effects depend on many factors including dose, duration of therapy, and individual susceptibility. Possible side effects include:

*Digestive Tract:* Nausea; vomiting; diarrhea.

*Skin:* Burning; stinging; itching (ointment only); rash.

*Other:* Headache; abnormal skin sensations; weakness; numbness or tingling; general body discomfort.

## Guidelines for Use:

- Dosage is individualized. Take exactly as prescribed. Do not exceed recommended dosage, frequency or length of treatment.
- Antiherpes virus agents are not cures for herpes simplex infections.
- Avoid sexual intercourse when lesions (sores) are present to prevent infecting your partner.
- Notify your doctor if lesions appear more frequently or become worse.
- *Oral* — Patient information from the manufacturer is included with product.
  If a dose is missed, take it as soon as possible. If several hours have passed or it is nearing time for the next dose, do not double the dose to catch up, unless advised to do so by your doctor. If more than one dose is missed or it is necessary to establish a new dosage schedule, contact your doctor or pharmacist.
- *Topical* —Begin therapy as early as possible following the onset of symptoms.
  Apply to all lesions every 3 hours, 6 times per day for 7 days.
  A one-half inch ribbon of ointment will generally cover about 4 square inches.
  If an application is missed, apply as soon as possible, but not if it is almost time for the next application.
  Ointment must thoroughly cover all lesions.
  To reduce the risk of spreading the infection, use a finger cot or rubber glove to apply the ointment.
  Some burning, stinging or itching may occur. If these symptoms are persistent, consult your doctor.
  Acyclovir ointment is of little benefit in treating recurrent attacks. Do not use chronically to prevent recurrences.
  Do not use in or near eyes.

*If you have any questions, consult your doctor, pharmacist, or health care provider.*

| Generic Name<br>*Brand Name Example* | Supplied As | Generic<br>Available |
|---|---|---|
| Rx **Amantadine HCl** | **Capsules:** 100 mg | Yes |
| *Symmetrel* | **Tablets**: 100 mg | No |
| *Symmetrel* | **Syrup:** 50 mg/5 mL | Yes |

## Type of Drug:

Antiviral drug for influenza A virus; antiparkinson agent.

## How the Drug Works:

It is not known exactly how amantadine acts to treat and prevent influenza A infection or symptoms of Parkinson disease.

## Uses:

To prevent and treat respiratory tract infections caused by influenza A virus (flu) in high-risk patients with heart, lung, muscle-nerve, or immunodeficiency diseases, and for people in close contact with patients with influenza type A illness.

A flu shot (immunization) is the best way to prevent influenza type A infection. Amantadine may be used when flu shots are not possible or unavailable.

Recommendations for amantadine use for prevention of influenza type A virus:
During an influenza A outbreak, when the flu shot may not be effective.
To aid late immunization of high-risk individuals.
To reduce the spread of the virus to high-risk persons during influenza type A outbreaks.
To treat high-risk patients during the flu season when a flu shot is not possible because of allergy to the vaccine.
To supplement vaccination protection in those with impaired immune responses.

To treat Parkinson disease and drug-induced extrapyramidal reactions (movement disorders). See the Antiparkinson-Dopaminergic Agents monograph in the CNS Drugs chapter.

## Precautions:

*Do not use in the following situations:* Allergy to amantadine or any of its ingredients.

*Use with caution in the following situations:*

congestive heart failure
eczema, recurrent, history of
edema (fluid retention)
elderly
glaucoma, narrow angle
kidney disease

liver disease
mental illness (eg, psychosis)
seizure conditions (eg, epilepsy)
substance abuse, current or
 history of

*Abrupt discontinuation:* Do not abruptly stop taking amantadine. A few patients with Parkinson disease have experienced a parkinsonian crisis (tremors, rigidity, etc.) when this drug was stopped suddenly.

*Mental problems:* Amantadine can exacerbate mental problems in patients with a history of psychiatric disorders or substance abuse. Suicide attempts have been reported in patients treated with amantadine. Discontinue use and immediately notify your doctor if mood or personality changes are noted.

*Other respiratory tract illnesses:* Amantidine is not effective for preventing or treating viral respiratory tract illnesses other than influenza A.

*Pregnancy:* There are no adequate and well-controlled studies in pregnant women. Use only if clearly needed and the potential benefits to the mother outweigh the possible hazards to the fetus.

*Breastfeeding:* Amantadine appears in breast milk. Consult your doctor before you begin breastfeeding.

*Children:* Safety and effectiveness in children younger than 1 year of age have not been established.

*Elderly:* Patients 65 years of age and older may need lower doses than other individuals.

## Drug Interactions:

Tell your doctor or pharmacist if you are taking or planning to take any over-the-counter or prescription medications or dietary supplements with amantadine. Doses of one or both drugs may need to be modified or a different drug may need to be prescribed. The following drugs and drug classes interact with amantadine:

anticholinergics (eg, trihexyphenidyl)
CNS stimulants (eg, phentermine)
quinidine (eg, *Quinora*)
quinine
thiazide diuretics (eg, hydrochlorothiazide)
triamterene (eg, *Dyrenium*)
trimethoprim/sulfamethoxazole (eg, *Bactrim*)

## Side Effects:

Every drug is capable of producing side effects. Many amantadine users experience no, or minor, side effects. The frequency and severity of side effects depend on many factors including dose, duration of therapy, and individual susceptibility. Possible side effects include:

*Digestive Tract:* Nausea; constipation; appetite loss; diarrhea.

*Nervous System:* Dizziness; lightheadedness; depression; hallucinations; confusion; abnormal dreams; anxiety; irritability; headache; incoordination; sleeplessness; drowsiness.

*Other:* Skin mottling; edema (fluid retention); dry mouth; fatigue; orthostatic hypotension (dizziness or lightheadedness when rising quickly from a sitting or lying position).

## Guidelines for Use:

- Dosage is individualized. Take exactly as prescribed.
- Do not stop taking or change the dose, unless directed by your doctor.
- May be taken without regard to food. Take with food if stomach upset occurs.
- *For treatment of symptoms of influenza A virus* — Start as soon as possible after onset of symptoms and continue for 24 to 48 hours after symptoms disappear.
- *For prevention of influenza A virus* — Start in anticipation of contact or as soon as possible after exposure. Continue daily for at least 10 days. The infectious period extends from shortly before to one week after the onset of symptoms.
- If used in combination with the influenza vaccine (flu shot), take amantadine for 2 to 4 weeks after the vaccine has been given (until protective antibody responses to the vaccine have developed).
- If the flu vaccine is unavailable or cannot be taken, amantadine should be taken for up to 90 days.
- Therapy may not result in protection for all individuals.
- If a dose is missed, take it as soon as possible. If several hours have passed or it is nearing time for the next dose, do not double the dose to catch up, unless advised to do so by your doctor. If more than one dose is missed or it is necessary to establish a new dosage schedule, contact your doctor or pharmacist.
- This medicine may cause drowsiness, dizziness, or blurred vision. Use caution while driving or performing other tasks requiring alertness, coordination, or physical dexterity.
- If dizziness or lightheadedness occurs, avoid sudden changes in posture. Notify your doctor of this effect if this continues.
- Contact your doctor if you experience mood changes, swelling of hands or feet, difficult urination, or shortness of breath.
- Avoid excessive alcohol intake while taking amantadine. It may increase potential for dizziness, confusion, and lightheadedness.
- Store at controlled room temperature (59° to 86°F) in a tightly closed container. Protect tablets and capsules from moisture.

*If you have any questions, consult your doctor, pharmacist, or health care provider.*

| Generic Name Brand Name Example | Supplied As | Generic Available |
|---|---|---|
| Rx **Cidofovir** | | |
| *Vistide* | **Injection:** 75 mg/mL | No |

## Type of Drug:
Antiviral drug to treat cytomegalovirus (CHV) infections.

## How the Drug Works:
Cidofovir interferes with the ability of cytomegalovirus (CMV) to reproduce by stopping the production of important proteins needed by the virus to grow.

## Uses:
To treat CMV retinitis (infection in lining of eyeball) in patients with acquired immunodeficency syndrome (AIDS). It must be used in combination with oral probenecid.

The safety and efficacy of cidofovir have not been established for the treatment of other CMV infections (such as pneumonitis or gastroenteritis), congenital or neonatal CMV disease, or CMV disease in non-HIV-infected individuals.

## Precautions:
*Do not use in the following situations:*
> allergy to cidofovir or any of its ingredients
> allergy to probenecid or other sulfa-containing medications
> direct intraocular injection (injection into eye)
> kidney disease, moderate to severe
> nephrotoxic agents (eg, gentamicin), concurrent use

*Use with caution in the following situations:*
> elderly
> kidney disease

*Kidney impairment:* Kidney toxicity has occurred with cidofovir. Intravenous prehydration with normal saline and oral administration of probenecid will be used with each cidofovir infusion. Blood and urine tests will be performed no more than 48 hours before each dose of cidofovir.

*Pregnancy:* There are no adequate and well-controlled studies in pregnant women. Use only if clearly needed and potential benefits outweigh the possible hazards to the fetus. Advise against pregnancy during and for at least 1 month following the use of this medicine.

*Breastfeeding:* The Centers for Disease Control and Prevention (CDC) recommends that HIV-infected mothers not breastfeed their infants to avoid risking postnatal transmission of HIV. It is not known if cidofovir appears in breast milk. Do not breastfeed while taking this medicine.

*Children:* Safety and effectiveness in children have not been established.

*Elderly:* Use with caution in elderly patients. Dosage adjustments may be necessary.

*Lab tests* will be required to monitor therapy. Lab tests will include blood counts, kidney function tests, urine protein tests, and eye exams.

## Drug Interactions:

Tell your doctor or pharmacist if you are taking or if you are planning to take any over-the-counter or prescription medications or dietary supplements while taking cidofovir. Doses of one or both drugs may need to be modified or a different drug may need to be prescribed. The following drugs and drug classes may interact with cidofovir:

amphotericin B (eg, *Fungizone*)
aminoglycosides (eg, genta-micin)
foscarnet (*Foscavir*)

NSAIDs (eg, ibuprofen)
pentamidine (eg, *Pentam 300*)
vancomycin (eg, *Vancocin*)

## Side Effects:

Every drug is capable of producing side effects. Many cidofovir users experience no, or minor, side effects. The frequency and severity of side effects depend on many factors including dose, duration of therapy, and individual susceptibility. Possible side effects include:

*Digestive Tract:* Nausea; vomiting; diarrhea; appetite loss; mouth sores.

*Urinary and Reproductive Tract:* Protein in urine; elevated serum creatinine.

*Other:* Rash; hair loss; headache; weakness; fever; infections; chills; difficulty breathing; pneumonia; anemia; decreased white blood cell counts; low intraocular pressure (pressure of fluid inside eye); increased cough.

## Guidelines for Use:

- This medication will be prepared and administered by your health care provider in a medical setting.
- Usual dose is administered once weekly for 2 consecutive weeks, and then once every 2 weeks. The dose may be changed by your doctor as a result of lab test results.
- Probenecid may cause headache, nausea, vomiting, or allergic reactions (eg, rash, fever, chills, difficulty breathing). Taking probenecid after a meal or using antiemetics may decrease the nausea. Antihistamines or acetaminophen (eg, *Tylenol*) may be used to lessen the allergic reactions.
- *Zidovudine (AZT; Retrovir)* — Patients taking AZT should temporarily discontinue its administration or decrease its dose by half (50%) on the days of the cidofovir administration. Talk with your doctor about which would be best for you.
- Cidofovir is not a cure for CMV retinitis. You may continue to experience effects of retinitis during or following treatment. Patients should remain under the care of a doctor.
- HIV-infected mothers should not breastfeed because of the risk of transmitting the HIV infection or this drug to the infant.
- Contraceptive (birth control) measures are recommended for men and women during therapy. Men should use barrier contraception during and for at least 90 days following treatment. Women should use effective contraception during and for 30 days following treatment. Inform your doctor if you are pregnant, suspect pregnancy, or are planning to become pregnant.
- Kidney impairment is the major toxicity of cidofovir. Have blood tests and kidney function tests performed at least 48 hours before each dose of cidofovir.
- Lab tests and eye exams will be required to monitor therapy. Be sure to keep appointments.

*If you have any questions, consult your doctor, pharmacist, or health care provider.*

| Generic Name<br>*Brand Name Examples* | Supplied As | Generic<br>Available |
|---|---|---|
| Rx  **Ribavirin** | | |
| *Rebetol* | **Capsules:** 200 mg | No |
| *Virazole* | **Powder for reconstitution,<br>aerosol:** 6 g/100 mL<br>(20 mg/mL when reconstituted) | No |

## Type of Drug:

Antiviral drug for inhalation treatment of respiratory syncytial virus (RSV) infections, anti-hepatitis C virus (HCV) drug.

## How the Drug Works:

Ribavirin inhibits the growth of the respiratory syncytial virus. The exact mechanism of action is not known.

## Uses:

*Rebetol* — To treat chronic hepatitis C in patients with compensated liver disease. Only use in combination with interferon alfa-2b (*Intron A*).

*Virazole* — To treat certain hospitalized infants and young children with severe lung infections due to RSV. Adults are rarely treated with ribavirin by inhalation. Treatment early in the course of RSV infection is desirable for optimal effect.

## Precautions:

*Do not use in the following situations:*
  adults (*Virazole* only)
  allergy to ribavirin or any of its ingredients
  heart disease, unstable (*Rebetol* only)
  hemoglobin abnormalities (eg, sickle cell anemia) (*Rebetol* only)
  hepatitis, autoimmune
  kidney disease, severe (*Rebetol* only)
  male partners of pregnant women
  pregnancy or during periods when one may become pregnant

*Use with caution in the following situations:*
  heart disease (*Rebetol* only)
  kidney disease (*Rebetol* only)
  mechanical ventilation (*Virazole* only)

*Other viral infections:* Ribavirin capsules are not effective for treating viral infections (eg, HIV, hepatitis B, influenza) other than hepatitis C.

*Secondary exposure hazard:* Avoid direct care of patient if you are a mother or health care provider who is pregnant or planning to become pregnant. Aerosolized ribavirin is given in rooms with special ventilation. Wear appropriate respirator masks. The aerosol machine should be turned off 5 to 10 minutes before prolonged patient contact.

*Pregnancy:* Do not use during pregnancy. The risk of use in pregnant women clearly outweighs any possible benefit. Women of child-bearing potential, including female partners of male patients, must take extreme care to avoid pregnancy during and for 6 months after treatment has been stopped. Two forms of effective contraception must be used.

*Breastfeeding:* It is not known if ribavirin appears in breast milk. Consult your doctor before you begin breastfeeding.

*Children:* Safety and effectiveness of ribavirin capsules have not been established.

*Elderly:* Use ribavirin capsules with caution in elderly patients. Dosage adjustments may be necessary.

*Lab tests* will be required to monitor therapy with ribavirin capsules. Tests include pregnancy tests, blood counts, and liver and thyroid function tests.

## Drug Interactions:

Tell your doctor or pharmacist if you are taking or planning to take any over-the-counter or prescription medications or dietary supplements with ribavirin. Doses of one or both drugs may be modified or a different drug may need to be prescribed. Antacids (eg *Mylanta*) interact with ribavirin.

## Side Effects:

Every drug is capable of producing side effects. Many ribavirin users experience no, or minor, side effects. The frequency and severity of side effects depend on many factors including dose, duration of therapy, and individual susceptibility. Possible side effects include:

*Aerosol only –*

*Respiratory System:* Difficulty breathing; worsening of breathing status; collapse of lung; bacterial pneumonia; fluid in the lungs.

*Other:* Abnormal blood tests; anemia; rash; eye redness and inflammation; decrease in blood pressure; changes in heart rate.

*Capsules only –*

*Nervous System:* Dizziness; sleeplessness; irritability; depression; nervousness; emotional lability.

*Digestive Tract:* Nausea; appetite loss; indigestion; abnormal taste sensation.

*Other:* Rash; itching; difficulty breathing; sinus inflammation; fatigue; rigors; weakness; muscle and joint pain; anemia.

## Guidelines for Use:

- *Capsules* — Review Medication Guide before using and after each refill of medication.

  Dosage is individualized. Take exactly as prescribed.

  Do not change the dose or stop taking unless directed by your doctor.

  *Intron A* injection must be used in conjunction with ribavarin capsules in order to provide the most effective therapy. Use of ribavirin without *Intron A* is not effective.

  Drink plenty of water while taking ribavirin.

  It is not known if ribavirin reduces the risk of transmitting hepatitis virus to others through sexual contact or blood transfusion. Appropriate precautions to prevent transmitting hepatitis C virus to others should be taken.

  Ribavirin is contraindicated in pregnant women, including partners of male patients. Therapy should not be started until a negative pregnancy test has been obtained.

  Women of child-bearing potential, including female partners of male patients, must use 2 forms of reliable contraception during treatment and for 6 months after treatment has been stopped.

  If a dose is missed, take it as soon as possible. If several hours have passed or it is nearing time for the next dose, do not double the dose to catch up, unless advised to do so by your doctor. If more than one dose is missed or it is necessary to establish a new dosage schedule, contact your doctor or pharmacist.

  Do not take any OTC or prescription medications or dietary supplements unless advised to do so by your doctor.

  Lab tests will be required to monitor therapy. Be sure to keep appointments.

  Store at room temperature (59° to 86°F).

- *Aerosol* — Ribavirin will be prepared and administered by your health care provider in a hospital setting.

  Hospital personnel will closely monitor the patient's status and responses to treatment.

  Ribavirin will be administered by a specially designed machine.

  Ribavirin treatment will be administered over 12 to 18 hours a day for 3 to 7 days.

  Ribavirin is not indicated for use by adults. It is never to be used in pregnant women or during times when pregnancy might occur.

  Avoid direct care of patient if you are a mother or health care provider who is pregnant or planning to become pregnant. Aerosol ribavirin is given in rooms with special ventilation. Wear appropriate respirator masks. The aerosol machine should be turned off 5 to 10 minutes before prolonged patient contact.

*If you have any questions, consult your doctor, pharmacist, or health care provider.*

| Generic Name<br>*Brand Name Example* | Supplied As | Generic<br>Available |
|---|---|---|
| *Rx* **Rimantadine HCl** | | |
| *Flumadine* | **Tablets**: 100 mg | No |
| *Flumadine* | **Syrup**: 50 mg/5 mL | No |

## Type of Drug:

Antiviral drug for influenza A virus.

## How the Drug Works:

It is not fully understood how rimantadine acts to inhibit the growth and spread of the influenza A virus.

## Uses:

To prevent the symptoms of infection caused by the influenza A virus in adults and children younger than 1 year of age.

To treat adults with illness caused by strains of the influenza A virus.

## Precautions:

*Do not use in the following situations:* Allergy to rimantadine or amantadine (eg, *Symmetrel*) or any of their ingredients.

*Use with caution in the following situations:*

epilepsy
kidney disease
liver disease

patients whose contacts are at high risk for influenza A illness

*Flu vaccine:* A yearly vaccination with the influenza vaccine ("flu shot") is still the best way to prevent influenza.

*Seizures:* Seizure-like activity has been reported in a small number of patients with a history of seizures who were not taking anticoagulant medication.

*Pregnancy:* There are no adequate and well-controlled studies in pregnant women. Use only if clearly needed and the potential benefits to the mother outweigh the possible hazards to the fetus.

*Breastfeeding:* It is not known if rimantadine appears in breast milk. Consult your doctor before you begin breastfeeding.

*Children:* The safety and effectiveness in the treatment of influenza symptoms have not been established in children. Prophylaxis studies have not been performed in children younger than 1 year of age.

*Elderly:* An increase in adverse reactions in persons older than 64 years of age has been shown. May need lower doses than other individuals.

## Drug Interactions:

Tell your doctor if you are taking or planning to take any over-the-counter or prescription medications or dietary supplements with rimantadine. Doses of one or both drugs may need to be modified or a different drug may need to be prescribed. The following drugs and drug classes interact with rimantadine:

acetaminophen (eg, *Tylenol*)
aspirin
cimetidine (eg, *Tagamet*)

## Side Effects:

Every drug is capable of producing side effects. Many rimantadine users experience no, or minor, side effects. The frequency and severity of side effects depend on many factors including dose, duration of therapy, and individual susceptibility. Possible side effects include:

*Digestive Tract:* Nausea; vomiting; stomach pain; appetite loss.

*Nervous System:* Sleeplessness; dizziness; headache; nervousness; fatigue.

*Other:* Weakness; dry mouth.

---

### Guidelines for Use:

- Dosage is individualized. Take exactly as prescribed.
- Do not change the dose or stop taking unless directed by your doctor.
- May be taken without regard to meals.
- Children 10 years of age and older should receive the adult dose.
- *For treatment in adults* — Start as soon as possible after onset of symptoms and continue for 7 days. Rimantadine is most effective when started 48 hours or less after the onset of "flu" symptoms.
- Stop taking and immediately contact your health care provider if you experience seizures.
- May cause dizziness. Use caution while driving or performing other tasks requiring alertness, coordination, or physical dexterity.
- Contact your doctor if you develop persistent sleeplessness, dizziness, nausea, or vomiting.
- Store at room temperature (59° to 86°F).

---

*If you have any questions, consult your doctor, pharmacist, or health care provider.*

| Generic Name | | Generic |
| Brand Name Example | Supplied As | Available |
| --- | --- | --- |
| *Rx* **Zanamivir** | | |
| *Relenza* | **Powder for inhalation**: 5 mg/blister | No |

## Type of Drug:

Antiviral drug used to treat influenza A and B virus.

## How the Drug Works:

Zanamivir interferes with viral enzymes (neuramindase) that allow respiratory viruses to grow and spread.

## Uses:

Indicated for the treatment of uncomplicated acute illness (flu symptoms) due to influenza virus A and B in adults and adolescents 7 years of age and older who have been symptomatic for 2 days or less.

## Precautions:

*Do not use in the following situations:* Allergy to zanamivir or any of its ingredients.

*Use with caution in the following situations:*
asthma
lung disease, chronic obstructive

*Pregnancy:* There are no adequate and well-controlled studies in pregnant women. Use only if clearly needed and the potential benefits to the mother outweigh the possible hazards to the fetus.

*Breastfeeding:* It is not known if zanamivir appears in breast milk. Consult your doctor before you begin breastfeeding.

*Children:* Safety and effectiveness in patients younger than 12 years of age have not been established.

## Drug Interactions:

Tell your doctor or pharmacist if you are taking or planning to take any over-the-counter or prescription medications or dietary supplements while taking zanamivir. Doses of one or both drugs may need to be modified or a different drug may need to be prescribed.

## Side Effects:

Every drug is capable of producing side effects. Many zanamivir users experience no, or minor, side effects. The frequency and severity of side effects depend on many factors including dose, duration of therapy, and individual susceptibility. Possible side effects include:

*Digestive Tract:* Diarrhea; nausea; vomiting; stomach pain.

*Nervous System:* Headache; dizziness; general body discomfort; fatigue; fever.

*Respiratory System:* Nasal signs and symptoms; bronchitis; broncho-spasm; difficulty breathing; cough; sinus infection; ear, nose, or throat infections.

*Other:* Muscle pain; joint pain; rash; hives.

---

### Guidelines for Use:

- Read and carefully follow the patient instructions for use provided with zanamivir. Safe and effective use of zanamivir requires proper use of the *Diskhaler* to inhale the drug.
- This medicine is for administration to the respiratory tract by inhalation through the mouth only, using the *Diskhaler* provided.
- The recommended dose for patients 7 years of age and older is 2 inhalations (one 5 mg blister per inhalation for a total dose of 10 mg) 2 times daily (approximately 12 hours apart) for 5 days. Take 2 doses on the first day of treatment whenever possible, provided there are at least 2 hours between doses. On subsequent days, take doses about 12 hours apart (eg, morning and evening) at approximately the same time each day.
- Complete the entire 5-day course of treatment even if you begin to feel better.
- If you are scheduled to take an inhaled bronchodilator at the same time as this medicine, take the bronchodilator first.
- There is no evidence of zanamivir's effectiveness when started less than 2 days after the onset of signs or symptoms of influenza, or in the treatment of any other illness caused by agents other than influenza virus A or B.
- Use of this medicine has not been shown to reduce the risk of transmission of influenza to others.
- Zanamivir does not cure patients of influenza. It reduces time for improvement by 1 to 1.5 days.
- Zanamivir does not eliminate the need for an annual influenza vaccine in high-risk patients (eg, patients with asthma, diabetes, or heart disease; elderly patients).
- If you have asthma or chronic lung disease, you must have a fast-acting bronchodilator available. Stop this medicine and notify your doctor if you experience worsening of respiratory symptoms.
- Do not puncture any blister until immediately before taking a dose with the *Diskhaler.*
- Store at room temperature (59° to 86°F). Keep out of the reach of children.

---

*If you have any questions, consult your doctor, pharmacist, or health care provider.*

| Generic Name<br>*Brand Name Example* | Supplied As | Generic<br>Available |
|---|---|---|
| *Rx* **Oseltamivir Phosphate** | | |
| *Tamiflu* | **Capsules**: 75 mg | No |
| *Tamiflu* | **Suspension, oral**: 12 mg/mL | No |

## Type of Drug:

Antiviral drug for influenza A and B virus.

## How the Drug Works:

Oseltamivir interferes with viral enzymes (neuramidase) that allow respiratory flu viruses to grow and spread. Oseltamivir is not active until after it has been absorbed into the body.

## Uses:

For the treatment of uncomplicated acute illness due to influenza A or B infection in adults and pediatric patients 1 year of age and older who have had flu symptoms for no more than 2 days, and for the prevention of influenza A or B in adults and adolescents 13 years of age and older.

## Precautions:

*Do not use in the following situations:* Allergy to oseltamivir phosphate or any of its ingredients.

*Use with caution in the following situations:*
kidney disease, severe
liver disease

*Flu vaccine:* A yearly vaccination with the influenza vaccine ("flu shot") is still the best way to prevent influenza.

*Pregnancy:* There are no adequate and well-controlled studies in pregnant women. Use only if clearly needed and the potential benefits to the mother outweigh the possible hazards to the fetus.

*Breastfeeding:* It is not known if oseltamivir appears in breast milk. Consult your doctor before you begin breastfeeding.

*Children:* Safety and effectiveness in children younger than 1 year of age have not been established.

## Drug Interactions:

Tell your doctor or pharmacist if you are taking or planning to take any over-the-counter or prescription medications or dietary supplements while taking oseltamivir phosphate. Doses of one or both drugs may need to be modified or a different drug may need to be prescribed.

## Side Effects:

Every drug is capable of producing side effects. Many oseltamivir phosphate users experience no, or minor, side effects. The frequency and severity of side effects depend on many factors including dose, duration of therapy, and individual susceptibility. Possible side effects include:

*Digestive Tract:* Nausea; vomiting; diarrhea; stomach pain.

*Other:* Cough; dizziness; headache; fatigue; bronchitis; sleeplessness; vertigo (feeling of whirling motion).

### Guidelines for Use:

- Dosage is individualized. Take exactly as prescribed.
- Do not stop taking or change the dose, unless directed by your doctor.
- Patients should begin treatment as soon as possible following the first appearance of flu symptoms or following close contact with an infected individual. This medicine is not beneficial if started more than 2 days after flu symptoms are first noticed or after 2 days following close contact with an infected individual.
- May be taken without regard to meals or snacks. Take with food if stomach upset occurs.
- Patients should take missed doses as soon as they remember, except within 2 hours of next scheduled dose, and then continue normal dosage intervals.
- May cause dizziness. Use caution while driving or performing other tasks requiring alertness, coordination, or physical dexterity.
- Store at room temperature (59° to 86°F).

*If you have any questions, consult your doctor, pharmacist, or health care provider.*

| Generic Name<br>*Brand Name Examples* | Supplied As | Generic<br>Available |
|---|---|---|
| *Rx* **Amprenavir** | | |
| *Agenerase* | **Capsules**: 50 mg, 150 mg | No |
| *Agenerase*[1] | **Solution, oral**: 15 mg/mL | No |
| *Rx* **Indinavir Sulfate** | | |
| *Crixivan* | **Capsules**: 100 mg, 200 mg,<br>333 mg, 400 mg | No |
| *Rx* **Nelfinavir Mesylate** | | |
| *Viracept* | **Tablets**: 250 mg | No |
| *Viracept*[2] | **Powder, oral**: 50 mg/g | No |
| *Rx* **Ritonavir** | | |
| *Norvir* | **Capsules**: 100 mg | No |
| *Norvir*[3] | **Solution, oral**: 80 mg/mL | No |
| *Rx* **Saquinavir** | | |
| *Invirase* | **Capsules**: 200 mg<br>(as mesylate) | No |
| *Fortovase* | **Capsules, soft gelatin**: 200 mg | No |
| *Rx* **Lopinavir/Ritonavir** | | |
| *Kaletra* | **Capsules**: 133.3 mg/33.3 mg | No |
| *Kaletra* | **Solution, oral**:<br>80 mg/20 mg/mL | No |

[1] Contains propylene glycol.
[2] Contains phenylalanine.
[3] Contains alcohol.

## Type of Drug:

Antiviral; protease inhibitor; AIDS drug.

## How the Drug Works:

Protease inhibitors inhibit the growth of the human immunodeficiency virus type 1 (HIV-1), the virus that causes acquired immunodeficiency syndrome (AIDS).

## Uses:

Used alone or in combination with other antiretroviral agents for treatment of HIV-1 infection.

## Precautions:

*Do not use in the following situations:*

allergy to the protease inhibitor or any of its ingredients
amiodarone therapy, concurrent (nelfinavir, ritonavir only)
bepridil therapy, concurrent
dihydroergotamine therapy, concurrent
ergotamine therapy, concurrent

HMG-CoA reductase inhibitor therapy, concurrent (nelfinavir, ritonavir, lopinavir/ritonavir only)
midazolam therapy, concurrent
pregnancy (amprenavir oral solution only)

quinidine therapy, concurrent (nelfinavir, ritonavir only)
rifampin therapy, concurrent (nelfinavir, saquinavir, lopinavir/ritonavir only)
St. John's wort use, concurrent
triazolam therapy, concurrent

*Use with caution in the following situations:*
allergy to sulfonamides (amprenavir only)
diabetes

hemophilia A or B
liver disease, moderate to severe

*Diabetes:* Exacerbation of preexisting diabetes mellitus and of hyperglycemia (high blood sugar) have been reported with protease inhibitor use. Some patients require initiation or dosage adjustments of insulin or hypoglycemic (blood sugar-lowering) agents.

*Fat redistribution:* Changes in body fat including central (stomach and chest) obesity, dorsocervical fat enlargement (buffalo hump), peripheral wasting (skinny arms and legs), and breast enlargement have occurred in patients receiving antiretrovial therapy. The cause of this and the long-term consequences of these changes are not known at this time.

*Phenylketonuria patients:* Nelfinavir powder contains phenylalanine. Consult your doctor or pharmacist.

*Vitamin E:* Amprenavir capsules and oral solution contain large amounts of vitamin E, exceeding the Reference Daily Intake. Adults and pediatric patients taking amprenavir should not take supplemental vitamin E.

*Pregnancy:* There are no adequate and well-controlled studies in pregnant women. Use only if clearly needed and the potential benefits to the mother outweigh the possible hazards to the fetus. Amprenavir oral solution is contraindicated in pregnant women.

*Breastfeeding:* The Centers for Disease Control and Prevention (CDC) recommends that HIV-infected mothers not breastfeed their infants to avoid risking postnatal transmission of HIV. It is not known if protease inhibitors appear in breast milk. Consult your doctor before you begin breastfeeding.

*Children:* Safety and effectiveness of amprenavir have not been established in patients younger than 4 years of age. Safety and effectiveness of indinavir have not been established in pediatric patients. Safety and effectiveness of nelfinavir and ritonavir have not been established in patients younger than 2 years of age. Safety and effectiveness of saquinavir have not been established in patients younger than 16 years of age. Safety and effectiveness of lopinavir/ritonavir have not been established in patients younger than 6 months of age.

*Elderly:* Administer with caution in elderly patients.

*Lab tests* will be required to monitor therapy. Tests include cholesterol and triglyceride levels, liver enzymes, and blood sugar levels.

## Drug Interactions:

Tell your doctor or pharmacist if you are taking or planning to take any over-the-counter or prescription medications or dietary supplements while taking a protease inhibitor. Doses of one or both drugs may need to be modified or a different drug may need to be prescribed. The following drugs and drug classes interact with protease inhibitors:

amiodarone (eg, *Cordarone*) (amprenavir only)
antacids (eg, *Maalox*) (amprenavir only)
anticoagulants (eg, warfarin)
anticonvulsants (eg, carbamazepine)
azole antifungals (eg, ketoconazole)
benzodiazepines (eg, midazolam, triazolam)
bepridil (*Vascor*)
contraceptives, oral (eg, *Ortho-Novum*)
didanosine (*Videx*) (amprenavir only)
ergot alkaloids (eg, ergotamine)
HMG-CoA reductase inhibitors (eg, lovastatin)
immunosuppressants (eg, cyclosporine)
lidocaine (eg, *Xylocaine*) (amprenavir only)
quinidine (eg, *Quinora*) (amprenavir only)
rifamycins (eg, rifampin)
sildenafil (*Viagra*)
St. John's wort
tricyclic antidepressants (eg, amitriptyline) (amprenavir only)
vitamin E

## Side Effects:

Every drug is capable of producing side effects. Many protease inhibitor users experience no, or minor, side effects. The frequency and severity of side effects depend on many factors including dose, duration of therapy, and individual susceptibility. Possible side effects include:

*Nervous System:* Depression; headache; sleeplessness; anxiety; sex drive changes; drowsiness; dizziness.

*Digestive Tract:* Nausea; vomiting; diarrhea; loose stools; stomach pain; taste disorders; acid regurgitation; dry mouth; indigestion; gas; constipation; appetite changes.

*Skin:* Severe and life-threatening skin reactions (eg, Stevens-Johnson syndrome); rash; itching; abnormal skin sensations; tingling or numb sensation around the mouth (amprenavir only); eczema; warts.

*Other:* Lab test abnormalities; new onset of diabetes mellitus; exacerbation of preexisting diabetes mellitus; high blood sugar; redistribution or accumulation of body fat; numbness in the arms or legs; fatigue; pain; weakness; back, muscle, or bone pain; kidney stones (indinavir only); weakness; general body discomfort.

## Guidelines for Use:

- Read the patient information handout provided with your medicine.
- Dosage is individualized. Take exactly as prescribed.
- Do not change the dose or stop taking, unless directed by your doctor. Continuous therapy and strict compliance is necessary to obtain the maximum benefit from therapy.

## Guidelines for Use (cont.):

- Amprenavir may be taken with or without food, but avoid taking with high-fat meals, which decrease absorption into the body.
- Take indinavir without food, but with water 1 hour before or 2 hours after a meal, or take with other liquids (eg, skim milk, juice) or a light meal (eg, cereal and skim milk, toast with jelly).
- Take nelfinavir with a meal or light snack. The oral powder may be mixed with a small amount of water, milk, formula, soy formula, soy milk, or dietary supplement (eg, *Ensure*). Once mixed, consume the entire contents within 6 hours to obtain the full dose. Acidic food or juice (eg, orange juice, apple juice, apple sauce) are not recommended because of the bitter taste. Do not mix in the original container.
- Take ritonavir with food, if possible. The taste of the oral solution may be improved by mixing it with 8 oz of chocolate milk, *Ensure*, or *Advera* and taking it within 1 hour of mixing.
- Saquinavir should be taken with a meal or up to 2 hours after a meal.
- Take lopinavir/ritonavir with food.
- *Indinavir* — To reduce the risk of kidney stones, drink at least 48 oz (6 to 8 oz glasses) of liquids daily.
- If a dose is missed by less than 4 hours (2 hours for indinavir), take it as soon as possible and then return to the normal schedule. If a dose is missed by greater than 4 hours (2 hours for indinavir), wait and take the next dose at the regularly scheduled time. Do not double the next dose to catch up.
- If you are taking estrogen-based oral contraceptives (eg, *Ortho-Novum*), you must use alternate or additional forms of contraception during amprenavir, nelfinavir, ritonavir, or lopinavir/ritonavir therapy.
- Amprenavir capsules and oral solution are not interchangeable on a mg-per-mg basis.
- Remain under the care of your doctor while taking a protease inhibitor.
- Protease inhibitors are not a cure for HIV infection. You may continue to develop opportunistic infections and other complications associated with HIV.
- Protease inhibitors do not reduce the risk of transmitting HIV to others through sexual contact or blood contamination.
- HIV-infected mothers should not breastfeed because of the risk of transmitting the HIV infection.
- Do not share this medication with anyone else.
- May cause drowsiness or dizziness. Use caution while driving or performing other tasks requiring alertness, coordination, and physical dexterity.
- Inform your doctor if you are pregnant, plan on becoming pregnant, or become pregnant while taking this medicine.
- *Saquinavir* — *Invirase* and *Fortovase* are not bioequivalent and cannot be used interchangeably.
- Long-term effects of protease inhibitors are not known at this time.
- Lab tests will be required to monitor therapy. Be sure to keep appointments.
- Store as directed by the package labeling.

*If you have any questions, consult your doctor, pharmacist, or health care provider.*

| Generic Name<br>*Brand Name Example* | Supplied As | Generic<br>Available |
|---|---|---|
| *Rx* **Tenofovir Disoproxil Fumarate** | | |
| *Viread* | **Tablets**: 300 mg (245 mg tenofovir disoproxil) | No |

## Type of Drug:

Antiretroviral; AIDS drug.

## How the Drug Works:

Tenofovir inhibits the growth of the human immunodeficiency virus type 1 (HIV-1), the virus that causes acquired immunodeficiency syndrome (AIDS).

## Uses:

Used in combination with other antiretroviral agents for the treatment of HIV-1 infection.

## Precautions:

*Do not use in the following situations:* Allergy to tenofovir or any of its ingredients.

*Use with caution in the following situations:*
>     kidney disease
>     liver disease

*Fat redistribution:* Changes in body fat including central (stomach and chest) obesity, dorsocervical fat enlargement (buffalo hump), peripheral wasting (skinny arms and legs), and breast enlargement have occurred in patients receiving antiretrovial therapy. The cause of this and the long-term consequences of these changes are not known at this time.

*Lactic acidosis:* Lactic acidosis (excessive acid in blood) and severe hepatomegaly (enlarged liver) with steatosis (fat deposits in liver) have been associated with nucleoside analog therapy. If lactic acidosis or hepatoxicity are suspected or confirmed, therapy will be stopped.

*Pregnancy:* There are no adequate and well-controlled studies in pregnant women. Use only if clearly needed and the potential benefits to the mother outweigh the possible hazards to the fetus.

*Breastfeeding:* The Centers for Disease Control and Prevention (CDC) recommends that HIV-infected mothers not breastfeed their infants to avoid risking postnatal transmission of HIV. It is not known if tenofovir appears in breast milk. Consult your doctor before you begin breastfeeding.

*Children:* Safety and effectiveness have not been established.

*Lab tests* may be required to monitor therapy. Tests include kidney and liver function.

## Drug Interactions:

Tell your doctor or pharmacist if you are taking or planning to take any over-the-counter or prescription medications or dietary supplements while taking tenofovir. Doses of one or both drugs may need to be modified or a different drug may need to be prescribed. The following drugs and drug classes interact with tenofovir:

acyclovir (*Zovirax*)              ganciclovir (*Cytovene*)
cidofovir (*Vistide*)              valciclovir (*Valtrex*)
didanosine (*Videx*)               valganciclovir (*Valcyte*)

## Side Effects:

Every drug is capable of producing side effects. Many tenofovir users experience no, or minor, side effects. The frequency and severity of side effects depend on many factors including dose, duration of therapy, and individual susceptibility. Possible side effects include:

*Digestive Tract:* Nausea; diarrhea; vomiting; gas; stomach pain; appetite loss.

*Other:* Redistribution and accumulation of body fat; abnormal lab tests; headache; weakness.

## Guidelines for Use:

- Read the patient information handout provided with this medicine.
- Dosage is individualized. Take exactly as prescribed.
- Do not change the dose or stop taking, unless directed by your doctor.
- Take with meals to increase effectiveness.
- If taking with didanosine (*Videx*), take tenofovir 2 hours before or 1 hour after didanosine.
- If a dose is missed, take it as soon as possible. If several hours have passed or it is nearing time for the next dose, do not double the dose to catch up, unless advised to do so by your doctor. If more than one dose is missed or it is necessary to establish a new dosage schedule, contact your doctor or pharmacist.
- Notify your health care provider immediately if you experience difficulty breathing, unexplained rapid breathing or shortness of breath, muscle pain, general body discomfort, unusual drowsiness, or swelling or pain in the upper right stomach area. These could be symptoms of a serious side effect such as lactic acidosis or an enlarged liver.
- Notify your health care provider if you experience intolerable gastrointestinal problems or changes in body fat distribution.
- Tenofovir is not a cure for HIV infection. You may continue to develop opportunistic infections and other complications associated with HIV.
- Tenofovir does not reduce the risk of transmitting HIV to others through sexual contact or blood contamination.
- To be effective, this medicine must be taken with other HIV medications.
- HIV-infected mothers should not breastfeed because of the risk of transmitting the HIV infection.
- Do not share your medicine with anyone else.
- The long-term effects of tenofovir are unknown at this time.
- Lab tests will be required to monitor therapy. Be sure to keep appointments.
- Store at room temperature (59° to 86°F).

*If you have any questions, consult your doctor, pharmacist, or health care provider.*

| Generic Name *Brand Name Examples* | Supplied As | Generic Available |
|---|---|---|
| Rx **Abacavir** | | |
| *Ziagen* | **Tablets**: 300 mg | No |
| *Ziagen* | **Solution, oral**: 20 mg/mL | No |
| Rx **Didanosine** | | |
| *Videx*[1] | **Tablets, buffered, chewable/ dispersible**: 25 mg, 50 mg, 100 mg, 150 mg, 200 mg | No |
| *Videx EC* | **Capsules, delayed-release (with enteric-coated beadlets)**: 125 mg, 200 mg, 250 mg, 400 mg | No |
| *Videx* | **Powder for oral solution, buffered**: 100 mg, 167 mg, 250 mg/packet | No |
| *Videx*[2] | **Powder for oral solution, pediatric**: 2 g, 4 g/bottle | No |
| Rx **Lamivudine** | | |
| *Epivir-HBV* | **Tablets**: 100 mg | No |
| *Epivir* | **Tablets**: 150 mg | No |
| *Epivir-HBV* | **Solution, oral**: 5 mg/mL | No |
| *Epivir* | **Solution, oral**: 10 mg/mL | No |
| Rx **Stavudine** | | |
| *Zerit* | **Capsules**: 15 mg, 20 mg, 30 mg, 40 mg | No |
| *Zerit* | **Powder for oral solution**: 1 mg/mL | No |
| Rx **Zalcitabine** | | |
| *Hivid* | **Tablets**: 0.375 mg, 0.75 mg | No |
| Rx **Zidovudine**[3] | | |
| *Retrovir* | **Tablets**: 300 mg | No |
| *Retrovir* | **Capsules**: 100 mg | No |
| *Retrovir* | **Syrup**: 50 mg/5 mL | No |
| Rx **Lamivudine/Zidovudine** | | |
| *Combivir* | **Tablets**: 150 mg/300 mg | No |
| Rx **Abacavir Sulfate/Lamivudine/Zidovudine** | | |
| *Trizivir* | **Tablets**: 300 mg/150 mg/300 mg | No |

[1] Contains phenylalanine.
[2] Contains 1380 mg sodium/packet.
[3] Also available as an intravenous injection.

## Type of Drug:

Antiretroviral agents for use in the treatment of human immunodeficiency virus type 1 (HIV-1) infection; nucleoside reverse transcriptase inhibitors (NRTIs).

## How the Drug Works:

NRTIs inhibit the growth of HIV-1, the virus that causes acquired immunodeficiency syndrome (AIDS) and hepatitis B virus (HBV).

## Uses:

Used in combination with other antiretroviral agents for the treatment of HIV-1 infection.

*Epivir-HBV:* For the treatment of chronic hepatitis B infection associated with evidence of hepatitis B viral replication and active liver inflammation.

## Precautions:

*Do not use in the following situations:* Allergy to the NRTI or any of its ingredients.

*Use with caution in the following situations:*

bone marrow suppression (zidovudine only)
cardiomyopathy (zalcitabine only)
concurrent hepatitis B and HIV infection (*Epivir—HBV* only)
congestive heart failure (zalcitabine only)
kidney disease
liver disease, current or risk factors for
pancreatitis in children, history or risk of
peripheral neuropathy, history or risk of
prolonged nucleoside (NRTI) exposure

*Epivir/Epivir-HBV interchangeability: Epivir* tablets and oral solution contain a higher dose of the same active ingredient (lamivudine) than *Epivir-HBV* tablets and solution. Therefore, *Epivir* and *Epivir-HBV* are not interchangeable.

*Fatal hypersensitivity reactions:* Fatal hypersensitivity (allergic) reactions have been associated with NRTI therapy. NRTIs must be stopped immediately in patients who develop signs or symptoms of hypersensitivity (eg, fever; rash; fatigue; dizziness; fainting; gastrointestinal symptoms such as nausea, vomiting, diarrhea, stomach pain; respiratory symptoms such as sore throat, shortness of breath, cough). Do not restart taking the NRTI because a more severe reaction could occur.

*Lactic acidosis:* Lactic acidosis (acid in the blood) and severe hepatomegaly (liver enlargement) with steatosis (fatty changes in the liver) have been associated with NRTI therapy. Symptoms include feeling very weak or tired, unusual or unexpected stomach discomfort, unexplained shortness of breath or rapid breathing, feeling cold, dizzy, or lightheaded, and slow or irregular heartbeat. If lactic acidosis or hepatoxicity are suspected or confirmed, NRTI therapy should be stopped.

*Pancreatitis:* Didanosine, lamivudine, stavudine, and zalcitabine have been associated with pancreatitis (inflammation of pancreas gland). Stop taking and notify your doctor immediately if you experience nausea, vomiting, or stomach pain or tenderness.

*Peripheral neuropathy:* Didanosine, lamivudine, stavudine, and zalcitabine have been associated with peripheral neuropathy (numbness, tingling, burning, or pain in the hands of feet). Stop using and notify your doctor immediately if symptoms develop.

*Phenylketonuria:* Some of these products contain phenylalanine. Consult your doctor or pharmacist.

*Pregnancy:* There are no adequate and well-controlled studies in pregnant women. Use only if clearly needed and the potential benefits to the mother outweigh the possible hazards to the fetus.

*Breastfeeding:* The Centers for Disease Control and Prevention (CDC) recommends that HIV-infected mothers not breastfeed their infants to avoid risking postnatal transmission of HIV. It is not known if NRTIs appear in breast milk. Consult your doctor before you begin breastfeeding.

*Children:* Safety and effectiveness of abacavir in patients 3 months to 13 years of age have been established. Didanosine delayed-release capsules have not been studied in children. Safety of *Epivir-HBV* has not been established in children younger than 2 years of age. Safety of lamivudine and zidovudine has been established in patients 3 months of age and older. Didanosine and stavudine use in children is supported by adequate and well-controlled studies. Safety of zalcitabine has not been established in children younger than 13 years of age. Abacavir/lamivudine/zidovudine is not intended for pediatric use.

*Elderly:* Use with caution in elderly patients. Dosage adjustments may be necessary.

*Lab tests* may be required to monitor therapy. Tests include liver, kidney, and pancreas function tests, blood counts, and eye exams.

## Drug Interactions:

Tell your doctor or pharmacist if you are taking or planning to take any over-the-counter or prescription medications while taking an NRTI. Doses of one or both drugs may need to be modified or a different drug may need to be prescribed. The following drugs and drug classes interact with NRTIs:

allopurinol (eg, *Zyloprim*) (didanosine only)
antacids (zalcitabine only)
atovaquone (*Mepron*) (zidovudine only)
azole antifungals (eg, ketoconazole) (didanosine only)
cimetidine (eg, *Tagamet*) (zalcitabine only)
doxorubicin (eg, *Adriamycin RDF*) (zidovudine only)

ethanol (abacavir only)
ganciclovir (*Cytovene*) (zidovudine only)
indinavir (*Crixivan*) (didanosine only)
methadone (eg, *Dolophine*) (abacavir, zidovudine only)
phenytoin (eg, *Dilantin*) (zidovudine only)
probenecid (zalcitabine, zidovudine only)

quinolones (eg, ciprofloxacin) (didanosine only)

stavudine (*Zerit*) (zidovudine only)

zalcitabine (*Hivid*) (lamivudine only)

zidovudine (*Retrovir*) (stavudine only)

## Side Effects:

Every drug is capable of producing side effects. Many NRTI users experience no, or minor, side effects. The frequency and severity of side effects depend on many factors including dose, duration of therapy, and individual susceptibility. Possible side effects include:

*Nervous System:* Dizziness; headache; depression; sleeplessness and other sleep disorders; convulsions.

*Digestive Tract:* Nausea; vomiting; diarrhea; appetite loss; stomach pain or cramps; indigestion; constipation.

*Skin:* Rash; itching; hives.

*Respiratory System:* Difficulty breathing; cough; nasal signs and symptoms (eg, discharge, congestion); wheezing.

*Other:* Numbness, tingling, or pain in the hands or feet; retinal changes; optic neuritis; abnormal lab tests; pancreatitis; liver damage; severe allergic reactions (eg, rash, low blood pressure, difficulty breathing); lactic acidosis; fever; muscle pain or weakness; bone pain; joint pain or swelling; sweating; chills; general body discomfort; fatigue; ear, nose, or throat infection; ear pain, discharge, redness, or swelling; taste sensation changes; sore throat; sores in mouth or esophagus (food pipe); redistribution or accumulation of body fat.

---

### Guidelines for Use:

- Review the Patient Package Insert each time you fill your prescription. There may be new information added since your last refill.
- Dosage is individualized. Take exactly as prescribed.
- Do not change the dose or stop taking unless directed by your doctor. Strict compliance is crucial to prevent the virus from becoming resistant to the medicine.
- Take didanosine and zalcitabine on an empty stomach, at least 30 minutes before or 2 hours after a meal. All other NRTIs may be taken with or without food.
- *Didanosine chewable/buffered tablets* — Do not swallow whole. Take at least 2, but no more than 4 tablets per dose. Thoroughly chew or disperse in 2 or more tablespoons of water prior to taking. Stir until a uniform dispersion forms and drink the entire mixture immediately. If additional flavoring is desired, the mixture may be diluted with 2 tablespoons of clear apple juice. Do not use any other type of juice. Stir just before taking. The dispersion may be stored at room temperature for up to 1 hour.
- *Didanosine delayed-release capsules* — Do not open, crush, or chew capsules. Swallow whole.

## Guidelines for Use (cont.):

- *Didanosine buffered powder for oral solution* — Open packet and pour into approximately 4 ounces of water. Do not mix with fruit juice or other acid-containing liquid. Stir until the powder dissolves completely (approximately 2 to 3 minutes). Drink entire solution right away.
- *Didanosine pediatric oral solution* — Shake well before each use. Throw away any unused solution after 30 days.
- If a dose is missed, take it as soon as possible. If several hours have passed or it is nearing time for the next dose, do not double the dose to catch up, unless advised by your doctor. If more than one dose is missed or it is necessary to establish a new dosage schedule, contact your doctor or pharmacist.
- Abacavir tablets and oral solution can be used interchangeably.
- Zidovudine tablets, capsules, and syrup can be used interchangeably.
- Stop using and notify your doctor immediately if you experience fever, rash, fatigue, dizziness, fainting, gastrointestinal symptoms (eg, nausea, vomiting, diarrhea, stomach pain), respiratory symptoms (eg, sore throat, shortness of breath, unexplained rapid breathing, cough), slow or irregular heartbeat, or changes in vision (eg, blurring, color changes). These could be symptoms of a potentially fatal allergic reaction or toxic reaction.
- Women of childbearing age should use effective contraception while taking zalcitabine.
- NRTIs are not cures for HIV infection. You may continue to develop opportunistic infections and other complications associated with HIV.
- NRTIs do not reduce the risk of transmitting HIV to others through sexual contact or blood contamination.
- NRTIs must be used in combination with other HIV drugs to prevent the virus from becoming resistant.
- *Epivir-HBV* is not a cure for hepatitis B infection. It does not reduce the risk of transmitting hepatitis B to others through sexual contact or blood transfusions.
- Do not share this medicine with anyone else.
- The long-term effects of NRTIs are unknown at this time.
- Lab tests may be required to monitor therapy. Be sure to keep appointments.
- Store as directed by the package labeling.

*If you have any questions, consult your doctor, pharmacist, or health care provider.*

| Generic Name<br>*Brand Name Examples* | Supplied As | Generic<br>Available |
|---|---|---|
| *Rx* **Delavirdine Mesylate** | | |
| *Rescriptor* | **Tablets**: 100 mg, 200 mg | No |
| *Rx* **Efavirenz** | | |
| *Sustiva* | **Capsules**: 50 mg, 100 mg, 200 mg | No |
| *Sustiva* | **Tablets**: 600 mg | No |
| *Rx* **Nevirapine** | | |
| *Viramune* | **Tablets**: 200 mg | No |
| *Viramune* | **Suspension, oral**: 50 mg (as nevirapine hemihydrate)/5 mL | No |

## Type of Drug:

Antiretrovirals; NNRTIs; AIDS drugs.

## How the Drug Works:

These non-nucleoside reverse transcriptase inhibitors (NNRTIs) inhibit the growth of the human immunodeficiency virus type 1 (HIV-1), the virus that causes acquired immunodeficiency syndrome (AIDS).

## Uses:

For use in combination with other appropriate antiretroviral agents, including nucleoside analogs (eg, zidovudine) to treat HIV-1-infected adults when therapy is warranted (eg, deterioration of health).

## Precautions:

*Do not use in the following situations:*

allergy to the NNRTI or any of its ingredients
alprazolam therapy, concurrent
ergot-derivative therapy, concurrent
midazolam therapy, concurrent
St. John's wort use, concurrent
triazolam therapy, concurrent

*Use with caution in the following situations:*

kidney disease
liver disease
mental illness, history of (efavirenz only)
rash
substance abuse, history of (efavirenz only)

*Pregnancy:* There are no adequate and well-controlled studies in pregnant women. Use only if clearly needed and the potential benefits to the mother outweigh the possible hazards to the fetus.

*Breastfeeding:* The Centers for Disease Control and Prevention (CDC) recommends that HIV-infected mothers not breastfeed their infants to avoid risking postnatal transmission of HIV. NNRTIs may appear in breast milk. Consult your doctor before you begin breastfeeding.

*Children:* Safety and effectiveness of delavirdine mesylate in children younger than 16 years of age have not been established. Safety and effectiveness of efavirenz in children younger 3 years of age or children who weigh less than 29 pounds have not been established. Nevirapine has been used in infants as young as 2 months of age.

*Elderly:* Use with caution. Safety and effectiveness of delavirdine mesylate and efavirenz have not been extensively studied in patients older than 65 years of age. Safety and effectiveness of nevirapine have not been extensively studied in patients older than 55 years of age.

*Lab tests* will be required to monitor therapy. Tests include kidney and liver function, blood counts, and cholesterol and triglyceride levels.

## Drug Interactions:

Tell your doctor or pharmacist if you are taking or planning to take any over-the-counter or prescription medications or dietary supplements while taking an NNRTI. Doses of one or both drugs may need to be modified or a different drug may need to be prescribed. The following drugs and drug classes interact with NNRTIs:

antacids (eg, *Maalox*) (delavirdine only)

antiarrythmics (eg, amiodarone)

benzodiazepines (eg, triazolam)

calcium channel blockers (eg, nifedipine)

carbamazepine (eg, *Tegretol*)

clarithromycin (*Biaxin*)

corticosteroids (eg, dexamethasone) (delavirdine only)

dapsone (delavirdine only)

ergot derivatives (eg, ergotamine)

fluoxetine (eg, *Prozac*) (delavirdine only)

$H_2$ receptor antagonists (eg, cimetidine) (delavirdine only)

HMG-CoA reductase inhibitors (eg, lovastatin)

hormonal contraceptives (eg, ethinyl estradiol) (efavirenz, nevirapine only)

ketoconazole (eg, *Nizoral*) (delavirdine only)

methadone (eg, *Dolophine*)

nucleoside reverse transcriptase inhibitors (eg, didanosine)

phenobarbital (eg, *Solfoton*)

phenytoin (eg, dilantin) (efavirenz, delavirdine only)

protease inhibitors (eg, ritonavir)

proton pump inhibitors (eg, omeprazole)

quinidine (eg, *Quinora*)

rifamycins (eg, rifabutin)

sildenafil (*Viagra*)

St. John's Wort

warfarin (eg, *Coumadin*)

## Side Effects:

Every drug is capable of producing side effects. Many NNRTI users experience no, or minor, side effects. The frequency and severity of side effects depend on many factors including dose, duration of therapy, and individual susceptibility. Possible side effects include:

*Nervous System:* Headache; dizziness; sleeplessness; impaired concentration; drowsiness; abnormal dreams; hallucinations; euphoria; confusion; agitation; memory loss; stupor; abnormal thinking; depersonalization; depression; anxiety; nervousness; diminished sensitivity to stimulation.

*Digestive Tract:* Nausea; diarrhea; stomach pain; vomiting; indigestion; gas; appetite loss.

*Other:* Rash; itching; fever; fatigue; numbness or tingling in the arms or legs; abnormal skin sensations; weakness; muscle pain; abnormal lab tests; hepatitis; increased sweating; flu-like symptoms; bronchitis; cough; sore throat; sinus inflammation; yellowing of skin or eyes; joint pain.

## Guidelines for Use:

- Read the patient information handout provided with your medication.
- Dosage is individualized. Take exactly as prescribed.
- Do not change the dose or stop taking, unless directed by your doctor.
- Take efavirenz on an empty stomach, preferably at bedtime, to reduce side effects.
- Take delavirdine or nevirapine without regard to food. Take delavirdine and antacids at least 1 hour apart.
- Take delavirdine tablets whole. Delavirdine 100 mg tablets may be dispersed in water prior to taking. To disperse, add four 100 mg tablets to at least 3 ounces of water, allow to stand for a few minutes and then stir gently. Take immediately after mixing. Rinse glass with water and swallow rinse to ensure entire dose is taken.
- Gently shake nevirapine suspension before taking. Use oral dosage syringe or dosing cup to measure the correct dose. Rinse the dosing cup with water and swallow the rinse to ensure entire dose is taken.
- If a dose is missed, take it as soon as possible. If several hours have passed or it is nearing time for the next dose, do not double the dose to catch up, unless advised to do so by your doctor. If more than one dose is missed or it is necessary to establish a new dosage schedule, contact your doctor or pharmacist.
- Severe and life-threatening skin reactions have occurred in patients using NNRTIs. Notify your doctor if you experience severe rash, rash with fever, blistering, peeling, scaling, mouth sores, eye infection, muscle or joint aches, or general body discomfort.
- May cause dizziness, drowsiness, or impaired concentration. Use caution while driving or performing other tasks that require alertness, coordination, and physical dexterity.
- *Efavirenz* — Inform your doctor immediately if you experience serious psychiatric symptoms (eg, depression, behavior or personality changes).
- *Nevirapine* — Inform your doctor if you experience persistent fatigue, appetite loss, nausea, right upper stomach pain, tenderness, or swelling, or if you notice yellowing of the skin or eyes.
- NNRTIs are not cures for HIV infection. You may continue to develop opportunistic infections and other complications associated with HIV.
- NNRTIs do not reduce the risk of transmitting HIV to others through sexual contact or blood contamination.
- Women of childbearing potential should not become pregnant while taking an NNRTI. Use nonestrogen-based contraceptives (eg, condoms) to prevent pregnancy.
- HIV-infected mothers should not breastfeed because of the risk of transmitting the HIV infection.
- Do not share your medicine with anyone else.
- To be effective, this medicine must be taken with other HIV medications.
- The duration of effectiveness of these agents is variable and unpredictable.
- Lab tests will be required to monitor therapy. Be sure to keep appointments.
- Store at room temperature in a tightly closed container. Protect from high humidity.

*If you have any questions, consult your doctor, pharmacist, or health care provider.*

| Generic Name<br>*Brand Name Example* | Supplied As | Generic<br>Available |
|---|---|---|
| *Rx* **Albendazole** | | |
| *Albenza* | **Tablets**: 200 mg | No |

## Type of Drug:
Drug for tapeworm infections.

## How the Drug Works:
Albendazole kills parasites (tapeworms) by interfering with their metabolism.

## Uses:
To treat parenchymal neurocysticercosis (cysts in the brain tissue) caused by larval forms of the pork tapeworm, *Taenia solium.*

To treat cystic hydatid disease of the liver, lung, and peritoneum (lining of abdominal cavity) caused by the larval form of the dog tapeworm, *Echinococcus granulosus.*

Surgery is considered the treatment of choice for hydatid disease if medically feasible. When administering albendazole in the pre- or postsurgical setting, optimal killing of cyst contents is achieved when 3 courses of therapy have been given.

## Precautions:
*Do not use in the following situations:* Allergy to albendazole, benzimidazoles (eg, mebendazole), or any of their ingredients.

*Use with caution in the following situations:* Liver disease.

*Pregnancy:* There are no adequate and well-controlled studies in pregnant women. Use in pregnant women only when no alternative therapy is available. If a patient becomes pregnant during therapy, discontinue albendazole immediately. Patients should not become pregnant for at least 1 month after stopping albendazole therapy.

*Breastfeeding:* It is not known if albendazole appears in breast milk. Consult your doctor before you begin breastfeeding.

*Children:* Safety and effectiveness in children younger than 6 years of age have not been established. Albendazole has been used safely and effectively in a small number of infants and children.

*Lab tests* will be required periodically during treatment. Tests may include white blood cell counts, liver function tests, and theophylline blood levels.

## Drug Interactions:

Tell your doctor or pharmacist if you are taking or planning to take any over-the-counter or prescription medications or dietary supplements with albendazole. Doses of one or both drugs may need to be modified or a different drug may need to be prescribed. The following drugs or drug classes interact with albendazole:

cimetidine (eg, *Tagamet*)
dexamethasone (eg, *Decadron*)
praziquantel (*Biltricide*)

## Side Effects:

Every drug is capable of producing side effects. Many albendazole users experience no, or minor, side effects. The frequency and severity of side effects depend on many factors including dose, duration of therapy, and individual susceptibility. Possible side effects include:

*Nervous System:* Headache; dizziness; vertigo (feeling of whirling motion).

*Digestive Tract:* Stomach pain; nausea; vomiting.

*Other:* Fever; hair loss (temporary); decreased white blood cell count; abnormal liver function tests; meningeal signs (eg, headache, stiff neck).

---

### Guidelines for Use:

- Dosage is individualized. Take exactly as prescribed.
- Do not change the dose or stop taking unless directed by your doctor.
- Usual dose is twice daily. Take with food to increase absorption and effectiveness.
- If a dose is missed, take it as soon as possible. If several hours have passed or it is nearing time for the next dose, do not double the dose to catch up, unless advised to do so by your doctor. If more than one dose is missed or it is necessary to establish a new dosage schedule, contact your doctor or pharmacist.
- Inform your doctor if you are pregnant, become pregnant, plan on becoming pregnant, or are breastfeeding before beginning therapy. Albendazole may cause fetal harm. Begin treatment only after a negative pregnancy test has been conducted in women of childbearing age. Patients should not become pregnant for at least 1 month following cessation of albendazole.
- Women of childbearing age should use effective contraception during therapy.
- May cause dizziness. Use caution while driving or performing other tasks requiring alertness, coordination, or physical dexterity.
- Patients being treated for neurocysticercosis may require oral or injectable steroid and anticonvulsant therapy.
- Lab tests will be required to monitor therapy. Blood counts and liver function tests will be performed at the start of each 28-day treatment cycle and every 2 weeks during each 28-day cycle. Be sure to keep appointments.
- Store at a controlled room temperature (68° to 77°F).

---

*If you have any questions, consult your doctor, pharmacist, or health care provider.*

| Generic Name *Brand Name Examples* | Supplied As | Generic Available |
|---|---|---|
| *Rx* **Mebendazole** *Vermox* | **Tablets, chewable:** 100 mg | Yes |

## Type of Drug:

Drug for intestinal worms.

## How the Drug Works:

Mebendazole kills parasitic worms by blocking glucose (sugar uptake), thus depleting glycogen stored in the parasite. Without glycogen as an energy source, the parasite cannot reproduce or survive.

## Uses:

To treat parasitic infections such as pinworm (Enterobiasis), common roundworm (Ascariasis), common hookworm (*Ancyclostoma duodenale*), American hookworm (*Necator americanus*) and whipworm (Trichuriasis).

Effectiveness depends on pre-existing diarrhea, gastrointestinal transit time, degree of infection and type of parasite.

## Precautions:

*Do not use in the following situations:* Allergy to this medicine.

*Pregnancy:* Adequate studies have not been done in pregnant women, or animal studies may have shown a risk to the fetus. This drug is not recommended for use in pregnant women, especially during the first trimester. Use only if clearly needed and potential benefits outweigh the possible hazards to the fetus.

*Breastfeeding:* It is not known if mebendazole appears in breast milk. Contact your doctor before beginning breastfeeding.

*Children:* Safety and effectiveness is not established for children under 2 years of age.

## Drug Interactions:

Tell your doctor or pharmacist if you are taking or if you are planning to take any over-the-counter or prescription medications. Doses of one or both drugs may need to be modified or a different drug may need to be prescribed. The following drugs and drug classes may interact with this medicine.

carbamazepine (eg, *Tegretol*)  hydantoins (eg, phenytoin)
cimetidine (eg, *Tagamet*)

## Side Effects:

Every drug is capable of producing side effects. Many patients experience no, or minor, side effects. The frequency and severity of side effects depend on many factors including dose, duration of therapy and individual susceptibility. Possible side effects include stomach pain and diarrhea.

## Guidelines for Use:

- Use exactly as prescribed. Doses vary according to type of parasite.
- The tablets may be chewed, swallowed or crushed and mixed with food.
- Parasite death may be slow. Removal from digestive tract may take up to 3 days after treatment. Effectiveness depends of factors such as degree of infection or resistance of parasites to treatment, presence of diarrhea and how quickly things pass through the digestive system.
- Laxative therapy and fasting are not necessary.
- *Adults and children* — One tablet morning and evening for 3 consecutive days when treating hookworm, roundworm, and whipworm. The pinworm dose is a single table given once.
- If a dose is missed, take it as soon as possible. If several hours have passed or if it is nearing time for the next dose, do not double the dose in order to "catch up" (unless advised to do so by your doctor). If more than one dose is missed or it is necessary to establish a new dosage schedule, contact your doctor or pharmacist.
- If not cured in 3 weeks, a second treatment is recommended.
- Inform your doctor if you are pregnant, become pregnant, are planning to become pregnant, or if you are breastfeeding.
- Pinworm infections are easily spread to others. If one family member has a pinworm infection, treat all family members in close contact with the patient. This decreases the chance of spreading the infection.
- Strict hygiene is essential to prevent reinfection. Disinfect toilets daily. Change and wash underwear, bed linens, towels and nightclothes daily. Wash hands before eating.
- Store at controlled room temperature (59° to 86°F).

*If you have any questions, consult your doctor, pharmacist, or health care provider.*

| Generic Name<br>*Brand Name Examples* | How Supplied | Generic<br>Available |
|---|---|---|
| *otc* **Pyrantel** | | |
| *Pin-Rid, Reese's Pinworm* | **Capsules, soft gel:** 180 mg | No |
| *Antiminth* | **Oral Suspension:** 50 mg/mL | No |
| *Pin-Rid, Pin-X, Reese's Pinworm* | **Liquid:** 50 mg/mL | No |

## Type of Drug:
Drug for intestinal worms.

## How the Drug Works:
Pyrantel paralyzes the nervous system of the intestinal parasites (worms). Muscles of the worm do not function properly and the worms separate from the intestine. The worms are then eliminated from the body during bowel movements.

## Uses:
To treat pinworm infection (enterobiasis).

## Precautions:
*Do not use in the following situations:*
    allergy to this medicine
    liver disease
    pregnancy

*Pregnancy:* Do not use during pregnancy unless otherwise directed by your doctor.

*Children:* Safety and effectiveness is not established for children under 2 years of age.

## Drug Interactions:
Tell your doctor or pharmacist if you are taking or are planning to take any over-the-counter or prescription medications while taking this medicine. Doses of one or both drugs may need to be modified or a different drug may need to be prescribed. Theophylline (eg, *Theo-Dur*) may interact with this medicine.

## Side Effects:
Every drug is capable of producing side effects. Many patients experience no, or minor, side effects. The frequency and severity of side effects depend on many factors including dose, duration of therapy and individual susceptibility. Possible side effects include:

*Digestive Tract:* Nausea; vomiting; diarrhea; stomach ache and cramps; appetite loss.

*Nervous System:* Headache; dizziness; drowsiness; sleeplessness.

*Other:* Rash; fever.

## Guidelines for Use:

- Use exactly as prescribed. Follow the guidelines in the patient information available with this medicine.
- A single dose is required. The dose is based on body weight.
- May be taken with food, milk, juice or on an empty stomach anytime during the day. Be certain to take the entire dose.
- Using a laxative after taking the drug to facilitate removal of the parasites is not necessary.
- Pinworm infections are easily spread to others. If one family member has a pinworm infection, treat all family member in close contact with the patient. This deceases the chance of spreading the infection.
- Strict hygiene is essential to prevent reinfection. Disinfect toilet seats and bath tubs daily. Change and wash underwear, bed linens, towels and nightclothes at the time of treatment.
- Children should take morning showers to remove any pinworm eggs deposited at night.
- Trim an infected child's nails and wash hands frequently, especially before meals and after using the toilet.
- Store at controlled room temperature (59° to 86°F).

*If you have any questions, consult your doctor, pharmacist, or health care provider.*

| Generic Name<br>*Brand Name Examples* | Supplied As | Generic<br>Available |
|---|---|---|
| *Rx* **Thiabendazole** | | |
| *Mintezol* | **Tablets, chewable:** 500 mg | No |
| *Mintezol* | **Oral Suspension:** 500 mg/tsp | No |

## Type of Drug:
Drug for intestinal worms.

## How the Drug Works:
The exact mechanism of thiabendazole is not known, but it kills intestinal parasites, suppresses egg or larvae production and may inhibit the subsequent development of those eggs or larvae that are passed in the stools.

## Uses:
To treat parasitic worms including pinworm (enterobiasis), threadworm (strongyloidiasis), large roundworm (ascariasis), hookworm (uncinariasis), whipworm (trichuriasis), creeping eruption (cutaneous larva migrans) and visceral larva migrans.

To alleviate symptoms of trichinosis during the invasion phase.

## Precautions:
*Do not use in the following situations:* Allergy to this medicine.

*Use with caution in the following situations:*

| | |
|---|---|
| anemia | liver disease |
| dehydration (fluid loss) | malnutrition |
| kidney disease | |

*Pregnancy:* Adequate studies have not been done in pregnant women. Use only if clearly needed and potential benefits outweigh the possible hazards to the fetus.

*Breastfeeding:* It is not known if thiabendazole appears in breast milk. Contact your doctor before you begin breastfeeding.

*Children:* Safety and effectiveness are not established in children weighing less than 30 pounds.

*Lab tests* may be required. Lab tests may include liver function tests.

## Drug Interactions:
Xanthines (eg, theophylline) interact with this medicine.

## Side Effects:

Every drug can produce side effects. The frequency or severity of side effects depend on dose, duration of therapy and individual susceptibility. Side effects may include:

*Digestive Tract:* Nausea; vomiting; diarrhea; stomach pain; appetite loss.

*Nervous System:* Dizziness; tiredness; drowsiness; giddiness; headache; numbness; irritability; convulsions; collapse; psychic disturbances.

*Skin:* Itching; rectal rash; hives; redness; facial flushing; yellowing of skin or eyes.

*Other:* Blood or crystals in urine; bedwetting; asparagus-like odor of urine; fever; chills; eye irritation; blurred vision; vision changes (objects appearing yellow); dry mouth and eyes; ringing in the ears; difficulty breathing; low blood pressure; high blood sugar levels.

## Guidelines for Use:

- Use exactly as prescribed.
- May cause stomach upset; take with food.
- Usual dose is twice daily. Dosage is determined by the patient's weight.
- *Tablets* — Chew thoroughly before swallowing.
- *Oral Suspension* — Shake well before use.
- Dietary restrictions or cleansing enemas are not needed.
- Duration of therapy varies from 2 or more days depending upon the condition being treated.
- If a dose is missed, take it as soon as possible. If several hours have passed or if it is nearing time for the next dose, do not double the dose in order to "catch up" (unless advised to do so by your doctor). If more than one dose is missed or it is necessary to establish a new dosage schedule, contact your doctor or pharmacist.
- Strict hygiene is essential to prevent reinfection. Disinfect toilets daily. Change and wash underwear, bed linens, towels and nightclothes daily.
- Pinworm infections are easily spread to others. If one family member has a pinworm infection, treat all family members in close contact with the patient. This decreases the chance of spreading the infection.
- *Pinworm infections* — Repeat therapy in 7 days to prevent reinfection.
- May produce drowsiness or dizziness. Use caution when driving or performing other tasks requiring alertness, coordination or physical dexterity.
- Store tablets and suspension in well closed containers at room temperature.

*If you have any questions, consult your doctor, pharmacist, or health care provider.*

| Generic Name Brand Name Examples | Supplied As | Generic Available |
|---|---|---|
| Rx **Ivermectin** | | |
| *Stromectol* | **Tablets:** 6 mg | No |

## Type of Drug:
Anthelmintic (antiparasitic) agent.

## How the Drug Works:
Ivermectin causes paralysis of the nerve and muscle cells of certain parasitic worms.

## Uses:
To treat strongyloidiasis of the intestinal tract and to treat onchocerciasis.

## Precautions:
*Do not use in the following situations:* allergy to drug or any ingredients

*Use with caution in the following situations:* immunocompromised hosts

*Pregnancy:* Adequate studies have not been done in pregnant women; animal studies may have shown a risk to the fetus. Use only if clearly needed and potential benefits outweigh the possible hazards to the fetus.

*Breastfeeding:* Ivermectin appears in breast milk. Consult your doctor before breastfeeding.

*Children:* Safety and effectiveness in children weighing less than 33 lbs is not established.

## Drug Interactions:
Tell your doctor or pharmacist if you are taking or planning to take any over-the-counter or prescription medications while taking this medicine. Doses of one or both drugs may need to be modified or a different drug may need to be prescribed.

## Side Effects:
Every drug is capable of producing side effects. Many patients experience no, or minor, side effects. The frequency and severity of side effects depend on many factors including dose, duration of therapy and individual susceptibility. Side effects may include: Fast heartbeat; itching; rash; skin disorder; abnormal sensation in eyes; swelling of eyelids; eye inflammation/redness; enlarged and tender lymph nodes; joint pain and swelling; fever; facial swelling; swelling of arms and legs; headache; muscle pain; diarrhea; nausea; dizziness; dizziness or lightheadedness when rising quickly from a sitting or lying position.

**Guidelines for Use:**

- Take as a single oral dose with a full glass of water.
- The dose is based on body weight. Take the prescribed number of tablets.
- *Strongyloidiasis* — Repeated stool examinations are recommended.
- *Onchocerciasis* — Treatment with ivermectin does not kill adult onchocerca parasites and repeated follow-up and retreatment is usually required.
- Lab tests will be required to monitor treatment. Be sure to keep appointments.
- Store at temperatures below 86°F.

*If you have any questions, consult your doctor, pharmacist, or health care provider.*

| Generic Name<br>*Brand Name Examples* | Supplied As | Generic<br>Available |
|---|---|---|
| Rx **Methenamine Hippurate** | | |
| *Hiprex*[1], *Urex* | **Tablets:** 1 g | No |
| Rx **Methenamine Mandelate** | | |
| *Mandelamine* | **Tablets, film coated:** 0.5 g, 1 g | Yes |

[1] Contains the dye tartrazine.

## Type of Drug:

Urinary anti-infective drugs.

## How the Drug Works:

Methenamine is broken down in acid urine to produce ammonia and formaldehyde. Formaldehyde kills certain bacteria in the urine. The salt forms of methenamine (mandelate and hippurate) are acid salts and help keep the urine acidic. An acid urine increases the effectiveness of methenamine.

## Uses:

For long-term therapy to suppress or eliminate bacteria in the urine that cause certain urinary tract infections after the use of other antimicrobial drugs.

## Precautions:

*Do not use in the following situations:*
>      allergy to the drug
>      concurrent use of sulfonamides
>      dehydration, severe (fluid loss)
>      kidney disease
>      liver disease

*Use with caution in the following situations:*
>      acid urine cannot be maintained
>      elderly, debilitated or people susceptible to lipid pneumonia

*Active infection:* Methenamine does not treat urinary tract infections; it only prevents recurrent infections. Use only after a urinary tract infection has been treated with other antibiotics.

*Pregnancy:* Adequate studies have not been done in pregnant women. Use only if clearly needed and potential benefits outweigh the possible hazards to the fetus.

*Breastfeeding:* Methenamine appears in breast milk. Consult your doctor before you begin breastfeeding.

*Lab tests* are required during therapy. Be sure to keep appointments. Tests will include liver function studies and repeated urine cultures.

*Tartrazine:* Some of these products may contain the dye tartrazine (FD&C Yellow No. 5) which can cause allergic reactions in certain individuals. Check package label when available or consult your doctor or pharmacist.

## Drug Interactions:

Tell your doctor or pharmacist if you are taking or if you are planning to take any over-the-counter or prescription medications with methenamine. Doses of one or both drugs may need to be modified or a different drug may need to be prescribed. The following drugs and drug classes interact with methenamine:

potassium citrate (eg, *Urocit-K*)
sodium acetate
sodium bicarbonate
sodium citrate

sodium lactate
sulfonamides (eg, sulfamethi-zole)
tromethamine (eg, *Tham*)

## Side Effects:

Every drug is capable of producing side effects. Many methenamine users experience no, or minor, side effects. The frequency and severity of side effects depend on many factors including dose, duration of therapy and individual susceptibility. Possible side effects include:

*Urinary and Reproductive Tract:* Urination problems; blood or protein in urine.

*Digestive Tract:* Nausea; upset stomach; vomiting; stomach cramps.

*Skin:* Rash; itching.

---

### Guidelines for Use:

- Take as directed by your doctor. The daily dose varies depending on individual needs. Do not adjust the dose without consulting your pharmacist or doctor.
- Take the full course of therapy to ensure best results. Do not stop the drug without consulting your doctor.
- It may be necessary to attempt to acidify the urine in order to get the best clinical response. Ascorbic acid (vitamin C) at doses of 2 g/day or administration of 8 to 12 g of ammonium chloride per day may acidify the urine. Intake of cranberries, plums, prunes, or cranberry juice may help slightly in producing an acid urine.
- Avoid heavy intake of medications such as bicarbonate and acetazolamide. They may change the urine from acid to alkaline.
- Large doses (up to 8 g/day for 3 to 4 weeks) may cause bladder irritation, painful and frequent urination, and protein or blood in the urine.
- Notify your doctor if rash, urination problems or severe stomach upset occurs.
- Lab tests will be required and may include urine cultures and liver enzymes. Keep appointments.
- Store at controlled room temperature (59° to 86°F). Protect from light.

---

*If you have any questions, consult your doctor, pharmacist, or health care provider.*

| Generic Name Brand Name Examples | Supplied As | Generic Available |
|---|---|---|
| Rx **Fosfomycin Trometh-amine** | | |
| *Monurol* | **Single-dose sachet:** 3 g | No |

## Type of Drug:
Urinary tract anti-infective.

## How the Drug Works:
Fosfomycin inhibits bacterial cell wall reproduction and reduces bacteria from adhering to cells lining the urinary tract.

## Uses:
To treat uncomplicated urinary tract infections in women caused by suscep-tible bacteria.

## Precautions:
*Do not use in the following situations:*
allergy to the drug

*Use with caution in the following situations:*
acute cystitis                          kidney disease

*Pregnancy:* Fosfomycin does cross the placenta. Studies in pregnant women or in animals have been judged not to show a risk to the fetus. However, no drug should be used during pregnancy unless clearly needed.

*Breastfeeding:* It is not known if fosfomycin tromethamine appears in breast milk. Consult your doctor before you begin breastfeeding.

*Children:* Safety and effectiveness in children less than 12 years of age have not been established.

## Drug Interactions:
Tell your doctor or pharmacist if you are taking or planning to take any over-the-counter or prescription medications while taking this medicine. Doses of one or both drugs may need to be modified or a different drug may need to be prescribed. Metoclopramide (eg, *Reglan*) may interact with this medicine.

## Side Effects:
Every drug is capable of producing side effects. Many patients experience no, or minor, side effects. The frequency and severity of side effects depend on many factors including dose, duration of therapy and indi-vidual susceptibility. Possible side effects include: Diarrhea; nausea; indi-gestion; sore throat; abdominal pain; dizziness; nasal congestion; runny nose; inflammation of the vagina; painful menstruation; rash; head-ache; weakness; back pain; pain.

## Guidelines for Use:

- May be taken with or without food.
- Recommended dosage is 1 packet.
- The packet should not be taken in its dry form. Mix with 3 to 4 oz of cold water before ingesting. (Do not use hot water.) Take immediately after dissolving in water.
- If symptoms do not improve 2 to 3 days after taking fosfomycin tromethamine, contact the healthcare provider.
- Do not use more than one single dose to treat a single occurrence of minor urinary tract infection. Repeated daily doses did not improve clinical success, but did increase the incidence of side effects.
- Store at controlled room temperature (59° to 86°F).

*If you have any questions, consult your doctor, pharmacist, or health care provider.*

| Generic Name<br>*Brand Name Examples* | Supplied As | Generic<br>Available |
|---|---|---|
| *Rx* **Nalidixic Acid** | | |
| *NegGram* | **Caplets:** 250 mg, 500 mg, 1 g | No |
| *NegGram* | **Suspension:** 250 mg/5 mL | No |

## Type of Drug:

Urinary tract anti-infection drug.

## How the Drug Works:

Nalidixic acid interferes with DNA formation in certain bacteria.

## Uses:

To treat urinary tract infections caused by susceptible bacteria.

## Precautions:

*Do not use in the following situations:*
> allergy to nalidixic acid
> seizures, history of

*Use with caution in the following situations:*
> cerebral arteriosclerosis (hardening of the arteries)
> epilepsy
> glucose-6-phosphate dehydrogenase (G-6-PD) deficiency
> insufficient blood flow to brain
> kidney disease
> liver disease
> parkinsonism
> photosensitivity to drugs, history (light sensitivity)

*Lab Tests:* Blood counts and liver and kidney function tests may be required periodically if treatment continues for more than 2 weeks.

*Pregnancy:* Adequate studies have not been done in pregnant women; animal studies may have shown a risk to the fetus. Use only if clearly needed and potential benefits outweigh possible hazards to the fetus.

*Breastfeeding:* It is not known if nalidixic acid appears in breast milk. Consult your doctor before you begin breastfeeding.

*Children:* Use with caution. Not recommended for children under 3 months of age.

## Drug Interactions:

Tell your doctor or pharmacist if you are taking or if you are planning to take any over-the-counter or prescription medications with nalidixic acid. Doses of one or both drugs may need to be modified or a different drug may need to be prescribed. Drugs that interact with nalidixic acid include:

> antacids (eg, *Maalox*)
> caffeine (eg, *NoDoz*)
> iron (eg, *Feosol*)
> nitrofurantoin (eg, *Macrodantin*)
> oral anticoagulants (eg, *Coumadin*)
> sucralfate (eg, *Carafate*)
> theophylline (eg, *TheoDur*)
> zinc

## Side Effects:

Every drug is capable of producing side effects. Many nalidixic acid users experience no, or minor, side effects. The frequency and severity of side effects depend on many factors including dose, duration of therapy and individual susceptibility. Possible side effects include:

*Digestive Tract:* Nausea; vomiting; diarrhea; stomachache; infectious colitis.

*Nervous System:* Drowsiness; weakness; dizziness; headache; feeling of whirling motion; convulsions.

*Skin:* Itching; rash; hives.

*Other:* Joint pain, swelling and stiffness; eye and skin sensitivity to light; difficulty focusing; double vision; decreased visual acuity; yellowing of skin or eyes; change in color perception; blood disorder.

---

### Guidelines for Use:

- May be taken with or without food. Take with food if GI upset occurs.
- Drink fluids liberally. Do not take with antacids.
- Administer to adults and children in 4 equally divided doses per day.
- May cause drowsiness, dizziness or lightheadedness, or blurred vision. Use caution when driving or performing other tasks requiring alertness, coordination, or physical dexterity.
- *Sensitivity to sunlight* — Nalidixic acid may cause sensitivity to the sun and other sources of ultraviolet light. Avoid prolonged exposure to the sun and artificial ultraviolet lights. Use sunscreens and wear protective clothing if exposure cannot be avoided. Discontinue therapy if phototoxicity occurs.
- If seizures, diarrhea (possible pseudomembranous colitis), skin rash or other signs of allergic reaction occur while taking nalidixic acid, contact your doctor immediately.
- Use OTC caffeine-containing products and caffeinated beverages cautiously while taking nalidixic acid. Increased caffeine effects (eg, tremors, rapid heartbeat, sleeplessness) may occur.
- Store at room temperature. While the suspension does not need to be refrigerated, it may be chilled to improve the taste. Avoid freezing the suspension.

---

*If you have any questions, consult your doctor, pharmacist, or health care provider.*

| Generic Name<br>*Brand Name Examples* | **Suplied As** | Generic<br>Available |
|---|---|---|
| *Rx* **Nitrofurantoin** | | |
| *Macrobid* | **Capsules:** 25 mg | No |
| *Furadantin* | **Oral Suspension:** 25 mg/tsp | No |
| *Rx* **Nitrofurantoin**<br>**Macrocrystals** | | |
| *Macrodantin* | **Capsules:** 25 mg, 50 mg,<br>100 mg | Yes |

## Type of Drug:

Urinary anti-infective.

## How the Drug Works:

Nitrofurantoin interferes with metabolism and protein synthesis, and may also disrupt cell wall formation in susceptible bacteria.

## Uses:

To treat urinary tract infections caused by susceptible bacteria.

## Precautions:

*Do not use in the following situations:*

allergy to nitrofurantoin
infants under 1 month of age
labor and delivery, during
kidney disease
pregnant women at term

*Use with caution in the following situations:*

anemia
diabetes
electrolyte imbalance
glucose-6-phosphate dehydrogenase (G-6-PD) deficiency
vitamin B deficiency

*Superinfection:* Use of antibiotics (especially prolonged or repeated therapy) may result in bacterial or fungal overgrowth. Such overgrowth may lead to a second infection. Nitrofurantoin may need to be stopped and another antibiotic prescribed for the second infection.

*Lab tests:* Lab tests may be required to monitor therapy. Be sure to keep appointments.

*Pregnancy:* Studies in pregnant woman or in animals have been judged not to show a risk to the fetus, except late in pregnancy. However, no drug should be used during pregnancy unless clearly needed. Do not use in pregnant women at term, or during labor and delivery.

*Breastfeeding:* Nitrofurantoin appears in breast milk. Consult your doctor before you begin breastfeeding.

*Children:* Safety and effectiveness have not been established for children under 12 years of age. Do not use in children less than 1 month old.

## Drug Interactions:

Tell your doctor or pharmacist if you are taking or if you are planning to take any over-the-counter or prescription medications while taking this medicine. Doses of one or both drugs may need to be modified or a different drug may need to be prescribed. The following drugs and drug classes interact with this medicine.

anticholinergics (eg, atropine)          probenecid (eg, *Benemid*)
magnesium salts (eg, antacids)       sulfinpyrazone (eg, *Anturane*)

## Side Effects:

Every drug is capable of producing side effects. Many patients experience no, or minor, side effects. The frequency and severity of side effects depend on many factors including dose, duration of therapy and individual susceptibility. Possible side effects include:

*Digestive Tract:* Nausea; vomiting; gas; appetite loss; stomach ache; indigestion; constipation; diarrhea; inflammation of the salivary glands or the mouth.

*Nervous System:* Headache; dizziness; drowsiness; weakness; vertigo (feeling of whirling motion); tingling or numbness in hands or feet; confusion; depression.

*Skin:* Rash; redness; itching; hives; temporary hair loss; light sensitivity.

*Other:* Asthma; difficult breathing; cough; fever; chills; muscle or joint pain; swelling; changes in heartbeat; vision problems; rapid eye movement; yellowing of eyes or skin; general body discomfort; anemia; abnormal lab and blood values.

## Guidelines for Use:

- *Macrodantin Capsules, Furadantin Oral Solution* - Usual dose is 4 times a day, with meals and at bedtime.
- *Macrobid Macrocrystals* - Usual dose is 1 capsule every 12 hours for 7 days.
- May cause stomach upset; take with food or milk.
- Shake suspension well before use.
- Many patients who cannot tolerate the macrocrystals *(Macrobid)* are able to take *Macrodantin* without nausea.
- Avoid antacids containing magnesium (eg, *Maalox*) while taking this medicine.
- If a dose is missed, take it as soon as possible. If several hours have passed or it is nearing time for the next dose, do not double the dose in order to "catch up," unless advised by your doctor. If more than one dose is missed, contact your doctor or pharmacist.
- Continue use until all of the prescribed medicine has been taken, even if fever or other symptoms of infection have disappeared. Failure to take all of the medicine may prevent complete elimination of bacteria, allowing the infection to return.
- Use of antibiotics (especially prolonged or repeated therapy) may result in bacterial or fungal overgrowth. Such overgrowth may lead to a second infection. Nitrofurantoin may need to be stopped and another antibiotic prescribed for the second infection.
- If severe diarrhea, stomach pain/cramps or bloody stools occur, contact your doctor immediately. This could be a sign of a serious side effect requiring immediate medical attention. Do not treat diarrhea without consulting your doctor.
- Contact your doctor immediately if numbness or tingling in feet or hands, fever, chills, cough, chest pain, difficulty breathing, skin rash, general body discomfort, or severe stomach upset occurs.
- A brownish discoloration of the urine may occur. This is normal.
- This medicine may cause a false-positive reaction for glucose in the urine.
- Lab tests may be required to monitor therapy. Be sure to keep appointments.
- Exposure to strong light may darken the oral solution. Protect from light.
- Store at room temperature (59° to 86°F), away from light.

*If you have any questions, consult your doctor, pharmacist, or health care provider.*

| Generic Name<br>*Brand Name Examples* | Supplied As | Generic<br>Available |
|---|---|---|
| *Rx* **Sulfonamide Combinations** | | |
| *Urobiotic-250* | **Capsules:** 250 mg sulfamethizole, 250 mg oxytetracycline, 50 mg phenazopyridine HCl | No |
| *Azo-Sulfisoxazole* | **Tablets:** 500 mg sulfisoxazole, 50 mg phenazopyridine HCl | Yes |
| *Bactrim[1], Cotrim, Septra[1]* | **Tablets:** 400 mg sulfamethoxazole, 80 mg trimethoprim | Yes |
| *Bactrim DS, Cotrim DS, Septra DS* | **Tablets, double strength:** 800 mg sulfamethoxazole, 160 mg trimethoprim | Yes |
| *Bactrim Pediatric, Cotrim Pediatric, Septra, Sulfatrim* | **Oral Suspension:** 200 mg sulfamethoxazole, 40 mg trimethoprim/tsp | Yes |
| *Rx* **Methenamine Combinations** | | |
| *Trac Tabs 2X* | **Tablets:** 120 mg methenamine, 30 mg phenyl salicylate, 0.06 mg atropine sulfate, 0.03 mg hyoscyamine sulfate, 7.5 mg benzoic acid, 6 mg methylene blue | No |
| *Prosed/DS* | **Tablets:** 81.6 mg methenamine, 36.2 mg phenyl salicylate, 10.8 mg methylene blue, 9 mg benzoic acid, 0.06 mg atropine sulfate, 0.06 mg hyoscyamine sulfate | No |
| *Urimar-T, Urogesic Blue* | **Tablets:** 81.6 mg methenamine, 40.8 mg sodium biphosphate, 36.2 mg phenyl salicylate, 10.8 mg methylene blue, 0.12 mg hyoscyamine sulfate | No |
| *Uro-Phosphate* | **Tablets:** 300 mg methenamine, 434.78 mg sodium biphosphate | No |
| *Uroquid-Acid No. 2* | **Tablets:** 500 mg methenamine mandelate, 500 mg sodium acid phosphate monohydrate | No |
| *Urisedamine* | **Tablets:** 500 mg methenamine mandelate, 0.15 mg hyoscyamine | No |

| Generic Name<br>*Brand Name Examples* | Supplied As | Generic<br>Available |
|---|---|---|
| **Methenamine Combinations (cont.)** | | |
| Rx *Atrosept, Dolsed, UAA, Uridon Modified, Urinary Antiseptic No. 2, Urised, Uritin* | **Tablets:** 40.8 mg methen-amine, 18.1 mg phenyl salicy-late, 0.03 mg atropine sulfate, 0.03 mg hyoscyamine (as sul-fate), 4.5 mg benzoic acid, 5.4 mg methylene blue | Yes |
| otc *Cystex* | **Tablets:** 162 mg methenamine, 162.5 mg sodium salicylate, benzoic acid | No |

[1] Also available as an injection.

For further information, see methenamine and methenamine salts; sulfon-amides; tetracycline and oxytetracycline; trimethoprim (TMP); sulfamethox-azole and trimethoprim combinations (TMP-SMZ).

## Type of Drug:

Urinary anti-infective combinations.

## Uses:

For relief of frequent, painful, or burning urination. To treat urinary tract infections caused by susceptible bacteria.

*Methenamine* is an anti-infective and acidifies the urine.

*Phenazopyridine HCl, sodium salicylate, and phenyl salicylate* are pain relievers.

*Belladonna alkaloids* (eg, atropine, hyoscyamine) relieve urinary tract spasms.

*Sodium biphosphate (sodium acid phosphate) and benzoic acid* acidify the urine.

## Guidelines for Use:

- Use exactly as prescribed.
- Take each dose with a full glass of water. Drink plenty of fluids while taking these drugs.
- *OTC Products* – Do not use without first talking to your doctor if you are pregnant or breastfeeding or if this is the first time you have had urinary tract infection symptoms (eg, frequent or burning urination). Discontinue use when symptoms subside. If symptoms do not get better in 5 days, discontinue use and consult your doctor.
- *Oral Suspension* – Shake well before use.
- If a dose is missed, take it as soon as possible. If several hours have passed or if it is nearing time for the next dose, do not double the dose in order to catch up, unless advised by your doctor. If more than one dose is missed, contact your doctor or pharmacist.
- Continue use until all of the prescribed medicine has been taken, even if fever or other symptoms have disappeared. Failure to take all of the medicine may prevent complete elimination of bacteria, allowing the infection to return.
- Notify your doctor if rash, hives, sore throat, fever, chills, pale skin, yellowing of skin or eyes, rash, or unusual bleeding or bruising occurs.
- *Superinfection* – Use of antibiotics (especially prolonged or repeated therapy) may result in bacterial or fungal overgrowth (secondary infections). This medicine may need to be stopped and another antibiotic prescribed for the second infection.
- Some of these products may cause sensitivity to sunlight. Avoid prolonged exposure to the sun or other forms of ultraviolet (UV) light (eg, tanning beds). Use sunscreens and wear protective clothing until tolerance is determined.
- Some of these products contain sulfonamides. Consult your doctor or pharmacist if you are allergic to sulfonamides.
- Lab tests may be required to monitor treatment. Be sure to keep appointments.
- Store at room temperature (59° to 86°F); protect from moisture and light.

*If you have any questions, consult your doctor, pharmacist, or health care provider.*

| Generic Name<br>*Brand Name Examples* | Supplied As | Generic<br>Available |
|---|---|---|
| Rx **Capreomycin** | | |
| *Capastat Sulfate* | **Powder for Injection:** 1 g/vial | No |
| Rx **Cycloserine** | | |
| *Seromycin Pulvules* | **Capsules:** 250 mg | No |
| Rx **Ethambutol Hydrochloride** | | |
| *Myambutol* | **Tablets:** 100 mg, 400 mg | No |
| Rx **Ethionamide** | | |
| *Trecator-SC* | **Tablets:** 250 mg | No |
| Rx **Isoniazid (INH)** | **Tablets:** 100 mg, 300 mg | Yes |
| | **Syrup:** 50 mg/5 mL | Yes |
| *Nydrazid* | **Injection:** 100 mg/mL | Yes |
| Rx **Isoniazid w/Rifampin** | | |
| *Rifamate* | **Capsules:** 150 mg isoniazid and 300 mg rifampin | No |
| Rx **Pyrazinamide** | **Tablets:** 500 mg | Yes |
| Rx **Rifabutin** | | |
| *Mycobutin* | **Capsules:** 150 mg | No |
| Rx **Rifampin** | | |
| *Rifadin* | **Capsules:** 150 mg, 300 mg | No |
| *Rimactane* | **Capsules:** 300 mg | No |
| *Rifadin* | **Injection:** 600 mg/vial | No |
| Rx **Rifampin w/Isoniazid and Pyrazinamide** | | |
| *Rifater* | **Tablets:** 120 mg rifampin, 50 mg isoniazid, 300 mg pyrazinamide | No |
| Rx **Rifapentine** | | |
| *Priftin* | **Tablets:** 150 mg | No |

## Type of Drug:
Drugs for treating tuberculosis (TB).

## How the Drug Works:
Antituberculosis agents kill or stop the growth of tuberculosis organisms. Many of these drugs must be used in combination with other antituberculosis drugs during therapy. Therapy with these agents is usually long-term.

## Uses:

*All (except Rifabutin):* To treat tuberculosis infections caused by susceptible organisms.

*Cycloserine:* To treat urinary tract infections caused by susceptible organisms when more conventional antibiotic therapy has failed.

*Isoniazid:* To prevent and to treat tuberculosis.

*Rifabutin:* To prevent spreading of *Mycobacterium avium* complex (MAC) disease in patients with advanced HIV infection.

*Rifampin:* To treat asymptomatic carriers of *Neisseria meningitidis.*

*Unlabeled Use(s):* Occasionally doctors may prescribe rifampin to treat certain infections (eg, Legionnaires' disease, leprosy, and to prevent meningitis due to *Haemophilus influenzae*). Isoniazid may be used to improve severe tremors in patients with multiple sclerosis.

## Precautions:

*Do not use in the following situations:*

> *All* — allergy to the drug or any of its ingredients
> *Cycloserine* — epilepsy; depression; severe anxiety; psychosis; severe kidney disease; excessive concurrent alcohol use
> *Ethambutol* — optic neuritis (inflammation of optic nerve)
> *Ethionamide* — severe liver disease and impairment
> *Isoniazid* — previous isoniazid-associated liver damage; other severe reactions to isoniazid (eg, fever, chills, arthritis); or liver disease of any etiology or cause
> *Pyrazinamide* — acute gout; severe liver damage
> *Rifabutin* — allergy to any other rifamycin; active tuberculosis
> *Rifapentine and Rifampin* — allergy to any other rifamycin

*Use with caution in the following situations:*

> *Capreomycin* – kidney disease; hearing impairment
> *Ethambutol* — kidney disease; cataracts, diabetic retinopathy, or other vision problems
> *Ethionamide* — diabetes mellitus
> *Isoniazid* — kidney or liver disease; daily users of alcohol; older than 35 years of age; chronically administered medicines, concurrent use; history of previous discontinuation of isoniazid; peripheral neuropathy, existence or conditions of; pregnancy; injectable drug abusers; post-partum women of minority groups; HIV-seropositive patients.
> *Pyrazinamide* — diabetes mellitus; liver disease; kidney disease; history of gout; increased risk of liver disease; elderly; daily users of alcohol
> *Rifampin* — liver disease
> *Rifapentine* — liver disease

*Hypersensitivity Reaction:* Allergic-type reactions may occur with the use of these drugs. Symptoms may include fever, rash, hives, swollen lymph nodes, itching, difficulty breathing, yellowing of the eyes or skin, and false blood or liver tests.

*Capreomycin:* Audiometric (hearing) measurements and assessments of vestibular function (balance) should be performed prior to initiation of therapy and at regular intervals during treatment.

*Cycloserine:* Patients receiving greater than 500 mg daily should be closely monitored. Anticonvulsant drugs or sedatives may be effective in controlling symptoms of CNS toxicity, such as convulsions, anxiety, and tremor. Toxicity is closely related to excessive blood levels. Risk of convulsions is increased in chronic alcoholics. Cycloserine blood level tests should be determined at least weekly for patients with kidney disease, individuals receiving daily dosage greater than 500 mg, and for those showing signs and symptoms of toxicity.

Vitamin $B_{12}$ and folic acid deficiencies and anemia have been associated with the use of cycloserine. Contact your doctor to determine if supplementation is required.

*Ethambutol:* Adverse effects on vision may occur with the use of ethambutol. Physical exams should include ophthalmoscopy, finger perimetry, and testing of color discrimination. Tests should be repeated periodically during therapy. Changes in visual activity may be in one or both eyes; therefore each eye must be tested separately and both eyes together. Any drug-induced changes in vision are generally reversible when the drug is discontinued. Changes in color perception are the first signs of toxicity. Contact your doctor if you experience any changes in vision. Renal function monitoring is encouraged.

*Ethionamide:* Diabetics may experience an increased difficulty in the management of diabetes. Adverse effects on vision may occur with use of ethionamide. Ophthalmic examinations should be performed before and periodically during therapy. Contact your doctor if you experience any changes in vision.

*Isoniazid:* Pyridoxine (vitamin $B_6$) deficiency is sometimes seen during treatment with isoniazid. Contact your doctor to determine if vitamin $B_6$ supplements are required. Ophthalmic examinations should be performed before and periodically during therapy. Contact your doctor if you experience any changes in vision.

*Pyrazinamide:* If high blood uric acid levels are accompanied by acute gouty arthritis, pyrazinamide should be discontinued. Diabetics may experience an increased difficulty in the management of diabetes.

*Rifabutin:* Rifabutin prophylaxis of MAC must not be used in patients with active tuberculosis. If active TB symptoms develop, contact your doctor immediately.

*Rifampin and Rifapentine:* If diarrhea develops during rifampin or rifapentine use, consider pseudomembranous colitis. This inflammatory condition of the colon is due to overgrowth of bacteria that are not killed by rifampin or rifapentine. The primary cause is a toxin produced by a bacteria known as *Clostridia difficile.* Colitis symptoms may range from mild to life-threatening. Mild cases usually respond by stopping the antibiotic. In more serious cases, another antibiotic may need to be prescribed.

*Rifapentine, rifabutin, and rifampin:* Urine, stool, saliva, sputum, sweat, and tears may be colored red-orange or reddish brown. This is not harmful. Soft contact lenses may be permanently stained.

*Pregnancy:* Safety for use during pregnancy has not been established for many of these medications. Therefore, routine use of these medications during pregnancy is not appropriate.

*Breastfeeding:* Isoniazid, pyrazinamide, and rifampin appear in breast milk. It is not known if other antituberculosis drugs appear in breast milk. Consult your doctor before you begin breastfeeding.

*Children:* Safety and effectiveness of capreomycin, cycloserine, and rifabutin have not been established. Rifampin with isoniazid and pyrazinamide is not recommended for use in children under 15 years of age. Ethambutol is not recommended for use in children under 13 years of age. Ethionamide and rifapentine is not recommended for use in children under 12 years of age. Isoniazid may be used in infants and children. Rifampin dosing is available for infants and children. Pyrazinamide appears to be well tolerated in children. Rifabutin has been used in a limited number of children (1 to 16 years of age) with HIV.

*Elderly:* Safety and dosage have not been sufficiently determined. However, in general, dose selection for elderly patients should be cautious, starting with the lowest effective dose.

*Lab tests* and periodic doctor visits may be required during treatment with these drugs. Tests may include eye examinations, liver and kidney function tests, blood counts, urine tests, blood electrolytes, uric acid tests, blood drug levels, and hearing and eye tests.

## Drug Interactions:

Tell your doctor or pharmacist if you are taking or if you are planning to take any over-the-counter or prescription medications with antituberculosis drugs. Doses of one or both drugs may need to be modified or a different drug may need to be prescribed. The following drugs and drug classes interact with antituberculosis drugs.

*All antituberculosis drugs* — alcohol

*Capreomycin* — injectable antituberculosis agents (eg, streptomycin, viomycin), nonantituberculosis antibiotics (eg, gentamicin)

*Cycloserine* — isoniazid (eg, *Nydrazid*), ethionamide

*Ethionamide* – isoniazid (eg, *Nydrazid*), cycloserine, excessive ethanol

*Isoniazid* —

acetaminophen (eg, *Tylenol*)
aluminum salts (eg, some antacids)
anticoagulants, oral (eg, warfarin)
benzodiazepines (eg, clonazepam)
carbamazepine (eg, *Tegretol*)
disulfiram (*Antabuse*)

enflurane (*Enthrane*)
hydantoins (eg, phenytoin)
ketoconazole *(Nizoral)*
meperidine (eg, *Demerol*)
primidone (eg, *Mysoline*)
rifampin (eg, *Rifadin*)
theophylline (eg, *Slo-Bid*)
valproate sodium (eg, *Depakote*)

*Pyrazinamide* — *Acetest* and *Ketostix* urine tests

*Rifabutin —*

cardiac glycosides (eg, digoxin)
narcotics (eg, methadone)

zidovudine (*Retrovir*)

Because of similarities between rifabutin, rifapentine, and rifampin, similar interactions may be expected. See rifampin interactions.

*Rifampin —*

analgesics, narcotics
(eg, methadone)
antacids (eg, *Maalox*)
antiarrhythmics (eg, disopyramide)
anticoagulants, oral (eg, warfarin)
anticonvulsants (eg, phenytoin)
azole antifungals (eg, fluconazole)
barbiturates (eg, phenobarbital)
benzodiazepines, (eg, diazepam)
beta blockers (eg, propranolol)
cardiac glycosides (eg, digoxin)
calcium channel blockers (eg,
diltiazem)
chloramphenicol (*Chloromycetin*)
clarithromycin (*Biaxin*)
clofibrate (eg, *Atromid-S*)
contraceptives, oral (eg, *Ortho-
Novum*)
corticosteroids (eg, prednisone)
co-trimoxazole (eg, *Bactrim*)
cyclosporine (eg, *Sandimmune*)

digitoxin (*Crystodigin*)
doxycycline (eg, *Vibramycin*)
enalapril (*Vasotec*)
estrogens (eg, estrone)
fluoroquinolones (eg, ciprofloxacin)
haloperidol (eg, *Haldol*)
halothane (eg, *Fluothane*)
hydantoins (eg, phenytoin)
isoniazid (eg, *Nydrazid*)
mexiletine *(Mexitil)*
probenecid
progestins (eg, *Provera*)
propafenone (*Rythmol*)
quinidine (eg, *Quinora*)
sulfasalazine (eg, *Azulfidine*)
sulfones (eg, dapsone)
sulfonylureas (eg, tolbutamide)
tacrolimus (*Prograf*)
theophylline (eg, *Theo-Dur*)
thyroid drugs (eg, levothyroxine)
tocainide *(Tonocard)*
tricyclic antidepressants
(eg, nortriptyline)
zidovudine (*Retrovir*)

*Rifapentine —*

contraceptives, oral (eg, *Ortho-
Novum*)
itraconazole (*Sporanox*)

nifidipine (eg, *Procardia*)
protease inhibitors
(eg, indinavir)

Because of similarities between rifabutin, rifapentine, and rifampin, similar interactions may be expected. See rifampin interactions.

## Side Effects:

Every drug is capable of producing side effects. Many antituberculosis drug users experience no, or minor, side effects. The frequency and severity of side effects depend on many factors including dose, duration of therapy, and individual susceptibility. Possible side effects include:

*Digestive Tract:* Nausea; vomiting; appetite loss; diarrhea; stomach pain; upset stomach.

*Nervous System:* Dizziness; unusual tiredness; weakness; drowsiness; confusion; headache.

*Skin:* Rash; itching; hives.

*Other:* Muscle or joint pain; vision problems; fever; abnormal lab tests (eg, liver function, blood count); numbness, pain, or tingling in hands or feet; general body discomfort.

In addition to the side effects listed, many of the drugs have specific side effects:

*Capreomycin* – Damage to kidney cells; hearing loss; ringing in ears; feeling of whirling motion; excessive bleeding at injection site; increased or decreased white blood counts; pain, hardness, or abscess at injection site; nerve damage; blood disorders.

*Cycloserine* – Slurred speech; tremor; sudden development of congestive heart failure; convulsions; behavioral changes; vitamin $B_{12}$ or folic acid deficiency; partial or complete paralysis; exaggerated reflexes; feeling of a whirling motion; disorientation with memory loss; psychosis (possibly with suicidal tendencies); hyperirritability; aggression; allergy; skin rash; coma; drowsiness; sleepiness; depression; confusion; headache; abnormal skin sensations; anemia; seizures; allergic reaction.

*Ethambutol* – Changes in vision (see Precautions); disorientation; hallucinations; gout; joint pain; elevated blood uric acid levels; liver impairment; allergic reactions; skin inflammation; headache; abnormal lung x-rays.

*Ethionamide* – Metallic taste; excessive salivation; yellowing of the eyes or skin; hepatitis; depression; difficulty managing diabetes; fainting; restlessness; sensitivity to light; low blood sugar levels; breast growth; impotence; acne; weight loss; decreased blood platelets; pellagra syndrome.

*Isoniazid* – Numbness, pain, or tingling in hands or feet; yellowing of the eyes or skin; increased blood sugar; breast enlargement; vitamin $B_6$ or pyridoxine deficiency; vision problems; swollen lymph nodes; inflammation of blood vessels; abnormal blood cell counts; general ill feeling; hepatitis; agranulocytosis; skin eruptions; niacin deficiency; rheumatic syndrome; peripheral neuropathy; pellagra; anemia; fever; blood disorders; convulsions; memory impairment; high blood sugar.

*Pyrazinamide* – Dark urine; gout; yellowing of the eyes or skin; joint pain; anemia; low platelet count; muscle pain or tenderness; difficult or painful urination; acne; porphyria; sensitivity to light; blood disorders.

*Rifabutin* – Chest pain; indigestion; belching; gas; sleeplessness; taste perversion; reddish discoloration of body fluids; muscle pain or tenderness; low white blood cell counts; lab test abnormalities.

*Rifampin* – Menstrual irregularities; reddish orange discoloration of body fluids; heartburn; gas; cramps; sore mouth and tongue; flushing; inability to concentrate; generalized numbness; behavioral changes; fluid retention; shortness of breath; wheezing; low blood pressure; liver dysfunction; yellowing of the eyes or skin; decreased platelets; blood cell disorders; hepatitis; conjunctivitis; anemia; leukopenia; decreased hemoglobin; clumsiness; allergic reaction; muscular weakness; flu-syndrome; myopathy; shock; visual disturbances; pain in hands or feet; injection site reaction; pemphigoid reaction; fever.

*Rifapentine* – Abnormal liver tests; pus in urine; excess protein in urine; blood in urine; acne; anemia; decreased white blood counts; joint pain; pain; high blood pressure; decreased platelet count; vomiting blood; abnormal urine tests; reddish orange discoloration of body fluids.

## Guidelines for Use:

- Generally two or more antituberculosis drugs are prescribed to treat active TB. All prescribed drugs must be taken as prescribed to reduce the chance of a resistant TB organism developing and to increase the chance of effectively treating the infection.
- Take as directed. Avoid missing doses. Do not stop taking this medicine before consulting your doctor. Failure to adhere to the drug regimen for the full duration of treatment can result in treatment failure and lead to other serious health risks. Treatment is often long-term.
- If a dose is missed, take it as soon as possible. If several hours have passed or if it is nearing time for the next dose, do not double the dose in order to catch up (unless advised to do so by your doctor). If more than one dose is missed, or if it is necessary to establish a new dosage schedule, contact your doctor or pharmacist. Use exactly as prescribed.
- Contact your doctor if any of the following occurs: Fever; rash; hives; swollen lymph nodes; itching; difficulty breathing; yellowing of skin or eyes.
- Lab tests will be required to monitor therapy. Be sure to keep appointments.
- *Capreomycin* —
  Usual dosage is 1 g/day (not to exceed 20 mg/kg day) given intramuscularly or by infusion intravenously for 60 to 120 days, followed by 1 g, 2 to 3 times weekly.
  Reduced dosage should be used for patients with known or suspected kidney impairment.
  Therapy for tuberculosis should be maintained for 12 to 24 months. If facilities for administering injectable medication are not available, change to appropriate oral therapy as indicated on patient's release from hospital.
  The solution may turn pale yellow and darken. After reconstitution, all solutions may be stored in a refrigerator up to 24 hours.
  Store at room temperature (59° to 86°F) before reconstitution.
- *Cycloserine* —
  Initial adult dosage is 250 mg twice daily at 12-hour intervals for the first 2 weeks. Usual dosage is 500 mg to 1 g daily in divided doses monitored by blood levels. Daily dose of 1 g should not be exceeded.
  May cause drowsiness. Use caution when driving or performing other tasks requiring alertness, coordination, or physical dexterity.
  Avoid excessive alcohol consumption.
  Contact your doctor if any of these symptoms occur: Convulsions; psychosis; excessive drowsiness; depression; confusion; exaggerated reflexes; headache; tremor; feeling of a whirling motion; partial or complete paralysis; slurred speech. These may be signs or symptoms of CNS toxicity. Cycloserine should be discontinued or the dosage reduced. Patients receiving more than 500 mg daily should be closely monitored.
  Store at room temperature (59° to 86°F).

## Guidelines for Use (cont.):

- *Ethambutol* —
  For initial treatment, usual dose is 7 mg per pound of body weight taken as a single oral dose once every 24 hours. For retreatment, the dose is 11 mg per pound of body weight, taken as a single oral dose once every 24 hours. After 60 days, the dose is decreased to 7 mg per pound of body weight taken as a single oral dose once every 24 hours. Proper dose may require combination of different sized tablets taken at the same time. Be sure to check tablets before each dose to make sure the proper number and strength are being taken.
  May cause stomach upset. Take with food if this occurs.
  Notify your doctor if changes in vision (eg, blurring, red-green color blindness) or skin rash occurs.
  Store at room temperature (59° to 86°F).

- *Ethionamide* —
  Usual adult dosage is 7 mg to 9 mg per pound of body weight taken once-daily. If stomach upset occurs with once daily administration, then divide into 2 to 3 doses. Concomitant administration of pyridoxine is recommended. Duration of treatment should be based on individual response.
  Avoid excessive alcohol consumption. Psychotic reactions have been reported.
  Take with food to reduce stomach upset.
  May cause stomach upset, appetite loss, metallic taste, or salivation. Notify your doctor if these effects persist or are severe.
  Notify your doctor of any changes in vision or eye pain during treatment.
  Store at room temperature (77°F) in a tight container.

- *Isoniazid* —
  Take on an empty stomach, at least 1 hour before or 2 hours after meals. Studies have shown the absorption of isoniazid is reduced significantly when administered with food. However, isoniazid may be taken with food if stomach upset occurs.
  Minimize alcohol use. Alcohol may increase the risk of hepatitis.
  Discontinue the drug and notify your doctor if any of the following occurs: Weakness; numbness or tingling of hands or feet; right upper quadrant discomfort; persistent fatigue or fever lasting longer than 3 days; general body discomfort; appetite loss; nausea; vomiting; yellowing of skin or eyes; dark urine; abdominal tenderness. Isoniazid should be discontinued promptly since continued use may cause more liver damage.
  Concomitant administration of vitamin $B_6$ (pyridoxine) is recommended in malnourished patients, patients at risk of developing neuropathy (eg, alcoholics, diabetics), and children.
  Store at room temperature (59° to 86°F) and protect from light. Injection may crystallize at low temperatures. If this occurs, warm the vial to room temperature before use to dissolve crystals.

- *Isoniazid w/ Rifampin* —
  Usual dosage is 2 capsules (600 mg rifampin, 300 mg isoniazid) once daily, 1 hour before or 2 hours after a meal. Concomitant administration of pyridoxine ($B_6$) is recommended in malnourished patients, those predisposed to neuropathy (eg, alcoholics, diabetics), and children.
  Also see isoniazid and rifampin.

## Guidelines for Use (cont.):

- *Pyrazinamide* —
Administer orally, 7 mg to 14 mg per pound of body weight, once daily. Do not exceed 3 g (6 tablets) per day. Alternatively, a twice-weekly dosage regimen has been developed on an outpatient basis.
In patients with concomitant HIV infection, a longer course of treatment may be required.
Notify your doctor if fever, appetite loss, general body discomfort, nausea, vomiting, dark urine, yellowing of the skin or eyes, or pain or swelling of the joints occurs.
Store at room temperature (59° to 86°F) in a tightly sealed container.

- *Rifabutin* —
Usual dosage is 300 mg once daily. If stomach upset occurs, taking 150 mg twice daily with food may help.
Contact your doctor if you develop symptoms or signs of either tuberculosis or *M. avium* complex (MAC). These may include persisent fever, weight loss, night sweats, or productive cough.
May cause a reddish orange discoloration of urine, stools, saliva, tears, sweat, sputum, and skin. This is not harmful. May also permanently discolor soft contact lenses.
Oral contraceptives may not be as effective while taking this medicine. Patients should use nonhormonal methods of birth control.
Store at room temperature (59° to 86°F) in a tightly sealed container.

- *Rifampin* —
A 3-drug regimen consisting of rifampin, isoniazid, and pyrazinamide is recommended in the initial phase of short–course therapy which is usually continued for 2 months. Treatment should be continued with rifampin and isoniazid for at least 4 months. Injection is indicated for initial treatment when oral dosage is not possible. Injection is for intravenous infusion only. Do not administer by intramuscular or subcutaneous route.
Usual adult dosage to treat TB is 10 mg per kg of body weight (not to exceed 600 mg) taken as a single daily dose.
Usual adult dosage to treat meningococcal carriers is 600 mg twice daily for 2 days.
Take on an empty stomach, at least 1 hour before or 2 hours after meals with a full glass of water. Food reduces absorption of rifampin.
Take rifampin at least 1 hour before any antacid.
May cause a reddish orange discoloration of urine, stools, saliva, tears, sweat, and sputum. This is not harmful. May also permanently discolor soft contact lenses.
Notify your doctor if fever, general body discomfort, nausea, vomiting, appetite loss, yellowing of the skin or eyes, dark urine, or pain or swelling of the joints occurs.
Oral contraceptives may not be as effective while taking this medicine. Patients should use nonhormonal methods of birth control.
Store capsules in a tightly closed container in a dry place. Avoid excessive heat. Do not store capsules above 86°F. Protect injection from light and do not store above 104°F.

## Guidelines for Use (cont.):

- *Rifampin w/Isoniazid and Pyrazinamide —*
Usual dose (based on weight) is given once daily, 1 hour before or 2 hours after a meal with a full glass of water: 4 tablets if less than 98 pounds; 5 tablets if 99 to 120 pounds; 6 tablets if more than 120 pounds. Initial phase therapy is usually continued for 2 months, followed by rifampin and isoniazid for at least 4 months.
Concomitant administration of vitamin $B_6$ (pyridoxine) is recommended in malnourished patients, patients at risk of developing neuropathy (eg, alcoholics, diabetics), and children.
Store at room temperature (59° to 86°F). Protect from excessive moisture.
Also see isoniazid, pyrazinamide, and rifampin.

- *Rifapentine —*
Intensive phase therapy lasts 2 months. Dosage is 600 mg (4 tablets) given twice weekly with intervals of 3 or more days (more than 72 hours) between doses. Following the intensive phase, treatment is usually continued at 600 mg once weekly for 4 or more months combined with other TB drugs.
Take on an empty stomach at least 1 hour before or 2 hours after meals. May be taken with food if stomach upset occurs.
May cause a reddish orange discoloration of urine, stools, saliva, tears, sweat, and sputum. This is not harmful. May also permanently discolor soft contact lenses.
Oral contraceptives may not be as effective while taking this medicine. Patients should use nonhormonal methods of birth control.
Notify your doctor if fever, appetite loss, general body discomfort, nausea, vomiting, dark urine, yellowing of skin or eyes, or pain or swelling of the joints occurs.
Concomitant administration of vitamin $B_6$ (pyridoxine) is recommended in malnourished patients, patients at risk of developing neuropathy (eg, alcoholics, diabetics), and children.
Store at room temperature (59° to 86°F). Protect from heat and humidity.

*If you have any questions, consult your doctor, pharmacist, or health care provider.*

| Generic Name<br>*Brand Name Examples* | Supplied As | Generic<br>Available |
|---|---|---|
| *Rx* **Atovaquone** | | |
| *Mepron*[1] | **Suspension:** 750 mg/5 mL | No |

[1] Contains benzyl alcohol.

## Type of Drug:

Antiprotozoal agent to treat *Pneumocystis carinii* pneumonia (PCP), a serious respiratory infection.

## How the Drug Works:

The mechanism of action is not fully known. Studies indicate that it may inhibit enzymes necessary for the organism to grow and reproduce.

## Uses:

To treat mild to moderate PCP infection in patients who cannot tolerate trimethoprim-sulfamethoxazole (TMP-SMZ) (eg, *Septra*). Atovaquone is not used to prevent PCP infection.

## Precautions:

*Do not use in the following situations:*
allergy to atovaquone or any of its ingredients

*Use with caution in the following situations:*
elderly
presence of other respiratory infections
stomach and intestinal disorders

*Pregnancy:* Adequate studies have not been done in pregnant women. Use only if clearly needed and potential benefits outweigh the possible hazards to the fetus.

*Breastfeeding:* It is not known if atovaquone appears in breast milk. Consult your doctor before you begin breastfeeding.

*Children:* Safety and effectiveness in children have not been established.

*Elderly:* Use with caution in the elderly.

*Lab tests* may be required to monitor therapy. Tests may include blood cell counts, liver and kidney function tests, x-rays, and blood gases.

## Drug Interactions:

Tell your doctor or pharmacist if you are taking or if you are planning to take any over-the-counter or prescription medications while taking atovaquone. Doses of one or both drugs may need to be modified or a different drug may need to be prescribed. The following drugs may interact with atovaquone:

rifabutin (*Mycobutin*)
rifampin (eg, *Rifadin*)

## Side Effects:

Every drug is capable of producing side effects. Many atovaquone users experience no, or minor, side effects. The frequency and severity of side effects depend on many factors including dose, duration of therapy, and individual susceptibility. Possible side effects include:

*Digestive Tract:* Nausea; diarrhea; vomiting; mouth sores; stomach pain; constipation; appetite loss; indigestion; taste changes; mouth infections; inflammation of the pancreas.

*Nervous System:* Headache; sleeplessness; dizziness; anxiety.

*Respiratory System:* Cough; sinus inflammation; runny nose.

*Other:* Pain; weakness; rash; itching; sweating; fever; low blood sugar; low blood pressure; abnormal liver function tests; abnormal blood cell counts; eye problems; sudden kidney failure.

---

### Guidelines for Use:

- Use exactly as prescribed.
- Shake gently before use.
- Recommended dose is 750 mg (1 teaspoonful) with meals twice daily for 21 days (total daily dose 1500 mg).
- Administration with meals enhances atovaquone's absorption. Failure to take with food may result in therapeutic failure.
- Continue to use medicine until all of it is gone. Failure to take all of the medicine may allow the infection to worsen or recur.
- If a dose is missed, take it as soon as possible. If several hours have passed or if it is nearing time for the next dose, do not double the dose to catch up. If more than one dose is missed, contact your doctor or pharmacist.
- Do not share your medication with anyone else.
- Atovaquone is not effective for existing pulmonary (lung) conditions such as bacterial, viral, or fungal pneumonia or mycobacterial (eg, tuberculosis) diseases. Another medicine may need to be prescribed to treat other lung conditions that are present.
- Stomach and intestinal disorders may limit absorption of atovaquone.
- Lab tests will be required to monitor therapy. Be sure to keep appointments.
- Store at room temperature (59° to 77°F) in a tightly sealed container. Do not freeze.

---

*If you have any questions, consult your doctor, pharmacist, or health care provider.*

| Generic Name<br>*Brand Name Example* | **Supplied As** | **Generic<br>Available** |
|---|---|---|
| *Rx* **Pentamidine Isethionate**[1]<br>*NebuPent* | **Aerosol:** 300 mg | No |

[1] This product is also available as an injection.

## Type of Drug:

Aerosolized pentamidine. Drug for prevention of *Pneumocystis carinii* pneumonia (PCP). Drug for HIV-infected patients.

## How the Drug Works:

The mechanism of action is not fully understood. Studies indicate that the drug interferes with the production of DNA, RNA, phospholipids and protein.

## Uses:

To prevent *Pneumocystis carinii* pneumonia (PCP) infection in high-risk HIV-infected patients who either have had a previous episode of PCP infection or whose T4 cell count is equal to or less than 200 cells/mm$^3$.

*Unlabeled Use(s):* Occasionally, doctors may prescribe pentamidine IV to treat trypanosomiasis and visceral leishmaniasis (serious infections caused by protozoa).

## Precautions:

*Do not use in the following situations:*
anaphylactic allergy to pentamidine isethionate in any dosage form

*Use with caution in the following situations:*

| | |
|---|---|
| abnormal ECG | liver disease |
| anemia | low blood pressure (hypoten- |
| asthma | sion) |
| blood count disorders | low blood sugar levels |
| diabetes | low calcium levels |
| heart rhythm disturbance | lung infection |
| high blood potassium levels | pancreatitis |
| hives | smoking |
| kidney disease | Stevens-Johnson syndrome |

*Pregnancy:* Adequate studies have not been done in pregnant women or animal studies may have shown a risk to the fetus. Use only if clearly needed and potential benefits outweigh the possible hazards to the fetus.

*Breastfeeding:* It is not known if pentamidine isethionate appears in breast milk. Consult your doctor before you begin breastfeeding.

*Children:* Safety and effectiveness in children less than 16 years of age have not been established.

*Lab tests* may be required because of limited experience with chronic (long-term) aerosolized pentamidine use. Tests that may be required include: Electrocardiogram; blood sugar; calcium; complete blood count and liver, kidney and pancreas function tests.

## Drug Interactions:

Tell your doctor or pharmacist if you are taking or planning to take any over-the-counter or prescription medications while taking pentamidine isethionate. Doses of one or both drugs may need to be modified or a different drug may need to be prescribed. The following drugs and drug classes interact with pentamidine isethionate:

> aminoglycosides (eg, neomycin sulfate)
> amphotericin B (eg, *Albecet*)
> cisplatin (*Platinol-AQ*)
> foscarnet (*Foscavir*)
> vancomycin (eg, *Vancocin*)

## Side Effects:

Every drug is capable of producing side effects. Many pentamidine isethionate aerosol users experience no, or minor, side effects. The frequency and severity of side effects depend on many factors including dose, duration of therapy and individual susceptibility. Possible side effects include:

*Digestive Tract:* Nausea; vomiting; appetite loss; diarrhea; stomach ache; colon inflammation; sore throat.

*Nervous System:* Dizziness; fatigue; headache; lightheadedness.

*Respiratory System:* Shortness of breath; chest pain; congestion; cough; bronchitis; wheezing; difficulty breathing; upper respiratory infection; sinus infection.

*Other:* Night sweats; bad taste; anemia; inflammation of pancreas; diabetes; throat irritation; herpes; flu; fever; infection; allergic reaction; rash; chills; blood in stool; abnormal blood counts; fast heartbeat; mouth infection; abnormal heart rhythms. The injection product may cause additional and more severe side effects.

## Guidelines for Use:

- Prepare and administer pentamidine aerosol solution as instructed by your healthcare provider.
- Administer 300 mg pentamidine isethionate only by the *Respigard* II nebulizer with a high-pressure compressor air or oxygen source at a flow rate of 5 to 7 L/min. Treatment usually takes 30 to 45 minutes and is given once every 4 weeks.
- Do not use more than once a month. Do not increase dose.
- Freshly prepared solutions for aerosol use are recommended. Reconstitute only with Sterile Water for Injection.
- Do not mix the pentamidine solution with any other drugs. Do not use the *Respigard* II nebulizer to administer a bronchodilator.
- If severe sudden abdominal pain, nausea or fever occur, contact your doctor immediately.
- If difficulty breathing, cough or fever develop, contact your doctor. This could indicate the presence of PCP.
- Use of a bronchodilator drug prior to treatment may reduce breathing side effects (bronchospasm, cough).
- Lab tests will be required. Be sure to keep appointments.
- Store at room temperature and protect from light. The reconstituted solution is stable for 48 hours if stored at room temperature and protected from light. Discard unused portion after this time.

*If you have any questions, consult your doctor, pharmacist, or health care provider.*

| Generic Name<br>*Brand Name Example* | Supplied As | Generic<br>Available |
|---|---|---|
| Rx **Interferon alfa-n3**<br>**(Human leukocyte**<br>**derived)** | | |
| *Alferon N* | **Injection**: 5 million IU/mL | No |

## Type of Drug:

Miscellaneous anti-infective; drug used to treat genital warts.

## How the Drug Works:

The specific mechanism of action is unknown. Interferon alfa-n3 binds to membranes on cell surfaces, which initiates a series of responses, including inhibition of virus replication, suppression of cell proliferation, and immunomodulation.

## Uses:

To treat refractory or recurring external condylomata acuminata (genital warts) in patients at least 18 years of age who have not satisfactorily responded to other treatments (eg, podophyllin resin, surgery, laser or cryo therapy).

## Precautions:

*Do not use in the following situations:* Allergy to interferon alfa-n3, other human interferon alpha proteins, mouse immunoglobulin (IgG), egg protein, neomycin, or any other ingredients.

*Use with caution in the following situations:*

| | |
|---|---|
| cardiovascular disease<br>(eg, CHF, angina)<br>coagulation disorders<br>diabetes mellitus with<br>ketoacidosis | fever<br>myelosuppression, severe<br>pulmonary disease, severe<br>seizure disorders |

*Fertility impairment:* Interferon alpha has been shown to affect the menstrual cycle and decrease serum estradiol and progesterone levels in adult females. Use interferon alfa-n3 with caution in fertile men.

*Pregnancy:* Abortions have occured in nonhuman primates receiving high doses of recombinant interferon alpha. There are no adaquate and well-controlled studies that determine whether interferon alfa-n3 can cause fetal harm or affect reproductive capacity. Fertile women should use effective contraception during therapy. Use only if clearly needed and the potential benefits to the mother outweigh possible hazards to the fetus.

*Breastfeeding:* It is not known if interferon alfa-n3 appears in breast milk. Consult your doctor before you begin breastfeeding.

*Children:* Safety and effectiveness have not been established in children under 18 years of age.

*Lab tests* may be required to monitor therapy. Tests may include white blood cell and platelet counts; hemoglobin, alkaline phosphatase, and bilirubin levels; and certain enzyme levels.

## Drug Interactions:

Tell your doctor or pharmacist if you are taking or planning to take any over-the-counter or prescription medications or dietary supplements with interferon alfa-n3. Doses of one or both drugs may need to be modified or a different drug may need to be prescribed. The following drugs and drug classes interact with interferon alfa-n3:

corticosteroids (eg, prednisone)           zidovudine (AZT; *Retrovir*)
melphalan (*Alkeran*)
theophyllines (eg, amino-
  phylline)

## Side Effects:

Every drug is capable of producing side effects. Many interferon alfa-n3 users experience no, or minor, side effects. The frequency and severity of side effects depend on many factors including dose, duration of therapy, and individual susceptibility. Possible side effects include:

*Digestive Tract:* Nausea; vomiting; heartburn; indigestion; diarrhea; appetite loss.

*Nervous System:* Headache; dizziness; light-headedness; numbness; stiffness; general body discomfort; insomnia; fatigue; depression; confusion.

*Other:* Fever; sweating; chills; muscle, chest, joint, or back pain; rash; hives; itching; runny nose; sinus congestion; blurred vision; sore mouth; low blood pressure; soreness at the injection site; abnormal blood counts.

---

### Guidelines for Use:

- This medicine will be prepared and administered by your health care provider in a medical setting. The dose is injected into the base of each wart.
- Interferon will be administered twice weekly for up to, but no more than, 8 weeks.
- Inform your doctor if you are pregnant, become pregnant, plan on becoming pregnant, or are breastfeeding.
- Female patients should use effective contraception during therapy.
- Inform your doctor if you experience any new symptoms or begin taking any other prescription or nonprescription medication.
- Contact your doctor immediately if you experience any signs of allergic reactions (eg, hives, itching, redness, rash, tightness of the chest, wheezing, hypotension).
- Lab tests may be required to monitor therapy. Be sure to keep appointments.

---

*If you have any questions, consult your doctor, pharmacist, or health care provider.*

| Generic Name<br>Brand Name Examples | Supplied As | Generic<br>Available |
|---|---|---|
| Rx **Interferon alfacon-1** | | |
| *Infergen*[1] | **Injection**: 9 mcg/0.3 mL;<br>15 mcg/0.5 mL | No |

[1] Preservative free.

## Type of Drug:

Miscellaneous anti-infective.

## How the Drug Works:

The exact mechanism of action of interferon alfacon-1 is unknown. It may directly destroy the virus, prevent viral reproduction or alter the body's natural defense against the virus.

## Uses:

To treat long-term (chronic) hepatitis C virus (HCV) infection in patients greater than 18 years of age with compensated (normal liver function) liver disease who have anti-HCV serum antibodies or the presence of HCV RNA.

*Unlabeled Use(s):* Doctors may occasionally prescribe interferon alfacon-1, along with other agents, for the treatment of hairy-cell leukemia. Further investigation is needed.

## Precautions:

*Do not use in the following situations:*
> allergy to alpha interferons
> allergy to any ingredient of the product
> allergy to *E. coli*-derived products
> autoimmune (active) liver disease
> severe mental disorders, history of

*Use with caution in the following situations:*

| | |
|---|---|
| autoimmune disorders (eg, systemic lupus erythematosis) | heart disease, pre-existing |
| | high blood pressure |
| bone marrow suppression agents, use with | high triglycerides |
| | immunosuppressive use (eg, azathioprine) |
| depression, history of | long-term illness |
| diabetes | low blood cell counts |
| endocrine disorders, history of (eg, low thyroid) | transplantation patients |

*Postadministration reaction:* Flu-like symptoms, such as headache, fatigue, rigors, muscle discomfort, sweating and joint pain, often occur shortly after the drug is given. These symptoms are usually mild and can be treated with acetaminophen.

*Pregnancy:* Adequate studies have not been done in pregnant women or animal studies may have shown a risk to the fetus. Use only if clearly needed and potential benefits outweigh the possible hazards to the fetus.

*Breastfeeding:* It is not known if interferon alfacon-1 appears in breast milk. Consult your doctor before you begin breastfeeding.

*Children:* Safety and effectiveness have not been established in patients less than 18 years of age. Not recommended in pediatric patients.

*Lab tests* will be required to monitor therapy. Be sure to keep appointments. Tests may include: Complete blood counts; blood cell differential; liver, kidney and thyroid function tests and blood lipids (or fats).

## Drug Interactions:

Tell your doctor or pharmacist if you are taking or planning to take any over-the-counter or prescription medications while taking interferon alfacon-1. Doses of one or both drugs may need to be modified or a different drug may need to be prescribed. The following drug classes interact with interferon alfacon-1:

agents known to cause bone marrow suppression (eg, azathioprine, immunosuppressant drugs)
agents metabolized by cytochrome P450 pathway (eg, theophylline, warfarin, diazepam, phenytoin)

## Side Effects:

Every drug is capable of producing side effects. Many patients experience side effects. The frequency and severity of side effects depend on many factors including dose, duration of therapy and individual susceptibility. Possible side effects include:

*Digestive Tract:* Stomach pain; nausea; diarrhea; appetite loss; indigestion; vomiting; constipation; gas; toothache; hemorrhoids; dry mouth.

*Nervous System:* Depression; sleeplessness; dizziness; abnormal skin sensations; memory loss; decreased sensitivity to touch; tense muscles; confusion; drowsiness; nervousness; anxiety; unstable emotions; abnormal thinking; agitation.

*Circulatory System:* High blood pressure; pounding in chest (palpitations); fast heartbeat.

*Respiratory System:* Upper respiratory infection; cough; sinus discomfort; nasal congestion; chest congestion; runny nose; nosebleed; difficulty breathing; bronchitis.

*Urinary and Reproductive Tract:* Painful menstruation; inflammation of the vagina; menstrual disorder; yeast infection.

*Skin:* Hair loss; itching; rash; redness; dry skin; wound; unusual bruising.

*Senses:* Earache; ear infection; ringing in the ears; taste perversion; eye pain; eye infection; abnormal vision.

*Other:* Flu-like symptoms (eg, headache, tiredness, fever, chills, increased sweating, muscle and joint pain); injection site reactions (redness, pain, bruising); body pain; hot flushes; general body discomfort; weakness; swelling of arms and legs; allergic reaction; weight loss; abnormal blood cell counts; back, chest, limb, neck and bone pain; muscle-bone disorder; decreased sex drive; sore throat; swollen lymph glands; liver tenderness/enlargement; infection; abnormal thyroid tests.

## Guidelines for Use:

- Follow the injection procedure taught to you by your health care provider. This drug must be given subcutaneously (SC) (beneath the skin).
- Inject this medicine as a single dose 3 times a week. At least 48 hours should elapse between doses. The dose varies depending on individual needs.
- Flu-like side effects may be treated with nonnarcotic analgesics (eg, ibuprofen).
- If flu-like side effects are bothersome, administration at bedtime may lessen the problem.
- Follow proper disposal procedure for used syringes and needles.
- May be warmed to room temperature before injecting.
- Do not use if contents of the vial are discolored or have particulate matter.
- Use each vial only once. Discard any unused solution. Do not save unused solution for later use.
- Do not stop taking this medicine or change the dose unless advised by your doctor.
- Do not use other forms of interferon without consulting your pharmacist or doctor. Products manufactured by different companies may not be equally effective.
- Temporarily discontinue the dosage if severe adverse reactions occur. If the reaction does not become tolerable, the dosage may be reduced or discontinued as recommended by your doctor.
- Notify your doctor immediately if you experience depression, unusual bleeding or bruising, fever, or infection.
- Lab tests are recommended to monitor treatment. Be sure to keep appointments.
- Visual exams are recommended before therapy begins in patients with diabetes mellitus or hypertension.
- Store in the refrigerator (36° to 46°F). Do not freeze. Avoid vigorous shaking.

*If you have any questions, consult your doctor, pharmacist, or health care provider.*

| Generic Name<br>*Brand Name Example* | Supplied As | Generic<br>Available |
|---|---|---|
| *Rx* **Interferon gamma-1b** | | |
| *Actimmune*[1] | **Injection:** 100 mcg<br>(2 million IU)/0.5 mL | No |

[1] Contains mannitol, sodium succinate, and polysorbate 20.

## Type of Drug:

Miscellaneous anti-infective; biologic response modifier.

## How the Drug Works:

Interferon gamma-1b appears to alter the body's natural defense against the causes of certain diseases.

## Uses:

For reducing the frequency and severity of serious infections associated with chronic granulomatous disease.

For delaying time to disease progression in patients with severe, malignant osteopetrosis (bone overgrowth).

## Precautions:

*Do not use in the following situations:* Allergy to interferon-gamma, *Escherichia coli*-derived products, or any component of this medicine.

*Use with caution in the following situations:*

| | |
|---|---|
| bone marrow suppression | heart disease |
| central nervous system disorders | seizure disorder |

*Pregnancy:* There are no adequate and well-controlled studies in pregnant women. Use only if clearly needed and the potential benefits to the mother outweigh the possible hazards to the fetus.

*Breastfeeding:* It is not known if interferon gamma-1b appears in breast milk. Consult your doctor before you begin breastfeeding.

*Children:* Safety and effectiveness for use in children under 1 year of age have not been established.

*Lab tests* will be required during treatment. Tests may include blood cell counts, liver and kidney function tests, and urinalysis.

## Drug Interactions:

Tell your doctor or pharmacist if you are taking or if you are planning to take any over-the-counter or prescription medications or dietary supplements while taking interferon gamma-1b. Doses of one or both drugs may need to be modified or a different drug may need to be prescribed. The following drugs and drug classes interact with interferon gamma-1b:

agents metabolized by cytochrome P450 pathway
(eg, theophylline)
bone marrow suppressants (eg, azathioprine)

## Side Effects:

Every drug is capable of producing side effects. Many interferon gamma-1b users experience no, or minor, side effects. The frequency and severity of side effects depend on many factors including dose, duration of therapy, and individual susceptibility. Possible side effects include:

*Digestive Tract:* Vomiting; nausea; diarrhea; stomach pain.

*Nervous System:* Depression; headache.

*Other:* Flu-like symptoms; fever; chills; rash; redness, tenderness, or pain at injection site; fatigue; joint or muscle pain.

---

### Guidelines for Use:

- Dosage is individualized. Take exactly as prescribed.
- For subcutaneous (beneath the skin) injection only.
- Visually inspect the solution for discoloration or particles. Do not use the solution if particles or discoloration are seen.
- Follow the preparation and injection procedures taught to you by your health care provider.
- If flu-like side effects are bothersome, administering your dose at bedtime may lessen the problem.
- Acetaminophen (eg, *Tylenol*) can be used before the injection to prevent or partially alleviate the fever and headache associated with therapy.
- Follow proper disposal procedures for used syringes and needles.
- Use each vial only once. Discard any unused solution. Do not save unused solution for later use.
- Lab tests will be required to monitor treatment. Be sure to keep appointments.
- Refrigerate immediately (36° to 46°F). Do not freeze or shake. If left at room temperature for more than 12 hours, discard the vial. Do not use after the expiration date stamped on the vial.

---

*If you have any questions, consult your doctor, pharmacist, or health care provider.*

| Generic Name<br>*Brand Name Examples* | Supplied As | Generic<br>Available |
|---|---|---|
| *Rx* **Crotamiton** | | |
| *Eurax* | **Cream:** 10% | No |
| *Eurax* | **Lotion:** 10% | No |
| *Rx* **Lindane (Gamma Benzene Hexachloride)** | **Lotion:** 1% | Yes |
| | **Shampoo:** 1% | Yes |
| *Rx* **Malathion** | | |
| *Ovide* | **Lotion:** 0.5% | No |
| *Rx/ otc[1]* **Permethrin[2]** | **Lotion:** 1% | Yes |
| *Rx* **Acticin,Elimite* | **Cream:** 5% | Yes |
| *otc* *Nix[2]* | **Liquid (cream rinse):** 1% | No |
| *otc* **Pyrethrins[3]** | | |
| *Tisit* | **Liquid:** 0.3% | No |
| *Tisit[4]* | **Shampoo:** 0.3% | No |
| *A-200[4], Clear Total Lice Elimination System[5], Pronto[6], Pyrinyl Plus[2], R&C[2], RID[7]* | **Shampoo:** 0.33% | No |
| *A-200[2]* | **Gel:** 0.33% | No |
| *RID* | **Mousse:** 0.33% | No |

[1] This product is available *Rx* or *otc*, depending on package labeling.
[2] In kit containing removal comb.
[3] Available only in combination with piperonyl butoxide.
[4] Available in kits containing comb or spray.
[5] In kit containing lice egg remover and comb.
[6] Available in kits containing comb, creme rinse, spray, disposable gloves, magnifying glass, or hair separators.
[7] Available in kits containing spray or gel.

## Type of Drug:

Scabicides; pediculicides; drugs for lice, crabs, and scabies.

## How the Drug Works:

It is not clear how these drugs kill lice. They may attack the nervous system of the adult parasite and the developing nervous system of the egg. Pyrethrins are used only in combination with piperonyl butoxide, a product that enhances the effectiveness.

## Uses:

*Crotamiton:* To treat scabies and relieve nonspecific itching of skin.

*Lindane:* To treat head lice and crab (pubic) lice and their eggs. The lotion is also indicated for scabies.

*Malathion:* To treat head lice and their eggs.

*Permethrin:* The cream is used to treat scabies. The lotion and liquid are used to treat head lice and their eggs.

*Pyrethrins:* To treat head, body, and crab (pubic) lice and their eggs.

## Precautions:

*Do not use in the following situations:*

allergy to any ingredient in the product

skin irritation, skin infection

primary irritation to topical medicines

*Use with caution in the following situations:*

allergy to ragweed (pyrethrins only)

asthma or breathing difficulty

*Pregnancy:* Adequate studies have not been done in pregnant women. Potential effects on the fetus are unknown. Studies in pregnant women or in animals have been judged not to show a risk to the fetus in individuals using permethrin. However, use during pregnancy only if clearly needed.

*Breastfeeding:* It is not known if these products appear in breast milk. Consult your doctor before you begin breastfeeding.

*Children: Crotamiton* - Safety and effectiveness in children have not been established.

*Permethrin* – Safety and effectiveness in children under 2 months have not been established.

## Drug Interactions:

Tell your doctor or pharmacist if you are using or if you are planning to use any over-the-counter or prescription medications. One or both drugs may need to be modified or a different drug may need to be prescribed.

## Side Effects:

Every drug is capable of producing side effects. Many scabicide/pediculicide users experience no, or minor, side effects. The frequency and severity of side effects depend on many factors including dose, duration of therapy, and individual susceptibility. Possible side effects include:

*Skin:* Allergic skin irritation; burning; itching; stinging; redness; tingling; numbness; swelling; rash; discomfort.

## Guidelines for Use:

- For external use only.
- Patient instructions and information are available with the product. Do not exceed the prescribed dosage.
- Avoid contact with open cuts, eyes, nose, mouth or other mucous membranes, acutely inflamed skin, or raw skin oozing a liquid.
- If contact occurs between the eye and the drug, flush the eye thoroughly with tap water for several minutes.
- Contact your doctor if the condition being treated worsens or if itching, stinging, redness, burning, swelling, or skin rash occurs.
- Discontinue use if severe irritation or sensitization develops.
- Consult a doctor if infestation of eyebrows or eyelashes occurs.
- Shake liquids and shampoos well before use.
- Change clothing and bed linens the morning following application. Patients should maintain proper hygiene (eg, routine bathing).
- Sexual partners of infected individuals should be treated to avoid infection.
- Frequency of application and length of treatment depends on the condition being treated, drug utilized, strength of the drug and dosage form employed. For assistance in product selection and dosage guidelines, consult your pharmacist or doctor.

*If you have any questions, consult your doctor, pharmacist, or health care provider.*

**Immune Globulins,** 1235

**Monoclonal Antibody**
Palivizumab, 1241

**Agents for Active Immunization,** 1243

**Vaccines**
Rabies, 1248
Diphtheria/Tetanus/Pertussis, 1250
Haemophilus b, 1254
Haemophilus b/Hepatitis B, 1257
Diphtheria/Tetanus/Pertussis/
  Haemophilus b, 1259
Polio, 1261
Measles, Mumps and Rubella
  Virus, 1265
Varicella, 1268
Influenza, 1270
Hepatitis A, 1275
Hepatitis B, 1278
Hepatitis A/Hepatitis B, 1282
Pneumococcal, 1285
Pneumococcal 7-Valent
  Conjugate, 1287

**Tuberculin Tests,** 1289

| | Generic Name<br>*Brand Name Examples* | Uses |
|---|---|---|
| *Rx* | **Antithymocyte Globulin (Rabbit) (ATG Rabbit)**<br>*Thymoglobulin* | *Kidney transplant rejection:* For treatment in conjunction with other immunosuppressant therapy. |
| *Rx* | **Cytomegalovirus Immune Globulin Intravenous (Human) (CMV-IGIV)**<br>*CytoGam* | *Cytomegalovirus (CMV):* To prevent CMV disease associated with kidney, lung, liver, pancreas, or heart transplantation. |
| *Rx* | **Hepatitis B Immune Globulin (Human) (HBIG)**<br>*BayHep B,*<br>*Nabi-HB* | *For postexposure:* Prevention of hepatitis B infection following exposure (eg, by accidental "needle-stick", splash, sexual exposure, oral ingestion) to hepatitis B-positive materials such as blood.<br><br>*For infants* born to hepatitis B-positive mothers.<br><br>*For individuals who are at high risk of hepatitis B infection:* Protection is achieved when HBIG is given before, or at the same time as, active immunization for hepatitis B with hepatitis B vaccine. |
| *Rx* | **Immune Globulin (Human) (IG; IGIM; Gamma Globulin; IgG)**<br>*BayGam* | *Hepatitis A:* To prevent hepatitis A when given before or within 2 weeks after exposure. Not for patients with symptoms of hepatitis or those exposed more than 2 weeks previously.<br><br>*Measles (Rubeola):* To prevent measles in patients (who have not been vaccinated or had measles previously) exposed < 6 days previously.<br><br>*Immunoglobulin deficiency:* May prevent serious infection in patients who are unable to produce sufficient amounts of protective antibodies (IgG antibodies).<br><br>*Varicella (chickenpox) in immunosuppressed patients:* If varicella-zoster immune globulin is unavailable, IGIM may be used for passive immunization.<br><br>*Rubella:* Some studies suggest use in susceptible pregnant women exposed to rubella can lessen the likelihood of infection and fetal damage. |

| | Generic Name *Brand Name Examples* | Uses |
|---|---|---|
| *Rx* | **Immune Globulin Intravenous (Human) (IGIV)** *Carimune, Gamimune N, Gammagard S/D, Gammar-P I.V., Iveegam, Panglobulin, Polygam S/D, Venoglobulin-S* | *Immunodeficiency syndrome:* For maintenance treatment of patients who are unable to produce sufficient amounts of protective antibodies (IgG antibodies) to prevent infection. *Idiopathic thrombocytopenic purpura (ITP), acute and chronic (Carimune, Gamimune N, Gammagard S/D, Panglobulin, Polygam S/D, Venoglobulin-S):* To create a rapid but temporary rise in the platelet count (platelets aid in clotting blood), to prevent or control bleeding, and to allow a patient with ITP to undergo surgery. Not all patients will respond. *B-cell chronic lymphocytic leukemia (CLL) (Gammagard S/D, Polygam S/D):* For prevention of bacterial infections in patients with hypogammaglobulinemia and/or recurrent bacterial infections associated with B-cell CLL. *Kawasaki syndrome (Gammagard S/D, Iveegam, Polygam S/D, Venoglobulin-S):* In conjunction with high dose aspirin for the prevention of coronary artery aneurysms associated with Kawasaki syndrome. *Bone marrow transplantation (Gamimune N):* Prevention of septicemia (blood poisoning), pneumonia, and acute graft-vs-host disease in transplant patients ≥ 20 years of age. *Pediatric HIV infection (Gamimune N):* To decrease the frequency of serious and minor bacterial infections, the frequency of hospitalization, and to increase the time free of serious bacterial infections in children with evidence of HIV disease. |
| *Rx* | **Lymphocyte Immune Globulin, Antithymocyte Globulin (Equine), (LIG, ATG)** *Atgam* | *Kidney transplant rejection:* To manage allograft rejection or as an adjunct to other immunosupressive therapy to delay onset of allograft rejection. *Aplastic anemia:* To treat moderate to severe cases in patients who are unsuitable for bone marrow transplantation. |

| | Generic Name<br>*Brand Name Examples* | Uses |
|---|---|---|
| *Rx* | **Rabies Immune Globulin (Human) (RIG)**<br>*BayRab,*<br>*Imogam Rabies-HT* | *Rabies exposure:* In conjunction with rabies vaccine to treat patients suspected of exposure to rabies, particularly severe exposure (but not people who have previously been immunized with HDCY rabies vaccine in a pre- or postexposure treatment series). |
| *Rx* | **Respiratory Syncytial Virus Immune Globulin Intravenous (Human) (RSV-IGIV)**<br>*RespiGam* | *Respiratory Syncytial Virus (RSV):* To prevent serious lower respiratory tract infection caused by RSV in children < 24 months of age with bronchopulmonary dysplasia (BPD) or a history of premature birth ($\leq$ 35 weeks gestation). |
| *Rx* | **$Rh_o$(D) Immune Globulin (Human)**<br>*BayRho-D Full Dose,*<br>*RhoGAM* | *Full-term delivery:* To prevent hemolytic disease of the newborn. Used within 72 hours of birth in a $Rh_o$(D)-negative mother not previously exposed to the $Rh_o$(D)-positive factor who has delivered a $Rh_o$(D)-positive baby.<br><br>Also used in certain $Rh_o$(D)-negative patients after incomplete pregnancy or transfusions of Rh incompatible blood or blood products. |
| *Rx* | **$Rh_o$(D) Immune Globulin Micro-Dose ($Rh_o$[D] IG Micro-dose)**<br>*BayRho-D Mini Dose,*<br>*MICRhoGAM* | *Incomplete pregnancy (of $\leq$ 12 weeks gestation) or transfusions:* Prevents isoimmunization of $Rh_o$(D)-negative women when the father is not known to be $Rh_o$(D) negative. |
| *Rx* | **$Rh_o$(D) Immune Globulin IV (Human)**<br>*WinRho SDF* | *Full-term delivery:* To prevent Rh isoimmunization of the mother when a $Rh_o$(D)-negative mother not previously exposed to the $Rh_o$(D)-positive factor has a $Rh_o$(D)-positive baby.<br><br>Also used in certain $Rh_o$(D)-negative women after incomplete pregnancy or transfusions with $Rh_o$(D)-positive blood or blood products.<br><br>*Immune Thrombocytopenic Purpura (ITP):* To increase platelet count and to control excessive bleeding in $Rh_o$(D)-positive children with chronic or acute ITP, adults with chronic ITP, or anyone with ITP secondary to HIV. |
| *Rx* | **Tetanus Immune Globulin (Human) (TIG)**<br>*BayTet* | *Tetanus:* Prevention of tetanus following injury in patients whose tetanus immunization is incomplete or uncertain. Also indicated in the regimen of treatment of active cases of tetanus. |

| Generic Name<br>*Brand Name Examples* | Uses |
|---|---|
| *Rx* **Varicella-Zoster Immune Globulin (Human) (VZIG)** | *Varicella-Zoster:* For passive immunization of exposed, susceptible patients who are at greater risk of complications from varicella (chickenpox or zoster) than healthy individuals (eg, immunocompromised patients, newborns of mothers with varicella shortly before or after delivery, premature infants, normal, susceptible adults, susceptible high-risk infants < 1 year of age). |

## Type of Drug:

Immune globulins; antibodies.

## How the Drug Works:

*Passive immunization:* Most immune globulins contain antibodies from plasma obtained from human blood donors. LIG, ATG contains antibodies derived from horse (equine) serum and ATG rabbit contains antibodies derived from rabbit serum. Administration of immune serums temporarily increases the antibody concentration in the person receiving the serum. Protection derived from these products will be of rapid onset, but will only protect for a short period of time (1 week to 3 months).

## Precautions:

*Do not use in the following situations:*

allergic response to antithymocyte globulin (equine) or other equine immunoglobulin preparations (LIG, ATG equine only)
allergic response to gamma globulin or anti-immunoglobulin A (IgA) antibodies
allergic response to human immunoglobulin preparation
allergic response to rabbit proteins (ATG rabbit only)
immunoglobulin A (IgA) deficiency
pregnancy after 12 weeks gestation (Rh$_o$(D) IG micro-dose only)
viral illness, acute (ATG rabbit only)

*Use with caution in the following situations:*

bleeding disorder (IM administration only)
cardiovascular disease, history of (IGIV products only)
diabetes mellitus (IGIV products only)
kidney disease, pre-existing (IGIV products only)
nephrotoxic drug therapy (IGIV products only)
older than 65 years of age (IGIV products only)
paraproteinemia (IGIV products only)
sepsis (IGIV products only)
thrombocytopenia (IGIV products only)
thrombotic episodes (IGIV products only)
volume depletion (IGIV products only)

*Infectious agents:* Products made from human plasma may contain infectious agents, such as viruses that can cause disease. Multiple steps are taken to remove all infectious agents from these products but there is a very small possibility that unknown infectious agents may still be present. Discuss the risks and benefits with your health care provider.

*Pregnancy:* There are no adequate and well-controlled studies in pregnant women. Use only if clearly needed and the potential benefits to the mother outweigh the possible hazards to the fetus. *BayRho-D Mini-Dose* is not indicated for use during pregnancy and it should be administered only postabortion or postmiscarriage of 12 weeks or less gestation.

*Breastfeeding:* It is not known if immune globulins appear in breast milk. Safety has not been established. Consult your doctor before you begin breastfeeding.

*Children:* Safety and effectiveness have not been established in children. Do not inject infants with $Rh_o(D)$ IGIV, $Rh_o(D)$ IGIM, or $Rh_o(D)$ IG microdose. RSV-IGIV is indicated for use in children under 24 months of age; however, safety and effectiveness in children with congenital heart disease have not been established.

*Lab tests* may be required to monitor therapy. Tests include kidney function, urine output, and blood counts.

## Drug Interactions:

Live virus vaccines are typically recommended for administration at least 2 weeks before or 3 months after administration of immune serums. The immune serum may reduce the effectiveness of the vaccine. It may be necessary to revaccinate people who received immune serums shortly after live virus vaccination. Consult the specific product information on guidelines for administering vaccines before or after use of an immune globulin.

## Side Effects:

Modern immune sera and immune globulins are generally safe and effective. Many immune globulin recipients experience no, or minor, local side effects. The severity of side effects depends on many factors including dose and individual susceptibility. Possible side effects include:

*Local:* Hives; swelling; itching; muscle stiffness; tenderness, pain, redness, heat, burning, ache, or irritation at injection site.

*Nervous System:* Headache; dizziness; anxiety; night sweats; lightheadedness; fatigue; shaking; agitation; lethargy; listlessness.

*Digestive Tract:* Vomiting; nausea; diarrhea; stomach pain; inflammation of the mouth; sore mouth or throat; mouth sores.

*Circulatory System:* Irregular heartbeat; inflammation of muscular walls of the heart; congestive heart failure; chest tightness; abnormal blood counts; clotted A/V fistula; change in blood pressure; change in heart rate; low oxygen concentration in blood.

*Other:* General body discomfort; enlarged liver or spleen; seizures; difficulty breathing; sweating; wheezing; pounding in the chest; joint stiffness; burning soles or palms; foot sole pain; abnormal liver or kidney function tests; serum sickness-like symptoms; nosebleed; tender or swollen lymph nodes; rash; pneumonia; fluid retention; urinary tract infection; vaginal infection; bluish discoloration of the skin; herpes simplex infection; weakness; fever; chills; flushing; swelling of feet and ankles; muscle cramps; back, joint, muscle, chest, hip, neck, flank, or leg pain.

---

## Guidelines for Use:

- These immune globulins will be prepared and administered by your health care provider in a medical setting.
- Live virus vaccines are not typically recommended for administration within 3 months of immune globulin administration. In some cases, this period may be longer. Consult the specific product information for administration guidelines. It may be necessary to revaccinate persons who received immune globulin shortly after live virus vaccination.
- Protection received from these immunizations will be of rapid onset, but short duration (generally 1 week to 3 months).
- Immediate allergic reactions (eg, anaphylaxis) are a possibility. If an allergic reaction occurs, your health care provider will discontinue the immune globulin and provide emergency treatment as indicated.
- Serum sickness-like reactions (skin rashes with inflammation, pain in the joints, and fever) have been reported in aplastic anemia patients administered *Atgam*. Resolution of symptoms is generally prompt and long-term sequelae have not been observed. Administration of corticosteroids may decrease the frequency of this reaction.
- Aseptic meningitis syndrome (AMS) has been reported to occur infrequently in association with Immune Globulin Intravenous (IGIV) treatment. The syndrome usually begins within several hours to 2 days following treatment. It is characterized by severe headache, neck stiffness, drowsiness, fever, eye sensitivity to light, painful eye movements, nausea, and vomiting. Contact your doctor immediately if you notice any of these symptoms. AMS may occur more frequently in association with high-dose treatment. Discontinuation of IGIV treatment has resulted in remission of AMS within several days.
- Kidney dysfunction has been reported in association with treatment with IGIV products. Notify your doctor immediately if you experience decreased urination, sudden weight gain, fluid retention or swelling, or shortness of breath.
- Local reactions to injections may occur (eg, tenderness, pain, burning, irritation). Application of a warm compress may alleviate symptoms. If these persist or become bothersome, contact your doctor.
- *LIG, ATG* — A skin test is usually performed before the first dose to check for possible allergy to serum.
- Lab tests will be required to monitor therapy. Be sure to keep appointments.

---

*If you have any questions, consult your doctor, pharmacist, or health care provider.*

| Generic Name<br>*Brand Name Example* | How Supplied | Generic<br>Available |
|---|---|---|
| *Rx* **Palivizumab** | | |
| *Synagis* | **Powder for injection:** 100 mg[1] | No |

[1] Lyophilized.

## Type of Drug:

Antiviral drug for treatment of respiratory syncytial virus (RSV) infection.

## How the Drug Works:

Palivizumab is an immune system protein which is designed to be highly specific for the RSV virus to inhibit viral replication.

## Uses:

For the prevention of serious lower respiratory tract disease caused by respiratory syncytial virus (RSV) in pediatric patients at high risk.

Safety and effectiveness were established in infants with bronchopulmonary dysplasia (BPD) and in infants with a history of prematurity (35 weeks gestational age or less).

## Precautions:

*Do not use in the following situations:*
allergy to this product or its components

*Use with caution in the following situations:*
abnormal blood clotting
low blood platelets

*Pregnancy:* It is not known if palivizumab causes fetal harm. Palivizumab is not indicated for use in adults.

## Drug Interactions:

Tell your doctor or pharmacist if you are giving or plan to give your baby any over-the-counter or prescription medications or dietary supplements while giving palivizumab. Doses of one or both drugs may need to be modified or a different drug may need to be prescribed.

## Side Effects:

Every drug is capable of producing side effects. Many palivizumab users experience no, or minor, side effects. The frequency and severity of side effects depend on many factors including dose, duration of therapy, and individual susceptibility. Possible side effects include:

*Digestive Tract:* Diarrhea; stomach irritation; vomiting.

*Respiratory System:* Upper respiratory tract infection due to other organisms; runny nose; asthma; sore throat; bronchitis; cough; wheezing; croup; pneumonia; difficulty breathing; sinus infection.

*Skin:* Fungal skin inflammation; itching; oily skin; rash; injection site redness and pain.

*Other:* Ear infection; hernia; failure to thrive; nervousness; abnormal liver function tests; eye redness or inflammation; other viral infections; mouth infection; anemia; flu-like syndrome; mouth sores.

## Guidelines for Use:

- Palivizumab is not indicated for adult use.
- Palivizumab will be administered by a health care professional and should be administered exactly as prescribed. It is for IM use only.
- *Preparation of solution* — Slowly add 1 mL Sterile Water for Injection to 100 mg vial. Gently swirl for 30 seconds; avoid foaming. Do not shake. Allow reconstituted solution to stand at room temperature for a minimum of 20 minutes until the solution becomes clear. Administer within 6 hours of reconstitution.
- This drug is for IM administration only, preferably injected in the front part of the thigh. The buttocks (gluteal region) should not be used as a regular injection site because of the risk of damage to the sciatic nerve.
- The recommended dose is 15 mg/kg body weight. The first dose should be administered IM prior to the beginning of the RSV season (November through April in the northern hemisphere). Patients, including those who develop an RSV infection, should receive monthly doses throughout the RSV season.
- This medication is designed to prevent RSV infection. It is not used to treat an established RSV infection.
- Store unreconstituted vial at 35° to 46°F. Do not freeze. Do not use after expiration date.

*If you have any questions, consult your doctor, pharmacist, or health care provider.*

## Recommended Childhood and Adolescent Immunization Schedule United States, 2003[1]

| Vaccine | Age | | | | | | | | | | | |
|---|---|---|---|---|---|---|---|---|---|---|---|---|
| | Birth | 1 mo | 2 mos | 4 mos | 6 mos | 12 mos | 15 mos | 18 mos | 24 mos | 4-6 yrs | 11-12 yrs | 13-18 yrs |
| Hepatitis B[2] | HepB #1 *only* if mother HBsAg(-) | | | | | | | | | | | |
| | | HepB #2 | | | HepB #3 | | | | | HepB series catch-up | | |
| Diphtheria, Tetanus, Pertussis[3] | | DTaP #1 | DTaP #2 | DTaP #3 | | DTaP #4 | | | | DTaP #5 | Td | |
| *Haemophilus influenzae* Type b[4] | | Hib #1 | Hib #2 | Hib #3 | Hib #4 | | | | | | | |
| Inactivated Polio | | IPV #1 | IPV #2 | IPV #3 | | | | | | IPV #4 | | |
| Measles, Mumps, Rubella[5] | | | | | | MMR #1 | | | | MMR #2 | MMR #2 catch-up | |
| Varicella[6] | | | | | | Varicella | | | | Varicella | | |
| Pneumococcal[7] | | PCV #1 | PCV #2 | PCV #3 | PCV #4 | | | | | | | |
| Vaccines below this line are for selected populations | | | | | | | | | | | | |
| | | | | | | | | | | PCV | | |
| | | | | | | | | | | PPV | | |
| Hepatitis A[8] | | | | | | | | | | Hep A series | | |
| Influenza[9] | | | | | Influenza (yearly) | | | | | | | |

■ Range of recommended ages

■ *Catch-up vaccination*

■ Preadolescent assessment

[1] This schedule indicates the recommended ages for routine administration of currently licensed childhood vaccines as of December 1, 2002, for children through 18 years of age. Any dose not given at the recommended age should be given at any subsequent visit when indicated and feasible.

▆ Indicates age groups that warrant special effort to administer those vaccines not given previously. Additional vaccines may be licensed and recommended during the year. Licensed combination vaccines may be used whenever any components of the combination are indicated and the vaccine's other components are not contraindicated. Providers should consult the manufacturers' package inserts for detailed recommendations.

[2] **Hepatitis B vaccine (HepB):** All infants should receive the first dose of HepB vaccine soon after birth and before hospital discharge; the first dose may also be given by 2 months of age if the infant's mother is HBsAg-negative. Only monovalent HepB can be used for the birth dose. Monovalent or combination vaccine containing HepB may be used to complete the series; 4 doses of vaccine may be administered when a birth dose is given. The second dose should be given at least 4 weeks after the first dose, except for combination vaccines, which cannot be administered before 6 weeks of age. The third dose should be given at least 16 weeks after the first dose and at least 8 weeks after the second dose. The last dose in the vaccination series (third or fourth dose) should not be administered before 6 months of age.
*Infants born to HBsAg-positive mothers* should receive HepB vaccine and 0.5 mL hepatitis B immune globulin (HBIG) within 12 hours of birth at separate sites. The second dose is recommended at 1 to 2 months of age. The last dose in the vaccination series should not be administered before 6 months of age. These infants should be tested for HBsAg and anti-HBs at 9 to 15 months of age.
*Infants born to mothers whose HBsAg status is unknown* should receive the first dose of HepB vaccine series within 12 hours of birth. Maternal blood should be drawn as soon as possible to determine the mother's HBsAg status; if the HBsAg test is positive, the infant should receive HBIG as soon as possible (no later than 1 week of age). The second dose is recommended at 1 to 2 months of age. The last dose in the vaccination series should not be administered before 6 months of age.

[3] **Diphtheria and tetanus toxoids and acellular pertussis vaccine (DTaP):** The fourth dose of DTaP may be administered at 12 months of age, provided that 6 months have elapsed since the third dose and the child is unlikely to return at 15 to 18 months of age. **Tetanus and diphtheria toxoids (Td)** is recommended at 11 to 12 years of age if at least 5 years have elapsed since the last dose of Td-containing vaccine. Subsequent routine Td boosters are recommended every 10 years.

[4] *Haemophilus influenzae* **type b (Hib) conjugate vaccine:** Three Hib conjugate vaccines are licensed for infant use. If PRP-OMP (*PedvaxHIB* or *ComVax* [Merck]) is administered at 2 and 4 months of age, a dose at 6 months of age is not required. DTaP/Hib combination products should not be used for primary vaccination in infants at 2, 4, or 6 months of age, but can be used as boosters following any Hib vaccine.

[5] **Measles, mumps, and rubella vaccine (MMR):** The second dose of MMR is recommended routinely at 4 to 6 years of age but may be administered during any visit, provided that at least 4 weeks have elapsed since the first dose and that both doses are administered beginning at or after 12 months of age. Those who have not received the second dose previously should complete the schedule by the visit at 11 to 12 years of age.

[6] **Varicella vaccine:** Varicella vaccine is recommended at any visit at or after 12 months of age for susceptible children (ie, those who lack a reliable history of chickenpox). Susceptible patients at least 13 years of age should receive 2 doses, given at least 4 weeks apart.

[7] **Pneumococcal vaccine:** The heptavalent **pneumococcal conjugate vaccine (PCV)** is recommended for all children 2 to 23 months of age. It also is recommended for certain children 24 to 59 months of age. **Pneumococcal polysaccharide vaccine (PPV)** is recommended in addition to PCV for certain high-risk groups. See *MMWR*. 2000;49(RR-9);1-37.

[8] **Hepatitis A vaccine:** Hepatitis A vaccine is recommended for children and adolescents in selected states and regions, and for certain high risk groups. Consult local public health authority and *MMWR*. 1999;48(RR-12);1-37. In addition, healthy children 6 to 23 months of age are encouraged to receive influenza vaccine if feasible because children in this age group are at substantially increased risk for influenza-related hospitalizations. Children and adolescents in these states, regions, and high-risk groups who have not been immunized against hepatitis A can begin the hepatitis A vaccination series during any visit. The two doses in the series should be administered at least 6 months apart.

[9] **Influenza vaccine:** Influenza vaccine is recommended annually for children at least 6 months of age with certain risk factors (including, but not limited to asthma, cardiac disease, sickle cell disease, HIV, and diabetes and household members of persons in groups at high risk [see *MMWR*. 2002;51(RR-30:1–30.]) and can be administered to all others wishing to obtain immunity. Children 12 years of age or younger should receive vaccine in a dosage appropriate for their age (0.25 mL if 6 to 35 months of age or 0.5 mL if 3 years of age or older). Children 8 years of age or younger who are receiving influenza vaccine for the first time should receive 2 doses separated by at least 4 weeks.

## Type of Drug:
Bacterial and viral vaccines and toxoid injections; immunizations.

## How the Drug Works:
Vaccines contain either killed or weakened viruses or bacteria that cause recipients to make their own protective antibodies against infection. Either partial or whole viruses and bacteria may be used. These viral or bacterial vaccines do not themselves cause disease, but are used to prevent disease. Toxoids are a kind of vaccine made by inactivating bacterial toxins. Toxoids are not toxic. Vaccines usually cause approximately 80% to 99% of recipients to make protective antibodies. Vaccines usually lower the risk of infection 60% to 99%, depending on the type.

Active immunization with bacterial and viral vaccines and toxoids provides long-term protection (immunity) against various infections.

## Uses:
See individual product descriptions.

## Precautions:
*Immune system diseases:* Do not give live, weakened virus vaccines to people with immune deficiency diseases (reduced ability to produce antibodies and fight infection), and those with decreased ability for immune response (eg, leukemia, lymphoma, cancer, or therapy with corticosteroids, cancer drugs, or radiation).

*Children with symptomatic AIDS:* Do not give live-virus and live-bacterial vaccines to children or young adults with AIDS unless specifically recommended by the Advisory Committee on Immunization Practices (ACIP). After exposure to measles or chicken pox, these patients may receive passive immunization with immune globulin or varicella-zoster immune globulin.

Immunization with DTP, inactivated polio vaccine (IPV), *Haemophilus influenzae* type b, pneumococcal, and influenza (flu) vaccines is recommended, although immunization may be less effective than it would be for children with a normal immune system. Immunization with influenza and pneumococcal vaccines for children over 2 years of age is recommended.

*Children with previously diagnosed asymptomatic AIDS:* Children with previously diagnosed AIDS, but without symptoms, have received live-virus vaccines without side effects. However, observe for possible side effects and for occurrence of vaccine-preventable diseases, because immunization may be less effective than for children with a normal immune system.

Do not use oral polio vaccine (OPV). Use IPV routinely to immunize these children or members of a household in which there is an HIV-positive patient. DTP, *Haemophilus influenzae* type b, and hepatitis B vaccines may be given in accordance with ACIP recommendations.

*Simultaneous vaccinations:* Most vaccines can be administered simultaneously at separate injection sites.

*Illnesses with fever:* Delay immunization of people with severe acute illness until the illness is treated.

*Vaccination during pregnancy:* Live, weakened virus vaccines are not generally given to pregnant women or to those likely to become pregnant within 3 months after receiving the vaccine(s). Do not give some of these vaccines during pregnancy, particularly rubella, measles, mumps, and varicella. When a vaccine is to be given during pregnancy, waiting until the second or third trimester to minimize any link to coincidental miscarriage is a reasonable precaution. However, there has been no evidence of congenital rubella syndrome in infants born to mothers who received rubella vaccine during pregnancy. Experience to date has not revealed any risks of other vaccines to the fetus.

Any vaccine may be given safely to children and other contacts of pregnant women.

Give vaccines against influenza, hepatitis B, meningococcal disease, tetanus, and diphtheria to pregnant women to adequately protect against these diseases in the mother or child.

*Allergy to vaccine components:* Vaccines produced in allergenic substances (eg, eggs) may cause allergic reactions. Therefore, do not give such vaccines (eg, influenza, yellow fever vaccines) to people with known allergy to these components. These vaccines are only rarely associated with serious allergic reactions.

Live virus vaccines prepared by growing viruses in cell cultures usually do not contain allergenic substances. On very rare occasions, allergic reactions to measles vaccine have been reported in persons with allergy to eggs. However, measles vaccine can be given safely to egg-allergic individuals provided the symptoms of the allergy are not severe. The same precautions apply to mumps vaccine.

Some vaccines contain preservatives (eg, thimerosal) or small amounts of antibiotics (eg, neomycin) to which patients may rarely be allergic.

*Immunization for other diseases:* Immunization for other diseases is recommended for people with a risk of exposure. Specific immunization requirements and recommendations for international travel can be obtained from the Superintendent of Documents, US Government Printing Office, Washington, DC, 20402 in the publication *Health Information for International Travel.*

*Centers for Disease Control and Prevention (CDC):*

| | |
|---|---|
| Information Hotline | 800–232–2522 |
| International Travel Hotline | 877–394–8747 |
| Spanish Hotline | 800–232–0233 |
| CDC Web site | www.cdc.gov |

Refer to the Immunization Gateway: Your Vaccine Fact-Finder at www.immunofacts.com for direct links to all the best vaccine resources on the Internet.

## Side Effects:

Modern vaccines are extremely safe and effective. Side effects following immunization have been reported with all vaccines. These range from frequent, minor, local reactions to extremely rare, severe, bodily illness such as paralysis associated with oral polio vaccine. See individual product descriptions for details.

*If you have any questions, consult your doctor, pharmacist, or health care provider.*

| Generic Name *Brand Name Example* | Uses |
|---|---|
| Rx **Rabies Vaccine** *RabAvert* | For pre- and postexposure immunization against rabies. Preexposure immunization should be boosted periodically to provide continuous protection. |

*Individuals at high risk include:* Veterinarians; animal handlers; wildlife officers; laboratory workers; travelers to high-risk areas; people whose activities bring them into contact with potentially rabid dogs, cats, foxes, skunks, bats or other species at risk of having rabies.

Carnivorous wild animals (especially skunks, raccoons, foxes and coyotes) and bats are the animals most commonly infected with rabies. Unless an animal is tested and shown not to be rabid, initiate postexposure vaccination.

The likelihood that a domestic dog or cat is infected with rabies varies from region to region; therefore so does the need for postexposure prophylaxis.

Rodents (eg, squirrels, hamsters, guinea pigs, gerbils, chipmunks, rats, mice) and lagomorphs (eg, rabbits, hares) are rarely infected with rabies and have not been shown to cause human rabies in the US. Contact the state and local health department before initiating postexposure antirabies prophylaxis.

An unprovoked attack is more likely than a provoked attack to indicate an animal is rabid. Consider bites inflicted when a person is attempting to feed or handle an apparently healthy animal to be "provoked."

Rabies is transmitted by introducing the virus into open cuts or wounds in skin or through mucous membranes. The likelihood of rabies infection varies with nature and extent of exposure. Consider two categories of exposure: 1) Bites, any penetration of the skin by teesth, to the face and hands have the highest risk, but the site of the bite should not influence the decision to begin treatment; 2) a non-bite can be scratches, abrasions, open wounds or mucous membranes contaminated with saliva or other potentially infectious material. Casual contact, such as petting, does not indicate prophylaxis.

Post-bite exposure may require use of both vaccine and immune globulin treatment.

## Type of Drug:
Active immunization for rabies virus.

## How the Drug Works:
Rabies vaccine provides long-term protection against rabies by stimulating the body to produce antibodies against the virus.

## Precautions:
*Do not use in the following situations:* Allergy to egg, immediate reaction.

*Use with caution in the following situations:*

allergy to bovine gelatin, chicken protein, neomycin, chlortetra-cycline and amphotericin B convalescent

infectious disease, active stage
sick
immunosuppressive illness

*Pregnancy:* Adequate studies have not been done pregnant women. Use only if clearly needed and potential benefits outweigh the possible risks.

## Drug Interactions:

Tell your doctor or pharmacist if you are taking or if you are planning to take any over-the-counter or prescription medications or dietary supplements with the rabies vaccine. Doses of one or both drugs may need to be modified or a different drug may need to be prescribed. The following drugs and drug classes interact with the rabies vaccine.

antimalarials (eg, chloroquin)
corticosteroids (eg, prednisone)

immunosuppressive agents
(eg, azathioprine, cyclosporine)

## Side Effects:

Every drug is capable of producing side effects. Many patients experience no, or minor, side effects. The frequency and severity of side effects depend on many factors including dose, duration of therapy and individual susceptibility. Possible side effects include:

*Local:* Swelling; reddening; hardening; pain at the injection site; swollen lymph nodes.

*Other:* Headache; dizziness; general body discomfort; muscle pain; fever; swollen lymph nodes; GI problems.

---

### Guidelines for Use:

- *Recommended vaccination schedule —*
  *Preexposure:* Usual regimen consists of three injections. The second and third doses are given 7 days and 21 or 28 days after the inital injection, respectively.
  *Postexposure:* Begin immunization as soon as possible after exposure. Usual regimen consists of five injections. The last four doses are given 3, 7, 14 and 28 days after the initial injection.
  *Postexposure therapy of previously immunized people:* Usual regimen consists of two injections, one immediately and one 3 days later.
- It is not guaranteed that the vaccine will protect everyone from rabies.
- *Booster doses:* Certain individuals who are at high risk of contracting rabies will need booster doses. Blood tests determine when the booster dose is due.
- The vaccine will be prepared and administered by a healthcare provider.

---

*If you have any questions, consult your doctor, pharmacist, or health care provider.*

| | Generic Name<br>*Brand Name Examples* | Uses |
|---|---|---|
| *Rx* | **Tetanus Toxoid Adsorbed**[1] | For active immunization against tetanus in adults and children 7 years of age or older. |
| *Rx* | **Diphtheria and Tetanus Toxoids Adsorbed** | |
| | *Pediatric (DT)*[1] | For active immunization against diphtheria and tetanus in infants and children between 6 weeks and 7 years of age. |
| | *Adult (Td)*[1] | For active immunization against diphtheria and tetanus in adults and children 7 years and older. |
| *Rx* | **Diphtheria and Tetanus Toxoids and Acellular Pertussis Vaccine Adsorbed (DTaP)** | |
| | *Daptacel, Infanrix, Tripedia*[1] | For active immunization of infants and children between 6 weeks and 7 years of age against diphtheria, tetanus, and pertussis (whooping cough).<br>*Unlabeled uses:* To immunize adults against pertussis. |

[1] Contains thimerosal.

## Type of Drug:

Diphtheria, tetanus, pertussis (whooping cough) vaccines; active immunization.

## How the Drug Works:

These vaccines provide long-term protection against diphtheria, tetanus, and pertussis by stimulating the body to produce antibodies against the organisms causing these infections.

## Precautions:

*Do not use in the following situations:*
adults (DT, DTaP only)
allergy to the vaccine or its components
allergy to thimerosal
children older than 7 years of age (DT, DTaP only)
children younger than 7 years of age (tetanus toxoid adsorbed only)
illness, acute with fever
polio outbreak
serious reaction (eg, seizure, unconsciousness, allergic reaction) after a previous dose

*Use with caution in the following situations:*

blood clotting (coagulation) disorder

chemotherapy (cancer drugs)

convulsions (within 3 days of prior vaccine) (DTaP only)

corticosteroid (eg, prednisone) use, current

fever, high (within 48 hours of prior vaccine) (DTaP only)

immune deficiency disorder (decreased antibody formation)

infection, active

low platelet count

nervous system disorder (DTaP only)

persistent crying, over 3 hours (within 48 hours of prior vaccine) (DTaP only)

pertussis infection, history of (DTaP only)

radiation therapy

seizures, family history of (DTaP only)

shock (within 48 hours of prior vaccine) (DTaP only)

*Fluid tetanus toxoid:* Use fluid tetanus toxoid to immunize patients who are allergic to the adsorbed tetanus toxoid.

*Immunodeficiency:* People receiving corticosteroids, chemotherapy, radiation therapy, those with a recent injection of immunoglobulin, or with an immunodeficiency disorder (eg, AIDS) may not respond well to these vaccines. Defer vaccination until immunosuppressive therapy has ended, or give another dose 1 month after therapy has ended. However, vaccination of AIDS patients is recommended.

*Nervous system complications:* Convulsions, Guillain-Barre Syndrome, and brachial neuritis may rarely be associated with tetanus toxoid. Degenerative diseases of the brain, other diseases affecting the nerves, and Sudden Infant Death Syndrome have been reported following administration of preparations containing diphtheria, tetanus, and/or pertussis antigens. No cause and effect relationships have been established for these effects.

*Toxoids:* Never use tetanus, pertussis, or diphtheria toxoids to treat actual infections, nor for immediate protection of unimmunized people.

*Pregnancy:* There are no adequate and well-controlled studies in pregnant women. Diphtheria and tetanus toxoid is the preferred vaccine for pregnant women. It has been administered safely to thousands of pregnant women in an effort to prevent tetanus in newborns considered to be at high risk. Use tetanus toxoid or diphtheria and tetanus toxoid only if clearly needed.

*Breastfeeding:* It is not known if these vaccines appear in breast milk. Consult your doctor before you begin breastfeeding.

*Children:* DTaP is the recommended immunization for most children younger than 7 years of age. Safety and effectiveness of DTaP in children younger than 6 weeks of age has not been established. Tetanus toxoid may be used in children. However, for children younger than 7 years of age, DT (for pediatric use) is preferred to tetanus toxoid alone if pertussis vaccine is not indicated. For children 7 years of age and older, tetanus and diphtheria toxoids (Td) (for adult use) is preferred to tetanus toxoid alone.

## Drug Interactions:

Tell your doctor or pharmacist if you are taking or if you are planning to take any over-the-counter or prescription medications or dietary supplements while receiving this vaccine. Doses of one or both drugs may need to be modified or a different drug may need to be prescribed. The following drugs and drug classes interact with this vaccine:

anticoagulants (eg, warfarin)

immunosuppressants (eg, cancer drugs, corticosteroids)

## Side Effects:

Every vaccine is capable of producing side effects. Many patients experience no, or minor, side effects. The frequency and severity of side effects depend on many factors including dose and individual susceptibility. Possible side effects include:

*Local:* Redness; warmth; pain; tenderness; swelling; nodules; abscess.

*Other: (Moderate):* Fever; chills; appetite loss; drowsiness; vomiting; diarrhea; fussiness; general body discomfort; joint, muscle, or body aches and pains; headache; flushing; rash; hives; itching; irritability; rapid heartbeat; low blood pressure; nasal congestion; nausea; degenerative brain disease; loss of consciousness; neurological problems.
*(Severe):* Fever of 105°F or higher; persistent crying lasting 3 hours or more; unusual high-pitched crying; collapse; shock-like state; seizures; convulsions with or without fever.

## Guidelines for Use:

- Immunizations will be prepared and administered by your health care provider in a medical setting.
- *Primary immunization (DTaP):* For children 6 weeks through 7 years of age (ideally beginning at age 6 weeks to 2 months). Given on three occasions at 4 to 8 week intervals with a fourth injection 6 to 12 months after the third injection.
- *Booster doses* are given when the child is 4 to 6 years of age (preferably prior to entering kindergarten or elementary school). However, if the fourth dose of the basic series was administered after the fourth birthday, a recall (booster) of DTaP or DT prior to school entry is not necessary.
- *Tetanus boosters:* After complete primary tetanus immunization, boosters — even for wound management — need to be given only every 10 years when wounds are minor and uncontaminated. For other wounds, a booster is appropriate if the patient has not received tetanus toxoid within the preceding 5 years. Administering booster doses more frequently than recommended may cause increased incidence and severity of reactions.
- Before the administration of any dose of vaccine, the parent, guardian, or adult patient will be asked about the recent health status and immunization history of the patient being immunized in order to determine whether any problems may exist that should prevent vaccination.

## Guidelines for Use (cont.):

- When the parent, guardian, or adult patient returns for the next dose in a series, he should be questioned concerning the occurrence of any symptoms or side effects after the previous dose.
- *Tetanus and Diphtheria Toxoids Adsorbed for Adult Use (Td)* is the preferred preparation for active tetanus immunization in wound management of patients 7 years of age or older. This is to enhance diphtheria protection. Given on two occasions at 4- to 8-week intervals with a third injection 6 to 12 months after the second injection.
- Delay vaccination when infections with fever are present. Only healthy individuals should be injected. Delay voluntary immunization of patients during a polio outbreak.
- Diphtheria, pertussis, or tetanus toxoids are not used to treat active infections with diphtheria, pertussis, or tetanus.
- Infection with tetanus or diphtheria does not ensure immunity; initiation or completion of vaccination is required at the time of recovery from these infections. However, children who have recovered from pertussis do not need further pertussis vaccination.
- Patients receiving corticosteroids, chemotherapy, or radiation therapy, and those with a recent injection of immune globulin or an immunodeficiency disorder (eg, AIDS) may not respond well to active immunization. When possible, interrupt treatment of these conditions when immunization is considered due to a tetanus-prone wound.
- If any of the following occurs after administration, contact your doctor immediately and avoid further use of this product: allergic reaction, fever of 105°F or greater within 48 hours of injection, collapse or shock, crying lasting 3 hours or more, unusual high-pitched crying occurring within 48 hours, seizures with or without fever within 3 days of injection, nervous system symptoms including unconsciousness within 7 days of injection.
- Fever, chills, crying, aching, and redness and tenderness at the injection site may occur following vaccination. Contact your doctor if these symptoms persist or become bothersome.
- Vaccination may not result in development of antibodies in all individuals.
- Acetaminophen (eg, *Tylenol*) may be given at time of vaccination and every 4 to 6 hours to reduce post-vaccination fever.

*If you have any questions, consult your doctor, pharmacist, or health care provider.*

| Generic Name Brand Name Examples | Uses |
|---|---|
| Rx **Haemophilus b Conjugate Vaccine** ActHIB, HibTITER[1], Liquid PedvaxHIB | For the routine immunization of children 2 to 71 months of age (HibTITER, PedvaxHIB), 2 to 18 months of age (ActHIB and ActHIB reconstituted with DTP), and 15 to 18 months of age (ActHIB reconstituted with TriHIBit [see Diphtheria/Tetanus/Pertussis/Haemophilus b monograph in this chapter]) against invasive diseases caused by Haemophilus influenzae type b. These vaccines will not protect against Hemophilus influenzae other than type b or other bacteria or viruses that cause meningitis or other infections. |

[1] Multidose vial contains thimerosal.

Haemophilus influenzae type b (Haemophilus b, Hib) is a leading cause of serious bacterial infections in the US. Most cases of H. influenzae meningitis among children are caused by type b H. influenzae. In addition to meningitis (infection of lining of brain and spinal cord), haemophilus b is responsible for other diseases, including epiglottitis (infection of flap at back of throat), sepsis (blood poisoning), septic arthritis (infection in joints), osteomyelitis (bone infection), pericarditis (infection around the heart), and pneumonia.

Approximately 17% of all cases of haemophilus b disease occur in infants less than 6 months of age, 47% by 1 year of age and the remaining 53% over the next 4 years. Peak incidence occurs between 6 and 11 months of age. Incidence rates of Hib disease are increased in high risk groups, such as Native Americans (ie, American Indians, Eskimos), blacks, low-income individuals, household contacts of cases, caucasians who lack the G2m (n or 23) immunoglobulin allotype and patients with asplenia, sickle cell disease, Hodgkin disease, and immune deficiency syndromes. Recent studies suggest that risk for children under 5 acquiring Hib disease appears greater for those who attend daycare facilities than for those who do not.

## Type of Drug:

Active immunization for Haemophilus influenzae type b infections.

## How the Drug Works:

Haemophilus b vaccine provides long-term protection against H. influenzae type b by stimulating the body to produce antibodies to the organism.

## Precautions:

Do not use in the following situations:

allergy to components of vaccine (eg, diphtheria toxoid, meningococcal proteins, pertussis vaccine)
allergy to thimerosal (HibTITER multidose vial only)

*Use with caution in the following situations:*

blood clotting (coagulation) disorders
chemotherapy (cancer drugs)
fever
immune deficiency disorders (decreased antibody production)
immunosuppressive therapy
infection, active
low platelet count
radiation therapy

*Immunodeficiency:* People receiving corticosteroids, chemotherapy, radiation therapy, those with a recent injection of immunoglobulin, or with an immunodeficiency disorder (eg, AIDS) may not respond well to these vaccines. Defer vaccination until immunosuppressive therapy has ended, or give another dose 1 month after therapy has ended. However, vaccination of AIDS patients is recommended.

*Pregnancy:* There are no adequate and well-controlled studies in pregnant women. Use is not recommended.

*Children:* Safety and effectiveness in infants younger than 6 weeks of age have not been established.

## Drug Interactions:

Tell your doctor or pharmacist if you are taking or planning to take any over-the-counter or prescription medication or dietary supplements while receiving this vaccine. Doses of one or both drugs may need to be modified or a different drug may need to be prescribed. The following drugs and drug classes interact with this vaccine:

anticoagulants (eg, warfarin)
immunosuppressive agents (eg, cancer drugs, corticosteroids)

## Side Effects:

Every vaccine is capable of producing side effects. Many patients experience no, or minor, side effects. The frequency and severity of side effects depend on many factors including dose and individual susceptibility. Possible side effects include:

*Local:* Redness; pain; swelling; tenderness; nodules; rash.

*Other:* Fever; crying; irritability; drowsiness; diarrhea; vomiting; appetite loss; lethargy.

## Guidelines for Use:

- This vaccine will be prepared and administered by your health care provider in a medical setting.
- For recommended immunization schedules, see the chart in this chapter.
- To obtain maximum protection, the entire immunizing series must be completed.
- If possible, delay the vaccine when there is fever or infection present.
- *Haemophilus b disease* may be contracted during the week after vaccination, prior to the onset of the protective effects of the vaccine.
- Before the administration of any dose of vaccine, the parent, guardian, or adult patient will be asked about the recent health status and immunization history of the patient being immunized in order to determine whether any problems may exist that should prevent vaccination.
- When the parent, guardian, or adult patient returns for the next dose in a series, he should be questioned concerning the occurrence of any symptoms or side effects after the previous dose.
- Fever, crying, or redness, hardness, or tenderness at the injection site may occur following vaccination. Contact your doctor if these symptoms persist or become bothersome.
- If any of the following occurs after administration, contact your doctor immediately and avoid further use of this product: allergic reaction, fever of 105°F or greater within 48 hours of injection, collapse or shock, crying lasting 3 hours or more, unusual high-pitched crying occurring within 48 hours, seizures with or without fever within 3 days of injection, nervous system symptoms including unconsciousness within 7 days of injection.
- These vaccines may not work for every patient.
- Acetaminophen (eg, *Tylenol*) may be given at time of vaccination and every 4 to 6 hours to reduce post-vaccination fever.

*If you have any questions, consult your doctor, pharmacist, or health care provider.*

| Generic Name<br>*Brand Name*<br>*Example* | Uses |
|---|---|
| *Rx*  **Haemophilus b Conjugate and Hepatitis B Vaccine**<br><br>*Comvax* | For vaccination against disease caused by *Haemophilus influenzae* type b and hepatitis B virus in infants 6 weeks to 15 months of age born of mothers who do not have evidence of hepatitis B infection. |

## Type of Drug:

Vaccine.

## How the Drug Works:

Produces immunity by fostering the production of antibodies.

## Precautions:

*Do not use in the following situations:*
> allergy to the vaccine or any of its ingredients
> acute febrile illness

*Use with caution in the following situations:*
> immunosuppression
> infants with bleeding disorders
> malignancy

*Children:* This drug should not be used in infants younger than 6 weeks of age.

## Drug Interactions:

Tell your doctor or pharmacist if you taking or planning to take any over-the-counter or prescription medications or dietary supplements while receiving this vaccine. Doses of one or both drugs may need to be modified or a different drug may need to be prescribed. Immunosuppressive drugs (eg, prednisone) interact with this vaccine.

## Side Effects:

Every vaccine is capable of producing side effects. Many patients experience no, or minor, side effects. The frequency and severity of side effects depend on many factors, including dose and individual susceptibility. Possible side effects include:

*Digestive Tract:* Loss of appetite; vomiting; diarrhea.

*Nervous System:* Irritability; agitation; sleepiness; crying.

*Respiratory System:* Cough; upper respiratory infection; runny nose; difficulty breathing.

*Other:* Pain at the injection site; swelling; fever; rash; seizures; joint pain; arthritis; visual disturbances; inflammation of the middle ear; rapid heartbeat; redness or indentation at injection site.

---

**Guidelines for Use:**

- This vaccine will be prepared and administered by your health care provider in a medical setting.
- Infants born to HBsAg negative monthers should be vaccinated with three 0.5 mL doses, ideally at 2, 4 and 12 to 15 months of age. If the recommended schedule cannot be followed, the interval between the first two doses should be at least six weeks and the interval between the second and the third dose should be as close as possible to 8 to 11 months.
- Not for use in any infant before the age of 6 weeks.

---

*If you have any questions, consult your doctor, pharmacist, or health care provider.*

| Generic Name<br>*Brand Name*<br>*Example* | Uses |
|---|---|
| *Rx* **Diphtheria and Tetanus Toxoids and Pertussis Vaccine Adsorbed and Haemophilus b Conjugate Vaccine**<br>*TriHIBit*[1] | For active immunization of children 15 to 18 months of age who have previously been immunized against diphtheria, tetanus, and pertussis with 3 doses consisting of either diphtheria and tetanus toxoids and whole cell pertussis (DTP) or DTaP vaccine and 3 or fewer doses of *ActHIB* within the first year of life for the prevention of invasive diseases caused by *Haemophilus influenzae* type b or by diphtheria, tetanus, and pertussis (refer to the separate monographs for these vaccines in this chapter). |

[1] Contains thimerosal.

## Type of Drug:

Active immunization against diphtheria, tetanus, pertussis, and haemophilus b.

## How the Drug Works:

This vaccine provides long-term protection against diphtheria, tetanus, pertussis, and haemophilus b by stimulating the body to produce antibodies against the organisms causing these infections.

## Precautions:

*Do not use in the following situations:*

allergy to the vaccine or any of its ingredients
allergy to thimerosal
fever
infection, acute or active
pertussis, history of
polio outbreak
seizures, history of
serious reaction after a previous dose of DTaP (eg, seizure, high fever, shock, unconsciousness, allergic reaction)

*Use with caution in the following situations:*

blood clotting (coagulation) disorder
chemotherapy (cancer drugs)
corticosteroid (eg, prednisone) use, current
immune deficiency disorders
low platelet count
nervous system disorders, history of
radiation therapy

*Immunodeficiency:* People receiving corticosteroids, chemotherapy, radiation therapy, those with a recent injection of immunoglobulin, or with an immunodeficiency disorder (eg, AIDS) may not respond well to these vaccines. Defer vaccination until immunosuppressive therapy has ended, or give another dose 1 month after therapy has ended. However, vaccination of AIDS patients is recommended.

*Pregnancy:* There are no adequate and well-controlled studies in pregnant women. Use is not recommended.

*Children:* Safety and effectiveness in children younger than 15 months of age have not been established.

## Drug Interactions:

Tell your doctor or pharmacist if you are taking or if you are planning to take any over-the-counter or prescription medications or dietary supplements while receiving this vaccine. Doses of one or both drugs may need to be modified or a different drug may need to be prescribed. The following drugs and drug classes interact with this vaccine:

anticoagulants (eg, warfarin)

immunosuppressive agents (eg, cancer drugs, corticosteroids)

## Side Effects:

Every vaccine is capable of producing side effects. Many patients experience no, or minor, side effects. The frequency and severity of side effects depend on many factors including dose and individual susceptibility. Possible side effects include:

Consider side effects of Diphtheria/Tetanus/Pertussis and Haemophilus b vaccines as well. Refer to the monographs in this chapter.

*Local:* Redness; pain or tenderness; swelling; warmth; nodules.

*Other:* Fever; irritability; drowsiness; restless sleep; appetite loss; vomiting; diarrhea; rash; crying; lethargy.

### Guidelines for Use:

- This vaccine will be prepared and administered by your health care provider in a medical setting.
- It is important that the patient complete the immunization series.
- Delay vaccination when fever or infection are present.
- Doses of the vaccine are generally given at 2 months, 4 months, 6 months, between 15 to 18 months, and between 4 to 6 years of age.
- Before the administration of any dose of vaccine, the parent, guardian, or adult patient will be asked about the recent health status and immunization history of the patient being immunized in order to determine whether any problems may exist that should prevent vaccination.
- When the parent, guardian, or adult patient returns for the next dose in a series, he should be questioned concerning the occurrence of any symptoms or side effects after the previous dose.
- Fever, crying, or redness, hardness, or tenderness at the injection site may occur following vaccination. Contact your doctor if these symptoms persist or become bothersome.
- If any of the following occurs after administration, contact your doctor immediately and avoid further use of this product: allergic reaction, fever of 105°F or greater within 48 hours of injection, collapse or shock, crying lasting 3 hours or more, unusual high-pitched crying occurring within 48 hours, seizures with or without fever within 3 days of injection, nervous system symptoms including unconsciousness within 7 days of injection.
- Acetaminophen (eg, *Tylenol*) may be given at time of vaccination and every 4 to 6 hours to reduce post-vaccination fever.
- This vaccine may not work for every patient.

*If you have any questions, consult your doctor, pharmacist, or health care provider.*

| | Generic Name<br>*Brand Name*<br>*Examples* | Uses |
|---|---|---|
| *Rx* | **Poliovirus Vaccine,<br>Live, Oral,<br>Trivalent (TOPV;<br>OPV; Sabin)**<br>*Orimune* | To prevent poliomyelitis caused by Poliovirus 1, 2 and 3. |
| *Rx* | **Poliovirus Vaccine,<br>Inactivated<br>(PIV; Salk)**<br>*IPOL, Poliovax* | To prevent poliomyelitis caused by Poliovirus 1, 2 and 3. |

Immunization is recommended for certain adults who are at greater risk of poliomyelitis (polio) than the general population, including: Travelers to areas or countries where polio immunization is needed, members of communities or specific population groups with disease caused by wild polioviruses, laboratory workers handling specimens which may contain poliovirus, healthcare workers in close contact with patients who may be excreting polioviruses and incompletely or unvaccinated adults in contact with children receiving OPV.

Persons with immune-deficiency diseases such as agammaglobulinemia, acquired immune deficiency syndrome (AIDS), or immune diseases or immunosuppressive therapy (eg, corticosteroids) as well as persons with close contacts or household members who have such conditions, should receive Poliovirus Vaccine Inactivated if immunization is indicated.

It is recommended that routine immunization of children against polio be accomplished using Poliovirus Vaccine Live Oral. However, Poliovirus Vaccine Inactivated is preferred in children with immunodeficiency or who have siblings with immunodeficiency until the immune status of the family can be documented.

## Type of Drug:
Active immunization against polio.

## How the Drug Works:
Poliovirus vaccine provides long-term protection against poliomyelitis by stimulating the body to produce antibodies against the virus causing the disease.

## Precautions:
*Do not use in the following situations:*

allergy to vaccine or any of its components, including streptomycin, poliomyxin B or neomycin (IPV only)

diarrhea (OPV only)
fever, severe
illness, acute
vomiting (OPV only)

*Use with caution in the following situations:*
immune globulin (IG) vaccine (OPV only)

*Immune diseases:* The oral vaccine (OPV) must not be given to people with immune deficiency diseases or those with altered immune states (eg, leukemia, lymphoma or generalized malignancy, HIV) or with immune systems compromised by therapy with corticosteroids, cancer chemotherapy or radiation. Because the vaccine virus may be spread by the vaccinated person (through feces), OPV should not be given to family members of people with altered immune status. IPV is the preferred method for immunizing these individuals.

*Vaccine-associated paralysis:* When the vaccine is introduced into a household with adults who have never been vaccinated or whose immune status cannot be determined, risk may be minimized by giving them 2 doses of IPV a month apart before the children receive OPV. The children may receive the first dose of OPV at the same time as the adults receiving the second dose of IPV. The adults should also take precautions, such as handwashing after diaper changes.

The Centers for Disease Control report that during the years 1973 through 1984 approximately 274 million doses of OPV were distributed in the US. During this same period, 105 vaccine-associated cases were reported. Of these, 35 "vaccine-associated" and 50 "contact vaccine-associated" paralytic cases were reported. Fourteen other "vaccine-associated" cases have been reported in persons (recipients or contacts) with immune deficiency conditions and 6 other cases occurred in persons with no history of vaccine exposure.

Recipients of the OPV should avoid close contact with all persons with altered immune status for 6 to 8 weeks.

*Pregnancy:* Safety for use during pregnancy has not been established, or animal studies may have shown a risk to the fetus. Use only when clearly needed and when potential benefits outweigh the possible hazards to the fetus. However, if immediate protection against poliomyelitis is needed, OPV is recommended.

*Breastfeeding:* Women should avoid breastfeeding for 2 to 3 hours before and after the infant is vaccinated so that it does not interfere with the vaccine.

*Children:* Safety and effectiveness for use in children under 6 weeks have not been established.

## Drug Interactions:

Tell your doctor or pharmacist if you are taking or planning to take any over-the-counter or prescription medications or dietary supplements while taking this medicine. Doses of one or both drugs may need to be modified or a different drug may need to be prescribed. The following drugs and drug classes interact with this medicine.

cholera vaccine
immunosuppressants (eg, corticosteroids)

## Side Effects:

Every vaccine is capable of producing side effects. Many patients experience no, or minor, side effects. The frequency and severity of side effects depend on many factors including dose and individual susceptibility. Possible side effects include:

*Oral – Vaccine-associated paralysis:* Paralysis following the use of live poliovirus vaccines have been reported in individuals given the vaccine and in persons who were in close contact with people who have recently been vaccinated.

The risk of vaccine-associated paralysis is extremely small for those vaccinated, susceptible family members and other close personal contacts.

*Injection –* Redness, hardness and pain or discomfort at injection site (within 6-12 hours of vaccination and lasting 1-3 days); fever; sleepiness; fussiness; reduced appetite; crying; spitting up feedings.

## Guidelines for Use:

- The polio vaccine series is three doses.

    *OPV* — The ACIP and the American Academy of Pediatrics recommend that the series be started at 6 to 12 weeks of age. The second dose should be given not less than 6, and preferably 8, weeks later. The third dose is given 8 to 12 months after the second dose. An optional dose may be given at 6 months.

    *IPV* — The first two doses are given at 2 and 4 months of age with an interval of not less than 4, and preferably 8, weeks, commonly with the first DTP immunization at 2 months of age. The third dose is given not less than 6, and preferably 12, months later.

    *School entrance* — When entering elementary school, all children who have completed the primary series should receive a single followup dose of OPV, unless they received the third dose on or after their fourth birthday. All others should complete the primary series. The ACIP does not recommend routine booster doses of vaccine beyond those given when entering school.

    *Older children, adolescents and adults* — Two doses of OPV, given not less than 6, and preferably 8, weeks apart and the third dose 6 to 12 months after the second dose. An optional third dose may be given 6 to 8 weeks after the second dose.

- Delay vaccination when vomiting, diarrhea, fever or infection are present.

- People allergic to neomycin, polymyxin B or streptomycin should not receive IPV vaccine.

- The vaccine will not change or prevent cases of existing or incubating poliomyelitis.

- *Vaccine-associated paralysis* — Paralytic disease following OPV vaccination has been reported in individuals receiving the vaccine and in persons who were in close contact with vaccines. The risk is greater in those with immune-deficiency diseases.

- *Guillain-Barre syndrome (GBS),* characterized by paralysis, has occurred rarely after the administration of the OPV vaccine. No cause and effect relationship has been established. Evaluate the possible risk of GBS against the risk of polio and its complications.

- Redness, hardness and tenderness at the injection site, sleepiness, fussiness, reduced appetite and crying may occur beginning 6 to 12 hours following vaccination. They will begin to disappear in 1 to 3 days. Contact your doctor if any of these symptoms persist or become bothersome.

- Vaccination may not work in everybody.

*If you have any questions, consult your doctor, pharmacist, or health care provider.*

| Generic Name<br>*Brand Name Examples* | Uses |
|---|---|
| *Rx* **Measles (Rubeola)<br>Virus Vaccine,<br>Live, Attenuated**<br>*Attenuvax* | For immunization against measles (rubeola) in children 15 months or older and adults. |
| *Rx* **Rubella Virus Vaccine,<br>Live**<br>*Meruvax II* | For immunization against rubella in children 12 months or older and adults. |
| *Rx* **Mumps Virus Vaccine,<br>Live**<br>*Mumpsvax* | For immunization against mumps in children 12 months or older and adults. |
| *Rx* **Rubella and Mumps<br>Virus<br>Vaccine, Live**<br>*Biavax II* | For simultaneous immunization against rubella and mumps in children 12 months or older and adults. |
| *Rx* **Measles (Rubeola) and<br>Rubella Virus Vaccine,<br>Live**<br>*M-R-Vax II* | For simultaneous immunization against measles and rubella in children 15 months or older and adults. |
| *Rx* **Measles, Mumps and<br>Rubella Virus Vaccine,<br>Live**<br>*M-M-R II* | For simultaneous immunization against measles, mumps and rubella in children 15 months or older and adults. |

Children in kindergarten and the first grades of elementary school may be required to have measles, mumps and rubella vaccinations because they are often the major source of infection in the community.

A two-dose schedule for MMR vaccination is now recommended to improve control of measles. When rubella vaccine is part of a combination that includes measles, give the combination to children at 15 months of age or older to maximize protection. A second dose of MMR is recommended at school entry. Vaccinate older children who have not received rubella vaccine promptly.

Strongly recommended for: Children living in schools, orphanages and similar institutions; malnourished children; those with inactive or active tuberculosis under treatment; those with chronic diseases such as cystic fibrosis, heart disease, asthma and other chronic lung diseases.

## Type of Drug:
Active immunization against measles, mumps and rubella.

## How the Drug Works:
Measles, mumps and rubella vaccines provide long-term protection against measles (rubeola), mumps or rubella by stimulating the body to produce antibodies to organisms causing these illnesses.

## 1271 Precautions:

*Do not use in the following situations:*

AIDS
allergy to eggs, severe
allergy to neomycin
blood diseases (eg, leukemia)
infection, with fever
immune deficiency disorders
  (decreased antibody production), including family history

immunosuppressive therapy
  (eg,chemotherapy)
infection with fever
pregnancy
tuberculosis, active, untreated

*Use with caution in the following situations:*

brain injury, history
conditions where stress due to fever should be avoided
seizures, individual or family history

*Pregnancy:* Do not use during pregnancy. Avoid pregnancy for 3 months following vaccination. Adequate studies of the vaccine strain of the measles virus have not been done in pregnant women. Contracting measles during pregnancy increases the possibility of fetal harm. Increased rates of miscarriage, stillbirth, congenital defects and prematurity have been reported after contracting natural measles. The vaccine may also be capable of inducing harm to the fetus for up to 3 months following vaccination. If measles exposure occurs during pregnancy, consider providing temporary protection with immune serum globulin (ISG).

*Breastfeeding:* It is not known if these vaccines appear in breast milk. Consult your doctor before you begin breastfeeding.

*Children:* Use with caution in children with a history of fever convulsions, head injury or conditions in which stress due to fever should be avoided. Fever may occur following vaccination. Children infected with immune deficiency disorders but without manifestations of the disorders should be monitored closely. Mumps and rubella vaccines are not recommended for children under 1 year of age.

## Side Effects:

Every vaccine is capable of producing side effects. Many patients experience no, or minor, local side effects. The frequency and severity of side effects depend on many factors including dose and individual susceptibility. Possible side effects include fever (up to 103° F for up to 1 month); rash (between 5th and 12th days); hives; swelling, redness, hardness, tenderness, burning or stinging at injection site; swollen glands; muscle and joint aches; general body discomfort; cough; nasal congestion; sore throat; headache; dizziness; nausea; vomiting; diarrhea; nerve inflammation; inflammation of the eye.

## Guidelines for Use:

- *MMR* is given after 15 months of age followed by a second dose at school entry.
- Children vaccinated when younger than 12 months of age should be revaccinated at 15 months of age.
- Do not administer within one month of DTaP, DTP or OPV.
- Delay vaccination when fever or infection is present.
- People who have had severe allergic reactions to eggs or neomycin should not receive these vaccines.
- Vaccination should be deferred for at least 3 months following blood or plasma transfusions, or administration of ISG.
- Fever (up to 103° F) may occur for up to 1 month following vaccination. A rash may appear between the 5th and 12th day following vaccination. Swelling, redness, burning or stinging at the injection site, swollen glands and muscle and joint aches may also occur. Contact your doctor if any of these symptoms persist or become bothersome.
- *Tuberculin skin test:* Measles, mumps and rubella vaccines may temporarily depress tuberculin skin reaction. Administer the test before or at the same time as the vaccine.
- *Measles: If immediate protection* against measles is required for persons in whom the vaccine is not recommended, passive immunization with ISG is recommended. Do not give ISG with measles vaccination.
- Giving the live virus vaccine immediately after exposure to natural measles may prevent illness. When in doubt, vaccination is recommended.
- The mumps vaccine does not give protection when given after exposure to natural mumps.
- *Guillain-Barre syndrome (GBS),* characterized by paralysis, has occurred rarely after administration of the live measles virus. No cause and effect relationship has been established. Evaluate the possible risk of GBS as compared with the risk of measles and its complications.
- These vaccinations may not result in development of antibodies in all individuals.

*If you have any questions, consult your doctor, pharmacist, or health care provider.*

| Generic Name *Brand Name Example* | Uses |
|---|---|
| Rx **Varicella Virus Vaccine, Live** *Varivax* | For immunization of persons over 12 months of age who have not yet had the varicella virus (chickenpox). |

## Type of Drug:
Active immunization against varicella.

## How the Drug Works:
The varicella vaccine provides protection against varicella (chickenpox) by stimulating the body to produce antibodies to the virus causing this illness.

## Precautions:
*Do not use in the following situations:*
> allergy to the vaccine or its ingredients, including gelatin
> allergy to neomycin
> acquired immunodeficiency syndrome (AIDS)
> blood, bone marrow or lymph system diseases
> immune deficiency disorders (deceased antibody production), including family history
> immunosuppressive therapy
> infection, active with fever
> pregnancy (or those attempting to become pregnant)
> respiratory illness, with fever
> tuberculosis, active, untreated

*Pregnancy:* Adequate studies have not been done in women, or animal studies may have shown a risk to the fetus. It is recommended that the vaccine not be administered during pregnancy. Contracting varicella during pregnancy (via the live vaccine) increases the possibility of fetal harm. Avoid pregnancy for 3 months following vaccination.

*Breastfeeding:* It is not known if this vaccine virus appears in breast milk. Consult your doctor before you begin breastfeeding.

*Children:* Safety and effectiveness in children younger than 1 year of age have not been established.

## Drug Interactions:
Tell your doctor or pharmacist if you are taking or if you are planning to take any over-the-counter or prescription medications or dietary supplements while taking this medicine. Doses of one or both drugs may need to be modified or a different drug may need to be prescribed. Immunosuppressants and salicylates (eg, aspirin) interact with this medicine.

## Side Effects:

Every drug is capable of producing side effects. Many patients experience no, or minor, side effects. The frequency and severity of side effects depend on many factors including dose, duration of therapy and individual susceptibility. Possible side effects include:

*Local:* Pain, swelling, rash, itching, stiffness, hardness, redness, numbness, bruising at injection site.

*Digestive Tract:* Diarrhea; appetite changes; vomiting; nausea; constipation; stomach pain.

*Nervous System:* Irritability; nervousness; tiredness; sleep disorders; headache.

*Respiratory System:* Runny nose; upper or lower respiratory illness; cough.

*Other:* Fever; chills; ear infection; teething; general body discomfort; eye problems; muscle or joint pain; stiff neck; dry skin; cold/canker sores.

---

### Guidelines for Use:

- *Recommended vaccination schedule* — 1 to 12 years of age: one dose; Over 12 years of age: two doses given 1-2 months apart.
- Contact your doctor if any of the following occurs: itching, rash, fever, difficulty breathing.
- Female patients should avoid becoming pregnant for 3 months after receiving this vaccine.
- Do not use salicylates (eg, aspirin) for 6 weeks after receiving this vaccine.
- Persons given this vaccine could pass the active vaccine virus to others. Therefore, avoid close contact with pregnant women, infants and people with low immune systems.
- Wait at least 5 months to receive this vaccine after blood/plasma transfusions, immune globulin or varicella zoster immune globulin (VZIG) therapy.
- Any immune globulin, including VZIG, should not be given for 2 months after administration of this vaccine.
- This vaccine may be given at the same time as the measles, mumps, rubella, diptheria, tetanus and pertussis vaccines.
- The length of protection from the virus is not known, nor is it a guarantee that the vaccine will protect everyone from the chickenpox virus.

---

*If you have any questions, consult your doctor, pharmacist, or health care provider.*

| Generic Name Brand Name Examples | Uses |
|---|---|
| Rx **Influenza Virus Vaccine**[1] *Fluogen*; *FluShield*; *Fluvirin*; *Fluzone (subvirion and whole virion)* | For high-risk persons 6 months of age or older; medical care personnel and primary providers of care in the home; children and teenagers (6 months to 18 years of age) receiving long-term aspirin therapy; persons infected with human immunodeficiency virus (HIV); and other persons who wish to reduce their chances for acquiring influenza. |

[1] Contains 0.01% thimerosal and sulfites.

*Groups at increased risk for influenza complications include:* Adults and children with chronic lung and heart disorders, including children with asthma; residents of nursing homes and other chronic care facilities housing patients of any age with chronic medical conditions; persons 65 years of age or older; adults and children who have required regular medical follow-up or hospitalization during the preceding year because of chronic metabolic diseases (including diabetes mellitus), kidney disease, blood disorders, or immunosuppression; children and teenagers (6 months to 18 years of age) who are receiving long-term aspirin therapy and therefore may be at risk of developing Reye's syndrome after influenza; and women who will be in the second or third trimester of pregnancy during the influenza season.

*Groups capable of transmitting influenza to high-risk persons include:* Doctors, nurses, and others in both hospital and outpatient care; employees of nursing homes and chronic care facilities who have contact with patients or residents; providers of home care to high-risk persons (eg, health care workers); and household members (including children) of high-risk persons.

*General population:* Any person who wishes to reduce the chance of acquiring influenza should be vaccinated. Persons who provide essential community services (eg, the military) and students or others in institutional settings (eg, those who reside in dormitories) may consider vaccination to prevent the disruption of routine activities during outbreaks.

*Pregnant women* who have other medical conditions that increase their risks for complications from influenza should be vaccinated. Although the vaccine is considered safe for pregnant women, the clinical judgement of the attending doctor should prevail at all times in determining whether to administer the vaccine to a pregnant woman.

*Persons infected with HIV:* Little information exists regarding the frequency and severity of influenza illness or benefits among persons infected with HIV. Because influenza may result in serious illness and complications, vaccination is recommended. However, response to the vaccine may be low in persons with advanced HIV-related illnesses and a second dose has not been shown to improve response.

*Travelers:* The risk of exposure to influenza during travel depends on the time of year and destination. Persons at high risk for complications of influenza should consider influenza vaccination before travel if they were not vaccinated with the influenza vaccine during the preceding fall or winter and they plan to travel to the Tropics, travel with large, organized tourist groups at any time of year, or travel to the Southern Hemisphere from April through September. Persons at high risk who received the previous season's vaccine before travel should be revaccinated with the current vaccine in the following fall or winter. Because the influenza vaccine might not be available during the summer in North America, persons 65 years of age or older and others at high risk should consult their doctors regarding symptoms and risks of influenza before embarking on travel during the summer.

## Type of Drug:

Flu vaccine (flu shot).

## How the Drug Works:

Injection of material from inactivated influenza virus stimulates the production of specific antibodies. Protection from this injection is only against those strains from which the vaccine is prepared, or against closely related strains. Having received a vaccination for one flu season does not prevent the need to be revaccinated for subsequent flu seasons to provide ideal protection.

## Precautions:

*Do not use in the following situations:*

allergy to any component of the vaccine

allergy to chicken eggs, chicken, chicken feathers, or chicken dander

allergy to thimerosal (eg, mercury)

children younger than 6 months of age

febrile illness, acute

Guillain-Barré syndrome, history

neurologic disorder, active

*Use with caution in the following situations:*

anticoagulant therapy, concurrent

children 6 to 35 months of age

coagulation disorder (eg, thrombocytopenia)

impaired immune response

*Other vaccinations:* Because children are accessible when pediatric vaccines are given, the influenza vaccine may be given with other routine pediatric vaccines, but at a different injection site.

Pneumococcal, measles-mumps-rubella, oral polio, and *Haemophilus* b vaccines can be given at the same time as the influenza vaccine. Vaccines should be given at different injection sites. Influenza vaccine is given annually; pneumococcal vaccine should be given only once.

*Guillain-Barré syndrome (GBS),* which causes paralysis, has occurred within 10 weeks following influenza vaccine. However, it is usually self-limited and reversible. Most persons recover without permanent weakness, although about 5% of cases are fatal. Current vaccines (since 1980) have not been associated with an increased frequency of GBS. Nonetheless, be aware of the possible risk as compared with the risk of influenza and its complications.

*Other neurologic disorders* Other neurologic disorders, including degenerative disease of the brain, have been temporarily associated with influenza vaccination.

*Immunosuppressed patients* (eg, persons with leukemia, lymphoma, cancer, or persons undergoing therapy with corticosteroids, cancer drugs, or radiation) may experience a lower than expected response to the vaccine. Oral amantadine may be given to supplement vaccination in high-risk patients.

*Pregnancy:* Pregnancy has not been demonstrated to be a risk factor for severe influenza infection. However, pregnant women with medical conditions that increase the risk of complications from influenza should be vaccinated. Influenza vaccine is considered safe for pregnant women without a severe egg allergy. Vaccination should be given after the first trimester. However, it may be undesirable to delay vaccinating a pregnant woman who has a high-risk condition and will still be in the first trimester of pregnancy when the influenza season usually begins. Influenza vaccine should be given to a pregnant woman only if clearly needed. The clinical judgement of the attending doctor should prevail at all times in determining whether to administer the vaccine to a pregnant woman.

*Breastfeeding:* Influenza vaccine does not affect the safety of mothers who are breastfeeding or their infants. Breastfeeding does not adversely affect immune response and is not a contraindication for vaccination.

*Children:* Influenza split virus vaccines (*Fluogen, FluShield, Fluzone, Fluvirin*) are not approved for infants under 6 months of age. The likelihood of fever-induced convulsions is greater in children 6 months through 35 months of age. Therefore, special care should be taken in weighing the risks and benefits of vaccination. The whole virus vaccine (*Fluzone*) should not be given to children under 13 years of age. The safety and effectiveness of *Fluvirin* in children between 6 months and 4 years of age has not been established. However, vaccination for children 6 months of age and older is strongly recommended because of the increased risk of complications from influenza.

*Elderly:* Elderly persons and persons with underlying health problems are at an increased risk of complications from influenza infection. Members of these high risk groups are more likely than the general population to require hospitalization if they become ill with influenza.

*Sulfites:* Some of these products may contain sulfite preservatives which can cause allergic reactions in certain individuals (eg, some asthmatics). Check package label when available, or consult your doctor or pharmacist.

## Drug Interactions:

Tell your doctor or pharmacist if you are taking or planning to take any over-the-counter or prescription medications or dietary supplements before being vaccinated against the influenza virus. Doses of one or both drugs may need to be modified or a different drug may need to be prescribed. The following drugs and drug classes interact with influenza virus vaccine:

carbamazepine (eg, *Tegretol*) (*Fluzone* only)

theophylline (eg, *Theo-Dur*) warfarin (eg, *Coumadin*)

## Side Effects:

Every vaccine is capable of producing side effects. Many patients experience no, or minor, side effects. The frequency and severity of side effects depend on many factors including dose and individual susceptibility. Possible side effects include soreness at the injection site (1 to 2 days), fever, general body discomfort, and muscle aches.

## Guidelines for Use:

- This vaccine will be prepared and administered by your health care provider in a medical setting.
- *Recommended vaccination schedule* — Beginning each September, influenza vaccine should be offered to persons at high risk when they are seen by health care providers for routine care or as a result of hospitalization. For organized vaccination campaigns, the optimal time to vaccinate persons in high-risk groups is usually from October through mid-November because influenza activity in the United States generally peaks between late December and early March. Administering vaccine too far in advance of the influenza season should be avoided in certain facilities (eg, nursing homes) because antibody levels may begin to decline within a few months following vaccination. Children younger than 9 years of age not previously vaccinated require 2 doses administered at least 1 month apart. The second dose should be given before December, if possible.
- People allergic to chicken eggs, chicken, chicken feathers, or chicken dander should not receive this vaccine. In addition, administer vaccine with caution in patients with latex sensitivity since packaging includes some dry natural rubber.
- In persons suspected of having an allergy to chicken eggs, chicken, chicken feathers, or chicken dander, a scratch test should be performed prior to immunization. The scratch test will determine sensitivity to the vaccine. If the reaction is positive, the vaccine is not recommended.
- Delay the vaccine in acute illness with fever.
- *Children* — Because children are accessible when pediatric vaccines are given, it may be desirable to give the influenza vaccine at the same time as routine pediatric vaccines, but at a different injection site.
- Talk to your doctor about the risks of developing Guillain-Barré syndrome.
- Soreness at the injection site, fever, and muscle aches may occur following vaccination. Consult your doctor if these persist or become bothersome.
- Vaccination may not result in development of antibodies in all individuals.
- Contact your doctor if you experience rash, hives, itching, difficulty breathing, or redness or swelling at the injection site.

*If you have any questions, consult your doctor, pharmacist, or health care provider.*

| **Generic Name** | |
| *Brand Name Examples* | **Uses** |

*Rx* **Hepatitis A Vaccine, Inactivated**

*Havrix, VAQTA* — For active immunization of people 2 years of age and older against infection caused by the hepatitis A virus (HAV). This vaccine will not prevent infections caused by other hepatitis viruses or other infectious agents that can infect the liver.

*Individuals at high risk include:*

*Travelers:* People living in or traveling to areas where hepatitis A is common. These areas include, but are not limited to, Africa, Asia (except Japan), the Mediterranean basin, Eastern Europe, the Middle East, Central and South America, Mexico, and parts of the Caribbean. Consult current Centers for Disease Control and Prevention (CDC) advisories with regard to specific locales.

*Certain ethnic and geographic populations that experience cyclic hepatitis A epidemics:* Native peoples of Alaska and the Americas.

*Certain institutional workers:* Caretakers for the developmentally challenged, employees of child daycare centers, laboratory workers who handle live HAV, and handlers of primates that may be harboring the HAV.

*Others:* Military personnel, persons involved in high-risk sexual activity (eg, homosexual males), users of illicit injectable drugs, residents of a community experiencing an outbreak of hepatitis A, people with chronic liver disease (eg, alcoholic cirrhosis, hepatitis B, hepatitis C) or clotting-factor disorders, hemophiliacs and other recipients of therapeutic blood products, and certain food handlers.

For persons requiring postexposure prophylaxis or needing immediate protection (eg, travel on short notice to endemic areas), the vaccine may be supplemented with an injection of immune globulin (IG).

## Type of Drug:

Vaccine to immunize against HAV infection.

## How the Drug Works:

Hepatitis A vaccine provides active protection (immunization) against HAV by stimulating the body to produce antibodies against the virus causing this illness.

Primary immunization should be completed 2 or more weeks prior to expected exposure to HAV.

## Precautions:

*Do not use in the following situations:* Allergy to hepatitis A vaccine or any of its ingredients.

*Use with caution in the following situations:*

anticoagulant (eg, warfarin) therapy, concurrent
bleeding disorders
fever
immune deficiency disorders (eg, HIV-positive patients)

immunosuppression (due to illness or drug therapy)
infection, acute
low platelet count

*Pregnancy:* There are no adequate or well-controlled studies in pregnant women. Use only if clearly needed and potential benefits to the mother outweigh the possible hazards to the fetus.

*Breastfeeding:* It is not known if hepatitis A vaccine appears in breast milk. Consult your doctor before you begin breastfeeding.

*Children:* Safety and effectiveness in children younger than 2 years of age have not been established.

## Drug Interactions:

Tell your doctor or pharmacist if you are taking or planning to take any over-the-counter or prescription medications or dietary supplements while receiving hepatitis A vaccine. Doses of one or both drugs may need to be modified or a different drug may need to be prescribed. Anticoagulants (eg, warfarin) may increase bleeding at the injection site.

## Side Effects:

Every vaccine is capable of producing side effects. Many patients experience no, or minor, side effects. The frequency and severity of side effects depend on many factors including dose and individual susceptibility. Most side effects are mild and do not last for longer than 24 hours. Possible side effects include:

*Local:* Soreness; swelling; redness; warmth; pain; tenderness; unusual bruising or swelling at injection site.

*Digestive Tract:* Stomach pain; appetite loss; nausea; diarrhea; vomiting.

*Other:* Headache; sleeplessness; fatigue; fever; general body discomfort; itching; rash; hives; congestion; sore throat; upper respiratory infection; back, arm, joint, or muscle pain; stiffness; menstruation disorder; weakness; dizziness; sensitivity to light.

## Guidelines for Use:

- This medicine will be prepared and administered by your health care provider in a medical setting. The vaccine must be administered intramuscularly (IM; into a muscle) in the deltoid region of the shoulder.
- *Recommended vaccination schedule* — People who wish to be protected against HAV should complete the primary immunization schedule at least 2 weeks before exposure to HAV if possible. Booster doses result in prolonged protection. Dosing regimens depend on the agent selected and the age of the patient.
- The vaccination may not be effective for several days (15 to 30), and it may not prevent unrecognized HAV infection that exists at the time of vaccination. Immune globulin, which is used to provide rapid but temporary protection against HAV, can be administered at the same time.
- Contact your doctor if you experience rash, hives, itching, or difficulty breathing.
- Inform you doctor if you are pregnant, become pregnant, plan on becoming pregnant, or are breastfeeding.
- This vaccine should not be given when a fever is present.
- Immunosuppressed people or those receiving immunosuppressive therapy may not be fully protected and acquire the virus even after vaccination.
- Travelers to areas where HAV is common should take all necessary precautions to avoid contact and ingestion of HAV-contaminated food and water. Contact the CDC for specific travel destination information.
- The length of protection from the virus following complete immunization is not known, but may persist for at least 10 years. There is no guarantee that the vaccine will protect everyone from the hepatitis A virus.

*If you have any questions, consult your doctor, pharmacist, or health care provider.*

| Generic Name Brand Name Examples | Uses |
|---|---|
| *Rx* **Hepatitis B Vaccine**[1] *Engerix-B, Recombivax HB*[2] | For immunization of adults, infants, and children at high risk against infection caused by all known types of the hepatitis B virus (HBV). Immunity to HBV also protects against the hepatitis D virus; hepatitis D can only infect and cause illness in people with HBV. This vaccine will not prevent infections caused by other hepatitis viruses or other diseases which can infect the liver. |

[1] Contains 0.005% thimerosal (mercury).
[2] Also available in dialysis formulation.

*Individuals at high risk include:*

*Health care personnel:* Doctors; podiatrists; surgeons; dentists; dental hygienists; oral surgeons; nurses; paramedics; blood bank and plasma fractionation workers; laboratory personnel who handle blood, blood products, and patient specimens; custodial staff who may be exposed to blood or patient specimens; dental, medical, and nursing students.

*Selected patients and patient contacts:* Patients and staff in hemodialysis and hematology/oncology units; patients requiring frequent or large-volume blood transfusions (eg, hemophiliacs); hemodialysis patients and patients with early renal failure before they require hemodialysis; residents and staff of institutions for the mentally handicapped; classroom contacts of deinstitutionalized mentally handicapped persons who exhibit aggressive behavior or have persistent HBV antigenemia; infants born to HBsAg-positive mothers; household and other intimate contacts with persons with persistent HBV type infections.

*Adolescents:* The Advisory Committee on Immunization Practices (ACIP) and the Committee on Infectious Diseases of the American Academy of Pediatrics (AAP) have endorsed universal infant immunization to lower the incidence of HBV. These advisory committees recommend vaccination of all adolescents at 11 to 12 years of age if previously unvaccinated. High-risk adolescents at older ages should also be vaccinated.

*Populations with high incidence of the disease:* Alaskan natives; Pacific islanders; Indochinese immigrants; Haitian or other immigrants from areas where there is a high rate of HBV; infants born in areas where HBV is prevalent.

*Persons at increased risk due to their sexual practices:* Homosexual males; prostitutes; persons who repeatedly contract sexually transmitted diseases; persons with multiple sex partners (eg, more than 1 partner in a 6-month period).

*Persons with chronic hepatitis C virus:* Risk factors for hepatitis C are similar to those for HBV. Immunization with hepatitis B vaccine is recommended for patients with chronic hepatitis C.

*Travelers to high-risk areas:* Contact the Centers for Disease Control and Prevention (CDC) with regard to such locales.

*Others:* Military personnel; international travelers; police and fire department personnel who render first aid or medical assistance; morticians; embalmers; prisoners; IV drug abusers; any others who may be exposed to HBV through work or personal lifestyle.

## Type of Drug:
Vaccine to prevent hepatitis B viral infection.

## How the Drug Works:
Hepatitis B vaccine provides active protection (immunization) against HBV by stimulating the body to produce antibodies against the virus causing the illness.

## Precautions:
*Do not use in the following situations:* Allergy to hepatitis B vaccine, thimerosal, yeast, or any other hepatitis B vaccine ingredients.

*Use with caution in the following situations:*

anticoagulant (eg, warfarin)
therapy, concurrent
fever
immune deficiency disorders
(eg, HIV-positive patients)

infection, active
radiation therapy, concurrent

*Pregnancy:* There are no adequate or well-controlled studies in pregnant women. Use only if clearly needed and potential benefits to the mother outweigh the possible hazards to the fetus.

*Breastfeeding:* It is not known if hepatitis B vaccine appears in breast milk. Empirical evidence suggests no harm. Consult your doctor before you begin breastfeeding.

*Children:* Hepatitis B vaccine is well-tolerated in infants and children of all ages. Newborns also respond well. However, the safety and effectiveness of the dialysis formulation in children have not been established.

*Elderly:* HBV immunity is somewhat reduced in patients 65 years of age and older.

## Drug Interactions:
Tell your doctor or pharmacist if you are taking or planning to take any over-the-counter or prescription medications or dietary supplements while receiving hepatitis B vaccine. Doses of one or both drugs may need to be modified or a different drug may need to be prescribed. Anticoagulants (eg, warfarin) and interleukin-2 (*Leuvectin*) interact with hepatitis B vaccine.

## Side Effects:

Every vaccine is capable of producing side effects. Many patients experience no, or minor, side effects. The frequency and severity of side effects depend on many factors including dose and individual susceptibility. Possible side effects include:

*Local:* Itching, pain, soreness, tenderness, redness, swelling, bruising, warmth, or nodule formation at injection site.

*Nervous System:* Headache; weakness; fatigue; dizziness; lightheadedness; feeling of whirling motion; fainting; sleeplessness; drowsiness.

*Digestive Tract:* Nausea; vomiting; appetite loss; stomach pain or cramps; indigestion; diarrhea.

*Respiratory System:* Sore throat; upper respiratory tract infection; asthma-like symptoms; cough.

*Skin:* Rash; hives; flushing; hair loss; unusual bleeding or bruising; flushing; abnormal skin sensations (eg, burning, prickling, tingling).

*Other:* General body discomfort; achiness; fatigue; joint, muscle, back, arm, or shoulder pain; neck stiffness or pain; facial swelling; low blood pressure; flu-like symptoms; fever; warmth; sweating; chills; earache; painful or difficult urination; abnormal liver function tests.

## Guidelines for Use:

- This medicine will be prepared and administered by your health care provider in a medical setting. For adults and adolescents, the preferred intramuscular (IM; into a muscle) injection site is the deltoid muscle of the shoulder. For infants and young children, the anterolateral thigh is the preferred site for injection. Patients at high risk of bleeding following an IM injection may receive the vaccine subcutaneously (SC; beneath the skin) but the response may be less than optimal.

- *Recommended vaccination schedule* – Usual regimen consists of 3 consecutive doses. The second and third doses are given at 1 month and 6 months after the initial vaccine, respectively. Alternate schedules may also be used.

- This vaccine should not be given when a fever is present, unless recommended by a doctor.

- The vaccination may not be effective for several days, and it may not prevent unrecognized HBV infections that exist at the time of vaccination.

- Soreness, tenderness, redness, and warmth at injection site, fever, or nausea may occur following vaccination. Contact your doctor if these symptoms persist or become bothersome.

- Contact your doctor if you experience rash, hives, itching, or difficulty breathing.

- Inform you doctor if you are pregnant, become pregnant, plan on becoming pregnant, or are breastfeeding.

- Immunosuppressed patients or those receiving immunosuppressive therapy may not be fully protected and acquire the virus even after vaccination.

- The length of protection against the virus following complete immunization is not known, nor is it a guarantee that the vaccine will protect everyone from HBV.

- Lab tests may be required to monitor therapy. Be sure to keep appointments.

*If you have any questions, consult your doctor, pharmacist, or health care provider.*

| Generic Name<br>*Brand Name Example* | Uses |
|---|---|
| *Rx* **Hepatitis A, Inactivated and Hepatitis B, Recombinant Vaccine**<br><br>*Twinrix*[1] | For immunization of people 18 years of age and older against infection caused by hepatitis A virus (HAV) and all known subtypes of hepatitis B virus (HBV). Immunity to HBV also protects against hepatitis D virus; hepatitis D can only infect and cause illness in people with HBV. This vaccine will not prevent infections caused by other hepatitis viruses or other diseases that can infect the liver. |

[1] Contains thimerosol (less than 1 mcg mercury per mL).

*Individuals at high risk:*

See the Hepatitis A and Hepatitis B monographs in this chapter for a complete listing of people at high risk of HAV and HBV infections.

## Type of Drug:

Vaccine to immunize against HAV and HBV-type infections.

## How the Drug Works:

Hepatitis A and hepatitis B vaccine provides protection against HAV and HBV by stimulating the body to produce antibodies against the virus causing the illness.

## Precautions:

*Do not use in the following situations:* Allergy to hepatitis A vaccine, hepatitis B vaccine, thimerosol, yeast, or any other ingredients within the vaccine.

*Use with caution in the following situations:*

anticoagulant (eg, warfarin) therapy, concurrent
Bell palsy
fever
immune deficiency disorders (eg, HIV-positive patients)
immunosuppressive therapy, concurrent
infection, acute, moderate to severe
low platelet count

*Patients 40 years of age and older:* Hepatitis B vaccine may not be as effective if given to patients 40 years of age and older. Consult you doctor.

*Pregnancy:* There are no adequate or well-controlled studies in pregnant women. Use only if clearly needed and the potential benefits to the mother outweigh the possible hazards to the fetus.

*Breastfeeding:* It is not known if hepatitis A and hepatitis B vaccine appears in breast milk. Consult your doctor before you begin breastfeeding.

*Children:* Safety and effectiveness in people under 18 years of age have not been established.

*Elderly:* There are no sufficient studies in patients 65 years of age and older. Use with caution in elderly patients.

## Drug Interactions:

Tell your doctor or pharmacist if you are taking or planning to take any over-the-counter or prescription medications or dietary supplements while receiving hepatitis A and hepatitis B vaccine. Doses of one or both drugs may need to be modified or a different drug may need to be prescribed. The following drugs or drug classes interact with hepatitis A and hepatitis B vaccine:

anticoagulants (eg, warfarin)
corticosteroids (eg, prednisone)
immunosuppressants
  (eg, cyclosporine)

interleukin-2 (*Leuvectin*)
yellow fever vaccine (*YF-Vax*)

## Side Effects:

Every vaccine is capable of producing side effects. Many patients experience no, or minor, side effects. The frequency and severity of side effects depend on many factors including dose and individual susceptibility. Possible side effects include:

*Local:* Soreness; tenderness; pain; redness; swelling; hardening; warmth; itching.

*Other:* Headache; fever; fatigue; diarrhea; nausea; vomiting; upper respiratory infection.

## Guidelines for Use:

- This medicine will be prepared and administered by your health care provider in a medical setting.
- *Recommended vaccination schedule* — Primary immunization for adults consists of 3 doses given at 1 month and 6 months after the initial vaccination. Alternate schedules may also be used.
- The vaccination may not be effective for several days, and it may not prevent unrecognized HAV or HBV infections that exist at the time of vaccination.
- This vaccine should not be administered when a fever is present, unless recommended by a doctor.
- Contact your doctor if you experience rash, hives, itching, or difficulty breathing.
- Inform your doctor if you are pregnant, become pregnant, plan on becoming pregnant, or are breastfeeding.
- Immunosuppressed people or those receiving immunosuppressive therapy may not be fully protected and acquire the virus even after vaccination.
- The length of protection against HAV and HBV following complete immunization is not known, nor is there a guarantee that the vaccine will protect everyone.
- Contact the Centers for Disease Control and Prevention for specific travel destination information concerning the prevalence of HAV and HBV if you are a world traveler.

*If you have any questions, consult your doctor, pharmacist, or health care provider.*

| Generic Name<br>*Brand Name Examples* | **Uses** |
|---|---|
| *Rx* **Pneumococcal Vaccine**<br>*Pneumovax 23*[1],<br>*Pnu-Imune 23*[2] | For high-risk people 2 years of age and older, certain population groups (eg, Native Americans), people in closed institutions (eg, residential schools, nursing homes), and during a general pneumonia outbreak. |

[1] Contains 0.25% phenol.
[2] Contains 0.01% thimerosal (mercury).

*Individuals at high risk include:*

Adults over 50 years of age; people 2 years of age and older at high risk due to chronic illnesses (eg, cardiovascular or pulmonary disease, diabetes, alcoholism, cirrhosis, CSF leaks) or compromised immune systems (eg, spleen, kidney, or liver disorders, organ transplantations, sickle cell disease, cancers, HIV infection); Hodgkin disease (if the vaccine can be given 10 days before treatment).

## Type of Drug:
Pneumococcal vaccine (pneumonia).

## How the Drug Works:
Injection of material from inactivated pneumococcal bacteria stimulates the production of specific antibodies. Protection from this injection is only against those strains from which the vaccine is prepared.

## Precautions:
*Do not use in the following situations:*

allergy to pneumococcal vaccine or any of its ingredients
fever
Hodgkin disease patients less than 14 days prior to immunosuppressive therapy

Hodgkin disease patients who have received chemotherapy or nodal irradiation
infection, acute respiratory or other

*Use with caution in the following situations:*

heart disease, severe
impaired immune responsiveness

lung disease, severe

*Revaccination:* Do not give a repeat (booster) injection to previously vaccinated patients, except for those at highest risk of pneumococcal infection. Revaccination may result in more frequent and severe local reactions at the injection site.

*Children at highest risk:* Children with asplenia, sickle cell disease, or splenectomy should be revaccinated after 3 to 5 years if they will be 10 years of age or younger.

*Antibiotic therapy:* Patients who require antibiotic therapy against possible pneumococcal infection should continue the antibiotic therapy after vaccination.

*Chemotherapy or immunosuppresion:* The interval between immunization and initiation of chemotherapy or immunosuppression should be 2 weeks or longer.

*Pregnancy:* There are no adequate or well-controlled studies in pregnant women. Use only if clearly needed and the potential benefits to the mother outweigh the possible hazards to the fetus.

*Breastfeeding:* It is not known if this drug appears in breast milk. Consult your doctor before you begin breastfeeding.

*Children:* Safety and effectiveness have not been established for children under 2 years of age.

## Drug Interactions:

Tell your doctor or pharmacist if you are taking or planning to take any over-the-counter or prescription medications or dietary supplements while taking this medicine. Doses of one or both drugs may need to be modified or a different drug may need to be prescribed. Immunosuppressants (eg, corticosteroids) interact with this vaccine.

## Side Effects:

Every vaccine is capable of producing side effects. Many patients experience no, or minor, side effects. The frequency and severity of side effects depend on many factors including dose, duration of therapy, and individual susceptibility. Possible side effects include: Soreness, hardness, warmth, redness, or swelling at the injection site (within 2 days of vaccination); fever; rash; muscle or joint pain; headache; nausea; vomiting; general body discomfort; weakness.

---

### Guidelines for Use:

- Delay the vaccine when respiratory illness with fever or infection is present.
- This vaccination may not work for everyone.
- Patients who require antibiotic therapy against possible pneumococcal infection should continue the antibiotic therapy after vaccination.
- *Guillain-Barré syndrome (GBS):* This syndrome, characterized by paralysis, has occurred rarely after the administration of the pneumococcal vaccination. No cause and effect relationship has been established. Evaluate the possible risk of GBS as compared with the risk of pneumonia and its complications.
- A single administration of the pneumoncoccal vaccine is generally adequate for a lifetime. The exception is those adults at highest risk for acquiring a pneumococcal infection (eg, splenic dysfunction, Hodgkin's disease, lymphoma, multiple myeloma, nephrotic syndrome, organ transplant recipients).
- This vaccine may be given at the same time as the flu vaccine.
- Store at 36° to 46°F. Do not freeze.

---

*If you have any questions, consult your doctor, pharmacist, or health care provider.*

| Generic Name<br>*Brand Name Example* | Supplied As | Generic<br>Available |
|---|---|---|
| *Rx* **Pneumococcal 7-Valent Conjugate Vaccine** | | |
| *Prevnar* | **Injection:** 2 mcg each of 6 polysaccharide isolates; 4 mcg of 1 polysaccharide isolate per 0.5 mL dose | No |

## Type of Drug:

Bacterial vaccines.

## How the Drug Works:

Pneumoccocal 7–valent conjugate vaccine provides long-term protection to infants and toddlers against 7 of the most common forms of serious bacterial infections caused by *Streptoccoccus pneumoniae*. Protection from this vaccine is only against those strains contained in the vaccine and not all causes of bacterial infection.

Approximately 80% of serious infections in children (eg, pneumonia, middle ear infections, meningitis, sinus infections, blood infections) are caused by these 7 types of *S. pneumoniae*.

## Uses:

To immunize infants and toddlers against bacterial infections caused by the 7 most common types of *S. pneumoniae*. This vaccine is not intended to be used for treatment of active infection.

## Precautions:

*Do not use in the following situations:*
> allergy to any component of the vaccine, including diphtheria toxoid
> fever, moderate to severe

*Use with caution in the following situations:*
> bleeding disorder (eg, thrombocytopenia)
> latex sensitivity, history of

*Impaired immune responsiveness:* Children with an impaired immune system (eg, immunosuppressive therapy, chemotherapy, HIV infection) may have a reduced response to the vaccine.

*Pregnancy:* It is not known whether pneumococcal 7–valent conjugate vaccine can cause fetal harm when administered to a pregant women or whether it can affect reproductive capacity. Pneumococcal 7–valent conjugate vaccine is not recommended for use in pregnant women.

*Breastfeeding:* It is not known whether vaccine antigens or antibodies are excreted in breast milk. This vaccine is not recommended for use in nursing mothers.

*Children:* The safety and efficacy of pneumococcal 7–valent conjugate vaccine in children under 6 weeks of age have not been established. Immune responses elicited by pneumococcal 7–valent conjugate vaccine among infants born prematurely have not been studied.

*Elderly:* This vaccine is not recommended for use in adult patients. Do not use as a substitute for the 23–valent pneumococcal polysaccharide vaccine used in elderly patients.

## Drug Interactions:

Tell your doctor or pharmacist if you are taking or if you are planning to take any over-the-counter or prescription medications or dietary supplements with pneumococcal 7–valent conjugated vaccine. Doses of one or both drugs may need to be modified or a different drug may need to be prescribed. The following drugs and drug classes interact with pneumococcal 7–valent conjugated vaccine:

> anticoagulants (eg, heparin)
> immunosuppressive agents (eg, corticosteroids)

## Side Effects:

Every drug is capable of producing side effects. Many pneumococcal 7–valent conjugate vaccine users experience no, or minor, side effects. The frequency and severity of side effects depend on many factors including dose, duration of therapy, and individual susceptibility. Possible side effects include:

*Digestive Tract:* Decreased appetite; vomiting; diarrhea.

*Other:* Fever; drowsiness; rash; hives; irritability; restless sleep; redness, swelling, or tenderness at injection site.

---

### Guidelines for Use:

- This medicine will be prepared and administered by your health care provider in a medical setting.
- Contact your doctor if any side effect becomes bothersome.

---

*If you have any questions, consult your doctor, pharmacist, or health care provider.*

| Generic Name<br>*Brand Name Examples* | Supplied As | Generic<br>Available |
|---|---|---|
| *Rx* **Tuberculin Purified<br>Protein Derivative** | | |
| *Tubersol* | 1 TU (tuberculin unit)/0.1 mL | No |
| *Aplisol, Tubersol* | 5 TU/0.1 mL | No |
| *Tubersol* | 250 TU/0.1 mL | No |
| *Rx* **Tuberculin PPD Multiple<br>Puncture Device** | | |
| *Aplitest, Tine Test PPD* | 5 TU/test | No |
| *Rx* **Old Tuberculin, Multiple<br>Puncture Devices** | | |
| *Mono-Vacc Test (O.T.);*<br>*Tuberculin, Old, Tine Test* | 5 TU/test | No |

## Type of Drug:

Skin test for tuberculosis (TB); Mantoux; Tine Test.

## How the Drug Works:

The test involves injecting inactive material from the tuberculosis organism just under the skin. People previously exposed to TB infection will develop a local skin reaction 2 to 3 days after the skin test is given.

## Uses:

To aid in diagnosing TB infection.

To determine risk of TB exposure in high-risk health care workers or institutionalized persons (eg, long-term hospital patients, prisoners, military personnel).

## Precautions:

*Repeated testing:* Repeated testing of the uninfected individual does not cause sensitivity to tuberculin.

*Tuberculin-positive reactors:* Not to be given to known tuberculin-positive reactors because of the severe reactions that may occur at the test site.

*Altered reactivity:* Reactivity to tuberculin may be reduced for as long as 4 weeks by bacterial or viral infections; live virus vaccines (eg, measles, smallpox, polio, rubella, mumps); severe fever, sarcoidosis, or cancer; overwhelming tuberculosis; use of corticosteroids or immunosuppressive drugs; immunosuppressive infections (eg, HIV); old age; and malnutrition. In most patients who are very sick with tuberculosis, the previously negative tuberculin test becomes positive after a few weeks of treatment. A positive reaction does not necessarily signify active disease. Further diagnostic procedures such as chest x-ray and bacteriologic examinations of sputum must be done before there is a diagnosis of tuberculosis.

*Pregnancy:* The risk of unrecognized tuberculosis and the close postpartum contact between a mother with active disease and her infant leaves the infant in grave danger of tuberculosis and complications such as tuberculous meningitis. No adverse effects upon the fetus recognized as being due to tuberculosis skin testing have been reported.

*Breastfeeding:* It is unlikely that tuberculin is excreted in breast milk. Consult your doctor before you begin breastfeeding.

*Children:* A child who has been exposed to a tuberculosis adult must not be judged free of infection until there is a negative tuberculin reaction at least 10 weeks after exposure to the tuberculosis person.

## Side Effects:

Every vaccine is capable of producing side effects. Many patients experience no, or minor, side effects. The frequency and severity of side effects depend on many factors including dose and individual susceptibility. Possible side effects include redness, swelling; ulceration; bleeding; pain, itching at injection site; dead skin organs; scarring.

---

### Guidelines for Use:

- *"Positive" skin test* — A blister or hardness develops at the site 48 to 72 (96 hours for Mono-Vacc) hours after it is given. The size of the affected area is also important in deciding test results.
- *"Positive" skin test* does not mean you have an active TB infection. Further tests will be needed.
- TB skin tests should not be given on areas affected by acne or hair.
- TB tests may be given first at 1 year of age before measles vaccination and every year or two thereafter.
- TB tests should not be given to persons who are known to have active TB, prior positive test reactions or known severe allergic reactions to it.
- Current infections, recent vaccination, certain drug use, serious illness or pregnancy may interfere with test results.

---

*If you have any questions, consult your doctor, pharmacist, or health care provider.*

**General Guidelines for Topical Ophthalmic Drug Therapy,** 1293

**Agents for Glaucoma**
Alpha-2 Adrenergic Agonists, 1295
Beta-Blockers, 1297
Miotics, Cholinesterase Inhibitors, 1300
Miotics, Direct-Acting, 1303
Prostaglandin Agonists, 1306
Sympathomimetics, 1309
Apraclonidine, 1312
Carbonic Anhydrase Inhibitors, 1314
Dorzolamide/Timolol, 1316
Combinations, 1319

**Alpha-Adrenergic Blocking Agents,** 1320

**Ophthalmic Vasoconstrictors**
Decongestants, 1322
Decongestant Combinations, 1326

**Cycloplegic Mydriatics,** 1328

**Ophthalmic Anti-inflammatory Agents**
Corticosteroids, 1331
Loteprednol, 1334
Mast Cell Stabilizers, 1336
Nonsteroidal Anti-inflammatory Agents, 1338

**Antihistamines**
Levocabastine, 1340
Azelastine, 1342
Olopatadine, 1344
Ketotifen, 1346

**Ophthalmic Anti-infectives**
Antibiotics, 1348
Steroid and Antibiotic Combinations, 1352
Natamycin, 1356
Antiviral Agents, 1358
Fomivirsen Sodium, 1360

**Ophthalmic Phototherapy**
Verteporfin, 1362

**Artificial Tears,** 1365

**Ocular Lubricants,** 1368

**Contact Lens Products**
Hard Contact Lens Products, 1369
Rigid Gas Permeable Contact Lens Products, 1372
Soft (Hydrogel) Contact Lens Products, 1375

**Otic Antibiotics,** 1379

**Otic Preparations, Miscellaneous,** 1382

Topical (surface) application is the most common way to administer ophthalmic drugs. Advantages of topical administration include convenience, simplicity, noninvasive nature, and the ability of the patient to self-administer the medication. Topical medications do not typically penetrate in useful concentrations into the internal eye structures. Therefore, they are of no therapeutic benefit for diseases of the retina, optic nerve, and other internal structures of the eye.

**Medications:**

*Solutions and Suspensions:* Most topical eye preparations are commercially available as solutions or suspensions that are applied directly to the eye from the bottle, which serves as the eye dropper. Avoid touching the dropper tip to the eye because this can lead to contamination of the medication and also may cause injury to the eye.

| Recommended Procedures for Administration of Solutions or Suspensions | |
|---|---|
| 1. | Wash hands thoroughly before use. |
| 2. | Shake suspensions well before using. |
| 3. | Tilt head backward or lie down and gaze upward. |
| 4. | Gently grasp lower eyelid below eyelashes and pull the eyelid away from the eye to form a pouch. |
| 5. | Place dropper directly over eye. Avoid contact of the dropper tip with the eye, finger, or any surface. |
| 6. | Look upward just before applying a drop. |
| 7. | After instilling (applying) the drop, look downward for several seconds. |
| 8. | Release the lid slowly and close eyes gently. |
| 9. | With eyes closed, apply gentle pressure with fingers to the inside corner of the eye (next to the bridge of the nose) for 3 to 5 minutes. This prevents drainage of solution from the intended area. |
| 10. | Do not rub the eye or squeeze the eyelid. Minimize blinking. |
| 11. | Do not rinse the dropper. |
| 12. | Do not use eye drops that have changed color or contain particles. |
| 13. | If more than one drop or type of eye drop is used, wait at least 5 minutes before using the second drop or drug. |
| 14. | When the instillation of eye drops is difficult (eg, children, adults with particularly strong blink reflex), the closed-eye method may be used. This involves lying down, placing the prescribed number of drops on the eyelid in the inner corner of the eye, then opening the eye so that drops will fall into the eye by gravity. |
| 15. | Temporary blurring of vision or irritation may occur after use. Contact your doctor or pharmacist with any concerns. |

*Lid Scrubs:* Commercially available eyelid cleansers or antibiotic solutions or ointments can be directly applied to the lid. This is best accomplished by applying the drug to the end of a cotton-tipped applicator and then scrubbing the eyelid margin several times daily. The gauze pads supplied with commercially available eyelid cleansers are also convenient.

*Ointments:* The primary purpose for an eye ointment is to prolong drug contact time with the surface of the eye. This is particularly useful for treating children, who may "cry out" topically applied solutions, and for medicating eye injuries, such as corneal abrasions, when the eye is to be patched.

| Recommended Procedures for Administration of Ointments | |
|---|---|
| 1. | Wash hands thoroughly before using. |
| 2. | Tilt head backward or lie down and gaze upward. |
| 3. | Gently pull down the lower lid to form a pouch. |
| 4. | Place 0.25 to 0.5 (¼ to ½) inch of ointment with a sweeping motion inside the lower lid by squeezing the tube gently and then slowly release the eyelid. |
| 5. | Close the eye for 1 to 2 minutes and roll the eyeball in all directions. |
| 6. | Temporary blurring of vision may occur. Avoid activities requiring clear vision until blurring clears. |
| 7. | Remove excessive ointment around the eye or ointment tube tip with a tissue. |
| 8. | If using more than one kind of ointment, wait about 10 minutes before applying the second drug. |
| 9. | If using eye drops and ointments, instill the drops first. Ointments prevent entry of drops. |

*Gels:* Ophthalmic gels are similar in thickness and clinical usage to eye ointments. Pilocarpine (*Pilopine HS*) and timolol maleate (*Timoptic-XE*) are currently the only eye preparations available in gel form. They are intended to serve as "sustained-release preparations," requiring only once-daily use (at bedtime).

*Sprays:* Although not commercially available, some practitioners use mydriatics or cycloplegics, alone or in combination, administered as a spray to the eye to dilate (open) the pupil or for cycloplegic examination. This is most often used for pediatric patients, and the solution is administered using a sterile atomizer or spray bottle.

Ophthalmic products contain a variety of preservatives, antioxidants, buffers, and other nontherapeutic formulation ingredients. Patients may be hypersensitive (allergic) to one or more of these agents. Any unexpected or discomforting itching, irritation, watering from the eye, redness, or sensitivity should be reported to a doctor or pharmacist.

*If you have any questions, consult your doctor, pharmacist, or health care provider.*

| Generic Name<br>*Brand Name Example* | Supplied As | Generic<br>Available |
|---|---|---|
| *Rx* **Brimonidine Tartrate** | | |
| *Alphagan* | **Solution:** 0.2% | No |

## Type of Drug:
Alpha-adrenergic receptor stimulator.

## How the Drug Works:
Ophthalmic receptor stimulators decrease fluid production and increases the outflow. They lower pressure in the eye.

## Uses:
To lower intraocular (fluid) pressure in open-angle glaucoma or ocular hypertension (pressure in the eye).

## Precautions:
*Do not use in the following situations:*
   allergy to the drug
   monoamine oxidase (MAOI) inhibitor therapy

*Use with caution in the following situations:*
   cardiovascular disease, severe       kidney impairment
   cerebral insufficiency               liver impairment
   contact lens wear                    orthostatic hypotension
   coronary insufficiency               Raynaud's phenomenon
   depression                           thromboangitis obliterans

*Pregnancy:* Studies in women or in animals have been judged not to show a risk to the fetus. However, no drug should be used during pregnancy unless clearly needed.

*Breastfeeding:* It is not known if brimonidine tartrate appears in breast milk. Consult your doctor before you begin breastfeeding.

*Children:* Safety and effectiveness in children have not been established.

## Drug Interactions:
Tell your doctor or pharmacist if you are taking or planning to take any over-the-counter or prescription medications or dietary supplements while taking this medicine. Doses of one or both drugs may need to be modified or a different drug may need to be prescribed. The following drugs and drug classes interact with this medicine.

   antihypertensives (eg, *hydro-*        IOP-lowering medication
   *chlorothiazide)*                      (eg, *pilocarpine)*
   beta-blockers, ophthalmic and          tricyclic antidepressants
   systemic (eg, *timolol,*               (eg, *amitriptyline)*
   *propranolol)*
   cardiac glycosides (eg, *digoxin)*
   CNS depressants (alcohol, barbiturates, opiates, sedatives,
   anesthetics)

## Side Effects:

Every drug is capable of producing side effects. Many patients experience no, or minor, side effects. The frequency and severity of side effects depend on many factors including dose, duration of therapy, and individual susceptibility. Possible side effects include the following:

*Nervous System:* Headache; fatigue/drowsiness; dizziness; depression; anxiety; sleeplessness.

*Circulatory System:* High blood pressure; pounding in the chest.

*Eyes or Ocular:* Red or blood shot eyes; burning/stinging; blurring; allergic reactions; itching; sensitive to light; redness of the eyelid; ache/pain; dryness; tearing; eyelid swelling; conjunctival edema; irritation; whitening; abnormal or change in vision; lid crusting; bleeding; discharge; conjunctival follicles.

*Other:* Muscular pain; abnormal taste; nasal dryness; fainting; weakness; dry mouth.

---

## Guidelines for Use:

- Usual dose is 1 drop 3 times daily, 8 hours apart.
- Soft contact wearers should wait 15 minutes after using this medication before inserting lenses.
- This medicine may cause drowsiness. Use caution while driving or performing other tasks requiring mental alertness, coordination, or physical dexterity.
- Store below 77°F.

---

*If you have any questions, consult your doctor, pharmacist, or health care provider.*

| Generic Name<br>*Brand Name Examples* | Supplied As | Generic<br>Available |
|---|---|---|
| *Rx* **Betaxolol HCl** | **Solution**: 0.5% | Yes |
| *Betoptic S* | **Suspension**: 0.25% | No |
| *Rx* **Carteolol HCl** | | |
| *Ocupress* | **Solution**: 1% | Yes |
| *Rx* **Levobetaxolol HCl** | | |
| *Betaxon* | **Suspension**: 0.5% | · No |
| *Rx* **Levobunolol HCl** | | |
| *Betagan Liquifilm*[1] | **Solution**: 0.25%, 0.5% | Yes |
| *Rx* **Metipranolol HCl** | | |
| *OptiPranolol* | **Solution**: 0.3% | No |
| *Rx* **Timolol Maleate** | | |
| *Timoptic*[1], *Timoptic in Ocudose* | **Solution**: 0.25%, 0.5% | Yes |
| *Timoptic-XE* | **Gel**: 0.25%, 0.5% | Yes |

[1] Contains sulfites.

## Type of Drug:

Nonselective beta-adrenergic blocking agents for the eye.

## How the Drug Works:

Ophthalmic beta-blockers decrease the fluid pressure in the eye. They may be used alone or in combination with other drugs.

## Uses:

To help lower intraocular (fluid) pressure (IOP) in chronic open-angle glaucoma. Also used to help manage ocular hypertension (high intraocular pressure).

## Precautions:

*Do not use in the following situations:*

allergy to the beta-blocker or any of its ingredients
bronchial asthma
cardiogenic shock
chronic obstructive pulmonary disease, severe
heart failure
slowed heart rate/heart block

*Use with caution in the following situations:*

decreased blood flow to brain
diabetes
heart disease
hyperthyroidism (overactive thyroid)
lung disease or breathing difficulties (eg, bronchitis, emphysema)
myasthenia gravis
surgery, with anesthesia

*Diabetes:* Diabetic patients and patients subject to hypoglycemia (low blood sugar) should use caution. Beta-blockers may mask the signs of hypoglycemia.

*Pregnancy:* There are no adequate and well-controlled studies in pregnant women. Use only if clearly needed and the potential benefits to the mother outweigh the possible hazards to the fetus.

*Breastfeeding:* Timolol maleate appears in breast milk. It is not known if betaxolol, carteolol, levobetaxolol, levobunolol, or metipranolol appear in breast milk. Consult your doctor before you begin breastfeeding.

*Children:* Safety and effectiveness in children have not been established.

*Sulfites:* Some of these products may contain sulfite preservatives, which can cause allergic reactions in certain individuals. Check package label when available or consult your doctor or pharmacist.

## Drug Interactions:

Tell your doctor or pharmacist if you are taking or if you are planning to take any over-the-counter or prescription medications or dietary supplements while taking a beta-blocker. Doses of one or both drugs may need to be modified or a different drug may need to be prescribed. The following drugs and drug classes interact with beta-blockers:

beta-blockers, oral
(eg, propranolol)
calcium antagonists
(eg, verapamil)
catecholamine-depleting drugs
(eg, reserpine)

digitalis (eg, *Lanoxin)*
epinephrine, topical and ophthalmic (eg, *Epifrin)*
phenothiazines (eg, promethazine)
quinidine (eg, *Quinora)*

Also consider all drug interactions reported for oral beta-blockers (eg, propranolol). (See the monograph in the Cardiovascular Drugs chapter.)

## Side Effects:

Every drug is capable of producing side effects. Many beta-blocker users experience no, or minor, side effects. The frequency and severity of side effects depend on many factors including dose, duration of therapy, and individual susceptibility. Possible side effects include the following:

*Eyes or Ocular:* Temporary stinging or pain when instilling drops; double vision; swelling; crusting; visual problems; irritation; blurred vision; burning; inflammation; tearing; dry eyes; foreign body sensation; itching eyes; cataracts; light sensitivity; drooping of upper eyelid; red eyes.

*Digestive Tract:* Appetite loss; taste changes; dry mouth; nausea; diarrhea; stomachache; constipation.

*Nervous System:* Depression; confusion; dizziness; headache; drowsiness; nervousness; nightmares; memory loss; hallucinations; sleeplessness; anxiety; vertigo (feeling of whirling motion).

*Circulatory System:* Abnormal heart rhythm; palpitations (pounding in the chest); congestive heart failure; chest pain; changes in blood pressure; worsening of angina.

*Respiratory System:* Difficulty breathing; cough; runny nose.

*Skin:* Rash; itching; hives; abnormal skin sensations; worsening of psoriasis.

*Other:* Weakness; fatigue; muscle pain; fainting; hair loss; nasal congestion; inflammation of the tongue; gout; increased blood lipids; arthritis; nosebleed; changes in sense of smell; sexual dysfuction (male); masked symptoms of hypoglycemia (low blood sugar); cold hands and feet; incoordination. Also consider the side effects associated with oral beta-blockers (eg, propranolol).

## Guidelines for Use:

- Dosage is indvidualized. Use exactly as prescribed. Do not skip doses.
- If a dose is missed, instill it as soon as possible. If several hours have passed or it is nearing time for the next dose, do not double the dose to catch up, unless advised by your doctor. If more than one dose is missed, contact your doctor or pharmacist.
- Take contact lenses out of your eyes prior to instilling this medicine. You may reinsert contact lenses 15 minutes following instillation.
- Avoid allowing the tip of the dispensing container to contact the eye or surrounding area to avoid contamination. Replace cap immediately after use.
- May cause stinging or pain when first instilled in the eye.
- Temporary blurred vision may occur for up to 5 minutes, impairing your ability to perform hazardous tasks. Use caution before operating machinery or driving a motor vehicle.
- Intraocular pressure will have to be monitored periodically by your doctor. Be sure to keep appointments.
- Notify your doctor if you plan to have eye surgery or if you experience an eye infection or trauma. You may have to stop using the drops.
- *Betaxolol, levobetaxolol* — Shake well before using.
- *Timolol maleate gel* — Invert the closed container and shake once before each use. Other eye medications should be used 10 minutes before the gel.
- Wait at least 5 minutes before using any other eye medications.
- Store upright at room temperature (59° to 86°F). Avoid freezing. Protect from light.

*If you have any questions, consult your doctor, pharmacist, or health care provider.*

| Generic Name<br>*Brand Name Examples* | Supplied As | Generic<br>Available |
|---|---|---|
| Rx **Demecarium Bromide** | | |
| *Humorsol* | **Solution:** 0.125%, 0.25% | No |
| Rx **Echothiophate Iodide** | | |
| *Phospholine Iodide* | **Powder for Reconstitution:** 1.5 mg (to make 0.03%); 3 mg (0.06%); 6.25 mg (0.125%); 12.5 mg (0.25%) | No |
| Rx **Physostigmine** | | |
| *Eserine Sulfate* | **Ointment:** 0.25% | No |

## Type of Drug:

Drugs that cause the pupil to constrict (decrease in size); glaucoma drugs.

## How the Drug Works:

Cholinesterase inhibitor miotics decrease the fluid pressure inside the eye by increasing the outflow of fluid (aqueous humor) from the eye. They cause the pupils to get smaller (miosis) and cause the ciliary muscle of the eye to contract.

## Uses:

To treat open-angle glaucoma.

*Demecarium* also is used after iridectomy (surgical removal of a portion of the iris) or to treat accommodative esotropia or certain conditions affecting aqueous (fluid) outflow.

*Echothiophate* also is used to treat some types of angle-closure glaucoma after iridectomy (surgical removal of a portion of the iris), strabismus, and esotropia.

## Precautions:

*Do not use in the following situations:*

allergy to these drugs or their ingredients
glaucoma, angle-closure (echothiophate only)
inflammation of the iris, choroid or ciliary body, with or without glaucoma
pregnancy (demecarium only)

*Use with caution in the following situations:*

asthma
epilepsy
heart attack, recent
low blood pressure, severe
myasthenia gravis (muscle weakness)
narrow-angle glaucoma, chronic
eye conditions/problems, other
parkinsonism
peptic ulcer
slow heart rate, severe
surgery, prior to
spastic GI conditions (stomach cramping)
vagotonia (irritability of the vagal nerve)

*Eye exams* will be required to monitor treatment. Be sure to keep appointments.

*Pregnancy:*

*Demecarium* – Do not use during pregnancy. The risk of use in a pregnant woman clearly outweighs any possible benefit.

*All others* – Adequate studies have not been done in pregnant women, or animal studies may have shown a risk to the fetus. Use only if clearly needed and potential benefits outweigh the possible hazards to the fetus.

*Breastfeeding:* It is not known if these drugs appear in breast milk. Because of the risk of serious reactions in infants, consult your doctor before breastfeeding.

*Children:* Safety and effectiveness of physostigmine have not been established. Use demecarium with extreme caution in children who may require general anesthesia.

## Drug Interactions:

Tell your doctor or pharmacist if you are taking or if you are planning to take any over-the-counter or prescription medications or dietary supplements while taking these medicines. Doses of one or both drugs may need to be modified or a different drug may need to be prescribed. Anticholinesterases (eg, ambenonium), insecticides/pesticides (carbamate or organophosphate) and succinylcholine (eg, *Sucostrin*) interact with these medicines.

## Side Effects:

Every drug is capable of producing side effects. Many patients experience no, or minor, side effects. The frequency and severity of side effects depend on many factors including dose, duration of therapy and individual susceptibility. Possible side effects include the following:

*Eyes or Ocular:* Tearing; burning; redness; lid twitching; nearsightedness; blurred vision; browache/headache; inflammation of iris; retinal detachment; cloudy lens; increase in intraocular pressure; cysts.

*Other:* Nausea; vomiting; stomach cramps; diarrhea; loss of bladder control; excessive salivation or sweating; fainting; muscle weakness; difficulty breathing; irregular heartbeat.

## Guidelines for Use:

- Use exactly as prescribed. Do not use more often than directed.
- Follow Administration Guidelines found at the beginning of this chapter.
- Wash hands before and immediately after instilling these drugs.
- If a dose is missed, instill it as soon as possible. If several hours have passed or if it is nearing time for the next dose, do not the double the dose in order to catch up (unless advised to do so by your doctor). If more than one dose is missed, contact your doctor or pharmacist.
- Local irritation and headache may occur when you first start using these drugs.
- May cause vision problems in poor light. Use caution while driving at night or performing tasks in poor lighting.
- Discontinue this medication and consult your doctor if any of the following occur: Excess sweating or mouth watering, loss of bladder control, stomach cramps, diarrhea, muscle weakness, difficulty breathing, or irregular heartbeat.
- Eye ointments may slow corneal healing.
- *Echothiophate* — Tolerance may develop after prolonged use; a rest period usually restores response to the medication.
- *Storage* — Store demecarium and physostigmine between 59° to 86° F, away from heat and cold. Keep tightly closed.
  After mixing echothiophate, store in refrigerator and use within 6 months. Use solution within 1 month if it is stored at room temperature (59° to 86° F).

*If you have any questions, consult your doctor, pharmacist, or health care provider.*

| Generic Name<br>*Brand Name Examples* | Supplied As | Generic<br>Available |
|---|---|---|
| *Rx* **Acetylcholine Chloride, Intraocular** | | |
| *Miochol-E* | **Solution**: 1% | No |
| *Rx* **Carbachol, Intraocular** | | |
| *Carbastat, Miostat* | **Solution**: 0.01% | No |
| *Rx* **Carbachol, Topical** | | |
| *Carboptic, Isopto Carbachol* | **Solution**: 0.75%, 1.5%, 2.25%, 3% | Yes |
| *Rx* **Pilocarpine HCl** | | |
| *Adsorbocarpine, Akarpine, Isopto Carpine, Pilocar, Piloptic, Pilopto-Carpine, Pilostat, Storzine 2* | **Solution**: 0.25%, 0.5%, 1%, 2%, 3%, 4%, 5%, 6%, 8%, 10% | Yes |
| *Pilopine HS* | **Gel**: 4% | No |
| *Ocusert Pilo* | **Ocular therapeutic system**: 20 mcg/hr, 40 mcg/hr | No |
| *Rx* **Pilocarpine Nitrate** | | |
| *Pilagan* | **Solution**: 1%, 2%, 4% | No |

## Type of Drug:

Drugs that cause the pupil to constrict (decrease in size); glaucoma drugs.

## How the Drug Works:

Direct-acting miotics decrease the fluid pressure inside the eye by increasing the outflow of fluid (aqueous humor) from the eye. They cause the pupils to get smaller (miosis) and cause the ciliary muscle of the eye to contract.

## Uses:

To decrease elevated intraocular (fluid) pressure in glaucoma.

*Acetylcholine, carbachol (intraocular):* To induce miosis (pupil constriction) during surgery.

*Pilocarpine HCl and nitrate:* To reverse mydriasis (pupil dilation).

## Precautions:

*Do not use in the following situations:*
allergy to any of these drugs
glaucoma, pupillary block or
  secondary

inflammation of eye interior or
  iris, severe

*Use with caution in the following situations:*

| | |
|---|---|
| asthma | hyperthyroidism |
| blood pressure, high or low | Parkinson disease |
| corneal abrasion (carbachol only) | peptic ulcer |
| | retinal disease, history |
| GI spasm (cramping) | urinary tract obstruction |
| heart problems | |

*Pregnancy:* Adequate studies have not been done in pregnant women, or animal studies may have shown a risk to the fetus. Use only if clearly needed and potential benefits outweigh the possible hazards to the fetus.

*Breastfeeding:* It is not known if these agents appear in breast milk. Consult your doctor before you begin breastfeeding.

*Children:* Safety and effectiveness have not been established.

## Drug Interactions:

Tell your doctor or pharmacist if you are taking or if you are planning to take any over-the-counter or prescription medications or dietary supplements while taking these medicines. Doses of one or both drugs may need to be modified or a different drug may need to be prescribed. Topical nonsteroidal anti-inflammatory drugs (NSAIDs, eg, suprofen, flurbiprofen) interact with these medicines.

## Side Effects:

Every drug is capable of producing side effects. Many patients experience no, or minor, side effects. The frequency and severity of side effects depend on many factors including dose, duration of therapy, and individual susceptibility. Possible side effects include the following:

*Eyes or Ocular:* Burning; stinging; tearing; blurring; redness; inflammation of cornea and conjunctiva (white of eyes); reduced vision in poor light; nearsightedness; detached retina (floaters, flashes of light).

*Other:* Stomach cramps; nausea; vomiting; diarrhea; flushing; fainting; excess salivation; sweating; headache; changes in blood pressure; bladder tightness; frequent urination; bronchial spasms; asthma; difficulty breathing; irregular heartbeat.

## Guidelines for Use:

- Use exactly as prescribed.
- Follow Administration Guidelines found at the beginning of this chapter.
- If a dose is missed, instill it as soon as possible. If several hours have passed or if it is nearing time for the next dose, do not double the dose in order to catch up. If more than one dose is missed, contact your doctor or pharmacist.
- If accidental overdosage occurs, flush eyes with water and contact your doctor.
- Report any changes in vision to your doctor immediately.
- May sting when used, especially the first few times. May also cause headache, browache, or decreased night vision. Use caution while driving at night or performing tasks in poor lighting.
- *Solution* — To avoid contamination, do not touch tip of container to any surface, including the eye. Wash hands before and immediately after use. Keep bottle tightly closed when not in use. Discard solution after expiration date. Store at room temperature. Do not freeze. Keep out of reach of children.
- *Gel* — Apply once daily at bedtime. If other glaucoma medications (drops) are also being used, use drops at least 5 minutes before the gel. Store at room temperature. Do not freeze.
- *Pilocarpine ocular systems (Ocusert Pilo)* —
  Follow the patient instructions provided in the package.
  Wash hands with soap and water before touching or manipulating the system. If a displaced system contacts unclean surfaces, rinse with cool tap water before replacing. Discard contaminated systems and replace with a fresh unit.
  Check for the presence of the system before retiring at night and upon arising. If keeping the unit in the eye is a problem, contact your doctor. Damaged or deformed systems should not be placed or retained in the eye. Store in the refrigerator (36° to 46°F).

*If you have any questions, consult your doctor, pharmacist, or health care provider.*

| Generic Name<br>*Brand Name Examples* | Supplied As | Generic<br>Available |
|---|---|---|
| Rx **Bimatoprost** | | |
| *Lumigan* | **Solution**: 0.03% | No |
| Rx **Latanoprost** | | |
| *Xalatan* | **Solution**: 0.005% | No |
| Rx **Travoprost** | | |
| *Travatan* | **Solution**: 0.004% | No |
| Rx **Unoprostone Isopropyl** | | |
| *Rescula* | **Solution**: 0.15% | No |

## Type of Drug:
Agents for glaucoma.

## How the Drug Works:
Prostaglandin agonists reduce pressure on the eye by increasing the outflow of aqueous humor (fluid) in the eye.

## Uses:
For the reduction of elevated intraocular pressure (IOP) in patients with open-angle glaucoma or ocular hypertension who are intolerant of other IOP-lowering medications or insufficiently responsive to another IOP-lowering medication.

## Precautions:
*Do not use in the following situations:* Allergy to the prostaglandin agonist, benzalkonium chloride (a preservative in the eye drop), or any other ingredients.

*Use with caution in the following situations:*

| | |
|---|---|
| absence of lens of the eye | liver impairment |
| contact lens wear | macular edema, risk factors for |
| intraocular inflammation, active | pseudophakic patients with a |
| (eg, uveitis) | torn posterior lens capsule |
| kidney impairment | |

*Eye changes:* Prostaglandin agonists may gradually change eye color, causing the irises to become more brown. This is more noticeable in green-brown, blue/gray-brown, or yellow-brown eyes. Eyelid skin darkening and gradual changes in the eyelashes (eg, length, thickness, pigmentation, number of lashes) also have been reported. These changes may be permanent. The long-term effects are currently unknown.

*Pregnancy:* There are no adequate and well-controlled studies in pregnant women. Use only if clearly needed and the potential benefits to the mother outweigh the possible hazards to the fetus. Travoprost may interfere with the maintenance of pregnancy and should not be used by women during pregnancy or by women attempting to become pregnant.

*Breastfeeding:* It is not known if prostaglandin agonists appear in breast milk. Consult your doctor before you begin breastfeeding.

*Children:* Safety and effectiveness in children have not been established.

## Drug Interactions:

Tell your doctor or pharmacist if you are taking or planning to take any over-the-counter or prescription medications or dietary supplements while using a prostaglandin agonist. Doses of one or both drugs may need to be modified or a different drug may need to be prescribed. Eye drops containing thimerosal may interact with prostaglandin agonists.

## Side Effects:

Every drug is capable of producing side effects. Many prostaglandin agonist users experience no, or minor, side effects. The frequency and severity of side effects depend on many factors including dose, duration of therapy, and individual susceptibility. Possible side effects include the following:

*Eyes or Ocular:* Changes in vision (eg, blurred vision, double vision); burning or stinging; red eyes; eye color change; dry eye; excessive tearing; eye pain; lid crusting; lid swelling; lid discomfort or pain; light sensitivity; foreign body sensation; eyelid itching; eyelash changes (eg, length, thickness, number of lashes, pigmentation); eye discharge.

*Nervous System:* Anxiety; depression; headache; weakness; dizziness.

*Respiratory System:* Upper respiratory tract infection; cold; flu; sinus inflammation; runny nose.

*Skin:* Rash; itching; excessive hair growth; eyelid skin darkening.

*Other:* Muscle, joint, back, or chest pain; indigestion; high cholesterol levels; changes in blood pressure; infection; pain; prostate disorder; urinary incontinence; urinary tract infection; abnormal liver function tests; diabetes mellitus; sore throat.

## Guidelines for Use:

- The recommended dose of bimatoprost, latanoprost, and travoprost is 1 drop in the affected eye(s) once daily in the evening. The recommended dose of unoprostone is 1 drop in the affected eye(s) twice daily.
- Wait at least 5 minutes between use of other eye drops or eye products.
- Do not use while wearing contact lenses; they may be reinserted 15 minutes after administration.
- Changes in eye or eyelid color and eyelash changes may occur in the treated eye(s). These changes may be permanent.
- To prevent contamination of the solution or dropper tip of the bottle, do not touch the eyelids or surrounding areas with the dropper tip.
- Contact your doctor if you experience eye trauma, infection, or surgery during treatment. Also contact your doctor if you experience eye inflammation, irritation, discharge, or lid reactions.
- Store as directed on the container. Protect from light.

*If you have any questions, consult your doctor, pharmacist, or health care provider.*

| Generic Name<br>*Brand Name Examples* | Supplied As | Generic<br>Available |
|---|---|---|
| *Rx* **Dipivefrin** | | |
| *AKPro, Propine* | **Solution**: 0.1% | Yes |
| *Rx* **Epinephrine (as HCl)** | | |
| *Epifrin, Glaucon*[1] | **Solution**: 0.1%, 0.5%, 1%, 2% | Yes |
| *Rx* **Epinephrine (as Borate)** | | |
| *Epinal* | **Solution**: 0.5%, 1% | No |

[1] Contains sulfites.

## Type of Drug:

Vasoconstrictors. Drugs that cause the pupil to dilate (widen) and intraocular pressure to decrease.

## How the Drug Works:

Sympathomimetics decrease the intraocular (fluid) pressure in the eye by decreasing formation of fluid (aqueous humor). They also relax the ciliary muscle, dilate the pupil, and increase aqueous humor flow out of the eye. May be used alone or in combination with other drugs.

## Uses:

To help manage open-angle (chronic simple) glaucoma.

## Precautions:

*Do not use in the following situations:*

absence of lens in the eye (epinephrine only)
allergy to these medicines or their ingredients
narrow-angle glaucoma
narrow-angles (but no glaucoma)
shallow-angle glaucoma
soft contact lens wear

*Use with caution in the following situations:*

anesthesia
absence of lens in the eye (dipivefrin only)
asthma
cerebral arteriosclerosis (hardening of the arteries)
diabetes
heart disease
high blood pressure
hyperthyroidism (overactive thyroid), untreated

*Pregnancy:*

*Epinephrine* – Adequate studies have not been done in pregnant women, or animal studies may have shown a risk to the fetus. Safety for use has not been established. Use only when clearly needed and potential benefits outweigh possible hazards to the fetus.

*Dipivefrin* – Studies in pregnant women or in animals have been judged not to show a risk to the fetus. However, no drug should be used during pregnancy unless clearly needed.

*Breastfeeding:* It is not known if these drugs appear in breast milk. Consult your doctor before you begin breastfeeding.

*Children:* Safety and effectiveness have not been established.

*Elderly:* Use with caution in elderly patients.

*Sulfites:* Some of these products contain sulfite preservatives, which can cause allergic reactions in certain individuals. Check package label when available or consult your doctor or pharmacist.

## Drug Interactions:
Tell your doctor or pharmacist if you are taking or if you are planning to take any over-the-counter or prescription medications or dietary supplements while taking these medicines. Doses of one or both drugs may need to be modified or a different drug may need to be prescribed. The following drugs and drug classes interact with these medicines.

anesthetics (eg, halothane)
beta-blockers (eg, propranolol)
bretylium (*Bretylol*)
ergotrate
guanethidine (*Ismelin*)

methylergonovine (*Methergine*)
oxytocin (eg, *Pitocin*)
tricyclic antidepressants
 (eg, amitriptyline)

## Side Effects:
Every drug is capable of producing side effects. Many patients experience no, or minor, side effects. The frequency and severity of side effects depend on many factors including dose, duration of therapy, and individual susceptibility. Possible side effects include:

*Eyes or Ocular:* Eyeache; stinging; burning; redness or irritation of eyelid; sensitivity to light; glare; changes in eye color.

*Nervous System:* Fainting; headache; browache.

*Circulatory System:* Heart pounding (palpitations); increased heart rate; abnormal heart rhythm; high blood pressure.

## Guidelines for Use:

- For use in eyes only.
- Do not use if solution is brown or contains particles.
- Follow Administration Guidelines found at the beginning of this chapter.
- To avoid contamination, do not touch tip of container to any surface. Replace cap after use.
- If a dose is missed, instill it as soon as possible. If several hours have passed or if it is nearing time for the next dose, do not double the dose to "catch up" (unless advised to do so by your doctor). If more than one dose is missed or it is necessary to establish a new dosage schedule, contact your doctor or pharmacist.
- Do not use while wearing soft contact lenses. Discoloration of lenses may occur.
- If overdosage occurs, flush eye(s) with water or normal saline.
- May cause stinging or burning when you first instill drops into the eyes. Headache or browache may occur.
- May cause a sensitivity to bright light. Protect eyes and wear sunglasses.
- Report any changes in vision to your doctor immediately.
- *Epinephrine* may cause temporary blurred or unstable vision after instillation. Use caution while driving, operating machinery, or performing other tasks requiring clear vision.
- *Storage* — Store in a cool place (36° to 75° F), away from light. Do not freeze. Keep container tightly sealed.

*If you have any questions, consult your doctor, pharmacist, or health care provider.*

| Generic Name Brand Name Example | Supplied As | Generic Available |
|---|---|---|
| Rx **Apraclonidine HCl** *Iopidine* | **Solution**: 0.5% | No |

## Type of Drug:

Vasoconstrictor. A drug that causes the pupil to dilate (widen).

## How the Drug Works:

Apraclonidine reduces intraocular (fluid) pressure, IOP, in the eye by decreasing the rate of fluid production.

## Uses:

For short-term therapy to lower intraocular (fluid) pressure in adults who are on the highest tolerated medical therapy.

## Precautions:

*Do not use in the following situations:*

allergy to apraclonidine or clonidine
monoamine oxidase inhibitor (MAOI) use

*Use with caution in the following situations:*

depression
heart attack, recent
heart disease
hypertension (high blood pressure)
kidney disease
liver disease
vascular disease (eg, Raynaud disease, thromboangiitis obliterans, cerebrovascular disease)

*Pregnancy:* Adequate studies have not been done in pregnant women, or animal studies may have shown a risk to the fetus. Use only if clearly needed and potential benefits outweigh possible hazards to the fetus.

*Breastfeeding:* It is not known if apraclonidine appears in breast milk. Consult your doctor before you begin breastfeeding.

*Children:* Safety and effectiveness in children have not been established.

*Lab tests* will be required periodically.

## Drug Interactions:

Tell your doctor or pharmacist if you are taking or if you are planning to take any over-the-counter or prescription medications or dietary supplements while taking this medicine. Doses of one or both drugs may need to be modified or a different drug may need to be prescribed. The following drugs and drug classes interact with this medicine.

alcohol
anesthetics (eg, halothane)
antihypertensives (eg, methyldopa)
barbiturates (eg, phenobarbital
beta-blockers (eg, propranolol)
cardiac glycosides (eg, digoxin)
MAO inhibitors (eg, phenelzine)
opiates (eg, morphine)
sedatives (eg, diazepam)
tricyclic antidepressants (eg, amitriptyline)

## Side Effects:

Every drug is capable of producing side effects. Many patients experience no, or minor, side effects. The frequency or severity depend on many factors, including dose, duration of therapy and individual susceptibility. Possible side effects include the following:

*Eyes or Ocular:* Blood-shot eyes; discomfort; tearing; itching; swelling of eyelid; feeling of a foreign body in the eye; dry eyes; blurred vision; discharge from the eyes; paleness of inner lining of eyelid.

*Other:* Dry mouth; dry nose; headache; weakness; changes in taste; dizziness; drowsiness.

---

### Guidelines for Use:

- Place 1 to 2 drops in the affected eye(s) 3 times daily. Wait 5 minutes before using any other eye medications.
- Do not touch the dropper tip to any surface, including your eye, because this may contaminate the contents or cause damage/infect the eye.
- *Soft contact lenses* — Do not wear during treatment.
- Do not increase or decrease this medicine without your doctor's approval. If a dose is missed, instill it as soon as possible. If several hours have passed or if it is within 2 hours of the next dose, do not double the dose to "catch up" unless advised to do so by your doctor). If more than one dose is missed or it is necessary to establish a new dosage schedule, contact your doctor or pharmacist. Use exactly as prescribed.
- Contact your doctor immediately if any of the following occurs: Blood-shot eyes; itching; discomfort; tearing; feeling of a foreign body in the eye; swelling of the eyelid. You may need to stop using the medicine.
- This medicine may cause drowsiness or dizziness. Avoid driving or performing other tasks requiring alertness or coordination until effects are known, then use caution.
- Lab and visual tests (especially for glaucoma patients) may be required to monitor therapy. Be sure to keep appointments.
- Do not share this medicine with anyone else.
- Store between 36° to 80°F. Protect from freezing and light.

---

*If you have any questions, consult your doctor, pharmacist, or health care provider.*

| Generic Name<br>*Brand Name Examples* | Supplied As | Generic<br>Available |
|---|---|---|
| Rx **Brinzolamide** | | |
| *Azopt* | **Suspension**: 1% | No |
| Rx **Dorzolamide HCl** | | |
| *Trusopt* [1] | **Solution**: 2% | No |

[1] Contains benzalkonium chloride.

## Type of Drug:

Carbonic anhydrase inhibitor.

## How the Drug Works:

Brinzolamide and dorzolamide reduce fluid pressure in the eye by decreasing the rate of fluid production.

## Uses:

Brinzolamide and dorzolamide lower fluid pressure in the eyeball in patients with ocular hypertension or open-angle glaucoma. Dorzolamide may be used in combination with other medications.

## Precautions:

*Do not use in the following situations:*

allergy to brinzolamide or dorzolamide, to any of its ingredients, or its relatives (eg, sulfa drugs)

kidney function, severely impaired

soft contact lens wear (dorzolamide)

*Use with caution in the following situations:*

oral carbonic anhydrase inhibitor use

soft contact lens wear (brinzolamide)

kidney function, reduced

liver disease

*Pregnancy:* Adequate studies have not been done in pregnant women, or animal studies may have shown a risk to the fetus. Use only if clearly needed and potential benefits outweight possible hazards to the fetus.

*Breastfeeding:* It is not known if brinzolamide and dorzolamide appear in breast milk. Consult your doctor before you begin breastfeeding.

*Children:* Safety and effectiveness in children have not been established.

## Drug Interactions:

Tell your doctor or pharmacist if you are taking or if you are planning to take any over-the-counter or prescription medications or dietary supplements while taking these medicines. Doses of one or both drugs may need to be modified or a different drug may need to be prescribed. High dose salicylates (eg, aspirin) and oral carbonic anhydrase inhibitors (acetazolamide, dichlorphenamide, methazolamide) may interact with brinzolamide and dorzolamide.

## Side Effects:

Every drug is capable of producing side effects. Many patients experience no, or minor, side effects. The frequency and severity of side effects depend on many factors including dose, duration of therapy, and individual susceptibility. Possible side effects include the following:

*Eyes or Ocular:* Burning, stinging or discomfort immediately following use; tearing; blurred vision; dryness; light sensitivity; skin or eyelid inflammation; dry eye; foreign body sensation; cornea inflammation; eye discharge, pain and itching.

*Other:* Bitter, sour or unusual taste; sinus infection; headache.

---

### Guidelines for Use:

- Shake brinzolamide suspension well before use.
- Place one drop in the affected eye(s) 3 times daily. Do not increase or decrease this medicine without your doctor's approval. Wait at least 10 minutes before using any other eye medications. Use exactly as prescribed
- Brief stinging or burning of the eye may occur after administration. This is normal. Contact your doctor if the symptom(s) continue or worsen.
- Do not touch the dropper tip to any surface, including your eye, because this may contaminate the contents or damage/infect the eye.
- Dorzolamide contains benzalkonium chloride, a preservative that may be absorbed by soft contact lenses.
- Soft contact lenses — Do not wear during treatment with dorzolamide. May be reinserted 15 minutes after brinzolamide use.
- Dorzolamide may cause sensitivity to bright light. Protect your eyes and wear sunglasses if this occurs.
- Temporary blurred vision is possible following use. Use caution when operating machinery or driving a motor vehicle.
- Contact your doctor if you receive an eye injury or undergo eye surgery; your medication may need to be changed.
- Discontinue this medicine immediately and contact your doctor if any of the following occurs: Swelling of the eyelids; redness; itching; discharge; tearing or any other signs of an infection or eye irritation.
- Brinzolamide and dorzolamide are sulfonamides and although administered topically, can be absorbed into the body. Therefore, the same types of side effects that can occur with sulfonamides can also occur with this drugs.
- Do not use either of these drugs if you are allergic to sulfonamides. Do not use with other carbonic anhydrase inhibitors.
- Store brinzolamide at controlled room temperature (36° to 86°F). Store dorzolamide at room temperature (59° to 86°F). Protect from light.

---

*If you have any questions, consult your doctor, pharmacist, or health care provider.*

| Generic Name<br>*Brand Name Examples* | Supplied As | Generic<br>Available |
|---|---|---|
| *Rx* **Dorzolamide HCl/Timolol Maleate** | | |
| *Cosopt* | **Solution**: 2% dorzolamide, 0.5% timolol | No |

## Type of Drug:

A combination of two drugs, a carbonic anhydrase inhibitor (dorzolamide HCl) and a beta–adrenergic receptor blocker (timolol maleate), each of which lowers pressure within the eye (intraocular). Antiglaucoma medicines.

## How the Drug Works:

Reduces fluid formation within eyeball resulting in lowering of intraocular pressure.

## Uses:

Reduction of elevated intraocular pressure (IOP) in patients with open-angle glaucoma or ocular hypertension who have not responded to beta blockers alone.

## Precautions:

*Do not use in the following situations:*

allergy to dorzolamide HCl or sulfa drugs
allergy to timolol maleate
bronchial asthma, current or history
heart conduction problems
heart failure, overt
sudden decreased heart function
chronic obstructive lung disease, severe
kidney impairment, severe
sinus bradycardia (slow heart rate)

*Use with caution in the following situations:*

bronchitis, chronic
chronic obstructive lung disease, mild to moderate
diabetes mellitus
emphysema, chronic
heart failure, history
hypoglycemia, spontaneous
liver impairment
major surgery
myasthenia gravis
surgical anesthesia
thyroid disorder

*Pregnancy:* Adequate studies have not been done in pregnant women. Use only if clearly needed and potential benefits outweigh the possible hazards to the fetus.

*Breastfeeding:* It is not known if dorzolamide appears in breast milk. Timolol appears in breast milk. Consult your doctor before you begin breastfeeding. A decision should be made whether to discontinue nursing or discontinue the drug, taking into account the importance of the drug to the mother.

*Children:* Safety and effectiveness in children have not been established.

*Lab tests* and eye examinations may be required during therapy.

## Drug Interactions:

Tell your doctor or pharmacist if you are taking or planning to take any over-the-counter or prescription medications or dietary supplements while taking this medicine. Doses of one or both drugs may need to be modified or a different drug may need to be prescribed. The following drugs and drug classes interact with this medicine:

beta-adrenergic blocking agents, oral or topical (eg, propranolol)
calcium antagonists, oral or intravenous (eg, verapamil)
carbonic anhydrase inhibitors, oral (eg, acetazolamide)

catecholamine-depleting drugs (eg, reserpine)
digitalis (eg, digoxin)
quinidine (eg, *Quinora*)

## Side Effects:

Every drug is capable of producing side effects. Many dorzolamide HCl/timolol maleate users experience no, or minor, side effects. The frequency and severity of side effects depend on many factors including dose, duration of therapy, and individual susceptibility. Possible side effects include the following:

*Eyes or Ocular:* Stinging, itching, or burning eyes; blurred vision; cloudy vision; dry eyes; eye debris; eye discharge; eye pain; eye tearing; eye swelling; eyelid pain, discomfort, or swelling; eyelid redness; eyelid discharge or scales; cataract; corneal staining; conjunctivitis; corneal erosion; lens opacity; decreased corneal sensitivity; visual disturbances including refractive changes and double vision; foreign body sensation.

*Digestive Tract:* Taste changes; stomach pain; indigestion; nausea; sore throat.

*Nervous System:* Bronchitis; cough; upper respiratory tract infection; sinus infection; bronchospasm.

*Other:* Back pain; urinary tract infection; influenza; dizziness; headache; high blood pressure.

## Guidelines for Use:

- Recommended dose is 1 drop in the affected eye(s) 2 times daily.
- Do not allow the tip of the dispensing container to contact the eye as it may become contaminated with bacteria known to cause eye infections. Serious eye damage and loss of vision can result.
- If more than 1 topical ophthalmic drug is being used, the drugs should be administered at least 10 minutes apart.
- Contact lenses should be removed prior to administration of the solution. Lenses may be reinserted 15 minutes following administration.
- Discontinue the drug and notify your doctor immediately if any of the following occurs: Hives; itching; rash; difficulty breathing; shortness of breath; swelling in feet or ankles; inflammation of eye or eyelids; changes in vision; muscle weakness.
- This drug may mask certain signs (eg, fast heartbeat) of hyperthyroidism. Hyperthyroid patients should be managed carefully by their doctor.
- Patients using this medication with a history of allergies or severe anaphylactic reactions to a variety of allergens may be unresponsive to the usual doses of epinephrine used to treat reactions.
- Your doctor may have you gradually stop this drug before elective surgery.
- Store between 59° and 77°F. Protect from light.

*If you have any questions, consult your doctor, pharmacist, or health care provider.*

| Generic Name Brand Name Examples | Supplied As | Generic Available |
|---|---|---|
| **Rx Pilocarpine and Epinephrine**[1] | | |
| *P₁E₁* | **Solution**: 1% pilocarpine HCl and 1% epinephrine bitartrate | No |
| *P₂E₁* | **Solution**: 2% pilocarpine HCl and 1% epinephrine bitartrate | No |
| *P₃E₁* | **Solution**: 3% pilocarpine HCl and 1% epinephrine bitartrate | No |
| *P₄E₁* | **Solution**: 4% pilocarpine HCl and 1% epinephrine bitartrate | No |
| *P₆E₁* | **Solution**: 4% pilocarpine HCl and 1% epinephrine bitartrate | No |
| **Rx Pilocarpine and Physostigmine** | | |
| *Isopto P-ES* | **Solution**: 2% pilocarpine HCl and 0.25% physotigmine salicylate | No |

[1] These products contain sulfites.

## Type of Drug:

Combination products to lower intraocular (fluid) pressure in the eye.

## How the Drug Works:

*Epinephrine* reduces pressure in the eye by decreasing the rate of fluid production. Improved fluid outflow has also been reported.

*Physostigmine* increases outflow of aqueous humor.

*Pilocarpine* lowers pressure in the eye by improving fluid (aqueous humor) outflow and, to a lesser extent, by decreasing aqueous humor production.

Combinations of pilocarpine and physostigmine have been used on the theory that improved response may result. Studies do not show that additive pressure lowering effects are achieved over either agent used alone. The combination of pilocarpine and epinephrine provides additive effects in lowering intraocular pressure. These fixed combinations do not permit the flexibility needed to adjust the dosage of each agent.

## Uses:

To lower intraocular (fluid) pressure in glaucoma.

### Guidelines for Use:

- May cause temporary blurred or unstable vision. Use caution while driving or performing other hazardous tasks.
- Do not use while wearing soft contact lenses. Lenses may become discolored.
- Report any vision changes to your doctor immediately.
- *Storage* — Store in a cool, dark place. Discard if solution becomes brown or discolors, becomes cloudy, or contains particles.

*If you have any questions, consult your doctor, pharmacist, or health care provider.*

| Generic Name<br>*Brand Name Example* | Supplied As | Generic<br>Available |
|---|---|---|
| *Rx* **Dapiprazole HCl** | | |
| *Rēv-Eyes* | **Ophthalmic powder for reconstitution**: 5 mg/mL | No |

## Type of Drug:
Pupil constrictor.

## How the Drug Works:
Dapiprazole produces pupil constriction by blocking the alpha-adrenergic receptors in the dilator muscle of the iris.

## Uses:
To reverse mydriasis (extreme dilation of the pupil) due to treatment with phenylephrine or tropicamide during eye examinations or surgery.

## Precautions:
*Do not use in the following situations:*
>    acute iritis
>    allergy to any component of the product
>    open-angle glaucoma, treatment of
>    reduction of intraocular pressure

*Pregnancy:* Adequate studies have not been done in pregnant women. Use only if clearly needed and potential benefits outweigh the possible hazards to the fetus.

*Breastfeeding:* It is not known if dapiprazole appears in the breast milk. Consult your doctor before you begin breastfeeding.

*Children:* Safety and effectiveness for use in children have not been established.

## Side Effects:
Every drug is capable of producing side effects. Many dapiprazole users experience no, or minor, side effects. The frequency and severity of side effects depend on many factors including dose, duration of therapy and individual susceptibility. Possible side effects include the following:

*Eyes or Ocular:* Burning when first instilled; drooping eyelids; eyelid redness; eyelid inflammation; edema (fluid retention) of eyelids; itching; inflammation and formation of deposits on cornea; conjunctival congestion and edema; sensitivity to light; dry eyes; tearing; blurred vision.

*Other:* Headache; browache.

## Guidelines for Use:

- For use in eyes only.
- Shake container for several minutes to ensure mixing.
- Instill 2 drops into each eye, followed 5 minutes later by an additional 2 drops.
- Do not touch dropper to lids or any surface, as this may contaminate the solution. Recap container after use.
- If a dose is missed, instill it as soon as possible. If several hours have passed or if it is nearing time for the next dose, do not double the dose in order to catch up (unless advised to do so by your doctor). If more than one dose is missed or it is necessary to establish a new dosage schedule, contact your doctor or pharmacist. Use exactly as prescribed.
- Do not use more than once a week.
- May cause stinging or burning when you first instill drops into the eyes.
- May cause vision problems in poor light. Use caution when driving at night or performing other tasks in poor lighting.
- May cause sensitivity to light. This may be reduced by wearing sunglasses.
- Store at room temperature (59° to 86°F) for 21 days after reconstitution. Discard any solution that is not clear and colorless.

*If you have any questions, consult your doctor, pharmacist, or health care provider.*

| Generic Name<br>*Brand Name Examples* | Supplied As | Generic Available |
|---|---|---|
| **Naphazoline HCl** | | |
| otc *Allerest Eye Drops, Allergy Drops, Clear Eyes, Clear Eyes ACR[1], Comfort Eye Drops, Degest 2, Maximum Strength Allergy Drops, Naphcon, VasoClear* | **Solution**: 0.012%, 0.02%, 0.03% | Yes |
| Rx *AK-Con, Albalon, Nafazair, Naphcon Forte* | **Solution**: 0.1% | Yes |
| **Oxymetazoline HCl** | | |
| otc *OcuClear, Visine L.R.* | **Solution**: 0.025% | No |
| **Phenylephrine HCl** | | |
| otc *AK-Nefrin, Prefrin Liquifilm, Relief* | **Solution**: 0.12% | Yes |
| Rx *AK-Dilate, Mydfrin 2.5%[1], Neo-Synephrine, Neo-Synephrine Viscous, Phenoptic* | **Solution**: 2.5%, 10% | Yes |
| **Tetrahydrozoline HCl** | | |
| otc *AR Eye Drops - Astringent Redness Reliever[1], Collyrium Fresh, Eye Drops, Eye Drops Extra, Eyesine, Geneye, Geneye Extra, Mallazine Eye Drops, Murine Plus, Optigene 3, Tetrasine, Tetrasine Extra, Visine, Visine Moisturizing* | **Solution**: 0.05% | Yes |

[1] Contains sulfites.

## Type of Drug:

Ophthalmic vasoconstrictors; drugs that reduce redness and cause the pupil to dilate (widen).

## How the Drug Works:

The effects of these agents on the eye include the following: Pupil dilation (widening), increase in outflow of fluid (aqueous humor) and vasoconstriction (narrowing of blood vessels).

The strong vasoconstrictors (phenylephrine 2.5% and 10%) are used to prepare the eye for diagnostic exams, during surgery, and to prevent scarring. Intermediate strength solutions (epinephrine 0.5% to 2%) are used in open-angle glaucoma, alone, or with other drugs. Weak solutions (phenylephrine 0.12%, naphazoline, tetrahydrozoline) are used as ophthalmic decongestants (that narrow conjunctival blood vessels) to relieve redness due to minor eye irritations.

## Uses:

To dilate the pupils (phenylephrine 2.5%, 10% only).

To temporarily reduce irritation and redness caused by minor eye irritations, such as smoke, smog, sunglare, contact lens wear, allergies, swimming, or wind.

## Precautions:

*Do not use in the following situations:*

allergy to any of these medicines

aneurysm (phenylephrine 10% only)

infants (phenylephrine 10% only)

iridectomy (surgical removal of a portion of the iris), prior to

narrow-angle glaucoma

narrow angles (but no glaucoma)

*Use with caution in the following situations:*

anesthetics (general), use

anesthetics, local (prior to use of phenylephrine)

arteriosclerosis (hardening of the arteries)

children, low body weight

diabetes

elderly

glaucoma, narrow-angle (to free adhesions)

heart disease, history (phenylephrine 10% only)

high blood pressure

hyperthyroidism (overactive thyroid), untreated

*Pigment floaters:* Phenylephrine may cause temporary pigment floaters ("black spots") in the visual field of older individuals.

*Rebound congestion* (redness or swelling of the eye surface) may occur with frequent or extended use of ophthalmic vasoconstrictors.

*Rebound miosis* (decrease in size of pupil) may occur in some patients 1 day after using phenylephrine.

*Pregnancy:* Adequate studies have not been done in pregnant women, or animal studies may have shown a risk to the fetus. Use only if clearly needed and potential benefits outweigh the possible hazards to the fetus.

*Breastfeeding:* Safety and effectiveness have not been established. Consult your doctor before you begin breastfeeding.

*Children:* Safety and effectiveness have not been established. Do not use phenylephrine 10% in infants. Use with caution in children of low body weight.

*Elderly:* Those with a history of heart problems should use caution when using phenylephrine 10%.

*Sulfites:* Some of these products may contain sulfite preservatives, which can cause allergic reactions in certain individuals. Check package label when available or consult your doctor or pharmacist.

## Drug Interactions:

Tell your doctor or pharmacist if you are taking or if you are planning to take any over-the-counter or prescription medications or dietary supplements while taking these medicines. Doses of one or both drugs may need to be modified or a different drug may need to be prescribed. The following drugs and drug classes interact with these medicines.

> anesthetics (eg, cyclopropane, halothane)
> beta-blockers (eg, propranolol)
> monoamine oxidase inhibitors (MAOIs, eg, phenelzine)

Also consider drug interactions that may occur with systemic sympatho-mimetics.

## Side Effects:

Every drug is capable of producing side effects. Many patients experience no, or minor, side effects. The frequency and severity of side effects depend on many factors including dose, duration of therapy and individual susceptibility. Possible side effects include the following:

*Eyes or Ocular:* Stinging; blurring; redness; eye discomfort; allergic reactions; inflammation of cornea; tearing; glaucoma; decrease in pupil size (phenylephrine).

*Circulatory System:* Palpitations (pounding in the chest); collapse; blood clots; high blood pressure; heart attack; stroke; irregular heartbeat.

*Other:* Pale skin; sweating; dizziness; nausea; nervousness; drowsiness; weakness; high blood sugar; headache; browache.

## Guidelines for Use:

- Use exactly as prescribed.
- Follow Administration Guidelines found at the beginning of this chapter.
- If a dose is missed, instill it as soon as possible. If several hours have passed or if it is nearing time for the next dose, do not double the dose in order to catch up (unless advised to do so by your doctor). If more than one dose is missed or it is necessary to establish a new dosage schedule, contact your doctor or pharmacist.
- Do not use for more than 48 to 72 hours (2 to 3 days) without contacting your doctor.
- Overuse may produce increased eye redness.
- *Phenylephrine* — May cause temporary blurred or unstable vision. Use caution when driving, operating machinery, or performing other tasks requiring clear vision.
- Discontinue use and contact your doctor if any of the following occur: Severe eye pain, headache, vision changes, floating spots, dizziness, decrease in body temperature, drowsiness, acute eye redness, or pain when exposed to light.
- Discontinue use and contact your doctor if any of the following persist: Irritation, blurring, redness.
- Do not use if you have glaucoma unless advised by your doctor.
- Some of these products may contain sulfite preservatives, which can cause allergic reactions in certain individuals. Check package label when available or consult your doctor or pharmacist.
- Do not use if solution changes color, becomes cloudy, or contains particles.
- Store in a cool place (36° to 75°F) away from light. Keep container tightly sealed. Avoid freezing.

*If you have any questions, consult your doctor, pharmacist, or health care provider.*

| Generic Name<br>*Brand Name Examples* | Supplied As | Generic<br>Available |
|---|---|---|
| **otc Phenylephrine-containing Solutions** | | |
| *Zincfrin* | **Solution**: 0.12% phenylephrine HCl and 0.25% zinc sulfate | No |
| **Naphazoline-containing Solutions** | | |
| *otc Vasocon-A* | **Solution**: 0.05% naphazoline HCl and 0.5% antazoline phosphate | Yes |
| *otc Naphazoline Plus, Naphcon-A* | **Solution**: 0.025% naphazoline HCl and 0.3% pheniramine maleate | Yes |
| *Rx Naphoptic-A* | **Solution**: 0.025% naphazoline HCl and 0.3% pheniramine maleate | Yes |
| *otc Opcon-A* | **Solution**: 0.027% naphazoline HCl and 0.315% pheniramine maleate | No |
| *otc Clear Eyes ACR* | **Solution**: 0.012% naphazoline HCl and 0.25% zinc sulfate | No |
| *otc VasoClear A* | **Solution**: 0.02% naphazoline HCl and 0.25% zinc sulfate | No |
| **Tetrahydrozoline-containing Solutions** | | |
| *otc Geneye AC Allergy Formula, Visine Allergy Relief* | **Solution**: 0.05% tetrahydrozoline HCl and 0.25% zinc sulfate | Yes |

## Type of Drug:

Ophthalmic decongestants; agents to reduce eye redness.

## How the Drug Works:

In these combinations:

*Phenylephrine HCl, naphazoline HCl, and tetrahydrozoline* are used for their decongestant actions. (See the Ophthalmic Vasoconstrictors — Decongestants monograph for complete information.)

*Zinc sulfate* is used as an astringent (agent that tightens the tissues).

*Pheniramine maleate and antazoline* are antihistamines.

## Uses:

Temporary relief of minor eye symptoms of itching and redness caused by pollen, animal hair, smoke, smog, contact lens wear, wind, sunglare, swimming, etc.

## Precautions:

*Use with caution in the following situations:*
narrow-angle glaucoma or a history of glaucoma

Also see precautions for ophthalmic decongestants.

---

### Guidelines for Use:

- Use exactly as prescribed.
- Follow Administration Guidelines found at the beginning of this chapter.
- If a dose is missed, instill it as soon as possible. If several hours have passed or if it is nearing time for the next dose, do not double the dose in order to catch up (unless advised to do so by your doctor). If more than one dose is missed or it is necessary to establish a new dosage schedule, contact your doctor or pharmacist.
- Do not use longer than 48 to 72 hours (2 to 3 days) without contacting your doctor.
- May cause temporary blurred or unstable vision. Use caution when driving, operating machinery, or performing other tasks requiring clear vision.
- Discontinue use and consult your doctor if any of the following occurs: Severe eye pain, headache, vision changes, floating spots, dizziness, decrease in body temperature, drowsiness, swelling, acute eye redness, pain when exposed to light.
- Discontinue use and consult your doctor if any of the following persist: Irritation, blurring, redness, or swelling.
- Do not use if solution changes color, becomes cloudy, or contains particles.
- Store in a cool place (36° to 75°F), away from light. Keep container tightly sealed. Avoid freezing.

---

*If you have any questions, consult your doctor, pharmacist, or health care provider.*

| Generic Name<br>*Brand Name Examples* | **Supplied As** | Generic<br>Available |
|---|---|---|
| *Rx* **Atropine Sulfate** | | |
| *Atropine Sulfate* | **Ointment**: 1% | Yes |
| *Atropine Care, Atropine-1,<br>Atropisol, Isopto Atropine* | **Solution**: 0.5%, 1%, 2% | Yes |
| *Rx* **Cyclopentolate HCl** | | |
| *AK-Pentolate, Cyclogyl,<br>Pentolair* | **Solution**: 0.5%, 1%, 2% | Yes |
| *Rx* **Homatropine HBr** | | |
| *AK-Homatropine, Isopto<br>Homatropine* | **Solution**: 2%, 5% | Yes |
| *Rx* **Scopolamine HBr<br>(Hyoscine HBr)** | | |
| *Isopto Hyoscine* | **Solution**: 0.25% | No |
| *Rx* **Tropicamide** | | |
| *Mydriacyl, Opticyl,<br>Tropicacyl* | **Solution**: 0.5%, 1% | Yes |
| *Rx* **Mydriatic Combinations** | | |
| *Cyclomydril* | **Solution**: 0.2% Cyclopentolate<br>HCl and 1% phenylephrine HCl | No |
| *Murocoll-2*[1] | **Drops**: 0.3% scopolamine HBr<br>and 10% phenylephrine HCl | No |
| *Paremyd* | **Solution**: 0.25% tropicamide<br>and 1% hydroxyamphetamine<br>HBr | No |

[1] Contains sulfites.

## Type of Drug:

Pupil dilators.

## How the Drug Works:

Cycloplegic mydriatics relax the muscles of the eye to cause the pupil to dilate (widen) and prevent the eye from focusing (cycloplegia) on near objects.

## Uses:

To dilate the pupil when there is eye inflammation or when an eye exam is performed.

## Precautions:

*Do not use in the following situations:*

adhesions (scarring) between iris and lens
allergy to belladonna alkaloids or any component of the
formulation
children, previous severe reaction to atropine
glaucoma, active or tendency toward

*Use with caution in the following situations:*

| | |
|---|---|
| brain damage, children | nursing women |
| Down syndrome | small children, infants |
| elderly | |

*Pregnancy:* Adequate studies have not been done in pregnant women, or animal studies may have shown a risk to the fetus. Use only if clearly needed and potential benefits outweigh the possible hazards to the fetus.

*Breastfeeding:* Atropine and homatropine appear in breast milk. It is not known if cyclopentolate appears in breast milk. Consult your doctor before you begin breastfeeding.

*Children:* Tropicamide and cyclopentolate may cause dangerous nervous system disturbances in infants and children. Infants, young children, and children with spastic paralysis or brain damage may be more susceptible to cyclopentolate. Feeding intolerance may follow use of cyclopentolate in newborns. Withhold feeding for 4 hours after examination.

*Sulfites:* Some of these products may contain sulfite preservatives, which can cause allergic reactions in certain individuals. Check package label when available or consult your doctor or pharmacist.

## Side Effects:

Every drug is capable of producing side effects. Many patients experience no, or minor, side effects. The frequency and severity of side effects depend on many factors including dose, duration of therapy, and individual susceptibility. Possible side effects include the following:

*Eyes or Ocular:* Increased intraocular (fluid) pressure; stinging; burning; irritation; sensitivity to light; blurred vision.

*Nervous System:* Headache; drowsiness; hallucinations; psychotic reaction or behavioral disturbance, usually in children (cyclopentolate and tropicamide).

*Other:* Flushing; rash; decreased sweating or salivation; dryness of mouth, sinuses and skin; stomach bloating (in infants); urinary retention; constipation; rapid heart rate; fever.

## Guidelines for Use:

- For use in eyes only. Use exactly as prescribed.
- Follow Administration Guidelines found at the beginning of this chapter.
- To avoid contamination, do not touch dropper tip to any surface. Replace cap after using.
- If instilling this medicine for someone else, wash your hands and theirs following administration.
- Avoid excessive systemic absorption by using your fingers to press on the corner of the eye next to the nose during use and for 2 to 3 minutes after use.
- Do not exceed recommended dosages. If overdosage occurs, flush eyes with water or normal saline.
- If a dose is missed, instill it as soon as possible. If several hours have passed or if it is nearing time for the next dose, do not double the dose in order to "catch up." If more than one dose is missed, contact your doctor or pharmacist.
- May cause drowsiness, blurred vision, or sensitivity to light (due to dilated pupils). Use caution while driving, operating machinery, or performing other tasks requiring clear vision and alertness. Protect eyes in bright sunlight or illumination.
- If eye pain occurs, discontinue use and contact your doctor immediately.
- Store at room temperature (46° to 75°F) away from heat and light.

*If you have any questions, consult your doctor, pharmacist, or health care provider.*

| Generic Name Brand Name Examples | Supplied As | Generic Available |
|---|---|---|
| Rx **Dexamethasone** | | |
| *Maxidex* | **Suspension**: 0.1% | Yes |
| Rx **Dexamethasone Sodium Phosphate** | | |
| *AK-Dex, Decadron Phosphate*[1] | **Solution**: 0.1% | Yes |
| *AK-Dex, Decadron Phosphate, Maxidex* | **Ointment**: 0.05% | Yes |
| Rx **Fluorometholone** | | |
| *Flarex, Fluor-Op, FML, FML Forte* | **Suspension**: 0.1%, 0.25% | No |
| *FML S.O.P.* | **Ointment**: 0.1% | No |
| Rx **Medrysone** | | |
| *HMS* | **Suspension**: 1% | No |
| Rx **Prednisolone Acetate** | | |
| *Pred Mild*[1], *Econopred, Econopred Plus, Pred Forte*[1] | **Suspension**: 0.12%, 0.125%, 1% | Yes |
| Rx **Prednisolone Sodium Phosphate** | | |
| *AK-Pred*[1], *Inflamase Forte, Inflamase Mild* | **Solution**: 0.125%, 1% | Yes |
| Rx **Rimexolone** | | |
| *Vexol* | **Suspension**: 1% | No |

[1] Contains sulfites

## Type of Drug:

Anti-inflammatory agents for the eye.

## How the Drug Works:

Corticosteroids inhibit the inflammatory response (redness, swelling, warmth, etc) of tissues to mechanical, chemical, or allergy-causing agents. Prostaglandins are chemicals produced by the body in response to irritating substances. The mechanism of action of corticosteroids, in part, is thought to be inhibition of the production of prostaglandins.

## Uses:

To treat inflammatory conditions of the eye, injuries to the cornea, anterior uveitis, and graft rejection after keratoplasty (corneal graft).

## Precautions:

*Do not use in the following situations:*

after removal of a minor corneal foreign body
allergy to the drug
fungal eye infections
herpes simplex inflammation of the cornea
inflammation of the iris (medrysone only)
inflammation of the uvea (medrysone only)

mustard gas keratitis
mycobacterial diseases of the eye
Sjogren's keratoconjunctivitis (dry eye, etc)
tuberculosis of the eye
viral infections of the eye

*Pregnancy:* Adequate studies have not been done in pregnant women, or animal studies may have shown a potential risk to the fetus. Use only if clearly needed and potential benefits outweigh the possible hazards to the fetus.

*Breastfeeding:* It is not known if topical steroids appear in breast milk. Consult your doctor before you begin breastfeeding.

*Children:* Safety and effectiveness have not been established.

*Sulfites:* Some of these products may contain sulfite preservatives, which can cause allergic reactions in certain individuals. Check package label when available or consult your doctor or pharmacist.

## Side Effects:

Every drug is capable of producing side effects. Many patients experience no, or minor, side effects. The frequency and severity of side effects depend on many factors including dose, duration of therapy, and individual susceptibility. Possible side effects include the following:

*Note:* Also consider all side effects reported for systemic corticosteroids (see Hormones chapter) when using ophthalmic corticosteroids.

*Eyes or Ocular:* Glaucoma with optic nerve damage; blurring; cataracts; eye infections; perforation of the eye; stinging; burning; discharge; discomfort; pain; foreign body sensation; engorgement of blood; itching (rimexolone only).

*Other:* Headache; low blood pressure; runny nose; sore throat; taste changes.

## Guidelines for Use:

- Use exactly as prescribed.
- Follow Administrative Guidelines found at the beginning of this chapter.
- To avoid contamination, do not touch applicator tip to any surface. Replace cap after use.
- If a dose is missed, instill it as soon as possible. If several hours have passed or if it is nearing time for the next dose, do not double the dose in order to "catch up" (unless advised to do so by your doctor). If more than one dose is missed or it is necessary to establish a new dosage schedule, contact your doctor or pharmacist.
- Prolonged use may result in glaucoma, optic nerve damage, blurred vision, cataracts, or infections. Frequent eye exams are required to monitor treatment. Be sure to keep appointments.
- If improvement does not occur within several days or if pain, itching or swelling of the eye occurs, contact your doctor. Do not stop using this drug without consulting your doctor.
- Store upright at room temperature (46° to 77° F). Do not freeze.

*If you have any questions, consult your doctor, pharmacist, or health care provider.*

| Generic Name<br>*Brand Name Example* | Supplied As | Generic<br>Available |
|---|---|---|
| *Rx* **Loteprednol Etabonate** | | |
| *Alrex* | **Suspension**: 0.2% | No |
| *Lotemax* | **Suspension**: 0.5% | No |

## Type of Drug:

Topical anti-inflammatory drug for treating symptoms involving the eye.

## How the Drug Works:

Corticosteroids inhibit the inflammatory response (swelling, redness, etc) of tissues to irritating agents. The mechanism of action of corticosteroids is thought to be due, in part, to the inhibition of the body's chemical response to irritating substances.

## Uses:

*Alrex:* For temporary relief of seasonal allergy eye symptoms.

*Lotemax:* To treat inflammatory conditions of the eye due to allergies, bacteria or virus (eg, iritis, acne rosacea, herpes zoster keratitis) and post-operative eye surgery inflammation.

## Precautions:

*Do not use in the following situations:*

allergy to this drug or to corticosteroids
fungal eye infections
mycobacterial eye infections

ocular herpes simplex, history
ocular viral infections
soft contact lens (*Lotemax* only)

*Use with caution in the following situations:*

contact lens use (*Alrex* only)
corneal thinning
eye discharge
eye infections (not included
above)

glaucoma
post cataract surgery (*Lotemax*
only) (may delay wound
healing)

*Pregnancy:* Adequate studies have not been done in pregnant women, or animal studies may have shown a risk to the fetus. Use only if clearly needed and potential benefits outweigh the possible hazards to the fetus.

*Breastfeeding:* It is not known if topical corticosteroids appear in breast milk. Consult your doctor before you begin breastfeeding.

*Children:* Safety and effectiveness in children have not been established.

*Lab tests* may be required with long-term steroid use. Tests may include fungal cultures and intraocular (fluid) pressure.

## Drug Interactions:

Tell your doctor or pharmacist if you are planning to take any over-the-counter or prescription medications or dietary supplements while taking loteprednol. Doses of one or both drugs may need to be modified or a different drug may need to be prescribed.

## Side Effects:

Every drug is capable of producing side effects. Many loteprednol users experience no, or minor, side effects. The frequency and severity of side effects depend on many factors including dose, duration of therapy, and individual susceptibility. Possible side effects include the following:

*Note:* Also consider all side effects reported for systemic corticosteroids (see Hormones chapter) when using ophthalmic corticosteroids.

*Eyes or Ocular:* Optic nerve damage; blurred vision; elevated intraocular pressure; cataracts; eye infections; secondary ocular infections (eg, herpes simplex); perforation of the eye; eyelid swelling; burning; discharge; dry eyes; foreign body sensation; itching; discomfort; pain; tearing; light sensitivity; redness; irritation; abnormal vision.

*Other:* Headache; rhinitis; sore or inflamed throat.

---

### Guidelines for Use:

- For ophthalmic use only.
- Shake well before using.
- *Lotemax* — Eye disease inflammation/allergies: Place 1 drop into the affected eye(s) 4 times daily. During first week of treatment, dosage may be increased up to 1 drop per hour if needed. Effectiveness depends on consistency of use.
- *Lotemax* — For postoperative inflammation apply 1 to 2 drops 4 times daily beginning 24 hours after surgery. Continue using regularly for 14 days after surgery.
- *Lotemax* – Do not wear soft contact lenses when using *Lotemax*.
- *Alrex* — Dosage is 1 drop 4 times daily.
- *Alrex* — Patients should be advised not to wear a contact lens if their eye is red.
- *Alrex* — Do not use this product to treat contact lens related irritations. The preservative benzalkonium chloride may be absorbed by soft contact lenses. Patients who wear soft contact lenses and whose eyes are not red, should wait 10 minutes after applying before inserting contact lenses.
- To avoid contamination do not touch dropper tip to any surface.
- Prolonged use may result in glaucoma, optic nerve damage, blurred vision, and cataracts or infections. Eye exams may be required to monitor treatment. Be sure to keep appointments.
- If improvements do not occur after 2 days, or eye redness or itching increases, contact your doctor.
- Store upright between 59° to 77°F. Do not freeze.

---

*If you have any questions, consult your doctor, pharmacist, or health care provider.*

| Generic Name<br>*Brand Name Examples* | Supplied As | Generic<br>Available |
|---|---|---|
| *Rx* **Cromolyn Sodium** | | |
| *Crolom* | **Solution, ophthalmic**: 4% | Yes |
| *Rx* **Lodoxamide Tromethamine** | | |
| *Alomide* | **Solution, ophthalmic**: 0.1% | No |
| *Rx* **Nedocromil Sodium** | | |
| *Alocril* | **Solution, ophthalmic**: 2% | No |
| *Rx* **Pemirolast Potassium** | | |
| *Alamast* | **Solution, ophthalmic**: 0.1% | No |

## Type of Drug:

Mast cell stabilizer; antiallergy agent for the eye.

## How the Drug Works:

Mast cell stabilizers prevent allergy symptoms (eg, itching, redness, tearing) that involve the eye by preventing the local release of histamine and other chemicals that cause allergic symptoms from mast cells.

## Uses:

For the prevention and treatment of eye itching caused by allergic reactions (allergic conjunctivitis).

*Lodoxamide tromethamine and cromolyn sodium* — For the treatment of vernal (occuring in the springtime) keratoconjunctivitis, vernal conjunctivitis, and vernal keratitis.

## Precautions:

*Do not use in the following situations:*

allergy to the mast cell stabilizer or any of its ingredients
soft contact lens wear (cromolyn sodium only)

*Pregnancy:* There are no adequate and well-controlled studies in pregnant women. Use only if clearly needed and the potential benefits to the mother outweigh the possible hazards to the fetus.

*Breastfeeding:* It is not known if mast cell stabilizers are excreted in breast milk. Consult your doctor before you begin breastfeeding.

*Children:* Safety and effectiveness of use of lodoxamide in children less than 2 years of age are not established. Safety and effectiveness of use of nedocromil and pemirolast in children less than 3 years of age are not established. Safety and effectiveness of use of cromolyn sodium in children less than 4 years of age are not established.

## Drug Interactions:

Tell your doctor or pharmacist if you are taking or if you are planning to take any over-the-counter or prescription medications or dietary supplements while using a mast cell stabilizer. Doses of one or both drugs may need to be modified or a different drug may need to be prescribed.

## Side Effects:

Every drug is capable of producing side effects. Many mast cell stabilizer users experience no, or minor, side effects. The frequency or severity of side effects depend on many factors including dose, duration of therapy, and individual susceptibility. Possible side effects include the following:

*Eyes or Ocular:* Burning; stinging; dry eye; foreign body sensation; redness; discomfort or irritation; tearing; discharge; styes; itching; watery eyes; puffy eyes; sensitivity to light; blurred vision.

*Respiratory System:* Runny nose; cold or flu symptoms; cough; bronchitis; sinus inflammation; sneezing; nasal congestion; asthma.

*Other:* Headache; allergy; back pain; painful menstruation; fever; unpleasant taste sensation.

---

### Guidelines for Use:

- Dosage is individualized. Use exactly as prescribed.
- Effectiveness of mast cell stabilizers is dependent on administration at regular intervals. They are not effective when used sporadically or "as needed."
- For topical ophthalmic use only. Not for injection or oral use.
- Review guidelines at the beginning of this chapter for proper technique for instilling eye drops.
- Temporary stinging or burning sensations may occur following application. Inform your doctor if this becomes bothersome or intolerable.
- If a dose is missed, take it as soon as possible. If several hours have passed or it is nearing time for the next dose, do not double the dose to "catch up" unless advised to do so by your doctor. If more than one dose is missed or it is necessary to establish a new dosage schedule, contact your doctor or pharmacist.
- To prevent contamination of the dropper tip and solution, do not touch the eyelids or surrounding areas with the dropper tip.
- *Contact lens wearers* — Do not wear contact lenses while you have signs and symptoms of allergic conjunctivitis. Do not wear soft contact lenses during treatment with cromolyn sodium, nedocromil, or lodoxamide. The preservative in pemirolast potassium, lauralkonium chloride, may be absorbed by soft contact lenses. If you wear soft contact lenses and your eyes are not red, wait at least 10 minutes after instilling pemirolast potassium before inserting contact lenses. Do not wear contact lens if your eye is red. Do not use to treat a contact lens-related irritation.
- Symptoms usually respond to therapy within a few days, but it may take up to 6 weeks. Once relief of symptoms has occurred, continue the medicine on a regular basis to prevent return of symptoms.
- Store at room temperature. Keep the bottle tightly closed. Replace cap immediately after use.

---

*If you have any questions, consult your doctor, pharmacist, or health care provider.*

| Generic Name<br>*Brand Name Examples* | Supplied As | Generic<br>Available |
|---|---|---|
| *Rx* **Diclofenac Sodium** | | |
| *Voltaren* | **Solution**: 0.1% | Yes |
| *Rx* **Flurbiprofen Sodium** | | |
| *Ocufen* | **Solution**: 0.03% | Yes |
| *Rx* **Ketorolac Tromethamine** | | |
| *Acular* | **Solution**: 0.5% | No |
| *Rx* **Suprofen** | | |
| *Profenal* | **Solution**: 1% | No |

## Type of Drug:

Nonsteroidal anti-inflammatory drugs for the eye; NSAIDs.

## How the Drug Works:

NSAIDs for the eye are thought to inhibit the inflammatory response (redness, itching, swelling, warmth, etc) of tissues to mechanical, chemical, or allergy-causing agents. Prostaglandins are chemicals produced by the body that respond to irritating substances and cause constriction (narrowing) of the pupil of the eye during cataract surgery. NSAIDs inhibit the production of prostaglandins.

## Uses:

*Diclofenac* — To treat eye inflammation after cataract surgery.

*Flurbiprofen and Suprofen* — To prevent pupil constriction (miosis) during surgery.

*Ketorolac* — For the relief of ocular itching due to seasonal allergic conjunctivitis.

*Unlabeled Use(s):* Occasionally doctors may prescribe flurbiprofen for eye inflammation after surgery, cystoid macular edema or uveitis (inflammation of the uvea) syndromes.

## Precautions:

*Do not use in the following situations:*
>allergy to any component of the formulation
>herpes simplex infection of the eye (flurbiprofen and suprofen only)
>soft contact lens wearers (diclofenac and ketorolac only)

*Use with caution in the following situations:*
>allergy to aspirin
>allergy to other NSAIDs
>bleeding tendency (ocular surgical patients)
>prolonged bleeding time or known bleeding tendencies

*Pregnancy:* Adequate studies have not been done in pregnant women. Use only if clearly needed and potential benefits outweigh the possible hazards to the fetus. Diclofenac use should be avoided in late stages of pregnancy.

*Breastfeeding:* Suprofen appears in breast milk after oral use. Eye drops may be absorbed into the body. It is not known if flurbiprofen or ketorolac appears in breast milk. Because of the potential for adverse effects, a decision should be made whether to discontinue nursing or the drug, taking into account the importance of the drug to the mother. Consult your doctor.

*Children:* Safety and effectiveness have not been established.

## Side Effects:

Every drug is capable of producing side effects. Many ophthalmic NSAID users experience no, or minor, side effects. The frequency and severity of side effects depend on many factors including dose, duration of therapy and individual susceptibility. Possible side effects include the following:

*Most frequent:* Temporary burning or stinging; irritation; redness/burning (contact lens wearers).

*Diclofenac and ketorolac:* Inflammation of cornea; ocular allergy.

*Diclofenac:* Nausea; vomiting; viral infections.

---

### Guidelines for Use:

- Consult your doctor if you have experienced bleeding tendencies, are on drugs that prolong bleeding time (eg, "blood thinners"), or have herpes simplex infection of the eye.
- *Flurbiprofen* — May delay wound healing.
- Use proper administration technique.
- Mild burning or stinging after instillation is no cause for alarm unless symptoms persist or worsen.

---

*If you have any questions, consult your doctor, pharmacist, or health care provider.*

| Generic Name Brand Name Example | Supplied As | Generic Available |
|---|---|---|
| Rx **Levocabastine HCl** | | |
| *Livostin* | **Suspension**: 2.5 mL, 5 mL, 10 mL | No |

## Type of Drug:

Antiallergy (antihistamine) for the eye.

## How the Drug Works:

Levocabastine is systemically absorbed and reduces itching in the eye due to seasonal allergies.

## Uses:

To relieve the symptoms of seasonal conjunctivitis.

## Precautions:

*Do not use in the following situations:*
> allergy to levocabastine
> soft contact lens use

*Pregnancy:* Adequate studies have not been done in pregnant women. Use only if clearly needed and potential benefits outweigh the possible hazards to the fetus.

*Breastfeeding:* Levocabastine appears in breast milk. Consult your doctor before you begin breastfeeding.

*Children:* Safety and effectiveness in children below the age of 12 have not been established.

## Drug Interactions:

Tell your doctor or pharmacist if you are taking or if you are planning to take any over-the-counter or prescription medications or dietary supplements with levocabastine. Doses of one or both drugs may need to be modified or a different drug may need to be prescribed.

## Side Effects:

Every drug is capable of producing side effects. Many levocabastine users experience no, or minor, side effects. The frequency and severity of side effects depend on many factors including dose, duration of therapy, and individual susceptibility. Possible side effects include the following:

*Nervous System:* Headache; sleepiness; fatigue.

*Respiratory System:* Difficulty breathing; cough; pharyngitis.

*Other:* Rash; nausea; dry mouth.

*Eyes or Ocular:* Visual disturbances; fluid retention in the eyelids; mild, transient stinging and burning; eye pain; dryness; red eyes; discharge from the eye.

## Guidelines for Use:

- For topical use only. Not for injection.
- Do not touch eyelids or surrounding areas with the dropper tip of the bottle.
- Do not use if the suspension has discolored.
- Store at room temperature. Protect from freezing.
- Shake well before using.

*If you have any questions, consult your doctor, pharmacist, or health care provider.*

| Generic Name Brand Name Example | Supplied As | Generic Available |
|---|---|---|
| Rx **Azelastine** | | |
| *Optivar* | **Solution, ophthalmic**: 0.05% | No |

## Type of Drug:
Antihistamine.

## How the Drug Works:
Azelastine inhibits the release of histamine and other chemicals from cells involved in the allergic response. It also antagonizes the effect of histamine.

## Uses:
For the treatment of itching of the eye associated with allergic conjunctivitis.

## Precautions:
*Do not use in the following situations:* Allergy to azelastine or any of its ingredients.

*Pregnancy:* There are no adequate and well-controlled studies in pregnant women. Use only if clearly needed and the potential benefits to the mother outweigh the possible hazards to the fetus.

*Breastfeeding:* It is not known if azelastine appears in breast milk. Consult your doctor before you begin breastfeeding.

*Children:* Safety and effectiveness in children less than 3 years of age have not been established.

## Drug Interactions:
Tell your doctor or pharmacist if you are taking or planning to take any over-the-counter or prescription medications or dietary supplements while using azelastine. Doses of one or both drugs may need to be modified or a different drug may need to be prescribed.

## Side Effects:
Every drug is capable of producing side effects. Many azelastine users experience no, or minor, side effects. The frequency or severity of side effects depend on many factors including dose, duration of therapy, and individual susceptibility. Possible side effects include the following:

*Eyes or Ocular:* Burning; stinging; pain; blurred vision.

*Other:* Headache; bitter taste sensation; asthma; runny nose; itching; sore throat; flu-like symptoms; fatigue; difficulty breathing.

## Guidelines for Use:

- The usual dose is 1 drop in the affected eye(s) twice daily.
- Do not change the dose or stop taking this medicine, unless advised to do so by your doctor.
- For topical ophthalmic use only; not for injection or oral use.
- To avoid contaminating the dropper tip and solution, do not touch any surface, the eyelids, or surrounding areas with the dropper tip of the bottle.
- *Contact lens wearers* — Do not wear a contact lens if your eye is red. Do not use azelastine to treat contact lens-related irritation. The preservative, benzalkonium chloride, may be absorbed by soft contact lenses. Wait at least 10 minutes after instilling azelastine before you insert a contact lens.
- Store upright between 36° and 77°F. Keep container tightly closed.

*If you have any questions, consult your doctor, pharmacist, or health care provider.*

| Generic Name<br>*Brand Name Example* | Supplied As | Generic<br>Available |
|---|---|---|
| *Rx* **Olopatadine** | | |
| *Patanol* | **Solution**: 0.1% | No |

## Type of Drug:
Topical antihistamine.

## How the Drug Works:
Olopatadine is an antihistamine that blocks the release of histamine.

## Uses:
To prevent itching of the eye due to allergic conjunctivitis or allergies.

## Precautions:
*Do not use in the following situations:*
> allergy to the drug
> soft contact lens wear

*Pregnancy:* Adequate studies have not been done in pregnant women, or animal studies may have shown a risk to the fetus. Use only if clearly needed and potential benefits outweigh the possible hazards to the fetus.

*Breastfeeding:* It is not known if olopatadine appears in breast milk. Consult your doctor before you begin breastfeeding.

*Children:* Safety and effectiveness in children under 3 years of age have not been established.

## Drug Interactions:
Tell your doctor or pharmacist if you are taking or planning to take any over-the-counter or prescription medications or dietary supplements while taking this medicine. Doses of one or both drugs may need to be modified or a different drug may need to be prescribed.

## Side Effects:
Every drug is capable of producing side effects. Many patients experience no, or minor, side effects. The frequency and severity of side effects depend on many factors including dose, duration of therapy, and individual susceptibility. Possible side effects include the following:

*Eyes or Ocular:* Burning/stinging; dry eye; foreign body sensation; congestion; irritation; swelling of the lid; itching.

*Other:* Headaches; weakness; cold syndrome; sore throat; nasal congestion; sinus infection; change in taste.

## Guidelines for Use:

- The recommended dose is 1 to 2 drops in the affected eye(s) twice daily every 6 to 8 hours.
- Olopatadine is for topical use only. Do not use as an injection.
- Do not use while wearing contact lenses.
- Do not touch the eyelids or surrounding areas with the dropper tip of the bottle to prevent contamination of the solution/dropper tip.
- Store at 39° to 86°F. Keep bottle tightly closed.

*If you have any questions, consult your doctor, pharmacist, or health care provider.*

| Generic Name<br>*Brand Name Example* | Supplied As | Generic<br>Available |
|---|---|---|
| Rx **Ketotifen Fumarate** | | |
| *Zaditor* | **Solution**: 0.025% | No |

## Type of Drug:

Antiallergy (antihistamine) for the eye.

## How the Drug Works:

Ketotifen prevents allergy symptoms (eg, itching, redness) that involve the eye by preventing the local release of histamine and other chemicals that cause allergic symptoms.

## Uses:

For the temporary prevention of itching of the eye due to allergic conjunctivitis.

## Precautions:

*Do not use in the following situations:*
allergy to ketotifen or any of its ingredients

*Pregnancy:* There are no adequate and well-controlled studies in pregnant women. Use only if clearly needed and the potential benefits to the mother outweigh the possible hazards to the fetus.

*Breastfeeding:* It is not known if ketotifen appears in breast milk. Consult your doctor before you begin breastfeeding.

*Children:* Safety and effectiveness in patients less than 3 years of age have not been established.

## Drug Interactions:

Tell your doctor or pharmacist if you are taking or planning to take any over-the-counter or prescription medications or dietary supplements while taking ketotifen. Doses of one or both drugs may need to be modified or a different drug may need to be prescribed.

## Side Effects:

Every drug is capable of producing side effects. Many ketotifen users experience no, or minor, side effects. The frequency and severity of side effects depend on many factors including dose, duration of therapy, and individual susceptibility. Possible side effects include the following:

*Eyes or Ocular:* Conjunctivitis; eye burning, stinging, discharge, pain, or rash; dry or itchy eyes; eyelid disorder; keratitis; lacrimation disorder; enlarged pupils; sensitivity to light; tearing.

*Other:* Headaches; runny nose; flu-like symptoms; sore throat; allergic reaction.

## Guidelines for Use:

- The recommended dosage is 1 drop in the affected eye(s) every 8 to 12 hours.
- For topical ophthalmic use only. Do not take by mouth or place in the ear.
- To prevent contamination of the dropper tip and solution, care should be taken not to touch the eyelids or surrounding area with the dropper tip of the bottle.
- Temporary burning or stinging of the eye may occur when instilled into the eye. If symptoms persist or are bothersome, contact your doctor.
- Do not wear contact lenses if your eyes are red.
- Do not use to treat contact lens irritation.
- Benzalkonium chloride, the preservative in ketotifen solution, may be absorbed by soft contact lenses. If you wear soft contact lenses and your eyes are not red, wait at least 10 minutes after instilling ketotifen before you insert your lenses.
- Store at 39° to 77°F. Keep bottle tightly closed when not in use.

*If you have any questions, consult your doctor, pharmacist, or health care provider.*

| Generic Name<br>*Brand Name Examples* | Supplied As | Generic<br>Available |
|---|---|---|
| *Rx* **Bacitracin** | | |
| *AK-Tracin* | **Ointment**: 500 units/g | Yes |
| *Rx* **Chloramphenicol** | | |
| *Chloromycetin, Chloroptic* | **Ointment**: 1% | Yes |
| *Chloromycetin* | **Powder for solution**: 25 mg/vial | No |
| *Chloroptic* | **Solution**: 0.5% | Yes |
| *Rx* **Ciprofloxacin HCl** | | |
| *Ciloxan* | **Ointment**: 0.3% | No |
| *Ciloxan*[1] | **Solution**: 3.5 mg/mL | No |
| *Rx* **Erythromycin** | **Ointment**: 0.5% | Yes |
| *Rx* **Gentamicin** | | |
| *Genoptic, Gentak* | **Ointment**: 0.3% | Yes |
| *Garamycin*[1], *Genoptic*[1], *Gentacidin*[1], *Gentak*[1] | **Solution**: 0.3% | Yes |
| *Rx* **Levofloxacin** | | |
| *Quixin*[1] | **Solution**: 0.5% | No |
| *Rx* **Ofloxacin** | | |
| *Ocuflox*[1] | **Solution**: 0.3% | No |
| *Rx* **Polymyxin B Sulfate Sterile** | **Powder for solution**: 6000 units/mg | Yes |
| *Rx* **Sulfacetamide Sodium** | | |
| *AK-Sulf*[1] | **Ointment**: 10% | Yes |
| *AK-Sulf*[2], *Bleph-10*[1], *Ocusulf-10*[2], *Sulf-10*[1,2] | **Solution**: 10%, 30% | Yes |
| *Rx* **Tobramycin** | | |
| *Tobrex* | **Ointment**: 0.3% | No |
| *AK-Tob*[1], *Tobrex*[1] | **Solution**: 0.3% | Yes |

[1] Contains benzalkonium chloride.
[2] Contains sulfites.

## Type of Drug:

Topical antibiotics for use in treating or preventing bacterial infections of the eye.

## How the Drug Works:

Ophthalmic antibiotics stop or prevent susceptible bacteria infections of the eyeball and eyelid by either killing or inhibiting the growth of susceptible bacteria.

## Uses:

To treat superficial eye infections caused by susceptible bacteria. The spectrum of antibacterial activity of the ophthalmic anti-infectives is variable. Consult specific product information to determine potential antibacterial susceptibility.

*Chloramphenicol* — Only for serious infections for which less potentially dangerous drugs are ineffective or not recommended.

*Erythromycin* — For the prevention of ophthalmia neonatorum (eye infection in newborn) due to *Neisseria gonorrhoeae* or *Chlamydia trachomatis.*

## Precautions:

*Do not use in the following situations:* Allergy to the antibiotic or any of its ingredients.

*Use with caution in the following situations:*
  corneal lesions
  pus in eye (sulfacetamide sodium only)

*Superinfection:* Use of antibiotics (especially prolonged or repeated therapy) may result in bacterial or fungal overgrowth. Such overgrowth may lead to a second infection. The first antibiotic may need to be stopped and another antibiotic may need to be prescribed for the second infection.

*Pregnancy:* Safety for use during pregnancy has not been established. Use only if clearly needed and if the potential benefits to the mother outweigh the possible hazards to the fetus.

*Breastfeeding:* Chloramphenicol and tobramycin appear in breast milk. It is not known if topical ciprofloxacin, levofloxacin, or ofloxacin appears in breast milk. Because of the potential for side effects in breastfed infants, decide whether to discontinue nursing or discontinue the drug, taking into account the importance of the drug to the mother. Consult your doctor before you begin breastfeeding.

*Children:* Gentamicin and tobramycin are safe and effective in children. Erythromycin is safe and effective in newborns and children. Safety and effectiveness of sulfacetamide sodium in infants less than 2 months of age have not been established. Safety and effectiveness of chloramphenicol, ciprofloxacin solution, levofloxacin, and ofloxacin in children less than 1 year of age have not been established. Safety and effectiveness of ciprofloxacin ointment in children less than 2 years of age have not been established.

*Lab tests* may be required during treatment. Tests may include bacterial culture and susceptibility testing.

*Sulfites:* Some of these products contain sulfite preservatives, which can cause allergic reactions in certain individuals. Check package label when available or consult your doctor or pharmacist.

## Drug Interactions:

Tell your doctor or pharmacist if you are taking or if you are planning to take any over-the-counter or prescription medications or dietary supplements with ophthalmic antibiotics. Doses of one or both drugs may need to be modified or a different drug may need to be prescribed. Silver preparations interact with sulfacetamide sodium.

Consider all drug interactions reported for oral anti-infectives when using ophthalmic anti-infectives. Refer to the individual drug monographs in the Anti-infectives chapter.

## Side Effects:

Every drug is capable of producing side effects. Many ophthalmic antibiotic uses experience no, or minor, side effects. The frequency and severity of side effects depend on many factors including dose, duration of therapy, and individual susceptibility. Possible side effects include the following:

*Eyes or Ocular:* Lid crusting, crystals/scales, foreign body sensation, corneal staining, decreased vision, tearing, sensitivity to light (ciprofloxacin, levofloxacin, and ofloxacin only); irritation; burning; stinging; pain; itching; lid swelling; redness; dryness; watering; blurred vision.

*Other:* Bad or abnormal taste sensation (ciprofloxacin, levofloxacin, and ofloxacin only); sore throat (ciprofloxacin, levofloxacin, and ofloxacin only); aplastic anemia (chloramphenicol only); rash; headache.

Oral anti-infective-associated side effects should be considered when using these agents in the eye. Refer to the individual drug monographs in the Anti-infectives chapter.

## Guidelines for Use:

- Dosage is individualized. Use exactly as prescribed.
- Do not change the dose or stop taking this medicine, unless advised to do so by your doctor.
- Review guidelines at the beginning of this chapter for proper technique for instilling eye drops or eye ointments.
- To avoid contamination, do not touch tip of container to any surface. Replace cap after using.
- May cause temporary stinging or blurring of vision following administration.
- Contact your doctor if stinging, burning, or itching becomes pronounced or if redness, irritation, swelling, decreasing vision, or pain persists or worsens.
- In general, patients being treated for bacterial conjunctivitis should not wear contact lenses; however, if your doctor considers contact lens use appropriate, wait at least 15 minutes after using any solutions containing benzalkonium chloride before inserting the lens, as it may be absorbed by the lens.
- *Ciprofloxacin, levofloxacin, and ofloxacin* — Discontinue use and notify your doctor if you experience skin rash or other signs of allergic reactions.
- Lab tests may be required to monitor therapy. Be sure to keep appointments.
- Store at controlled room temperature (59° to 86°F). Keep bottles and tubes tightly closed. Protect from light.
- Polymyxin B ophthalmic solution must be stored in a refrigerator (36° to 46°F). Discard unused solution after 72 hours.

*If you have any questions, consult your doctor, pharmacist, or health care provider.*

| Generic Name *Brand Name Examples* | Steroid | Antibiotic | Generic Available |
|---|---|---|---|
| **Rx** | | | |
| **Steroid and Antibiotic Suspensions and Solutions** | | | |
| *Chloromycetin/ Hydrocortisone for Suspension* | 0.5% hydro-cortisone acetate | 0.25% chloram-phenicol | Yes |
| *AK-Spore H.C. Ophthalmic Suspension, Cortisporin Suspension* | 1% hydro-cortisone | Neomycin sulfate equivalent to 0.35% neo-mycin base and 10,000 units polymyxin B sulfate/mL | Yes |
| *Terra-Cortril Suspension* | 1.5% hydro-cortisone acetate | 0.5% oxyte-tracycline | No |
| *Poly-Pred Suspension* | 0.5% pred-nisolone ace-tate | Neomycin sulfate equivalent to 0.35% neo-mycin base and 10,000 units polymyxin B sulfate/mL | No |
| *Pred-G Suspension* | 1% predniso-lone acetate | Gentamycin sulfate equiva-lent to 0.3% gentamicin base | No |
| *AK-Neo-Dex Solution, Neo-Dexameth, Neodecadron Solution* | 0.1% dexa-methasone phosphate | Neomycin sulfate equiva-lent to 0.35% neomycin base | Yes |
| *TobraDex Suspension* | 0.1% dexa-methasone | 0.3% tobra-mycin | No |

| Generic Name Brand Name Examples | Steroid | Antibiotic | Generic Available |
|---|---|---|---|
| AK-Trol Suspension, Dexacine Suspension, Maxitrol Suspension | 0.1% dexamethasone | Neomycin sulfate equivalent to 0.35% neomycin base and 10,000 units polymyxin B sulfate/mL | Yes |

Rx **Steroid and Antibiotic Ointments**

| | | | |
|---|---|---|---|
| Ophthocort[1] | 0.5% hydrocortisone acetate | 1% chloramphenicol, 10,000 units polymyxin B/g | No |
| AK-Spore H.C.[1], Cortisporin | 1% hydrocortisone | Neomycin sulfate equivalent to 0.35% neomycin base, 400 units bacitracin zinc, 10,000 units polymyxin B sulfate/g | Yes |
| Neotricin HC | 1% hydrocortisone acetate | Neomycin sulfate equivalent to 0.35% neomycin base, 400 units bacitracin zinc, 10,000 units polymyxin B sulfate/g | No |
| Pred-G S.O.P. | 0.6% prednisolone acetate | Gentamicin sulfate equivalent to 0.3% gentamicin base | No |
| Neodecadron | 0.05% dexamethasone phosphate | Neomycin sulfate equivalent to 0.35% neomycin base | No |
| TobraDex | 0.1% dexamethasone | 0.3% tobramycin | No |

| | Generic Name<br>*Brand Name*<br>*Examples* | **Steroid** | **Antibiotic** | Generic<br>Avail-<br>able |
|---|---|---|---|---|
| | *AK-Trol,*<br>*Dexacidin,*<br>*Dexasporin,*<br>*Maxitrol* | 0.1% dexa-<br>methasone | Neomycin<br>sulfate equiva-<br>lent to 0.35%<br>neomycin base,<br>10,000 units<br>polymyxin B<br>sulfate/g | Yes |
| *Rx* | **Steroid and**<br>**Sulfonamide,**<br>**Suspensions**<br>**and Solutions** | | | |
| | *FML-S*<br>*Suspension* | 0.1% fluoro-<br>metholone | 10% sodium<br>sulfacetamide | No |
| | *Blephamide*<br>*Suspension* | 0.2% pred-<br>nisolone ace-<br>tate | 10% sodium<br>sulfacetamide | No |
| | *Isopto Ceta-*<br>*pred Suspen-*<br>*sion* | 0.25% pred-<br>nisolone ace-<br>tate | 10% sodium<br>sulfacetamide | No |
| | *AK-Cide*<br>*Suspension,*<br>*Metimyd*<br>*Suspension* | 0.5% pred-<br>nisolone ace-<br>tate | 10% sodium<br>sulfacetamide | No |
| | *Sulster*<br>*Solution,*<br>*Vasocidin*<br>*Solution* | 0.25% pred-<br>nisolone<br>sodium<br>phosphate | 10% sodium<br>sulfacetamide | Yes |
| *Rx* | **Steroid and**<br>**Sulfonamide,**<br>**Ointments** | | | |
| | *Blephamide* | 0.2% pred-<br>nisolone ace-<br>tate | 10% sodium<br>sulfacetamide | No |
| | *Cetapred* | 0.25% pred-<br>nisolone ace-<br>tate | 10% sodium<br>sulfacetamide | No |
| | *AK-Cide,*<br>*Vasocidin* | 0.5% pred-<br>nisolone ace-<br>tate | 10% sodium<br>sulfacetamide | No |

[1] Preservative free.

For more information, see the Ophthalmic Antibiotic monograph and Steroid monograph.

## Type of Drug:

Antibiotic/anti-inflammatory combinations for use in the eye.

## Uses:

To treat eye infections or inflammatory conditions of the eye in which bacterial infection or risk of infection exists.

To treat chronic anterior uveitis and corneal injury from chemical, radiation or heat burns, or from penetration of foreign bodies.

---

### Guidelines for Use:

- Use exactly as prescribed.
- Follow the Administration Guidelines found at the beginning of this chapter.
- Shake suspensions well before use.
- If a dose is missed, instill it as soon as possible. If several hours have passed or if it is nearing time for the next dose, do not double the dose in order to "catch up" (unless advised to do so by your doctor). If more than one dose is missed or it is necessary to establish a new dosage schedule, contact your doctor or pharmacist.
- May cause temporary blurring of vision or stinging following administration.
- Contact your doctor if stinging, burning, itching, redness, irritation, swelling, decreasing vision, or pain persists or worsens.
- Continue use until all of the prescribed medicine has been used, even if redness or other symptoms have disappeared. Failure to use all of the medicine may prevent complete elimination of bacteria, allowing the infection to return.
- *Superinfection* – Use of antibiotics (especially prolonged or repeated therapy) may result in bacterial or fungal overgrowth. Such overgrowth may lead to a second infection. This medicine may need to be stopped and another antibiotic may need to be prescribed for the second infection.
- Some of these products may contain sulfite preservatives, which can cause allergic reactions in certain individuals (eg, asthmatics). Check package label when available or consult your doctor or pharmacist.
- Do not use with contact lenses unless advised to do so by your eye doctor.
- Do not use if solution has particles or discoloration.
- Store at room temperature (59° to 86°F), away from heat and light. Do not freeze.

---

*If you have any questions, consult your doctor, pharmacist, or health care provider.*

| Generic Name<br>*Brand Name Examples* | Supplied As | Generic<br>Available |
|---|---|---|
| *Rx* **Natamycin** | | |
| *Natacyn* | **Suspension**: 5% | No |

## Type of Drug:

Topical antifungal.

## How the Drug Works:

Natamycin appears to bind to the cell membrane of susceptible fungi. This alters the cell wall and allows essential elements of the fungus to leak out of the cell. This results in cell death.

## Uses:

To treat fungal eye infections caused by susceptible fungi.

## Precautions:

*Do not use in the following situations:*

allergy to natamycin or any component of the product

*Pregnancy:* Adequate studies have not been done in pregnant women, or animal studies may have shown a risk to the fetus. Use only if clearly needed and the potential benefits outweigh the possible hazards to the fetus.

*Breastfeeding:* It is not known if natamycin appears in breast milk. Consult your doctor before you begin breastfeeding.

*Children:* Safety and effectiveness in children have not been established.

*Lab tests* may be required to monitor therapy. Be sure to keep appointments.

## Side Effects:

Every drug is capable of producing side effects. Many natamycin users experience no, or minor, side effects. The frequency and severity of side effects depend on many factors including dose, duration of therapy, and individual susceptibility. Possible side effects include redness and swelling.

## Guidelines for Use:

- Follow Administration Guidelines found at the beginning of this chapter.
- Shake well before mixing.
- For topical use only. Not for injection.
- Continue therapy for 14 to 21 days or until the fungal infection disappears.
- Notify your doctor if improvement does not occur within 7 to 10 days.
- Do not use with contact lenses without first consulting with your eye doctor.
- Lab tests or exams may be required to monitor therapy. Be sure to keep appointments.
- Store at room temperature (46° to 75° F) or in the refrigerator (36° to 46° F). Do not freeze. Avoid exposure to sunlight and excessive heat.

*If you have any questions, consult your doctor, pharmacist, or health care provider.*

| Generic Name Brand Name Examples | Supplied As | Generic Available |
|---|---|---|
| Rx **Trifluridine (Trifluorothymidine)** | | |
| *Viroptic* | **Solution**: 1% | No |
| Rx **Vidarabine (Adenine Arabinoside; Ara-A)** | | |
| *Vira-A* | **Ointment**: 3% | No |

## Type of Drug:

Topical ophthalmic antiviral.

## How the Drug Works:

Ophthalmic antivirals kill susceptible viruses by preventing viral cell reproduction that may result in eye infections.

## Uses:

To treat herpes simplex keratitis (viral inflammation of the cornea of the
eye).

## Precautions:

*Do not use in the following situations:* Allergy to this medicine or any of
its ingredients.

*Corticosteroids* may accelerate the spread of viral infections and are usually not to be used in herpes simplex infections. If corticosteroid (eg,
prednisolone) therapy is used with this medicine, corticosteroid-induced
side effects (eg, glaucoma, cataract formation, worsening of bacterial
or viral infection) also may occur.

*Pregnancy:* Adequate studies have not been done in pregnant women. Use
only if clearly needed and the potential benefits outweigh the possible
hazards to the fetus.

*Breastfeeding:* It is not known if these medicines appear in breast milk.
Consult your doctor before you begin breastfeeding.

*Children:* Safety and effectiveness have not been established for children
less than 2 years of age for vidarabine and for children less than 6 years
of age for trifluridine.

## Drug Interactions:

Tell your doctor or pharmacist if you are taking or if you are planning to
take any over-the-counter or prescription medications or dietary
supplements while taking an ophthalmic antiviral agent. Doses of one
or both drugs may need to be modified or a different drug may need to
be prescribed.

## Side Effects:

Every drug is capable of producing side effects. Many ophthalmic antiviral agent users experience no, or minor, side effects. The frequency and severity of side effects depend on many factors including dose, duration of therapy, and individual susceptibility. Possible side effects include the following: Irritation; pain; swelling of the eye or lids; increased tearing; sensitivity to light; clouding of vision; allergic reaction; foreign body sensation; increased fluid pressure in the eye; inflammation; red eye; dry eye; corneal changes; mild transient burning or stinging upon instillation.

---

## Guidelines for Use:

- Use exactly as prescribed. Follow administration and dosing guidelines provided by your doctor or pharmacist.
- *Trifluridine* — Instill 1 drop onto cornea of affected eye(s) every 2 hours while awake for a maximum daily dose of 9 drops. After apparent healing, instill 1 drop every 4 hours while awake for a minimum daily dose of 5 drops for an additional 7 days to prevent recurrence. Temporary burning or stinging may occur upon administration.
- *Vidarabine* — Administer approximately ½ inch of ointment into the lower conjunctival sac of the affected eye(s) 5 times daily at 3-hour intervals. After apparent healing, administer twice daily for an additional 7 days to prevent recurrence.
- If both eye drops and eye ointment are used, instill eye drops at least 10 minutes before instilling the ointment.
- A temporary visual haze may occur upon administration.
- Other forms of therapy may be needed if there are no signs of improvement after 7 to 14 days or complete healing has not occurred by 14 days for trifluridine or 21 days for vidarabine. Some severe cases may require longer treatment. Continued use of trifluridine for more than 21 days is not recommended due to potential toxicity to the eye.
- May cause sensitivity to light. This may be minimized by wearing sunglasses.
- Do not stop using this medicine unless instructed to do so by your doctor. Use for the full course of therapy as directed by your doctor.
- Do not use more often or for a longer period of time than prescribed.
- Do not use with contact lenses without first consulting your eye doctor.
- If used with a corticosteroid (eg, prednisolone), corticosteroid-induced side effects (eg, glaucoma, cataract formation, worsening of bacterial or viral infections) may occur.
- Notify your doctor if condition worsens or if decreased vision, pain, itching, or swelling of the eye occurs.
- Recurrence of infection may be seen if medication is not used exactly as prescribed.
- *Trifluridine* — Store in the refrigerator (36° to 46°F).
- *Vidarabine* — Store at room temperature (59° to 86°F).

---

*If you have any questions, consult your doctor, pharmacist, or health care provider.*

| Generic Name<br>*Brand Name Example* | **Supplied As** | **Generic<br>Available** |
|---|---|---|
| Rx **Fomivirsen Sodium** | | |
| *Vitravene* | **Intravitreal injection**:<br>6.6 mg/mL | No |

## Type of Drug:

Injectable ophthalmic antiviral.

## How the Drug Works:

Ophthalmic antivirals kill susceptible viruses by preventing viral cell reproduction that may result in eye infections.

## Uses:

Fomivirsen sodium is indicated for the local treatment of cytomegalovirus
(CMV) retinitis in patients with acquired immunodeficiency syndrome
(AIDS) who are intolerant of or have a contraindication to other treat-
ment(s) for CMV retinitis or who were insufficiently responsive to previous treatment(s) for CMV retinitis.

## Precautions:

*Do not use in the following situations:* Allergy to this medicine or any of
its ingredients.

*Corticosteroids* may accelerate the spread of viral infections and are usually not to be used in herpes simplex infections. If corticosteroid
(eg, prednisolone) therapy is used with this medicine, corticosteroid-
induced side effects (eg, glaucoma, cataract formation, worsening of bacterial or viral infection) also may occur.

*Pregnancy:* Adequate studies have not been done in pregnant women. Use
only if clearly needed and the potential benefits to the mother outweigh
the possible hazards to the fetus.

*Breastfeeding:* It is not known if these medicines appear in breast milk.
Consult your doctor before you begin breastfeeding.

*Children:* Safety and effectiveness in children have not been established.

## Drug Interactions:

Tell your doctor of pharmacist if you are taking or if you are planning to
take any over-the-counter or prescription medications or dietary
supplements with fomivirsen. Doses of one or both drugs may need to
be modified or a different drug may need to be prescribed.

## Side Effects:

Every drug is capable of producing side effects. Many fomivirsen users experience no, or minor, side effects. The frequency and severity of side effects depend on many factors including dose, duration of therapy, and individual susceptibility. Possible side effects include the following:

*Eyes or Ocular:* Abnormal vision; blurred vision; cataract; vision changes; pain; floaters; increased fluid pressure in eye; sensitivity to light; retinal detachment; bleeding in eye; eye inflammation; application site reaction; bloodshot eye; eye swelling; eye irritation; low fluid pressure in eye; retinal edema; retinal pigment changes.

*Other:* Stomach pain; weakness; diarrhea; fever; headache; nausea; pneumonia; rash; infection; vomiting; sinus infection; abnormal thinking; allergic reactions; appetite loss; back pain; chest pain; weight loss; dehydration; depression; dizziness; difficulty breathing; flu syndrome; increased cough; abnormal nerve sensations; sweating; abnormal blood cell count; anemia; abnormal liver tests; infection; systemic CMV; bronchitis; catheter infection; kidney failure; pain; pancreas infection; oral fungus.

---

### Guidelines for Use:

- Use exactly as prescribed. Follow administration and dosage guidelines provided by your doctor or pharmacist.
- The diagnosis and evaluation of CMV retinitis is ophthalmologic and should be made by comprehensive retinal examination by a physician.
- Fomivirsen is for direct injection into the eye by a medical professional. It is not for topical administration.
- Other forms of therapy may be needed if there are no signs of improvement after 7 to 14 days or complete healing has not occurred by 14 to 21 days. Severe cases may require longer treatment.
- May cause sensitivity to light. This may be minimized by wearing sunglasses.
- Do not use with contact lenses without first consulting your eye doctor.
- If used with a corticosteroid (eg, prednisolone), corticosteroid-induced side effects (eg, glaucoma, cataract formation, worsening of bacterial or viral infections) may occur.
- Notify your doctor if condition worsens or if decreased vision, pain, itching, or swelling of the eye occurs.

---

*If you have any questions, consult your doctor, pharmacist, or health care provider.*

| Generic Name *Brand Name Example* | Supplied As | Generic Available |
|---|---|---|
| *Rx* **Verteporfin** | | |
| *Visudyne* | **Lyophilized cake**: 15 mg (reconstituted to 2 mg/mL) | No |

## Type of Drug:

Photosensitizing agent; light-activated drug used in photodynamic therapy.

## How the Drug Works:

Verteporfin therapy is a 2-step process requiring administration of drug and light. The first step is an IV infusion of verteporfin; the second is the activation of verteporfin with light from a nonthermal diode laser.

Verteporfin accumulates in abnormal blood vessels in the eye. In the presence of light, verteporfin produces short-lived radicals, which damage the blood vessels, temporarily blocking them.

## Uses:

For the treatment of age-related macular degeneration in patients with predominantly classic subfoveal choroidal neovascularization (CNV).

During clinical studies, older patients (approximately 75 years of age), patients with dark irides, patients with occult lesions, or patients with less than 50% classic CNV were less likely to benefit from verteporfin therapy.

## Precautions:

*Do not use in the following situations:*
    allergy to verteporfin or any component of the preparation
    porphyria

*Use with caution in the following situations:*
    liver disease, moderate to severe

*Pregnancy:* There are no adequate and well-controlled studies in pregnant women. Use during pregnancy only if clearly needed and the potential benefits outweigh the possible hazards to the fetus.

*Breastfeeding:* It is not known whether verteporfin is excreted in breast milk. Use caution when verteporfin is administered to a woman who is breastfeeding. Consult your doctor.

*Children:* Safety and efficacy of verteporfin in children have not been established.

*Elderly:* A reduced treatment effect was seen with increasing age.

*Lab tests* will be required periodically during treatment with verteporfin. Liver function tests will be conducted.

## Drug Interactions:

Tell your doctor or pharmacist if you are taking or if you are planning to take any over-the-counter or prescription medications or dietary supplements with verteporfin. Doses of one or both drugs may need to be modified or a different drug may need to be prescribed. The following drugs and drug classes interact with verteporfin:

β-carotene
calcium channel blockers
 (eg, nifedipine)
dimethyl sulfoxide
 (eg, *Rimso 50*)
diuretics (eg, hydrochlorothiazide)
ethanol
griseofulvin (*Fulvicin*)
hypoglycemic agents (eg, sulfonylureas)

mannitol (*Resectisol*)
phenothiazines (eg, cholor-
 promazine)
polymyxin B
sulfonamides (eg, sulfanilamide)
tetracyclines (eg, oxytetracycline)
thromboxane $A_2$ inhibitors
 (eg, dipyridamole)

## Side Effects:

Every drug is capable of producing side effects. Many verteporfin users experience no, or minor, side effects. The frequency and severity of side effects depend on many factors including dose, duration of therapy, and individual susceptibility. Possible side effects include the following:

*Digestive Tract:* Constipation; gastrointestinal cancer; nausea.

*Nervous System:* Headache; diminished sensitivity to stimuli; sleep disorder; feeling of whirling motion.

*Circulatory System:* Abnormal heart rhythms; high blood pressure; blood vessel disorders; varicose veins; anemia; decreased white blood count; increased white blood count.

*Respiratory System:* Sore throat; pneumonia.

*Skin:* Rash; injection-site reactions; itching; skin inflammation; eczema; sunburn.

*Eyes or Ocular:* Severe vision decrease; blurred vision; decreased visual acuity; visual field defects; cataracts; eye inflammation; double vision; dry eyes; ocular itching; eye muscle spasms; excessive tearing of eyes; bleeding.

*Other:* Protein in the urine; increased creatinine; decreased hearing; joint pain or dysfunction; muscle weakness; back pain; fever; flu syndrome; sensitivity to light; prostatic disorder; abnormal liver function tests.

## Guidelines for Use:

- This medicine will be prepared and administered by your health care provider in a medical setting.
- Treatment is a 2-step process. The first step is the intravenous (into a vein) administration of verteporfin. The second step is the activation of verteporfin with light from a laser. Therapy may be repeated depending on the results.
- Avoid exposure of unprotected skin, eyes, or other body organs to direct sunlight or bright indoor light (eg, tanning beds, bright halogen lighting) for 5 days after treatment.
- Wear protective clothing and dark sunglasses if you must go outdoors in daylight during the first 5 days after treatment. Ultraviolet (UV) sunscreens are not effective in protecting the skin.
- Expose skin to ambient indoor light. Do not stay in the dark. This will help inactivate the drug in the skin.

*If you have any questions, consult your doctor, pharmacist, or health care provider.*

| Generic Name Brand Name Examples | Supplied As | Generic Available |
|---|---|---|
| *otc* **Artificial Tear Solutions** | | |
| *Akwa Tears, AquaSite[1], Artificial Tears, Artificial Tears Plus, Celluvisc[1], Dry Eyes, Dry Eye Therapy, Duratears Naturale, Gen-Teal Multidose, HypoTears, HypoTears PF[1], Isopto Plain, Isopto Tears, Just Tears, Liquifilm Tears, Moisture Eyes, Murocel, Muro 128 2%, Muro 128 5%, Preservative Free Moisture Eyes[1], Puralube, Refresh[1], Refresh Plus[1], Refresh Tears, Teargen, Teargen II, Tearisol, Tears Naturale, Tears Naturale II, Tears Naturale Free[1], Tears Plus, Tears Renewed, Ultra Tears* | **Solution** | Yes |
| *Rx* **Artificial Tear Insert** | | |
| *Lacrisert[1]* | **Insert:** 5 mg hydroxypropyl cellulose | No |

[1] Preservative free.

## Type of Drug:

Artificial tear solutions and device.

The artificial tear solutions contain a diverse group of chemicals. This monograph does not follow the typical format due to the lack of consistency of information from product to product. Also, products may not share the same inactive ingredients. For additional information about a specific product, consult the product package labeling or your doctor or pharmacist.

## How the Drug Works:

Provide tear-like lubrication for relief of dry eyes and eye irritation. Components of these products include:

*Boric acid* is a buffering agent that adjusts pH.

*Methylcellulose, hydroxyethylcellulose, hydroxypropyl methylcellulose, hydroxypropyl cellulose, propylene glycol, gelatin, dextran, povidone, polyvinyl alcohol, and polyethylene glycol* are thickening agents that prolong eye contact time.

*Benzalkonium chloride, methyl- and propylparabens, chlorobutanol, and thimerosal* are preservatives that maintain sterility.

*Balanced amounts of salts* help to maintain isotonicity (0.9% NaCl equivalent).

## Uses:

*Solution* — For relief of dry eyes and eye irritation that are generally associated with reduced tear production. Also used as lubricants for artificial eyes. Some of these products can be used with hard contact lenses.

*Insert* — To treat moderate to severe dry eye syndromes including keratoconjunctivitis sicca (inflammation of the cornea and conjunctiva), exposure keratitis (inflammation of the cornea), decreased corneal sensitivity, and recurrent corneal erosions.

## Precautions:

*Do not use in the following situations:* Allergy to any ingredient of the medicine.

## Side Effects:

Every drug is capable of producing side effects. Many artificial tears solution and device users experience no, or minor, side effects. The frequency and severity of side effects depend on many factors including dose, duration of therapy, and individual susceptibility. Possible side effects include the following:

*Inserts:* Transient blurring of vision; eye discomfort or irritation; matting or stickiness of eyelashes; sensitivity to light; allergic reaction; swelling of eyelids; red eyes.

## Guidelines for Use:

- For use in eyes only.
- May produce temporary blurring of vision. Use caution while driving or performing other hazardous tasks.
- Remove contact lenses before use.

*Solutions —*

- Wash hands thoroughly before use.
- Pull down the lower lid of the affected eye, forming a "V" pocket.
- Instill 1 to 2 drops into eye(s) 3 to 4 times daily. Repeat as needed or as advised by your doctor.
- Do not use if solution changes color or becomes cloudy.
- Do not use *Liquifilm Tears*, *Teargen II*, or *Tearisol* on or with soft contact lenses.
- If headache, eye pain, changes in vision, continued redness, or irritation occurs, or if condition worsens or persists for more than 72 hours, discontinue use and consult your doctor.
- For single-dose applications, use immediately after opening. Do not store open containers. Discard single-dose applicator/container after installation of solution.
- To avoid contamination, do not touch the tip of the container or dropper to any surface. Close multi-use container immediately after each use.
- Store at room temperature (59° to 86°F) and keep tightly closed and out of the reach of children.

*Inserts —*

- Wash hands thoroughly before use.
- Use 1 insert daily.
- If insert is placed improperly in the eye, a corneal abrasion (scrape) may result. Practice insertion and removal of insert while in your doctor's office until the technique is mastered. Illustrated instructions are included in each package. Follow instructions carefully.
- Occasionally, the insert is expelled from the eye. To avoid displacement of insert, do not rub the eye(s), especially when awakening. Another insert may be used if the initial insert is expelled.
- To avoid transient blurred vision, the insert may be removed a few hours after insertion. Another insert may be used if needed.
- If symptoms worsen or persist, remove insert and notify your doctor.
- Store at room temperature (59° to 86°F) and out of the reach of children. Do not remove from storage blister until just prior to insertion.

*If you have any questions, consult your doctor, pharmacist, or health care provider.*

| Generic Name<br>*Brand Name Examples* | Supplied As | Generic<br>Available |
|---|---|---|
| *otc* **Ocular Lubricants** | | |
| *Akwa Tears*[1], *Artificial Tears, Dry Eyes, Duratears Naturale*[1], *HypoTears, Lacri-Lube S.O.P., Moisture Eyes PM, Refresh PM* | **Ointment** | Yes |
| *Tears Naturale II*[1], *Dry Eyes*[1] | **Drops** | Yes |

[1] Preservative free.

## Type of Drug:

Ocular lubricants. Most products contain white petrolatum and mineral oil to lubricate the eye.

## How the Drug Works:

Forms a smooth, comfortable protective film to protect and lubricate the cornea and conjunctiva (eye).

## Precautions:

*Do not use in the following situations:* If you are allergic to the medicine or any of its ingredients.

---

### Guidelines for Use:

- For use in eyes only.
- Remove contact lenses before using.
- Pull down the lower lid of the affected eye forming a "V" pocket. Apply 1 drop of solution or a small amount (¼ inch) of ointment to the inside of the eyelid, 1 or more times daily, or as directed by your doctor. Look downward before closing the eye(s).
- Generally, tear substitute drops are used during the day and ointments at nighttime.
- To avoid contamination, do not touch tip to any surface. Replace the cap immediately after each use.
- If eye pain, change in vision, continued redness, or irritation occurs, or if condition worsens or persists for more than 72 hours, discontinue use and consult your doctor.
- Ointment may cause a visual "haze" or blurring of vision. Use caution while driving or performing hazardous tasks.
- Store at room temperature (59° to 86°F), and keep tightly closed and out of the reach of children.

---

*If you have any questions, consult your doctor, pharmacist, or health care provider.*

| **Generic Name**<br>*Brand Name Examples* | **Uses** |
|---|---|
| *otc* **Wetting Solutions** | |
| *Liquifilm Wetting*[1],<br>*Sereine*[1] | Wetting solutions contain surfactants to maintain the water content of the hard lens surface. These solutions include methylcellulose and derivatives, polyvinyl alcohol, povidone, some newer polymers, preservatives, and buffering agents. These agents increase solution thickness and act as a physical cushioning agent between the lens and cornea. |
| *otc* **Wetting/Soaking Solutions** | |
| *Soac-Lens*,<br>*Wetting & Soaking*,<br>*Wet-N-Soak Plus* | These solutions, in addition to wetting the lens surface, also can be used as soaking solutions. |
| *otc* **Cleaning, Soaking, and Wetting Solution** | |
| *Total*[1] | This solution, in addition to wetting and soaking, also can be used as a cleaning solution. |
| *otc* **Rewetting Solutions** | |
| *Boston Rewetting Drops*,<br>*Clerz 2*[1], *Lens Drops*[1],<br>*Opti-Tears Soothing Drops*[1] | Rewetting solutions are intended for use directly in the eye with a contact lens. These products improve wearing time by rewetting the eye and the lens, which may become dry and contaminated during wear. |
| *otc* **Cleaning Solutions and Gels** | |
| *LC-65, MiraFlow Extra Strength*[2],<br>*Opti-Clean Daily Cleaner*,<br>*Opti-Clean II*[1],<br>*Opti-Free Daily Cleaner* | Cleaning solutions and gels contain surfactant cleaners to ease removal of debris from lens surface. To adequately clean, physically rub lens with solution or gel and rinse with water or sterile saline solution. |

| Generic Name<br>*Brand Name Examples* | Uses |
|---|---|
| *otc* **Cleaning and Soaking Solution** | |
| *Clean-N-Soak*[1] | This solution eases removal of debris from the lens surface. |
| *otc* **Enzymatic Cleaner** | |
| *Opti-Free Enzymatic Cleaner Especially for Sensitive Eyes* | Enzymatic cleaning, by soaking the lens in a solution prepared from enzyme tablets, is recommended once weekly. This is intended to remove protein and other lens deposits. Contact lens must be rinsed and disinfected before wearing. |

[1] Thimerosal free.
[2] Preservative free.

For optimum comfort and to minimize problems, conventional hard lenses require care with separate wetting, cleaning, and soaking solutions.

## Type of Drug:
Hard contact lens products.

## How the Drug Works:
Contact lens products are sterile, isotonic, and free of particulate matter. They contain various chemical ingredients to achieve specific goals of contact lens care.

## Precautions:
*Do not use in the following situations:* Allergy to the product or any of its ingredients.

## Side Effects:
These products are capable of producing side effects. Many contact lens users experience no, or minor side effects. The frequency and severity of side effects depend on many factors including individual suscepti-bility and adherence to instructions for proper lens care. Possible side effects include the following:

*Eyes or Ocular:* Stinging, burning, or itching of eye(s); excessive tearing; unusual eye secretions; redness of eye(s); reduced sharpness of vision; blurred vision; sensitivity to light; dry eyes; infection.

## Guidelines for Use:

- Proper contact lens care will increase success and decrease complications.
- See individual product information for detailed directions and safety information. Problems with contact lens and lens care products could result in serious injury to the eye. Always follow label directions and your doctor's recommendations.
- Cleaning does not disinfect lenses. Disinfecting does not clean lenses.
- Wash and rinse hands thoroughly before handling contact lenses.
- Do not take enzymatic tablets internally.
- Do not use enzymatic tablets that are soft and sticky or irregular in appearance.
- Weekly enzymatic/disinfection cycle is not a substitute for daily cleaning and disinfecting.
- Do not insert contact lenses if eyes are red or irritated.
- Do not wear contact lenses while sleeping.
- For hard contact lens care, use only products designed for hard contact lenses. Because many of these products can only be used with certain lens types, consult your eye doctor before using any product if you are uncertain which type of lens you wear.
- If cleaner or disinfectant gets in eye(s), remove lens immediately and flush eye(s) with water or saline for several minutes.
- Do not change or substitute products from a different manufacturer without consulting your doctor.
- Do not store lenses in tap water.
- Never use saliva to wet contact lenses.
- Never reuse the solution in your lens case.
- To avoid contamination, do not touch tip of container to any surface. Replace cap and keep tightly closed when not in use.
- Do not instill topical medications while contact lenses are being worn unless directed to do so by your doctor.
- Eye problems, including corneal ulcers, can develop rapidly and lead to loss of vision. If eye discomfort; excessive tearing; vision changes; or eye redness, burning, or irritation occur, immediately remove your lenses. If the problem stops and the lenses appear to be undamaged, thoroughly clean, rinse, and disinfect the lenses and reinsert them. If the problem continues or a lens appears damaged, remove the lens and contact your eye care practitioner immediately.
- It is recommended that contact lens wearers see their eye doctor twice a year, or more frequently if directed.
- Use before the expiration date marked on the carton and bottle, or within the time indicated on the package (usually within 60 to 90 days).
- Keep contact lens care products out of the reach of children.
- Store tablets in a dry place. Do not remove from foil pouch until just prior to use.
- Do not use solution if it becomes cloudy or discolored.
- Store at room temperature.

*If you have any questions, consult your doctor, pharmacist, or health care provider.*

| Generic Name<br>*Brand Name Examples* | Uses |
|---|---|
| *otc* **Disinfecting/Wetting/ Soaking Solutions** | |
| *Boston Advance Comfort[1], Boston Advance Comfort Formula Convenience Pack, Boston Condition- ing[1], Boston Simplicity Multi-Action, Wet-N-Soak, Wet-N-Soak Plus[1]* | These solutions are used for disinfecting and help to main- tain the water content of the lens. |
| *otc* **Cleaning/Soaking Solution** | |
| *Boston Reconditioning Drops* | This solution eases removal of debris from the lens surface. For use with the *Boston Lens*. |
| *otc* **Cleaning Solutions** | |
| *Boston Advance Cleaner[1], Boston Cleaner (original formula), LC-65 Daily Cleaner[1], Opti-Clean Daily Cleaner, Opti- Clean II[1], Opti-Free Daily Cleaner, Opti- Free Supra Clens Daily Protein Remover[2]* | These solutions are used for daily cleaning to prevent the accumulation of deposits and to remove other debris. |
| *otc* **Enzymatic Cleaners** | |
| *Boston One Step Liquid, Opti-Zyme Enzymatic Cleaner, Opti-Zyme Espe- cially for Sensitive Eyes, ProFree/GP Weekly Enzy- matic Cleaner Tablets* | Enzymatic cleaning, by soaking in a solution prepared from enzyme tablets, is recommended once weekly. This is intended to remove protein and other lens deposits. Contact lenses must be rinsed and disinfected before wearing. |
| *otc* **Rewetting Solutions** | |
| *Wet-N-Soak[1], Opti-Tears Soothing Drops[1], Lens Drops[1], Boston Rewetting Drops[1]* | Rewetting solutions may be used directly in the eye to wet and improve lens comfort. |

[1] Thimerosal free.
[2] Preservative free.

Rigid gas (oxygen) permeable contact lens (RGP) care regimens include use of a surfactant cleaner and storage in a chemical disinfecting solution. Follow the lens care procedure provided by the lens manufacturer. The advantages of RGP lenses are that they maintain the natural state of the cornea, preventing complications. However, they are predisposed to drying and accumulating protein and lipid deposits.

## Type of Drug:

Rigid gas permeable contact lens products.

## How the Drug Works:

Contact lens products are sterile, isotonic, and free of particulate matter. They contain various chemical ingredients to achieve specific goals of contact lens care.

## Precautions:

*Do not use in the following situations:* Allergy to the product or any of its ingredients.

## Side Effects:

These products are capable of producing side effects. Many contact lens users experience no, or minor side effects. The frequency and severity of side effects depend on many factors including individual susceptibility and adherence to instructions for proper lens care. Possible side effects include the following:

*Eyes or Ocular:* Stinging, burning, or itching of eye(s); excessive tearing; unusual eye secretions; redness of eye(s); reduced sharpness of vision; blurred vision; sensitivity to light; dry eyes; infection.

## Guidelines for Use:

- Proper contact lens care will increase success and decrease complications.
- See individual product information for detailed directions and safety information. Problems with contact lens and lens care products could result in serious injury to the eye. Always follow label directions and your doctor's recommendations.
- Cleaning does not disinfect lenses. Disinfecting does not clean lenses.
- Wash and rinse hands thoroughly before handling contact lenses.
- Do not take enzymatic tablets internally.
- Do not use enzymatic tablets that are soft and sticky or irregular in appearance.
- Weekly enzymatic/disinfection cycle is not a substitute for daily cleaning and disinfecting.
- Do not insert contact lenses if eyes are red or irritated.
- Do not wear contact lenses while sleeping.
- For rigid gas permeable lens care, use only products designed for rigid gas permeable lenses. Because many of these products can only be used with certain lens types, consult your eye doctor before using any product if you are uncertain of which type of lens you wear.
- If cleaner or disinfectant gets in eye(s), remove lens immediately and flush eye(s) with water or saline for several minutes.
- Do not change or substitute products from a different manufacturer without consulting your doctor.
- Do not store lenses in tap water.
- Never use saliva to wet contact lenses.
- Never reuse the solution in your lens case.
- To avoid contamination, do not touch tip of container to any surface. Replace cap and keep tightly closed when not in use.
- Do not instill topical medications while contact lenses are being worn unless directed by your doctor.
- Eye problems, including corneal ulcers, can develop rapidly and lead to loss of vision. If eye discomfort; excessive tearing; vision changes; eye redness, burning, or irritation occur, immediately remove your lenses. If the problem stops and the lenses appear to be undamaged, thoroughly clean, rinse, and disinfect the lenses and reinsert them. If the problem continues or a lens appears damaged, remove the lens and contact your eye care practitioner immediately.
- It is recommended that contact lens wearers see their eye doctor twice a year, or more frequently if directed.
- Use before the expiration date marked on the carton and bottle, or within the time indicated on the package (usually within 60 to 90 days).
- Keep contact lens care products out of the reach of children.
- Store tablets in a dry place. Do not remove from foil packet until just prior to use.
- Do not use solution if it becomes cloudy or discolored.
- Store at room temperature.

*If you have any questions, consult your doctor, pharmacist, or health care provider.*

| | Generic Name<br>*Brand Name Examples* | **Uses** |
|---|---|---|
| *otc* | **Preserved Saline Solutions**<br><br>*Opti-Soft[1], Saline Solution[1], Sensitive Eyes Saline[1], Sensitive Eyes Plus Saline* | These solutions are for rinsing and storage of soft lenses in conjunction with heat disinfection. Thimerosal-free preserved saline solutions may be used by patients sensitive to thimerosal or mercury-containing compounds. |
| *otc* | **Preservative Free Saline Solutions[2]**<br><br>*Blairex Sterile Saline, Ciba Vision Saline, Lens Plus, Sensitive Eyes Sterile Saline Spray, Unisol, Unisol 4* | These solutions are for patients intolerant to preservatives. Use them for rinsing or storage and to help minimize mucus accumulation. |
| *otc* | **Surfactant Cleaning Solutions**<br><br>*Ciba Vision Daily Cleaner[1], Daily Cleaner[1], LC-65, Lens Plus Daily Cleaner[2], MiraFlow Extra Strength[2], Opti-Clean II[1], Opti-Clean Daily Cleaner, Opti-Free Daily Cleaner[1], Opti-Free Supra Clens Daily Protein Remover[1], Pliagel[1], Pure Eyes Cleaner/Rinse[1,2], Pure Eyes Disinfecting/Soaking[1,2], Sensitive Eyes Daily Cleaner[1], Sensitive Eyes Saline/ Cleaning Solution[1]* | Cleaning solutions are used for daily cleaning to prevent the accumulation of deposits and to remove other debris. |
| *otc* | **Enzymatic Tablet Cleaners**<br><br>*Allergan Enzymatic, Opti-Free Enzymatic Cleaner, Opti-Zyme Enzymatic Cleaner Especially for Sensitive Eyes[2], ReNu 1 Step, ReNu Effervescent, Sensitive Eyes Enzymatic Cleaner, Ultrazyme* | Enzymatic cleaning, by soaking in a solution prepared from enzyme tablets, is recommended once weekly. This is intended to remove protein and other deposits from the lens. Contact lens must be rinsed and disinfected before wearing. |

| Generic Name *Brand Name Examples* | Uses |
|---|---|
| *otc* **Rewetting Solutions** | |
| *Clerz 2 Lubricating and Rewetting Drops, Lens Drops, Lens Plus Rewetting Drops[2], Opti-Free Rewetting Drops[1], Opti-Tears Soothing Drops[1], ReNu Lubricating and Rewetting Drops[1], Sensitive Eyes Drops[1]* | Rewetting solutions may be used directly in the eye to wet and improve comfort of soft lenses. |
| *otc* **Chemical Disinfection Systems** | |
| **One-solution systems** | |
| *AOSEPT[1], Disinfecting Solution, Opti-Free, Opti-Free Express, Opti-Soft Disinfecting[1], ReNu Multi-Purpose[1], ReNu MultiPlus[1]* | Chemical disinfection is an alternative to heat. One-solution systems use the same solution for rinsing and storing. Two-solution systems use separate disinfecting and rinsing solutions. |
| **Two-solution systems** | |
| *AOSept Disinfecting, Oxysept Disinfection System, Quick Care Starting Solution[1,2]* | **Warning:** Lenses must not be disinfected by heating when using most of these solutions. See individual label for restrictions. |

[1] Thimerosal free.
[2] Preservative free.

Soft (hydrogel) contact lenses must be maintained in a wet state in saline to prevent them from becoming brittle. Soft lenses will absorb many substances; therefore, use only solutions specifically formulated for soft lenses. In addition, these lenses must be disinfected either by heating or by soaking in a chemical solution. *Heating lenses in solutions used for chemical disinfection may cause them to become opaque.*

Soft lens solutions are especially made to be compatible with, and to meet the particular needs of, soft contact lenses. Of particular importance to soft lens care is the need for thorough cleaning to remove deposits that coat and may discolor the lens, especially when subjected to disinfection by heating.

**WARNING:** DO NOT use conventional (hard) lens solutions on soft contact lenses. Consult your eye doctor for product selection. Not all products are intended for use in all types of soft lenses.

## Type of Drug:
Soft contact lens products.

## How the Drug Works:

Contact lens products are sterile, isotonic, and free of particulate matter. They contain various chemical ingredients to achieve specific goals of contact lens care.

## Precautions:

*Do not use in the following situations:* If you are allergic to the product or any of its ingredients

## Side Effects:

These products are capable of producing side effects. Many contact lens users experience no, or minor side effects. The frequency and severity of side effects depend on many factors including individual suscepti- bility, length of wear, and adherence to instructions for proper lens care. Possible side effects include the following:

*Eyes or Ocular:* Stinging, burning, or itching of eye(s); excessive tearing; unusual eye secretions; redness of eye(s); reduced sharpness of vision; blurred vision; sensitivity to light; dry eyes; infection.

---

## Guidelines for Use:

- Proper contact lens care will increase success and decrease complications.
- See individual product information for detailed direction and safety infor- mation. Always follow label directions and your doctor's recommenda- tions. Problems with contact lens and lens care products could result in serious injury to the eye.
- Cleaning does not disinfect lenses. Disinfecting does not clean lenses.
- Wash and rinse hands thoroughly before handling contact lenses.
- Do not take enzymatic tablets internally.
- Do not use enzymatic tablets that are soft and sticky or irregular in appearance.
- Weekly enzymatic/disinfection cycle is not a substitute for cleaning and disinfecting.
- Do not insert contact lenses if eyes are red or irritated.
- Do not wear contact lenses while sleeping unless they have been pre- scribed for extended wear. Daily wear lenses are not indicated for over- night wear and should not be worn while sleeping because this may cause serious side effects.
- Remove extended-wear lenses regularly for cleaning and disinfecting or for disposal and replacement on the schedule prescribed by your doctor to avoid serious side effects. The risk of serious side effects increases the longer extended-wear lenses are worn before removal for cleaning and disinfecting or for disposal and replacement. Smokers have a higher incidence of side effects.
- For soft lens care, use only products designed for soft lenses. Because many of these products can only be used with certain lens types, con- sult your eye doctor before using any product if you are uncertain which type of lens you wear.

## Guidelines for Use (cont.):

- *Homemade saline solution* — Soft contact lens wearers who use home-made saline (salt) solutions are at risk of developing *Acanthamoeba keratitis*, a serious and painful corneal infection. This infection may cause impaired vision or blindness. Homemade saline solution is not recommended. Use commercial sterile saline solutions.
- If cleaner or disinfectant gets in eye(s), remove lens immediately and flush eye(s) with water or saline for several minutes.
- Do not put lens in eye(s) until rinsed with a neutralizer or saline unless it is a one-solution system.
- Do not change or substitute products from a different manufacturer without consulting your doctor.
- Do not store lenses in tap water.
- Never use saliva to wet contact lenses.
- Never reuse the solution in your lens case. To prevent contamination and to avoid eye injury, always empty and rinse lens case with fresh rinsing solution and allow to air dry. Do not use tap water, soap, or detergent.
- To avoid contamination, do not touch tip of container to any surface. Replace cap and keep tightly closed when not in use.
- Do not transfer saline to another container since the packaged container keeps the saline sterile.
- *Perservative Free Salines* — Discard bottle and contents 30 days after opening. Because the preservative free salines have no strong preservatives, they will not remain sterile indefinitely after opening and therefore should not be used as an eye drop.
- Do not instill topical medications while contact lenses are being worn unless directed to do so by your doctor.
- Eye problems, including corneal ulcers, can develop rapidly and lead to loss of vision. If eye discomfort; excessive tearing; vision changes; eye redness, burning, or irritation occur, immediately remove your lenses. If the problem stops and the lenses appear to be undamaged, thoroughly clean, rinse, and disinfect the lenses and reinsert them. If the problem continues or a lens appears damaged, remove the lenses and contact your eye care practitioner immediately.
- It is recommended that contact lens wearers see their eye doctor twice a year, or more frequently if directed.
- Use before the expiration date marked on the carton and bottle, or within the time indicated on the package (usually within 60 to 90 days).
- Keep contact lens care products out of the reach of children.
- Do not use solution if it becomes cloudy or discolored.
- Store tablets in a dry place. Do not open foil packets until just prior to use.
- Store tablets and solutions at room temperature.

*If you have any questions, consult your doctor, pharmacist, or health care provider.*

| | Brand Name Examples | Antibiotic | Steroid |
|---|---|---|---|
| Rx | Chloromycetin Otic | **Solution**: 0.5% chloramphenicol/mL | |
| Rx | AK-Spore H.C. Otic[1], Cortisporin Otic[1] | **Solution**: 3.5 mg neomycin sulfate, 10,000 units polymyxin B sulfate/mL | 1% hydrocortisone/mL |
| Rx | AK-Spore H.C. Otic, Cortisporin Otic | **Suspension**: 3.5 mg neomycin sulfate, 10,000 units polymyxin B sulfate/mL | 1% hydrocortisone/mL |
| Rx | Coly-Mycin S Otic, Cortisporin-TC | **Suspension**: 3.3 mg neomycin sulfate, 3 mg colistin, 0.05% thonzonium bromide/mL | 1% hydrocortisone/mL |

[1] Contains sulfites.

## Type of Drug:

Antibiotic and antibiotic-steroid combinations for the ear. Used to treat superficial bacterial infections of the outer ear.

## How the Drug Works:

Antibiotics interfere with protein production and cellular activity of susceptible bacteria. This interference may impair reproductive ability or kill the bacteria. Steroids inhibit the inflammatory response (eg, redness, swelling) of tissues due to mechanical, chemical, or allergy-causing agents, and infectious processes.

## Uses:

To treat susceptible bacterial infections of the outer ear. The steroid ingredient (usually hydrocortisone) has an anti-inflammatory effect.

## Precautions:

*Do not use in the following situations:*

allergy to these drugs or any of their ingredients
fungal infections of the ear
perforated eardrum (solutions only)
viral infections of the ear (eg, herpes simplex, varicella-zoster)

*Use with caution in the following situations:*

chronic otitis media (middle ear infection)
perforated eardrum (suspensions only)

*Superinfection:* Use of antibiotics (especially prolonged or repeated therapy) may result in resistant bacterial or fungal overgrowth. Such overgrowth may lead to a second infection. The medication may need to be stopped and another antibiotic may need to be prescribed for the second infection.

*Neomycin sensitization:* When using neomycin-containing products to control secondary infection in the chronic dermatoses (eg, chronic otitis externa, stasis dermatitis), keep in mind that the skin in these conditions is more liable than healthy skin to become sensitized to many substances, including neomycin.

*Pregnancy:* No adequate and well-controlled studies have been done in pregnant women. Use only if clearly needed and potential benefits to the mother outweigh the possible hazards to the fetus.

*Breastfeeding:* Otic antibiotics and hydrocortisone appear in breast milk. Consult your doctor before you begin breastfeeding.

*Children:* Contact your doctor or pharmacist before using in children less than 12 years of age.

*Lab tests* may be required to verify the identification of the organism. Tests include cultures and susceptibility tests.

*Sulfites:* Some of these products may contain sulfite preservatives that can cause allergic reactions in certain individuals. Check package label when available or consult your doctor or pharmacist.

## Side Effects:

Every drug is capable of producing side effects. Many users of topical antibiotic combinations for the ear experience no, or minor, side effects. The frequency and severity of side effects depend on many factors including dose, duration of therapy, and individual susceptibility. Possible side effects include the following:

*Skin:* Irritation; itching; burning; redness; rash; hives; stinging; dryness; allergic skin reaction; tearing of skin.

*Other:* Secondary infection.

## Guidelines for Use:

- *Suspension* — Shake the container for 10 seconds before using.
- *Suspension and Solution* — To warm the medication before use, hold the container in the hand for a few minutes. To avoid loss of potency, do not heat above body temperature .
- *AK-Spore H.C., Cortisporin* — Instill 4 drops in the affected ear(s) 3 to 4 times daily. Instill 3 drops 3 to 4 times daily for infants and children.
- *Coly-Mycin S and Cortisporin-TC* — Instill 5 drops in the affected ear(s) 3 times daily. Instill 4 drops 3 times daily for infants and children.
- *Chloromycetin* — Instill 2 to 3 drops in the affected ear(s) 3 times daily.
- *Drops* — Administer the prescribed number of drops using the calibrated dropper included with each bottle of drops.
- Do not use in eyes.
- Clean the outer ear canal thoroughly and dry with a sterile cotton applicator before using the medicine.
- Avoid touching the dropper to the ear, fingers, counter top, or other surfaces.
- Lie on your side or tilt the affected ear up prior to administering the drug.
- Keep the ear tilted for about 5 minutes after administration. To assist the drops in running into the external ear canal, hold the earlobe up and back in adults and down and back in children.
- If preferred, insert a cotton wick into the ear canal and saturate it with solution. Keep wick moist by adding solution every 4 hours. Replace the wick at least once every 24 hours.
- If reddening with swelling, dry scaling, burning, or itching occurs or persists after use, contact your doctor.
- Duration of therapy should be limited to no more than 10 consecutive days.
- If infection is not improved after 1 week, your doctor will repeat the cultures and susceptibility tests to verify the identity of the infecting organism and to determine whether therapy should be changed.
- Allergic cross-reactions may occur with neomycin which could prevent the use of any or all of the following antibiotics for the treatment of future infections: Kanamycin, paromomycin, streptomycin, and possibly gentamicin.
- Store between 59° to 86°F. Store *Cortisporin* between 59° and 77°F. Store *Otobiotic* between 36° and 86°F.

*If you have any questions, consult your doctor, pharmacist, or health care provider.*

| | Brand Name Examples | Supplied As | Generic Available |
|---|---|---|---|
| Rx | Acetasol, Borofair Otic, VōSol Otic | **Solution**: 2% acetic acid | Yes |
| Rx | Americaine Otic, Otocain | **Solution**: 20% benzocaine | No |
| Rx | Tympagesic[1] | **Solution**: 5% benzocaine, 5% antipyrine, 0.25% phenylephrine HCl | No |
| Rx | Allergen Ear Drops, Auroto Otic | **Solution**: 1.4% benzocaine, 5.4% antipyrine, glycerin | Yes |
| otc | Aurocaine 2 | **Solution**: 2.75% boric acid, 97.25% isopropyl alcohol | No |
| otc | Auro Ear Drops, Aurocaine Ear Drops, Debrox Drops, E•R•O Ear Drops, Mollifene Ear Wax Removal Aid, Murine Ear Drops, Murine Ear Wax Removal System | **Solution**: 6.5% carbamide peroxide | No |
| Rx | Cortic Ear Drops, Zōtō-HC Ear Drops | **Solution**: 0.1% chloroxylenol, 1% hydrocortisone, 1% pramoxine HCl | No |
| Rx | Cresylate | **Solution**: 25% m-cresyl acetate, 0.5% acetic acid | No |
| Rx | EarSol-HC | **Solution**: 1% hydrocortisone | No |
| Rx | Acetasol-HC, VōSol HC Otic | **Solution**: 1% hydrocortisone, 2% acetic acid | No |
| otc | Auro-Dri, Dri/Ear, Ear-Dry, Swim Ear | **Solution**: 95% isopropyl alcohol, 5% anhydrous glycerin | No |
| otc | Star-Otic | **Solution**: Modified Burow's solution (aluminum acetate), acetic acid, boric acid | No |
| Rx | Cerumenex Drops | **Solution**: 10% triethanolamine polypeptide oleate-condensate | No |

[1] Contains metabisulfite.

## Type of Drug:

Drugs used to treat various external ear conditions.

## Uses:

In these combinations:

*Acetic acid, aluminum acetate, boric acid, chloroxylenol,* and *m-cresyl acetate* provide antibacterial or antifungal action.

*Antipyrine* is a pain reliever with local anesthetic action.

*Benzocaine and pramoxine HCl* are local anesthetics that provide relief from pain or itching.

*Carbamide peroxide and triethanolamine* dissolve ear wax.

*Glycerin* is a solvent.

*Hydrocortisone* is a steroid used for its anti-inflammatory and antipruritic (anti-itch) effects.

*Isopropyl alcohol* is an antiseptic in topical anti-infective products.

*Phenylephrine HCl* is a vasoconstrictor, which may be a decongestant, and is used to decrease swelling.

## Precautions:

*Do not use in the following situations:*

allergy to the medicine or any of its ingredients
chickenpox (steroid only)
ear discharge (benzocaine, antipyrine, phenylephrine only)
herpes simplex (steroid only)
perforated eardrum
vaccine (steroid only)

*Use with caution in the following situations:*

dizziness
ear pain, severe
otitis media, severe

*Pregnancy:* There are no adequate and well-controlled studies in pregnant women. Use only if clearly needed and potential benefits to the mother outweigh the possible risks to the fetus.

*Breastfeeding:* It is not known if these otic preparations appear in breast milk. Consult your doctor before you begin breastfeeding.

*Children:* Consult your doctor about dosing and safety in children. Safety and effectiveness have not been established for *Cerumenex.* Do not use *Americaine Otic* in children less than 1 year of age. Do not use *Ear-sol-HC* in children less than 2 years of age except under the advice and supervision of your doctor. Safety and effectiveness have not been established for children less than 3 years of age for *Acetasol,* , *Acetasol-HC, VōSol* and *VōSol HC.* Safety and effectiveness have not been established for children less than 12 years of age for *Tympagesic.*

*Sulfites:* Some of these products may contain sulfite preservatives, which can cause allergic reactions in certain individuals (eg, asthmatics). Check package label when available or consult your doctor or pharmacist.

## Drug Interactions:

Tell your doctor or pharmacist if you are taking or if you are planning to take any over-the-counter or prescription medications or dietary supplements with otic preparations. Doses of one or both drugs may need to be modified or a different drug may need to be prescribed.

## Side Effects:

Every drug is capable of producing side effects. Many otic preparation users experience no, or minor, side effects. The frequency and severity of side effects depend on many factors including dose, duration of therapy, and individual susceptibility. Possible side effects include the following:

*Local:* Stinging; burning; irritation; skin inflammation; swelling; flushing; redness of the outer ear canal; itching; pain; rash; hives; dryness; inflammation of the hair follicles; excess hair growth; acne-like eruptions; decrease in skin or tissue coloration; tenderness.

*Other:* Headache; dizziness; restlessness; anxiety.

---

### Guidelines for Use:

- For use in the ear only. Avoid contact with eyes. Do not use in eyes or take internally.
- To properly administer ear drops, observe the following steps: Avoid touching the dropper to the ear. Hold the container in the hand for a few minutes to warm it if it has been refrigerated.
  Lie on your side or tilt the affected ear(s) up prior to administering the drug. Administer the prescribed number of drops. Keep the ear(s) tilted up for about 2 minutes. To assist the drops in running into the outer ear canal, hold the earlobe up and back in adults and down and back in children. Cotton may be placed in the ear to prevent drops from escaping.
- If problem persists or worsens after recommended treatment period, consult your doctor.
- Discontinue use and contact your doctor promptly if sensitization or irritation occurs after use.
- *Allergen, Auralgan,* and *Tympagesic* — Do not rinse dropper after use. Discard the solution 6 months after the dropper is first placed into the solution. Do not use if solution is brown or contains solid particles floating in the solution.
- Do not use wax-removing solutions if you have ear drainage or discharge, ear pain, irritation, rash in the ear, or if you are dizzy.
- Indiscriminate use of anesthetic ear drops may mask symptoms of an infection in the middle ear.
- *Debrox Drops* foam on contact with ear wax due to release of oxygen. There may be an associated crackling sound.
- Store at room temperature (59° to 86°F). Protect from freezing, direct sunlight, and excessive heat. Keep container tightly closed and out of the reach of children. Store *VōSol, VōSol-HC,* and *Acetasol HC* between 68° and 77°F.

---

*If you have any questions, consult your doctor, pharmacist, or health care provider.*

## Mouth and Throat Products
Carbamide Peroxide, 1387
Chlorhexidine, 1389
Saliva Substitutes, 1391
Tetracycline, 1394
Amlexanox, 1396
Benzyl Alcohol, 1398
Mouth and Throat Products, 1399

## Vaginal Preparations
Douche Products, 1407

## Spermicides, 1409

## Anorectal Preparations, 1411

## Acne Products
Benzoyl Peroxide, 1416
Azelaic Acid, 1419
Sulfur, 1421

## Retinoids
Adapalene, 1422
Altretinoin, 1425
Tretinoin, 1427

## Miscellaneous Acne Combinations, 1430

## Agents for Psoriasis
Anthralin, 1437
Calcipotriene, 1439
Acitretin, 1441
Methotrexate, 1444
Psoralens, 1447

## Antiacne, Antipsoriatic
Tazarotene, 1451

## Diabetic Ulcer Agent
Becaplermin, 1454

## Burn Preparations
Mafenide, 1456
Silver Sulfadiazine, 1458

## Antiseborrheics
Selenium Sulfide, 1460
Miscellaneous, 1462
Combinations, 1466

## Anesthetics
For Mucous Membranes, 1468
For Skin Disorders, 1472

## Keratolytics
Diclofenac, 1476
Podofilox, 1478
Salicylic Acid, 1480

## Emollients, 1483
Miscellaneous, 1486

## Analgesics
Capsaicin, 1489

## Antihistamines, 1491

## Antiseptics and Germicides, 1494

## Diaper Rash Products, 1497

## Minoxidil, 1499

## Poison Ivy Treatment Products, 1502

## Rubs and Liniments, 1504

## Sunscreens, 1506

## Skin Cleansers, 1516

## Astringents
Aluminum Acetate, 1517

## Miscellaneous Topical Agents, 1518

## Eflornithine, 1525

| Generic Name<br>*Brand Name Examples* | Supplied As | Generic<br>Available |
|---|---|---|
| *otc* **Carbamide Peroxide** | | |
| *Orajel Perioseptic* | **Liquid**: 15% | No |
| *Cankaid, Gly-Oxide Liquid* | **Solution**: 10% | No |
| *Proxigel* | **Gel**: 10% | No |

## Type of Drug:

Antiseptic mouth-cleansing agent for irritated and inflamed areas.

## How the Drug Works:

Carbamide peroxide releases oxygen into irritated mouth tissue to provide a cleansing effect. This helps reduce inflammation, relieve pain and inhibit growth of odor-forming bacteria so that healing can begin.

## Uses:

To treat and prevent minor mouth and gum irritation or inflammation (eg, canker sores, accidental injuries, dentures, orthodontic appliances, postdental procedures).

Aid to oral hygiene when normal cleansing measures are inadequate or impossible (eg, total care geriatrics or when patient wears orthodontic or dental appliances).

## Precautions:

*Use with caution in the following situations:*
    dental irritation or oral inflammation, severe or persistant gingivitis

*Children:* Do not use in children under 2 years of age (*Cankaid* — under 3 years of age) unless directed by a doctor or dentist.

## Side Effects:

Every drug is capable of producing side effects. Most carbamide peroxide users experience no, or minor, side effects. Possible side effects include irritation; rash; inflammation; gingivitis; swelling; fever.

## Guidelines for Use:

- Do not swallow.
- *Liquid and Solution* — Do not dilute. Apply 4 times daily after meals and at bedtime or as directed. Place several drops directly on the affected area; expectorate (spit out) after 2 to 3 minutes or place 10 drops on the tongue, mix with saliva, swish thoroughly and expectorate (spit out).
- *Gel* — Do not dilute. Use 4 times daily or as directed. Massage gently on the affected area. Allow medicine to remain in place for 1 minute then spit out. Do not drink or rinse mouth for 5 minutes after use. Replace bottle tip after each use.
- Avoid contact with eyes.
- Do not use for more than 7 days.
- Severe or persistant oral inflammation, dental irritation or gingivitis may be serious. Consult your doctor or dentist immediately.
- If condition persists or worsens, or if irritation, redness, swelling or fever occurs, stop using this medication and contact your doctor or dentist.
- Do not use for children under 2 years of age (*Cankaid* — under 3 years of age) unless directed by a doctor or dentist.
- Cap tightly. Protect from heat and light.

*If you have any questions, consult your doctor, pharmacist, or health care provider.*

| Generic Name<br>*Brand Name Example* | Supplied As | Generic<br>Available |
|---|---|---|
| *Rx* **Chlorhexidine Gluconate** | | |
| *Peridex*[1] | **Oral rinse**: 0.12% | No |

[1] Contains alcohol.

## Type of Drug:

Antibacterial oral rinse for treating inflamed gingiva (gums).

## How the Drug Works:

Chlorhexidine gluconate is an oral rinse that decreases bacteria in the mouth.

## Uses:

To treat gingivitis (redness and swelling of the gums) characterized by redness, swelling, and bleeding of the gums upon probing.

## Precautions:

*Do not use in the following situations:*

allergy to the drug or any ingredient

*Staining of oral surfaces* (eg, teeth, restorations, tongue) may occur. Stains will be more pronounced in patients with heavy plaque accumulations.

Stains resulting from use does not adversely affect health of the gums or other oral tissues. Stains can be removed from most tooth surfaces by conventional dental cleaning techniques (make take longer). Patients who have restorations with rough surfaces or margins should use with caution; stains in these areas may be difficult to remove.

*Changes in taste perception* may occur while undergoing treatment. Most patients indicate it is less noticeable with continued use.

*Pregnancy:* Studies in pregnant women have not shown a risk to the fetus. However, no drug should be used during pregnancy unless clearly needed.

*Breastfeeding:* It is not known if chlorhexidine gluconate appears in breast milk. Consult your doctor before you begin breastfeeding.

*Children:* Safety and effectiveness in children under 18 years of age have not been established.

## Side Effects:

Every drug is capable of producing side effects. Many chlorhexidine gluconate users experience no, or minor, side effects. Possible side effects include:

*Mouth:* Staining of teeth and other oral surfaces (eg, restorations, tongue); tartar increase; altered taste perception; minor sloughing of the oral mucosa (especially in children); dry mouth; mouth inflammation; gingivitis; red, inflamed tongue; mouth ulcers; diminished sensitivity; swelling; abnormal sensations in the mouth.

*Other:* Stomach upset or nausea (if swallowed); allergy symptoms.

---

### Guidelines for Use:

- Begin therapy after a thorough cleaning of teeth by a dentist or dental hygienist.
- Usual dose is 15 mL (undiluted) twice daily, morning and evening, after brushing the teeth.
- Do not dilute.
- Do not rinse mouth with water or other mouthwash, brush teeth or eat immediately after rinsing with *Peridex*.
- To minimize discoloration, brush and floss daily emphasizing areas that begin to stain.
- To avoid taste interference, rinse with *Peridex* after meals.
- Tooth staining may occur.
- Taste changes may occur during use.
- Do not swallow the drug. Spit out after rinsing.
- Dental checkups are necessary every 6 months.
- Store above freezing.

---

*If you have any questions, consult your doctor, pharmacist, or health care provider.*

| Generic Name<br>*Brand Name Example* | Supplied As | Generic<br>Available |
|---|---|---|
| otc *Entertainer's Secret, Moi-<br>Stir, Moi-Stir 10, Mouth-<br>Kote[1], Optimoist, Saliva<br>Substitute[2]* | **Solution**: Contains a variety of<br>lubricants | No |
| otc *Moi-Stir Swabsticks* | **Swabsticks**: Contains a variety<br>of lubricants | No |
| otc *Salivart[1,2]* | **Aerosol spray**: Contains a<br>variety of lubricants | No |
| otc *Salix* | **Tablets**: Contains a variety of<br>lubricants | No |

[1] Sugar free.
[2] Dye free.

## Type of Drug:

Saliva substitute.

## Uses:

To relieve dry mouth and throat caused by xerostomia (dry mouth) after surgery or from some illnesses (eg, Sjögren's syndrome, Bell's Palsy), some medications (eg, antidepressants, tranquilizers, antihistamines) and aging.

To aid healing after medical or surgical procedures (eg, chemotherapy, radiation, tracheotomy) that adversely affect the throat.

## Guidelines for Use:

- Dosing varies. Be sure to read package insert for instructions.
- *Solution* — Squirt or spray a small quantity into the mouth as often as needed to moisten and lubricate.
- Solution may be swallowed or expectorated (spit out).
- *Tablets* — Allow to move around and slowly dissolve in mouth. Repeat one tablet per hour as necessary.
- *Entertainer's Secret* — Can spray into each nostril while inhaling to apply drug to upper throat.
- Do not drink water immediately after use.
- *Solutions* — Close container between uses.
- Store at room temperature.

*If you have any questions, consult your doctor, pharmacist, or health care provider.*

| Generic Name
Brand Name Example | Supplied As | Generic
Available |
|---|---|---|
| Rx  Pilocarpine HCl | | |
| Salagen | Tablets: 5 mg | No |

## Type of Drug:

Salivary gland stimulator.

## How the Drug Works:

Pilocarpine increases the production of saliva by stimulating muscles found in salivary glands.

## Uses:

To treat xerostomia (dry mouth) in patients with malfunctioning salivary glands due to cancer radiotherapy of the head and neck.

To treat the symptoms of dry mouth caused by Sjögren's syndrome.

## Precautions:

*Do not use in the following situations:*

allergy to pilocarpine
asthma, uncontrolled

glaucoma, narrow-angle
iritis, acute

*Use with caution in the following situations:*

asthma, controlled
bronchitis, chronic
chronic obstructive lung disease,
 requiring drug therapy
gall bladder disease
heart disease, significant
high blood pressure

kidney disease
liver disease
mental illness
nephrolithiasis
retinal disease
visual problems (eg, night
 blindness)

*Pregnancy:* Adequate studies have not been done in pregnant women. Use only if potential benefits outweigh possible hazards to the fetus.

*Breastfeeding:* It is not known if pilocarpine appears in breast milk. Consult your doctor before you begin breastfeeding.

*Children:* Safety and effectiveness in children have not been established.

## Drug Interactions:

Tell your doctor or pharmacist if you are taking or if you are planning to take any over-the-counter or prescription medications or dietary supplements with pilocarpine. Doses of one or both drugs may need to be modified or a different drug may need to be prescribed. The following drugs and drug classes interact with pilocarpine:

anticholinergic agents (eg, atropine, inhaled ipratropium bromide)
beta-adrenergic blockers (eg, propranolol)

## Side Effects:

Every drug is capable of producing side effects. Many pilocarpine users experience no, or minor, side effects. The frequency and severity of side effects depend on many factors including dose, duration of therapy and individual susceptibility. Possible side effects include:

*Digestive Tract:* Nausea; vomiting; diarrhea; gas; indigestion; stomach ache; difficulty swallowing; taste distortion.

*Nervous System:* Dizziness; headache; tremor.

*Circulatory System:* Edema (fluid retention); high blood pressure; rapid or slow heart beat; flushing; low blood pressure.

*Respiratory System:* Nasal congestion; sore throat; runny nose; sinus pain.

*Skin:* Sweating; chills; rash; itching.

*Other:* Urinary frequency; vaginitis (itching, inflammation or abnormal discharge); weakness; abnormal vision; eye inflammation; excess tears; nosebleed; ringing in ears; voice alteration; back pain; blurred vision; impaired depth perception.

---

### Guidelines for Use:

- Take 1 tablet 3 times daily.
- *Sjögren's syndrome:* Take 1 tablet 4 times daily.
- If a dose is missed, take it as soon as possible. If several hours have passed or if it is nearing time for the next dose, do not double the dose in order to catch up (unless advised to do so by your doctor). If more than one dose is missed or it is necessary to establish a new dosage schedule, contact your doctor or pharmacist. Use exactly as prescribed.
- Maximum benefit may not be reached for several weeks.
- The lowest tolerable yet effective dose should be used for maintenance as adverse effects may increase with higher doses.
- Patients should have eye examinations before beginning treatment with pilocarpine.
- May cause visual problems. Use caution while driving, especially at night or when performing hazardous activities in reduced lighting.
- Notify your doctor if any of the following occurs: Headache, visual problems, tearing, excessive sweating, difficulty breathing, stomach cramps, nausea, vomiting, diarrhea, fast or slow pulse, blood pressure changes, confusion, tremor or irregular heartbeat.
- Store at room temperature (59° to 86°F).

---

*If you have any questions, consult your doctor, pharmacist, or health care provider.*

| Generic Name *Brand Name Example* | Supplied As | Generic Available |
|---|---|---|
| *Rx* **Tetracycline HCl** | | |
| *Actisite* | **Fiber**: 12.7 mg/23 cm | No |

## Type of Drug:
Topical antibiotic.

## How the Drug Works:
Tetracycline reduces bacterial infections by inhibiting protein synthesis.

## Uses:
Topical treatment for gum disease (periodontitis) in adults. It is used in combination with good hygiene, scaling, and root planing.

## Precautions:
*Do not use in the following situations:*
allergy to any tetracyclines

*Use with caution in the following situations:*
abscess, acute
candidiasis, oral
kidney disease
medical disorders, contributing

*Superinfection* – Use of antibiotics (especially prolonged or repeated therapy) may result in bacterial or fungal overgrowth. Such overgrowth may lead to a second infection. Tetracycline may need to be stopped and another antibiotic may need to be prescribed for the second infection.

*Photosensitivity* – May cause photosensitivity (tendency to sunburn). Avoid prolonged exposure to the sun or other forms of ultraviolet light (eg, tanning beds). Use sunscreens and wear protective clothing until tolerance is determined. Discontinue use at the first sign of redness of the skin.

*Pregnancy:* Adequate studies have not been done in pregnant women, or studies in animals may have shown a risk to the fetus. Use only if clearly needed and the potential benefits outweigh the possible hazards to the fetus (See Children).

*Breastfeeding:* Tetracycline appears in breast milk. Because of the potential for serious side effects in nursing infants, use in a nursing woman only if clearly needed. Consult your doctor before you begin breastfeeding.

*Children:* Safety and effectiveness in children have not been established. The use of tetracycline class drugs during tooth development (last half of pregnancy, infancy and childhood to 8 years of age) may cause permanent discoloration of the teeth. Tetracycline drugs should not be used in these age groups unless other treatment is not likely to be effective or if alternative therapy is contraindicated.

## Side Effects:

Every drug is capable of producing side effects. Many patients experience no, or minor, side effects. The frequency and severity of side effects depend on many factors including dose, duration of therapy and individual susceptibility. Possible side effects include discomfort on fiber placement and redness following removal.

### Guidelines for Use:

- Avoid actions which may dislodge the fiber. Do not chew hard, crusty or sticky foods; do not brush or floss near any treated areas (continue to clean other teeth); do not engage in any other hygienic practices that could dislodge the fibers and do not probe at the treated area with tongue or fingers.
- The antibiotic-containing fiber provides continuous release of tetracycline for 10 days. At the end of 10 days of treatment, all fibers must removed by the dentist. Any fibers lost before the end of 7 days must be replaced by the dentist.
- Notify the dentist promptly if the fiber is dislodged or falls out before the scheduled visit, or if pain, swelling or other problems occur.
- May cause photosensitivity (tendency to sunburn). Avoid prolonged exposure to the sun or other forms of ultraviolet light (eg, tanning beds). Use sunscreen and wear protective clothing until tolerance is determined. Discontinue use at first sign of redness of the skin.
- Store at room temperature (59° to 86° F).

*If you have any questions, consult your doctor, pharmacist, or health care provider.*

| Generic Name<br>*Brand Name Example* | Supplied As | Generic<br>Available |
|---|---|---|
| *Rx* **Amlexanox** | | |
| *Aphthasol* | **Paste, oral**: 5% | No |

## Type of Drug:

Mouth ulcer ("canker sore") treatment.

## How the Drug Works:

The mechanism of action is unknown. The drug seems to inhibit inflammatory reactions.

## Uses:

For the treatment of mouth ulcers ("canker sores") in patients with normal immune systems.

## Precautions:

*Do not use in the following situations:* Allergy to amlexanox or any of its ingredients.

*Pregnancy:* Studies in pregnant women or in animals have been judged not to show a risk to the fetus. However, no drug should be used during pregnancy unless clearly needed.

*Breastfeeding:* It is not known if amlexanox appears in breast milk. Consult your doctor before you begin breastfeeding.

*Children:* Safety and effectiveness of amlexanox in children have not been established.

## Drug Interactions:

Tell your doctor or pharmacist if you are taking or planning to take any over-the-counter or prescription medications or dietary supplements while taking amlexanox. Doses of one or both drugs may need to be modified or a different drug may need to be prescribed.

## Side Effects:

Every drug is capable of producing side effects. Many amlexanox users experience no, or minor, side effects. The frequency and severity of side effects depend on many factors including dose, duration of therapy, and individual susceptibility. Possible side effects include: Transient pain; stinging or burning at the application site.

## Guidelines for Use:

- Apply the paste 4 times a day following oral hygiene after breakfast, lunch, dinner, and at bedtime as directed by your doctor. Begin therapy as soon as you notice symptoms of a mouth ulcer.
- Squeeze a dab (¼ inch) of paste onto fingertip. Dab the paste onto each ulcer in the mouth using gentle pressure.
- Wash hands immediately after applying amlexanox. In the event of rash or contact irritation, discontinue use and contact your doctor.
- Wash eyes promptly if there is contact with the paste.
- Use the paste until the ulcers heal. If significant healing or pain reduction has not occurred in 10 days, consult your dentist or doctor.
- Keep out of the reach of children.
- Store at controlled room temperature (59° to 86°F).

*If you have any questions, consult your doctor, pharmacist, or health care provider.*

| Generic Name<br>*Brand Name Example* | Supplied As | Generic<br>Available |
|---|---|---|
| *otc* **Benzyl Alcohol** | | |
| *Zilactin*[1] | **Gel**: 10% | No |

[1] Contains tannic acid.

## Type of Drug:
Soft tissue protectant.

## How the Drug Works:
Benzyl alcohol reduces sensory stimulation to relieve pain, burning, and itching.

## Uses:
To provide temporary relief of pain, burning and itching in cold sores, canker sores, and fever blisters.

## Side Effects:
Every drug is capable of producing side effects. Most benzyl alcohol users experience no, or minor, side effects. Possible side effects include temporary burning upon application (short duration) and allergic reactions.

---

### Guidelines for Use:

- Apply this product 4 times daily for a minimum of 2 days. Use every 4 to 6 hours as needed. Wipe the affected area dry before applying the gel. Hold the affected area away from the other elements of the oral cavity for 30 to 60 seconds after application to maximize tissue binding.
- Do not use in or around eyes. If contact with eyes occurs, flush the eye(s) immediately and continuously with clean tap water for 10 minutes. Consult your doctor if pain or irritation persists.
- Burning of a temporary nature when applied to an open sore or blister is normal and no cause for concern.
- Do not peel off protective film. Attempting to peel off film may result in skin irritation or tenderness. To remove film, first apply another coat of *Zilactin* to film, then immediately wipe the area with a gauze pad or tissue.
- If inflammation persists beyond 10 days or worsens, stop using and consult your doctor.

---

*If you have any questions, consult your doctor, pharmacist, or health care provider.*

**Generic Name**
*Brand Name Examples*  Supplied As

*otc* **Lozenges**

*Cēpastat Fast-Acting*[5]  **Lozenges**: 14.5% phenol, menthol

*Cēpacol ColdCare*
(Peppermint)[1,2]  **Lozenges**: 9 mg zinc

*Cēpacol* [3] (Cherry)  **Lozenges**: 3.6 mg menthol,
cetylpyridinium chloride

*Cēpacol*[3] (Mint)  **Lozenges**: 2 mg menthol,
cetylpyridinium chloride

*Cēpacol Maximum
Strength*[3] (Mint)  **Lozenges**: 10 mg benzocaine,
2 mg menthol, cetylpyridinium
chloride

*Cēpacol Maximum
Strength*[3] (Cherry)  **Lozenges**: 10 mg benzocaine,
3.6 mg menthol, cetylpyridinium
chloride

*Cēpacol Sugar Free*[4],
Maximum Strength
(Cherry)  **Lozenges**: 10 mg benzocaine,
4.5 mg menthol, cetylpyridinium
chloride

*Cēpacol Sugar Free*[4],
Maximum Strength
(Mint)  **Lozenges**: 10 mg benzocaine,
2.5 mg menthol, cetylpyridinium
chloride

*Cēpastat Cherry*[4,5]  **Lozenges**: 14.5 mg phenol,
menthol

*Cēpastat Extra Strength*[4,5]  **Lozenges**: 29 mg phenol,
menthol

*Vicks Chloraseptic*  **Lozenges**: 6 mg benzocaine,
10 mg menthol

*Hall's Mentho-Lyptus*[6]  **Lozenges**: 7 mg menthol and
eucalyptus oil

*Mycinettes*[4,5]  **Lozenges**: 15 mg benzocaine,
cetylpyridinium chloride

*N'ice*[4,5]  **Lozenges**: 5 mg menthol

*Spec-T* [1,3,7]
(Rasping Coughs)  **Lozenges**: 10 mg benzocaine,
10 mg dextromethorphan HCl

*Spec-T* [1,3,7]
(Nasal Congestion)  **Lozenges**: 10 mg benzocaine,
5 mg phenylephrine HCl,
10.5 mg phenylpropanolamine
HCl

*Spec-T* [3] (Sore Throat)  **Lozenges**: 10 mg benzocaine

*Sucrets* (Wild Cherry)  **Lozenges**: 2 mg dyclonine HCl

*Sucrets* (Original Mint)  **Lozenges** : 2 mg dyclonine HCl

*Sucrets* (Assorted Flavors)  **Lozenges**: 2 mg dyclonine HCl

*Sucrets* (Vapor Lemon)[6]  **Lozenges**: 2 mg dyclonine HCl

*Sucrets, Children's* (Cherry)  **Lozenges**: 1.2 mg dyclonine HCl

| **Generic Name**<br>*Brand Name Examples* | **Supplied As** |
| --- | --- |
| *Sucrets Maximum Strength*[6]<br>(Cherry) | **Lozenges**: 3 mg dyclonine HCl, menthol |
| *Sucrets Maximum Strength*[6]<br>(Wintergreen) | **Lozenges**: 2 mg dyclonine HCl |
| *Trocaine*[7] | **Lozenges**: 10 mg benzocaine |

*otc* **Mouthwashes and Sprays**

| | |
| --- | --- |
| *Cēpacol*[7,8,9] | **Mouthwash/Gargle**:<br>0.05% cetylpyridinium chloride |
| *Cēpacol Maximum Strength* [4] | **Throat spray**: 0.1% dyclonine HCl, cetylpyridinium chloride |
| *Listerine*[8] | **Mouthwash**: 0.064% thymol,<br>0.092% eucalyptol,<br>0.060% methyl salicylate,<br>0.042% menthol |
| *Scope*[8] | **Mouthwash**: cetylpyridinium chloride |

*otc* **Preparations for Sensitive Teeth**

| | |
| --- | --- |
| *Aquafresh Sensitive Teeth* | **Toothpaste**: 0.243% sodium fluoride, 5% potassium nitrate |
| *De-Sensitize Plus*[5] | **Toothpaste**: 5% potassium nitrate, sodium fluoride |
| *Oral-B Sensitive with Fluoride* | **Toothpaste**: 5% potassium nitrate, 0.225% sodium fluoride |
| *Promise Sensitive* | **Toothpaste**: Potassium nitrate |
| *Crest Sensitivity Protection*[5], *Sensodyne Cool Gel for Sensitive Teeth and Cavity Prevention*[5], *Sensodyne w/ Baking Soda for Sensitive Teeth and Cavity Prevention*[5], *Sensodyne-SC Original Formula for Sensitive Teeth*[5], *Sensodyne Extra Whitening for Sensitive Teeth*[4] | **Toothpaste**: Potassium nitrate, sodium fluoride |

[1] Contains dextrose.
[2] Dietary supplement to promote general well being during cold season.
[3] Contains glucose, sucrose.
[4] Sugar free.
[5] Contains sorbitol.
[6] Contains sucrose.
[7] Contains the dye tartrazine.
[8] Contains alcohol.
[9] Contains edetate disodium, polysorbate 80, saccharin.

## Type of Drug:

Mouth and throat products used to treat a variety of product specific conditions.

## Uses:

In these combinations:

*Benzocaine* is a local anesthetic.

*Cetylpyridinium chloride, eucalyptus oil, thymol, benzalkonium chloride, and hexylresorcinol* have mild antiseptic activity.

*Menthol, dyclonine, clove oil, phenol and methylsalicylate* are used for their anti-itch, mild local anesthetic and counterirritant activities.

*Sodium fluoride* is used to prevent cavities and *potassium nitrate* is a desensitizing agent.

*Zinc* is considered a dietary supplement and is not approved by the FDA for any other uses.

## Precautions:

*Tartrazine:* Some of these products may contain the dye tartrazine (FD&C Yellow No. 5), which can cause allergic reactions in certain individuals. Check package label when available or consult your pharmacist or doctor.

---

### Guidelines for Use:

- Do not exceed recommended dosage.
- Dosing and symptoms treated by these products vary. Please read the instructions on the packaging carefully before using any of these products.
- *Lozenges* — Allow lozenge to dissolve slowly in mouth.
- If sore mouth or throat is severe, if irritation, redness or pain persists or worsens or it is accompanied by high fever, headache, swelling, rash, nausea or vomiting, contact your doctor or dentist promptly.
- Do not use products containing benzocaine if you are allergic to procaine, butacaine, benzocaine or other "-caine" anesthetics.
- Do not take throat lozenges for ongoing cough such as occurs with smoking, asthma or emphysema, or if cough is accompanied by a lot of mucous unless directed by your doctor.
- Sensitive teeth may mean that there is a serious problem that requires care by a dentist. See your dentist if the problem is ongoing or worsens. Do not use toothpaste for sensitive teeth longer than 4 weeks unless recommended by a dentist or doctor.
- A persistent cough could be a sign of a serious condition. If cough persists greater than 1 week, tends to recur or is accompanied by rash, fever or persistent headache, contact your doctor.

---

*If you have any questions, consult your doctor, pharmacist, or health care provider.*

| Brand Name Examples | Supplied As | Use |
|---|---|---|
| otc Amosan | **Powder**: Sodium peroxyborate mono-hydrate | Soothes sore gums, canker sore pain, denture and orthodontic irritation and oral injuries after dental procedures |
| otc Anbesol[2] | **Liquid**: 6.3% benzocaine, 0.5% phenol, menthol, camphor<br><br>**Gel:** 6.3% benzocaine, 0.5% phenol, camphor | For relief of denture or orthodontic appliance irritation, toothache, sore gums, cold sores, fever blisters, braces, canker sores and minor dental procedure pain |
| otc Anbesol Cool Mint | **Gel**: 10% benzocaine | |
| otc Anbesol Maximum Strength | **Gel**[3,4] and **Liquid**:[2,3] 20% benzocaine | |
| otc Babee Teething[1,2] | **Lotion**: 2.5% benzocaine, 0.02% cetalkonium chloride, thymol, urea, eucaplyptol, menthol, camphor | For teething discomfort or the pain of children's braces |
| otc Baby Numz•it[3] | **Gel**: 7.5% benzocaine, clove and peppermint oil | For temporary relief of sore gums due to teething in children at least 4 months of age |
| otc Baby Orajel [3,8] (Cherry Flavored) | **Gel**: 7.5% benzocaine | For the relief of teething pain in children at least 4 months of age |
| otc Benzodent | **Cream**: 20% benzocaine, petrolatum | For relief of denture pain or discomfort |
| otc Blistex Lip[2] | **Ointment**: 1% allantoin, 0.6% menthol, 0.5% phenol, 0.5% camphor | For dry, chapped lips, pain and itching caused by cold sores and fever blisters |

| | Brand Name Examples | Supplied As | Use |
|---|---|---|---|
| otc | Blistex Lip Medex | **Ointment**: Petrolatum, 1% camphor, 1% menthol, 0.5% phenol, cocoa butter, lanolin, oil of cloves | For treatment of fever blisters and sore, dry and cracked lips |
| otc | Kanka[2,3] | **Liquid**: 20% benzocaine, cetylpyridinium chloride, benzyl alcohol tincture compound, tannic acid | To relieve pain of mouth and canker sores and brace irritation |
| Rx | Kenalog in Orabase | **Paste**: 0.1% triamcinolone acetonide, mineral oil gel base | To aid in treating and relieving inflamed mouth sores and ulcers resulting from trauma |
| otc | Orabase-B | **Gel**: 20% benzocaine in plasticized hydrocarbon gel | For fast, temporary relief of canker sore pain, denture and orthodontic appliance irritations and mouth and gum sores |
| otc | Orabase Gel [3,6] | **Gel**: 15% benzocaine, salicylic acid | To relieve pain, itching and burning associated with canker sores, cold sores and fever blisters |
| otc | Orabase-Plain | **Paste**: Plasticized hydrocarbon gel | For temporary relief from minor irritations of the mouth and gums and denture discomfort, mouth sores, orthodontic appliance irritations, toothbrush abrasions and minor mouth surgery |
| otc | Orajel [3] | **Gel**: 10% benzocaine | For temporary relief of toothache pain until dentist is consulted |
| otc | Orajel Denture[3] | **Gel**: 20% benzocaine, menthol | To relieve pain and discomfort from dentures and minor irritation from orthodontic appliances |
| otc | Orajel, Maximum Strength | **Gel**,[3] **Liquid**:[2,3,5] 20% benzocaine | For temporary relief of toothache until medical attention is available |

| | Brand Name<br>Examples | Supplied As | Use |
|---|---|---|---|
| otc | Orajel Mouth-Aid | **Liquid**:[3,5,6] 20% benzocaine<br><br>**Gel**:[3,7] 20% benzocaine, 0.02% benzalkonium chloride, 0.1% zinc chloride, peppermint oil | To relieve pain and inflammation of cold sores, fever blisters, canker sores, mouth and gum sores and other minor mouth irritations |
| otc | Peroxyl | **Gel**: 1.5% hydrogen peroxide in mint flavored gel base | For canker sores and cleaning minor wounds or gum inflammation from minor dental procedures, braces, dentures, mouth and gum irritations |
| otc | Peroxyl [3,6,9] | **Solution**: 1.5% hydrogen peroxide, menthol | To cleanse canker sores, gum irritations, dental and mouth sores, orthodontic irritations, mouth burns and cheek bites and toothbrush abrasions |
| otc | Pfeiffer's Cold Sore[2] | **Lotion**: 7% gum benzoin, camphor, menthol, thymol and eucalyptol | For cold sores, fever blisters and cracked lips |
| otc | Rid-A-Pain Dental [2] | **Drops**: 6.3% benzocaine, 0.5% phenol, camphor, menthol | For temporary relief of toothache, brace and denture pain, orthodontic device irritation, sore gums, cold and canker sores and fever blisters |
| otc | Tanac[3] | **Liquid**: 10% benzocaine, 0.12% benzalkonium chloride and tannic acid | For the pain relief of mouth sores, canker sores, gum irritations and fever blisters |

[1] Sugar free.
[2] Contains alcohol.
[3] Contains saccharin.
[4] Contains methylparaben.
[5] Contains tartrazine.
[6] Contains ethyl alcohol.
[7] Contains edetate disodium.
[8] Contains sorbitol.

## Type of Drug:

Mouth and throat products. Ingredient(s) determine use.

## Uses:

In these products:

*Benzocaine* is a local anesthetic.

*Cetylpyridinium chloride, hydrogen peroxide* and *eucalyptus oil* have mild antiseptic activity.

*Menthol, camphor* and *phenol* are used for their antipruritic, mild local anesthetic and counterirritant activities.

*Eugenol* is a mild pain reliever.

*Tannic acid* protects oral tissue and possesses astringent (drying) properties.

*Triamcinolone acetonide* and *hydrocortisone acetate* have anti-inflammatory action.

## Precautions:

*Do not use in the following situations:*
    allergy to any ingredient of the drug
    fungal, viral or bacterial infections of mouth or throat (*Kenalog in Orabase* only)

*Use with caution in the following situations:*
    diabetes
    peptic ulcer
    pregnancy (*Kenalog in Orabase* only)
    tuberculosis

*Tartrazine:* Some of these products many contain the dye tartrazine (FD&C Yellow No. 5), which can cause allergic reactions in certain individuals. Check package label when available or consult your pharmacist or doctor.

## Guidelines for Use:

- Dosing and uses for products vary. Carefully read the instructions on the packaging before using any of these medications.
- Do not exceed recommended dosage.
- Do not swallow products.
- Do not use benzocaine-containing products if there is a history of allergy to local anesthetics such as procaine, butacaine, benzocaine or other "-caine" anesthetics. Do not use if there is an allergy to any other ingredients.
- Do not use for fungal, viral or bacterial infections of the mouth or throat.
- If sore mouth conditions last for more than 7 days; if irritation, pain and redness persists or worsens; or if swelling, rash or fever develops, see your doctor or dentist.
- Do not use for longer than 5 to 7 days unless directed by your doctor or dentist. Do not use *Tanac* for longer than 5 consecutive days.
- Fever and nasal congestion are not symptoms of teething and may indicate an infection.
- Mild burning may occur at application site.
- Allergic reactions at place of application may occur after prolonged or repeated use; discontinue use and contact your doctor if this occurs.
- Benzocaine products may make swallowing difficult or inhibit gag reflexes in infants and children.
- Avoid contact with eyes.
- Keep away from flame.
- Do not apply over large areas of the body or cover with a bandage.
- Inform your doctor if you are pregnant, become pregnant, are planning to become pregnant or if you are breasfeeding.
- Do not use in young children (ages are specified on packaging).

*If you have any questions, consult your doctor, pharmacist, or health care provider.*

| | Brand Name Examples | Supplied As |
|---|---|---|
| otc | Massengill Douche | **Powder**: Sodium chloride, ammonium alum, phenol, methyl salicylate, eucalyptus oil, menthol, thymol |
| otc | Trichotine Douche | **Powder**: Sodium lauryl sulfate, sodium perborate monohydrate, silica |
| | Trichotine Liquid Douche Concentrate[1] | **Liquid concentrate**: Sodium lauryl sulfate |
| otc | Massengill Disposable Douche, Summer's Eve Disposable Douche, Summer's Eve Post-Menstrual Disposable Douche | **Solution**: Contents of these products vary by manufacturer. See package labels for complete product contents. |
| otc | Massengill Extra Mild Disposable Douche, Summer's Eve Douche[2] | **Solution**: Purified water, vinegar |
| otc | Massengill Extra Cleansing Disposable Douche[1] | **Solution**: Purified water, vinegar, cetylpyridinium chloride, diazolidinyl urea |
| otc | Massengill Baking Soda and Water Disposable Douche | **Solution**: Sanitized water, sodium bicarbonate |
| otc | Massengill "Scented" Disposable Douches[1,3] | **Solution**: Water, SD alcohol 40, lactic acid, sodium lactate, octoxynol-9, cetylpyridinium chloride, propylene glycol, diazolidinyl urea |
| otc | Zonite Douche[1] | **Liquid concentrate**: Benzalkonium chloride, menthol, thymol, acetic acid |
| otc | Massengill Douche | **Liquid concentrate**: Lactic acid, sodium bicarbonate, SD alcohol 40 and octoxynol 9, eucalyptol, menthol, thymol |
| otc | Massengill Medicated Disposable Douche | **Solution**: Povidone-iodine |
| otc | Betadine Medicated Disposable Douche, Summer's Eve Medicated Disposable Douche | **Solution**: 0.3% povidone-iodine |

[1] Contains EDTA.
[2] Contains benzoic acid.
[3] Contains parabens, fragrance, coloring.

## Type of Drug:

Vaginal cleansing agents; douches.

## How the Drug Works:

*Povidine-iodine, eucalyptol, menthol, phenol, sodium perborate and thymol* may have antiseptic or germicidal activity.

Povidine-iodine also relieves minor irritation. It may be absorbed from the vagina. Patients with thyroid disorders and pregnant patients should avoid iodine-containing douches.

*Eucalyptol, menthol, phenol, methyl salicylate and thymol* are counterirritants used for their anesthetic or antipruritic effects.

*Ammonium alum* is an astringent that reduces local edema and inflammation; high concentrations can be irritating.

*Octoxynol 9, sodium lauryl sulfate and benzalkonium chloride* are surfactants that facilitate douche spread over vaginal mucosa.

*Sodium perborate and lactic acid* affect pH.

## Uses:

For general cleansing of the vaginal and genital area.

For deodorizing vaginal area.

To relieve minor vaginal itching and irritation.

To remove vaginal discharge, secretions and mucus.

To alter vaginal acidity.

---

### Guidelines for Use:

- For external use only. See packaging for instructions.
- Consult manufacturer's recommendations for proper dilution and use of these products. Follow instructions carefully.
- Avoid contact with eyes.
- *Iodine-containing products* — Do not use if allergic to iodine, or if you are pregnant or breastfeeding.
- Vaginal douches are not contraceptive agents. Also, do not use for the treatment or prevention of pelvic inflammatory disease or sexually transmitted diseases. Do no use as a contraceptive or to self-treat or prevent sexually transmitted diseases or pelvic inflammatory disease.
- Do not douche for at least 6 hours after use of a vaginal spermicide.
- Do not use douche products during pregnancy unless instructed to do so by your doctor.
- If you have pelvic or stomach pain, fever, chills, nausea, vomiting, pus-like yellow cervical discharge with an odor, painful or frequent urination, genital sores or vaginal bleeding, contact your doctor immediately.
- If pain, soreness, swelling, redness, itching, excessive dryness, irritation, odor or discharge occurs or persists, or if symptoms continue after 7 days, discontinue use and call your doctor.
- An association has been reported between excessive douching and pelvic inflammatory disease, ectopic pregnancy and infertility.

---

*If you have any questions, consult your doctor, pharmacist, or health care provider.*

| Brand Name Examples | Supplied As |
|---|---|
| otc Conceptrol | **Vaginal gel**: 100 mg nonoxynol-9 |
| otc Conceptrol Contraceptive Inserts | **Vaginal suppositories**: 100 mg nonoxynol-9 |
| otc Delfen Contraceptive | **Vaginal foam**: 100 mg nonoxynol-9 |
| otc Encare | **Vaginal insert**: 100 mg nonoxynol-9 |
| otc Gynol II Original Formula | **Vaginal jelly**: 2% nonoxynol-9 |
| otc Gynol II Extra Strength, Koromex | **Vaginal jelly**: 3% nonoxynol-9 |
| otc Koromex Clear | **Vaginal gel**: 30% nonoxynol-9 |
| otc Ortho-Gynol Contraceptive | **Vaginal jelly**: 100 mg octoxynol 9 |
| otc Semicid [1] | **Vaginal suppositories**: 100 mg nonoxynol-9 |
| otc Milex Shur-Seal | **Vaginal gel**: 2% nonoxynol-9 |
| otc Durex | **Spermicide-containing condom**: 5% nonoxynol-9 |

[1] Contains methylparaben.

Topical contraceptive agents provide spermicidal action that is generally reliable when properly used either with a vaginal diaphragm or as the sole method of contraception. These agents are generally less effective than oral contraceptives. To reduce the potential for conception (pregnancy), follow directions for use carefully.

## Type of Drug:

Vaginal contraceptive.

## How the Drug Works:

Spermicides (nonoxynol-9, octoxynol) are agents that immobilize and inactivate sperm cells by rupturing or removing their outer membrane. The gel, cream, foam or jelly vehicle which carries the spermicide also serves as a partial barrier to the union of sperm with an egg by adhering to the opening of the cervix.

## Uses:

To prevent pregnancy. Can be used alone (at high concentrations [eg, at least 8%] or in large amounts) or with other contraceptive methods (eg, diaphragm, cervical cap, contraceptive sponge, condoms).

## Precautions:

*Do not use in the following situations:*
allergy to the active drug or any ingredient of the formulation

*Use with caution in the following situations:*
burning or irritation of vagina, penis or genital area following use
inability to understand directions for proper use

*Condom use and sexually transmitted diseases (STDs):* The CDC advises using condoms to prevent STDs. If used properly, condoms may help prevent infection by *Chlamydia trachomatis, Ureaplasma urealyticum, Trichomonas vaginalis, Candida albicans,* herpes simplex 1 and 2 (when lesions are on penis or female genital area), human papilloma virus, *Treponema pallidum, Haemophilus ducreyi* and AIDS.

*Nonoxynol-9* has been shown to inhibit or reduce the risk of chlamydia and, to a lesser degree, gonorrhea. Use of nonoxynol-9 has been shown to increase the risk of developing a yeast infection.

## Side Effects:

Every drug is capable of producing side effects. Most spermicide users experience no. or minor, side effects. Possible side effects include burning, irritation and itching.

---

### Guidelines for Use:

- Strictly follow manufacturer's instructions for proper use of these products in order to achieve maximum protection.
- *Contraceptive foam* — Thoroughly shake the aerosol canister before use.
- *Vaginal spermicides* — Apply at least 10 minutes (but no more than 1 hour) before intercourse to ensure effectiveness. Products provide 1 hour of protection and should be reapplied for repeated intercourse.
- Apply high in the vagina, near the cervix.
- One applicatorful of spermicide is enough for only one act of intercourse. A new dose is required prior to each act of intercourse.
- Do not douche for 6 or more hours after intercourse. Premature douching may dilute the spermicide and may propel sperm into the uterus.
- *Diaphragm* — For contraceptive effectiveness, leave the diaphragm in place for 6 hours after intercourse, but remove it as soon as possible thereafter. Toxic shock syndrome, which can be fatal, has been reported with the use of diaphragms.
- *Vaginal suppositories* must melt and be dispersed before intercourse. Suppositories may not be as effective a mechanical barrier over the cervical opening as foams, creams, jellies and gels. Do not insert suppositories into the urinary opening.
- Contact your doctor if vaginal, penile, or genital burning, itching, irritation or painful urination follows use.
- These agents are not as effective as oral contraceptives or certain combination methods of contraception (eg, condom plus spermicide).
- These products are inserted into the vagina only, not into the urethra or rectum.
- If pregnancy is medically contraindicated, consult your doctor for a contraception program.
- These products have not been shown to protect against STDs.

---

*If you have any questions, consult your doctor, pharmacist, or health care provider.*

| Generic Name<br>*Brand Name Examples* | Supplied As |
|---|---|
| **Rx** **Steroid-Containing Products** | |
| *Carmol HC* | **Cream**: 1% hydrocortisone acetate, 10% urea, sodium bisulfite, propylene glycol, alcohol, EDTA |
| *Proctocort* | **Cream**: 1% hydrocortisone, propylene glycol, benzyl alcohol |
| | **Suppositories**: 30 mg hydrocortisone acetate |
| *ProctoFoam-HC* | **Aerosol foam**: 1% hydrocortisone acetate, 1% pramoxine HCl, propylene glycol, parabens, alcohol |
| *Anucort-HC, Anumed-HC, Hemorrhoidal HC* | **Suppositories**: 25 mg hydrocortisone acetate |
| otc *Nupercainal* | **Cream**: 1% hydrocortisone cream, white petrolatum, propylene glycol, alcohol |
| otc *Corticaine* | **Cream**: 0.5% hydrocortisone acetate, propylene glycol, methylparaben |
| otc *Anusol HC-1* | **Ointment**: 1% hydrocortisone, mineral oil, propylene glycol, white petrolatum, parabens |
| otc **Local Anesthetic-Containing Products** | |
| *Medicone* | **Ointment**: 20% benzocaine, methylparaben |
| *Nupercainal* | **Ointment**: Dibucaine |
| *Anusol* | **Ointment**: 1% pramoxine HCl, benzyl benzoate, Peruvian balsam, 12.5% zinc oxide with mineral oil, cocoa butter |
| *Tronolane* | **Cream**: 1% pramoxine HCl in zinc oxide, glycerin, parabens, beeswax, alcohol |
| *ProctoFoam* | **Aerosol foam**: 1% pramoxine HCl, propylene glycol, parabens, alcohol |

| Generic Name<br>*Brand Name Examples* | Supplied As |
|---|---|
| *otc* **Local Vasoconstrictor-Containing Products** | |
| *Pazo Hemorrhoid* | **Ointment**: 0.2% ephedrine sulfate, 2% camphor and 5% zinc oxide with lanolin and petrolatum |
| *Preparation H* | **Ointment**: 71.9% petrolatum, 14% mineral oil, 3% shark liver oil and 0.25% phenylephrine HCl, glycerin, parabens, beeswax, lanolin |
| | **Suppositories**: 85.5% cocoa butter, 0.25% phenylephrine HCl, 3% shark liver oil, parabens |
| *Tronolane* | **Suppositories**: 5% zinc oxide, 95% hard fat |
| *Medicone* | **Suppositories**: 0.25% phenylephrine HCl, 88.7% hard fat, mineral oil, white petrolatum, propylene glycol, parabens |
| *Hem-Prep* | **Suppositories**: 0.25% phenylephrine HCl, 11% zinc oxide, hard fat |
| *otc* **Miscellaneous Combinations** | |
| *Rectagene Medicated Rectal Balm* | **Ointment**: Live yeast cell derivative that suppplies 2000 units of skin respiratory factor per ounce, 3% shark liver oil, 1:10,000 phenylmerconic nitrate, white petrolatum, lanolin |
| *Calmol 4* | **Suppositories**: 80% cocoa butter, 10% zinc oxide, parabens |
| *Nupercainal* | **Suppositories**: 2.1 g cocoa butter, 0.25 g zinc oxide, bismuth subgallate and sodium bisulfite |
| *Anusol* | **Suppositories**: 51% topical starch, benzyl alcohol |
| *otc* **Perianal Hygiene Products** | |
| *Tucks, Tucks Take-Alongs* | **Pads**: 50% witch hazel, glycerin, propylene glycol, parabens, alcohol |
| *Balneol Perianal Cleansing* | **Lotion**: Mineral oil, propylene glycol, glyceryl stearate, lanolin oil, sodium acetate and acetic acid, methylparaben |
| *ConvaTec Aloe Vesta Perineal* | **Solution**: Sodium $C_{12-14}$ olefin sulfonate, disodium cocoamphodiacetate, propylene glycol, aloe vera, sorbitol, DMDM hydantoin, cetethyl morpholinium ethosulfate and citric acid |

The anorectal (anus and rectum) preparations are used primarily for the symptomatic relief of the discomfort associated with hemorrhoids and peri-anal itching or irritation. In addition to the products listed in this section, many of the Topical Local Anesthetics and Topical Corticosteroids may also be used in anorectal therapy.

## Type of Drug:

Preparations used for minor disorders of the anus and rectum region.

## Uses:

The various components of these products are briefly discussed below. For complete information on these ingredients, refer to the appropriate monographs.

*Hydrocortisone* reduces inflammation, itching and swelling. Steroids are not recommended in fungal and most viral infections of the skin, including herpes, vaccinia, and varicella.

*Local anesthetics* (eg, benzocaine, dibucaine, pramoxine) temporarily relieve pain, itching and irritation. The most frequent side effects of topical local anesthetic use are allergic reactions (eg, burning, rash, itching).

*Vasoconstrictors* (eg, ephedrine or phenylephrine) reduce swelling and congestion of anorectal tissues. They relieve local itching by a slight anesthetic effect. These agents are not effective in stopping bleeding from tissues.

*Astringents* (eg, witch hazel, zinc oxide) shrink skin cells, protecting the underlying tissue and decreasing the cell volume. They lessen mucus and other secretions and relieve anorectal irritation and inflammation.

*Antiseptics* (eg, phenylmercuric nitrate, zinc oxide) are not of value when applied to the anorectal area. There is no convincing evidence that they prevent infection in the anorectal area. Many are present as preservatives.

*Emollients/protectants* (eg, cod liver oil, hard fat, glycerin, lanolin, mineral oil, petrolatum, zinc oxide, cocoa butter, shark liver oil, bismuth salts) form a physical barrier on the skin and lubricate tissues, preventing irritation of the anorectal area and water loss from the tissues. Many of these substances are used as bases and carriers of active ingredients.

*Humectants* (eg, propylene glycol) are water absorbing to blot and dry moisture from affected tissue.

*Counterirritants* (eg, menthol, camphor) evoke a feeling of comfort, cooling, tingling or warmth and diminish the perception of pain and itching.

*Keratolytics* (eg, resorcinol) cause shedding and sloughing of surface cells and may help to expose underlying tissue to therapeutic agents.

*Wound-healing agents* (eg, balsam Peru, skin respiratory factor [SRF]), yeast-cell derivative) are claimed to promote wound healing or tissue repair. Effectiveness of these compounds has not been demonstrated.

## Precautions:

*Do not use in the following situations:*

allergy to any ingredient in the
 preparations
diabetes
enlarged prostate gland

heart disease
high blood pressure
thyroid disease

*Use with caution in the following situations:*

children
infections, dermatological
occlusive dressings

*Pregnancy:* Adequate studies have not been done in pregnant women. Use only if clearly needed and potential benefits outweigh the possible hazards to the fetus.

*Breastfeeding:* It is not known if topical administration of corticosteroids subsequently appears in breast milk. Consult your doctor before you begin breastfeeding.

*Children:* Use steroid-containing agents with caution as children may demonstrate greater susceptibility to topical corticosteroid-induced HPA axis suppression due to a larger skin surface area-to-body weight ratio. Chronic cortiosteroid therapy may interfere with growth development.

## Side Effects:

Every drug is capable of producing side effects. Many anorectal preparations users experience no, or minor side effects. The frequency and severity of side effects depend on many factors including dose, duration of therapy and individual susceptibility. Possible side effects include:

*Skin:* Burning; itching; irritation; dryness; inflammation of follicles or skin; acne; allergic contact dermatitis; skin disorder; loss of pigmentation; allergic reaction; flaking of the skin; secondary infection.

## Guidelines for Use:

- Avoid contact with eyes.
- Dosage and uses vary. Please read the instructions for use on the packaging before using any of these medications.
- Creams, ointments and foams are for external use only.
- Do not use if you are allergic to any ingredient in these products.
- Do not use in young children (ages vary depending on product) unless instructed by your doctor.
- Maintain normal bowel movements by proper diet, adequate fluid intake and regular exercise.
- Avoid excessive laxative use.
- Stool softeners or bulk laxatives may be useful as an aid to some therapies.
- Avoid scratching or rubbing area; washing with strong or scented soaps; or eating spicy foods, peppers or tomatoes.
- Notify your doctor if symptoms do not improve in 7 days, or if bleeding, protrusion or seepage occurs. *Hydrocortisone-containing products* may cause the following side effects: Burning; itching; irritation; dryness; flaking of the skin; loss of pigment; allergic reaction; infection; blistering; abnormal hair growth; swelling of skin; skin disorder.
- Tell your doctor if you are pregnant, become pregnant, planning to become pregnant or are breastfeeding.
- *Hydrocortisone-containing products* — Do not bandage or cover with plastic dressings unless directed by your doctor. Do not use with tight-fitting diapers or plastic pants.
- *Products containing vasoconstrictors (eg, ephedrine, phenylephrine)* — Do not use if you have heart disease, high blood pressure, thyroid disease, diabetes or enlarged prostate with difficulty urinating unless directed by your doctor. Also, do not use if currently taking medications for high blood pressure or depression unless directed by your doctor.

*If you have any questions, consult your doctor, pharmacist, or health care provider.*

| Generic Name<br>*Brand Name Examples* | Supplied As | Generic<br>Available |
|---|---|---|
| **Benzoyl Peroxide, Cleansers** | | |
| *Rx* *Benzac W Wash 5 and 10, Desquam-X Wash* | **Liquid**: 5%, 10% | No |
| *otc* *Fostex 10% Wash* | **Liquid**: 10% | No |
| *otc* *PanOxyl* | **Bar**: 5%, 10% | No |
| *otc* **Benzoyl Peroxide, Lotions** | | |
| *Benoxyl 5,*[3,4] *Benoxyl 10,*[3,4] *Clearasil 10%, Loroxide* | **Lotion**: 5%, 5.5%, 10% | Yes |
| *otc* **Benzoyl Peroxide, Creams** | | |
| *Clearasil Maximum Strength,*[3,4] *Fostex*[5] | **Cream**: 5%, 10% | No |
| **Benzoyl Peroxide, Gels** | | |
| *otc* *Del Aqua-5, Del Aqua-10, Fostex, Oxy Balance, Oxy 10 Balance, Persa-Gel W* | **Gel**: 5%, 10% | No |
| *Rx* *Benzac 5 and 10,*[1] *Benzac W 2.5, 5 and 10, Benzagel,*[1] *Desquam-E, Desquam-X 5 and 10, PanOxyl 5 and 10,*[1] *PanOxyl AQ 2.5, 5 and 10*[3] | **Gel**: 2.5%, 5%, 10% | Yes |
| *Rx* **Benzoyl Peroxide Combinations** | | |
| *Benzamycin*[1,2] | **Gel**: 5% benzoyl peroxide and 3% erythromycin | No |
| *Sulfoxyl Regular* | **Lotion**: 5% benzoyl peroxide and 2% sulfur, propylene glycol | No |
| *Sulfoxyl Strong* | **Lotion**: 10% benzoyl peroxide and 5% sulfur, propylene glycol | No |
| *Vanoxide-HC* | **Lotion**: 5% benzyl peroxide, 0.5% hydrocortisone, mineral oil, lanolin, propylene glycol, parabens | No |

[1] Contains alcohol.
[2] For more information, see Erythromycin monograph.
[3] Contains methyparaben.
[4] Contains propylparaben.
[5] Contains salicylic acid.

## Type of Drug:

Acne products.

## How the Drug Works:

The effectiveness of benzoyl peroxide is related primarily to its keratolytic (skin sloughing) and antibacterial action, especially against *Propionibacterium acnes,* which is the predominant bacteria in sebaceous follicles and comedones (blackheads). The antibacterial activity is most likely related to its effects on bacterial proteins. Benzoyl peroxide's action is also aided by a drying action, removal of excess sebum (oil) and decreased sebum formation.

## Uses:

To treat mild to moderate acne vulgaris and oily skin. These medications can be used alone or in combination with other acne medications, including antibiotics. These agents should not be used to treat acne rosacea.

## Precautions:

*Do not use in the following situations:*

allergy to benzoyl peroxide, benzoic acid, cinnamon or any ingredients of the medications
hypersensitive skin

*Pseudomembranous colitis* may occur with the long-term use of *Benzamycin.* If severe diarrhea, stomach pain/cramps or bloody stools occur, contact your doctor immediately. This could be a symptom of a serious side effect requiring immediate medical attention. Do not treat diarrhea associated with *Benzamycin* use without consulting your doctor.

*Pregnancy:* Adequate studies have not been done in pregnant women. Use only if clearly needed and potential benefits outweigh the possible hazards to the fetus.

*Breastfeeding:* It is not known if benzoyl peroxide appears in breast milk. Consult your doctor before you begin breastfeeding.

*Children:* Safety and effectiveness in children under 12 years of age have not been established.

## Drug Interactions:

Tell your doctor or pharmacist if you are taking or if you are planning to take any over-the-counter or prescription medications or dietary supplements with benzoyl peroxide.

## Side Effects:

Every drug is capable of producing side effects. Many benzoyl peroxide users experience no, or minor, side effects. The frequency and severity of side effects depend on many factors including dose, duration of therapy and individual susceptibility. Possible side effects include: Excessive dryness, peeling, facial swelling, oiliness, redness, tenderness of skin; sloughing of skin; local irritation; edema (fluid accumulation in the treated area); stinging and burning on application; itching; blistering; excessive hair growth; loss of skin pigment; skin disorder; photosensitivity to sunlight or tanning beds.

## Guidelines for Use:

- Directions for use vary. Read instructions for medications carefully.
- For external use only. Keep away from eyes, eyelids, mouth, lips, inside the nose, any mucous membrane, and highly inflamed or damaged skin. If contact with eyes occurs, flush with water.
- May produce a temporary feeling of warmth or slight stinging. Expect dryness and peeling.
- If dryness, itching, swelling, redness, or peeling becomes excessive, reduce the frequency of application or discontinue use temporarily and contact your doctor.
- Adjust applications on a given day from no application to 2 applications. Eventually a routine schedule can be established.
- If irritation continues or becomes severe, discontinue use and consult your doctor.
- Use of other topical acne medications at the same time or following each other may increase dryness and irritation of the skin. If this occurs, use one medicine at a time unless directed by your doctor.
- Use moisturizers, cool compresses, or topical steroids (eg, hydrocortisone) to treat the side effects of excessive sensitivity, drying, redness, or peeling.
- Use a sunscreen and avoid sunlight, sunlamps, or other topical acne medications and sources of skin irritation unless directed by your doctor.
- Concurrent use of some of these products and PABA-containing sunscreens may result in temporary skin discoloration.
- May bleach hair or colored fabric. Avoid contact with hair and fabric if possible.
- Water-based cosmetics may be used after benzoyl peroxide use. Thoroughly remove prior to application of benzoyl peroxide.
- *Cleansers* (washes and bar soaps) — Use once or twice daily on the affected skin. Wet area prior to application and thoroughly rinse after application.
- *Creams, lotions, gels* — Apply once daily for the first few days. If dryness, redness, or peeling does not occur, increase frequency of application to 2 to 3 times daily.

*If you have any questions, consult your doctor, pharmacist, or health care provider.*

| Generic Name<br>*Brand Name Examples* | Supplied As | Generic<br>Available |
|---|---|---|
| *Rx* **Azelaic Acid** | | |
| *Azelex, Finevin* | **Cream**: 20% | No |

## Type of Drug:

Acne product.

## How the Drug Works:

The exact mechanism of action is not known. This medicine has been shown to have antibacterial action against certain bacteria when applied to the skin.

## Uses:

A skin cream used to treat mild to moderate acne in patients older than 12 years of age.

## Precautions:

*Do not use in the following situations:* Allergy to azelaic acid or any of its ingredients.

*Use with caution in the following situations:* Persons with dark complexions.

*Pregnancy:* Studies in pregnant women or in animals have been judged not to show a risk to the fetus. However, no drug should be used during pregnancy unless clearly needed.

*Breastfeeding:* Azelaic acid may appear in breast milk. Consult your doctor before you begin breastfeeding.

*Children:* Safety and effectiveness in children under 12 years of age have not been established.

## Side Effects:

Every drug is capable of producing side effects. Many azelaic acid users experience no, or minor, side effects. The frequency and severity of side effects depend on many factors including dose, duration of therapy, and individual susceptibility. Possible side effects include:

*Skin:* Itching; burning; stinging; tingling; rash; irritation; redness; dryness; peeling; skin color changes.

## Guidelines for Use:

- Dosage is individualized. Use exactly as prescribed.
- Continue use until all of the prescribed medicine has been used. Failure to use a full course of therapy may prevent complete elimination of bacteria.
- For use on the skin only. Do not use in eyes.
- Wash skin thoroughly and pat dry. Gently, but thoroughly, massage a thin film of the medicine into the affected area twice a day (morning and evening). Wash hands following use. Length of treatment may vary depending upon the severity of the acne. Improvement usually occurs within 4 weeks.
- If a dose is missed, apply it as soon as possible. If several hours have passed or if it is nearing time for the next dose, do not double the dose to catch up, unless advised to do so by your doctor. Of more than one dose is missed or it is necessary to establish a new dosage schedule, contact your doctor or pharmacist.
- If sensitivity or severe irritation develops with the use of this medicine, discontinue use and contact your doctor.
- Do not use tight dressings or wrappings on the affected areas.
- Do not use near mouth, eyes, or other mucous membranes (eg, nose). If this medicine does come into contact with eyes, wash eyes with large amounts of tap water. Contact your doctor if eye irritation persists.
- If you have a dark complexion, contact your doctor if you have any changes in skin color (eg, light spots).
- Temporary skin irritation (ie, itching, burning, stinging) may occur when this medicine is applied to broken or inflamed skin, usually at the beginning of treatment. This irritation usually subsides with continued use. If irritation continues, use only once-a-day, or stop using this medicine until the side effects have subsided. If irritation persists, stop using this medicine and contact your doctor.
- Store at room temperature (59° to 86°F). Do not freeze.

*If you have any questions, consult your doctor, pharmacist, or health care provider.*

| Generic Name<br>*Brand Name Examples* | Supplied As | Generic<br>Available |
|---|---|---|
| **Sulfur Preparations** | | |
| otc *Fostex Medicated Cover-Up* | **Cream**: 2% sulfur | No |
| otc *Transact* | **Gel**: 2% sulfur, 40% alcohol and laureth-4 | No |
| otc *Xerac* | **Gel**: 4% microcrystalline sulfur and 44% isopropyl alcohol | No |
| otc *Liquimat* | **Lotion**: 5% sulfur and 22% alcohol | No |
| otc *Sulpho-Lac* | **Soap**: 5% sulfur | No |
| Rx *Bensulfoid*[1] | **Powder**: Highly reactive sulfur on colloidal bentonite | No |

[1] For compounding prescriptions.

## Type of Drug:
Acne product.

## How the Drug Works:
Sulfur provides antibacterial, peeling and drying actions. Although it may help to clear up comedones ("blackheads"), it may also promote the development of new ones.

## Uses:
To aid in the treatment of mild acne and oily skin.

## Guidelines for Use:
- For external use only.
- Apply a thin film 1 to 3 times daily. Cleanse skin thoroughly with a mild cleanser prior to use.
- Avoid overuse and contact with the eyes. Certain people may be allergic to one or more ingredients. If skin irritation develops or becomes excessive, discontinue use and consult your doctor.

*If you have any questions, consult your doctor, pharmacist, or health care provider.*

| Generic Name *Brand Name Example* | Supplied As | Generic Available |
|---|---|---|
| Rx **Adapalene** | | |
| *Differin* | **Cream:** 0.1% | No |
| *Differin* | **Gel:** 0.1% | No |
| *Differin* | **Solution:** 0.1% | No |

## Type of Drug:
Retinoid; acne agent.

## How the Drug Works:
How adapalene works on acne is not fully known. Adapalene appears to reduce the abnormal skin cell formation and inflammation (ie, redness, swelling) that are thought to cause acne.

## Uses:
For the topical treatment of acne vulgaris.

## Precautions:
*Do not use in the following situations:*
allergy to the drug or any of its ingredients
eczematous skin
skin cuts or abrasions
sunburned skin

*Use with caution in the following situations:*
skin sensitivity or chemical irritation
sun or extreme weather exposure (eg, wind, cold)

*Photosensitivity:* Minimize exposure to sunlight and sunlamps. Use effective sunscreen (at least SPF 15) any time you are outside. For extended sun exposure, wear protective clothing. If sunburn occurs, stop therapy until skin has recovered.

*Pregnancy:* There are no adequate and well-controlled studies in pregnant women. Use only if clearly needed and potential benefits outweigh potential risks to the fetus.

*Breastfeeding:* It is not known if adalapene is excreted in breast milk. Consult your doctor before you begin breastfeeding.

*Children:* Safety and effectiveness in children younger than 12 years of age have not been established.

## Drug Interactions:
Tell your doctor or pharmacist if you are taking or planning to take any over-the-counter or prescription medications or dietary supplements with this drug. Drug doses may need to be modified or a different drug prescribed. Potentially irritating topical products (eg, sulfur, resorcinol, salicylic acid) interact with this drug.

## Side Effects:

Every drug is capable of producing side effects. Many patients experience no, or minor, side effects. The frequency and severity of side effects depend on many factors including dose, duration of therapy, and individual susceptibility. Possible side effects include skin redness, dryness, scaling, itching, burning, or irritation, sunburn, acne flares, or stinging.

### Guidelines for Use:

- Dosage is individualized. Use exactly as prescribed.
- Read patient instructions provided with the product before starting therapy and with each refill.
- Cleanse area with a mild or soapless cleanser before applying medication.
- Apply a thin film once a day to affected areas in the evening before bedtime.
- *Pledgets* — Remove pledget from foil packet just before using. Discard pledget after using once. Do not reuse pledget. Do not use if seal is broken.
- *Solution* — Apply solution directly to affected skin using applicator in bottle.
- Moisturizers may be used if necessary; however, avoid products containing alpha hydroxy or glycolic acids.
- For external use only. Avoid contact with eyes, lips, angles of the nose, and mucous membranes. Exposure of the eye to this medication may result in swelling, conjunctivitis, and eye irritation.
- Do not apply to cuts, abrasions, or eczematous or sunburned skin.
- Concomitant use of other potentially-irritating topical products (eg, medicated or abrasive soaps and cleansers, soaps and cosmetics that have a strong drying effect, products with a high concentration of alcohol, astringents, spices, or lime) should be approached with caution. Exercise particular caution in using preparations containing sulfur, resorcinol, or salicylic acid. If these preparations have been used, it is advisable not to start therapy with adapalene until the effects on the skin have subsided.
- Application may cause a feeling of warmth and slight stinging. This is normal.
- Use may cause redness, dryness, scaling, burning, or itching at site of application. These reactions are most likely to occur during the first 2 to 4 weeks of therapy, are mostly mild to moderate in intensity, and will usually lessen with continued medication. If symptoms persist or worsen, use the medication less frequently, stop use temporarily, or stop use altogether, as recommended by your doctor.
- Avoid prolonged exposure to the sun and other sources of ultraviolet (UV) light (eg, tanning beds). Use sunscreens and wear protective clothing.
- May cause an unusual sensitivity to wind and cold. Avoid when possible.
- Avoid the use of waxing as a depilatory method on skin because of the potential for skin erosions.

## Guidelines for Use (cont.):

- If excessive medication is applied, redness, peeling, or discomfort may occur. Excessive application does not improve results.
- Early in treatment, acne may appear to worsen. Do not stop therapy. Positive effects may be seen after 2 weeks, but at least 8 weeks are required to obtain consistent beneficial effects.
- Inform your doctor if you are pregnant, become pregnant, plan on becoming pregnant, or are breastfeeding.
- Store at controlled room temperature (68° to 77°F). Protect from freezing. Keep solution bottle tightly closed and store upright.

*If you have any questions, consult your doctor, pharmacist, or health care provider.*

| Generic Name<br>*Brand Name Example* | Supplied As | Generic<br>Available |
|---|---|---|
| Rx **Alitretinoin** | | |
| *Panretin* | **Gel:** 0.1% | No |

## Type of Drug:
Second generation retinoid.

## How the Drug Works:
Alitretinoin alters skin cell growth and development and appears to be able to stop the growth of Kaposi sarcoma (KS) cells.

## Uses:
For the topical treatment of skin lesions in patients with AIDS-related Kaposi sarcoma (KS).

## Precautions:
*Do not use in the following situations:*
> allergy to the drug or any of its ingredients
> systemic KS therapy

*Use with caution in the following situations:* Cutaneous T-cell lymphoma.

*Photosensitivity:* Retinoids as a class have been associated with photosensitivity. Minimize exposure of treated areas to sunlight and sunlamps.

*Pregnancy:* Studies have shown a potential adverse effect on the fetus. Use only if clearly needed and potential benefits outweigh the possible risks to the fetus.

*Breastfeeding:* It is not known if alitretinoin is excreted in breast milk. Because of the potential adverse reactions in nursing infants, mothers should discontinue breastfeeding prior to using the drug. Consult your doctor before you begin breastfeeding.

*Children:* Safety and effectiveness have not been established.

*Elderly:* Inadequate information is available to assess safety and effectiveness in patients 65 years of age and older.

## Drug Interactions:
Tell your doctor or pharmacist if you are taking or planning to take any over-the-counter or prescription medications or dietary supplements with this drug. Drug doses may need to be modified or a different drug prescribed. DEET (N, N-diethyl-m-toluamide) (eg, *Deep Woods OFF*) interacts with this drug.

## Side Effects:

Every drug is capable of producing side effects. Many patients experience no, or minor, side effects. The frequency and severity of side effects depend on many factors including dose, duration of therapy, and individual susceptibility. Possible side effects include skin rash, irritation, scaling, redness, inflammation, itching, burning, pain, flaking, peeling, exfoliation, cracking, scabbing, crusting, drainage, oozing, fissure, abnormal skin sensations (eg, stinging, tingling), or swelling.

---

### Guidelines for Use:

- Dosage is individualized. Use exactly as prescribed.
- Initially apply 2 times/day to lesions. The application frequency can be gradually increased to 3 or 4 times/day, depending on response to medication. If irritation occurs, reduce frequency of application. If severe irritation occurs, discontinue applications for a few days until symptoms subside.
- Do not stop taking or change the dose, unless instructed by your doctor.
- For external use only. Avoid gel application to normal skin surrounding lesions. Do not apply gel on or near mucosal surfaces of the body.
- Cover lesions with generous gel coating. Allow gel to dry 3 to 5 minutes before covering with clothing.
- Do not use occlusive dressings with gel.
- This is not a systemic therapy. It cannot treat visceral KS or prevent development of new lesions where it has not been applied.
- May cause sensitivity to sunlight. Avoid prolonged exposure to the sun or other forms of ultraviolet (UV) light (eg, tanning beds). Use sunscreens and wear protective clothing until tolerance is determined.
- Many insect repellent products contain DEET, which produces adverse reactions when used concurrently with alitretinoin. Do not use without consulting your doctor.
- Inform your doctor if you are pregnant, become pregnant, are planning to become pregnant, or are breastfeeding.
- Improvement of lesions may be seen as soon as 2 weeks after starting therapy, but most patients require longer application (4 to 14 weeks). Further benefit may be attained with continued application.
- Store at room temperature (59° to 86°F). Keep tube tightly capped.

---

*If you have any questions, consult your doctor, pharmacist, or health care provider.*

| Generic Name<br>*Brand Name Examples* | Supplied As | Generic<br>Available |
|---|---|---|
| *Rx* **Tretinoin** | | |
| *Avita*[1] | **Cream**: 0.025% | No |
| *Altinac, Retin-A* | **Cream**: 0.025%, 0.05%, 0.1% | No |
| *Renova*[1] | **Cream**: 0.02%, 0.05% | No |
| *Avita,*[1] *Retin-A*[1] | **Gel**: 0.025%, | No |
| *Retin-A Micro* | **Gel**: 0.04%, 0.1% | No |
| *Retin-A*[1] | **Gel**: 0.01% | No |
| *Retin-A*[1] | **Liquid**: 0.05% | No |

[1] Contains alcohol.

## Type of Drug:
Acne agent; trans-retinoic acid; vitamin A acid.

## How the Drug Works:
The exact mechanism of action is not known. Tretinoin appears to increase skin-cell turnover and reduce the tendency for skin cells to stick together. This reduces the formation of pimples and allows quicker healing of pimples that do develop.

## Uses:
To treat mild to moderate acne vulgaris.

As an adjunct to a comprehensive skin care program to reduce fine facial wrinkles.

*Unlabeled Use(s):* Occasionally doctors may prescribe tretinoin to treat several different forms of skin cancer, lamellar ichthyosis, mollusca contagiosa, verrucae plantaris, verrucae planae juveniles, ichthyosis vulgaris, bullous congenital ichthyosiform, and pityriasis rubra pilaris. Tretinoin also has been used to reduce liver spots associated with aging and to enhance the absorption of topical minoxidil.

## Precautions:
*Do not use in the following situations:*
allergy to the drug or any of its ingredients
eczematous skin
photosensitizing drug therapy (eg, tetracycline), current
skin irritation, severe or persistant
sunburn

*Use with caution in the following situations:*
skin irritation, redness, or dryness
sun or extreme weather exposure

*Photosensitivity:* Minimize exposure to sunlight and sunlamps. Use effective sunscreen (at least SPF 15) any time you are outside, even on hazy days. For extended sun exposure, wear protective clothing. Do not use artificial sunlamps or UV tanning booths while using tretinoin. If sunburn occurs, stop therapy until skin has recovered.

*Pregnancy:* There are no adequate and well-controlled studies in pregnant women. Use only if clearly needed and potential benefits outweigh the possible risks to the fetus.

*Breastfeeding:* It is not known if tretinoin appears in breast milk. Consult your doctor before you begin breastfeeding.

## Drug Interactions:

Tell your doctor or pharmacist if you are taking or planning to take any over-the-counter or prescription medications or dietary supplements with this drug. Drug doses may need to be modified or a different drug prescribed. The following drugs and drug classes interact with this drug:

fluoroquinolones (eg, ciprofloxacin)
phenothiazines (eg, promethazine HCl)
sulfonamides (eg, sulfadiazine)
tetracyclines (eg, doxycycline)
thiazides (eg, chlorothiazide)

## Side Effects:

Every drug is capable of producing side effects. Many patients experience no, or minor, side effects. The frequency and severity of side effects depend on many factors, including dose, duration of therapy, and individual susceptibility. Possible side effects include: Red, swollen, irritated skin; blistered or crusted skin; increased or decreased skin pigmentation (color); increased sensitivity to sunlight; itching; peeling; stinging.

## Guidelines for Use:

- Dosage is individualized. Use exactly as prescribed.
- For external use only.
- Read patient instructions provided with the product.
- Wash area to be treated thoroughly with a mild soap before use and dry skin gently. Wait 20 to 30 minutes for skin to dry before applying medication.
- Lightly apply to affected area once a day at bedtime. Wash hands immediately after use.
- Keep away from eyes, mouth, angles of the nose, mucous membranes, and open wounds.
- *Liquid* — Apply with fingertip, gauze pad, or cotton swab. Do not overwet. Liquid may run into uneffected areas.
- *Gel* — Excessive application results in "pilling" of the gel.
- Application may cause a feeling of warmth and slight stinging. This is normal.
- Use may cause severe redness and peeling at the site of application. If these symptoms persist, use the medication less frequently, stop use temporarily, or stop use altogether, if recommended by your doctor.
- Tretinoin may cause sensitivity to sunlight and other sources of ultraviolet light. Avoid prolonged exposure to the sun. Use sunscreens and wear protective clothing until tolerance is determined.
- May cause an unusual sensitivity to wind and cold. Avoid when possible.
- Use of other agents to promote sloughing of skin (eg, sulfur, resorcinol, salicylic acid), use of another topical medication at the same time, medicated or abrasive soaps, and cleansers with a strong drying effect (eg, alcohol, astringents, spices, lime) are not recommended. "Rest" the skin for a few days before beginning tretinoin.
- If excessive medication is applied, redness, peeling, and pain may occur. Excessive application does not improve results.
- Every morning after washing the affected area apply a moisturizer with sunscreen (at least SPF 15) that will not aggravate your acne.
- Cosmetics may be used; however, thoroughly remove cosmetics before applying tretinoin.
- Early in treatment, acne may appear worse due to the action of the drug. Do not stop therapy. Positive effects should be seen in 2 to 3 weeks but may not be optimal for 6 weeks or more. Many users see improvement by 12 weeks.
- Once tolerance is determined, the frequency of application may be increased. Application procedures, drug concentration, and dose frequency will be closely monitored by your doctor.
- Once a good response is seen, therapy may be maintained with less frequent application or lower concentrations.
- Do not allow anyone else to use this medication.
- Store the liquid and gel below 86°F and the cream below 80°F. Avoid freezing. The gel is flammable. Keep away from heat and flame.

*If you have any questions, consult your doctor, pharmacist, or health care provider.*

| Brand Name Examples | Sulfur | Salicylic Acid | Other Content |
|---|---|---|---|
| **Creams, Lotions and Gels** | | | |
| *otc* *Acno Lotion* | 3% | | |
| *otc* *Acnomel Cream* | 8% | | 11% alcohol, 2% resorcinol |
| *otc* *Acnotex Lotion* | 8% | | 20% isopropyl alcohol, 2% resorcinol |
| *Rx* *Bensulfoid Cream* | 8%[1] | | 12% alcohol, 2% resorcinol |
| *otc* *Clearasil Adult Care Cream* | † | | Resorcinol, 10% alcohol, parabens |
| *otc* *Clearasil Clearstick Maximum Strength* | | 2% | 39% alcohol, menthol, EDTA |
| *otc* *Clearasil Clearstick Regular Strength* | | 1.25% | 39% alcohol, aloe vera gel, menthol, disodium, EDTA |
| *otc* *Clearasil Double Clear Maximum Strength Pads* | | 2% | 40% alcohol, witch hazel distillate, menthol |
| *otc* *Clearasil Double Clear Regular Strength Pads* | | 1.25% | 40% alcohol, witch hazel distillate, menthol |
| *otc* *Cuticura Ointment* | 0.5%[2] | | 0.1% phenol, 0.05% oxyquinoline |
| *otc* *Finac Lotion* | | 2% | 22.5% isopropyl alcohol, propylene glycol, acetone |
| *otc* *Fostex Acne Cleansing Cream* | | 2% | Stearyl alcohol, EDTA |
| *otc* *Fostril Lotion* | † | | Zinc oxide, parabens, EDTA |
| *otc* *Medicated Acne Cleanser* | 4% | | 2% resorcinol |
| *otc* *Neutrogena Drying Gel* | | | Isopropyl alcohol, witch hazel, EDTA, parabens, tartrazine |

| Brand Name Examples | Sulfur | Salicylic Acid | Other Content |
|---|---|---|---|
| Rx Novacet Lotion | 5% | | 10% sodium sulfacetamide, cetyl alcohol, benzyl alcohol, EDTA, sodium thiosulfate |
| otc Oxy Night Watch Maximum Strength Lotion | | 2% | Cetyl alcohol, EDTA, parabens, stearyl alcohol |
| otc Oxy Night Watch Sensitive Skin Lotion | | 1% | Cetyl alcohol, EDTA, stearyl alcohol, parabens |
| otc PROPApH Acne Maximum Strength Cream | | 2% | Lanolin alcohol, cetearyl alcohol, stearyl alcohol, menthol, EDTA |
| otc PROPApH Cleansing Lotion for Normal/ Combination Skin | | 0.5% | SD alcohol 40, menthol, EDTA |
| otc PROPApH Cleansing Pads | | | |
| otc PROPApH Cleansing for Oily Skin Lotion | | 0.6% | SD alcohol 40, EDTA, menthol |
| otc RA Lotion | | | 43% alcohol, 3% resorcinol |
| otc Rezamid Lotion | 5% | | 28% alcohol, 2% resorcinol |
| otc R/S Lotion | | | |
| otc Sal-Clens Acne Cleanser Gel | | 2% | |
| otc Seale's Lotion Modified | 6.4% | | |
| otc Sebasorb Lotion | | 2% | 10% attapulgite |
| Rx Sodium Sulfacetamide 10% and Sulfur 5% | 5% | | 10% sodium sulfacetamide, cetyl alcohol, benzyl alcohol, EDTA |
| otc Stridex Clear Gel | | 2% | 9.3% SD alcohol |
| Rx Sulfacet-R Lotion | 5% | | 10% sodium sulfacetamide, parabens |

| Brand Name Examples | Sulfur | Salicylic Acid | Other Content |
|---|---|---|---|
| otc  Sulforcin Lotion | 5% | | 11.65% SD alcohol, 2% resorcinol, methylparaben |
| otc  Therac Lotion | 10%[1] | | |
| **Medicated Bar Cleansers** | | | |
| otc  Aveeno Cleansing for Acne-Prone Skin[3] | | † | Colliodal oatmeal, glycerin, titanium dioxide |
| otc  Buf-Puf Acne Cleansing | | 2% | Vitamin E acetate, EDTA |
| otc  Clearasil Antibacterial Soap | | | triclosan |
| otc  Fostex Acne Medication Cleansing Bar | | 2% | EDTA |
| otc  Oxy Medicated Soap | | | 1% triclosan, EDTA |
| otc  Salicylic Acid Cleansing Bar | | 2% | EDTA |
| otc  Salicylic Acid and Sulfur Soap | 10% | 3% | |
| otc  SAStid Soap | 10% | | EDTA |
| otc  Sulfur Soap | | | |
| otc  Stri-Dex Cleansing Bar | | | 1% triclosan, lanolin, alcohol, EDTA |
| **Abrasive Cleansers** | | | |
| otc  Brasivol | | | Aluminum oxide in a surfactant cleansing base |
| otc  Ionax | | | Benzalkonium Cl, SD alcohol 40 |
| otc  Listerex Scrub | | 2% | Methylparaben, tartrazine |

| Brand Name Examples | Sulfur | Salicylic Acid | Other Content |
|---|---|---|---|
| otc  Pernox Lathering Abradant Scrub Lotion | † | † | |
| otc  Pernox Scrub for Oily Skin | † | † | EDTA |
| otc  PROPApH Peel-Off Acne Mask | | 2% | Polyvinyl alcohol, parabens, SD alcohol 40, vitamin E acetate |
| otc  Seba-Nil Cleansing Mask | | | SD alcohol 40, castor oil, methylparaben |
| **Liquid Cleansers** | | | |
| otc  Acno Cleanser | | | 60% isopropyl alcohol, EDTA |
| otc  Clearasil Double Textured Pads Maximum Strength | | 2% | 40% alcohol, aloe vera gel, menthol, EDTA |
| otc  Clearasil Double Textured Pads Regular Strength | | 2% | 40% alcohol, glycerin, aloe vera gel, EDTA |
| otc  Clearasil Medicated Deep Cleaner | | 0.5% | 42% alcohol, menthol, EDTA, aloe vera gel, castor oil |
| otc  Drytex Lotion | | † | 40% isopropyl alcohol, 10% acetone, tartrazine |
| otc  Exact | | 2% | Propylene glycol, parabens, aloe vera gel, EDTA, menthol, glycerin, diazolidinyl urea |
| otc  Ionax Astringent Cleanser | | † | EDTA, isopropyl alcohol |
| otc  Ionax Foam | | | Benzalkonium Cl, propylene glycol |
| otc  Neutrogena Antiseptic Cleanser for Acne-Prone Skin | | | Benzethonium chloride, butylene glycol, menthol, methylparaben, witch hazel, camphor, peppermint oil, eucalyptus oil, cornmint oil |

| Brand Name Examples | Sulfur | Salicylic Acid | Other Content |
|---|---|---|---|
| otc Neutrogena Oil-Free Acne Wash | | 2% | EDTA, propylene glycol, aloe, tartrazine |
| otc Oil of Olay Foaming Face Wash Liquid | | | Potassium cocoyl, collagen, glycerin, EDTA |
| otc Oxy Medicated Cleanser & Pads Regular Strength | | 0.5% | 40% alcohol, citric acid, menthol, propylene glycol |
| otc Oxy Medicated Pads Maximum Strength | | 2% | 50% alcohol, propylene glycol, citric acid, menthol |
| otc Oxy Medicated Pads Sensitive Skin | | 0.5% | 22% alcohol, disodium lauryl sulfosuccinate, menthol, trisodium EDTA |
| otc Oxy ResiDON'T Medicated Face Wash | | | Cocamidopropyl betaine, sodium laureth sulfate, sodium cocoyl isethionate, triclosan, diazolidinyl urea |
| otc PROPApH Cleansing Maximum Strength Pads | | 2% | SD alcohol 40, EDTA, propylene glycol, menthol, aloe vera gel |
| otc PROPApH Cleansing for Sensitive Skin Pads | | 0.5% | SD alcohol 40, EDTA, menthol, aloe vera gel |
| otc PROPApH Foaming Face Wash | | 2% | EDTA, menthol, aloe vera gel |
| otc SalAc Cleanser | 2% | | Benzyl alcohol, glyceryl cocoate |
| otc Seba-Nil Oily Skin Cleanser | | | SD alcohol 40, acetone |
| otc Stri-Dex Pads Oil Fighting Formula | | 2% | citric acid, 54% SD alcohol, menthol |
| otc Stri-Dex Pads Maximum Strength | | 2% | 44% SD alcohol, citric acid, menthol |

| Brand Name Examples | Sulfur | Salicylic Acid | Other Content |
|---|---|---|---|
| otc Stri-Dex Pads Regular Strength | | 0.5% | 28% SD alcohol, citric acid, menthol |
| otc Stri-Dex Pads Sensitive Skin | | 0.5% | Citric acid, menthol, aloe vera gel, 28% SD alcohol |
| otc Tyrosum Cleanser Liquid and Packets | | | 50% isopropanol, 2% polysorbate 80, 10% acetone |
| Rx Xerac AC | | | 6.25% aluminum chloride hexahydrate in 96% anhy-drous ethyl alcohol |

[1] As colloidal sulfur.
[2] As precipitated sulfur.
[3] Soap free.
† Percentage not listed in manufacturer insert.

## Type of Drug:

Acne products.

## How the Drug Works:

These products contain keratolytics (peeling agents) and astringents (shrinking agents) to aid in removing keratin and to dry the skin. Many products also contain water, alcohol or organic solvent bases to aid in the removal of sebum (oil).

## Uses:

*Parachlorometaxylenol, sodium thiosulfate* and *sodium sulfacetamide* have antimicrobial activity (treat or prevent infection).

*Benzalkonium chloride, oxyquinoline, methylbenethzonium chloride, ethanol, isopropyl alcohol, phenol, triclosan, thymol* and *sulfur* are antiseptics (prevent infection).

*Zinc oxide* and *calamine* are astringents.

*Methylsalicylate* is a local anesthetic and counterirritant.

*Salicylic acid, resorcinol* and *sulfur* are keratolytics.

*Titanium dioxide* and *zinc oxide* are protectives and absorbants.

---

### Guidelines for Use:

- Use exactly as prescribed or directed.
- For external use only.
- *Lotions* — Shake well before using.
- Apply a thin film 1 to 3 times daily. Cleanse the skin thoroughly with a mild cleanser and dry the skin before applying the medication.
- Avoid overuse.
- Avoid contact with eyes, mouth, nose or other mucous membranes. If contact occurs, bathe the area with large amounts of tap water for several minutes.
- Certain people may be sensitive to one or more ingredients. If skin irritation develops or becomes excessive, discontinue use and consult your doctor.

---

*If you have any questions, consult your doctor, pharmacist, or health care provider.*

| Generic Name<br>*Brand Name Examples* | Supplied As | Generic<br>Available |
|---|---|---|
| *Rx* **Anthralin**<br>*Anthra-Derm,*<br>*Drithocreme,*<br>*Drithocreme HP 1%,*<br>*Dritho-Scalp* | **Ointment**: 0.1, 0.25, 0.5, 1%<br>**Cream:** 0.1, 0.25, 0.5, 1% | No<br>No |

## Type of Drug:

Agent for psoriasis.

## How the Drug Works:

Anthralin apparently slows the rate of skin cell growth by inhibiting forma-tion of DNA.

## Uses:

To treat psoriasis.

## Precautions:

*Do not use in the following situations:* Allergy to anthralin, acute or inflamed psoriasis, or use on face.

*Use with caution in the following situations:* Kidney disease or long-term anthralin use.

*Pregnancy:* Adequate studies have not been done in pregnant women, or animal studies may have shown a risk to the fetus. Use only if clearly needed and potential benefits outweigh the possible hazards to the fetus.

*Breastfeeding:* It is not known if anthralin appears in breast milk. Consult your doctor before you begin breastfeeding.

*Children:* Safety and effectiveness have not been established.

*Lab tests or exams* may be required to monitor therapy. Keep appointments.

## Side Effects:

Every drug is capable of producing side effects. Many patients experience no, or minor, side effects. The frequency and severity of side effects depend on many factors including dose, duration of therapy and indi-vidual susceptibility. Possible side effects include: Irritation of normal skin, discoloration of fingernails and hair.

## Guidelines for Use:

- Use exactly as prescribed.
- For external use only. Remove by washing. Rinse tub with hot water after use.
- Apply with plastic gloves. Wash hands after use. May stain fabrics, skin or hair.
- Apply a thin layer as directed to psoriatic lesions only. Rub gently until absorbed.
- Therapy may be gradually increased. High concentrations may cause irritation.
- Keep away from eyes. Do not use on face, genitalia, folds or creases of skin. Remove any residue from behind ears. Stop use if allergic reactions or if skin irritation develops. If excessive soreness occurs or lesions spread, reduce application frequency; if severe, stop using and consult your doctor.
- Wait at least 1 week between discontinuing topical steroids and starting anthralin therapy. Continue treatment until skin is entirely clear.
- Store at room temperature (59° to 88° F) in a tightly sealed container.

*If you have any questions, consult your doctor, pharmacist, or health care provider.*

| Generic Name
*Brand Name Example* | Supplied As | Generic Available |
|---|---|---|
| *Rx* **Calcipotriene**
*Dovonex* | **Ointment**: 0.005% | No |

## Type of Drug:
Agent for psoriasis.

## How the Drug Works:
Calcipotriene is a synthetic vitamin $D_3$ derivative.

## Uses:
To treat psoriasis.

## Precautions:
*Do not use in the following situations:*
allergy to calcipotriene or any of its components
evidence of vitamin D poisoning
excess calcium in the blood

*Use with caution in the following situations:*
elevated calcium levels in the blood.
irritation of psoriasis lesions and surrounding skin.

*Pregnancy:* Adequate studies have not been done in pregnant women. Use only if clearly needed and potential benefits outweigh the possible hazards to the fetus.

*Breastfeeding:* It is not known if calcipotriene appears in breast milk. Consult your doctor before you begin breastfeeding.

*Children:* Safety and effectiveness have not been established.

*Elderly:* Side effects may be more severe.

## Side Effects:
Every drug is capable of producing side effects. Many calcipotriene users experience no, or minor, side effects. The frequency and severity of side effects depend on many factors including dose, duration of therapy and individual susceptibility. Possible side effects include: Burning; itching; irritation; redness; inflammation; dry skin; peeling; rash and worsening of psoriasis; including development of facial or scalp psoriasis.

## Guidelines for Use:

- For external use only.
- Use only as directed by your physician. Keep away from eyes; do not apply to face. Wash hands after using.
- Apply a thin layer to the affected skin twice daily and rub in gently and completely.
- Do not use this medication for any disorder other than that for which it was prescribed.
- Report to your physician any signs of local adverse reactions. If irritation develops, discontinue use.

*If you have any questions, consult your doctor, pharmacist, or health care provider.*

| Generic Name<br>*Brand Name Example* | Supplied As | Generic<br>Available |
|---|---|---|
| Rx **Acitretin** | | |
| *Soriatane*[1] | **Capsules**: 10 mg, 25 mg | No |

[1] Contains gelatin, methyl- and propylparabens, benzyl alcohol and edetate calcium disodium.

## Type of Drug:

A retinoid. Related to retinoic acid and retinol (vitamin A).

## How the Drug Works:

The mechanism of action is unknown.

## Uses:

To treat severe psoriasis unresponsive to other therapies or when other treatments are contraindicated in adults.

## Precautions:

*Do not use in the following situations:*

alcohol consumption
allergy to any ingredient in the product
benign intracranial hypertension
blood donor
breastfeeding
paraben sensitivity
pregnancy
visual difficulties

*Use with caution in the following situations:*

diabetes
kidney disease, severe
lipid disturbance, family history
liver disease, severe
obesity
spine, bone, joint problems
triglyceride increases
vitamin A use
women of childbearing potential

*Pseudotumor cerebri* (benign intracranial hypertension) has occurred with acitretin. Early signs and symptoms include pain behind the eyes, headache, nausea, vomiting and visual disturbances. If present, discontinue the drug immediately and consult your doctor.

*Pregnancy:* Women who are pregnant or who may become pregnant must not use acitretin. There is an extremely high risk that a deformed infant will result if pregnancy occurs while taking this drug in any amount, even for short periods. Potentially all exposed fetuses can be affected.

*Breastfeeding:* It is not known if acetretin appears in breast milk. However, nursing mothers should not take acitretin because of the potential for excretion in milk and the serious adverse reactions that may have on the infant.

*Children:* Safety and effectiveness in children have not been established.

*Lab tests* are required to monitor treatment. Tests may include blood lipid, triglycerides, cholesterol, liver function and pregnancy. Be sure to keep appointments.

## Drug Interactions:

Tell your doctor or pharmacist if you are taking or planning to take any over-the-counter or prescription medications or dietary supplements while taking acitretin. Doses of one or both drugs may need to be modified or a different drug may need to be prescribed. The following drugs and drug classes interact with acitretin:

alcohol
methotrexate (eg, *Rheumatrex*)

progestin microdosed "minipill"
vitamin A

## Side Effects:

Every drug is capable of producing side effects. Most acitretin users experience side effects. The frequency and severity of side effects depend on many factors including dose, duration of therapy and individual susceptibility. Possible side effects include:

*Digestive Tract:* Nausea; vomiting; swollen and bleeding gums; increased saliva; bloating; stomach ulcer/pain; diarrhea; tongue disorder; increased/decreased appetite.

*Nervous System:* Depression; sleeplessness; drowsiness; tiredness.

*Skin:* Peeling skin; dry skin; itching; nail disorder; red rash; diminished sensitivity to stimulation; abnormal skin sensation; sticky skin; loss of skin elasticity (atrophy); abnormal skin odor; abnormal hair texture; blisters; cold, clammy skin; swollen skin; increased sweating; infection; psoriasis-like rash; red/purple spots; pus-filled sores; excessively oily skin; cracking of skin; sunburn; flushing.

*Senses:* Dry eyes; eye irritation; brow and lash loss; Bell's Palsy; swollen and crusting eyelids; blurred vision; eye infection; cataracts; decreased night vision; double vision; itchy eyes or eyelids; sore eyes; visual disturbance; sensitivity to light; earache; taste perversion; ringing in the ears.

*Other:* Flushing; congested or runny nose; headache; bone abnormality; swollen lips; nosebleed; dry mouth; hair loss; joint, back, muscle or bone pain/disorder; chills; thirst; pain; muscle stiffness; swelling; hot flashes; arthritis.

## Guidelines for Use:

- Individualize dosage. Initial dosage is 25 or 50 mg/day as a single dose given with the main meal.
- Therapy should be terminated when sores have healed and when directed by your doctor.
- If a dose is missed, take it as soon as possible. If several hours have passed or it is nearing time for the next dose, do not double the dose to catch up (unless advised by your doctor). If more than one dose is missed or it is necessary to establish a new dosage schedule, contact your doctor or pharmacist. Use exactly as prescribed.
- A prescription will not be given until a report of a negative pregnancy test has been received by your doctor. Pregnancy testing and counseling will be done on a regular basis.
- Sexually active women of childbearing potential should practice contraception 1 month before starting therapy, during therapy and for at least 3 years after therapy has been stopped.
- Two reliable forms of contraception should be used at the same time unless abstinence is the chosen method.
- Contact your doctor immediately if pregnancy is suspected during therapy. Major birth defects have been associated with acitretin use. Discuss continuation of the pregnancy with your doctor.
- Discontinue the drug and contact your doctor immediately if pain behind the eyes, headache, nausea, vomiting, visual disturbances and decreased tolerance of contact lens wear occurs.
- Women of childbearing potential should be advised to not drink beverages or take products containing alcohol while taking acetretin and for 2 months after treatment has been stopped.
- Most patients experience a relapse of psoriasis after stopping therapy. Other courses of therapy have produced similar results to the first course.
- Do not take vitamin A supplements while taking acitretin.
- Worsening of psoriasis may be seen during initial treatment and it may be 2 to 3 months before the full benefit of acitretin is seen.
- If you experience visual difficulties, discontinue use and contact your doctor.
- Do not donate blood during and for 3 years following therapy.
- Avoid the use of sun lamps and excessive exposure to sunlight. Use appropriate sunscreen and wear protective clothing.
- Regularly scheduled appointments will be made to check your response to the medication and lab tests are required. Tests include: Blood lipid, triglycerides, cholesterol, liver function and pregnancy. Be sure to keep appointments.
- Store between 59° and 77°F. Protect from light, high temperatures and moisture.

*If you have any questions, consult your doctor, pharmacist, or health care provider.*

| Generic Name<br>*Brand Name Examples* | Supplied As | Generic<br>Available |
|---|---|---|
| *Rx* **Methotrexate (MTX)** | | |
| *Rheumatrex Dose Pack[1]* | **Tablets**: 2.5 mg | Yes |
| *Methotrexate Sodium Injection[2], Methotrexate LPF Sodium[3]* | **Injection**: 25 mg/mL | Yes |
| *Methotrexate Sodium For Injection[3]* | **Powder for injection**: 20 mg/vial, 1 g/vial | Yes |

[1] Contains lactose.
[2] Contains benzyl alcohol.
[3] Preservative free.

## Type of Drug:

Agent for psoriasis, rheumatoid arthritis, and certain types of cancer.

## How the Drug Works:

Methotrexate (MTX) is an antimetabolite which interferes with folic acid production, DNA production, and cellular reproduction. It is used in conditions involving rapidly growing tissue (eg, psoriasis, cancer). Methotrexate inhibits cell production.

## Uses:

To treat severe, disabling psoriasis when other therapy fails.

To treat certain types of cancer, alone or with other anticancer agents (see Antimetabolites monograph).

To treat severe, disabling rheumatoid arthritis when other therapy fails.

*Unlabeled Use(s):* Occasionally doctors may prescribe methotrexate for Reiter disease.

## Precautions:

*Do not use in the following situations:*

abnormal blood counts (eg, low platelet and white-cell count)
alcoholism
allergy to the drug or any ingredients
anemia
blood disorders before MTX therapy

breastfeeding
immunodeficiency syndrome
liver disease
pregnancy
women of childbearing potential

*Use with caution in the following situations:*

bone marrow depression
infection, active
kidney disease
liver damage

peptic ulcer, active
poor health and debility
ulcerative colitis

*Liver:* Methotrexate may be highly toxic to the liver, particularly at high doses or with prolonged therapy. Liver atrophy, necrosis, cirrhosis, fatty liver and liver fibrosis may occur. Liver function should be determined before methotrexate therapy begins and monitored regularly.

*Pregnancy:* Methotrexate has caused fetal death and severe birth defects. Defective egg (ovum) or sperm formation caused by methotrexate has been reported. Women of childbearing potential should not use MTX unless benefits outweigh the risks. Not generally recommended for pregnant psoriasis or rheumatoid arthritis patients.

*Breastfeeding:* Methotrexate appears in breast milk. Since the drug may accumulate in the newborn, breastfeeding is not recommended. Decide whether to discontinue breastfeeding or to discontinue the drug, taking into account the importance of the drug to the mother.

*Children:* Safety and effectiveness in children have not been established other than in cancer chemotherapy.

*Lab tests* will be required during treatment with MTX. Tests will include: Blood counts, urine tests, kidney, liver and pulmonary function tests and chest x-rays. When high dose or long-term therapy is used, a liver biopsy or bone marrow sample may be needed.

## Drug Interactions:

Tell your doctor or pharmacist if you are taking or if you are planning to take any over-the-counter or prescription medications or dietary supplements with methotrexate. Doses of one or both drugs may need to be modified or a different drug may need to be prescribed. The following drugs and drug classes interact with methotrexate:

bismuth subsalicylate
charcoal
chloramphenicol
 (eg, *Chloromycetin Kapseals)*
cisplatin (*Platinol-AQ)*
digoxin (eg, *Lanoxin)*
folic acid (eg, *Folvite)*
nonsteroidal anti-inflammatory
 agents (eg, indomethacin, ketoprofen, naproxen)
penicillins
phenylbutazone
 (eg, *Azolid)*

phenytoin (eg, *Dilantin)*
probenecid (eg, *Benemid)*
salicylates (eg, aspirin)
sulfonamides
 (eg, *Sulfisoxazole)*
tetracycline
 (eg, *Achromycin V)*
theophylline
 (eg, *Slo-Phyllin)*
trimethoprim-sulfamethoxazole
 (eg, *Bactrim)*

## Side Effects:

Every drug is capable of producing side effects. Many methotrexate users experience no, or minor, side effects. The frequency and severity of side effects depend on many factors including dose, duration of therapy and individual susceptibility. Possible side effects include:

*Digestive Tract:* Nausea; vomiting; appetite loss; diarrhea; mouth ulcers.

*Hematologic:* Decreased platelet count; decreased white blood count; decreased other cell count.

*Nervous System:* Dizziness; headache.

*Respiratory System:* Lung disease; cough; nasal congestion; nosebleed.

*Skin:* Rash; itching; sensitivity to sunlight and tanning lamps; "burning" of skin lesions; sweating.

*Urinary and Reproductive Tract:* Vaginal discharge; painful urination.

*Other:* Fever; joint pain; decreased resistance to infection; liver disease; chest pain; hair loss; eye discomfort.

---

### Guidelines for Use:

- Dosing and administration vary depending on disease; follow the directions given to you by your doctor and read all package insert materials before taking this drug.
- Deaths have been reported from MTX use for treating psoriasis and rheumatoid arthritis. Patients given MTX must receive close medical supervision. Risks of therapy must be fully understood.
- Avoid alcohol, aspirin, other salicylates, NSAIDs and prolonged exposure to sunlight or sunlamps.
- Contact your doctor if nausea, vomiting, appetite loss, infection, hair loss, skin rash, boils or acne occurs or persists.
- Discontinue the drug and contact your doctor if any of the following symptoms occur: Diarrhea, abdominal pain, black sticky stools, fever, chills, sore throat, unusual bruising or bleeding, sores in or around the mouth, cough, shortness of breath, yellow discoloration of the skin or eyes, dark urine, bloody urine, swelling of the feet or legs, or joint pain.
- Rule out pregnancy at least 2 weeks before beginning therapy with MTX. Use contraceptive measures for at least 8 weeks after stopping therapy to decrease the risk of severe birth defects or fetal death if pregnancy should occur.
- Avoid pregnancy if either partner is using methotrexate.
- *Conception* — Men should wait at least 3 months and women should wait at least 1 ovulatory cycle after stopping use of MTX before attempting conception.
- Prior to therapy, a complete blood workup, urinalysis, chest x-ray and kidney and liver function tests are required. Follow-up tests will also be required.

---

*If you have any questions, consult your doctor, pharmacist, or health care provider.*

| Generic Name<br>*Brand Name Examples* | Supplied As | Generic<br>Available |
|---|---|---|
| *Rx* **Methoxsalen**<br>**(8-Methoxypsoralen)** | | |
| *Oxsoralen-Ultra*[1] | **Capsules**: 10 mg | No |
| *Rx* **Methoxsalen** | | |
| *Oxsoralen* [2,3] | **Lotion**: 1% | No |
| *Rx* **Trioxsalen** | | |
| *Trisoralen* [1] | **Tablets**: 5 mg | No |

[1] Contains the dye tartrazine.
[2] For office use only; never dispensed to a patient.
[3] Contains alcohol.

## Type of Drug:

Photosensitizing drugs used in combination with ultraviolet (UV) light for the treatment of psoriasis, vitiligo and other skin disorders.

## How the Drug Works:

Psoralens act as "photosensitizers." Oral psoralens reach the skin by the bloodstream. When the skin is exposed to UV light, an inflammatory reaction occurs. The inflammation is followed over several days to weeks by repair which is seen as increased darkening and thickening of the skin layers.

## Uses:

*Oxsoralen-Ultra:* To control symptoms of severe resistant disabling psoriasis not responsive to other therapy when the diagnosis has been supported by biopsy. Used only with long wave UV radiation. *Oxsoralen-Ultra* should not be interchanged with *Oxsoralen* lotion.

*Oxsoralen (topical), trioxsalen:* Used with long wave UV radiation or sunlight. For repigmentation (darkening) of idiopathic vitiligo.

*Trioxsalen:* For increasing tolerance to sunlight and for enhancing pigmentation.

## Precautions:

*Do not use in the following situations:*

absence of lens of eye (aphakia)
adverse reaction to psoralen compounds, history
albinism
allergy to psoralens
children under 12 years of age (*Oxsoralen* lotion and trioxsalen)
diseases associated with light sensitivity (porphyria, acute lupus erythematosus, leukoderma)
melanoma, history
squamous cell cancer
use of other photosensitizing drugs
xeroderma pigmentosum

*Use with caution in the following situations:*

| | |
|---|---|
| arsenic therapy, history | grenz or x-ray therapy, history |
| basal cell carcinoma, history | heart disease |
| cataracts | liver disease |
| fair-skinned individuals | tar or UVB treatment, prolonged |

*Photosensitizing (light sensitizing) agents:* Exercise special care in treating patients who are receiving therapy (either topically or systemically) with other known photosensitizing agents such as:

| | |
|---|---|
| anthralin | griseofulvin |
| bacteriostatic soaps | nalidixic acid |
| coal tar (and derivatives) | phenothiazines |
| dyes (eg methylene blue, toluidine blue, rose bengal, methyl orange) | sulfonamides |
| | tetracycline |
| | thiazide diuretics |

*Furocoumarin-containing foods:* No clinical reports or tests show that serious reactions may result, but eating the following while on psoralen therapy may be dangerous: Limes, figs, parsley, parsnips, mustard, carrots and celery.

*Skin cancer:* Studies have shown an increased risk of squamous cell and basal cell carcinoma among patients receiving psoralens and (UV) radiation.

*Cataracts:* Like the skin, psoralens reach the lens of the eye by the bloodstream. If the eye is exposed to UVA while methoxsalen is in the lens, cataracts may appear. However, if the lens is shielded from UVA, the methoxsalen will leave the eye in 24 hours. Wear UVA-absorbing, wraparound sunglasses for the 24 hours following oral use of methoxsalen, whether exposed to direct or indirect sunlight in the open, or through window glass.

*Oxsoralen-Ultra* should not be substituted for regular *Oxsoralen*.

*Pregnancy:* Adequate studies have not been done in pregnant women. Use only if clearly needed and potential benefits outweigh the possible hazards to the fetus.

*Breastfeeding:* It is not known if psoralens appear in breast milk. Consult your doctor before you begin breastfeeding.

*Children:* Safety of methoxsalen use in children has not been established. Potential hazards include possible cancer, cataracts and premature aging of skin. Oral trioxsalen and methoxsalen lotion are not recommended in children under 12 years of age.

*Lab tests* are required before and at regular intervals during therapy with psoralens. Tests may include: Blood counts, antinuclear antibodies, liver and kidney function tests and eye exams.

*Tartrazine:* Some of these products may contain the dye tartrazine (FD&C Yellow No. 5) which can cause allergic reactions in certain individuals. Check package label when available or consult your pharmacist or doctor.

## Drug Interactions:

Tell your doctor or pharmacist if you are taking or planning to take any over-the-counter or prescription medications or dietary supplements while taking this medicine. Doses of one or both drugs may need to be modified or a different drug may need to be prescribed. Photosensitizing agents (see Precautions) interact with psoriasis agents.

## Side Effects:

Every drug is capable of producing side effects. Many psoralen users experience side effects. The frequency and severity of side effects depend on many factors including dose, duration of therapy and individual susceptibility. Possible side effects include:

*Skin:* Burns (from excessive sunlight or sunlamp UV exposure); skin cancer; decreased pigmentation; skin rash; herpes simplex; hives; itching; redness; swelling; blisters.

*Nervous System:* Nervousness; sleeplessness; depression; lethargy; dizziness; headache.

*Other:* Fluid retention (edema); leg cramps; general body discomfort; low blood pressure; spread of psoriasis; tenderness or aging of the skin; herpes simplex eruptions; nausea.

*Combined methoxsalen/UVA therapy* – Itching may be lessened with frequent application of bland emollients or other topical agents. Severe itching may require oral treatment. If itching is unresponsive, shield itching areas from further UVA exposure until the condition improves. If itching is "all over," discontinue UVA treatment until itching disappears. Mild, transient redness 24 to 48 hours after PUVA therapy is expected. It indicates a therapeutic interaction between methoxsalen and UVA. Shield any area showing moderate redness during future UVA exposures until the redness is gone. Discuss all symptoms with your doctor.

*Serious burns* from either UVA or sunlight (even through window glass) may occur if recommended dosage of the drug or exposure schedules are exceeded.

---

### Guidelines for Use:

- Individualize treatment. Take self-administered products exactly as prescribed.
- Do not stop taking this medicine or change the dose without checking with your doctor; this could have serious adverse effects.
- *Use topical methoxsalen* only on small, well defined lesions which can be protected by clothing from exposure to sunlight. If used to treat vitiligo of face or hands, keep the treated area protected from sunlight or other UV light exposure by use of protective clothing or sunscreens. The area of application may be highly photosensitive (light-sensitive) for several days and may result in severe burns if exposed to additional UV or sunlight. This medicine is only applied by a doctor under controlled lighting conditions.

## Guidelines for Use (cont.):

- *Use topical methoxsalen* (cont.)
  Treatment frequency is generally once a week or less, depending on the results, but should never be given more than once every other day. Significant repigmentation may require 6 to 9 months of treatment. Retreatment may be required. Repigmentation occurs less rapidly over less fleshy areas such as the back of the hands or tops of the feet.

- *Before use* — Do not sunbathe during the 24 hours prior to methoxsalen ingestion and UV exposure. Sunburn may prevent an accurate evaluation of the patient's response to photochemotherapy.

- *After use* — Wear UVA-absorbing, wraparound sunglasses during daylight for 24 hours to prevent cataracts (see Precautions). The protective eyewear must prevent entry of stray radiation to the eyes, including that which may enter from the sides of the eyewear.

- *Avoid sun exposure,* even through window glass or cloud cover, for at least 8 hours after use. If sun exposure cannot be avoided, wear protective devices such as a hat and gloves, or apply sunscreens that filter out UVA radiation (eg, sunscreens with SPF 15 or more). Apply sunscreens to all areas that might be exposed to the sun (including lips). Do not apply sunscreens to areas affected by psoriasis until after treatment in the UVA chamber.

- *During PUVA therapy,* wear total UVA-absorbing/blocking goggles mechanically designed to give maximal protection. Failure to do so may increase the risk of cataract formation. A radiometer can verify elimination of UVA transmission through the goggles. Protect lips with light-screening lipstick.

- Protect abdominal skin, breasts, genital organs and other sensitive areas for approximately one-third of the initial exposure time until tanning occurs. Unless affected by disease, shield male genital organs.

- *After combined methoxsalen/UVA therapy:* Wear UVA-absorbing, wraparound sunglasses during the daylight for 24 hours after therapy. Do not sunbathe for 48 hours after therapy. Redness or burning due to photochemotherapy and sunburn are additive.

- Minimize or avoid nausea by taking the drug with milk or food, or by dividing into two doses, taken 1/2 hour apart.

- Do not exceed prescribed dosage or exposure time. Serious burns may result.

- Avoid furocoumarin-containing foods (eg, limes, figs, parsley, parsnips, mustard, carrots, celery).

- *Oxsoralen-Ultra* should not be substituted for regular *Oxsoralen.*

- Use of methoxsalen with UV light should only occur when a doctor experienced in diagnosis and treatment of psoriasis and vitiligo is involved.

- UVA therapy may cause ocular damage, skin aging and skin cancer. The safe total dose of UVA given over a long period of time has not been established.

- Eye exams are recommended before the start of therapy and then every year. Periodic lab tests are required, as well. Be sure to keep appointments.

*If you have any questions, consult your doctor, pharmacist, or health care provider.*

| Generic Name<br>*Brand Name Example* | Supplied As | Generic<br>Available |
|---|---|---|
| *Rx* **Tazarotene** | | |
| *Tazorac*[1] | **Gel, topical**: 0.05%; 0.1% | No |

[1] Contains benzyl alcohol as a preservative.

## Type of Drug:

Topical psoriasis drug; antiacne medicine.

## How the Drug Works:

The exact mechanism of drug action is unknown. The drug reduces skin inflammation and changes associated with the development of psoriasis and acne.

## Uses:

For the topical treatment of psoriasis of up to 20% of the body surface. For the topical treatment of mild-to-moderate acne.

## Precautions:

*Do not use in the following situations:*

> allergy to the drug or any of its ingredients
> application to eyes, eyelids and mouth
> eczema
> itching, burning, redness or peeling of the skin
> pregnancy
> skin medications causing strong drying effects

*Use with caution in the following situations:*

> concurrent administration of other photosensitizing drugs (eg, tetracyclines, thiazides, quinolones, sulfonamides)
>
> exposure to sunlight or sun lamps
> extreme weather conditions (wind or cold)

*Pregnancy:* Do not use during pregnancy. The risk of use in a pregnant woman clearly outweighs any possible benefit.

*Breastfeeding:* It is not known if tazarotene appears in breast milk. Consult your doctor before you begin breastfeeding.

*Children:* Safety and effectiveness have not been established in children under 12 years of age.

## Drug Interactions:

Tell your doctor or pharmacist if you are taking or planning to take any over-the-counter or prescription medications or dietary supplements while taking tazarotene. Doses of one or both drugs may need to be modified or a different drug may need to be prescribed. The following drugs and drug classes interact with tazarotene:

> thiazides (eg, chlorthalidone, hydrochlorothiazide)
> tetracyclines (eg, doxycycline)
> fluoroquinolones (eg, ciprofloxacin)
> phenothiazines (eg, promethazine)
> sulfonamides (eg, sulfamethoxazole)

## Side Effects:

Every drug is capable of producing side effects. Many tazarotene users experience no, or minor, side effects. The frequency and severity of side effects depend on many factors including dose, duration of therapy and individual susceptibility. Possible side effects include:

*Skin:* Itching; burning; stinging; redness; worsening of psoriasis; irritation; skin pain; rash; peeling of skin; contact skin inflammation; cracking, splitting of skin; bleeding; dry skin; localized swelling; skin discoloration.

## Guidelines for Use:

- For external use only. Keep away from eyes, mouth and nose.
- Apply this medication as directed by your doctor. Contact your doctor if the psoriasis or acne becomes worse.
- If itching, burning, redness, peeling or stinging occurs, discontinue use and contact your doctor immediately. If irritation is excessive, application should be discontinued.
- *For psoriasis:*
  - Apply once a day in the evening to lesions on no more than 20% of the body surface using enough to cover only the lesion with a thin film.
  - Skin should be clean and dry before applying gel.
  - Avoid application to unaffected skin, because it may be more susceptible to irritation. Avoid eyes and mouth.
- *For acne:*
  - Cleanse face gently.
  - After the skin is dry, apply a thin film once a day in the evening where lesions appear.
  - Use enough to cover the entire affected area.
- If you become pregnant while using tazarotene, immediately discontinue use and contact your doctor.
- Women of child-bearing potential who use tazarotene should use contraceptive measures while using this medicine.
- If you use a cream or lotion to soften or lubricate your skin, remove the cream or lotion first and then apply tazarotene after ensuring that there is no more cream or lotion on the skin.
- Do not cover the treated areas with dressings or bandages.
- Wash hands after applying the medication unless you are treating your hands for psoriasis. If the gel accidently gets on areas you do not need to treat, wash it off.
- If tazarotene comes in contact with your eyes, wash your eyes with large amounts of cool water and contact a doctor if eye irritation persists.
- If a dose is missed, apply it as soon as possible. If several hours have passed or it is nearing time for the next application, do not double the application to catch up (unless advised by your doctor). If more than one application is missed or it is necessary to establish a new application schedule, contact your doctor or pharmacist. Use exactly as prescribed.
- Use with caution on eczema (dry scaly skin).
- Avoid, if possible, any topical medication or cosmetic that has a strong drying effect.
- May cause photosensitivity (sensitivity to sunlight). Avoid prolonged exposure to the sun or other forms of ultraviolet light (eg, tanning beds). Use sunscreens and wear protective clothing.
- Store at 59° to 86°F.

*If you have any questions, consult your doctor, pharmacist, or health care provider.*

| Generic Name<br>*Brand Name Example* | Supplied As | Generic<br>Available |
|---|---|---|
| *Rx* **Becaplermin** | | |
| *Regranex* | **Gel**: 100 mcg/g | No |

## Type of Drug:

Biologic; human platelet-derived growth factor.

## How the Drug Works:

Stimulates the body to grow new tissue in areas of tissue damage (ulcer site) where it is applied.

## Uses:

For the treatment of lower-extremity (limb) diabetic neuropathic ulcers that extend under the skin or deeper and have adequate blood supply. It is used along with proper ulcer care and infection treatment.

## Precautions:

*Do not use in the following situations:*

> allergy to drug or any of its ingredients
> tumors at site of application
> wounds that are likely to heal by themselves

*Pregnancy:* Adequate studies have not been done in pregnant women. Use only if clearly needed and potential benefits outweigh the possible hazard to the fetus.

*Breastfeeding:* It is not known if becaplermin appears in breast milk. Consult your doctor before you begin breastfeeding.

*Children:* Safety and effectiveness in children less than 16 years of age have not been established.

## Drug Interactions:

Tell your doctor or pharmacist if you are taking or planning to take any over-the-counter or prescription medications or dietary supplements while taking becaplermin. Doses of one or both drugs may need to be modified or a different drug may need to be prescribed.

## Side Effects:

Every drug is capable of producing side effects. Many becaplermin users experience no, or minor, side effects. The frequency and severity of side effects depend on many factors including dose, duration of therapy and individual susceptibility. Possible side effects include:

*Other:* Infection; inflammation of tissue; bone infection; red rash; tissue irritation.

## Guidelines for Use:

- For external use only.
- Apply amount once a day as prescribed by your doctor. The amount varies depending on individual needs and should be re-evaluated periodically by a doctor.
- Directions for use:
  - Wash hands thoroughly before applying.
  - Squeeze gel on to a clean, firm, non-absorbable surface (eg, wax paper).
  - With a clean cotton swab, tongue depressor or similar application aid, spread measured gel over ulcer surface in an even layer.
  - Cover with a saline-moistened gauze dressing.
  - After about 12 hours, rinse the ulcer with saline or water to remove residual gel and cover with a saline-moistened gauze dressing without the gel.
- The tip of the tube should not come into contact with the ulcer or any other surface. Recap tube tightly after each use.
- Use the gel with a strict non-weight-bearing program.
- Applying more gel than prescribed does not increase healing rate.
- Do not apply other topical products to the ulcer site.
- Becaplermin does not replace good ulcer care practices. It is used in addition to good ulcer care practices.
- If a dose is missed, apply it as soon as possible. If several hours have passed or if it is nearing time for the next dose, do not double the dose to "catch up" (unless advised by your doctor). If more than one dose is missed or it is necessary to adjust the dosage schedule, contact your doctor or pharmacist.
- Do not stop applying this medicine without consulting your doctor.
- Notify your doctor if a reaction at the ulcer site occurs while applying becaplermin.
- Store in refrigerator (36° to 46°F). Do not freeze.
- Use this medication by the expiration date noted on bottom of tube.

*If you have any questions, consult your doctor, pharmacist, or health care provider.*

| Generic Name<br>*Brand Name Example* | Supplied As | Generic<br>Available |
|---|---|---|
| *Rx* **Mafenide** | | |
| *Sulfamylon*[1] | **Cream** : 85 mg/g | No |

[1] Contains sulfites and parabens.

## Type of Drug:
Antibacterial burn agent.

## How the Drug Works:
Mafenide reduces the number of bacteria in second- and third-degree burn wounds. This permits healing. It is active even when pus and blood serum are present.

## Uses:
To treat and prevent bacterial infection in second- and third-degree burns. Used in combination with other treatments.

## Precautions:
*Do not use in the following situations:*
>allergy to mafenide
>sulfite sensitivity
>G6PD deficiency

*Use with caution in the following situations:*
>kidney or lung disease

*Superinfection:* Use of antibiotics (especially prolonged or repeated therapy) may result in overgrowth of nonsusceptible bacteria or fungi. Such overgrowth may lead to a second infection. Mafenide may need to be stopped and another antibiotic prescribed for the nonsusceptible secondary infection.

*Pregnancy:* Adequate studies have not been done in pregnant women. Use only if clearly needed and potential benefits outweigh the possible hazards to the fetus.

*Breastfeeding:* It is not known if mafenide appears in breast milk. Because of the potential for serious side effects in nursing infants, decide whether to discontinue the drug or discontinue breastfeeding. Consult your doctor.

*Children:* Use for children is the same as for adults.

*Lab tests* will be required to monitor therapy. Tests may include acid base balance.

*Sulfites:* This product may contain sulfite preservatives which can cause allergic reactions in certain individuals. Check package label when available or consult your doctor or pharmacist.

## Drug Interactions:

Tell your doctor or pharmacist if you are taking or if you are planning to take any over-the-counter or prescription medications or dietary supplements with mafenide. Doses of one or both drugs may need to be modified or a different drug may need to be prescribed.

## Side Effects:

Every drug is capable of producing side effects. Many mafenide users experience no, or minor, side effects. The frequency and severity of side effects depend on many factors including dose, duration of therapy and individual susceptibility. Possible side effects include:

*Skin:* Pain or burning sensation on application; rash; itching; hives; blisters; redness of skin.

*Other:* Fluid retention (edema); facial swelling; rapid breathing; swelling; increase in serum chloride.

---

### Guidelines for Use:

- For external use only. Use exactly as prescribed.
- Using a sterile glove, apply once or twice daily to burned areas to a thickness of about inch. Whenever necessary, reapply the cream to any areas from which it has been removed (eg, by patient activity).
- The treated area may be covered by a dressing, but this is not required.
- Bathe the burned area daily. A whirlpool bath is particularly helpful.
- Continue treatment until healing occurs or until the site is ready for grafting. Treatment may have to be discontinued if significant side effects occur.
- Do not stop using while there is the possibility of infection.
- Contact your doctor if hyperventilation (rapid breathing) or burn irritation occurs or if condition worsens.

---

*If you have any questions, consult your doctor, pharmacist, or health care provider.*

| Generic Name<br>*Brand Name Examples* | Supplied As | Generic<br>Available |
|---|---|---|
| Rx **Silver sulfadiazine** | | |
| *SSD,*[1] *SSD AF,*[1]<br>*Silvadene*[1] | **Cream**: 1% | No |

[1] Contains petrolatum and methylparaben

## Type of Drug:
Antibacterial burn agent.

## How the Drug Works:
Silver sulfadiazine reduces the number of bacteria in second-and third-degree burn wounds.

## Uses:
To help prevent and treat bacterial burn wound infections in second- and third-degree burns. Also used in combination with other medicines.

## Precautions:
*Do not use in the following situations:*
>        allergy to silver sulfadiazine or any ingredient in the preparation
>        allergy to sulfonamides (sulfa drugs)
>        infants less than 2 months old
>        pregnant women at or near delivery date
>        premature infants

*Use with caution in the following situations:*
>        fungal growth in burn
>        glucose-6-phosphate dehydrogenase (G-6-PD) deficiency
>        kidney disease
>        liver disease
>        topical proteolytic enzyme use

*Superinfection:* Use of antibiotics (especially prolonged or repeated therapy) may result in bacterial or fungal overgrowth. Such overgrowth may lead to a second infection. Silver sulfadiazine may need to be stopped and another antibiotic may need to be prescribed for the second infection.

*Pregnancy:* Safety for use during pregnancy has not been established. Use during pregnancy only if clearly justified, especially in women approaching or at delivery date.

*Breastfeeding:* It is not known if silver sulfadiazine cream appears in breast milk. Sulfonamides are known to be excreted in breast milk and since all sulfonamide derivatives have the potential to cause problems in the nursing infant, consult your doctor before you begin breastfeeding.

*Children:* Safety and effectiveness in children have not been established.

*Lab tests* are recommended during treatment. Tests may include blood drug concentrations, kidney function tests (blood and urine) and white blood cell counts. Be sure to keep appointments.

## Drug Interactions:

Tell your doctor or pharmacist if you are taking or if you are planning to take any over-the-counter or prescription medications or dietary supplements with silver sulfadiazine cream. Doses of one or both drugs may need to be modified or a different drug may need to be prescribed. Topical proteolytic enzymes interact with silver sulfadiazine cream.

## Side Effects:

Every drug is capable of producing side effects. Many silver sulfadiazine users experience no, or minor, side effects. The frequency and severity of side effects depend on many factors including dose, duration of therapy and individual susceptibility. Possible side effects include:

*Other:* Burning; rash; itching; dead skin; hives, redness; skin discoloration; decrease in white blood cell count. Because sulfadiazine may be absorbed, it is possible that any of the side effects of sulfonamides may occur (see sulfonamide monograph).

*Use of Silvadene* may delay the separation of the dead skin from the new skin, requiring a procedure involving scraping of the wound (escharotomy) in order to prevent abnormal skin development.

---

### Guidelines for Use:

- For external use only. Use exactly as prescribed.
- Apply once or twice daily to a thickness of about 1/16 of an inch. Apply using a sterile glove. Wash hands before and after application.
- Burn areas should be covered with silver sulfadiazine cream at all times.
- Reapply immediately after bathing and to any areas from which it has been removed by activity.
- May be covered by a dressing, but this is not required.
- Bathe the burned area daily. A whirlpool bath is particularly helpful.
- Continue treatment until healing occurs, until the site is ready for grafting or unless a significant side effect occurs.
- *Sulfonamide allergy* — If you are allergic to other sulfa drugs, you may react to silver sulfadiazine.
- If burn wounds involve extensive areas of the body, the sulfa drug may be absorbed to a significant extent. This could lead to systemic side effects.

---

*If you have any questions, consult your doctor, pharmacist, or health care provider.*

| Generic Name<br>*Brand Name Examples* | Supplied As | Generic<br>Available |
|---|---|---|
| **Selenium Sulfide** | | |
| *otc Selsun Blue (Regular, pH*<br>*Balanced,[1] Medicated[1]),*<br>*Head and Shoulders*<br>*Intensive Treatment* | **Lotion shampoo**: 1% | Yes |
| *Rx Selsun* | **Lotion shampoo**: 2.5% | Yes |

[1] Contains menthol.

## Type of Drug:

Controls dandruff flaking and itching.

## How the Drug Works:

Selenium sulfide reduces growth and multiplication of skin cells.

## Uses:

For treatment of dandruff, seborrheic dermatitis of the scalp and tinea versicolor (a fungal infection, *2.5% selenium sulfide only*).

## Precautions:

*Do not use in the following situations:*

allergy to any ingredient of the product
inflamed, broken skin

*Pregnancy:* Adequate studies have not been done in pregnant women. Use only if clearly needed and potential benefits outweigh the possible hazards to the fetus.

*Children:* Safety and effectiveness in infants have not been established.

## Side Effects:

Every drug is capable of producing side effects. Many selenium sulfide users experience no, or minor, side effects. The frequency and severity of side effects depend on many factors including dose, duration of therapy and individual susceptibility. Possible side effects include: Skin irritation; hair discoloration (minimize by thorough rinsing); oiliness or dryness of hair and scalp; hair loss.

## Guidelines for Use:

- *For dandruff, seborrheic dermatitis* — Shake well. Shampoo and rinse thoroughly. Use regularly for best results, at least twice a week as directed by your doctor.
- *For fungal infection* — Apply to affected areas and lather with a small amount of water. Allow to remain on skin for 10 minutes. Rinse thoroughly. Repeat daily for 7 days.
- For external use only.
- Avoid contact with the eyes. If contact occurs, rinse eye(s) thoroughly with water.
- If irritation occurs, discontinue use.
- Thoroughly rinse after application.
- Wash hands thoroughly after treatment.
- If condition worsens or does not improve after regular use of this product as directed, contact your doctor or pharmacist.
- Do not use on broken or inflamed skin.
- If using on bleached, tinted, gray or permed hair, rinse hair for at least 5 minutes.
- May damage jewelry; remove before using.
- Avoid contact of the shampoo in the genital area and skin folds as it may cause irritation and burning. Thoroughly rinse these areas after use.

*If you have any questions, consult your doctor, pharmacist, or health care provider.*

| Generic Name<br>*Brand Name Examples* | Supplied As | Generic<br>Available |
|---|---|---|
| *Rx* **Chloroxine** | | |
| *Capitrol* [2,7] | **Shampoo**: 2% | No |
| *otc* **Pyrithione Zinc** | | |
| *DHS Zinc, Head and Shoulders Dandruff, Sebulon, Zincon* | **Shampoo**: 1%, 2% | Yes |
| *Rx* **Sulfacetamide Sodium** | | |
| *Sebizon* | **Lotion**: 10% | No |
| *otc* **Tar Derivatives, Shampoos** | | |
| *DHS Tar* | **Shampoo**: 0.5% coal tar | No |
| *Neutrogena T/Gel* [6] | **Shampoo**: 0.5% coal tar | Yes |
| *Polytar* [2,3] | **Shampoo**: 0.5% coal tar | |
| *Neutrogena T/Gel Extra Strength* [5] | **Shampoo**: 1% coal tar | |
| *Zetar* [6] | **Shampoo**: 1% coal tar | Yes |
| *Tegrin Medicated Advanced Formula* [1,5] | **Shampoo**: 1.1% coal tar | No |
| *Denorex Medicated* [1] | **Shampoo**: 1.8% coal tar | No |
| *Denorex Medicated* | **Shampoo and Conditioner**: 1.8% coal tar | No |
| *Duplex T* | **Shampoo**: 2% coal tar | Yes |
| *Pentrax Gold* [6] | **Shampoo**: 2% coal tar | |
| *Duplex T* [1] | **Shampoo and Conditioner**: 2% coal tar | No |
| *Denorex Extra Strength* [1,4] | **Shampoo**: 2.5% coal tar | No |
| *Denorex Extra Strength* | **Shampoo and Conditioner**: 2.5% coal tar | No |
| *MG217* | **Shampoo**: 3% coal tar | No |
| *Pentrax* | **Shampoo**: 4.3% coal tar | No |
| **Tar Derivatives, Bath Products** | | |
| *otc* *Balnetar* | **Oil**: 0.5% coal tar | No |
| *otc* *Polytar* [2] | **Soap**: 0.5% coal tar | No |
| *otc* *Cutar Bath Oil* [6] | **Emulsion**: 1.5% coal tar | No |
| *Rx* *Zetar* [8] | **Emulsion**: 30% coal tar | No |

**Tar Derivatives, Emollients**

| | | |
|---|---|---|
| *otc Tegrin*[1] | **Cream**: 0.8% coal tar | No |
| *otc Medotar* | **Ointment**: 1% coal tar | No |
| *otc T/Derm* | **Emollient**: 1.2% coal tar | No |
| *otc PsoriGel* | **Gel**: 1.75% coal tar | No |
| *otc Fototar*[1] | **Cream**: 2% coal tar | No |
| *otc MG217 Medicated Intensive Strength* | **Ointment**: 2% coal tar | No |
| *otc Oxipor VHC*[1] | **Lotion**: 5% coal tar | No |
| *otc Estar*[1,7] | **Gel**: 5% coal tar | No |

[1] Contains alcohol.
[2] Contains edetate disodium.
[3] Contains lanolin.
[4] Contains menthol.
[5] Contains parabens.
[6] Contains parachlorometaxylenol 0.5%.
[7] Contains benzyl alcohol.
[8] Requires dilution prior to use.

## Type of Drug:

Antiseborrheic products.

## How the Drug Works:

*Chloroxine* reduces excess scaling and inhibits growth of bacteria and some fungi.

*Pyrithione zinc* reduces skin cell growth, flaking, itching and inhibits fungal growth.

*Selenium sulfide* reduces skin cell growth and inhibits growth of organisms associated with chronic flaking and itching.

*Sulfacetamide sodium* inhibits bacterial growth and reproduction.

*Tar derivatives* help correct abnormalities in the formation of keratin. Keratin is a protein found in skin (epidermis), hair and nails. Inhibits bacterial and fungal growth and helps control itching, flaking, scaling, irritation and redness.

## Uses:

*Shampoos:* To treat chronic scalp psoriasis, seborrhea, dandruff, eczema, cradle cap and other oily conditions of the scalp.

*Bath products, solutions, lotions, gels, creams:* To treat psoriasis, seborrheic dermatitis, atopic dermatitis, eczema and other chronic skin disorders.

## Precautions:

*Do not use in the following situations:*
> allergy to any of ingredients in product
> allergy to sulfonamides (sulfacetamide sodium only)
> open, inflamed, or infected lesions (chloroxine and tar derivatives)
> photosensitive (light sensitive) people (tar derivatives only)

*Use with caution in the following situations:*
> sun or ultraviolet light exposure (tar derivatives only)

*Superinfection:* Use of antibiotics (especially prolonged or repeated therapy) may result in bacterial or fungal overgrowth. Such overgrowth may lead to a second infection. Antiseborrheic products may need to be stopped and another antibiotic prescribed for the second infection.

*Pregnancy:* Adequate studies of these products have not been done in pregnant women. Use only if clearly needed and potential benefits outweigh the possible hazards to the fetus.

*Breastfeeding:* Safety for use of these products while breastfeeding has not been established. Consult your doctor before you begin breast-feeding.

*Children:* Safety and effectiveness of sulfacetamide sodium in children under 12 have not been established.

## Drug Interactions:

Tell your doctor or pharmacist if you are using or if you are planning to use any over-the-counter or prescription medications or dietary supplements with these medicines. Silver preparations interact with sulfacetamide sodium. Tetracyclines, psoralens and topical retinoic acid may interact with tar.

## Side Effects:

Every drug is capable of producing side effects. Many antiseborrheic product users experience no, or minor, side effects. The frequency and severity of side effects depend on many factors including dose, duration of therapy and individual susceptibility. Possible side effects include: Minor irritation; inflammation of follicles (after long-term use); allergic rash; sensitivity to light; blisters, swelling of skin.

## Guidelines for Use:

- For external use only.
- Directions for use vary from product to product. Read and follow instructions for use carefully.
- Avoid contact with eyes. If contact occurs, rinse thoroughly with water.
- *Chloroxine* — May discolor blond, gray or bleached hair.If irritation, burning or rash occurs, discontinue use and contact your doctor.Massage thoroughly into wet scalp. Allow lather to remain on scalp for 3 minutes; rinse. Repeat. Two treatments per week are usually sufficient.
- *Pyrithione zinc* — If condition worsens or does not improve with regular use as directed, see your doctor. May temporarily discolor blond, gray, bleached or tinted hair.
- *Selenium sulfide* — May discolor bleached, tinted, gray or permed hair; rinse for 5 minutes.
  If condition worsens or does not improve after regular use, discontinue use and notify your doctor.
- *Sulfacetamide sodium* — If irritation occurs or continues, or if rash develops, discontinue use and notify your doctor. Discontinue promptly if any arthritis, fever or sores in the mouth develop.
  Do not use with silver-containing medications (eg, *Silvadene*).
- *Tar derivatives* — If condition covers a large area of the body, worsens or does not improve, or if irritation develops after regular use as directed, consult your doctor. Do not use for prolonged periods or with other psoriasis therapy such as ultraviolet light or prescription drugs unless directed by your doctor.
  May stain clothing or temporarily discolor white, blond, gray, bleached or tinted hair. Skin may tingle during treatment.
  *Sensitivity to sunlight* — Avoid prolonged exposure to direct sunlight. Topical tar plus ultraviolet light may increase tendency to sunburn for 24 to 72 hours. Do not apply to genital or rectal area.
- *Seborrheic dermatitis* — In mild cases involving the scalp and skin, apply at bedtime and allow to remain overnight. Shampoo first if the hair and scalp are oily or greasy or if there is considerable debris. In severe cases, apply twice daily. Initially, and as frequently as needed thereafter, clean the hair and scalp with a nonirritating shampoo before using the medication.
- Contact your doctor if you notice any unusual side effects after using any of these medications.

*If you have any questions, consult your doctor, pharmacist, or health care provider.*

| Generic Name<br>*Brand Name Examples* | **Supplied As** |
|---|---|
| *otc* **Antiseborrheic Shampoos** | |
| *Sebulex, Sebulex with Conditioners* | **Shampoo**: 2% sulfur and<br>2% salicylic acid |
| *Ionil* | **Shampoo**: 2% salicylic acid,<br>benzalkonium chloride<br>and 12% SD alcohol 40 |
| *Ionil T* | **Shampoo**: 5% coal tar solution,<br>benzalkonium chloride,<br>4% isopropyl alcohol<br>and 12% alcohol |
| *Meted, Maximum Strength* | **Shampoo**: 5% sulfur and<br>3% salicylic acid |
| *P & S* | **Shampoo**: 2% salicylic acid |
| *Sebex* | **Shampoo**: 2% salicylic acid,<br>2% colloidal sulfur |
| *SLT Lotion* | **Lotion**: 2.5% coal tar solution,<br>isopropyl alcohol, benzalkonium<br>chloride |
| *Tarsum* | **Shampoo/Gel**: 10% coal tar<br>solution |
| *X-Seb T Plus, X-Seb T Pearl* | **Shampoo**: 10% coal tar solution |
| *otc* **Medicated Hair Dressings** | |
| *P & S* | **Liquid**: Phenol, mineral oil<br>and glycerin |
| *Sebucare* | **Lotion**: 1.8% salicylic acid<br>with 61% alcohol |

## Type of Drug:

Drugs used to treat seborrhea, dandruff, psoriasis and related skin conditions.

## Uses:

In these combinations:

*Salicylic acid and sulfur:* Used for sebum (oil)-reducing and skin-sloughing actions.

*Tar preparations:* Used for their anti-itch, antibacterial and antiseborrheic actions.

*Benzalkonium chloride* and *phenol:* Used as antiseptics.

## Guidelines for Use:

- For external use only.
- Avoid contact with eyes or mucous membranes. Flush with water if contact occurs.
- Discontinue use and consult your doctor if skin irritation develops or worsens.
- Tar increases sensitivity to the sun and may increase tendency to sunburn for up to 24 hours after use.
- Do not use for prolonged periods without consulting a doctor.
- Do not use on large areas of the body.
- If condition does not improve or worsens, see your doctor.
- Do not use these products with other psoriasis therapy such as ultraviolet light or prescription drugs unless directed by your doctor.
- Do not use on broken skin or around the genital area unless directed by your doctor.
- Do not use on children under 2 years of age.
- Products containing tar may temporarily discolor blond, gray, bleached or tinted hair, or cause slight staining of clothing.

*If you have any questions, consult your doctor, pharmacist, or health care provider.*

| Generic Name<br>*Brand Name Examples* | Supplied As | Generic<br>Available |
|---|---|---|
| **Benzocaine** | | |
| *otc Anbesol, Hurricaine,*[6] *Maximum Strength Anbesol,*[6] *Orabase-B Gel,*[3] *Orajel Mouth-Aid*[5] | **Gel**: 6.3%, 10%, 15%, 20% | Yes |
| *Anbesol, Hurricaine, Maximum Strength Anbesol, Orajel Mouth-Aid*[3,4] | **Liquid**: 6.3%, 20% | Yes |
| *Hurricaine* | **Spray**: 20% | No |
| *c-II* **Cocaine HCl** | **Solution**: 4% 10% | Yes |
| | **Powder**[1] | Yes |
| *Rx* **Dyclonine HCl** | | |
| *Dyclone* | **Solution**: 0.5%, 1% | No |
| *Rx* **Lidocaine HCl** | | |
| *Xylocaine* | **Ointment**: 2.5%, 5% | No |
| *Anestacon, Xylocaine* | **Jelly**: 2% | No |
| *Xylocaine* | **Liquid**: 5% | No |
| *Xylocaine, Xylocaine Viscous, Xylocaine-MPF* | **Solution**: 2%, 4% | Yes |
| *Xylocaine 10% Oral* | **Spray**: 10% | No |
| *Rx* **Tetracaine HCl** | | |
| *Pontocaine HCl* | **Solution**: 0.5% | No |
| *otc* **Topical Anesthetic Combinations** | | |
| *Vagisil, New Improved*[2] | **Cream**: 5% benzocaine and 1% dimethicone | No |
| *Vagisil, Maximum Strength* | **Cream**: 20% benzocaine, 1% dimethicone | No |

[1] Amount of anesthetic in the product is unknown.
[2] Contains methyl- and propylparabens.
[3] Contains ethyl alcohol.
[4] Contains tartrazine.
[5] Contains edetate disodium.
[6] Contains methylparaben and saccharin.

## Type of Drug:

Topical anesthetics for mucous membrane pain and discomfort.

## How the Drug Works:

Topical anesthetics applied externally inhibit conduction of nerve impulses from sensory nerves, thereby producing anesthesia (lack of feeling, numbness). Abrasions or ulcers of the membrane increase absorption and thus increase the effectiveness of the drug (however, side effects could be increased).

## Uses:

Local anesthesia for the examination of mucous membranes including: Oral, nasal and throat membranes; respiratory tract; digestive tract; and urinary tract.

To treat itching due to hemorrhoids or an inflamed anal or vaginal area.

*Cocaine:* Should only be used for office and surgical procedures.

## Precautions:

*Do not use in the following situations:*
> allergy to any component of the product
> eyes, use in or around

*Use with caution in the following situations:*

| | |
|---|---|
| allergy to externally applied drugs | infants less than 1 year of age |
| | infection at site of use |
| blood disorder | liver disease, severe |
| (eg, methoglobinemia) | severely injured or damaged |
| children | skin |
| ear problems | shock or heart block (lidocaine |
| elderly | and dyclonine only) |
| illness, acute | |

*Chronic use:* Do not apply to large areas of the body or use for prolonged periods of time. Chronic use may result in tissue irritation, breathing difficulties, seizures, low blood pressure, mental confusion, ringing in the ears and blurred or poor vision.

*Dependence:* Cocaine is addicting. Continual use of cocaine creates an excessively strong dependence and, sometimes, depression. Chronic use may cause progression from euphoria to paranoid psychosis; included may be perceptual changes (halo lights) and intense itching ("cocaine bugs"). This drug produces the highest degree of dependence seen among abused drugs.

*Pregnancy:*

*Lidocaine* – Studies in pregnant women or in animals have been judged not to show a risk to the fetus. However, no drug should be used during pregnancy unless clearly needed.

*Cocaine* – Adequate studies have not been done in pregnant women, or animal studies may have shown a risk to the fetus. Use only if clearly needed and potential benefits outweigh the possible hazards to the fetus. Women who use cocaine during pregnancy are at significant risk for complications such as shorter gestation, premature delivery and spontaneous abortion.

*Other Anesthetics* – Adequate studies have not been done in pregnant women, or animal studie may have shown a risk to the fetus. Use only if clearly needed and potential benefits outweigh the possible hazards to the fetus.

*Breastfeeding:* Lidocaine appears in breast milk. Safety for use of any of these medicines during breastfeeding has not been established. The American Academy of Pediatrics recommends that cocaine never be used during breastfeeding. Consult your doctor.

*Children:* Safety and effectiveness for use of cocaine in children have not been established. Safety and effectiveness for use of dyclonine and tetracaine in children less than 12 years of age have not been established. Safety and effectiveness of other topical anesthetics have not been established in children less than 1 year of age.

*Elderly:* Dosage adjustments may be necessary for elderly patients.

*Tartrazine:* Some of these products may contain the dye tartrazine (FD&C Yellow No. 5) which can cause allergic reactions in certain individuals. Check package label when available or consult your doctor or pharmacist.

*Sulfites:* Some of these products may contain sulfite preservatives which can cause allergic reactions in certain individuals. Check package labels when available or consult your doctor or pharmacist.

## Drug Interactions:

Tell your doctor or pharmacist if you are taking or if you are planning to take any over-the-counter or prescription medications or dietary supplements while using these medicines. One or both drugs may need to be modified or a different drug may need to be prescribed. The following drugs and drug classes interact with these medicines: Class I antiarrhythmic agents (eg, tocainide, mexiletine).

## Side Effects:

Every drug is capable of producing side effects. Many patients experience no, or minor, side effects. The frequency and severity of side effects depend on many factors including dose, duration of therapy and individual susceptibility. Possible side effects include:

*Cocaine:*

*Nervous System:* Nervousness; restlessness; exaggerated sense of well-being; excitement; tremor; seizures; shock; depression; paranoia.

*Circulatory System:* Changes in heart rate; increased blood pressure.

*Other:* Damage to nasal tissues and to nasal septum (abuse); withdrawal symptoms.

*Other Topical Anesthetics:*

*Skin:* Allergic contact dermatitis; hives; redness; rash; swelling; burning; stinging; irritation; tenderness; skin sloughing; lesions; bluish discoloration.

*Other:* Difficulty breathing; painful urination; blood in urine; seizures.

## Guidelines for Use:

- For external use only. Do not use in or around eyes.
- Do not eat, drink, or chew gum for at least 1 hour after use in mouth or throat, or if the mouth or throat area still feels numb. This is especially important for children who eat more frequently.
- Topical anesthetics can impair the ability to swallow and increase risk of choking (especially when eating or drinking), injury (eg, biting tongue), or vocal damage in singers who use these products to mask vocal discomfort during performances.
- Use lowest dose possible that still provides adequate pain relief.
- Doses and frequency of use depend on the condition, area being treated, blood supply in the area, individual tolerance and dosage form. Individual products should be reviewed for their use and dosage guidelines. Consult your pharmacist or doctor for product-specific information.
- A thin layer of solution, cream, lotion or ointment is all that is necessary. Additional doses can cause severe side effects. Do not use for an extended period of time.
- Stop therapy if irritation, rash or redness develops. Consult your doctor.
- Dosage adjustments may be necessary for the elderly, severely ill patients or children.
- When lidocaine is used, all feeling in the treated skin may be blocked. Avoid accidental injury to the skin by not scratching, rubbing or exposing the skin to extreme hot or cold temperatures until all feeling has returned.
- Store these products at room temperature unless otherwise instructed by specific product label guidelines. Avoid extreme heat, cold, sunlight or moisture.

*If you have any questions, consult your doctor, pharmacist, or health care provider.*

| Generic Name<br>*Brand Name Examples* | Supplied As | Generic<br>Available |
|---|---|---|
| *otc* **Benzocaine** | | |
| *Bicozene, Lanacane* | **Cream**: 5%, 6% | Yes |
| *Detane* | **Gel**: 7.5% | No |
| *Americaine First Aid, Boil-Ease, Foille Medicated First Aid, Chiggerex*[1] | **Ointment**: 5%, 20% | No |
| *Dermoplast, Solarcaine* | **Lotion**: 8%, 20% | No |
| *Chigger-Tox,*[1] *Sting-Kill* | **Liquid**: 20% | No |
| *Aerocaine, Aerotherm, Dermacoat, Dermoplast, Foille Plus, Foille Medicated FirstAid, Lanacane, Solarcaine* | **Aerosol/Spray**: 4.5%, 5%, 13.6%, 20% | No |
| *otc* **Butamben Picrate** | | |
| *Butesin Picrate* | **Ointment:** 1% | No |
| *otc* **Dibucaine** | | |
| *Nupercainal* | **Cream**: 0.5% | No |
| *Nupercainal* | **Ointment**: 1% | Yes |
| *otc* **Lidocaine HCl** | | |
| *Dr. Scholl's Cracked Heel Relief, Solarcaine Aloe Extra Burn Relief, Unguentine Plus* | **Cream**: 0.5%, 2% | No |
| *Solarcaine Aloe Extra Burn Relief, DermaFlex* | **Gel**: 0.5%, 2.5% | No |
| *Xylocaine* | **Ointment:** 2.5%, 5% | Yes |
| *Bactine Antiseptic Anesthetic, ProTech First-Aid Stik, Skeeter Stik, Zilactin-L* | **Liquid**: 2.5%, 4% | No |
| *Bactine Antiseptic Anesthetic, Medi-Quik, Solarcaine Aloe ExtraBurn Relief* | **Spray**: 0.5%, 2%, 2.5% | No |
| *otc* **Pramoxine HCl** | | |
| *Prax, Tronothane HCl* | **Cream**: 1% | No |
| *Itch-X, PrameGel* | **Gel**: 1% | No |
| *Prax* | **Lotion**: 1% | No |
| *Itch-X* | **Spray**: 1% | No |

| Generic Name<br>*Brand Name Examples* | Supplied As | Generic<br>Available |
|---|---|---|
| *otc* **Tetracaine** | | |
| *Pontocaine* | **Cream**: 1% | No |
| *Pontocaine* | **Ointment**: 0.5% | No |
| **Topical Anesthetic Combinations** | | |
| *Rx* **Cetacaine** | **Aerosol, Gel, Liquid,<br>Ointment**:14% benzocaine,<br>2% tetracaine | No |
| *Rx* **EMLA** | **Cream**: 2.5% lidocaine, 2.5%<br>prilocaine | No |

[1] Amount of anesthetic in the product is unknown.

Similar products of equal strengths are listed together in this table. However, they may not share the same inactive ingredients. For further information about the ingredients in these products, check individual package labels.

## Type of Drug:
Topical anesthetics for skin discomfort and pain.

## How the Drug Works:
Topical local anesthetics applied externally inhibit conduction of nerve impulses from sensory nerves, thereby producing anesthesia (lack of feeling, numbness). Abrasions or skin ulcers increase the absorption of the drug and therefore increase its effectiveness; however, side effects can also be increased.

## Uses:
To relieve skin pain, itching and discomfort associated with minor burns, scalds, prickly heat, abrasions, sunburn, allergy to certain plants (such as poison ivy), insect bites, eczema and other skin conditions.

*Lidocaine/Prilocaine:* To ease the pain of some injections.

## Precautions:
*Do not use in the following situations:*
allergy to any component of the product
bacterial infection
eyes, use in or around

*Use with caution in the following situations:*

| | |
|---|---|
| allergy to externally applied drugs | infection or damaged skin at site of use |
| children | liver disease |
| elderly | blood disorders (eg, methemo- |
| illness, acute | globinemia) |

*Chronic use:* Do not apply to large areas of the body or use for prolonged periods of time. Chronic use may result in tissue irritation, breathing difficulties, seizures, low blood pressure, mental confusion, ringing in the ears and blurred or poor vision.

*Pregnancy:*

*Lidocaine* – Studies in pregnant women or in animals have been judged not to show a risk to the fetus. However, no drug should be used during pregnancy unless clearly needed.

*Other anesthetics* – There are no adequate and well-controlled studies in pregnant women. Use only if clearly needed and the potential benefits outweigh the possible risks to the fetus.

*Breastfeeding:* Lidocaine appears in breast milk. It is not known if other anesthetics appear in breast milk. Consult your doctor before you begin breastfeeding.

*Children:* Safety and effectiveness of tetracaine in children younger than 12 years of age have not been established. Safety and effectiveness of the other anesthetics have not been established in children younger than 1 year of age.

*Elderly:* Dosages may need to be adjusted according to age, size, and physical condition.

*Tartrazine:* Some of these products may contain the dye tartrazine (FD&C Yellow No. 5), which can cause allergic reactions in certain individuals. Check package label when available or consult your doctor or pharmacist.

*Sulfites:* Some of these products may contain sulfite preservatives that can cause allergic reactions in certain individuals. Check package label when available or consult your doctor or pharmacist.

## Drug Interactions:

Tell your doctor or pharmacist if you are taking or planning to take any over-the-counter or prescription medications or dietary supplements while taking this drug. Drug doses may need to be modified or a different drug prescribed. Class I antiarrhythmic drugs (eg, tocainide, mexiletine) interact with this drug.

## Side Effects:

Every drug is capable of producing side effects. Many patients experience no, or minor, side effects. The frequency and severity of side effects depend on many factors including dose, duration of therapy, and individual susceptibility. Possible side effects include: Allergic contact dermatitis; redness; rash; swelling; burning; stinging; irritation; lesions; sloughing of skin.

## Guidelines for Use:

- Dosage is individualized. Take exactly as prescribed.
- Do not stop taking or change the dose, unless instructed by your doctor.
- For external use only. Do not use in or around the eyes.
- Topical anesthetics only relieve pain. They do not promote healing or prevent infection.
- Discontinue therapy and contact your doctor if you experience irritation, rash, redness, blisters, or swelling.
- Use the minimal effective dose. Doses and frequency of use depend on the condition, area being treated, blood supply in the area, individual tolerance, and dosage form.
- A thin layer of solution, cream, lotion, or ointment is all that is necessary. Additional benefit will not be achieved with larger amounts.
- Apply to the affected area as needed. Ointments and creams may be applied to gauze or a bandage before applying to skin.
- When lidocaine/prilocaine is used, all feeling in the treated skin may be blocked. Avoid accidental injury to the skin by not scratching, rubbing, or exposing the skin to extreme hot or cold temperatures until all feeling has returned.
- Store at room temperature (59° to 86°F.)

*If you have any questions, consult your doctor, pharmacist, or health care provider.*

| Generic Name<br>*Brand Name Example* | Supplied As | Generic<br>Available |
|---|---|---|
| *Rx* **Diclofenac Sodium** | | |
| *Solaraze* | **Gel**: 3% | No |

## Type of Drug:
Topical keratolytic

## How the Drug Works:
The mechanism of this drug in treating actinic keratosis is unknown.

## Uses:
To treat actinic keratosis (premalignant warts, skin lesions).

## Precautions:
*Do not use in the following situations:*

allergy to the drug or any of its ingredients
exfoliative dermatitis
open skin wounds
topical infection

*Use with caution in the following situations:*

allergy to aspirin
dermatitis, severe
hepatic impairment, severe
intestinal ulcers or bleeding
kidney impairment, severe
stomach ulcers or bleeding

*Pregnancy:* There are no adequate and well-controlled studies in pregnant women. Use only if clearly needed and the potential benefits outweigh the possible risks to the fetus.

*Breastfeeding:* It is not known if diclofenac sodium appears in breast milk. Consult your doctor before you begin breastfeeding.

*Children:* Diclofenac sodium should not be used by children.

## Drug Interactions:
Tell your doctor or pharmacist if you are taking or planning to take any over-the-counter or prescription medications or dietary supplements while taking this drug. Drug doses may need to be modified or a different drug prescribed. The following drugs and drug classes interact with this drug:

aspirin (at analgesic/ anti-inflammatory doses)
other NSAIDs (eg, ibuprofen, naproxen)

## Side Effects:

Every drug is capable of producing side effects. Many patients experience no, or minor, side effects. The frequency and severity of side effects depend on many factors including dose, duration of therapy, and individual susceptibility. Possible side effects include:

*Digestive Tract:* Constipation; diarrhea; upset stomach.

*Nervous System:* Anxiety; dizziness; slow movement.

*Circulatory System:* High blood pressure; vein inflammation.

*Skin:* Acne; hair loss; dry skin; swelling; scaling; pain; itching; rash; burning sensation; skin cancer; skin ulcer.

*Other:* Chest, neck, back, and joint pain; weakness; chills; flu-like syndrome; headache; infection; asthma; sore throat; pneumonia; runny nose; eye pain; red eyes; blood in urine.

---

## Guidelines for Use:

- Dosage is individualized. Use exactly as prescribed.
- Do not stop applying or change the dose, unless instructed by your doctor.
- If a dose is missed, apply it as soon as possible. If several hours have passed or it is nearing time for the next dose, do not double the dose to catch up, unless instructed by your doctor. If more than one dose is missed or it is necessary to establish a new dosage schedule, contact your doctor or pharmacist.
- The recommended duration of therapy is 60 to 90 days. Complete healing may not be evident for up to 30 days following the end of therapy.
- Do not apply to open skin wounds, infections, or exfoliative dermatitis.
- Do not let the gel come in contact with the eyes.
- Avoid exposure to sunlight and sunlamps.
- Inform your doctor if you are pregnant, become pregnant, plan to become pregnant, or are breastfeeding.
- Store at controlled room temperature (59° to 86°F). Protect from heat and freezing.

---

*If you have any questions, consult your doctor, pharmacist, or health care provider.*

| Generic Name Brand Name Examples | Supplied As | Generic Available |
|---|---|---|
| Rx **Podofilox** | | |
| Condylox | **Gel**: 0.5% | No |
| Condylox | **Solution**: 0.5% | No |

## Type of Drug:

An agent that promotes cell death of ano-genital wart tissue.

## How the Drug Works:

The exact mechanism of action is unknown. Podofilox prevents cell growth, resulting in the destruction of the visible wart tissue.

## Uses:

To treat external warts of the genital area.

*Gel:* To treat external warts of the anal area (perianal).

## Precautions:

*Do not use in the following situations:*
> allergy to the drug or any of its ingredients
> perianal warts (solution only)
> warts on mucous membranes

*Correct diagnosis* of warts is essential. Certain types of genital warts are not to be treated with podofilox.

*Pregnancy:* There are no adequate and well-controlled studies in pregnant women. Use only if clearly needed and the potential benefits outweigh the possible risks to the fetus.

*Breastfeeding:* It is not known if podofilox appears in breast milk. Consult your doctor before you begin breastfeeding.

*Children:* Safety and effectiveness have not been established.

## Drug Interactions:

Tell your doctor or pharmacist if you are taking or planning to take any over-the-counter or prescription medications or dietary supplements while taking this drug. Drug doses may need to be modified or a different drug prescribed.

## Side Effects:

Every drug is capable of producing side effects. Many patients experience no, or minor, side effects. The frequency and severity of side effects depend on many factors including dose, duration of therapy, and individual susceptibility. Possible side effects include:

*Skin:* Burning; pain; inflammation; stinging; scabbing; discoloration; rash; skin splitting; ulceration; itching; chafing; blistering; crusting; dryness; peeling; tingling; bleeding; tenderness; erosion; scarring.

*Other:* Headache; pain with intercourse; sleeplessness; offensive odor; dizziness; blood in the urine; vomiting.

## Guidelines for Use:

- External use only. Use exactly as prescribed.
- Patient package insert available with product.
- Apply twice daily morning and evening (every 12 hours) for 3 consecutive days, then withhold use for 4 consecutive days. This 1-week treatment cycle may be repeated up to 4 times until there is no visible wart tissue. If the response is incomplete after 4 treatment weeks, stop using and consider an alternative treatment. Safety and effectiveness of more than 4 treatment weeks have not been established. There is no evidence to suggest that more frequent applications will increase effectiveness.
- Wash hands thoroughly before each application. Apply podofilox with the applicator tip (supplied with the drug). Use the minimum amount of medicine necessary to cover the wart. The gel may also be applied with the finger.
- Allow the solution to dry before returning skin surfaces to their normal positions.
- After each treatment, the used applicator should be carefully disposed of and patients should wash their hands.
- Do not alter recommended method of application, frequency of application, and duration of usage.
- Podofilox is not indicated in the treatment of internal mucous membrane warts (including those of the urethra, rectum and vagina).
- If you miss a dose of this drug, wait until the next scheduled dose and extend treatment accordingly.
- Avoid contact with the eyes. If contact occurs, immediately flush the eye(s) thoroughly with water and contact your doctor.
- *Storage* — Avoid excessive heat. Keep product away from open flame. Store at controlled room temperature (59° to 86°F). Do not freeze.

*If you have any questions, consult your doctor, pharmacist, or health care provider.*

| | Brand Name Examples | Supplied As |
|---|---|---|
| otc | Calicylic Creme[2,3,4] | **Cream**: 5%, 10% |
| otc | Compound W,[1,9] Duoplant Gel | **Gel**: 17% |
| otc | Hydrisalic [1] | **Gel**: 5% |
| otc | Compound W,[1,5,8,9] Off-Ezy Wart Remover,[1,8,9] Wart-Off Maximum Strength,[1,7] Occlusal-HP, Duofilm[1,7] | **Liquid**: 17% |
| otc | Gordofilm | **Liquid**: 16.7% |
| otc | Compound W, Compound W Wart Remover for Kids | **Pad**: 40% |
| otc | Salactic Film[5,8] | **Film**: 17% |
| otc | Mediplast | **Plaster**: 40% |
| Rx | Trans-Ver-Sal | **Transdermal patch**: 15% |
| otc | Gets-It [6] | **Liquid**: 12% |

[1] Contains alcohol.
[2] Contains cetyl alcohol.
[3] Contains urea.
[4] Contains methyl- and propylparabens.
[5] Contains isopropyl alcohol.
[6] Collodion base contains ether.
[7] Flexible collodion.
[8] Contains ether.
[9] Collodion.

## Type of Drug:
An agent that promotes sloughing or peeling of skin; skin softening or dissolving.

## How the Drug Works:
Salicylic acid produces sloughing of the horny layer of skin (keratin) by dissolving the "cement" between skin cells. This causes the thickened epithelium to swell, soften and slough off.

## Uses:
To treat common warts and dry, scaly or calloused skin. Some products (not all) are approved for use in treating plantar warts. Read individual product labels carefully. Common warts have a rough, "cauliflower-like" appearance on the surface. Plantar warts are tender and located on the bottom of the foot.

## Precautions:
*Do not use in the following situations:*

allergy to salicylic acid or its ingredients
birthmarks
diabetes
irritated, infected, reddened skin
genital warts
large areas, especially children
moles
breastfeeding
open wounds
poor circulation
pregnancy
warts on face or mucous membranes (inside mouth, nose, lips, anus, genitals)
warts with hair growing from them, red edges or unusual color

*Use with caution in the following situations:*
    kidney disease
    liver disease

*Salicylic poisoning:* Prolonged use over large areas has caused salicylic poisoning. Symptoms include nausea; vomiting; dizziness; ringing in ears; hearing loss; diarrhea. For additional information on salicylate side effects, see the salicylate monograph.

*Pregnancy:* Adequate studies have not been done in pregnant women. Do not use during pregnancy without consulting your doctor.

*Breastfeeding:* Salicylic acid appears in breast milk. Because of the potential for serious side effects in breastfed infants, decide whether to discontinue breastfeeding or discontinue the drug. Consult your doctor.

*Children:* Do not use in young children (ages are specified in the product packaging).

## Drug Interactions:
Tell your doctor or pharmacist if you are using or if you are planning to use any topical over-the-counter or prescription medications or dietary supplements with salicylic acid (including bismuth subsalicylate). One or both drugs may need to be modified or a different drug may need to be prescribed. Tretinoin (eg, *Retin-A*) interacts with topical salicylic acid.

Consider all drug interactions reported for salicylates (see monograph) when using this drug.

## Side Effects:
Every drug is capable of producing side effects. Many topical salicylic acid users experience no, or minor, side effects. The frequency and severity of side effects depend on many factors including dose, duration of therapy and individual susceptibility. Possible side effects include:

*Skin:* Excessive redness; excessive sloughing and scaling; localized irritation.

## Guidelines for Use:

- For external use only. Use exactly as instructed.
- Apply once or twice daily as needed for 12 weeks.
- *Hydrisalic Gel* and *Trans-Ver-Sal* — Apply medicine at night and cover area. Wash off in the morning.
- Avoid contact with eyes, face, genitals, rectum, mucous membranes (eg, mouth, nose, genitals, lips) and normal skin.
- May produce reddening or scaling of skin when used on open skin lesions.
- Wash affected area. Soak skin in warm water 5 minutes before applying salicylic acid to enhance the effect. Remove loose tissue with brush, wash cloth or emery board and dry skin thoroughly.
- Wash hands thoroughly after use.
- Discontinue treatment if excessive irritation or discomfort persists and consult your doctor.
- Do not use on irritated, infected or reddened skin, if you are a diabetic, or if you have poor blood circulation.
- Do not use on moles, birthmarks, warts with hair growing from them, genital warts, warts on face or mucous membranes.
- If contact with eyes or mucous membranes occurs, flush thoroughly with water for 15 minutes and contact your doctor.
- Avoid inhaling the vapors of the medicine.
- Prolonged use over large areas may cause salicylism. This is most likely in children and in patients with liver or kidney damage.
- Medicine should not come into contact with normal skin surrounding warts.
- Keep away from fire and flame. Contents are flammable.

*If you have any questions, consult your doctor, pharmacist, or health care provider.*

| | Generic Name<br>*Brand Name*<br>*Examples* | Supplied As | Use |
|---|---|---|---|
| *otc* | **Dexpanthenol** | | |
| | *Panthoderm*[1] | **Cream**: 2% | To relieve itching and aid healing of skin in mild eczemas, minor wounds, insect bites, poison ivy, poison oak, minor skin irritations, diaper rash and chafing |
| | **Urea** | | |
| *Rx* | *Carmol 40* | **Cream**: 40% | To slough off dead skin or scabbed from burns and promote healing of infected skin sores |
| *otc* | *Nutraplus,*[1]<br>*Rea-Lo,*[2,5]<br>*Ureacin-20,*[1,4]<br>*Carmol 20* | **Cream**: 10%, 20%, 30% | To moisturize skin in dry skin conditions and to treat very dry, rough, cracked, hardened or calloused skin |
| | *Aquacare,*[5]<br>*Carmol 10,*<br>*Rea-Lo, Ultra*<br>*Mide 25,*<br>*Ureacin-10*[1,4,5] | **Lotion**: 10%, 15%, 25% | |
| *otc* | **Petrolatum and Lanolin** | | |
| | *A and D*[3] | **Ointment** | To treat and prevent diaper rash; heal dry, flaky and chafed skin; protects and soothes minor cuts and burns |

| Generic Name<br>*Brand Name*<br>*Examples* | **Supplied As** | **Use** |
|---|---|---|
| *otc* **Vitamin A and D** | | |
| *Lobana Derm-Ade*[1,5] | **Cream** | To provide relief of discomfort due to minor skin irritations including burns, sunburn, windburn, cuts and scrapes, bed sores and |
| *Lobana Peri-Garde*[5] | **Ointment** | chapped skin; to treat and prevent diaper rash; ointment protects skin against wetness from urine, feces and other skin irritants |
| *otc* **Vitamin E** | | |
| *Vite E,*[1] *Vitec* | **Cream, Lotion** | For control of dry or chapped skin. Also for temporary relief of minor skin disorders such as burns, sunburn and irritated skin |
| *otc* **Zinc Oxide** | | |
| *Balmex,*<br>*Desitin*[1,2,3] | **Ointment** | To treat and prevent diaper rash; protects against wetness from urine, feces and other skin irritants |

[1] Contains parabens.
[2] Contains talc.
[3] Contains lanolin.
[4] Contains EDTA.
[5] Contains alcohol.

The emollients contain a diverse group of chemicals. This monograph does not follow the typical format due to the lack of consistency of information from product to product. Primary ingredients and their uses are listed. However, they may not share the same inactive ingredients. For additional information about a particular product, consult your pharmacist or doctor.

## Type of Drug:

A variety of agents with differing primary uses (eg, skin softening, moisturizing, healing, soothing).

## Uses:

Uses are indicated in the preceding table.

### Guidelines for Use:

- For external use only.
- Do not use in eyes or allow to come in contact with the eye(s).
- Do not use if you are allergic to any ingredient of the products.
- Do not use on irritated or broken skin without consulting your doctor or pharmacist.
- If the condition for which these preparations is used persists or worsens or if irritation, develops, discontinue use and consult your doctor.
- Apply locally to affected skin with gentle massage. For minor burns and other minor skin irritations, the affected area may be covered with a loose layer of gauze or other suitable dressing. This is not required.
- These products do not contain antibiotic ingredients. Do not use to treat infection.
- *Vitamin A & D* — Do not apply over deep or puncture wounds, infections or lacerations.
- Stinging, burning, itching or irritation may develop with the use of these products.

*If you have any questions, consult your doctor, pharmacist, or health care provider.*

| Generic Name<br>*Brand Name*<br>*Examples* | **Supplied As** | **Other** |
|---|---|---|
| **Emollients** | | **Uses:** To lubricate and moisturize skin. To reduce dryness and itching. |
| *Rx*    *Lac-Hydrin* | **Lotion** | |
| *otc*    *Allercreme Ultra, Aveeno, Catrix, Complex 15, Curel Moisturizing, Cutemol, Hydrisinol, Keri Creme, Lubriderm, Masse Breast, Neutrogena Norwegian Formula, Nivea Moisturizing, Nutraderm, Pedi-Vit A, Pen-Kera, Purpose DrySkin, Shepard's Skin* | **Cream** | **Guidelines for Use:**<br>•For external use only.<br>•Do not use in eyes.<br>•If the condition for which these preparations are used persists, or if irritation develops, discontinue use and consult your doctor.<br>•Apply locally to affected skin with gentle massage. |
| *Balmex* | **Ointment** | For minor burns and other minor skin irritations, cover affected area with a layer of gauze or other suitable dressing. |
| *Neutrogena Body, NiveaMoisturizing, Nivea Skin* | **Oil** | |
| *Allercreme Skin, Aveeno, Balmex, Complex 15, Corn Huskers, Curel, Derma Viva, DML, Epilyt, Esoterica, Eucerin, Keri, Keri-Light, Lac-Hydrin Five, LactiCare, Lobana Body, Lubriderm, Moisturel, Neutrogena Body, Nivea, Moisturizing, Nutraderm, Pro-Cute, Ultra Derm, Wondra* | **Lotion** | |

| | Generic Name<br>*Brand Name*<br>*Examples* | Supplied As | Other |
|---|---|---|---|
| *otc* | **Skin Protectants** | | **Uses:** To protect skin against contact irritants and to coat minor sores. |
| | *Covicone, Kerodex* | **Cream** | |
| | *BlisterGard, New-Skin* | **Liquid** | |
| | *Hydropel, Silicone No. 2, White Cloverine Salve* | **Ointment** | **Guidelines for Use:**<br>•For external use only.<br>•Do not use silicone-containing preparations on rash or wet, oozing lesions. |
| | *New-Skin Antiseptic* | **Spray liquid** | |
| | *Aerozoin* | **Spray** | |
| | *Benzoin, TinBen, TinCoBen* | **Tincture** | |
| *otc* | **Bath Oils** | | **Uses:** To relieve minor skin irritations and itching of common skin problems and dry skin. |
| | *Alpha Keri Therapeutic, Aveeno Oilated Bath, Aveeno Regular, Cameo, Domol Bath and Shower, Lubriderm, LubraSol, Nutraderm, Nutra-Soothe, Therapeutic Bath, Ultra Derm* | **Oil** | |

| **Generic Name** *Brand Name Examples* | **Supplied As** | **Other** |
| --- | --- | --- |
| *Pedi-Bath Salts* | **Salts** | **Guidelines for Use:** •For external use only. •Use caution to avoid slipping in the tub. |
| *Alpha Keri* | **Spray** | •Do not use on raw skin. •Avoid contact with the eyes; flush with clear water |

*If you have any questions, consult your doctor, pharmacist, or health care provider.*

| Generic Name Brand Name Examples | Supplied As | Generic Available |
|---|---|---|
| otc **Capsaicin** | | |
| *Zostrix* | **Cream**: 0.025% | No |
| *Zostrix-HP* | **Cream**: 0.075% | No |

## Type of Drug:

Topical analgesic (pain relieving) cream.

## How the Drug Works:

Capsaicin is a natural chemical derived from plants. It is believed that capsaicin causes the skin to become insensitive to pain by causing the removal of substance P, a pain-transmitting compound from the nerve endings. With the lowered amount of substance P at the nerve endings, pain impulses cannot be transmitted to the brain. The active ingredient is found in red chili peppers.

## Uses:

For temporary relief of pain from rheumatoid arthritis, osteoarthritis, painful diabetic neuropathy or following shingles (herpes zoster).

## Precautions:

*Do not use in the following situations:*

allergy to any ingredient in the products
in or around the eyes or other mucous membranes
open wounds or damaged skin

*Children:* Do not use in children under 2 except with the supervision of a doctor.

## Side Effects:

Every drug is capable of producing side effects. Many capsaicin users experience no, or minor, side effects. The frequency and severity of side effects depend on many factors including dose, duration of therapy and individual susceptibility. Possible side effects include a burning sensation upon application (usually temporary).

## Guidelines for Use:

- For external use only.
- Onset of relief may take several weeks.
- Apply to affected area 3 to 4 times daily to achieve maximum pain relief. Thoroughly rub into the area so no residue is left on the skin surface. Wash hands after application.
- Avoid contact with eyes or other mucous membranes. If contact occurs, flush the affected area thoroughly with water.
- Do not use on children under 2 unless directed by a doctor.
- Do not apply to open wounds, damaged or irritated skin.
- Do not bandage tightly.
- Discontinue use if condition worsens or does not improve after 28 days. Consult a doctor.
- Warm water or excessive sweating may intensify burning sensation.
- Keep this and all medications out of the reach of children.

*If you have any questions, consult your doctor, pharmacist, or health care provider.*

|     | Brand Name Examples | Supplied As |
| --- | --- | --- |
| otc | Benadryl, Maximum Strength Benadryl 2% | **Cream or spray**: 1% or 2% diphenhydramine HCl |
| otc | Cala-gen | **Lotion**: 1% diphenhydramine HCl, camphor, 2% alcohol |
| otc | Calamycin | **Lotion**: Pyrilamine maleate, 10% zinc oxide, 10%calamine, benzocaine, chloroxylenol, zirconium oxide |
| otc | Clearly Cala-gel | **Gel**: Diphenhydramine HCl, menthol, zinc acetate, benzethonium chloride |
| otc | Dermamycin | **Cream**: 2% diphenhydramine HCl |
| otc | Derma-Pax | **Lotion**: 0.22% pyrilamine maleate, 0.22% pheniramine maleate, 0.06% chlorpheniramine maleate |
| otc | Dermarest | **Gel**: 2% diphenhydramine HCl, 2% resorcinol |
| otc | Dermarest Plus | **Gel or spray**: 2% diphenhydramine HCl, 1% menthol |
| otc | Di-Delamine | **Gel or spray**: 1% diphenhydramine HCl, 0.5% tripelennamine HCl, 0.12% benzalkonium chloride and 1% menthol |
| otc | Sting-Eze | **Concentrate**: Diphenhydramine HCl, camphor, phenol, benzocaine and eucalyptol |
| otc | Ziradryl | **Lotion**: 2% diphenhydramine HCl and 2% zinc oxide |
| otc | Zonalon | **Cream**: 5% doxepin HCl |

## Type of Drug:

Topical antihistamines.

## How the Drug Works:

The topical antihistamines counteract the effects of histamine. Histamine is the chemical in the body which causes blood vessels to dilate (widen), smooth muscle to contract, and heart rate and stomach secretions to increase. These effects play a role in allergic reactions.

Topical antihistamines have some local anesthetic activity and relieve itching.

Other ingredients which may be combined with the antihistamines include benzocaine (local anesthetic); camphor, menthol or phenol (anti-itching and anesthetic action); and calamine, titanium dioxide, zirconium oxide and zinc oxide (astringents).

## Uses:

To treat hives, insect bites or stings, and itching due to minor skin disorders, poison ivy, poison oak or sumac; mild sunburn.

## Precautions:

*Do not use in the following situations:*
allergy to this medicine or any of its ingredients
narrow angle glaucoma, untreated (doxepin only)
history of urinary retention, history of (doxepin only)

*Use with caution in the following situations:* Redness, swelling, inflammation, or pain.

*Pregnancy:* There are no adequate and well-controlled studies of doxepin in pregnant women. Use during pregnancy only if clearly needed.

*Breastfeeding:* It is not known if topical doxepin appears in breastmilk. Consult your doctor before you begin breastfeeding.

*Children:* Do not use on children less than 2 years of age. Safety and effectiveness of doxepin in children have not been established. Consult a doctor before treating chlidren less than 12 years of age with *Benadryl*.

## Drug Interactions:

Tell your doctor or pharmacist if you are taking or planning to take any over-the-counter or prescription medications or dietary supplements while using topical antihistamines. Doses of one or both drugs may need to be modified or a different drug may need to be prescribed. The following drugs and drug classes interact with doxepin only:

alcohol
antiarrhythmic drugs (eg, *Quinidine*)
carbamazepine (eg, *Tegretol*)

cimetidine (eg, *Tagamet)*
MAO inhibitors (eg, *Parnate)*
phenothiazines (eg, *Thorazine)*

## Side Effects:

Every drug is capable of producing side effects. Many topical antihistamine users experience no, or minor, side effects. The frequency and severity of side effects depend on many factors including dose, duration of therapy, and individual susceptibility. Possible side effects include:

*Doxepin only:* Drowsiness; headache; fatigue; dizziness; emotional changes; dry mouth or lips; fluid retention; thirst; taste changes.

*Skin:* Dry skin; abnormal skin sensation; burning and stinging; increased itching or aggravation of skin disorder; local irritation; rash; redness.

## Guidelines for Use:

- For external use only. Do not use in or near eyes.
- Do not apply to mucous membranes or to skin which is blistered, raw, or oozing a liquid.
- Do not use occlusive dressings unless directed by your doctor.
- If rash, burning, or irritation develops or worsens where the medicine is applied, stop using the medicine. Wash area with soap and water and contact your doctor.
- Avoid prolonged use or use on extensive skin areas, especially in infants.
- Do not use on chickenpox or measles unless supervised by your doctor.
- *Doxepin* — Allow an interval of 3 to 4 hours between applications. Do not bandage area being treated. May cause drowsiness. Use caution while driving or performing other tasks requiring alertness, coordination, or physical dexterity. Alcohol may cause added drowsiness. Do not use for more than 8 days.

*If you have any questions, consult your doctor, pharmacist, or health care provider.*

| Generic Name *Brand Name Examples* | Use(s) |
|---|---|
| *otc* **Iodine** *Iodex* | For external use against bacteria, fungi, viruses, spores, protozoa, and yeasts. Available as an ointment, solution, and tincture. |
| *otc* **Povidone-Iodine** *ACU-dyne*, Betadine, *Iodex, Operand, Pharmadine, Polydine* | Povidone-iodine liberates about 9% to 12% free iodine. It is bactericidal but does not irritate skin and mucous membranes (unless one is allergic to iodine). Also cleanses and deodorizes. Available as an ointment, solution, liquid, gauze pads, swabs, swabsticks, skin cleanser, surgical scrub solution, spray, cream, shampoo, perineal wash, mouthwash, vaginal suppositories, foil, douche, foam, pad, and stick. |
| *otc* **Thimerosal** | To treat contaminated wounds and disinfect healthy skin prior to surgery. Contains 49% mercury and has activity against bacteria and fungus. Available as a tincture, solution, and swabs. |
| *Rx* **Hexachlorophene** *pHisoHex, Septi-Soft* | For use as a surgical scrub and skin cleanser. Hexachlorophene is an antibacterial agent with activity against bacteria. Available as a foam, liquid skin cleanser, detergent cleaner, wash, shampoo, and sponge. |
| *otc* **Chlorhexidine Gluconate** *Chlorostat, Hibiclens Antiseptic/Antimicrobial Skin, Hibiclens, Hibistat Germicidal Hand* | For use as a surgical scrub, preoperative skin cleanser, skin wound cleanser, and hand rinse. Chlorhexidine gluconate is an antibacterial agent effective against a wide range of bacteria (including *Pseudomonas aeruginosa*). Available as a skin cleanser, sponge, liquid, towlettes, and rinse. |

| | Generic Name<br>*Brand Name Examples* | Use(s) |
|---|---|---|
| *otc* | **Benzalkonium Chloride**<br>*Benza, Benz-all,*<br>*Zephiran* | For disinfection of skin, mucous membranes, and small wounds; preoperative preparation of skin; surgeons' hand and arm soaks; treatment of wounds; preservation of ophthalmic solutions; irrigations of the eye, body cavities, bladder, and urethra; and vaginal douching. An anti-rust factor in this agent has been shown to be effective in the chemical disinfection of professional and hospital instruments and equipment. Benzalkonium chloride is a rapidly-acting anti-infective with a long duration of action. It is active against bacteria, some viruses, fungi, and protozoa. Available as a solution, tincture, and spray. |
| *otc* | **Glutaraldehyde**<br>*Cidex, Cidex For-*<br>*mula-7, Cidex Plus* | To disinfect and sterilize certain types of plastic, metal, or rubber respiratory or anesthesia equipment against vegetative bacteria (eg, *Pseudomonas aeruginosa*, pathogenic fungi, and certain viruses). Glutaraldehyde is mildly acidic. Do not use on skin or mucous membranes. Available as a 2.4% and 3.4% solution and test strips. |
| *otc* | **Peracetic Acid**<br>*Cidex PA* | To disinfect and sterilize metals (stainless steel and aluminium alloy), plastics, and elastomers. Do not use with brass or copper. Avoid contact with eyes. Available as a 0.08% solution. |
| *otc* | **Sodium Hypochlorite**<br>*Dakin's Solution Half*<br>*Strength, Dakin's*<br>*Solution Full Strength* | To disinfect skin against vegetative bacteria and viruses and, to some degree, against spores and fungi. It has germicidal, deodorizing, and bleaching properties. Sodium hypochlorite is bleach and is not to be used on skin or wounds. Sodium hypochlorite may produce chemical burns if it comes in contact with skin or eyes. Available as a solution. |

| Generic Name Brand Name Examples | Use(s) |
|---|---|
| otc **Oxychlorosene Sodium** *Clorpactin WCS-90* | To treat localized infections, remove dead tissue, counteract odorous discharges; for use as a pre- and postoperative irrigant; and for cleansing and disinfecting fistulas, the sinus tract, empyemas, and wounds.Available as a powder for solution or a concentrate. |

## Type of Drug:

Antiseptics and germicides (topical); agents that prevent or arrest the spread of disease-causing microorganisms.

## Uses:

Selected products and their primary use(s) are included in the table above.

---

### Guidelines for Use:

- Doses and frequency of use depend on the condition, area to be treated, individual tolerance, and dosage form. Individual products should be reviewed for their use and dosage guidelines. Consult your pharmacist or doctor for product-specific information.
- Discontinue use and consult your doctor if redness, irritation, swelling, or pain increases.
- *Sodium hypochlorite* is toxic to fish. Do not dispose product where it will drain into lakes, streams, or public water.
- *Benzalkonium chloride's* effects are deactivated by soap.

---

*If you have any questions, consult your doctor, pharmacist, or health care provider.*

| Generic Name<br>*Brand Name Examples* | Supplied As | Generic<br>Available |
|---|---|---|
| *otc* **Methionine** | **Tablets**: 500 mg | Yes |
| | **Powder**: 200 mg/tsp | Yes |
| *Pedameth, Uracid* | **Capsules**: 200 mg | No |
| *Pedameth* | **Liquid**: 75 mg/5 mL | No |
| *otc* **Miscellaneous Diaper Rash Products** | | |
| *Balmex Diaper Rash* | **Ointment**: 11.3% zinc oxide, aloe vera gel, balsam peru | No |
| *Desitin* | **Ointment**: 40% zinc oxide, cod liver oil, talc, petrolatum, lanolin | No |
| *Desitin Creamy* | **Ointment**: 10% zinc oxide | No |
| *Desitin with Zinc Oxide* | **Powder**: 88.2% corn starch, 10% zinc oxide | No |
| *Diaparene* | **Powder**: Methylbenzethonium chloride, corn starch | No |
| *Diaparene Medicated* | **Cream**: 0.1% methylbenze-thonium chloride, white petrola-tum, glycerin | No |
| *Diaparene Peri-Anal Medicated* | **Ointment**: 0.1% methylbenze-thonium chloride, zinc oxide, cod liver oil, white petrolatum, starch, lanolin calcium caseinate | No |
| *Flanders Buttocks* | **Ointment**: Zinc oxide, balsam peru | No |
| *Mexsana Medicated* | **Powder**: Corn starch, zinc oxide, kaolin, benzethonium chloride | No |

## Type of Drug:
Diaper rash products.

## How the Drug Works:
Methionine (for oral ingestion) creates an acid condition in the urine that results in an ammonia-free urine, and therefore, less diaper rash, odor, skin inflammation, and ulceration by urine.

The agents applied externally as ointment, cream, or powder contain a variety of ingredients:

*Antimicrobial agents* (benzethonium chloride, methylbenzethonium chloride) minimize bacterial growth.

*Balsam peru* is claimed to promote wound healing and tissue repair but its effectiveness has not been documented.

*Corn starch, kaolin, and talc* absorb moisture.

*Protectants (petrolatum, lanolin) and lubricants (glycerin, cod liver oil)* minimize chafing and irritation.

*Zinc oxide* is an astringent that dries the skin.

## Uses:
Methionine —

To prevent or treat diaper rash, urine odor, ammonia dermatitis (inflammation), and skin ulcers caused by excess ammonia in urine.

Topical products —

To provide a protective barrier against wetness and soothe and moisturize skin.

## Precautions:
*Do not use in the following situations:*
> liver disease, active (methionine only)
> liver disease, history of (methionine only)

## Side Effects:
Every drug is capable of producing side effects. Many diaper rash product users experience no, or minor, side effects. The frequency and severity of side effects depend on many factors including dose, duration of therapy, and individual susceptibility. Possible side effects related to topical diaper rash products include: Rash; irritation; itching; burning.

---

### Guidelines for Use:
- *Methionine* —
  Dosage will be individualized. Do not exceed recommended dosage.
  Take with meals.
  Do not take with dairy products.
  Capsules may be opened and the contents mixed with food, formula, juice, or water.
  Adequate protein intake must be maintained during therapy to prevent below normal weight gain.
- *Ointments, creams, or powders* —
  For external use only.
  Apply to the affected area several times daily as needed, especially at bedtime or any time when exposure to wet diapers may be prolonged.
  Cleanse the affected area and allow it to dry before application.
  Do not use on broken skin.
  Avoid contact with the eyes.
  Keep powder away from child's face to avoid inhalation, which can cause breathing problems.
  Consult a doctor if condition worsens or symptoms do not improve within 7 days.

---

*If you have any questions, consult your doctor, pharmacist, or health care provider.*

| Generic Name *Brand Name Examples* | Supplied As | Generic Available |
|---|---|---|
| *otc* **Minoxidil** | | |
| *Rogaine for Men,*[1] *Rogaine for Women*[1] | **Solution**: 2% | Yes |
| *Rogaine Extra Strength for Men*[1] | **Solution**: 5% | No |

[1] Contains alcohol.

## Type of Drug:

Topical scalp agent. Promotes hair growth.

## How the Drug Works:

It is not known how minoxidil stimulates scalp hair growth. It is possible that it dilates blood vessels in the scalp, which may improve hair follicle function and stimulate scalp hair growth.

## Uses:

To treat male pattern baldness in men and diffuse hair loss or thinnning of hair on forehead or temples in females. There is no effect in men with predominantly frontal hair loss.

*Unlabeled Use(s):* Occasionally, doctors may prescribe minoxidil for alopecia areata (a disease in which patches of hair fall out over a period of a few days on any part of the body).

## Precautions:

*Do not use in the following situations:*
allergy to minoxidil or any of its ingredients
childbirth-associated hair loss
no family history of hair loss
patients less than 18 years of age
red, inflamed, infected, irritated, or painful scalp
sudden or patchy hair loss
undergoing therapy with another topical scalp medication
unknown reason for hair loss
women (*Rogaine Extra Strength* only)

*Use with caution in the following situations:*
heart disease
inflamed or diseased scalp

*Results:* At least 4 months of continuous use is generally required before evidence of hair growth can be expected. Further growth continues through 1 year of treatment. The new growth of hair is not permanent. Continued use is necessary to increase and keep hair growth or hair loss will begin again.

*Pregnancy:* Adequate studies have not been conducted in pregnant women. Do not use if you are pregnant.

*Breastfeeding:* Because of the potential for adverse effects, do not use when breastfeeding.

*Children:* Safety and effectiveness in patients less than 18 years of age have not been established. Do not use on babies and children.

## Side Effects:

Every drug is capable of producing side effects. Many minoxidil users experience no, or minor, side effects. The frequency and severity of side effects depend upon many factors including dose, duration of therapy, and individual susceptibility. Possible side effects include:

*Digestive Tract:* Nausea; vomiting; diarrhea.

*Nervous System:* Headache; dizziness; faintness; lightheadedness; feeling of whirling motion.

*Circulatory System:* Blood pressure changes; changes in heart rate; chest pain; pounding in chest.

*Other:* Aches or pain; fluid retention; ear infections; weight gain; sinus infection; skin irritation or inflammation; hives.

## Guidelines for Use:

- For external use only.
- Minoxidil is indicated for patients who have a general thinning of hair on the top of the scalp. It is not intended for frontal baldness or a receding hairline.
- *Rogaine Extra Strength* is not for use by women. It may cause facial hair growth and be harmful during pregnancy or breastfeeding.
- Dry hair and scalp prior to application.
- Apply 1 mL (or 6 sprays if using *Extra Strength for Men*) 2 times a day directly onto the scalp in the hair loss area. Do not apply to other parts of the body.
- Do not exceed 2 mL daily. Larger or more frequent doses do not speed up or increase hair growth, but do increase the chance of side effects.
- If applied with fingertips, wash hands afterwards.
- First hair growth may be soft, downy, colorless, and barely visible. After further treatment, the new hair should be the color and thickness of other scalp hair.
- Apply to a healthy scalp only. Inflammation or disease of the scalp (eg, abrasions, severe sunburn, psoriasis, dermatitis) may increase absorption of the drug and increase the risk of side effects. Be alert for a rapid heart rate, weight gain, edema (fluid retention), and other side effects.
- *Contains alcohol* — May cause burning or irritation of sensitive skin, eyes, and mucous membranes. If the drug comes in contact with the eyes, mucous membranes, or sensitive skin areas, bathe the area with large amounts of cool tap water. Consult your doctor if irritation continues.
- Do not use with other topical scalp medications.
- Discontinue use and consult your doctor if you experience chest pain, rapid heartbeat, faintness, dizziness, sudden unexplained weight gain, swollen hands or feet, redness, or irritation at application site.
- Evidence of hair growth usually takes at least 4 months. If you do not see hair regrowth in 4 months with *Extra Strength for Men*, 8 months with *Rogaine for Women*, or 12 months with *Rogaine for Men*, stop treatment and contact your doctor.
- Use continuously to increase and keep your hair regrowth. If treatment is stopped, new hair will probably be shed within a few months.
- If a treatment is missed, do not attempt to make it up. Apply next treatment at regularly scheduled time.
- *Caution* — Accidental oral ingestion could produce significant side effects. Avoid inhalation of the spray mist.
- Store at controlled room temperature (68° to 77°F).

*If you have any questions, consult your doctor, pharmacist, or health care provider.*

| Brand Name Examples | Supplied As | Generic Available |
|---|---|---|
| otc Aveeno | **Cream, Lotion, Powder**: Colloidal oatmeal | No |
| otc Cala-gen, Calagesic | **Lotion**: 8% calamine, 1% pramoxine HCl | No |
| otc Calaclear | **Lotion**: 1% pramoxine HCl, 0.1% zinc acetate | No |
| otc Calamine | **Lotion**: 6.97% calamine, 6.97% zinc oxide, glycerin, bentonite magma in calcium hydroxide solution | Yes |
| otc Ivy-Rid | **Spray**: Isobutane, methylene chloride, benzalkonium chloride, alcohol, isopropyl myristate | No |
| otc Phenolated Calamine | **Lotion**: 8% calamine, 8% zinc oxide, 2% glycerin, bentonite magma, 1% phenol in calcium hydroxide solution | Yes |
| otc Rhuli Aerosol | **Solution**: 0.67% phenylcarbinol, 4.7% calamine, 0.025% menthol, 0.25% camphor, 1.15% benzocaine, 28.8% alcohol | No |
| otc Rhuli Gel | **Gel**: 2% phenylcarbinol, 0.3% menthol, 0.3% camphor, 31% SD alcohol | No |
| otc Rhuli Spray | **Spray**: 0.67% phenylcarbinol, 4.7% calamine, 0.025% menthol, 0.25% camphor, 1.15% benzocaine, 28.8% alcohol | No |

## Type of Drug:
Poison ivy treatment products.

## Uses:
To relieve itching, pain, and discomfort due to ivy, oak, and sumac poisoning. Some products are also recommended for nonpoisonous insect bites, sunburn, prickly heat, and other minor skin irritations.

In these products:

*Benzalkonium chloride* is used for its antimicrobial activity.

*Benzocaine, phenylcarbinol, and pramoxine HCl* are local anesthetics that temporarily relieve pain, itching, and irritation.

*Calamine, zinc oxide, and zirconium oxide* are used to shrink skin cells, thereby tightening skin.

*Camphor, menthol, and methyl salicylate* are counterirritants.

*Colloidal oatmeal* is a demulcent (soothing agent).

*Isopropyl alcohol, phenol, and phenylcarbinol* are antiseptics.

## Precautions:

*Children:* Do not use on children less than 2 years of age without consulting your doctor.

---

### Guidelines for Use:

- For external use only.
- Shake well before use.
- Before each use cleanse the skin with soap and water and dry the affected area.
- Apply to affected area 3 to 4 times daily.
- A cotton pledget or soft cloth may be used for ease of application.
- Avoid contact with the eyes and mucous membranes.
- If the condition for which these products are used worsens or does not improve within 7 days, or if rash, irritation, or allergy develops, discontinue use and consult your doctor.
- Store at room temperature (59° to 86°F).

---

*If you have any questions, consult your doctor, pharmacist, or health care provider.*

| Generic Name *Brand Name Examples* | Supplied As |
|---|---|
| otc **Menthol** | |
| *Absorbine Jr., Cool'n Hot Gel, Cool Hot Gel, Eucalyptamint* | **Gel, cream, ointment** |
| otc **Methyl Salicylate** | |
| *Exocaine Plus Rub, Gordogesic Creme* | **Gel, cream, ointment** |
| otc **Methyl Salicylate** and **Menthol** | |
| *Analgesic Balm, Ben Gay, Icy Hot, Pain Bust-R II Cream, Podiacin Soak'n Massage Gel, Thera-gesic* | **Gel, cream, ointment** |
| *Banalg Hospital Strength Lotion* | **Lotion, liniment** |
| otc **Methyl Salicylate**, **Menthol**, and **Camphor** | |
| *Ben Gay Ultra Strength Cream, Panalgesic Gold Cream* | **Gel, cream, ointment** |
| *Banalg Muscle Pain Reliever* | **Lotion, liniment** |
| otc **Methyl Salicylate**, **Methyl Nicotinate**, and **Menthol** | |
| *ArthriCare Rub* | **Gel, cream, ointment** |
| otc **Methyl Salicylate**, **Methyl Nicotinate**, **Camphor**, and **Menthol** | |
| *Deep-Down Rub* | **Gel, cream, ointment** |
| otc **Triethanolamine Salicylate** | |
| *Aspercreme, Exocaine Odor Free Creme, Mobisyl Creme, Sportscreme* | **Gel, cream, ointment** |
| *Aspercreme Rub* | **Lotion, liniment** |

| Generic Name<br>*Brand Name Examples* | Supplied As |
|---|---|
| *otc* **Miscellaneous Combinations** | |
| *Heet Spray* | **Aerosol** |
| *Argesic Cream, Arthro-Therapy Gel, Eucalyptamint 2000 Gel, Iodex w/Methyl Salicylate Ointment, Methagual, Myoflex Creme, Pain Relief Cream, Rid-A-Pain Cream, Rid-a-Pain HP Cream, Soltice Quick-Rub, Vicks Vapo Rub* | **Gel, cream, ointment** |
| *Arth-Rx Lotion, ArthriCare Lotion, ArthriCare Ultra Rub, Capsin Lotion, Sloan's Liniment* | **Lotion, liniment** |

Rubs and liniments contain a diverse group of chemicals. This monograph does not follow the usual format seen in this book due to the lack of consistency of information from product to product. For additional information about a particular product, consult your pharmacist or doctor.

## Uses:

To relieve pain of muscular aches, nerve pain, rheumatism, arthritis, sprains, and similar conditions when skin is intact.

## Precautions:

*Do not use in the following situations:*
allergy to any ingredient in the formulation
allergy to salicylates (eg, aspirin)

*Tartrazine:* Some of these products may contain the dye tartrazine (FD&C Yellow No. 5), which can cause allergic reactions in certain individuals. Check package label when available or consult your pharmacist or doctor.

## Guidelines for Use:

- For external use only.
- Avoid contact with eyes and mucous membranes.
- Apply only to affected areas. Do not apply to irritated skin. Discontinue use if excessive irritation occurs.
- Consult your doctor if pain persists for more than 7 to 10 days, if redness is present, or if the condition affects a child younger than 12 years of age.
- If applied to large skin areas, salicylate side effects (eg, ringing in the ears, nausea, vomiting) may occur. May be toxic if ingested.
- May cause local irritation in patients with sensitive skin.

*If you have any questions, consult your doctor, pharmacist, or health care provider.*

| Generic Name<br>*Brand Name Examples* | Supplied As | SPF |
|---|---|---|
| *otc* **Creams, Foams, Gels, Lotions, Oils, and Sprays** | | |
| *SolBar PF* | **Cream**: Oxybenzone, octyl methoxycinnamate, octocrylene | 50 |
| *Banana Boat Baby, Banana Boat Maximum, Banana Boat Sport* | **Lotion**: Octocrylene, octyl methoxycinnamate, oxybenzone, octyl salicylate | |
| *Hawaiian Tropic Baby Faces* | **Lotion**: Octyl methoxycinnamate, octyl salicylate, titanium dioxide | |
| *Coppertone Sport* | **Lotion**: Octyl methoxycinnamate, oxybenzone, homosalate, octyl salicylate | 48 |
| *Biosun Professional Sun Protection* | **Lotion**: Octyl methoxycinnamate, octocrylene, oxybenzone, octyl salicylate | 45 |
| *Bullfrog for Babies* | **Lotion**: Octocrylene, octyl methoxycinnamate, benzophenone-3, titanium dioxide, menthyl anthranilate, octyl salicylate | |
| *Bullfrog SuperBlock* | **Lotion**: Octocrylene, octyl methoxycinnamate, oxybenzone, menthyl anthranilate, octyl salicylate, titanium dioxide | |
| *Coppertone All Day, Coppertone Oil-Free, Coppertone Shade* | **Lotion**: Ethylhexyl p-methoxycinnamate, 2-ethylhexyl salicylate, oxybenzone, homosalate | |
| *Coppertone Water Babies* | **Lotion**: Octyl methoxycinnamate, oxybenzone, octyl salicylate, homosalate | |
| *Hawaiian Tropic 45 Plus* | **Lotion**: Octyl methoxycinnamate, octyl salicylate, titanium dioxide | |
| *Neutrogena Sunblock* | **Lotion**: Homosalate, octyl methoxycinnamate, benzophenone-3, octyl salicylate | |
| *Coppertone Water Babies Lotion* | **Spray**: Octyl methoxycinnamate, oxybenzone, octyl salicylate, homosalate | |

| | | |
|---|---|---|
| *Coppertone Kids Wacky Foam* | **Foam**: Octyl methoxycinnamate, oxybenzone, octyl salicylate, octocrylene | 40 |
| *Coppertone Kids, Coppertone Kids Colorblock* | **Lotion**: Octyl methoxycinnamate, octyl salicylate, oxybenzone, homosalate | |
| *Bullfrog Body Gel* | **Gel**: Octocrylene, octyl methoxycinnamate, oxybenzone | 36 |
| *Bullfrog for Kids* | **Gel**: Benzophenone-3, octocrylene, octyl methoxycinnamate | |
| *Bullfrog Quik Stick* | **Stick**: Octyl methoxycinnamate, octocrylene, oxybenzone, octyl salicylate | |
| *Elta Block* | **Cream**: Octyl methoxycinnamate, octyl salicylate, zinc oxide, titanium dioxide | 32 |
| *PreSun Ultra* | **Cream**: Avobenzone, octyl methoxycinnamate, octyl salicylate, oxybenzone | 30 |
| *Coppertone Shade* | **Gel**: Ethylhexyl p-methoxycinnamate, homosalate, oxybenzone | |
| *Kiss My Face* | **Gel**: Titanium dioxide, octyl methoxycinnamate | |
| *Fisher-Price Sunscreen for Kids, PreSun Ultra* | **Gel**: Avobenzone, octyl methoxycinnamate, octyl salicylate, oxybenzone | |
| *SolBar PF* | **Liquid**: Octocrylene | |
| *Bain de Soleil All Day Extended Protection, Bain de Soleil GentleBlock, Bain de Soleil Kids* | **Lotion**: Octyl methoxycinnamate, octocrylene, oxybenzone, titanium dioxide | |
| *Banana Boat Kids, Banana Boat Ultra* | **Lotion**: Octyl methoxycinnamate, oxybenzone, octyl salicylate | |
| *Bullfrog Body Lotion, Bullfrog Magic Block, Bullfrog Sport Lotion* | **Lotion**: Octocrylene, octyl methoxycinnamate, oxybenzone, octyl salicylate | |
| *Coppertone All Day, Coppertone Kids, Coppertone Kids Colorblock, Coppertone Oil-Free* | **Lotion**: Ethylhexyl p-methoxycinnamate, 2-ethylexyl salicylate, homosalate, oxybenzone | |
| *Coppertone Bug & Sun* | **Lotion**: Octocrylene, ethylhexyl p-methoxycinnamate, oxybenzone, n,n-diethyl m-toluamide | |

| | | |
|---|---|---|
| *Coppertone Shade UVA Guard* | **Lotion**: Ethylhexyl p-methoxy-cinnamate, oxybenzone, 2-eth-ylhexyl salicylate, homosalate, avobenzone | 30 |
| *Coppertone Sport, Coppertone Water Babies* | **Lotion**: Octyl methoxycinna-mate, oxybenzone, homosalate, octyl salicylate | |
| *DuraScreen* | **Lotion**: Octyl methoxycinna-mate, octyl salicylate, benzo-phenone-3, phenylbenzimidazole sulfonic acid, titanium dioxide | |
| *Hawaiian Tropic 30 Plus, Hawaiian Tropic Super Waterproof* | **Lotion**: Octyl salicylate, octyl methoxycinnamate, titanium dioxide | |
| *Neutrogena Sunblock* | **Lotion**: Octyl methoxycinna-mate, homosalate, octyl salicy-late, benzolphenone-3, avobenzone | |
| *Neutrogena Kids, Neutro-gena Oil-Free* | **Lotion**: Homosalate, octyl methoxycinnamate, benzophe-none-3, octyl salicylate | |
| *Ti•Screen* | **Lotion**: Octocrylene, octyl methoxycinnamate, benzophe-none-3, octyl salicylate, avobenzone | |
| *Coppertone Kids Spray 'n Splash* | **Spray**: Ethylhexyl p-methoxy-cinnamate, oxybenzone, 2-eth-ylhexyl salicylate, homosalate | |
| *Coppertone Shade* | **Spray**: Octyl methoxycinna-mate, octyl salicylate, homo-salate, oxybenzone, avobenzone | |
| *Coppertone Sport, Coppertone to Go, Coppertone Water Babies* | **Spray**: Octyl methoxycinna-mate, octyl salicylate, homo-salate, oxybenzone | |
| *Kiss My Face, Sun Splash* | **Spray**: Octyl methoxycinna-mate, octyl salicylate, benzo-phenone-3 | |
| *Coppertone Kids, Coppertone Shade* | **Stick**: Ethylhexyl p-methoxycin-namate, oxybenzone, 2-ethyl-hexyl salicylate, homosalate | |
| *Coppertone Sport* | **Stick**: Octyl methoxycinnamate, oxybenzone, octyl salicylate, homosalate | |

| Fisher-Price Sensitive Skin Sunblock for Kids, PreSun Sensitive | **Cream**: Titanium dioxide | 28 |
|---|---|---|
| Fisher-Price Spray Mist Sunscreen for Kids, Pre-Sun Ultra | **Spray**: Avobenzone, octyl methoxycinnamate, octyl salicylate, oxybenzone | 27 |
| Biosun Faces | **Lotion**: Octyl methoxycinnamate, oxybenzone, octyl salicylate | 25 |
| Banana Boat Action Sport | **Spray**: Octyl methoxycinnamate, octyl salicylate, homosalate, oxybenzone | |
| RVPaque | **Cream**: Red petrolatum, zinc oxide, cinoxate | 24 |
| Banana Boat Faces Plus | **Lotion**: Octyl methoxycinnamate, oxybenzone, octyl salicylate | 23 |
| Ti•Screen | **Spray**: Octyl methoxycinnamate, octocrylene, menthyl anthranilate, benzophenone-3 | |
| Ti•Screen Sports Gel | **Gel**: Octyl methoxycinnamate, benzophenone-3, octyl salicylate, avobenzone | 20 |
| Neutrogena Oil-Free | **Spray**: Homosalate, octyl methoxycinnamate, octyl salicylate, menthyl anthranilate | |
| Bullfrog Quik Gel | **Gel**: Benzophenone-3, octyl methoxycinnamate, octyl salicylate | 18 |
| Kiss My Face | **Gel**: Titanium dioxide | |
| Neutrogena Sensitive Skin | **Lotion**: Titanium dioxide | 17 |
| Ti•Baby Natural, Ti•Screen Natural | **Lotion**: Titanium dioxide | 16 |
| PreSun Ultra | **Cream**: Avobenzone, octyl methoxycinnamate, octyl salicylate, oxybenzone | 15 |
| Bain de Soleil Orange Gelee | **Gel**: Octyl methoxycinnamate, octocrylene, octyl salicylate, oxybenzone | |
| PreSun Ultra | **Gel**: Avobenzone, octyl methoxycinnamate, octyl salicylate, oxybenzone | |
| Abuval Sport | **Lotion**: Octyl methoxycinnamate, octyl salicylate | |

| | | |
|---|---|---|
| *Bain de Soleil All Day Extended Protection, Bain de Soleil Mademoiselle* | **Lotion**: Octyl methoxycinnamate, octocrylene, titanium dioxide, oxybenzone | 15 |
| *Banana Boat Sport, Coppertone Sport* | **Lotion**: Octyl methoxycinnamate, oxybenzone, octyl salicylate | |
| *Coppertone All Day, Coppertone Oil-Free* | **Lotion**: Ethylhexyl p-methoxycinnamate, oxybenzone | |
| *Coppertone Bug & Sun* | **Lotion**: Ethylhexyl p-methoxycinnamate, oxybenzone, 2-ethylhexyl salicylate, homosalate, n,n diethyl m-toluamide | |
| *DuraScreen* | **Lotion**: Octyl methoxycinnamate, octyl salicylate, benzophenone-3, titanium dioxide | |
| *Hawaiian Tropic 15 Plus, Hawaiian Tropic Super Waterproof* | **Lotion**: Octyl methoxycinnamate, octyl salicylate, titanium dioxide | |
| *Neutrogena Moisture* | **Lotion**: Octyl methoxycinnamate, octyl salicylate, benzophenone-3 | |
| *Neutrogena Sunblock* | **Lotion**: Octyl methoxycinnamate | |
| *Ray Block* | **Lotion**: Octyl dimethyl PABA, benzophenone-3 | |
| *Ti•Screen* | **Lotion**: Octyl methoxycinnamate, benzophenone-3 | |
| *Abuval Sport* | **Spray**: Octyl methoxycinnamate, oxybenzone, octyl salicylate | |
| *Coppertone Sport, Coppertone to Go* | **Spray**: Octyl methoxycinnamate, octyl salicylate, homosalate, oxybenzone | |
| *Bain de Soleil Orange Gelee* | **Gel**: Octyl methoxycinnamate, octocrylene, octyl salicylate, oxybenzone | 8 |
| *Bain de Soleil Mademoiselle* | **Lotion**: Octyl methoxycinnamate, octocrylene, titanium dioxide | |
| *Coppertone All Day, Coppertone Oil-Free* | **Lotion**: Ethylhexyl p-methoxycinnamate, oxybenzone | |
| *Coppertone Sport* | **Lotion**: Octyl methoxycinnamate, oxybenzone | |

| | | |
|---|---|---|
| *Panama Jack* | **Lotion**: Ethylhexyl p-methoxy-cinnamate, 2-ethylhexyl salicy-late | 8 |
| *Bain de Soleil Tanning Mist* | **Spray**: Octyl methoxycinna-mate, octocrylene, oxybenzone | |
| *Bain de Soleil Orange Gelee* | **Gel**: Octyl methoxycinnamate, octyl salicylate | 4 |
| *Bain de Soleil Mega Tan* | **Lotion**: Octyl methoxycinna-mate, octocrylene | |
| *Bain de Soleil Tropical Deluxe* | **Lotion**: Octyl methoxycinna-mate, octyl salicylate | |
| *Banana Boat Dark Tannning* | **Lotion**: Padimate O | |
| *Coppertone Moisturizing Suntan* | **Lotion**: Ethylhexyl p-methoxy-cinnamate, oxybenzone | |
| *Hawaiian Tropic Dark Tanning* | **Lotion**: 2-ethylhexyl p-methoxy-cinnamate, menthyl anthranilate | |
| *Panama Jack Dark Tanning* | **Lotion**: Octyl methoxycinna-mate | |
| *Coppertone Gold Dark Tanning* | **Oil**: Homosalate, oxybenzone | |
| *Panama Jack Dark Tanning* | **Oil**: Octyl dimethyl PABA | |
| *Banana Boat Dark Tanning* | **Oil**: Padimate O, octyl methoxy-cinnamate | |
| *Bain de Soleil Tanning Mist* | **Spray**: Octyl methoxycinna-mate, octocrylene | |
| *Banana Boat Dark Tanning* | **Oil**: Padimate O, octyl methoxy-cinnamate | 2 |
| *Coppertone Gold Tan Magnifier* | **Oil**: Triethanolamine salicylate | |
| *Coppertone Gold Dark Tanning Dry Oil* | **Spray**: Homosalate | |

*otc* **Lip Protectants**

| | | |
|---|---|---|
| *Coppertone Water Babies Little Licks* | **Lip Balm**: Ethylhexyl p-me-thoxycinnamate, oxybenzone, 2-ethylhexyl salicylate | 30 |
| *Chapstick Ultra* | **Lip Balm**: Octocrylene, octyl methoxycinnamate, octyl salicy-late, oxybenzone | |
| *Blistex DCT* | **Lip Balm**: Octyl methoxycinna-mate, oxybenzone | 20 |

| | | |
|---|---|---|
| *Chapstick Flava-Craze* | **Lip Balm**: Octyl methoxycinnamate, oxybenzone | 15 |
| *Coppertone Aloe and Vitamin E, Coppertone Natural Fruit Flavor, Ti•Screen* | **Lip Balm**: Ethylhexyl p-methoxycinnamate, oxybenzone | |
| *Blistex* | **Lip Balm**: Padimate O, oxybenzone | |

## Type of Drug:

Suntan and sunscreen topical agents.

## How the Drug Works:

Sunscreens provide either a chemical or physical barrier to sunlight by absorbing or reflecting harmful ultraviolet (UV) radiation (UVA and UVB rays). UVB rays cause sunburn and UVA and UVB rays both cause photoaging. Sunscreens help prevent sunburn, premature aging, actinic keratosis, and reduce incidences of skin cancer. Chemical sunscreens act by absorbing UV light rays responsible for sunburning and suntanning. Physical sunscreens reflect or scatter light, preventing penetration of the skin.

Sunscreen effectiveness is dependent on UV absorption, concentration, vehicle, and ability to withstand swimming or sweating.

Examples of chemical barrier and physical barrier sunscreens are listed below:

*Chemical Barriers:*

Benzophenones (avobenzone, oxybenzone, benzophenone-3)
P-amino benzoic acid (PABA) and PABA esters (padimate O)
Cinnamates (cinoxate, ethylhexyl p-methoxycinnamate, octocrylene, octyl methoxycinnamate)
Salicylates (2–ethylhexyl salicylate, octyl salicylate, homosalate, triethanolamine salicylate)
Miscellaneous (menthyl anthranilate, phenylbenzimidazole sulfonic acid)

*Physical Barriers:*

Titanium dioxide, red petrolatum, zinc oxide

## Uses:

To prevent sunburn. Overexposure to the sun may cause premature skin aging and skin cancer. The liberal and regular use of these products may help reduce the occurrence of these harmful effects.

For persons with conditions such as systemic lupus erythematosus, solar urticaria (hives), erythropoietic protoporphyria, or those taking photosensitizing drugs. A brief list of drugs that may cause photosensitivity includes:

antidepressants (eg, amitripty-line, doxepin, trazodone)
antihistamines (eg, diphenhydra-mine)
antihypertensives (eg, captopril, diltiazem)
anti-infectives (eg, tetracyclines)
antineoplastic agents (eg, fluorouracil)
antipsychotic agents (eg, pheno-thiazines)

diuretics (eg, thiazides)
hypoglycemic agents (eg, sulfo-nylureas)
nonsteroidal anti-inflammatory drugs (eg, naproxen)
miscellaneous (eg, cosmetics, coal tar, psoralens, amiodarone, oral contraceptives, quinidine, disopyramide, gold salts, isotretinoin, carbamazepine)

## Precautions:

*Do not use in the following situations:* Allergy to the sunscreen or any of its ingredients.

*Use with caution in the following situations:*
diseased or inflamed skin
rash, itching, burning, or irritation during or after application of the sunscreen
sensitivity to benzocaine, procaine, sulfonamides, thiazide diuretics, aniline dyes, paraphenylenediamine (an ingredient in hair dyes), PABA, or PABA esters

*SPF (Sun Protection Factor):* SPF reveals the amount of protection from sunburn the product provides compared to unprotected skin. For example, use of a product with an SPF value of 6 would permit 6 times more sun exposure before burning when compared to unprotected skin of the same type. Determine your skin type (see chart) and then select a product with the appropriate SPF factor.

| Skin Type | Skin Characteristics[1] | Suggested Product SPF |
|-----------|------------------------|----------------------|
| I | Always burns easily; never tans (sensitive) | 15+ |
| II | Always burns easily; tans minimally (sensitive) | 15+ |
| III | Burns moderately; tans gradually (light brown, normal) | 10 to 15 |
| IV | Burns minimally; always tans well (moderate brown, normal) | 6 to 10 |
| V | Rarely burns; tans easily (dark brown, insensitive) | 4 to 6 |
| VI | Never burns; dark skin (insensitive) | None indicated |

[1] Based on first 45 to 60 minutes of sun exposure after winter season or no sun exposure.

The value of an SPF greater than 15 is unknown. An SPF of 15 or more is recommended for most individuals by the Skin Cancer Foundation.

*Children:* Consult your doctor when using sunscreens on children less than 6 months of age.

*Elderly:* Vitamin D deficiency may occur in the elderly. Sunscreens that block certain types of UV light may block the synthesis of vitamin D by the skin.

*Tartrazine:* Some of these products may contain the dye tartrazine (FD&C Yellow No. 5), which can cause allergic reactions in certain individuals. Check package label when available or consult your pharmacist or doctor.

## Side Effects:

Every drug is capable of producing side effects. Many sunscreen users experience no, or minor, side effects. The frequency and severity of side effects depend on many factors including dose, duration of therapy, and individual susceptibility. Possible side effects include: Burning; rash; itching; inflammation; unexpected sensitivity to UV light (photosensitivity).

## Guidelines for Use:

- *Regular sunscreens* may need to be reapplied after swimming or excessive perspiration. *Water-resistant* formulas maintain sunburn protection after being in the water up to 40 minutes. *Waterproof* formulas are designed to maintain sunburn protection after being in the water up to 80 minutes. Check individual package labeling for instructions.
- Apply liberally to exposed areas at least 30 minutes prior to sun exposure (up to 2 hours for PABA and its esters) to allow for penetration into the skin. Reapply every 1 to 2 hours after swimming or excessive sweating. Reapplication does not extend the protection period.
- Reapply sun protection every 2 hours, even on cloudy days.
- Consult your doctor when using sunscreens on children less than 6 months of age.
- For external use only. Do not swallow. Avoid contact with the eyes.
- Avoid prolonged exposure to sun and to tanning lamps. Sun-sensitive persons in particular should exercise caution.
- If signs of irritation or rash occur, wash off the sunscreen and do not use again.
- PABA may produce a permanent yellow stain on clothing.
- Do not use sunscreens that contain alcohol on skin that is inflamed or eczematous.
- Be aware of the following facts related to sun exposure:
  The sun's rays are strongest and most direct between 10 am and 2 pm daily.
  Each 1000-foot increase in altitude adds 4% to light intensity.
  Reflection of light off water is almost 100% when the sun is directly overhead.
  Fresh snow reflects approximately 85% of light.
  Sand reflects approximately 20% to 25% of light.

*If you have any questions, consult your doctor, pharmacist, or health care provider.*

| Generic Name<br>*Brand Name Examples* | Supplied As |
|---|---|
| *otc* **Soap-Free Cleansers** | |
| *Aquanil, Cetaphil, Nivea Visage* | **Cream, lotion** |
| *Basis Cleaner Clean Face Wash, Basis Comfortably Clean Face Wash, Cetaphil, Cetaphil Oily Skin, Formula 405 AHA, Neutrogena, Neutrogena Oil-Free Acne Wash, Neutrogena Antiseptic Cleanser for Acne-Prone Skin, pHisoDerm Acne, pHisoDerm Baby, pHisoDerm Normal to Dry, pHisoDerm Normal to Oily, pHisoDerm Sensitive Skin, Spectro-Jel* | **Liquid** |
| *Ceta Cleanser, Neutrogena Non-Drying, Oilatum-AD, SFC* | **Lotion** |
| *Sulfoil, Teraseptic* | **Shampoo/ Liquid** |
| *Lowila Cake* | **Cleanser** |
| *otc* **Modified Bar Soaps** | |
| *Alpha Keri Shower and Bath, Aveeno Acne Treatment, Aveeno Combination Skin, Aveeno Dry Skin, Basis All Clear, Basis Sensitive Skin, Cuticura Medicated Antibacterial, Formula 405 Mois-turizing, Lubiderm, Neutrogena, Neutrogena Acne-Prone Skin, Neutrogena Dry Skin, Neutrogena Oily Skin, Nivea Creme, Oilatum, Purpose, Teraseptic* | **Bar** |

## Type of Drug:

Therapeutic skin cleansers. Soap-free and modified bar soap products.

## How the Drug Works:

Soap-free therapeutic cleansers are less irritating to sensitive skin than regular soap-containing cleansing products. Modified bar soap products contain emollient components or are adjusted to a neutral or slightly acidic PH.

## Uses:

For patients with sensitive, dry, or irritated skin who may react to soap products.

---

### Guidelines for Use:

- For external use only.
- Follow package instructions exactly.
- Avoid overuse and contact with the eyes.
- Certain people may be sensitive to one or more ingredients. If skin irritation develops or becomes excessive, discontinue use and consult your doctor.

---

*If you have any questions, consult your doctor, pharmacist, or health care provider.*

| Generic Name<br>*Brand Name Examples* | Supplied As | Generic<br>Available |
|---|---|---|
| *otc* **Aluminum Acetate Solution<br>(Burow's or Modified<br>Burow's Solution)** | | |
| *Burow's Solution* | **Solution**: Aluminum acetate | Yes |
| *Bluboro Powder, Boropak,<br>Buro-Sol, Domeboro<br>Powder Packets, Pedi-<br>Boro Soak Paks* | **Powder packets**: Aluminum<br>sulfate, calcium acetate | No |
| *Domeboro Tablets* | **Tablets, effervescent**: Alumi-<br>num sulfate, calcium acetate | No |

## Type of Drug:
Astringent.

## Uses:
To aid in the relief of inflammation and irritation of the skin due to allergies, contact dermatitis, insect bites, poison ivy, poison oak, poison
sumac, or athlete's foot. Also aids in the relief of swelling associated with
minor bruises.

## Drug Interactions:
The activity of the topical enzyme collagenase may be inhibited by Burow's
solution. Cleanse the site with repeated washings of normal saline
between applications of Burow's solution and the collagenase ointment.

## Guidelines for Use:
- For external use only. Keep away from eyes.
- Follow individual product instructions.
- *Powder Packets* - Dissolve packets in required amount of cool or warm
  water. Stir solution until fully dissolved. Do not strain or filter. Discard
  used solution after each use. Prepare fresh solution daily.
- *Effervescent Tablets* - Dissolve 1 or 2 tablets in required amount of cool
  or warm water. Stir solution until fully dissolved. Do not strain or filter
  the solution. Discard used solution after each use. Unused solution may
  be stored at room temperature in a clean, capped container for up to
  7 days.
- Discontinue use and contact your doctor if symptoms persist for more
  than 7 days or if irritation or worsening of condition occurs.
- Do not cover wet dressing with plastic or other materials that prevent
  evaporation.
- Remove, remoisten, and reapply dressing every 15 to 30 minutes for
  4 to 8 hours or as directed by your doctor.
- Do not allow dressing to dry out.
- Do not use over a large area of the body.
- Store at room temperature.

*If you have any questions, consult your doctor, pharmacist, or health care provider.*

| | Generic Name<br>*Brand Name*<br>*Examples* | **Supplied As** | **Uses** |
|---|---|---|---|
| *Rx* | **Aluminum Chloride Hexahydrate** | | |
| | *Drysol* | **Solution:** 20% | To aid in the management of excessive sweating. |
| *otc* | **Arnica** | **Tincture:** 20% | To relieve pain from sprains and bruises (of doubtful value) |
| *otc* | **Boric Acid Ointment** | | |
| | *Boric Acid, Borofax* | **Ointment:** 5%, 10% | To soothe chafed skin, abrasions, burns and other skin irritations. |
| *otc* | **Chlorophyll Derivatives** | | |
| | *Chloresium* | **Ointment:** 0.5% | To treat various skin ulcers, malignant lesions, traumatic injuries, skin grafting, skin defects and other skin disorders. |
| | *Chloresiom* | **Solution:** 0.2% | |
| *otc* | **Dihydroxyacetone** | | |
| | *Chromelin Complexion Blender* | 5% | To treat vitiligo and hyper-pigmented skin |

| | Generic Name<br>*Brand Name*<br>*Examples* | Supplied As | Uses |
|---|---|---|---|
| *otc* | **Hamamelis Water (Witch Hazel)** | **Liquid** | For temporary relief of anal or vaginal irritation and itching, hemorrhoids, postepisiotomy discomfort and anorectal surgical discomfort |
| | *Tucks Hemor-rhoidal* | **Cream:** 50% | |
| | *A•E•R* | **Pads:** 50% | |
| *Rx* | **Masoprocol** | | |
| | *Actinex* | **Cream:** 10% | To treat actinic (solar) keratoses (sun induced skin growths that may develop into skin cancer). |
| *Rx* | **Monobenzone** | | |
| | *Benoquin* | **Cream:** 20% | To treat light patches of the skin caused by extensive vitiligo |
| *otc* | **Zinc Oxide** | **Ointment:** 20% | To treat minor skin irritations, abrasions, chafed skin and diaper rash |

| Generic Name<br>*Brand Name*<br>*Examples* | Supplied As | Uses |
|---|---|---|
| **Combinations** | | |
| *otc*    *Aluminum*<br>*Paste* | **Ointment:** 10%<br>metallic aluminum | An occlusive<br>skin protectant. |
| *otc*    *Boil-Ease* | **Salve**: 5% benzo-<br>caine, 0.44% sulfur,<br>1.86% ichthammol,<br>camphor, anhy-<br>drous lanolin, euca-<br>lyptus oil, liquified<br>phenol, juniper tar,<br>menthol, paraffin,<br>petrolatum, rosin,<br>sexadecyl alcohol,<br>thymol, yellow wax<br>and zinc oxide | |
| *otc*    *Campho-*<br>*Phenique* | **Liquid**: 10.8% cam-<br>phor, 4.7% phenol,<br>eucalyptus oil and<br>light mineral oil | For relief of<br>pain and to<br>combat minor<br>infections. |
| *otc*    *Dome-Paste* | **Wound dressing**:<br>Zinc oxide, cala-<br>mine and gelatin | For conditions<br>of the arms and<br>legs (eg, vari-<br>cose ulcers)<br>requiring pro-<br>tection and<br>support. |
| *otc*    *Dr. Dermi-Heal* | **Ointment**: 1%<br>allantoin, zinc<br>oxide, balsam Peru,<br>castor oil and petro-<br>latum | For relief of<br>diaper rash,<br>chafing, minor<br>burns, bed<br>sores, external<br>vaginal itching<br>and irritation,<br>ostomy irritation<br>and heat rash |
| *otc*    *Mammol* | **Ointment**: 40% bis-<br>muth subnitrate,<br>30% castor oil, 22%<br>anhydrous lanolin,<br>7% ceresin wax<br>and 1% balsam<br>Peru | For prevention<br>of sore,<br>cracked nipples<br>during breast-<br>feeding. |

| | Generic Name<br>*Brand Name*<br>*Examples* | **Supplied As** | **Uses** |
|---|---|---|---|
| *otc* | *Ostiderm* | **Lotion**: 14.5 mg aluminum sulfate, 10 mg phenol per g, glycerin, zinc oxide, bentonite, silica, propylene glycol alginate, camphor and iron oxides | For the relief of bromhidrosis and hyperhidrosis, dermatitis, itching and poison ivy. |
| *otc* | *Outgro* | **Solution**: 25% tannic acid, 5% chlorbutanol and 83% isopropyl alcohol | For temporary pain relief of ingrown toenails |
| *otc* | *Oxyzal Wet Dressing* | **Liquid**: Oxyquinolone sulfate and benzalkonium chloride 1:2000 | For minor infections |
| *otc* | *Proderm Topical* | **Dressing**: 650 mg castor oil and 72.5 mg balsam Peru per 0.82 mL | For prevention and management of decubitus ulvers. |
| *otc* | *ProTech First-Aid Stik* | **Liquid**: 10% povidone iodine, 2.5% lidocaine | For cleaning and pain relief of cuts, scrapes and burns. |
| *otc* | *Saratoga* | **Ointment**: Zinc oxide, boric acid, eucalyptol, acetylated lanolin alcohols, white petrolatum and white beeswax | For temporary relief of itching and minor skin irritations, chapped and chafed skin, diaper rash, bed sores and mild burns. |
| *otc* | *Sarna Anti-Itch* | **Lotion and Foam**: 0.5% camphor, 0.5% menthol, carbomer 940, DMDM hydantoin, glyceryl stearate, PEG-8 and PEG-100 stea-rate and petrolatum | For relief of dry, itching skin. |

|  | **Generic Name** *Brand Name* *Examples* | **Supplied As** | **Uses** |
|---|---|---|---|
| *Rx* | *Scarlet Red Ointment Dressings* | **Wound dressings**: 5% scarlet red, lanolin, olive oil and petrolatum in fine mesh absorbent gauze | For healing of donor sites, burns and wounds |
| *otc* | *Schamberg* | **Lotion**: 8.25% zinc oxide, 0.25% menthol, 1.5% phenol, 30% cottonseed oil, 15% olive oil and lime water | For itchy eczema. |
| *otc* | *Schamberg's* | **Lotion**: Zinc oxide, 0.15% menthol, 1% phenol, peanut oil and lime water | For temporary relief of itching. |
| *otc* | *Soothaderm* | **Lotion**: 2.07 mg pyrilamine maleate, 2.08 mg benzo-caine and 41.35 mg zinc oxide per mL with simethicone, parabens, propy-lene glycol, wisteria oil, apple blossom oil, camphor and menthol | For relief of itching. |
| *otc* | *Stypto-Caine* | **Solution**: 250 mg aluminum chloride, 2.5 mg tetracaine HCl and 1 mg oxy-quinolone sulfate per g with glycerin | To stop bleed-ing in minor cuts. |
| *otc* | *Topic* | **Gel**: 5% benzyl alcohol, camphor, menthol and 30% isopropyl alcohol | For temporary relief of itching. |

| Generic Name<br>*Brand Name*<br>*Examples* | | **Supplied As** | **Uses** |
|---|---|---|---|
| *otc* | *Unguentine* | **Solution**: Benzo-<br>caine in alcohol | For pain relief<br>in minor burns. |
| | | **Ointment**: 1% phe-<br>nol petrolatum,<br>oleostearine, zinc<br>oxide, eucalyptus<br>oil and thyme oil | |

## Type of Drug:
Miscellaneous topical agents.

### Guidelines for Use:
- For external use only. Avoid contact with eyes.
- Cleanse affected area before application.
- Apply to affected area as directed. Check individual package labels for directions.
- Do not use tight-fitting dressings.
- Hands should be washed after use.
- May stain clothing or fabrics.

*If you have any questions, consult your doctor, pharmacist, or health care provider.*

Product is used following treatment with a pediculicide. For additional information about pediculices, see the Miscellaneous Anti-infectives — Scabicides/Pediculicides monograph in the Anti-infectives chapter.

| Generic Name Brand Name Example | Supplied As | Generic Available |
|---|---|---|
| *otc* **Nit Removal System** *Step 2* | **Creme rinse**: Benzyl alcohol, cetyl alcohol, 8% formic acid, glyceryl stearate, PEG-100 staerate, polyquaternium-10 | No |

## Type of Drug:

Adjunctive treatment for use with pediculicides.

## How the Drug Works:

It appears to loosen the bond that continues to hold both live and dead lice eggs to the hair shaft after pediculicide treatment. Surviving eggs can cause reinfestation if not removed. It does not kill head lice or its eggs.

## Uses:

For use following a pediculicide to aid in cleansing lice eggs from the hair shaft.

## Side Effects:

Every drug is capable of producing side effects. Many nit removal system users experience no, or minor, side effects. The frequency and severity of side effects depend on many factors including dose, duration of therapy and individual susceptibility. Possible side effects include itching, redness and swelling of the scalp.

## Guidelines for Use:

- For external use only. Avoid contact with eyes. If contact occurs, immediately fluch with water.
- Shake well before using.
- Protect eyes with a dry towel.
- Apply to wet hair after rinsing out the pediculicide. Apply enough to saturate each hair shaft and cover the entire scalp, making sure to cover the area around the ears and back of neck. Do not apply to eyelashes or eyebrows. Leave on the hair for approximately 10 minutes. Rinse with lukewarm water and dry with a hair dryer.
- May cause itching, redness or swelling of the scalp. Notify your doctor if these symptoms persist.
- In order to prevent accidental ingestion by children, the remaining contents should be discarded after use.

*If you have any questions, consult your doctor, pharmacist, or health care provider.*

| Generic Name Brand Name Example | Supplied As | Generic Available |
|---|---|---|
| Rx **Eflornithine HCl** | | |
| *Vaniqa* | **Cream**: 13.9% | No |

## Type of Drug:
Agent for reducing facial hair.

## How the Drug Works:
Eflornithine irreversibly inhibits ornithine decarboxylase with an enzyme found in the hair follicle of the skin needed for hair growth.

## Uses:
To retard growth of unwanted facial hair in women.

## Precautions:
*Do not use in the following situations:* Allergy to eflornithine or any of its ingredients.

*Use with caution in the following situations:* Irritated or broken skin.

*Pregnancy:* There are no adequate and well-controlled studies in pregnant women. Use only if clearly needed and the potential benefits to the mother outweigh the possible hazards to the fetus.

*Breastfeeding:* It is not known if eflornithine appears in breast milk. Consult your doctor before you begin breastfeeding.

*Children:* Safety and effectiveness in children less than 12 years of age have not been established.

## Drug Interactions:
Tell your doctor or pharmacist if you are taking or if you are planning to take any over-the-counter or prescription medications or dietary supplements with eflornithine. Doses of one or both drugs may need to be modified or a different drug may need to be prescribed. It is not known if eflornithine interacts with other topically applied drugs.

## Side Effects:
Every drug is capable of producing side effects. Many eflornithine users experience no, or minor, side effects. The frequency and severity of side effects depend on many factors including dose, duration of therapy, and individual susceptibility. Possible side effects include:

*Digestive Tract:* Indigestion; appetite loss; nausea.

*Nervous System:* Headache; dizziness; weakness.

*Skin:* Acne; ingrown hair; hair bumps; inflamed hair follicles; rosacea; tingling, stinging, or burning skin; rash; dry, red, or itchy skin; skin irritation; facial swelling; activation of herpes simplex.

## Guidelines for Use:

- Dosage is individualized. Use exactly as prescribed.
- Apply a thin layer of eflornithine to the affected areas of the face and adjacent involved areas under the chin. Rub in thoroughly. You should not wash the treated areas for at least 4 hours after application.
- For external use only. Avoid getting this medicine in your eyes or inside your nose or mouth. If it gets in your eyes, rinse thoroughly with water and contact your doctor.
- Wait a few minutes after applying eflornithine before you apply cosmetics or sunscreen.
- If you miss a dose, apply it as soon as possible. If several hours have passed, or if it is nearing time for the next application, do not double the dose to catch up, unless advised by your doctor.
- Eflornithine may cause temporary redness, rash, burning, stinging, or tingling, especially when the skin is damaged. If irritation continues, stop taking this medicine and contact your doctor.
- Improvement in the condition occurs gradually, taking 4 to 8 weeks. You will need to continue your normal procedures for hair removal until desired results have been achieved.
- Check with your doctor before using any facial or skin creams, or before taking any over-the-counter medicines, prescription medicines, or dietary supplements.
- This medicine is not a depilatory. It does not permanently remove hair or "cure" unwanted hair.
- Inform your doctor is you are pregnant, become pregnant, are planning to become pregnant, or if you are breastfeeding.
- Store at controlled room temperature (59° to 86°F). Do not freeze.

*If you have any questions, consult your doctor, pharmacist, or health care provider.*

**General Information,** 1529

**Antimetabolites**
Folic Acid Analogs, 1533
Purine Analogs and Related
Agents, 1536
Pyrimidine Analogs, 1539

**Camptothecins,** 1542

**Busulfan,** 1545

**Etoposide,** 1547

**Mitotic Inhibitors**
Vinorelbine Tartrate, 1549

**Anthracyclines**
Daunorubicin, 1551
Doxorubicin, 1553
Epirubicin, 1556
Idarubicin, 1558
Valrubicin, 1560

**Hormones**
Androgens, 1562
Antiandrogens, 1564
Progestins, 1567
Estrogens, 1569
Antiestrogens, 1571
Aromatase Inhibitors, 1574
Gonadotropin-Releasing Hormone
Analogs, 1577

**Alkylating Agents**
Carmustine, 1581
Lomustine, 1584
Streptozocin, 1586
Estrogen/Nitrogen Mustard, 1588
Nitrogen Mustards, 1590

**Immunologic Agents**
Interferons, 1594

**Retinoids**
Tretinoin, 1598

**Miscellaneous
Preparations,** 1601

**Enzymes,** 1607

**Porfimer Sodium,** 1610

**Monoclonal Antibodies**
Alemtuzumab, 1613
Gemtuzumab, 1615
Ibritumomab Tiuxetan, 1617
Rituximab, 1619
Trastuzumab, 1621

## Type of Drug:

Chemotherapy, "chemo," cancer drugs.

## How the Drug Works:

Cancer drugs include a wide range of drugs that work by various mechanisms. Although development has been directed toward agents that work only on cancer cells, those presently available cause significant toxicity in normal tissues.

Combinations of cancer drugs are superior to single drug therapy in the management of many diseases, leading to higher response rates and increased length of remissions. Improved response may be due to the use of agents that work by differing mechanisms. Cancer cells that acquire rapid resistance to a single agent develop resistance less rapidly when treated with a combination of agents.

Selection of agents for combination cancer drug therapy is based on: Mechanism of drug action; specificity of action; responsiveness to dosage schedules; and drug toxicity. Increased responsiveness to combination therapy may permit reduction in dose and, therefore, decreased toxicity.

The mechanism of action by which these agents slow the growth of cancer cells is not fully understood. Generally, they affect one or more stages of cell growth or reproduction. Major side effects on normal tissues include bone marrow, blood, hair follicles and mucous membranes of the digestive tract.

*Alkylating agents* alter DNA. The defective DNA molecules are unable to carry out normal cell reproduction. Alkylating agents include: Busulfan, carboplatin, carmustine, chlorambucil, cisplatin, cyclophosphamide, dacarbazine, estramustine, ifosfamide, lomustine, mechlorethamine, melphalan, pipobroman, streptozocin, thiotepa and uracil mustard.

*Antimetabolites* include a group of compounds that interfere with various metabolic processes, thereby disrupting normal cellular functions. These agents may act by: Incorporating the drug into an essential chemical compound; or inhibiting a key enzyme from functioning normally. Antimetabolites include: Cytarabine, floxuridine, 5-fluorouracil, fludarabine, gemcitabine, hydroxyurea, mercaptopurine, methotrexate and thioguanine

*Hormones* have been used to treat several types of cancer cells. Hormonal therapy interferes at the cell membrane. The mechanism of action, however, is still unclear. Corticosteroids are used primarily for their effects on blood cells in leukemia and lymphomas (tumors in lymph glands) and as a component in many combination regimens. The effect of androgens, estrogens and progestins has been used in the therapy of cancer of tissues dependent upon these sex-related hormones (eg, tumors of the breast, endometrium and prostate). These agents have the advantage of being more specific for tissues responsive to their effects, thus inhibiting cell growth without a direct toxic action. Hormones include: Aminoglutethimide, anastrozole, bicalutamide, diethylstilbestrol, estramustine, flutamide, goserelin, leuprolide, medroxyprogesterone, megestrol, mitotane, polyestradiol, tamoxifen and testolactone.

*Antibiotic* type agents are capable of disrupting cellular functions of tissues. Their primary mechanisms of action are to delay or inhibit cell division. Antibiotics include: Bleomycin, dactinomycin, daunorubicin, doxorubicin, idarubicin, mitomycin, mitoxantrone, pentostatin and plicamycin.

*Mitotic inhibitors* prevent cell division. These agents are derived from plants, eg, the periwinkle plant (vincristine, vinblastine and vinoreletoposide) or the May-apple plant (etoposide and teniposide). Another class of mitotic inhibitors called taxanes include paclitaxel and docetaxel.

*Radioactive* molecules (chromic phosphate, sodium iodide and strontium-89) exert a direct effect on exposed tissue via radiation. Use is restricted to doctors licensed by the Nuclear Regulatory Commission.

*Biological response modifiers* have complex antineoplastic, antiviral and immunomodulating activities. It is believed that direct action against tumor cells and modification of immune response (ability to produce antibodies) play important roles in the antitumor activity of interferon alfa-2a, recombinant and interferon alfa-2b, recombinant. Examples of biological agents are: Aldesleukin (human interleukin-2), interferon alfa-2a (recombinant DNA), interferon alfa-2b (recombinant DNA), interferon alfa-n3 (human leukocyte) and interferon gamma-1B (recombinant DNA).

*Miscellaneous:* Metabolism of altretamine is required for cytotoxicity, although the mechanisms are not clear. L-asparaginase is an enzyme that inhibits protein production in cancer cells. BCG promotes a local inflammatory reaction in the urinary bladder and reduces cancerous lesion. Cladribine inhibits DNA synthesis and repair through a complex mechanism. Levamisole is an immunomodulator with complex effects. Porfimer is a photsensitivity agent. Procarbazine produces toxic metabolites that cause chromosomal breakage. Topotecan and irinotecan are topoisomerase inhibitors. Tretinoin is related to vitamin A which induces cytodifferentiation.

## Side Effects:

*Extravasation* (loss of drug from blood vessel) occurs when IV fluid and medication leak into tissue. Damage resulting from extravasation of certain cancer drugs can range from painful red swelling to deep lesions, requiring surgical removal of dead and contaminated tissue and skin grafting.

*Prevention* of extravasation injury is based on careful and accurate administration of IV drugs. Areas of previous radiation (x-ray) therapy and arms and legs with poor circulation for IV placement must be avoided.

*Treatment* of extravasation includes stopping the drug immediately and appropriate use of an antidote. Goals of treatment are prevention of tissue damage. Immediate removal of the IV followed by application of ice has been recommended for all agents except etoposide, vinblastine and vincristine (warm compresses are recommended for these agents).

*Hydrocortisone sodium succinate or dexamethasone sodium phosphate* have been used for their anti-inflammatory activity. However, the use of these agents as well as other drugs such as sodium bicarbonate and dimethyl sulfoxide (DMSO) is unproven for antidote use.

The following drugs are associated with severe local tissue damage and cell death when extravasation occurs:

dacarbazine
dactinomycin
daunorubicin
doxorubicin
idarubicin
mechlorethamine

mitomycin
streptozocin
vinblastine
vincristine
vinorelbine

*Nausea and vomiting* may be the most prominent side effects of cancer treatment from the patient's perspective, with 30% or more of patients experiencing some degree of vomiting. The cancer drugs with the highest potential to cause vomiting are:

carboplatin
carmustine
cisplatin
cyclophosphamide
cytarabine
dacarbazine

dactinomycin
doxorubicin
mechlorethamine
methotrexate
procarbazine
streptozocin

The agents with moderate ability to cause vomiting are:

asparaginase
daunorubicin
etoposide
fluorouracil
hexamethylmelamine
idarubicin
ifosfamide

lomustine
mitomycin
mitoxantrone
paclitaxel
plicamycin
vinblastine
vinorelbine

The incidence of vomiting with these and other agents varies greatly among individuals. Dose, schedule, other medications, other medical complications and psychological conditions may affect the incidence as well.

*Treatment* of nausea and vomiting should include measures such as dietary adjustment, restriction of activity and positive support. However, if drug management is necessary, several agents or groups of agents may prove useful. Some drugs that have been used with varying degrees of success, either alone or in combination, include phenothiazines, butyrophenones, cannabinoids, corticosteroids, antihistamines, benzodiazepines, metoclopramide, ACTH, selective 5-HT$_3$ receptor antagonist and scopolamine. Since only 30% to 40% of patients are effectively treated with a single agent, studies using combination therapy have increased.

## Guidelines for Use:

- Because of the complexities and dangers in cancer chemotherapy, use should be restricted to, or under the direct supervision of, doctors experienced in their use. In addition to drug therapy, surgery and radiation are also employed when appropriate.
- *Handling of Antineoplastic Agents* — Direct contact may cause irritation of the skin, eyes and mucous membranes. Safe handling of parenteral (intravenous, IV; intramuscular, IM) cancer drugs by medical personnel involved in preparation and administration of these agents is mandatory. Potential risks from repeated contact with cancer drugs can be controlled by a combination of special equipment and proper work techniques.

*If you have any questions, consult your doctor, pharmacist, or health care provider.*

| Generic Name<br>*Brand Name Example* | Supplied As | Generic<br>Available |
|---|---|---|
| *Rx* **Methotrexate (MTX)** | **Injection**: 25 mg/mL[1] | Yes |
| *Rheumatrex Dose Pack* | **Tablets**: 2.5 mg | Yes |

[1] Also available in a preservative free formulation.

## Type of Drug:

Antimetabolite.

## How the Drug Works:

Methotrexate interferes with DNA synthesis, repair, and cellular replication. Actively multiplying cells, such as malignant cells, are more sensitive to this effect than other cells in the body.

## Uses:

To treat cancer of the breast, cervix, head and neck, lung, colon, ovary, prostate, stomach and pancreas, sarcomas, acute lymphocytic leukemia, lymphoma, and choriocarcinoma.

To control severe disabling psoriasis and rheumatoid arthritis unresponsive to other drug therapy. See the full monographs in the CNS Drugs and Topicals chapters.

*Unlabeled Use(s):* Occasionally, doctors may prescribe methotrexate to reduce corticosteroid requirements in patients with severe corticosteroid-dependent asthma, or as a high-dose regimen followed by leucovorin rescue for adjuvant therapy of bone cancer.

## Precautions:

*Do not use in the following situations:*

allergy to the drug or any of its
 ingredients
blood disorders
breastfeeding

immunodeficiency
pregnancy with psoriasis or
 rheumatoid arthritis

*Use with caution in the following situations:*

anemia
debilitation
decreased blood cell count
fever, severe
immunosuppression
infection

kidney disease
liver disease
lung disease
pleural effusion
vaccines

*Pregnancy:* Studies have shown that methotrexate can harm the fetus. Do not use during pregnancy unless the potential benefits outweigh the possible risks to the fetus. Women of childbearing potential should avoid becoming pregnant during therapy. Do not use in pregnant psoriatic or rheumatoid arthritis patients.

*Breastfeeding:* Methotrexate appears in breast milk. Because of the potential for serious adverse effects in a nursing infant, decide whether to discontinue nursing or discontinue the drug, taking into account the importance of the drug to the mother.

*Children:* Safety and effectiveness in children, other than in cancer chemo-therapy, have not been established.

*Lab tests* will be required to monitor therapy. Tests include complete blood and platelet counts, liver, lung, and kidney function tests, chest X-rays, and drug levels in the blood.

## Drug Interactions:

Tell your doctor or pharmacist if you are taking or planning to take any over-the-counter or prescription medications or dietary supplements with this drug. Drug doses may need to be modified or a different drug pre-scribed. The following drugs and drug classes interact with this drug:

alcohol
aminoglycosides, oral (eg, neo-mycin)
azathioprine (eg, *Imuran*)
charcoal
etretinate (eg, acitretin)
folic acid
hydantoins (eg, phenytoin)
NSAIDs (eg, ibuprofen)

penicillins (eg, amoxicillin)
probenecid
procarbazine (eg, *Matulane*)
retinoids (eg, tretinoin)
salicylates (eg, aspirin)
sulfasalazine (eg, *Azulfidine*)
sulfonamides (eg, sulfisoxazole)
theophylline (eg, *Theo-Dur*)
trimethoprim (eg, *Proloprim*)

## Side Effects:

Every drug is capable of producing side effects. Most patients experience side effects. The frequency and severity of side effects depend on many factors including dose, duration of therapy, and individual susceptibil-ity. Possible side effects include:

*Nervous System:* Headache; drowsiness; blurred vision; convulsions; dizzi-ness; confusion; speech impairment; impaired coordination.

*Skin:* Rash; itching; hives; pigment changes; hair loss; acne; lesions; bruising.

*Digestive Tract:* Stomach pain; nausea; gum inflammation; sore throat; appetite loss; vomiting; diarrhea; blood in the stool; mouth ulcers.

*Urinary and Reproductive Tract:* Kidney failure; blood in the urine; men-strual problems; vaginal discharge; infertility; bladder inflammation.

*Other:* Sensitivity to light; abnormal blood counts; general body discom-fort; fatigue; chills; fever; infection; slight or partial paralysis; bone mar-row depression; bleeding; lung disease; vision changes.

## Guidelines for Use:

- Dosage is individualized. Take exactly as prescribed.
- Do not stop taking or change the dose, unless instructed by your doctor.
- May cause sensitivity to light. Avoid prolonged exposure to the sun and other sources of UV light (eg, tanning beds). Use sunscreens and wear protective clothing until tolerance is determined.
- Avoid alcohol while taking this medicine.
- May cause nausea, vomiting, appetite loss, hair loss, rash, boils, or acne. Notify your doctor if these effects persist or become bothersome.
- Notify your doctor if you experience diarrhea, stomach pain, black tarry stools, seizures, fever and chills, sore throat, unusual bleeding or bruising, sores in or around the mouth, cough or shortness of breath, yellow discoloration of the skin or eyes, darkened urine, bloody urine, swelling of the feet or legs, or joint pain.
- Use contraceptive measures during and for at least 3 months (males) or 1 ovulatory cycle (females) after you stop taking this medicine.
- Store at controlled room temperature (59° to 86°F)

*If you have any questions, consult your doctor, pharmacist, or health care provider.*

| Generic Name<br>*Brand Name Examples* | Supplied As | Generic<br>Available |
|---|---|---|
| Rx **Allopurinol**[1] | | |
| *Zyloprim* | **Tablets**: 100 mg, 300 mg | Yes |
| Rx **Mercaptopurine** | | |
| *Purinethol* | **Tablets**: 50 mg | No |
| Rx **Thioguanine** | | |
| *Tabloid* | **Tablets**: 40 mg | No |

[1] Also available as an injection.

Cladribine, fludarabine, pentostatin, and rasburicase, purine analogs available as injections, are not included in this monograph. For more information on chemotherapy treatment, see the introduction to this chapter.

## Type of Drug:

*Allopurinol:* Xanthine oxidase inhibitor; uric acid-reducing agent.

*Mercaptopurine, thioguanine:* Chemotherapy drugs; anticancer drugs; antimetabolites.

## How the Drug Works:

*Allopurinol:* Certain cancer therapy (eg, antimetabolite) causes large numbers of cancer cells to die quickly. When these cells die, they release substances that are changed into uric acid by the enzyme xanthine oxidase. This can result in very high levels of uric acid in the blood and urine and can cause kidney damage. Allopurinol blocks the action of xanthine oxidase and prevents high blood and urine levels of uric acid caused by chemotherapy.

*Mercaptopurine, thioguanine:* Mercaptopurine and thioguanine are antimetabolites that are similar to naturally-occuring nutrients needed by the cells of the body for growth and reproduction. Cells, including cancer cells, use the antimetabolites instead of the naturally-occuring nutrients. Once inside the cell, the antimetabolites work by blocking normal metabolism, which causes the cells to die. Certain cancer cells may be more sensitive to this action than normal cells of the body.

## Uses:

*Allopurinol:* To manage uric acid elevation in blood (hyperuricemia) and urine (uricosuria) in patients being treated for leukemia, lymphomas, and other malignancies.

Also used in the treatment of gout. See the complete monograph in the CNS Drugs chapter.

*Mercaptopurine:* For remission induction and maintenance therapy of acute lymphatic leukemia and remission induction of acute myelogenous leukemia.

*Thioguanine:* For remission induction, consolidation, and maintenance therapy of acute nonlymphocytic leukemias. Also used to treat chronic myelogenous leukemia.

## Precautions:

*Do not use in the following situations:*
> allergy to the drug or any of its ingredients
> liver disease (mercaptopurine, thioguanine only)
> prior resistance to mercaptopurine or thioguanine (mercaptopurine, thioguanine only)

*Use with caution in the following situations:*
> kidney disease
> liver disease (allopurinol only)

*Pregnancy:* Studies have shown that mercaptopurine and thioguanine can harm the fetus. Do not use during pregnancy unless the potential benefits to outweigh the possible risks to the fetus. Women of childbearing potential should avoid becoming pregnant during therapy. There are no adequate and well-controlled studies of allopurinol in pregnant women. Use only if clearly needed and the potential benefits outweigh the possible risks to the fetus.

*Breastfeeding:* It is not known if mercaptopurine or thioguanine appear in breast milk. Allopurinol appears in breast milk. Because of the potential for serious side effects, decide whether to discontinue breastfeeding or discontinue the drug, taking into account the importance of the drug to the mother.

*Children:* These drugs have been administered to children with leukemia.

*Elderly:* Due to poor liver and kidney function in the elderly, lower doses may be used.

*Lab tests* will be required frequently during treatment. Tests may include complete blood and platelet counts, and liver, pancreas, and kidney function tests.

## Drug Interactions:

Tell your doctor or pharmacist if you are taking or planning to take any over-the-counter or prescription medications or dietary supplements with these drugs. Drug doses may need to be modified or a different drug prescribed. The following drugs and drug classes interact with these drugs:

allopurinol (eg, *Zyloprim)* (mercaptopurine only)
aminosalicylate derivatives (eg, olsalazine) (mercaptopurine, thioguanine only)
anticoagulants, oral (eg, warfarin) (mercaptopurine only)
cyclosporine (eg, *Neoral*) (allopurinol only)
penicillins (eg, amoxicillin) (allopurinol only)
thiopurines (eg, mercaptopurine) (allopurinol only)
trimethoprim/sulfamethoxazole (eg, *Septra)* (mercaptopurine only)
uricosuric agents (eg, sulfinpyrazone) (alopurinol only)

## Side Effects:

Every drug is capable of producing side effecrs. Most patients experience side effects. The frequency and severity of side effects depend on many factors including dose, duration of therapy, and individual susceptibility. Possible side effects include:

*Digestive Tract:* Nausea; vomiting, appetite loss; stomach pain; diarrhea.

*Skin:* Rash; skin pigment changes.

*Other:* Bone marrow suppression; immunosuppression; liver toxicity (eg, yellowing of the skin or eyes, diarrhea, appetite loss).

---

### Guidelines for Use:

• Dosage is individualized. Take exactly as prescribed.
• Do not stop taking or change the dose, unless instructed by your doctor.
• Drink plenty of liquids (10 to 12 eight ounce glasses a day) while taking these drugs.
• If a dose is missed, take it as soon as possible. If several hours have passed or it is nearing time for the next dose, do not double the dose to catch up, unless instructed by your doctor. If more than one dose is missed, or it is necessary to establish a new dosage schedule, contact your doctor or pharmacist.
• Lab tests will be required to monitor therapy. Be sure to keep appointments.
• Store at controlled room temperature (59° to 77°F). Protect from light and moisture.
• *Allopurinol* — Stop taking and notify your doctor if you develop a rash or other signs of an allergic reaction, painful urination, blood in the urine, irritation of the eyes, or swelling of the lips or mouth.
May cause drowsiness. Use caution while driving or performing other tasks requiring alertness, coordination, or physical dexterity until tolerance is determined.
• *Mercaptopurine, thioguanine* — Notify your doctor if you experience diarrhea, yellowing of the skin or eyes, appetite loss, nausea, vomiting, unusual bleeding or bruising, stomach or flank pain, swelling or the feet or legs, or symptoms suggestive of anemia (eg, easy fatigability, pounding in the chest [palpitations], increased heart rate, fast breathing with exertion).
Contraceptive (birth control) measures are recommended for men and women during therapy.
These drugs may lower your body's ability to fight infection. Notify your doctor immediately if you experience any signs of infection, including fever, sore throat, rash, or chills.

---

*If you have any questions, consult your doctor, pharmacist, or health care provider.*

| Generic Name<br>*Brand Name Example* | Supplied As | Generic<br>Available |
|---|---|---|
| Rx **Capecitabine** | | |
| *Xeloda* | **Tablets**: 150 mg, 500 mg | No |

Cytarabine, fluorouracil, floxuridine, and gemcitabine, pyrimidine analogs available as injections, are not included in this monograph. For more information on chemotherapy treatment, see the introduction to this chapter.

## Type of Drug:

Anticancer drug; antimetabolite.

## How the Drug Works:

Capecitabine is converted in the body to the anticancer drug 5-fluorouracil (5-FU) that kills certain types of cancer cells and decreases the size of some tumors.

## Uses:

For the treatment of breast cancer that has spread to other parts of the body and is resistant to treatment with paclitaxel and an anthracycline-containing chemotherapy regimen, and for patients for whom further anthracycline therapy is not indicated.

For first-line treatment of cancer of the colon or rectum that has spread to other parts of the body when treatment with fluoropyrimidine therapy alone is preferred.

## Precautions:

*Do not use in the following situations:*
allergy to capecitabine, 5-fluorouracil, or any of its ingredients
kidney disease, severe

*Use with caution in the following situations:*
coronary artery disease
kidney disease, mild to moderate
liver dysfunction due to cancer in the liver
pregnancy

*Diarrhea:* Capecitabine can cause severe diarrhea. Fluid and mineral (electrolyte) replacement may be needed.

*Pregnancy:* There are no adequate or well-controlled studies in pregnant women. Be aware of the potential hazard to the fetus if you become pregnant while taking this medicine. Women of childbearing potential should avoid becoming pregnant while taking capecitabine.

*Breastfeeding:* It is not known if capecitabine appears in breast milk. Consult your doctor before you begin breastfeeding.

*Children:* Safety and effectiveness in children younger than 18 years of age have not been established.

*Elderly:* Patients older than 80 years of age may experience gastrointestinal side effects (eg, diarrhea, nausea, vomiting) more frequently than younger patients.

*Lab tests* will be required to monitor therapy. Tests may include kidney and liver function, blood counts, and toxicity monitoring.

## Drug Interactions:

Tell your doctor if you are taking or planning to take any over-the-counter or prescription medications or dietary supplements with this drug. Drug doses may need to be modified or a different drug prescribed. The following drugs and drug classes interact with this drug:

antacids, aluminum hydroxide- and magnesium hydroxide- containing (eg, *Maalox*) anticoagulants, oral (eg, warfarin)

folic acid leucovorin (eg, *Wellcovorin*) phenytoin (eg, *Dilantin*)

## Side Effects:

Every drug is capable of producing side effects. Many patients experience side effects. The frequency and severity of side effects depend on many factors including dose, duration of therapy, and individual susceptibility. Possible side effects include:

*Nervous System:* Abnormal skin sensations; dizziness; sleeplessness; headache; depression; mood changes.

*Circulatory System:* Decreased white blood cells; decreased blood platelets; anemia; increased bilirubin; chest pain.

*Skin:* Nail disorder; numb, painful, swollen, or red palms of the hands or soles of the feet (hand-and-foot syndrome); rash; dry, itchy, or discolored skin; hair loss.

*Digestive Tract:* Diarrhea; nausea; vomiting; appetite loss or decreased appetite; mouth or throat sores; stomach pain; constipation; indigestion; intestinal obstruction; taste changes; dry mouth.

*Respiratory System:* Difficulty breathing; cough; sore throat; nosebleed; runny nose.

*Other:* Fatigue; fever; dehydration; eye irritation; weakness; joint, limb, muscle, or bone pain; swelling (edema); abnormal vision.

## Guidelines for Use:

- Read Patient Information Sheet before starting therapy and each time you refill your prescription.
- Dosage is individualized. Take exactly as prescribed.
- Do not stop taking or change the dose, unless instructed by your doctor.
- Specific dosage will be determined by your doctor. Take daily in 2 divided doses (morning and evening) within 30 minutes after the end of meals for 2 weeks, followed by a 1-week rest period, given as 3-week cycles.
- Tablets should be swallowed with water.
- Your doctor may want you to take a combination of 150 mg and 500 mg tablets for each dose. If a combination is prescribed, it is very important to correctly identify the tablets. Taking the wrong tablets could result in an over- or underdose.
- If you miss a dose, do not take the missed dose and do not double the dose to catch up. Continue your regular dosing schedule and contact your doctor.
- May cause photosensitivity (sensitivity to sunlight). Avoid prolonged exposure to the sun or other forms of ultraviolet (UV) light (eg, tanning beds). Use sunscreens and wear protective clothing until tolerance is determined.
- Stop taking and notify your doctor immediately if you experience severe diarrhea (more than 4 bowel movements each day or any diarrhea at night); vomiting more than once per day; loss of appetite; pain, redness, swelling, or sores in the mouth; pain, swelling, or redness of the hands or feet; or a temperature of 100.5°F or greater or other evidence of infection.
- Do not take aluminum hydroxide- and magnesium hydroxide-containing antacids (eg, *Maalox*) while undergoing therapy with this medicine.
- If you are taking the vitamin folic acid, inform your doctor.
- Lab tests will be required. Be sure to keep appointments.
- Store at room temperature (59° to 86°F) in a tightly sealed container.

*If you have any questions, consult your doctor, pharmacist, or health care provider.*

| Generic Name<br>*Brand Name Examples* | Supplied As | Generic<br>Available |
|---|---|---|
| Rx **Topotecan** | | |
| *Hycamtin* | **Injection:** 1 mg/mL after reconstitution in 4 mg vials | No |
| Rx **Irinotecan** | | |
| *Camptosar* | **Injection:** 20 mg/mL in 5 mL vials | No |

For more information on chemotherapy treatment, see the introduction to this chapter.

## Type of Drug:
Chemotherapy agents; anticancer drugs.

## How the Drug Works:
Works on an enzyme affecting DNA synthesis in cells by causing small breaks in DNA. The agents then bind to the DNA and prevent the closing of these breaks. Human and tumor cells are affected by this action.

## Uses:
*Irinotecan:* To treat cancer of the colon or rectum when disease has recurred or progressed following 5–FU therapy.

*Topotecan:* To treat cancer of the ovary after failure of initial or subsequent chemotherapy.

## Precautions:
*Do not use in the following situations:*
>    allergy to camptothecins or any of their ingredients
>    nursing mothers
>    pregnancy
>    severe bone marrow depression (topotecan only)

*Use with caution in the following situations:*

*irinotecan only-*
| | |
|---|---|
| decreased ability to fight infection | elderly |
| diarrhea | pelvic/abdominal irradiation |

*topotecan only-*
| | |
|---|---|
| anemia | decreased blood platelets |
| blood disorder | inadequate bone marrow |
| bone marrow suppression | reserves |

*Diarrhea:* Irinotecan can induce diarrhea, possibly preceded by stomach cramps and profuse sweating. Patients with severe diarrhea should be carefully watched and given fluids to avoid dehydration. Late diarrhea (developing 24 hours or more after administration) should be treated promptly with loperamide.

*Pregnancy:* Studies have shown a potential adverse effect on the fetus. Use only if clearly needed and potential benefits outweigh the possible risks.

*Breastfeeding:* Irinotecan appears in breast milk. Because of the potential for serious adverse reactions in nursing infants, it is recommended that nursing be discontinued when receiving therapy with irinotecan. It is not known if topotecan appears in breast milk. Consult your doctor before you begin breastfeeding.

*Children:* Safety and effectiveness in children under 16 years of age have not been established.

*Elderly:* No change in dosage and administration is recommended for elderly patients, other than adjustments related to renal function.

*Lab tests* are recommended before each dose of irinotecan. Be sure to keep appointments. Tests may include white blood cell count with differential, hemoglobin, and platelet count.

## Drug Interactions:
Tell your doctor or pharmacist if you are taking or planning to take any over-the-counter or prescription medications or dietary supplements while taking this medicine. Doses of one or both drugs may need to be modified or a different drug may need to be prescribed. The following drugs and drug classes interact with this medicine:

cisplatin (*Platinol*) (topotecan only)

dexamethasone (eg, *Decadron*) (irinotecan only)

diuretics (irinotecan only)

filgrastim (*Neupogen*) (topotecan only)

prochlorperazine (*Compazine*) (irinotecan only)

## Side Effects:
Every drug is capable of producing side effects. Many patients experience no, or minor, side effects. The frequency and severity of side effects depend on many factors including dose, duration of therapy, and individual susceptibility. Possible side effects include:

*Irinotecan only* —

*Digestive Tract:* Diarrhea; nausea; vomiting; appetite loss; constipation; gas; inflammation of the mouth; indigestion.

*Circulatory System:* Abnormal blood counts; anemia; blood disorder; flushing.

*Body As A Whole:* Weakness, stomach cramping or pain; fever; pain; headache; back pain; chills; minor infection; fluid retention; swelling of the stomach.

*Skin:* Hair loss; sweating; rash.

*Respiratory:* Difficulty breathing; increased coughing; sinus infection or congestion.

*Nervous System:* Sleeplessness; dizziness.

*Topotecan only* —

*Digestive Tract:* Nausea; vomiting; diarrhea; constipation; stomach pain; inflammation of the mouth; appetite loss.

*Circulatory System:* Blood disorder; abnormal blood counts: decreased platelets; anemia.

*Body As A Whole:* Fatigue; fever; infection; weakness.

*Skin:* Hair loss.

*Respiratory:* Difficulty breathing.

*Nervous System:* Headache; abnormal skin sensations (eg, burning, prickling).

---

### Guidelines for Use:

- These drugs may lower your body's ability to fight infection. Notify your doctor of signs of infection including fever, sore throat, rashes or chills.
- Patients should be informed of the expected toxic effects of these drugs, especially nausea, vomiting and diarrhea.
- The use of laxatives should be avoided, discuss any laxative use with your doctor.
- Patients should be alerted to the possibility of hair loss.
- These medications will be prepared and administered by your health care provider.
- Appointments for lab tests to monitor treatment are required.
- Store at room temperature in the original carton. Keep protected from light.

---

*If you have any questions, consult your doctor, pharmacist, or health care provider.*

| Generic Name<br>*Brand Name Example* | Supplied As | Generic<br>Available |
|---|---|---|
| *Rx* **Busulfan** | | |
| *Myleran* | **Tablets:** 2 mg | No |

For more information on chemotherapy treatment, see the introduction to this chapter.

## Type of Drug:
Chemotherapy drug; anticancer drug; alkylating agent.

## How the Drug Works:
Busulfan slows down reproduction and growth of certain white blood cells. It is used to control, not cure, certain types of leukemia. Leukemia is a disease in which the body makes too many white blood cells.

## Uses:
To control, not cure, chronic myelogenous leukemia.

## Precautions:
*Do not use in the following situations:*
　　acute leukemia
　　chronic lymphocytic leukemia
　　chronic myelogenous leukemia ("blastic crisis")
　　prior resistance to therapy

*Use with caution in the following situations:*

| | |
|---|---|
| history of seizures or head trauma | bone marrow depression from radiation or chemotherapy |

*Lung dysplasia:* A rare but serious complication of busulfan therapy. Symptoms have occurred within 8 months to 10 years after beginning therapy. Symptoms include: Harmful cough, difficulty breathing and low-grade fever.

*Pregnancy:* Studies have shown busulfan may cause harm to the fetus. Avoid use during pregnancy if possible.

*Breastfeeding:* It is not known if busulfan appears in breast milk. Consult your doctor before you begin breastfeeding.

*Lab tests* including blood and platelet counts are necessary and should be performed weekly to monitor for toxicity.

## Drug Interactions:
Tell your doctor or pharmacist if you are taking or planning to take any over-the-counter or prescription medications or dietary supplements with busulfan. Doses of one or both drugs may need to be modified or a different drug may need to be prescribed. Thioguanine interacts with busulfan.

## Side Effects:

Most busulfan users experience side effects. The frequency and severity of side effects depend on many factors including dose, duration of therapy, and individual susceptibility. Possible side effects include:

*Blood:* Severely decreased blood and platelet counts.

*Digestive Tract:* Diarrhea; appetite loss; nausea; vomiting.

*Nervous System:* Weakness; dizziness; confusion; fatigue; seizures.

*Respiratory System:* Shortness of breath; cough.

*Skin:* Unusual bleeding or bruising; hair loss; darkening of the skin; redness; hives; dry skin and mucous membranes.

*Other:* Fever; sore throat; lower back pain; joint pain; stomach ache; cataracts (long term use); weight loss.

---

### Guidelines for Use:

- Take this medication at the same time every day.
- Drink plenty of fluids while taking this drug.
- If a dose is missed, take it as soon as possible. If several hours have passed or it is nearing time for the next dose, do not double the dose to catch up, unless advised to do so by your doctor. If more than one dose is missed or it is necessary to establish a new dosage schedule, contact your doctor or pharmacist. Use exactly as prescribed.
- If nausea or vomiting occurs, it may help to take the drug on an empty stomach.
- Contraception (birth control) is recommended while taking this drug.
- Notify your doctor if unusual bleeding or bruising, fever, seizures, cough, shortness of breath, flank, stomach or joint pain occurs.
- May cause darkening of skin, diarrhea, dizziness, fatigue, appetite loss, mental confusion, nausea and vomiting. Notify your doctor if these become pronounced.
- These drugs may lower your body's ability to fight infection. Notify your doctor of any signs of infection including fever, sore throat, rashes or chills.

---

*If you have any questions, consult your doctor, pharmacist, or health care provider.*

| Generic Name<br>*Brand Name Example* | Supplied As | Generic<br>Available |
|---|---|---|
| Rx **Etoposide** | | |
| *VePesid*[1] | **Capsules:** 50 mg | No |

[1] Also available as an injection.

Vincristine sulfate and vinblastine sulfate, mitotic inhibitors available only as injections, are not incuded in this monograph. For more information on chemotherapy treatment, see the introduction to this chapter.

## Type of Drug:
Chemotherapy agent; anticancer drug; mitotic inhibitor.

## How the Drug Works:
Etoposide inhibits tumor cells from dividing (mitosis), thereby preventing the spread of certain types of cancer. Often used with other anticancer drugs.

## Uses:
To treat cancer of the testicles when other treatments are not working.

To treat small cell lung cancer.

*Unlabeled Use(s):* Occasionally doctors may prescribe etoposide to treat certain types of lymphomas and leukemias, including Hodgkin disease and Kaposi sarcoma.

## Precautions:
*Do not use in the following situations:*
    allergy to etoposide or any of its ingredients
    allergy to podophyllum

*Pregnancy:* Studies have shown a potential adverse effect to the fetus. Use only if clearly needed and potential benefits outweigh the possible risks.

*Breastfeeding:* It is not known if etoposide appears in breast milk. Consult your doctor before you begin breastfeeding.

*Children:* Safety and effectiveness have not been established.

*Lab tests* may be required during treatment with etoposide. Tests may include complete blood counts and platelet counts.

## Drug Interactions:
Tell your doctor or pharmacist if you are taking or planning to take any over-the-counter or prescription medications or dietary supplements with etoposide. Doses of one or both drugs may need to be modified or a different drug may need to be prescribed. Warfarin (eg, *Coumadin*) interacts with etoposide.

## Side Effects:

Every drug is capable of producing side effects. Most etoposide users experience no, or minor, side effects. The frequency and severity of side effects depend on many factors including dose, duration of therapy, and individual susceptibility. Possible side effects include:

*Allergic Reactions:* Chills; fever; rapid heart rate; painful or difficult breathing; decreased blood pressure.

*Digestive Tract:* Nausea; vomiting; appetite loss; diarrhea; constipation; stomach ache; difficulty swallowing.

*Skin:* Hair loss; rash; itching; skin discoloration.

*Other:* Short-term blindness; changes in blood pressure; aftertaste; fever; inflammation of the mouth; decrease in blood counts.

---

### Guidelines for Use:

- If a dose is missed, take it as soon as possible. If several hours have passed or it is nearing time for the next dose, do not double the dose to catch up, unless advised to do so by your doctor. If more than one dose is missed, or it is necessary to establish a new dosage schedule, contact your doctor or pharmacist. Use exactly as prescribed.
- Consult your doctor if chills, fever, rapid heartbeat, lightheadedness, flushing or difficult breathing occurs.
- Contraceptive measures (birth control) are recommended during treatment with etoposide.
- *Infections* — These drugs may lower your body's ability to fight infection. Notify your doctor of any signs of infection including fever, sore throat, rashes, or chills.
- Lab tests may be required to monitor therapy. Be sure to keep appointments.
- Capsules must be stored at 36° to 46°F. They will retain their effectiveness for 2 years under refrigeration, 3 months at room temperature. Do not freeze.

---

*If you have any questions, consult your doctor, pharmacist, or health care provider.*

| Generic Name Brand Name Example | Supplied As | Generic Available |
|---|---|---|
| Rx **Vinorelbine Tartrate** | | |
| *Navelbine*[1] | **Injection:** 10 mg/mL | No |

[1] Preservative free.

For more information on chemotherapy treatment, see the introduction to this chapter.

## Type of Drug:

Chemotherapy agent; anticancer drug; mitotic inhibitor.

## How the Drug Works:

Vinorelbine prevents tumor cells from dividing (mitosis), which slows or stops tumor growth.

## Uses:

To treat advanced non-small-cell lung cancer that cannot be surgically removed. May be used in combination with cisplatin.

*Unlabeled Use(s):* Occasionally doctors may prescribe vinorelbine for other forms of cancer, desmoid tumors and fibromatosis, advanced Kaposi sarcoma, and and Hodgkin disease.

## Precautions:

*Do not use in the following situations:*
    allergy to vinorelbine or any of its ingredients
    low blood (granulocyte) counts (less than 1000 cells/mm$^3$)

*Use with caution in the following situations:*

| | |
|---|---|
| bone marrow, compromised | liver disease |
| bronchospasm | lung disease |
| chemotherapy, recovery from | neuropathy, active or history of |
| constipation | radiation therapy, prior |
| infection | |
| intestinal disorder (eg, ileus, obstruction, perforation) | |

*Pregnancy:* Studies have shown a potential adverse effect to the fetus. Use only if clearly needed and the potential benefits to the mother outweigh the possible hazards to the fetus. Women of childbearing potential should avoid becoming pregnant during vinorelbine treatment.

*Breastfeeding:* It is not known if vinorelbine appears in breast milk. Consult your doctor before you begin breastfeeding.

*Children:* Safety and effectiveness in children have not been established.

*Lab tests* may be required to monitor therapy. Tests include frequent blood counts.

## Drug Interactions:

Tell your doctor or pharmacist if you are taking or if you are planning to take any over-the-counter or prescription medications or dietary supplements while taking vinorelbine. Doses of one or both drugs may need to be modified or a different drug may need to be prescribed. The Following drugs or drug classes interact with vinorelbine:

> cisplatin (*Platinol*)
> mitomycin (*Mutamycin*)
> P450 (CYP 3A) isoenzyme inhibitors (eg, zafirlukast)
> paclitaxel (eg, *Taxol*)

## Side Effects:

Every drug is capable of producing side effects. Many vinorelbine users experience no, or minor, side effects. The frequency and severity of side effects depend on many factors including dose, duration of therapy, and individual susceptibility. Possible side effects include:

*Digestive Tract:* Nausea; vomiting; mild to severe constipation; diarrhea; appetite loss; mouth soreness; stomach pain; bowel obstruction or disorder.

*Skin:* Hair loss; vein discoloration; pain or reactions at injection site; flushing; rash; itching; decreased sensitivity to touch; asbnormal sensitivity to touch, pain, or other stimuli; blisters; hives; skin sloughing; abnormal skin sensations (eg, burning, tingling, prickling).

*Other:* Headache; weakness; fatigue; back, jaw, joint, or muscle pain; fever; infection; incoordination; abnormal blood counts; difficulty breathing; abnormal liver function tests; chills; anemia; low white blood cell counts; decreased blood platelets; loss of tendon reflexes; abnormal gait; bladder inflammation; nerve damage; chest pain.

---

### Guidelines for Use:

- This medicine will be prepared and administered by your health care provider in a medical setting.
- For intravenous (IV; into a vein) use only.
- Avoid contact with skin and eyes. If the solution contacts the skin, wash immediately with soap and water. If the solution contacts the eyes, immediately and thoroughly flush with water.
- *Infections* — These drugs reduce your body's ability to fight infection. Notify your doctor of any signs of infection including fever, sore throat, rashes, or chills.
- Contraceptive measures (birth control) are recommended during treatment with vinorelbine in patients who are sexually active.
- Notify your doctor immediately if you experience chills, fever, difficulty breathing, cough, chest or stomach pain, hives, rash, or constipation.
- Lab tests will be required to monitor therapy. Be sure to keep appointments.

---

*If you have any questions, consult your doctor, pharmacist, or health care provider.*

| Generic Name<br>*Brand Name Examples* | Supplied As | Generic<br>Available |
|---|---|---|
| *Rx* **Daunorubicin HCl** | **Injection**: 5 mg/mL (equal to 5.34 mg daunorubicin HCl)[1] | Yes |
| *Rx* **Daunorubicin Citrate Liposome** | | |
| *DaunoXome* | **Injection**: 2 mg/mL (equal to 50 mg daunorubicin base) | No |

[1] Contains sodium chloride.

For more information on chemotherapy treatment, see the introduction to this chapter.

## Type of Drug:

Antineoplastic; anticancer drug; antitumor drug.

## How the Drug Works:

Daunorubicin interferes with cancer cell division and can produce cancer cell death, primarily by interfering with the normal functioning of the genetic material (eg, DNA) of cancer cells.

## Uses:

*Daunorubicin HCl* — In combination with other approved anticancer drugs, for remission induction in acute nonlymphocytic (myelogenous, monocytic, erythroid) of adults and for remission induction in acute lymphocytic leukemia in children and adults.

*Daunorubicin citrate liposome* — First-line cytotoxic therapy for advanced HIV-associated Kaposi sarcoma.

## Precautions:

*Do not use in the following situations:*
allergy to daunorubicin or any of its ingredients
bone marrow suppression, drug-induced preexisting
previously received the highest cumulative dose of either doxorubicin or daunorubicin

*Use with caution in the following situations:*

| | |
|---|---|
| doxorubicin therapy, previous | liver disease |
| heart disease, preexisting | myelosuppression |
| kidney disease | systemic infection, uncontrolled |

*Secondary leukemias:* There have been reports of secondary leukemias in patients exposed to topoisomerase II inhibitors when used in combination with other antineoplastic agents or radiation therapy.

*Pregnancy:* There are no adequate and well-controlled studies in pregnant women. Use only if clearly needed and the potential benefits to the mother outweigh the possible hazards to the fetus.

*Breastfeeding:* It is not known if daunorubicin appears in breast milk. However, mothers should be advised to discontinue breastfeeding during therapy. Consult your doctor before breastfeeding is resumed.

*Children:* Safety and effectiveness in children have not been established. Cardiac toxicity may be more frequent and occur at lower doses in children.

*Elderly:* Safety and effectiveness in elderly patients have not been established. Cardiac toxicity may be more frequent in the elderly. Use caution in patients who have inadequate bone marrow reserves or kidney function impaiment because of age.

*Lab tests* will be required to monitor therapy. Tests include blood, heart, kidney, and liver function.

## Drug Interactions:

Tell your doctor or pharmacist if you are taking or planning to take any over-the-counter or prescription medicines or dietary supplements while taking daunorubicin. Doses of one or both drugs may need to be modified or a different drug may need to be prescribed. The following drugs and drug classes interact with daunorubicin:

cyclophosphamide (eg, *Cytoxan*)
hepatoxic medications (eg, methotrexate)

myelosuppressive agents (eg, mitomycin)

## Side Effects:

Every drug is capable of producing side effects. Many daunorubicin users experience side effects. The frequency and severity of side effects depend on many factors including dose, duration of therapy, and individual susceptibility. Possible side effects include:

*Daunorubicin HCl* — Acute nausea and vomiting (usually mild); diarrhea; stomach pain; injection site reaction; reversible hair loss; rash; hives; itching; fever; chills; bone marrow suppression; secondary leukemia.

*Daunorubicin citrate liposomal* — Stomach pain; appetite loss; constipation; diarrhea; nausea; vomiting; depression; dizziness; fatigue; headache; sleeplessness; general body discomfort; nerve disease; chest tightness; flushing; hair loss; itching; back, joint, or muscle pain; rigors; cough; difficulty breathing; runny nose; sinus irritation.

---

## Guidelines for Use:

- This medicine will be prepared and administered by your health care provider in a medical setting.
- Dosage is individualized.
- Your urine may become reddish-colored while you are undergoing therapy. This is not cause for concern.
- Lab tests will be required to monitor therapy. Be sure to keep appointments.

---

*If you have any questions, consult your doctor, pharmacist, or health care provider.*

| Generic Name<br>*Brand Name Examples* | Supplied As | Generic<br>Available |
|---|---|---|
| *Rx* **Doxorubicin,<br>conventional** | | |
| *Adriamycin RDF* | **Powder for injection<br>(lyophilized)**: 10 mg, 20 mg,<br>50 mg, 150 mg | Yes |
| *Rubex* | **Powder for injection<br>(lyophilized)**: 50 mg, 100 mg | No |
| *Adriamycin PFS* | **Injection**: 10 mg, 20 mg,<br>50 mg, 75 mg | No |
| *Rx* **Doxorubicin, liposome** | | |
| *Doxil* | **Injection**: 20 mg | No |

## Type of Drug:

Antineoplastic; anticancer drug; antitumor drug.

## How the Drug Works:

This drug is toxic to cells, particularly rapidly-dividing cancer cells, by a variety of mechanisms.

## Uses:

*Doxorubicin, conventional* — To produce regression in disseminated neoplastic conditions such as the following: Acute lymphoblastic leukemia, acute myeloblastic leukemia, Wilms' tumor, neuroblastoma, soft tissue and bone sarcomas, breast carcinoma, ovarian carcinoma, transitional cell bladder carcinoma, thyroid carcinoma, Hodgkin and non-Hodgkin lymphomas, bronchogenic carcinoma (the small-cell histologic type is the most responsive), and gastric carcinoma.

*Doxorubicin, liposome* — For treatment of AIDS-related Kaposi sarcoma in patients with disease that has progressed on prior combination chemotherapy or in patients who are intolerant to such therapy.

## Precautions:

*Do not use in the following situations:*

allergy to doxorubicin or any of its ingredients

myelosuppression, marked and induced by previous treatment with other antitumor agents or by radiotherapy (conventional only)

nonresponsive neoplastic conditions (eg, malignant melanoma, kidney carcinoma, large bowel carcinoma, brain tumors, metastases to the central nervous system)

previous treatment with the complete cumulative doses of doxorubicin, daunorubicin, idarubicin, or other anthracyclines and anthracenes

*Use with caution in the following situations:*

elderly

heart disease, history of

high blood pressure

liver disease

*Pregnancy:* Safety for use during pregnancy has not been established. Fetal harm can occur if used in a pregnant woman. Use only if clearly needed and the potential benefits to the mother outweigh the possible hazards to the fetus.

*Breastfeeding:* Conventional doxorubicin appears in breast milk. It is not known if liposomal doxorubicin appears in breast milk. Mothers should, however, be advised to discontinue breastfeeding during therapy. Consult your doctor before breastfeeding is resumed.

*Children:* Doxorubicin may contribute to delayed cardiac toxicity, prepubertal growth failure, and gonadal impairment. Use with extreme caution in pediatric patients.

*Elderly:* Elderly patients may have an increased risk for cardiac toxicity.

*Lab tests* will be required to monitor therapy. Tests include blood counts, heart and liver function, and blood uric acid level.

## Drug Interactions:

Tell your doctor or pharmacist if you are taking or planning to take any over-the-counter or prescription medicines or dietary supplements while taking doxorubicin. Doses of one or both drugs may need to be modified or a different drug may need to be prescribed. The following drugs and drug classes interact with doxorubicin:

actinomycin-D
cyclophosphamide (eg, *Cytoxan*)
cyclosporine (eg, *Neoral*)
digoxin (eg, *Lanoxin*)
mercaptopurine (*Purinethol*)
paclitaxel (eg, *Taxol*)

phenobarbital (eg, *Solfoton*)
phenytoin (eg, *Dilantin*)
progesterone (eg, *Prometrium*)
radiation therapy
streptozocin (*Zanosar*)
verapamil (eg, *Calan*)

## Side Effects:

Every drug is capable of producing side effects. Many doxorubicin users experience side effects. The frequency and severity of side effects depend on many factors including dose, duration of therapy, and individual susceptibility. Possible side effects include:

*Doxorubicin, conventional* — Nausea; vomiting; sensory or motor disturbances; appetite loss; diarrhea; fever; chills; reversible, complete hair loss; hyperpigmentation of nail beds and skin creases (primarily in children); loosening of the nails; skin reaction; hives; injection site reaction; facial flushing; myelosuppression; abnormal blood counts; eye inflammation; infection (eg, candidiasis, cytomegalovirus, herpes simplex, Pneumocystis carinii pneumonia, mycobacterium avium).

*Doxorubicin, liposome* — Skin flushing; palmar or plantar skin eruptions (eg, swelling, pain, redness, shedding or scaling of skin on hands or feet); hair loss; rash; itching; shortness of breath; difficulty breathing; pneumonia; facial swelling; back pain; tightness in chest or throat; abnormal blood counts; joint pain; oral fungal infection; opportunistic viral or bacterial infection; headache; chills; fever; dizziness; drowsiness; low blood pressure; chest pain; fast heartbeat; abnormal heart rhythm; diarrhea; nausea; stomach pain; vomiting; mouth ulcer; inflammation or redness of the tongue; constipation; appetite loss; difficulty swallowing; herpes simplex; weight loss; infection; inflammation of the retina; watery eyes; emotional instability.

## Guidelines for Use:

- This medicine will be prepared and administered intravenously (IV; into a vein) by your health care provider in a medical setting.
- Dosage is individualized.
- Nausea and vomiting associated with therapy may be severe. Antiemetic medications may be necessary.
- You will almost certainly experience hair loss.
- Notify your doctor if you experience bloody stools.
- Your urine may turn reddish-colored for 1 to 2 days following therapy. This is not cause for concern.
- *Doxorubicin, liposome* — Notify your doctor if you experience an acute infusion-related reaction (eg, flushing, shortness of breath, facial swelling, headache, chills, back pain, tightness in the chest or throat, low blood pressure). This effect is more common with the first infusion and usually resolves in about a day.
- Do not undergo any vaccinations with live vaccines during doxorubicin therapy.
- Lab tests will be required to monitor therapy. Be sure to keep appointments.

*If you have any questions, consult your doctor, pharmacist, or health care provider.*

| Generic Name<br>*Brand Name Example* | Supplied As | Generic<br>Available |
|---|---|---|
| *Rx* **Epirubicin HCl** | | |
| *Ellence* | **Injection**: 2 mg/mL | No |

For more information on chemotherapy treatment, see the introduction to this chapter.

## Type of Drug:
Antineoplastic; anticancer drug; antitumor drug.

## How the Drug Works:
This drug interferes with a number of biochemical and biological cellular functions to slow or stop cancer cell growth.

## Uses:
As a component of adjuvant therapy in patients with evidence of axillary node tumor involvement following resection of primary breast cancer.

## Precautions:
*Do not use in the following situations:*
> allergy to epirubicin or any of its ingredients
> allergy to other anthracyclines or anthracenediones
> liver dysfunction, severe
> myocardial infarction, recent
> myocardial insufficiency, severe
> previous treatment with other anthracyclines up to the maximum cumulative dose
> severely reduced neutrophil count, preexisting

*Use with caution in the following situations:*
> bone marrow suppression, preexisting
> kidney disease
> liver disease
> radiation therapy, previous

*Pregnancy:* There are no adequate and well-controlled studies in pregnant women. Fetal harm can occur if used in a pregnant woman. Use only if clearly needed and the potential benefits to the mother outweigh the possible hazards to the fetus.

*Breastfeeding:* It is not known if epirubicin appears in breast milk. Mothers should, however, discontinue breastfeeding during therapy. Consult your doctor before resuming breastfeeding.

*Children:* Safety and effectiveness in children have not been established. Pediatric patients have a greater risk for anthracycline-induced acute manifestations of cardiotoxicity and for chronic congestive heart failure.

*Elderly:* Female patients 70 years of age and older are at an increased risk of drug accumulation and must be monitored closely.

*Lab tests* will be required to monitor therapy. Tests include blood counts and heart, liver, and kidney function tests.

## Drug Interactions:

Tell your doctor or pharmacist if you are taking or planning to take any over-the-counter or prescription medicines or dietary supplements while taking epirubicin. Doses of one or both drugs may need to be modified or a different drug may need to be prescribed. Cimetidine (eg, *Tagamet*) interacts with epirubicin.

## Side Effects:

Every drug is capable of producing side effects. Many epirubicin users experience side effects. The frequency and severity of side effects depend on many factors including dose, duration of therapy, and individual susceptibility. Possible side effects include:

*Digestive Tract:* Nausea; vomiting; diarrhea; appetite loss.

*Skin:* Injection site reaction (possibly severe); hair loss; rash; itching; skin changes.

*Other:* Secondary leukemia; myelosuppression; absence of menstrual bleeding; hot flashes; abnormal blood counts; infection; fever; lethargy; eye inflammation.

---

### Guidelines for Use:

- This medicine will be administered intravenously (IV; into a vein) by your health care provider in a medical setting.
- Dosage is individualized.
- Epirubicin can cause nausea, vomiting, and diarrhea. Antiemetic medications administered before therapy may reduce these side effects.
- Notify your doctor if you experience vomiting, dehydration, fever, evidence of infection, symptoms of congestive heart failure (eg, difficult or labored breathing, swelling of lower legs, fast heartbeat), or injection site pain.
- You will almost certainly experience hair loss. Hair usually starts to regrow within 2 to 3 months after therapy has ended.
- Your urine may turn reddish-colored for 1 to 2 days following therapy. This is not cause for concern.
- There is a risk of irreversible heart damage associated with treatment, as well as treatment-related leukemia.
- Epirubicin may cause chromosomal damage in sperm. Men undergoing treatment should use effective contraceptive methods.
- Women treated with epirubicin may develop irreversible absence of menstruation or premature menopause.
- Lab tests will be required to monitor therapy. Be sure to keep appointments.

---

*If you have any questions, consult your doctor, pharmacist, or health care provider.*

| Generic Name Brand Name Examples | Supplied As | Generic Available |
|---|---|---|
| Rx **Idarubicin HCl** | | |
| *Idamycin* | **Powder for injection (lyophilized)**: 20 mg | No |
| *Idamycin PFS* | **Injection**: 5 mg, 10 mg, 20 mg | No |

For more information on chemotherapy treatment, see the introduction to this chapter.

## Type of Drug:

Antineoplastic; anticancer drug; antileukemic drug.

## How the Drug Works:

Leukemia is a disease in which the body makes too many white blood cells. Idarubicin interferes with the reproduction (growth) of white blood cells as well as other cells formed in the bone marrow.

## Uses:

Used in combination with other approved antileukemic drugs for the treatment of acute myeloid leukemia (AML) in adults.

## Precautions:

*Do not use in the following situations:*
        allergy to idarubicin or any of its ingredients
        bone marrow suppression, preexisting

*Use with caution in the following situations:*
        heart disease
        kidney disease
        liver disease

*Pregnancy:* There are no adequate and well-controlled studies in pregnant women. Use only if clearly needed and the potential benefits outweigh the possible hazards to the fetus.

*Breastfeeding:* It is not known if idarubicin appears in breast milk. Consult your doctor before you begin breastfeeding.

*Children:* Safety and effectiveness in children have not been established.

*Lab tests* will be required to monitor therapy. Tests include blood cell counts and liver and kidney function.

## Drug Interactions:

Tell your doctor or pharmacist if you are taking or planning to take any over-the-counter or prescription medicines or dietary supplements while taking idarubicin. Doses of one or both drugs may need to be modified or a different drug may need to be prescribed.

## Side Effects:

Every drug is capable of producing side effects. Many idarubicin users experience side effects. The frequency and severity of side effects depend on many factors including dose, duration of therapy, and individual susceptibility. Possible side effects include:

*Digestive Tract:* Nausea; vomiting; stomach cramps or pain; diarrhea; inflammation of the lining of the mouth.

*Circulatory System:* Chest pain; irregular heart rhythm; congestive heart failure.

*Skin:* Hair loss; rash; hives.

*Other:* Infection; bleeding; abnormal lab tests; bone marrow suppression; fever; headache; seizure; nerve pain; difficulty breathing; psychological changes.

---

### Guidelines for Use:

- This medicine will be prepared and administered intravenously (IV; into a vein) by your health care provider in a medical setting.
- Dosage is individualized.
- Notify your doctor if you experience sore throat, fever, irregular heartbeat, difficulty breathing, or unusual bleeding or bruising.
- Lab tests will be required to monitor therapy. Be sure to keep appointments.

---

*If you have any questions, consult your doctor, pharmacist, or health care provider.*

| Generic Name Brand Name Example | Supplied As | Generic Available |
|---|---|---|
| Rx **Valrubicin** | | |
| Valstar | **Solution for intravesical instillation**: 40 mg/mL | No |

For more information on chemotherapy treatment, see the introduction to this chapter.

## Type of Drug:

Antineoplastic; anticancer drug.

## How the Drug Works:

This drug penetrates rapidly-dividing cancer cells, interfering with nucleic acid metabolism, which leads to extensive chromosomal damage, DNA damage, and arrested cancer cell growth in a significant percentage of patients.

## Uses:

For intravesical therapy of BCG-refractory carcinoma in situ (CIS) of the urinary bladder in patients for whom immediate cystectomy would be associated with morbidity or mortality.

## Precautions:

*Do not use in the following situations:*
> allergy to any anthracycline
> allergy to valrubicin or any of its ingredients
> > (eg, polyoxyethyleneglycol triricinoleate [*Cremophor EL*])
> perforated bladder or compromised integrity of bladder mucosa
> small bladder capacity (ie, unable to tolerate a 75 mL instillation)
> urinary tract infection, concurrent

*Use with caution in the following situations:* Severe irritable bladder symptoms.

*Pregnancy:* There are no adequate and well-controlled studies in pregnant women. Fetal harm can occur if a pregnant woman is exposed to valrubicin systemically. Use only if clearly needed and the potential benefits to the mother outweigh the possible hazards to the fetus.

*Breastfeeding:* It is not known if valrubicin appears in breast milk. However, any exposure of infants to this drug could pose sevre health risks. Consult your doctor before you begin breastfeeding.

*Children:* Safety and effectiveness in children have not been established.

*Lab tests* will be required to monitor therapy. Tests include bladder function, cystoscopy, biopsy, and urine cytology.

## Drug Interactions:

Tell your doctor or pharmacist if you are taking or planning to take any over-the-counter or prescription medicines or dietary supplements while taking valrubicin. Doses of one or both drugs may need to be modified or a different drug may need to be prescribed.

## Side Effects:

Every drug is capable of producing side effects. Many valrubicin users experience side effects. The frequency and severity of side effects depend on many factors including dose, duration of therapy, and individual susceptibility. Possible side effects include:

*Urinary and Reproductive Tract:* Increased urination; painful or difficult urination; urinary urgency; bladder spasm; blood in the urine; bladder pain; urinary incontinence; excessive urination at night; procedure-related local burning symptoms; urethral pain; pelvic pain; urinary tract infection; urinary retention.

*Digestive Tract:* Stomach pain; nausea; diarrhea; vomiting; gas.

*Other:* High blood sugar; swelling of the arms or legs; weakness; headache; general body discomfort; back, muscle, or chest pain; dizziness; rash; abnormal blood counts; fever; pneumonia; flushing.

---

### Guidelines for Use:

- This medicine will be prepared and administered by your health care provider in a medical setting.
- Dosage is individualized.
- Your urine may become reddish-colored for the first 24 hours after administration. This is not cause for concern.
- Notify your doctor if you experience prolonged reddish-colored urine or prolonged irritable bladder symptoms (eg, bladder spasm, spontaneous discharge of the drug).
- Women should not become pregnant and men should refrain from engaging in procreative activities during treatment. Use an effective contraception method during treatment.
- Lab tests will be required to monitor therapy. Be sure to keep appointments.

---

*If you have any questions, consult your doctor, pharmacist, or health care provider.*

| Generic Name<br>*Brand Name Example* | Supplied As | Generic<br>Available |
|---|---|---|
| *Rx* **Testolactone** | | |
| *Teslac* | **Tablets:** 50 mg | No |

For more information on chemotherapy treatment, see the introduction to this chapter.

## Type of Drug:
Chemotherapy agent; anticancer drug.

## How the Drug Works:
Testolactone is produced synthetically; it is related to testosterone but does not have the masculine effects of testosterone. It blocks the production of estrogen and helps to prevent the growth of breast cancers that are activated by estrogens. It may also protect tumor cells from being activated by other steroid hormones.

## Uses:
Used with other anticancer drugs to treat symptoms of breast cancer in women after menopause.

## Precautions:
*Do not use in the following situations:*
> allergy to testolactone or any if its ingredients
> breast cancer in men

*Pregnancy:* Adequate studies have not been done in pregnant women, or animal studies may have shown a risk to the fetus. Use only if clearly needed and potential benefits outweight the possible hazards to the fetus.

*Breastfeeding:* It is not known if testolactone appears in breast milk. Consult your doctor before you begin breastfeeding.

*Children:* Safety and effectiveness in children have not been established.

*Lab tests* may be required to monitor therapy. Tests may include calcium blood levels.

## Drug Interactions:
Tell your doctor or pharmacist if you are taking or if you are planning to take, any over-the-counter or prescription medications or dietary supplements while taking testolactone. Doses of one or both drugs may need to be modified or a different drug may need to be prescribed. Testolactone interacts with oral anticoagulants (eg, warfarin).

## Side Effects:

Every drug is capable of producing side effects. Many testolactone users experience side effects. The frequency and severity of side effects depend on many factors including dose, duration of therapy, and individual susceptibility. Possible side effects include:

*Digestive Tract:* Inflammation of the tongue; nausea; vomiting; appetite loss.

*Other:* Abnormal skin sensations; aches and swelling of the hands or feet; high blood pressure; hair loss.

### Guidelines for Use:

- Contraceptive (birth control) measures are recommended during treatment. Contact your doctor if pregnancy is suspected.
- If a dose is missed, take or inject as soon as possible. If several hours have passed or it is nearing time for the next dose, do not double the dose to catch up, unless advised to do so by your doctor. If more than one dose is missed, contact your doctor or pharmacist.
- The usual dose is five tablets 4 times daily.
- Notify your doctor if appetite loss, nausea, vomiting, hair loss or swelling of the hands or feet occur.
- Lab tests are required to monitor treatment. Be sure to keep appointments.
- Store at room temperature.

*If you have any questions, consult your doctor, pharmacist, or health care provider.*

| Generic Name<br>*Brand Name Examples* | Supplied As | Generic<br>Available |
|---|---|---|
| Rx **Bicalutamide** | | |
| *Casodex* | **Tablets:** 50 mg | No |
| Rx **Flutamide** | | |
| *Eulexin* | **Capsules:** 125 mg | No |
| Rx **Nilutamide** | | |
| *Nilandron* | **Tablets:** 50 mg | No |

For more information on chemotherapy treatment, see the introduction to this chapter.

## Type of Drug:
Chemotherapy agents; anticancer drugs.

## How the Drug Works:
Antiandrogens prevent androgens (eg, testosterone) from binding to and activating tumor cells of the prostate.

## Uses:
Bicalutamide and flutamide are for use in combination with other anticancer drugs to treat prostate cancer. Nilutamide is for use with surgical castration for the treatment of prostate cancer.

## Precautions:
*Do not use in the following situations:*
> allergy to the antiandrogen or any of its ingredients
> liver disease, severe (nilutamide only)
> respiratory insufficiency, severe (nilutamide only)

*Use with caution in the following situations:* Liver disease.

*Vision changes* may occur. Report any changes to your doctor.

*Flutamide and bicalutamide* should always be administered with other drugs (eg, leuprolide acetate). Do not stop or interrupt dosing without first consulting your doctor.

*Tumors:* Nilutamide has been associated with the development of benign tumors and bicalutamide has been associated with the development of both benign and cancerous tumors in animals. Bicalutamide may lead to male infertility, although long-term studies have not been conducted. Discuss any concerns with your doctor.

*Children:* Safety and effectiveness in children have not been established.

*Lab tests* will be required frequently during treatment. Tests may include liver function tests, PSA levels, and blood clotting tests.

## Drug Interactions:

Tell your doctor or pharmacist if you are taking or if you are planning to take any over-the-counter or prescription medications or dietary supplements while taking antiandrogens. Doses of one or both drugs may need to be modified or a different drug may need to be prescribed. The following drugs and drug classes interact with antiandrogens:

anticoagulants, oral (eg, warfarin)

phenytoin (eg, *Dilantin*) (nilutamide only)

theophylline (eg, *Theo-Dur*) (nilutamide only)

## Side Effects:

Every drug is capable of producing side effects. Many antiandrogen users experience side effects. The frequency and severity of side effects depend on many factors including dose, duration of therapy, and individual susceptibility. Possible side effects include:

*Digestive Tract:* Constipation; nausea; diarrhea; vomiting; black vomit; gas; weight changes; dry mouth; black, bloody stools; appetite loss; stomach pain or problem; indigestion.

*Nervous System:* Dizziness; abnormal skin sensations; sleeplessness; anxiety; depression; confusion; nervousness; drowsiness; headache; weakness; decreased sensitivity; disease of the nerves.

*Circulatory System:* High blood pressure; hot flashes; chest pain; heart failure.

*Respiratory System:* Difficulty breathing; cough; sore throat; upper respiratory infection; pneumonia; bronchitis; sinus infection; congestion.

*Skin:* Rash; itching; hair loss; sweating; dry skin; injection site reaction; body hair loss.

*Urinary and Reproductive Tract:* Urination problems; blood in the urine; discolored urine; urinary tract infection or disorder; excessive urination at night; bladder inflammation or problems; rectal bleeding; inflammation.

*Other:* Swelling of hands or lower legs; general body, back, neck, breast, bone, pelvic, stomach, muscle or joint pain; leg cramps; fever; chills; high blood sugar; dehydration; gout; weakness; infections; flu syndrome; impotence; breast growth in males; anemia; impaired visual adaptation to light or dark; atrophy of testicles; sensitivity to light; fainting; cataract; soreness or stiffness; diabetes; sweating; abnormal vision; changes in sex drive; abnormal coloring; bone fracture; loss of libido; abnormal blood counts; decreased blood platelets; arthritis; increased liver function tests; intolerance to alcohol.

## Guidelines for Use:
- Use exactly as prescribed.
- If a dose is missed, take it as soon as possible. If several hours have passed or it is nearing time for the next dose, do not double the dose to catch up, unless advised to do so by your doctor. If more than one dose is missed or it is necessary to establish a new dosage schedule, contact your doctor or pharmacist.
- Do not stop or interrupt dosing without first consulting your doctor.
- Lab tests/exams are required to monitor treatment. Be sure to keep appointments.
- Store at room temperature in a tightly sealed container. Avoid moisture and light.

*Bicalutamide:*
- Usual dose is one tablet daily (morning or evening) with or without food. If possible, try to take the tablet at the same time each day.
- Medicine may cause hot flashes, breast growth or breast pain.

*Flutamide:*
- Usual dose is two capsules 3 times daily, 8 hours apart.
- Notify your doctor if any of the following occurs: Itching, dark urine, appetite loss, yellowing skin or eyes, stomach pain/tenderness or flu-like symptoms.

*Bicalutamide and Flutamide:*
- Be sure to take this medicine in combination with your LHRH agonist analog (eg, leuprolide acetate) for proper treatment.

*Nilutamide:*
- May cause a delay in visual adaptation to the dark, ranging from seconds to a few minutes. Exercise caution in night driving or driving through tunnels. Wear tinted glasses.
- Notify your doctor if any of the following occurs: Difficulty in breathing, nausea/vomiting, abdominal pain or yellowing of the skin or eyes.
- Avoid alcohol.

*If you have any questions, consult your doctor, pharmacist, or health care provider.*

| Generic Name<br>*Brand Name Example* | Supplied As | Generic<br>Available |
|---|---|---|
| Rx **Megestrol Acetate** | | |
| *Megace* | **Tablets:** 20 mg, 40 mg | Yes |
| *Megace* | **Suspension, oral:** 40 mg/mL | No |

For more information on chemotherapy treatment, see the introduction to this chapter.

## Type of Drug:
Chemotherapy agents; anticancer drugs.

## How the Drug Works:
Progestins can interfere with the way that estrogen and other steroid hormones activate tumor cells of the breast and endometrium.

## Uses:
*Tablet:* To treat the symptoms of breast and endometrial cancers.

*Oral suspension:* To treat loss of appetite, weight loss or an unexplained, significant weight loss in patients with a diagnosis of AIDS.

## Precautions:
*Do not use in the following situations:*

allergy to megestrol or any of its ingredients
diagnostic test for pregnancy
neoplastic disease, other
pregnancy
pregnancy, first trimester

*Use with caution in the following situations:*

blood clotting disorders, history of
diabetes

*HIV infected women (oral suspension only)* have reported breakthrough bleeding with the use of megesterol acetate.

*Diabetics* should monitor glucose more frequently; insulin requirements may increase.

*Pregnancy:*

*Tablet* – Studies have shown a potential adverse effect on the fetus. Use only if clearly needed and potential benefits outweigh the possible risks. Megestrol is not recommended for use during the first four months of pregnancy.

*Oral suspension* – Do not use during pregnancy. The risk of use in a pregnant woman clearly outweights any possible benefit. Megestrol is not recommended for use during the first four months of pregnancy.

*Breastfeeding:* Because of the potential for adverse effects on newborns, nursing should be discontinued if the patient is taking megesterol acetate. Consult your doctor before you begin breastfeeding.

*Children:* Safety and effectiveness in children have not been established.

## Drug Interactions:

Tell your doctor if you are taking or if you are planning to take any over-the-counter or prescription medications or dietary supplements with progestins. Doses of one or both drugs may need to be modified or a different drug may need to be prescribed.

## Side Effects:

Every drug is capable of producing side effects. Many patients experience side effects. The frequency and severity of side effects depend on many factors including dose, duration of therapy and individual susceptibility. Possible side effects include:

*Digestive Tract:* Nausea; vomiting; diarrhea; indigestion; constipation; dry mouth; weight changes; increased salivation; mouth sores and infection; gas; stomach pain.

*Nervous System:* Weakness; sleeplessness; confusion; convulsions; depression; abnormal skin sensations; headache; chest or general body pain; mood changes; abnormal thinking; disease of the nerves.

*Circulatory System:* High blood pressure; pounding in the chest; heart failure; enlargement of the heart.

*Respiratory System:* Difficulty breathing; cough; sore throat; lung disorder.

*Skin:* Rash; itching; hair loss; sweating; decreased sensitivity to touch; skin disorder; herpes.

*Other:* Carpal tunnel syndrome; swelling; high blood sugar levels; fever; urinary changes; breast growth in males; breakthrough menstrual bleeding; hot flashes; glucose intolerance; impotence; anemia; infection; enlargement of the liver; abnormal blood counts; protein in the urine; urinary incontinence; urinary tract infection; decreased sex drive.

---

### Guidelines for Use:

- Contraceptive (birth control) measures are recommended during treatment. Contact your doctor if pregnancy is suspected.
- If a dose is missed, take or inject it at soon as possible. If several hours have passed or it is nearing time for the next dose, do not double the dose to catch up, unless advised to do so by your doctor. If more than one dose is missed, contact your doctor or pharmacist.
- Shake suspension well before using.
- Contact your doctor if chest or stomach pain, headache, nausea, vomiting or other adverse reactions occur.
- Store suspension at 59° to 77°F in a tight container. Protect from heat.
- Lab tests/exams are required to monitor treatment. Be sure to keep appointments.
- Store tablets at room temperature away from heat.

---

*If you have any questions, consult your doctor, pharmacist, or health care provider.*

| Generic Name *Brand Name Example* | Supplied As | Generic Available |
|---|---|---|
| *Rx* **Diethylstilbestrol Diphosphate** | | |
| *Stilphostrol* | **Tablets:** 50 mg | Yes |
| *Stilphostrol* | **Injection:** 0.25 g (as sodium salt) | No |

For more information on chemotherapy treatment, see the introduction to this chapter.

## Type of Drug:
Chemotherapy agents; anticancer drugs.

## How the Drug Works:
Diethylstilbestrol diphosphate increases estrogen levels in the body that prevent the formation of androgens that stimulate tumor cells of the prostate.

## Uses:
To treat symptoms of progressing prostate cancer where surgery is not possible.

## Precautions:
*Do not use in the following situations:*
> blood clotting disorders
> breast cancer (except for metastatic disease)
> estrogen-dependent tumors
> women

*Use with caution in the following situations:*

| | |
|---|---|
| asthma | heart problems |
| bone diseases | kidney disease |
| depression | liver disease, history of |
| diabetes | migraines |
| epilepsy | surgery, prior to |
| gallbladder disease | |

*Estrogen use in men:* Diethylstilbestrol should not be used in men with breast cancer (unless advised by a doctor), estrogen-dependent tumors or blood clots.

*Diabetes:* Diethylstilbestrol may decrease glucose (sugar) tolerance. Test blood sugar often.

*High blood pressure:* Diethylstilbestrol may increase blood pressure. Blood pressure should be checked frequently.

*Vision changes* may occur. Report any changes to your doctor.

*Children:* Use diethylstilbestrol with extreme caution in young patients who are still growing, because it may interfere with normal bone development.

*Lab tests* may be required to monitor therapy. Tests may include eye exams, complete blood counts, liver and kidney function tests, calcium blood levels, cholesterol and triglyceride blood levels, prostate specific antigen (PSA) levels, glucose (sugar) blood levels (diabetics), blood clotting tests, folic acid levels, blood pressure and heart rate.

## Drug Interactions:

Tell your doctor or pharmacist if you are taking or planning to take any over-the-counter or prescription medications or dietary supplements while taking an estrogen. Doses of one or both drugs may need to be modified or a different drug may need to be prescribed.

## Side Effects:

Every drug is capable of producing side effects. Many estrogen users experience side effects. The frequency and severity of side effects depend on many factors including dose, duration of therapy, and individual susceptibility. Possible side effects include:

*Digestive Tract:* Nausea; vomiting; stomach cramps; appetite loss; weight changes; bloating.

*Nervous System:* Headache; migraine; nervousness; dizziness; mood changes; depression; fatigue; involuntary movements; numbness/tingling around nose or mouth.

*Skin:* Unusual hair growth or loss; itching or burning in the rectal area; rash; skin discoloration; yellowing of eyes or skin.

*Other:* Intolerance to contact lenses; backache; breast tenderness or enlargement; changes in sex drive; vision problems; swelling of hands or feet; shortness of breath; chest pain; painful, difficult and frequent urination.

---

## Guidelines for Use:

- If a dose is missed, take or inject it as soon as possible. If several more hours have passed or it is nearing time for the next dose, do not double the dose to catch up, unless advised to do so by your doctor. If more than one dose is missed, contact your doctor or pharmacist.
- Diabetic patients should be prepared to monitor their blood sugar levels more frequently. Loss of glucose control may occur.
- Promptly report any of the following symptoms to your doctor: Bloating, nausea, vomiting, stomach cramps, loss of appetite, fluid retention, swelling/tenderness of breasts, rash, mood changes, depression, nervousness, dizziness, chest pain, shortness of breath, numbness or tingling around nose or mouth, vision changes, swelling, painful or frequent urination, yellowing of skin or eyes.
- Those who wear contact lenses may notice a change in their eyes or vision. Lens wear may not be possible.
- Lab tests and exams are required to monitor treatment. Be sure to keep appointments.
- Store tablets and injection at room temperature (59° to 86°F). Protect from light.

---

*If you have any questions, consult your doctor, pharmacist, or health care provider.*

| Generic Name<br>*Brand Name Examples* | Supplied As | Generic<br>Available |
|---|---|---|
| Rx **Tamoxifen Citrate** | | |
| *Nolvadex* | **Tablets**: 10 mg, 20 mg | Yes |
| Rx **Toremifene Citrate** | | |
| *Fareston* | **Tablets**: 60 mg | No |

## Type of Drug:

Antiestrogen; anticancer drug.

## How the Drug Works:

Estrogens may cause the growth of some types of breast tumors. Antiestrogens block the effects of estrogen on certain tissues in the body, including breast tissue. Antiestrogens may block the growth of breast tumors that are activated by estrogens.

## Uses:

*Tamoxifen:* For the treatment of metastatic breast cancer in men and women.

For the treatment of breast cancer in postmenopausal women following surgery and breast irradiation.

To reduce the rick of invasive breast cancer in women with ductal carcinoma in situ (DCIS) following breast surgery and radiation.

To reduce the incidence of breast cancer in women at high risk for developing breast cancer.

*Toremifene:* For the treatment of metastatic breast cancer in postmenopausal women with estrogen-receptor (ER) positive or ER-unknown tumors.

*Unlabeled Use(s):* Occasionally doctors may prescribe tamoxifen for treatment of breast pain and enlargement.

## Precautions:

*Do not use in the following situations:*

allergy to the antiestrogen or any of its ingredients

deep-vein thrombosis, history of (tamoxifen only when used to reduce the incidence of breast cancer)

oral anticoagulant therapy, concomitant (tamoxifen only when used to reduce the incidence of breast cancer)

pulmonary embolus, history of (tamoxifen only when used to reduce the incidence of breast cancer)

thromboembolic disease (toremifene only)

*Use with caution in the following situations:*

calcium blood levels, increased
cataracts (tamoxifen only)
cholesterol or triglyceride levels,
increased (tamoxifen only)
deep-vein thrombosis (following
surgery for breast cancer)
(tamoxifen only when used to
treat metastatic breast cancer
or breast cancer following
surgery and breast irradiation)

liver disease (tamoxifen only)
platelet count decreased (tamoxifen only)
pulmonary embolus (tamoxifen
only when used to treat metastatic breast cancer or breast
cancer following surgery and
breast irradiation)
white blood cells decreased
(tamoxifen only)

*Vision changes* may occur. Report any changes to your doctor.

*Pregnancy:* There are no adequate and well-controlled studies in pregnant women. Antiestrogens may cause fetal harm when administered
to a pregnant woman. Use only if clearly needed and potential benefits
to the mother outweigh the possible hazards to the fetus.

*Breastfeeding:* It is not known if antiestrogens appear in breast milk. A decision must be made whether to discontinue nursing or discontinue the
drug, taking into account the importance of the drug to the mother. Consult your doctor before you begin breastfeeding.

*Children:* Safety and effectiveness in children have not been established
Antiestrogens are not indicated for use in children.

*Lab tests* will be required to monitor therapy. Tests may include complete
blood counts, calcium levels, white blood cell counts, liver function tests,
platelet counts, breast examinations, mammograms, gynecological
exams, and cholesterol and triglyceride blood levels.

## Drug Interactions:

Tell your doctor or pharmacist if you are taking or if you are planning to
take any over-the-counter or prescription medications or dietary
supplements while taking an antiestrogen. Doses of one or both drugs
may need to be modified or a different drug may need to be prescribed.
The following drugs and drug classes interact with antiestrogens:

anticoagulants, oral (eg, warfarin)
bromocriptine (*Parlodel*)
chemotherapeutic agents (eg, methotrexate)
cytochrome P450 3A4 enzyme inducers (eg, phenobarbital,
phenytoin, carbamazepine)
rifamycins (eg, rifampin)

## Side Effects:

Every drug is capable of producing side effects. Many antiestrogen users
experience side effects. The frequency and severity of side effects
depend on many factors including dose, duration of therapy, and individual susceptibility. Possible side effects include:

*Eyes or Ocular:* Corneal changes; cataracts; need for cataract surgery;
decline in color vision perception; retinal vein thrombosis; retinopathy;
dry eyes; abnormal visual fields.

*Digestive Tract:* Nausea; vomiting; appetite loss; weight loss; stomach cramps; constipation.

*Nervous System:* Fatigue; depression; dizziness; light-headedness; headache.

*Skin:* Rash; skin changes; hair thinning or partial hair loss; flushing; sweating.

*Urinary and Reproductive Tract:* Abnormal vaginal bleeding and discharge; menstrual irregularities; ovarian cysts; vaginal itching; vaginal dryness; pelvic pain or pressure.

*Other:* Hot flashes; difficulty breathing; cough; pain; bone, tumor, or muscle pain; local disease flare; lesion size increase in soft tissue disease; new lesions; flushing or redness around the lesion; high blood calcium levels; elevated liver enzymes; decreased white blood cell counts; decreased platelet count; changes in triglyceride blood levels; changes in cholesterol levels; swelling of the arms or legs; distaste for food; fluid retention; increased creatinine; loss of sex drive; impotence; blood clot in lungs; blood clot in legs; endometrial cancer; heart failure.

## Guidelines for Use:

- Dosage is individualized. Take exactly as prescribed.
- Do not change the dose or stop taking, unless advised by your doctor.
- Swallow tablets whole with a glass of water.
- May be taken without regard to meals.
- Do not become pregnant during therapy. If you are sexually active, barrier or nonhormonal contraceptive (birth control) measures are recommended during treatment and for 2 months following the discontinuation of treatment. Contact your doctor if pregnancy is suspected.
- Notify your doctor immediately if you experience marked weakness, sleepiness, mental confusion, difficulty talking, numbness, pain or swelling of legs, unexplained shortness of breath, coughing up blood, sudden chest pain, changes in vision, new breast lumps, vaginal bleeding, gynecological symptoms (eg, menstrual irregularities, changes in vaginal discharge, pelvic pain or pressure), bone pain, hot flashes, nausea, vomiting, weight gain, dizziness, headache, or loss of appetite.
- If a dose is missed, take it as soon as possible. If several hours have passed or it is nearing time for the next dose, do not double the dose to catch up, unless advised to do so by your doctor. If more than one dose is missed, contact your doctor or pharmacist.
- Bone or tumor pain may occur shortly after starting tamoxifen and usually subsides rapidly.
- Lab tests and exams will be required to monitor therapy. Be sure to keep appointments. Women who receive long-term tamoxifen therapy should have regular gynecological and vision exams.
- Store at room temperature (68° to 77°F) in a tightly closed container. Protect from heat and light. Do not use after the expiration date.

*If you have any questions, consult your doctor, pharmacist, or health care provider.*

| Generic Name<br>*Brand Name Example* | Supplied As | Generic<br>Available |
|---|---|---|
| *Rx* **Anastrozole** | | |
| *Arimidex* | **Tablets**: 1 mg | No |
| *Rx* **Exemestane** | | |
| *Aromasin* | **Tablets**: 25 mg | No |
| *Rx* **Letrozole** | | |
| *Femara* | **Tablets**: 2.5 mg | No |

## Type of Drug:

Anticancer drug; antihormone; aromatase inhibitor.

## How the Drug Works:

Aromatase inhibitors lower estrone and estradiol (female sex hormones) levels, reducing or delaying the growth of tumors that are stimulated or maintained by female sex hormones in breast cancer patients.

## Uses:

To treat advanced breast cancer in postmenopausal women whose disease continues to grow after tamoxifen therapy.

*Anastrozole:* To treat postmenopausal women with hormone receptor positive early breast cancer.

*Anastrozole, letrozole:* For first-line treatment of postmenopausal women with hormone receptor positive or hormone receptor unknown locally advanced or metastatic breast cancer.

## Precautions:

*Do not use in the following situations:* Allergy to the drug or any of its ingredients.

*Use with caution in the following situations:*
    liver disease, severe
    pregnancy
    premenopausal women

*Pregnancy:* Studies have shown a potential adverse effect on the fetus. Aromatase inhibitors should only be used on postmenopausal women.

*Breastfeeding:* It is not known if aromatase inhibitors appear in breast milk. Consult your doctor before you begin breastfeeding.

*Children:* Safety and effectiveness have not been established.

*Lab tests* may be required to monitor therapy.

## Drug Interactions:

Tell your doctor or pharmacist if you are taking or planning to take any over-the-counter or prescription medications or dietary supplements while taking these drugs. Drug doses may need to be modified or a different drug prescribed. The following drugs or drug classes interact with these drugs:

> estrogen-containing agents (eg, *Estratest*)
> tamoxifen (eg, *Nolvadex*) (anastrozole, letrozole only)

## Side Effects:

Every drug is capable of producing side effects. Many patients experience no, or minor, side effects. The frequency and severity of side effects depend on many factors including dose, duration of therapy, and individual susceptibility. Possible side effects include:

*Digestive Tract:* Nausea; vomiting; diarrhea; constipation; stomach pain; appetite changes.

*Nervous System:* Headache; dizziness; depression; abnormal skin sensations; drowsiness; sleeplessness; confusion; anxiety; nervousness.

*Respiratory System:* Difficulty breathing; increased cough; sore throat; sinus infection; bronchitis; congestion.

*Skin:* Rash; itching; sweating; thinning hair.

*Other:* Hot flushes; pain; muscle, joint, back, bone, pelvic, neck, breast, or chest pain; general body discomfort; dry mouth; swelling of hands or feet; vaginal bleeding; weight gain; flu syndrome; fever; injury; infection; urinary tract infection; abnormal blood counts; anemia; abnormal lab tests; weight loss; fracture; feeling of whirling motion (vertigo); high blood pressure; fatigue; weakness; flushing; vaginal inflammation or discharge; osteoporosis.

## Guidelines for Use:

- Dosage is individualized. Take exactly as prescribed.
- Do not stop taking or change the dose, unless instructed by your doctor.
- Take exemestane after a meal. Anastrozole and letrozole may be taken without regard to food.
- If a dose is missed, take it as soon as possible. If several hours have passed or it is nearing time for the next dose, do not double the dose to catch up, unless instructed by your doctor. If more than one dose is missed or it is necessary to establish a new dosage schedule, contact your doctor or pharmacist.
- May cause dizziness or drowsiness. Use caution while driving or performing other tasks requiring mental alertness, coordination, or physical dexterity until tolerance is determined.
- Inform your doctor if your are pregnant, become pregnant, are planning to become pregnant, or if you are breastfeeding.
- Lab tests may be required to monitor therapy. Be sure to keep appointments.
- Store at room temperature (59° to 86°F). Store anastrozole at 68° to 77°F.

*If you have any questions, consult your doctor, pharmacist, or health care provider.*

| Generic Name<br>*Brand Name Example* | Supplied As | Generic<br>Available |
|---|---|---|
| *Rx* **Goserelin Acetate** | | |
| *Zoladex* | **Implant:** 3.6 mg, 10.8 mg | No |
| *Rx* **Leuprolide Acetate**[1] | | |
| *Lupron, Lupron for Pediatric Use* | **Injection**: 5 mg/mL | Yes |
| *Lupron Depot* | **Microspheres for injection**: 3.75 mg, 7.5 mg | No |
| *Lupron Depot-Ped* | **Microspheres for injection**: 7.5 mg, 11.25 mg, 15 mg | No |
| *Lupron Depot-3 Month* | **Microspheres for injection**: 11.25 mg, 22.5 mg | No |
| *Lupron Depot-4 Month* | **Microspheres for injection**: 30 mg | No |
| *Eligard* | **Powder for injection**: 7.5 mg, 22.5 mg | No |
| *Viadur* | **Implant**: 72 mg | No |

[1] Also available as microspheres for injection.

Triptorelin pamoate, a gonadotropin-releasing hormone analog available as an injection administered in a medical setting only, is not included in this monograph. For more information on chemotherapy treatment, see the introduction to this chapter.

## Type of Drug:

Synthetic hormones; luteinizing hormone-releasing hormone (LHRH) agonists; gonadotropin-releasing hormone (GnRH) agonist analogs.

## How the Drug Works:

Some diseases (eg, endometriosis) and cancers (eg, breast cancer, prostate cancer) are stimulated by sex hormones (estrogen in women, testosterone in men) produced by the body's sex organs (ovaries in women, testicles in men). Gonadotropin-releasing hormone analogs block the chemicals that stimulate the sex organs to produce sex hormones. As a result, the function of the sex organs are decreased and blood levels and actions of sex hormones are decreased. Lower blood levels of estrogens may improve symptoms of endometriosis and breast cancer in women. Lower levels of testosterone may improve symptoms of prostate cancer in men.

## Uses:

*Goserelin implant; leuprolide injection, implant:* To treat the symptoms of advanced prostate cancer when orchiectomy (castration) or estrogen administration is either not indicated or unacceptable to the patient.

*Goserelin 3.6 mg implant:* To manage endometriosis, including pain relief and lesion reduction.

To treat symptoms of advanced breast cancer in pre- and perimeno-pausal women.

To thin the endometrium prior to ablation procedures for dysfunc-tional uterine bleeding.

*Goserelin 10.8 mg implant:* Used in combination with flutamide to manage locally confined stage T2b-T4 (Stage B2-C) prostate cancer. Treatment should begin 8 weeks prior to initiating radiation therapy and should be continued during radiation therapy.

*Leuprolide pediatric injection:* For treatment of children with central preco-cious puberty (CPP).

## Precautions:

*Do not use in the following situations:*

allergy to the drug, any of its ingredients, or other gonado-tropin-releasing hormone ana-logs

breastfeeding
pregnancy
vaginal bleeding, abnormal women (10.8 mg implant only)

*Use with caution in the following situations:*

bone density-reducing drug (eg, anticonvulsants, corticoste-roids) therapy , current, chronic chronic alcohol abuse

osteoporosis, family history of risk of ureteral obstruction or spi-nal cord compression, males tobacco use

*Bone density:* Taking these drugs may result in decrease or loss of bone mineral density. Bone mineral loss may be greatest in patients with major risk factors such as chronic alcohol abuse, tobacco abuse, signifi-cant family history of osteoporosis, or chronic use of bone density reducing drugs (eg, anticonvulsants, corticosteroids). Benefits must be weighed carefully before therapy with goserelin is instituted.

*Contraception:* Effective non-hormonal contraception must be used by all women of childbearing potential while using goserelin and for 12 weeks following discontinuation of therapy.

*Diagnostic test interference:* These drugs will interfere with diagnostic tests of pituitary-gonadotropic and gonadal function.

*Pregnancy:* Do not use during pregnancy. The risk of use in a pregnant woman clearly outweighs any possible benefit. These drugs can cause fetal harm when administered to a pregnant woman. There is a risk for pregnancy termination (miscarriage) due to possible hormonal imbal-ances as a result of therapy.

*Breastfeeding:* It is not known if these drugs appear in breast milk. There is a potential for serious adverse reactions in nursing infants of moth-ers receiving these drugs. Consult your doctor before you begin breast-feeding.

*Children:* Safety and effectiveness have not been established for agents other than leuprolide pediatric injection.

*Lab tests* will be required to monitor therapy. Tests may include testosterone, estradiol, PSA, or prostatic acid phosphatase blood levels, pregnancy testing, and bone age testing.

## Drug Interactions:

Tell your doctor or pharmacist if you are taking or planning to take any over-the-counter or prescription medications or dietary supplements while taking this drug. Drug doses may need to be modified or a different drug prescribed.

## Side Effects:

Every drug is capable of producing side effects. Many patients experience side effects. The frequency and severity of side effects depend on many factors including dose, duration of therapy, and individual susceptibility. Possible side effects include:

*Digestive Tract:* Diarrhea; nausea; constipation; appetite changes; ulcer; vomiting; stomach pain.

*Nervous System:* Headache; migraine; emotional instability; depression; lethargy; dizziness; sleeplessness; nervousness; light-headedness.

*Circulatory System:* Chest pain; high blood pressure; fast or irregular heartbeat; congestive heart failure; vein irritation.

*Urinary and Reproductive Tract:* Sexual dysfunction; change in sex drive; decreased erections; ureteral or bladder obstruction; change in breast size; pelvic pain; breast pain; blood in urine; impotence; changes in urinary frequency; urinary tract infection; vaginal dryness, inflammation, bleeding, or discharge; painful or heavy menstruation; decreased testicular size; painful intercourse; testicular pain.

*Skin:* Hair loss; hives; itching; rash; sweating; acne; excessively oily skin; abnormal skin sensations; abnormal hair growth.

*Other:* Hot flashes; weakness; back, joint, bone, or muscle pain; flu-like syndrome; loss of bone mineral density; upper respiratory tract infection; injection or implant site reaction; voice alterations; leg cramps; swelling; sore throat; sinus infection; chronic obstructive lung disease; general pain; abnormal lab tests; difficulty breathing; weight changes; dehydration; gout; changes in blood sugar; infection; osteoporosis; tumor flare.

## Guidelines for Use:

- Notify your doctor if you experience irritation at the injection site or any other unusual signs or symptoms.
- During the first two months of therapy, a female may experience menses or spotting. If bleeding continues beyond the second month, notify your doctor.
- *Goserelin* — Implants will be implanted subcutaneously (SC; beneath the skin) into the upper abdominal wall by your health care provider in a medical setting every 28 days (3.6 mg dose) or every 12 weeks (10.8 mg dose).

  *3.6 mg* — Every effort should be made to adhere to the 28-day schedule. A missed dose may cause breakthrough bleeding and pregnancy (females).

  *10.8 mg* — Every effort should be made to adhere to the 12-week schedule.

  Menstruation should stop with therapy. If regular menstruation persists, notify your doctor.

  A nonhormonal method of contraception should be used by all premenopausal women during and for 12 weeks following treatment. If pregnancy occurs during treatment, discontinue use and be aware of the possible risks to the fetus.

  *Prostate cancer patients* — May cause increased bone pain and increased difficulty urinating during the first few weeks of treatment. May cause hot flashes, injection site irritation (eg, burning, itching, swelling), and may cause or aggravate nerve symptoms. Notify your doctor if these become pronounced.

  *CPP patients* — Prior to starting therapy, the parent or guardian must be aware of the importance of continuous therapy. Adherence to 4-week drug administration schedules must be accepted if therapy is to be successful.

- *Leuprolide* — Injection is administered subcutaneously (SC; beneath the skin) every day. Vary the injection site daily.

  A patient package insert is available with each leuprolide injection kit. Read carefully before the first dose and with each refill or injection/implantation.

  Carefully follow the instructions given to you for storage, preparation, administration, and disposal of used equipment.

  Do not stop taking or change the dose, unless instructed by your doctor.

  Store at room temperature (below 77°F). Do not freeze. Protect from light.

  Leuprolide powder for injection, microspheres for injection, and implants will be prepared and administered by your health care provider in a medical setting. The 7.5 mg powder for injection should be administered every month, the 22.5 mg powder for injection every 3 months, and the 72 mg implant every 12 months.

*If you have any questions, consult your doctor, pharmacist, or health care provider.*

| Generic Name<br>*Brand Name Examples* | Supplied As | Generic<br>Available |
|---|---|---|
| *Rx* **Carmustine** | | |
| *BiCNU* | **Powder for Injection:** 100 mg | No |
| *Gliadel* | **Wafer:** 7.7 mg | No |

For more information on chemotherapy treatment, see the introduction to this chapter.

## Type of Drug:

Anticancer agent; alkylating agent; nitrosourea.

## How the Drug Works:

Carmustine stops or slows the growth of cancerous cells by interfering with their reproduction.

## Uses:

*Injection:* To treat brain tumors, cancer of the bone marrow, Hodgkin disease and non-Hodgkin lymphoma (as a secondary therapy in combination with other drugs in failure of response to primary therapy).

*Wafer:* Used as an adjunct to surgery or used after surgery to prolong survival after removal of certain brain tumors.

## Precautions:

*Do not use in the following situations:* Allergy to carmustine or any of its ingredients.

*Use with caution in the following situations:*
bone marrow suppression (injection only)
complications of brain surgery (eg, seizures, abnormal wound healing) (wafer only)
lung disease (injection only)

*Long-term use* may cause secondary cancer.

*Pregnancy:* Studies have shown a potential effect to the fetus. Use only if clearly needed and potential benefits outweigh the possible risks.

*Breastfeeding:* It is not known if carmustine appears in breast milk. Either breastfeeding or drug therapy should be stopped, taking into account the importance of the drug to the mother. Consult your doctor before you begin breastfeeding.

*Children:* Safety and effectiveness in children have not been established.

*Lab tests* will be required frequently during treatment with carmustine. Be sure to keep appointments. Tests may include kidney, liver and lung function tests and blood counts.

## Drug Interactions:

Tell your doctor or pharmacist if you are taking or if you are planning to take any over-the-counter or prescription medications or dietary supplements with carmustine. Doses of one or both drugs may need to be modified or a different drug may need to be prescribed. The following drugs interact with injectable carmustine:

cimetidine (eg, *Tagamet*)          phenytoin (eg, *Dilantin*)
mitomycin (*Mutamycin*)

## Side Effects:

Every drug is capable of producing side effects. Many carmustine users experience no, or minor, side effects. The frequency and severity of side effects depend on many factors including dose, duration of therapy, and individual susceptibility. Possible side effects include:

*Injection -*

*Circulatory System:* Decreased blood platelets; abnormal blood counts; anemia.

*Skin:* Burning; excessive pigmentation; flushing; injection site burning.

*Other:* Nausea; vomiting; lowered ability to fight infection; liver toxicity; kidney abnormalities and damage; swelling of the retina and optic nerve (of the eye); watery eyes; lung toxicity.

*Wafer -*

*Digestive Tract:* Nausea; vomiting; diarrhea; constipation; bleeding.

*Nervous System:* Brain damage; brain or spinal cord swelling; brain infection; confusion; seizures; headache; one-sided paralysis; elevated brain pressure; drowsiness; acting unsensible; depression; abnormal thinking; clumsiness; dizziness; sleeplessness; coma; amnesia; paranoid reaction.

*Circulatory System:* Anemia; blood clots; high blood pressure; low blood pressure; decreased blood platelets; abnormal blood count; high blood sugar; low potassium count; salt depletion in blood.

*Respiratory System:* Pneumonia; lung clot; infection.

*Other:* Rash; fever; pain; abnormal healing; urinary tract infection; mouth infection; neck pain; accidental injury; back pain; allergic reaction; swelling of the arms and legs; weakness; chest pain; infection; eye pain; vision problems; double vision; difficulty in swallowing.

## Guidelines for Use:

- This medicine will be prepared and administered by your health care provider.
- Carmustine injection is administered every 6 weeks and should be monitored weekly for at least 6 weeks after a dose.
- Carmustine injection contains no preservatives.
- *Injection* — Nausea and vomiting may occur. Use of drugs for nausea before dosing may help reduce and sometimes prevent these side effects.
- *Infections* — This drug may lower your body's ability to fight infection. Notify your doctor of any signs of infection, including fever, sore throat, rashes or chills.
- Contraceptive measures should be used during therapy.
- Lab tests or exams will be required to monitor treatment. Be sure to keep appointments.
- Store dry powder for injection in refrigerator (36° to 46°F).
- Store wafers at or below −4°F.

*If you have any questions, consult your doctor, pharmacist, or health care provider.*

| Generic Name<br>*Brand Name Example* | Supplied As | Generic<br>Available |
|---|---|---|
| *Rx* **Lomustine (CCNU)** | | |
| *CeeNu* | **Capsules:** 10 mg, 40 mg, 100 mg | No |
| *CeeNu* | **Dose pack:** Two 10 mg capsules, two 40 mg capsules, two 100 mg capsules | No |

For more information on chemotherapy treatment, see the introduction of this chapter.

## Type of Drug:

Chemotherapy drug; anticancer drug; alkylating agent; CCNU; nitrosourea.

## How the Drug Works:

Lomustine stops the spread or growth of cancerous cells by interfering with their reproduction. This drug is often used with other anticancer drugs.

## Uses:

To treat brain tumors in patients who have had surgery and/or radiation treatment.

To treat Hodgkin disease when other drugs have failed.

## Precautions:

*Do not use in the following situations:* Allergy to lomustine or any of its ingredients.

*Breathing:* Lomustine can affect the lungs. Report any breathing difficulty to your doctor immediately.

*Long-term use* may cause secondary cancer.

*Pregnancy:* Studies have shown a potential adverse effect on the fetus. Use only if clearly needed and potential benefits outweigh the possible risks.

*Breastfeeding:* It is not known if lomustine appears in breast milk. Either breastfeeding or drug therapy should be stopped, taking into account the importance of the drug to the mother. Consult your doctor before you begin breastfeeding.

*Lab tests* will be required during treatment with lomustine. Blood counts should be monitored weekly for at least 6 weeks following a dose. Liver, kidney and lung function tests must be done periodically. Dosage adjustments may be necessary.

## Drug Interactions:

Tell your doctor or pharmacist if you are taking or planning to take any over-the-counter or prescription medications or dietary supplements while taking this medicine. Doses of one or both drugs may need to be modified or a different drug may need to be prescribed.

## Side Effects:

Most lomustine users experience side effects. The frequency and severity of side effects depend on many factors including dose, duration of therapy, and individual susceptibility. Possible side effects include:

*Digestive Tract:* Nausea; vomiting; appetite loss; sore throat.

*Nervous System:* Unusual tiredness; disorientation; clumsiness; slurred speech.

*Respiratory System:* Shortness of breath; dry cough; lung fibrosis.

*Skin:* Yellowing of the skin or eyes; unusual bleeding or bruising; hair loss.

*Other:* Fever; chills; sore throat; swelling of the lower legs or feet; sores on mouth or lips; kidney damage; abnormal liver and kidney function tests; abnormal blood counts; inflammation of the mouth; lowered ability to fight infection; anemia; visual disturbances; acute leukemia; bone marrow dysplasia.

## Guidelines for Use:

- Take on an empty stomach to reduce nausea. Nausea and vomiting may occur 3 to 6 hours after an oral dose and usually lasts less than 24 hours, although loss of appetite may last for several days. Use of drugs for nausea before dosing may help reduce and sometimes prevent these side effects.
- Lomustine is given as a single oral dose and will not be repeated for at least 6 weeks.
- *Infections* — These drugs may lower your body's ability to fight infection. Notify your doctor of any signs of infection, including fever, sore throat, rashes or chills.
- Notify your doctor if unusual bleeding or bruising, shortness of breath, dry cough, swelling of feet or lower legs, yellowing of eyes and skin, confusion, inflammation of the mouth or unusual tiredness occurs.
- May cause appetite loss, nausea and vomiting and, less frequently, hair loss. Notify your doctor if these reactions become pronounced.
- Avoid alcohol for short periods after taking a dose of lomustine.
- Contraceptive (birth control) measures are recommended during therapy.
- Patients should be aware that lomustine is an anticancer drug and belongs to the group of medicines known as alkylating agents.
- Patients should be aware that there may be 2 or more different types and colors of capsules in the container in order to provide the proper dose.
- Lab tests/exams will be required to monitor treatment. Be sure to keep appointments.
- Store at room temperature (68° to 77°F) in a tightly sealed container.

*If you have any questions, consult your doctor, pharmacist, or health care provider.*

| Generic Name<br>*Brand Name Example* | **Supplied As** | Generic<br>Available |
|---|---|---|
| *Rx* **Streptozocin** | | |
| *Zanosar* | **Powder for Injection:** 1 g | No |

For more information on chemotherapy treatment, see the introduction to this chapter.

## Type of Drug:

Anticancer agent.

## How the Drug Works:

Streptozocin stops or slows the spread of cancerous cells by disrupting the growth of DNA.

## Uses:

To treat cancer of the pancreas.

## Precautions:

*Do not use in the following situations:* Allergy to streptozocin or any of its ingredients.

*Use with caution in the following situations:*

| development of tumors at the | kidney disease |
| injection site | use with other kidney toxic drugs |

*Pregnancy:* Adequate studies have not been done in pregnant women. Use only if clearly needed and potential benefits outweigh the possible hazards to the fetus.

*Breastfeeding:* It is not known if streptozocin appears in breast milk. Consult your doctor before you begin breastfeeding.

*Lab tests* will be required frequently during treatment with streptozocin. Tests may include kidney and liver function tests, blood counts and urinalysis.

## Drug Interactions:

Tell your doctor or pharmacist if you are taking or planning to take any over-the-counter or prescription medications or dietary supplements with streptozocin. Doses of one or both drugs may need to be modified or a different drug may need to be prescribed. The use of other drugs toxic to the kidney should be used with caution or not at all with this drug.

## Side Effects:

Every drug is capable of producing side effects. Many streptozocin users experience no, or minor, side effects. The frequency and severity of side effects depend on many factors including the dose, duration of therapy, and individual susceptibility. Possible side effects include:

*Digestive Tract:* Nausea; vomiting; diarrhea; liver toxicity; elevated liver enzyme levels; low amounts of albumin in the blood.

*Circulatory System:* Blood toxicity; reduction in red and white blood cells; reduction in platelet count; abnormal glucose (sugar) tolerance.

*Other:* Kidney toxicity; excess urea in the blood; low amounts of phosphate in the blood; glucose in the urine.

### Guidelines for Use:

- This medicine will be prepared and administered by your healthcare provider.
- Streptozocin injection contains no preservatives.
- Use gloves during preparation and administration.
- If streptozocin powder or solution contacts the skin, wash with soap and water.
- Inform your doctor if you are pregnant, become pregnant, are planning to become pregnant or if you are breastfeeding.
- Lab tests or exams will be required to monitor treatment. Be sure to keep appointments.
- Store in refrigerator (35° to 46°F) and protect from light.

*If you have any questions, consult your doctor, pharmacist, or health care provider.*

| Generic Name Brand Name Example | Supplied As | Generic Available |
|---|---|---|
| **Estramustine Phosphate Sodium** | | |
| Rx  Emcyt | **Capsules:** Equivalent to 140 mg estramustine phosphate | No |

For more information on chemotherapy treatment, see the introduction to this chapter.

## Type of Drug:

Chemotherapy agents; anticancer drugs.

## How the Drug Works:

Estramustine increases estrogen levels in the body that prevent the formation of androgens that stimulate tumor cells of the prostate.

## Uses:

To treat the symptoms of prostate cancer.

## Precautions:

*Do not use in the following situations:*
>    allergy to estradiol or nitrogen mustard
>    blood clotting disorder, active

*Use with caution in the following situations:*
>    blood clotting disorders, history      epilepsy
>    calcium blood levels, increased      high blood pressure
>    cerebrovascular disease      kidney disease
>    congestive heart disease      liver disease
>    coronary artery disease      migraines
>    diabetes      stroke
>    edema (fluid retention)

*Estrogen use in men:* Estramustine should not be used in men with blood clots.

*Diabetes:* Estramustine may decrease glucose (sugar) tolerance. Test blood sugar often.

*High blood pressure:* Estramustine may increase blood pressure. Blood pressure should be checked frequently.

*Lab tests* may be required to monitor therapy. Be sure to keep appointments. Tests may include: Liver function tests, calcium blood levels, total bilirubin.

## Drug Interactions:

Tell your doctor or pharmacist if you are taking or planning to take any over-the-counter or prescription medications or dietary supplements while taking these medicines. Doses of one or both drugs may need to be modified or a different drug may need to be prescribed. The following drugs, drug classes and foods interact with this medicine:

calcium-containing antacids

milk, dairy products and calcium-rich foods

## Side Effects:

Every drug is capable of producing side effects. Many patients experience side effects. The frequency and severity of side effects depend on many factors including dose, duration of therapy, and individual susceptibility. Possible side effects include:

*Digestive Tract:* Nausea; vomiting; diarrhea; appetite loss; gas; burning throat; thirst; bleeding; stomach ache.

*Nervous System:* Headache; anxiety; sleeplessness; mood changes; drowsiness; depression.

*Circulatory System:* Chest pain; heart failure; stroke; heart attack; difficulty breathing; hoarseness; upper respiratory discharge; swelling.

*Skin:* Rash; itching; dry skin; peeling skin at fingertips; easy bruising; flushing; hair loss; thinning hair; skin color changes.

*Other:* Watery eyes; breast tenderness or enlargement; hot flashes; pain in eyes; ringing in the ears; abnormal blood counts; leg cramps; night sweats.

## Guidelines for Use:

- Contraceptive (birth control) measures are recommended during treatment. Contact your doctor if pregnancy is suspected.
- If a dose is missed, take it as soon as possible. If several hours have passed or it is nearing time for the next dose, do not double the dose to catch up, unless advised to do so by your doctor. If more than one dose is missed, contact your doctor or pharmacist.
- Take 3 to 4 times daily with water and at least 1 hour before or 2 hours after meals.
- Do not take milk, dairy products and calcium-rich foods or drugs (such as antacids) at the same time as estramustine.
- Prepare diabetic patients to monitor their blood sugar levels more frequently. Loss of glucose control may occur.
- Lab tests/exams are required to monitor treatment. Be sure to keep appointments.
- Store at 36° to 46°F.

*If you have any questions, consult your doctor, pharmacist, or health care provider.*

| Generic Name<br>*Brand Name Examples* | Supplied As | Generic<br>Available |
|---|---|---|
| *Rx* **Chlorambucil** | | |
| *Leukeran* | **Tablets:** 2 mg | No |
| *Rx* **Cyclophosphamide** | | |
| *Cytoxan* | **Tablets:** 25 mg, 50 mg | No |
| *Cytoxan* | **Powder for Injection:** 75 mg mannitol/100 mg cyclophospha-mide | No |
| *Rx* **Ifosfamide** | | |
| *Ifex* | **Powder for injection:** 1 g, 3 g | No |
| *Rx* **Mechlorethamine HCl** | | |
| *Mustargen* | **Powder for injection:** 10 mg | No |
| *Rx* **Melphalan**[1] | | |
| *Alkeran* | **Tablets:** 2 mg | No |

[1] Some of these products are available as an injection.

For more information on chemotherapy treatment, see the introduction to this chapter.

## Type of Drug:
Anticancer drugs.

## How the Drug Works:
Nitrogen mustard anticancer drugs interfere with the function of DNA, disrupting the reproduction of the cancer cells. They are often used in combination with other drugs.

## Uses:
*Chlorambucil:* To treat malignant lymphomas, a certain type of leukemia and Hodgkin disease.

*Cyclophosphamide:* To treat cancer of the breast and ovaries, lymphomas, certain leukemias, multiple myeloma and Hodgkin disease. Also used for advanced mycosis fungoides (cancer of skin and lymph nodes), neuroblastoma (malignant tumor of embryonic ganglion cells), adenocarcinoma (malignant tumor originating from glandular cells) and retinoblastoma (malignant tumor of the retina). To treat nephrotic syndrome in children when other treatment regimens have failed.

*Ifosfamide:* To treat testicular cancer in combination with other approved anticancer drugs.

*Mechlorethamine:* To treat Hodgkin's disease (Stages III and IV), lymphosarcoma, chronic myelocytic or chronic lymphocytic leukemia, polycythemia vera, mycosis fungoides, bronchogenic cancer and metastatic cancer causing effusions.

*Melphalan:* To treat cancer of the ovaries and multiple myeloma.

*Unlabeled Use(s):* Occasionally doctors may prescribe chlorambucil for uveitis, inflammation of the brain caused by Behcet disease, and for treating certain types of nephropathy and rheumatoid arthritis. Cyclophosphamide has been prescribed for rheumatoid conditions (eg, arthritis, systemic lupus erythematous), Wegener granulomatosis, other steroid-resistant vasculidites, multiple sclerosis, polyarteritis nodosa and polymyositis.

## Precautions:

*Do not use in the following situations:*

allergy to the drug or to other nitrogen mustard drugs
bone marrow depression, severe (cyclophosphamide and ifosfamide only)
infectious diseases (mechlorethamine only)
prior resistance to the drug

*Use with caution in the following situations:*

abnormal blood counts
abnormal uric acid levels (mechlorethamine)
adrenal surgery
anemia
anesthesia use
blood disorders (eg, decreased blood counts)
bone marrow depression
chemotherapy
decreased blood platelets
development of bleeding cysts, urinary (cyclophosphamide)
infection, recent
kidney disease
liver disease
pregnancy
radiation
tumor of the bone marrow
tumors of the bone and nervous tissues (mechlorethamine)
wounds

*Fertility impairment:* Nitrogen mustard agents may cause temporary or permanent infertility. These drugs can cause chromosome damage and can interfere with formation of sperm in males and eggs in females. They may also cause menstruation to stop.

*Infections:* These drugs may impair your body's ability to fight infection. Notify your doctor of any signs of infection including fever, sore throat, rashes or chills.

*Long-term use* may cause secondary cancer.

*Pregnancy:* Studies have shown a potential adverse effect to the fetus. Use only if clearly needed and potential benefits outweigh the possible risks. Women should avoid becoming pregnant and proper birth control should be used. Contact your doctor immediately if pregnancy is suspected.

*Breastfeeding:* Cyclophosphamide and ifosfamide appear in breast milk. It is not known if the other nitrogen mustards appear in breast milk. Use during breastfeeding is not recommended. Consult your doctor before you begin breastfeeding.

*Children:* Safety and effectiveness in children have not been established.

*Lab tests* will be required during treatment.

## Drug Interactions:

Tell your doctor or pharmacist if you are taking or planning to take any over-the-counter or prescription medications or dietary supplements with cyclophosphamide. Doses of one or both drugs may need to be modified or a different drug may need to be prescribed. The following drugs and drug classes interact with cyclophosphamide:

allopurinol (eg, *Zyloprim*)
anticoagulants (eg, warfarin)
chloramphenicol (eg, *Chloromy-cetin)*
corticosteroids (eg, *Prednisone)*
digoxin (eg, *Lanoxin)*
doxorubicin (eg, *Adriamycin)*

methotrexate (eg, *Folex)*
phenobarbital (eg, *Solfoton)*
quinolone antibiotics (eg, *Cipro)*
succinylcholine (eg, *Anectine)*
sulfonamides (eg, sulfisoxazole)
thiazide diuretics (eg, hydro-chlorothiazide)

## Side Effects:

Most nitrogen mustard users experience side effects. The frequency and severity of side effects depend on many factors including dose, duration of therapy, and individual susceptibility. Possible side effects include:

*Blood:* Bone marrow depression; decreased blood cell and platelet counts; anemias; abnormal red and white blood cell counts.

*Skin:* Unusual skin sensitivity; hair loss; discoloration (eg, yellowing of skin); rash.

*Digestive Tract:* Nausea; vomiting; diarrhea; mouth sores.

*Urinary and Reproductive Tract:* Prolonged or permanent infertility; cessation of menstruation; decreased sperm count; lesions.

*Other:* Allergic reaction; lung fibrosis; inflammation of the lungs.

*Other:*

*Chlorambucil* – Tremors; confusion; agitation; incoordination; seizures; inflammation of the corneas; inflammation of the bladder; fever; twitching; hallucinations; liver toxicity; pneumonia; leukemia; secondary cancer.

*Cyclophosphamide* – Stomach ache; appetite loss; colitis; new tumor growth; inflammation of the bladder; pigmentation of the skin; changes in nails.

*Ifosfamide* – Blood in the urine; infection; kidney impairment; liver dysfunction; pain at injection site.

*Mechlorethamine* – Blood clot; vein clot; allergic reaction; dizziness; ringing in the ears; diminished hearing; herpes zoster.

*Melphalan* – Allergy symptoms; inflamed blood vessels.

## Guidelines for Use:

- Notify your doctor of unusual bleeding or bruising, black tarry stools, nausea, vomiting, weight loss, fever, chills, sore throat, cough, shortness of breath, seizures, lack of menstrual flow, unusual lumps or masses, flank or stomach pain, joint pain, sores in the mouth or on the lips, yellow discoloration of the skin or eyes, skin rash or pain of unknown origin.
- Contraceptive (birth control) measures are recommended during therapy for both men and women.
- *Cyclophosphamide* — May cause darkening of skin and changes in fingernails. Contact your doctor if these become pronounced.
  Take tablets on an empty stomach. If stomach upset is severe, take with food. Oral solution may be made from injectable cyclophosphamide and Aromatic Elixir. Store in refrigerator and use within 14 days.
- *Mechlorethamine* — May cause potential risk to reproductive capacity.
- *Melphalan* — Take under close medical supervision.
  Response may be gradual over many months; repeated courses or continuous therapy are important. The maximum benefit may be missed if treatment is ended too soon.
  Long term use may produce secondary cancers and infertility.
  Protect tablets from light. Dispense in glass container.
- These medicines may cause drowsiness and/or dizziness. Use caution while driving or performing other tasks requiring mental alertness, coordination or physical dexterity.
- Inform your doctor if you are pregnant, become pregnant, are planning to become pregnant or if you are breastfeeding.
- *Infections*—These drugs may lower your body's ability to fight infection. Notify your doctor of any signs of infection, including fever, sore throat, rashes or chills.
- Lab tests will be required during treatment with these medications. Be sure to keep appointments.
- Store at controlled room temperature (59° to 77°F).

*If you have any questions, consult your doctor, pharmacist, or health care provider.*

| Generic Name<br>*Brand Name Examples* | Supplied As | Generic<br>Available |
|---|---|---|
| *Rx* **Interferon Alfa-2a** | | |
| *Roferon-A* | **Solution for Injection:** 3 million IU/vial, 9 million IU/vial, 18 million IU/vial, 36 million IU/vial | No |
| *Roferon-A* | **Powder for Injection:** 18 million IU/vial (3 million IU/0.5 mL when reconstituted) | No |
| *Rx* **Interferon Alfa-2b** | | |
| *Intron A* | **Solution for Injection:** 3 million IU/vial, 5 million IU/vial, 10 million IU/vial, 18 million IU/vial, 25 million IU/vial | No |
| *Intron A* | **Powder for Injection:** 3 million IU/vial, 5 million IU/vial, 10 million IU/vial, 18 million IU/vial, 25 million IU/vial, 50 miliion IU/vial | No |

## Type of Drug:

Chemotherapy agents; anticancer drugs.

## How the Drug Works:

This group of cancer drugs prevents cancer cell growth by unknown mechanisms or by directly destroying cancer cells. These agents are often used with other cancer drugs.

## Uses:

*Interferon Alfa-2a:* To treat hairy-cell leukemia and AIDS-related Kaposi sarcoma in selected patients.

*Interferon Alfa-2b:* To treat hairy-cell leukemia, condylomata acuminata (venereal warts) and AIDS-related Kaposi sarcoma in selected patients, skin cancer and chronic hepatitis C.

*Unlabeled Use(s):* Occasionally doctors may prescribe alpha interferons for a wide range of cancer types and viral infections.

## Precautions:

*Do not use in the following situations:*
allergy to the drug or any of its components
allergy to human interferon alpha
allergy to mouse immunoglobulin (IgG) (interferon alfa-2a only)
bone marrow depression (decreased blood cell counts and platelets)

*Use with caution in the following situations:*

AIDS-related Kaposi sarcoma, rapidly progressive or life-threatening
blood clotting disorders
bone marrow disorders
diabetes mellitus
heart disease or conditions, history of
kidney disease
liver disease
lung disease (eg, chronic obstructive pulmonary disease)
neurologic disorders
psoriasis (eg, skin dryness, flaking)
psychiatric disorders (eg, depression)
seizure disorders (epilepsy)
thyroid disease

*Sensitivity to sunlight:* Interferon Alfa-n3 may cause sensitivity to light. Avoid prolonged exposure to the sun. Use sunscreens and wear protective clothing until tolerance is determined.

*Infections:* These drugs may lower your body's ability to fight infection. Notify your doctor immediately of any signs of infection (fever, sore throat, rash or chills).

*Pregnancy:* Adequate studies have not been done in pregnant women, or animal studies may have shown a risk to the fetus. Use only if clearly needed and potential benefits outweigh the possible hazards to the fetus.

*Breastfeeding:* It is not known if these drugs appear in breast milk. Use is not recommended. A decision should be made whether to discontinue nursing or the drug, taking into account the importance of the drug to the mother. Consult your doctor.

*Children:* Safety and effectiveness in persons under 18 years of age have not been established.

*Lab tests* will be required to monitor treatment. Tests may include: Complete blood counts and platelet counts, liver function tests, bone marrow aspirations and electrocardiograms (EKG).

## Drug Interactions:

Tell your doctor or pharmacist if you are taking or planning to take any over-the-counter or prescription medications or dietary supplements while taking this medicine. Doses of one or both drugs may need to be modified or a different drug may need to be prescribed.The following drugs and drug classes interact with this medicine:

myelosupressives (eg, zidovudine)
theophylline (eg, *Theo-Dur)*

## Side Effects:

Every drug is capable of producing side effects. Most patients experience side effects. The frequency and severity of side effects depend on many factors including dose, duration of therapy, and individual susceptibility. Possible side effects include:

*Interferon Alfa-n3 only:* Impaired concentration; sensitivity to sunlight; increased salivation; hot feet; heat intolerance.

*Interferon Alfa-2b only:* Decreased sex drive; menstrual changes; leg cramps.

*Flu-like Symptoms (common):* Fever; drowsiness; chills; tiredness; sore throat; joint and muscle aches/pain; headache.

*Digestive Tract:* Appetite loss; diarrhea; constipation; stomach pain; indigestion; nausea; vomiting; gas; heartburn; inflammation of or dry/swollen mouth; taste changes; tongue sensitivity; thirst.

*Nervous System:* Dizziness; confusion; forgetfulness; incoordination; nervousness; drowsiness; sleep problems; anxiety; fatigue; mood disorders; emotional instability; depression; abnormal thinking; abnormal skin sensations; general body discomfort; rigidity; vertigo (feeling of whirling motion); numbness or tingling of hands or feet.

*Circulatory System:* Chest pain; abnormal heart rhythm; changes in blood pressure; abnormal blood counts; palpitations (pounding in the chest).

*Respiratory System:* Painful or difficult breathing; pneumonia; coughing; sinusitis; runny nose; chest congestion; nasal congestion; sore throat.

*Skin:* Hair loss; itching; rash; hives; flushing; dry skin; sweating; pain at injection site; yellowing of skin or eyes.

*Other:* Allergic reaction; swelling of hands or feet; back pain; night sweats; weight loss; inflammation of mucous membranes; hot flashes; cold sores; nosebleed; abnormal lab tests; lymph node swelling; abnormal vision; ear and eye pain; painful or difficult urination; temporary impotence.

## Guidelines for Use:

- Therapy should begin in the hospital where you can be closely observed.
- Use exactly as prescribed.
- Read patient information sheet carefully. Follow the administration and preparation instructions (of injections) as outlined by your doctor.
- Drink plenty of fluids, especially during the initial stages of treatment.
- Do not change brands of interferon. Changes in dosage may be necessary when changing from one brand to another.
- If a dose is missed, inject it as soon as possible. If several hours have passed or it is nearing time for the next dose, do not double the dose to catch up, unless advised to do so by your doctor. If more than one dose is missed or it is necessary to establish a new dosage schedule, contact your doctor or pharmacist.
- The most common side effects are "flu-like" symptoms, such as fever, chills, drowsiness, fatigue, headache, sore throat, appetite loss, nausea, vomiting, muscle aches and joint pain. These appear to lessen over time. Some symptoms may be minimized by bedtime doses. Use acetaminophen (eg, *Tylenol*) to prevent or lessen fever and headache. Notify your doctor if these symptoms become pronounced during therapy.
- May cause drowsiness or dizziness. Use caution while driving or performing other tasks requiring alertness, coordination or physical dexterity.
- Notify your doctor if hives, itching, tightness in the chest, cough, difficulty breathing, visual problems, wheezing, low blood pressure or light-headedness occurs.
- Contraceptive measures (birth control) are recommended during therapy with these drugs. Notify your doctor immediately if you suspect pregnancy.
- *Infections* — These drugs may lower your body's ability to fight infection. Notify your doctor immediately of any signs of infection (fever, sore throat, rash or chills).
- Avoid prolonged exposure to sunlight. Photosensitivity (sensitivity to sunlight) may occur. Wear protective clothing and use sunscreens until tolerance is determined (interferon alfa-n3 only).
- Lab tests will be required to monitor treatment. Be sure to keep appointments.
- Store in the refrigerator (36° to 46°F). Do not freeze or shake.

*If you have any questions, consult your doctor, pharmacist, or health care provider.*

| Generic Name<br>*Brand Name Example* | Supplied As | Generic<br>Available |
|---|---|---|
| Rx **Tretinoin** | | |
| *Vesanoid* | **Capsules:** 10 mg | No |

## Type of Drug:

Antineoplastic; anticancer drug; chemotherapy agent.

## How the Drug Works:

The exact mechanism of action is not known, but it appears that tretinoin decreases the growth (reproduction) of leukemia cells (acute promyelocytic leukemia cells) and promotes the growth of normal cells.

## Uses:

To induce remission of acute promyelocytic leukemia (APL). Further therapy with other medications usually will be necessary.

## Precautions:

*Do not use in the following situations:* Allergy to retinoids, its components or parabens.

*Use with caution in the following situations:*
high cholesterol or triglycerides
leukocytosis (high white blood cell count)
pregnancy

*Retinoic acid-APL syndrome:* A potentially serious drug reaction has occurred in patients given tretinoin to treat APL. Symptoms include: Fever, difficulty breathing or weight gain. Report these symptoms to your doctor immediately.

*Pseudotumor cerebri (pressure in brain/head):* High doses of tretinoin could produce symptoms such as: Headaches, nausea, vomiting or visual problems. Report these symptoms to your doctor immediately.

*Pregnancy:* Studies have shown a potential adverse effect on the fetus. Use only if clearly needed and potential benefits outweigh the possible risks.

*Breastfeeding:* It is not known if tretinoin appears in breast milk. Consult your doctor before you begin breastfeeding.

*Children:* Safety and effectiveness in children under 1 year of age have not been established.

*Lab tests* will be required to monitor therapy. Tests may include complete blood counts, coagulation profiles, liver function tests, triglyceride levels and cholesterol levels.

## Drug Interactions:

Tell your doctor or pharmacist if you are taking or planning to take any over-the-counter or prescription medications or dietary supplements while taking this medicine. Doses of one or both drugs may need to be modified or a different drug may need to be prescribed. The following drugs and drug classes interact with this medicine:

> cytochrome P-450 inducers or inhibitors (eg, phenobarbital, cimetidine)
> ketoconazole (eg, *Nizoral*)

## Side Effects:

Every drug is capable of producing side effects. Most patients experience side effects. The frequency and severity of side effects depend on many factors including dose, duration of therapy and individual susceptibility. Possible side effects include:

*Typical Retinoid Toxicity:* Headache; fever; skin/mucous membrane dryness; bone pain/inflammation; nausea; vomiting; rash; irritation of mucous membranes (eg, eye, nose); itching; increased sweating; abnormal vision/eye disorders; hair loss; skin changes; fatigue; weakness.

*Digestive Tract:* Appetite loss; bleeding; stomach pain/bloating; diarrhea; constipation; indigestion; enlargement of liver and spleen; ulcers; liver disorders.

*Nervous System:* Dizziness; abnormal skin sensations; anxiety; sleep changes; depression; confusion; agitation; hallucinations; difficulty walking (unsteady); tremors; convulsions; slow/slurred speech; facial paralysis; paralysis of one side of the body; weak reflexes; visual sensitivity to light; leg weakness; forgetfulness; drowsiness; unconsciousness.

*Circulatory System:* Abnormal heart rate; flushing; changes in blood pressure; vein inflammation/redness; blood clotting disorders; pressure in head; heart attack/failure; stroke.

*Respiratory System:* Breathing difficulties; pneumonia; bronchial asthma; swelling of the lungs/larynx; lung disease.

*Other:* Earache or feeling of fullness in the ears; hearing loss/disorders; general body discomfort; shivering; bleeding; infections; swelling of arms and legs; pain; chest discomfort; swelling; weight changes; muscle pain; facial swelling; pale skin; low body temperature; difficult or frequent urination; enlarged prostate; abnormal lab tests.

## Guidelines for Use:

- Use exactly as prescribed.
- Take each dose with fluids (6 to 8 oz) at evenly spaced intervals through-out the day, preferably every 12 hours.
- May be taken with food. Drug absorption is enhanced when taken with food.
- If a dose is missed, take it as soon as possible. If several hours have passed or it is nearing time for the next dose, do not double the dose to catch up, unless advised to do so by your doctor. If more than one dose is missed or it is necessary to establish a new dosage sched-ule, contact your doctor or pharmacist.
- Notify your doctor immediately if you experience fever, difficulty breath-ing or weight gain. These can be signs of a serious medical condition.
- Notify your doctor if you experience eye pain, headache, nausea, vom-iting, dizziness or abnormal vision. This especially applies to children.
- Notify your doctor if you are pregnant, become pregnant, are planning to become pregnant or if you are breastfeeding.
- Contraceptive measures (birth control) are recommended during therapy with this medicine and for 1 month after therapy.
- May cause sensitivity to bright light. Protect eyes and wear sunglasses.
- Lab tests will be required to monitor therapy. Be sure to keep appointments.
- Store at room temperature (59° to 86°F) in a tightly sealed container.

*If you have any questions, consult your doctor, pharmacist, or health care provider.*

| Generic Name<br>*Brand Name Examples* | Supplied As | Generic<br>Available |
|---|---|---|
| *Rx* **Altretamine** | | |
| *Hexalen* | **Capsules:** 50 mg | No |
| *Rx* **Hydroxyurea** | | |
| *Hydrea* | **Capsules:** 500 mg | No |
| *Rx* **Mitotane** | | |
| *Lysodren* | **Tablets:** 500 mg | No |
| *Rx* **Paclitaxel** | | |
| *Taxol* | **Injection:** 30 mg/5 mL single-dose vial | No |
| *Rx* **Pentostatin** | | |
| *Nipent* | **Powder for injection:** 10 mg/vial | No |
| *Rx* **Procarbazine** | | |
| *Matulane* | **Capsules:** 50 mg | No |

## Type of Drug:

Chemotherapy agents; anticancer drugs.

## How the Drug Works:

This miscellaneous group of cancer drugs prevents cancer cell growth by stopping the adrenal gland from working or directly destroying cancer cells. These agents are often used with other cancer drugs.

## Uses:

*Altretamine:* To treat ovarian cancer.

*Hydroxyurea:* To treat certain types of skin cancer (melanoma, primary squamous cell carcinoma), resistant chronic myelocytic leukemia and inoperable cancer of the ovary.

*Mitotane:* To treat inoperable cancer of the adrenal gland.

*Paclitaxel:* To treat ovarian cancer after failure of first-line or subsequent chemotherapy and to treat breast cancer after failure of combination chemotherapy or relapse within 6 months of adjuvant chemotherapy.

*Pentostatin:* To treat hairy cell leukemia.

*Procarbazine:* To treat Stage III and IV Hodgkin disease in combination with other anti-cancer drugs.

*Unlabeled Use(s):* Occasionally doctors may prescribe paclitaxel for a wide range of cancer types.

## Precautions:

*Do not use in the following situations:*

allergy to the drug or any of its components
allergy to polyoxyethylated castor oil (paclitaxel only)
bone marrow depression (decreased blood cell counts and
platelets)
CNS toxicity, severe (altretamine only)
severe neutropenia/low white blood cell count (paclitaxel only)

*Use with caution in the following situations:*

*altretamine — pregnancy*

*hydroxyurea —*

anemia, severe
bone marrow depressant
agents, use

kidney disease
pregnancy
radiation, recent

*mitotane —*
liver disease
long-term use

shock
trauma, severe

*paclitaxel —*
heart disease
liver disease
low blood pressure

peripheral neuropathy (burning
or numbness in hands or feet)
pregnancy

*pentostatin —*
infections
nervous system, kidney, liver or
lung toxicity

pregnancy
rash, severe

*procarbazine —*
bone marrow depressant
agents, use
kidney disease

liver disease
pregnancy
radiation, recent

*Infections:* These drugs may lower your body's ability to fight infection. Notify your doctor immediately of any signs of infection (eg, fever, sore throat, rash, chills).

*Mitotane long-term use:* Continuous use of high doses may lead to brain or nervous system damage.

*Paclitaxel allergy:* All patients should be premedicated with corticosteroids, diphenhydramine and $H_2$ antagonists to avoid the occurrence of severe hypersensitivity reactions. Severe reactions such as low blood pressure, labored breathing requiring bronchodilators, edema (swelling) or severe hives require immediate discontinuation of the drug and aggressive symptomatic therapy.

*Pregnancy:* There are no adequate studies and well-controlled studies of mittane in pregnant women. Studies have shown all others agents have a potential adverse effect on the fetus. Use only if clearly needed and the potential benefits to the mother outweigh the possible hazards to the fetus.

*Breastfeeding:* It is not known if these drugs appear in breast milk. Use is not recommended. A decision should be made whether to discontinue nursing or the drug, taking into account the importance of the drug to the mother. Consult your doctor.

*Children:* Safety and effectiveness in children have not been established.

*Elderly:* Elderly patients may be more sensitive to the effects of hydroxyurea and may require a lower dose.

*Lab tests* will be required to monitor treatment. Be sure to keep appointments. Tests may include: Complete blood and platelet counts, liver and kidney function tests, or bone marrow aspirations. Neurologic exams should be performed regularly with altretamine use.

## Drug Interactions:
Tell your doctor or pharmacist if you are taking or planning to take any over-the-counter or prescription medications or dietary supplements while taking one of these preparations Doses of one or both drugs may need to be modified or a different drug may need to be prescribed.The following drugs and drug classes interact with these preparations:

*altretamine* —

antidepressants, MAO inhibitor class (eg, phenelzine)
cisplatin (eg, *Platinol)*

histamine $H_2$ antagonists (eg, cimetidine)
pyridoxine (eg, *Nestrex)*

*mitotane* —

cytochrome P-450 inducers or inhibitors (eg, phenobarbital, cimetidine)

warfarin (eg, *Coumadin)*
spironolactone (eg, *Aldactone)*

*paclitaxel* —

cisplatin (eg, *Platinol)*

ketoconazole *(Nizoral)*

*pentostatin* —

fludarabine *(Fludara)*

vidarabine *(Vira-A)*

*procarbazine* —

antihistamines (eg, diphenhydramine)
barbiturates (eg, phenobarbital)
digoxin (eg, *Lanoxin)*
ethyl alcohol
foods containing tyramine
hypotensive agents
levodopa (eg, *Larodopa)*

narcotics (eg, codeine)
phenothiazines (eg, chlorpromazine)
sympathomimetics (eg, pseudoephedrine)
tricyclic antidepressants (eg, amitriptyline)

## Side Effects:
Every drug is capable of producing side effects. Most patients experience side effects. The frequency and severity of side effects depend on many factors including dose, duration of therapy, and individual susceptibility. Possible side effects include:

*Flu-like Symptoms (common):* Fever; chills; joint and muscle aches/pain; headache.

*Digestive Tract:* Appetite loss; diarrhea; constipation; stomach pain; indigestion; nausea; vomiting; gas; inflammation of mouth.

*Nervous System:* Dizziness; confusion; incoordination; mood disorders; disorders of consciousness; nervousness; drowsiness; anxiety; fatigue; weakness; abnormal skin sensations; sleepiness; depression; vertigo (feeling of whirling motion); numbness or tingling of hands or feet; seizures (altretamine only); CNS toxicity (pentostatin only).

*Circulatory System:* Chest pain; rapid heart rate; abnormal heart rhythm; changes in blood pressure; abnormal blood counts; anemia; bleeding; blood clots; slowed heart rate (paclitaxel only).

*Respiratory System:* Difficult breathing, upper respiratory infection; pneumonia; coughing; bronchitis; sinusitis; runny nose; sore throat; asthma (pentostatin only).

*Skin:* Hair loss; itching; redness; rash; hives; flushing; dry skin; skin disorders; sweating; skin discoloration or swelling at injection site (paciitaxel only); boils (pentostatin only).

*Other:* Allergic reaction; swelling of hands or feet; inflammation of mucous membranes; bone marrow suppression; pain; infections; abnormal lab tests; painful or difficult urination; blood in urine; bone pain; blood poisoning; fainting; facial swelling; blurred or double vision; discoloration of nails (paclitaxel oniy); herpes zosterlshingles (pentostatin only); urinary tract infection (pentostatin oniy); eye irritation (pentostatin only); dental abnormalities (pentostatin only); swollen gums (pentostatin only); over-development of mammary glands in prepubertal and early pubertal boys (procarbazine only).

---

## Guidelines for Use:

- Use exactly as prescribed.
- If a dose is missed, take or inject it as soon as possible. If several hours have passed or it is nearing time for the next dose, do not double the dose to catch up, unless advised to do so by your doctor. If more than one dose is missed or it is necessary to establish a new dosage schedule, contact your doctor or pharmacist.
- Flu-like symptoms (fever, drowsiness, chills, tiredness, sore throat, muscle aches, headache, joint pain) are common with these drugs. Notify your doctor if these become pronounced during therapy.
- Contraceptive measures (birth control) are recommended during therapy with these drugs. Notify your doctor immediately if you suspect pregnancy.
- May cause drowsiness or dizziness. Use caution whiie driving or performing other tasks requiring alertness, coordination or physical dexterity.
- *Infections* — These drugs may lower your body's ability to fight infection. Notify your doctor immediately of any signs of infection (fever, sore throat, rash or chills).

## Guidelines for Use (cont.):

- *Altretamine —*
  Avoid taking altretamine at the same time as antidepressants such as phenelzine and tranylcypromine (MAO inhibitors), as this may result in severe orthostatic hypotension (dizziness, lightheadedness or fainting when rising quickly from a sitting or lying position).
  May cause nausea, vomiting, incoordination, dizziness, vertigo (feeling of whirling motion) or fatigue. Notify your doctor if these become pronounced.
  Store at room temperature (59° to 86°F).

- *Hydroxyurea —*
  Notify your doctor if fever, chills, sore throat, nausea, vomiting, appetite loss, diarrhea, sores in the mouth and on the lips, unusual bleeding or bruising occurs.
  Contents of the capsule may be emptied into a glass of water and taken immediately. Some material from the capsule contents may not dissolve and may float on the surface of the water. This is a potent medication and should be handled with care. Do not allow powder to come in contact with the skin, eyes or mucous membranes.
  May cause drowsiness, constipation, redness of the face, rash, itching, nausea, vomiting, appetite loss, pain or inflammation at irradiation site or hair loss.
  Notify your doctor if these become pronounced.
  Drink plenty of fluids.

- *Hydroxyurea (cont.) —*
  Store at room temperature (59° to 86°F) in a tightly-closed container. Avoid excessive heat.

- *Mitotane —*
  Notify your doctor if you experience difficulty breathing, dizziness, lightheadedness, swelling, nausea, vomiting, appetite loss, diarrhea, depression, rash, darkening of the skin, or hives.
  May cause muscle aches, fever, flushing, or muscle twitching. Notify your doctor if these become pronounced.
  Store at room temperature (59° to 86°F).

- *Paclitaxel —*
  Read patient information sheet carefully. Follow the injection administration and preparation instructions as outlined by your doctor.
  Before treatment with paclitaxel, you must be pretreated with medication to prevent serious allergic reactions.
  Notify your doctor if you experience difficulty breathing, dizziness, lightheadedness, swelling (edema), or severe hives.
  Store in the refrigerator (36° to 46°F). Freezing does not harm the drug. Keep in original package to protect from light. Reconstituted solution will keep for 27 hours at room temperature (77°F).

- *Pentostatin —*
  Read patient information sheet carefully. Follow the injection administration and preparation instructions as outlined by your doctor.
  Notify your doctor if you experience severe rash or signs of nervous system toxicity (eg, drowsiness, weakness).
  Store vials in the refrigerator (36° to 46°F). Reconstituted solution will only keep for 8 hours since it does not contain any preservatives.

## Guidelines for Use (cont.):

• *Procarbazine* —
Avoid the following during treatment: tyramine-containing foods, alcohol, antihistamines, and sympathomimetics (eg, stimulant drugs or decongestants).

Notify your doctor if you experience cough, shortness of breath, thickened bronchial secretions, fever, chills, sore throat, unusual bleeding or bruising, vomiting of blood, or black tarry stools.

May cause muscle or joint pain, nausea, vomiting, sweating, tiredness, weakness, constipation, headache, difficulty swallowing, appetite loss, hair loss, or depression. Notify your doctor if these become pronounced. Store below 104°F, preferably between 59° to 86°F. Protect from light and moisture.

*If you have any questions, consult your doctor, pharmacist, or health care provider.*

| Generic Name<br>*Brand Name Example* | Supplied As | Generic<br>Available |
|---|---|---|
| *Rx* **Asparaginase** | | |
| *Elspar* | **Powder for injection**:<br>10,000 IU | No |
| *Rx* **Pegaspargase** | | |
| *Oncaspar* | **Injection**: 750 IU/mL | No |

## Type of Drug:

Chemotherapy agents; anticancer drugs.

## How the Drug Works:

Leukemic cells need asparagine to survive. These enzymes rapidly reduce the amount of asparaginase in the body. Without asparaginase, the leukemic cells die. Normal cells can make their own asparaginase and are less affected by these enzymes than leukemic cells.

## Uses:

To induce remissions of acute lymphoblastic leukemia (ALL), usually used in combination with other anticancer drugs.

## Precautions:

*Do not use in the following situations:*
    allergy to the drug or any of its ingredients
    bleeding problems after previously taking this medicine
    pancreatitis, current or history of

*Use with caution in the following situations:*
    hepatotoxic drugs (eg, chemotherapy)
    liver disease

*Bleeding:* Patients taking enzymes are at higher than usual risk for bleeding problems, especially if used with other drugs that may cause bleeding (eg, aspirin, NSAIDs, anticoagulants).

*Infections:* Enzymes may lower your body's ability to fight infection. Notify your doctor immediately of any signs of infections (eg, fever, sore throat, rash, chills).

*Pregnancy:* There are no adequate and well-controlled studies in pregnant women. Use only if clearly needed and potential benefits outweigh the possible hazards to the fetus.

*Breastfeeding:* It is not known if enzymes appear in breast milk; use is not recommended. A decision should be made whether to discontinue nursing or the drug, taking into account the importance of the drug to the mother. Consult your doctor before you being breastfeeding.

*Children:* Asparaginase toxicity is reported to be greater in children.

*Lab tests* will be required to monitor treatment. Tests may include complete blood counts (CBC) and platelet counts, blood sugar, bone marrow aspirations, skin tests, and liver function tests.

## Drug Interactions:

Tell your doctor or pharmacist if you are taking or planning to take any over-the-counter or prescription medications or dietary supplements while taking these drugs. Doses of one or both drugs may need to be modified or a different drug may need to be prescribed. The following drugs and drug classes interact with these drugs:

anticoagulants (eg, warfarin)
aspirin
dipyridamole (eg, *Persantine*)

methotrexate (eg, *Rheumatrex)*
NSAIDs (eg, ibuprofen)

## Side Effects:

Every drug is capable of producing side effects. Most patients experience side effects. The frequency and severity of side effects depend on many factors including dose, duration of therapy, and individual susceptibility. Possible side effects include:

*Digestive Tract:* Nausea; vomiting; diarrhea; stomach cramps; constipation; gas; indigestion; lip numbness or swelling; stomach pain; mouth or lip sores; appetite changes; difficulty swallowing; mouth tenderness; pancreatitis.

*Nervous System:* Headache; abnormal skin sensations; convulsions; depression; drowsiness; confusion; agitation or hallucinations (mild to severe); irritability; emotional instability; mood changes; disorientation; Parkinson-like symptoms.

*Circulatory System:* Changes in blood pressure; rapid heartbeat; chest pain; stroke; blood clots.

*Skin:* Rash; redness; swelling, hardness or pain at injection site; hives; itching; fever blister; hand whiteness; nail whiteness or ridging.

*Other:* Swelling or pain in the hands or feet; cough; difficulty breathing; jaundice (yellowing of skin or eyes); changes in blood sugar levels; unusual bleeding or bruising; night sweats; muscle or joint pain or stiffness; chills; fever; general body discomfort; anemia; abnormal blood or lab values; weight loss; fatigue; kidney dysfunction; increased thirst; coma; increased urination.

## Guidelines for Use:

- This medicine will be prepared and administered by your health care provider in a medical setting.
- Dosage is individualized.
- Contact your doctor immediately if you experience rash, redness, swelling, pain, hives, or difficulty breathing.
- May lower your body's ability to fight infection. Notify your doctor of any signs of infection, including fever, sore throat, rashes, or chills.
- Enzymes raise the risks of bleeding problems. Avoid the use of aspirin or nonsteroidal anti-inflammatory agents (NSAIDs) while taking this medicine.
- May affect the ability of the liver to function normally in some patients. Therapy with this medicine may increase the toxicity of other medications. Contact your doctor if there is any yellowing of the skin or eyes.
- *Diabetes* — Diabetic patients may experience loss of glucose control. Be prepared to monitor blood sugar more often.
- Lab tests will be required to monitor treatment. Be sure to keep appointments.

*If you have any questions, consult your doctor, pharmacist, or health care provider.*

| Generic Name<br>*Brand Name Example* | Supplied As | Generic<br>Available |
|---|---|---|
| *Rx* **Porfimer Sodium** | | |
| *Photofrin* | **Cake or powder for injection:** 75 mg/vial | No |

## Type of Drug:

Chemotherapy agent; anticancer drug.

## How the Drug Works:

Porfimer is a photosensitizing agent (drug activated by light) used in laser therapy or photodynamic therapy (PDT) of tumors.

## Uses:

To treat esophageal (food pipe) cancers in adults.

## Precautions:

*Do not use in the following situations:*

allergy to the drug or related medications
bronchoesophageal or tracheoesophageal fistula
porphyria or allergy to porphyrins
tumors eroding into a major blood vessel

*Use with caution in the following situations:* Esophageal varices.

*Chest Pain:* Some patients may experience chest pain because of inflammation of the area being treated. This pain may be strong enough to warrant treatment. Contact your doctor if severe chest pain occurs.

*Light Sensitivity:* Will cause sensitivity to the sun, bright indoor lights, or car headlights. For 30 days, avoid exposure of skin and eyes to direct sunlight or bright indoor light (eg, examination lights, including dental lamps, operating room lamps, unshaded light bulbs at close proximity). Wear dark sunglasses and cover exposed skin when outside.

*Pregnancy:* There are no adequate and well-controlled studies in pregnant women. Use only if clearly needed and potential benefits outweigh the possible hazards to the fetus. Women of childbearing potential should practice an effective method of contraception during therapy with this drug.

*Breastfeeding:* It is not known if porfimer appears in breast milk. Mothers taking porfimer should not breastfeed. Consult your doctor.

*Children:* Safety and effectiveness have not been established.

*Lab tests* may be required to monitor therapy.

## Drug Interactions:

Tell your doctor or pharmacist if you are taking or planning to take any over-the-counter or prescription medications or dietary supplements while taking this drug. Doses of one or both drugs may need to be modified or a different drug may need to be prescribed. The following drugs and drug classes interact with this drug:

alcohol
allopurinol (eg, *Zyloprim)*
beta-carotene (eg, *Max-Caro)*
calcium channel blockers
 (eg, nifedipine)
dimethyl sulfoxide *(Rimso-50)*
glucocorticoid hormones
 (eg, hydrocortisone)
mannitol (eg, *Osmitrol)*

photosensitizing agents
 (eg, fluoroquinolones, griseofulvin, hypoglycemic agents, phenothiazines, sulfonamides, tetracyclines, thiazide diuretics)
prostaglandin synthesis inhibitors (eg, NSAIDs)
thromboxane $A_2$ inhibitors
 (eg, aspirin)

## Side Effects:

Every drug is capable of producing side effects. Most patients experience side effects. The frequency and severity of side effects depend on many factors including dose, duration of therapy, and individual susceptibility. Possible side effects include:

*Skin:* Sensitivity to light; redness; swelling; itching; burning; discoloration; blisters.

*Digestive Tract:* Nausea; vomiting; constipation; diarrhea; indigestion; belching; appetite loss; weight loss; dark, bloody stools; vomiting of blood; stomach pain; difficulty swallowing; mouth sores; swelling of the esophagus.

*Other:* Dehydration; fever; cough; sore throat; general or back pain; difficulty breathing; pneumonia; unusual bleeding or bruising; difficult or painful urination; anemia; swelling of the hands or feet; swelling; weakness; tiredness; anxiety; confusion; sleeplessness; chest pain; rapid or unusual heartbeat; changes in blood pressure; heart failure; weight gain.

## Guidelines for Use:

- This medicine will be prepared and administered by your health care provider in a medical setting.
- Contact your doctor if you experience severe chest pain, difficulty breathing, or abnormal blood loss.
- *Light sensitivity* — Will cause sensitivity to the sun, bright lights or car headlights. For 30 days, avoid exposure of skin and eyes to direct sunlight from skylights or undraped windows or bright indoor light (eg, examination lights, including dental lamps, unshaded light bulbs at close proximity). Do not stay in a darkened room during this period, because exposure to indoor light is helpful in inactivating this medicine. Before exposing skin to bright indoor light or direct sunlight, test it for sensitivity. Expose a small skin area to sunlight for 10 minutes. If no sensitivity reactions (eg, rash, swelling, blistering) occur within 24 hours, gradually resume normal outdoor activities. If a sensitivity reaction occurs with the skin test, continue precautions for another 2 weeks before retesting.
  If you must go out during daylight hours, cover the skin as much as possible (long-sleeved shirts, slacks, gloves, socks, wide-brimmed hat) and wear dark sunglasses even on cloudy days or when in a car.
  The skin around the eyes may be most sensitive, so do not use the face for testing.
  UV (ultraviolet) sunscreens do not protect against sensitivity reactions.
- Contraceptive measures (birth control) are recommended during treatment to avoid birth defects. Inform your doctor if you are pregnant, become pregnant, are planning to become pregnant, or if you are breastfeeding.
- Lab tests may be required to monitor treatment. Be sure to keep appointments.

*If you have any questions, consult your doctor, pharmacist, or health care provider.*

| Generic Name<br>*Brand Name Example* | Supplied As | Generic<br>Available |
|---|---|---|
| *Rx* **Alemtuzumab** | | |
| *Campath* | **Solution for injection:**<br>30 mg/mL | No |

## Type of Drug:
Monoclonal antibody; anticancer drug.

## How the Drug Works:
Alemtuzumab is a synthetic antibody that attaches to and kills lymphocyte cells that cause leukemia.

## Uses:
Used for the treatment of B-cell chronic lymphocytic leukemia (B-CLL) in patients who have been treated with alkylating agents and who have failed fludarabine therapy.

## Precautions:
*Do not use in the following situations:*
allergy to the drug or any of its ingredients
immunodeficiency (eg, HIV)
live vaccines, administration of
systemic infections, active

*Use with caution in the following situations:*
blood pressure medication use, current
ischemic heart disease (eg, angina)

*Immunizations:* Patients who are receiving or have recently completed alemtuzumab therapy should not be vaccinated with live vaccines.

*Pregnancy:* There are no adequate and well-controlled studies in pregnant women. Use only if clearly needed and potential benefits outweigh the possible hazards to the fetus.

*Breastfeeding:* It is not known if alemtuzumab appears in breast milk. Consult your doctor before you begin breastfeeding.

*Children:* Safety and effectiveness have not been established.

*Lab tests* will be required to monitor therapy. Tests may include complete blood counts (CBC), platelet counts, and CD4.

## Drug Interactions:
Tell your doctor or pharmacist if you are taking or planning to take any over-the-counter or prescription medications or dietary supplements while taking this drug. Doses of one or both drugs may need to be modified or a different drug may need to be prescribed. Immunosuppressants (eg, prednisone, cancer drugs) interact with this drug.

## Side Effects:

Every drug is capable of producing side effects. Many patients experience side effects. The frequency and severity of side effects depend on many factors including dose, duration of therapy, and individual susceptibility. Possible side effects include:

*Circulatory System:* Changes in blood pressure; rapid heartbeat.

*Respiratory System:* Cough; difficulty breathing; sore throat; pneumonia; sinus infection; bronchitis; runny nose.

*Digestive Tract:* Inflammation of the mouth; diarrhea; nausea; vomiting; constipation; stomach pain; indigestion; sore throat.

*Nervous System:* Dizziness; sleeplessness; headache; depression; drowsiness; tremors; changes in skin sensations.

*Skin:* Itching; rash; hives; increased sweating.

*Other:* Chills; fever; fatigue; bone, muscle, back, or chest pain; loss of appetite; infection of blood; weakness; swelling; herpes simplex; general body discomfort; bruising; bleeding; infection; anemia; abnormal blood counts.

---

### Guidelines for Use:

- This medicine will be prepared and administered by your health care provider in a medical setting.
- Dosage is individualized.
- Premedication with acetaminophen (eg, *Tylenol*) and diphenhydramine (eg, *Benadryl*) are recommended before each infusion to reduce infusion-related side effects. Occasionally, hydrocortisone may be used by injection into a vein (IV; intravenous) before the infusion.
- Anti-infective (eg, antiviral, antibiotic) medications may be used during, and for 2 or more months after completing, therapy in an effort to reduce infections.
- Maintenance therapy is administered 3 times a week.
- Notify your doctor immediately if you experience rash, hives, unusual bruising, bleeding, fever or other signs of an infection, or difficulty breathing.
- Women of childbearing potential and men of reproductive potential should use effective contraceptive methods during treatment and for a minimum of 6 months following therapy.
- Lab tests will be required to monitor therapy. Be sure to keep appointments.

---

*If you have any questions, consult your doctor, pharmacist, or health care provider.*

| Generic Name<br>*Brand Name Example* | Supplied As | Generic<br>Available |
|---|---|---|
| *Rx* **Gemtuzumab Ozogamicin** | | |
| *Mylotarg*[1] | **Powder for injection:** 5 mg | No |

[1] Preservative free.

## Type of Drug:

Monoclonal antibody; antileukemia drug.

## How the Drug Works:

Gemtuzumab is a synthetic antibody that can attach to and kill certain types of leukemia cells.

## Uses:

For the treatment of patients with CD33 positive acute myeloid leukemia in first relapse who are 60 years of age and older and who are not considered candidates for other cytotoxic chemotherapy.

## Precautions:

*Do not use in the following situations:* Allergy to the drug or any of its ingredients.

*Use with caution in the following situations:*
combination therapy with other          liver disease
  chemotherapy agents

*Pregnancy:* There are no adequate and well-controlled studies in pregnant women. Women of childbearing potential should avoid becoming pregnant while receiving treatment.

*Breastfeeding:* It is not known if gemtuzumab appears in breast milk. Consult your doctor before you begin breastfeeding.

*Children:* Safety and effectiveness have not been established.

*Lab tests* will be required to monitor treatment.

## Drug Interactions:

Tell your doctor or pharmacist if you are taking or planning to take any over-the-counter or prescription medications or dietary supplements while taking this drug. Doses of one or both drugs may need to be modified or a different drug may need to be prescribed.

## Side Effects:

Every drug is capable of producing side effects. Many patients experience no, or minor, side effects. The frequency and severity of side effects depend on many factors including dose, duration of therapy, and individual susceptibility. Possible side effects include:

*Digestive Tract:* Appetite loss; constipation; diarrhea; indigestion; nausea; stomach pain; vomiting; mouth sores; bloating.

*Nervous System:* Depression; dizziness; sleeplessness; headache.

*Circulatory System:* Changes in blood pressure; rapid heartbeat.

*Respiratory System:* Increased cough; difficulty breathing; sore throat; pneumonia; runny nose.

*Skin:* Rash; swelling.

*Other:* Pain; chills; fever; weakness; back pain; joint pain; elevated blood sugar; abnormal lab tests; blood poisoning; bleeding; bruising; blood in the urine.

---

### Guidelines for Use:

- This medicine will be prepared and administered by your health care provider in a medical setting. It is administered as 2 separate doses by intravenous (IV; into a vein) infusion 14 days apart.
- Premedication with acetaminophen (eg, *Tylenol*) and diphenhydramine (eg, *Benadryl*) is recommended before each infusion to reduce infusion-related side effects.
- Notify your doctor if you experience upper-right stomach pain, unexplained shortness of breath, difficulty breathing, unusual bruising, bleeding, fever or other signs of infection, sore throat, yellowing of the skin or eyes, or rapid weight gain.
- Lab tests will be required to monitor therapy. Be sure to keep appointments.

---

*If you have any questions, consult your doctor, pharmacist, or health care provider.*

| Generic Name<br>*Brand Name Example* | Supplied As | Generic<br>Available |
|---|---|---|
| *Rx* **Ibritumomab Tiuxetan** | | |
| *Zevalin* | **Injection:** 3.2 mg | No |

## Type of Drug:
Monoclonal antibody; two-step regimen given with rituximab.

## How the Drug Works:
Ibritumomab is an antibody that binds to the CD20 antigen on normal and malignant B-lymphocytes. Tiuxetan binds Indium-111 or Yttrium-90 to the B-lymphocytes. Radiation from Indium-111 or Yttrium-90 kills the B-lymphocytes.

## Uses:
Used to treat patients with relapsed or refractory low-grade, follicular, or transformed B-cell non-Hodgkin lymphoma (NHL), including patients with rituximab-refractory follicular NHL.

## Precautions:
*Do not use in the following situations:*

allergy to indium chloride
allergy to murine proteins
allergy to rituximab
allergy to the drug or any of its ingredients
allergy to yttrium chloride
failed stem cell collection, history of
impaired bone marrow reserve

*Use with caution in the following situations:*

altered biodistribution
bleeding disorder
liver disease
neutropenia
thrombocytopenia

*Pregnancy:* Studies have shown a potential effect on the fetus. Use only if clearly needed and potential benefits outweigh the possible risks to the fetus.

*Breastfeeding:* It is not known if ibritumomab appears in breast milk. Consult your doctor before you begin breastfeeding.

*Children:* Safety and effectiveness have not been established.

*Lab tests* will be required to monitor therapy. Tests may include complete blood counts (CBC) and platelet counts.

## Drug Interactions:
Tell your doctor or pharmacist if you are taking or planning to take any over-the-counter or prescription medications or dietary supplements while taking this drug. Doses of one or both drugs may need to be modified or a different drug may need to be prescribed.

## Side Effects:

Every drug is capable of producing side effects. Many patients experience side effects. The frequency and severity of side effects depend on many factors including dose, duration of therapy, and individual susceptibility. Possible side effects include:

*Digestive Tract:* Nausea; stomach pain; vomiting; throat irritation; diarrhea; loss of appetite; stomach enlargement; constipation.

*Nervous System:* Headache; dizziness; sleeplessness; anxiety.

*Skin:* Itching; rash; flushing; hives.

*Hematologic/Lymphatic:* Decreased blood platelets; low white blood cells; unusual bruising.

*Respiratory System:* Difficulty breathing; increased cough; inflammed sinuses; bronchospasm.

*Other:* Low blood pressure; hives; joint pain; muscle pain; weakness; infection; chills; fever; back pain.

### Guidelines for Use:

- This medicine will be prepared and administered by your healthcare provider in a medical setting.
- Dosage is individualized.
- Lab tests will be required. Be sure to keep appointments.

*If you have any questions, consult your doctor, pharmacist, or health care provider.*

| Generic Name Brand Name Example | Supplied As | Generic Available |
|---|---|---|
| *Rx* **Rituximab** | | |
| *Rituxan*[1] | **Injection:** 10 mg/mL | No |

[1] Preservative free.

## Type of Drug:
Monoclonal antibody.

## How the Drug Works:
Rituximab is a synthetic monoclonal antibody directed against the CD20 antigen found on the surface of normal malignant B lymphocytes associated with non-Hodgkin lymphoma. It attaches to the antigen and kills the cell.

## Uses:
For recurring or untreatable low-grade or follicular, CD20–positive, B-cell non-Hodgkin lymphoma.

## Precautions:
*Do not use in the following situations:* Allergy to murine (rats, mice) proteins or any of the drug's ingredients.

*Use with caution in the following situations:*

| | |
|---|---|
| coronary artery disease | low blood pressure |
| heart rhythm disturbance, current or history of | |

*Pregnancy:* There are no adequate or well-controlled studies in pregnant women. Use only if clearly needed and potential benefits outweigh the possible hazards to the fetus.

*Breastfeeding:* It is not known if rituximab appears in breast milk. Consult your doctor before you begin breastfeeding or discontinue nursing until rituximab blood levels are no longer detectable.

*Children:* Safety and effectiveness have not been established.

*Lab tests* will be required to monitor treatment. Tests may include complete blood counts (CBC) and platelet counts.

## Drug Interactions:
Tell your doctor or pharmacist if you are taking or planning to take any over-the-counter or prescription medications or dietary supplements with this drug. Doses of one or both drugs may need to be modified or a different drug may need to be prescribed. Blood pressure medicine (eg, valsartan) interacts with this drug.

## Side Effects:

Every drug is capable of producing side effects. Many patients experience side effects. The frequency and severity of side effects depend on many factors including dose, duration of therapy, and individual susceptibility. Possible side effects include:

*Digestive Tract:* Nausea; vomiting; throat irritation; stomach pain; diarrhea; indigestion; loss of appetite.

*Nervous System:* Headache; dizziness; anxiety; nervousness; agitation; sleeplessness; depression; drowsiness; feeling of whirling motion (vertigo).

*Circulatory System:* Changes in blood pressure; chest pain; fast or irregular heartbeat.

*Respiratory System:* Difficulty breathing; nasal congestion; runny nose; sinus infection; increased cough.

*Skin:* Hives; rash; itching; abnormal skin sensations; herpes simplex; pain at injection site.

*Senses:* Eye infection; watery eyes.

*Other:* Weakness; back, muscle or joint pain; pain; high blood sugar; fluid retention; swelling of arms and legs; general body discomfort; tight muscles; fever; chills; flushing; night sweats; abnormal blood cell counts

---

## Guidelines for Use:

- This medicine will be prepared and administered by your health care provider in a medical setting.
- This medicine will be given as an intravenous (IV; into a vein) infusion once weekly for 4 or 8 doses.
- Premedication with acetaminophen (eg, *Tylenol*) and diphenhydramine (eg, *Benadryl*) is recommended before each infusion to reduce infusion-related side effects.
- Infusion reactions (eg, chills, fever) occur commonly with the first doses, but become less frequent with subsequent doses.
- Notify your doctor if you experience severe skin rash, unexplained shortness of breath, difficulty breathing, unusual bruising, fever, or other signs of infection, sore throat, abnormal heart rhythm, or pounding in the chest (palpitations).
- Withhold high blood pressure medications 12 hours before therapy because short-lived low blood pressure may occur during the infusion.
- Lab tests will be required to monitor treatment. Be sure to keep appointments.

---

*If you have any questions, consult your doctor, pharmacist, or health care provider.*

| Generic Name Brand Name Example | Supplied As | Generic Available |
|---|---|---|
| Rx **Trastuzumab** | | |
| *Herceptin* | **Powder for injection**: 440 mg/vial | No |

## Type of Drug:
Monoclonal antibody.

## How the Drug Works:
Trastuzumab is a synthetic antibody that attaches to and inhibits the growth of tumor cells that over-produce a specific protein (HER2 protein).

## Uses:
For the treatment of patients with metastatic breast cancer whose tumors over-produce the HER2 protein. Trastuzumab is used as a single agent for patients who have received one or more chemotherapy treatments or in combination with paclitaxel for patients who have not received chemotherapy for their metastatic disease.

## Precautions:
*Do not use in the following situations:* Allergy to the drug, any of its ingredients, or Chinese hamster ovary cell proteins.

*Use with caution in the following situations:*

anthracyclines (eg, doxorubicin), current of previous use cardiac disease, history of cardiac dysfunction, preexisting heart failure, congestive radiation therapy to chest, history of

*Congestive heart failure* associated with trastuzumab may be severe and has been associated with disabling cardiac failure, death, and stroke. Candidates for treatment should undergo thorough baseline cardiac assessment including history and physical exam and one or more of the following tests: EKG, echocardiogram, and MUGA scan. Monitoring may not identify all patients who will develop cardiac dysfunction.

*Pregnancy:* There are no adequate or well-controlled studies in pregnant women. Use only if clearly needed and potential benefits outweigh the possible hazards to the fetus.

*Breastfeeding:* It is not known if trastuzumab appears in breast milk. Consult your doctor before you begin breastfeeding. Because the potential for absorption and harm is unknown, women should be advised to discontinue nursing during trastuzumab therapy and for 6 months after the last dose of trastuzumab.

*Children:* Safety and effectiveness have not been established.

*Elderly:* Advanced age may increase the risk of heart problems. Because clinical experience is limited, it is not known if older patients respond differently than younger patients.

*Lab tests* and exams will be required to monitor therapy. Tests may include cardiac (heart) function tests and blood counts.

## Drug Interactions:

Tell your doctor or pharmacist if you are taking or planning to take any over-the-counter or prescription medications or dietary supplements while taking this drug. Doses of one or both drugs may need to be modified or a different drug may need to be prescribed. The following drugs and drug classes interact with this drug:

anthracyclines (eg, doxorubicin)        cyclophosphamide (eg, *Cytoxan)*

## Side Effects:

Every drug is capable of producing side effects. Many patients experience side effects. The frequency and severity of side effects depend on many factors including dose, duration of therapy, and individual susceptibility. Possible side effects include:

*Circulatory System:* Heart failure (eg, shortness of breath, increased cough, sudden nighttime shortness of breath, ankle and leg swelling); fast heartbeat.

*Digestive Tract:* Diarrhea; nausea; vomiting; stomach pain; loss of appetite.

*Nervous System:* Sleeplessness; dizziness; abnormal skin sensations; depression; inflammation of nerves; nerve pain; numbness; headache.

*Respiratory System:* Increased cough; sinus infection or inflammation; congested or runny nose; sore throat; difficulty breathing.

*Skin:* Rash; itching; hives; acne; herpes simplex.

*Other:* Infection; body, back, bone, or joint pain; pain at tumor sites; weakness; fever; chills; headache; flu syndrome; accidental injury; allergic reaction; urinary tract infection; swelling of hands or feet; anemia; low white blood cell count.

---

### Guidelines for Use:

- This medicine will be prepared and administered by your health care provider in a medical setting. It is given as an intravenous (IV; into a vein) infusion once weekly.
- Chills and fever frequently occur with the first dose, but are infrequent with subsequent doses.
- Notify your doctor if you experience difficulty breathing, increased cough, shortness of breath while lying down, or swelling in the ankles or feet.
- Lab tests and exams will be required to monitor therapy. Be sure to keep appointments.

---

*If you have any questions, consult your doctor, pharmacist, or health care provider.*

**Antidotes**
Charcoal, Activated, 1625
Flumazenil, 1627
Ipecac, 1629
Dexrazoxane, 1631
Nalmefene, 1633
Naloxone, 1635

**Chelating Agents**
Succimer, 1637

**Anticholinesterase Muscle Stimulants, 1639**

**Urinary Tract Products**
Acetohydroxamic Acid, 1642
Acidifiers, 1644
Alkalinizers, 1647
Bethanechol Chloride, 1650
Cellulose Sodium
   Phosphate, 1652
Cysteamine Bitartrate, 1654
Dimethyl Sulfoxide, 1656
Flavoxate, 1658
Oxybutynin Chloride, 1660
Tolterodine Tartrate, 1662
Phenazopyridine, 1664

**Immunosuppressives**
Azathioprine, 1666
Cyclosporine, 1668
Mycophenolate Mofetil, 1672
Muromonab-CD3, 1675
Tacrolimus, 1678

**Retinoids**
Isotretinoin, 1681

**Antirheumatic Agents**
Leflunomide, 1685

**Bromocriptine Mesylate, 1688**

**Cabergoline, 1691**

**Chymopapain, 1693**

**Cromolyn Sodium, Oral, 1695**

**Disulfiram, 1697**

**Naltrexone, 1700**

**Levomethadyl Acetate, 1703**

**Penicillamine, 1706**

**Immunomodulators**
Anakinra, 1709
Etanercept, 1711
Peginterferon Alfa-2a, 1714
Peginterferon Alfa-2b, 1717

**Smoking Deterrents**
Bupropion, 1720
Nicotine, 1724

**Agents for Impotence**
Alprostradil, 1729
Sildenafil Citrate, 1732

**Yohimbine, 1736**

**Interferon Beta, 1738**

**Riluzole, 1741**

**Glatiramer Acetate, 1743**

**Thalidomide, 1745**

| Generic Name<br>*Brand Name Examples* | Supplied As | Generic<br>Available |
|---|---|---|
| *otc* **Charcoal, Activated** | **Powder** | Yes |
| *Actidose-Aqua, Actidose with Sorbitol, CharcoAid, Liqui-Char, Superchar* | **Liquid** | Yes |

## Type of Drug:
Poisoning antidote.

## How the Drug Works:
Charcoal adsorbs (attaches to) toxic substances (eg, drugs, chemicals, poisons), forming a barrier between the particles and the stomach lining, thus preventing absorption of the toxic substance into the body.

*Sorbitol* may be added to some activated charcoal products because it improves the taste and does not leave a gritty residue.

## Uses:
To treat poisonings and drug overdoses caused by swallowing.

## Precautions:
Do not use when there is an overdose of cyanide, mineral acids and alkalies. Although not contraindicated, it is not effective for use in poisonings of alcohol or iron.

## Drug Interactions:
Tell your doctor or pharmacist if you are taking or if you are planning to take any over-the-counter or prescription medications or dietary supplements with activated charcoal. Doses of one or both drugs may need to be modified or a different drug may need to be prescribed. Ipecac interacts with activated charcoal. Do not take concomitantly. Charcoal will decrease the effectiveness of any medication taken at the same time.

## Side Effects:
Every drug is capable of producing side effects. Many activated charcoal users experience no, or minor, side effects. The frequency and severity of side effects depend on many factors including dose, duration of therapy and individual susceptibility. Possible side effects include constipation, diarrhea, black stools and vomiting.

## Guidelines for Use:
- Use exactly as prescribed.
- Contact your doctor or poison control center for all poisonings or suspected poisonings.
- Give only to conscious (alert) persons.
- If ipecac syrup is also given, give the ipecac first; give activated charcoal after vomiting occurs.
- Do not mix charcoal with milk, ice cream or sherbet since they will decrease the effectiveness of the activated charcoal.
- Keep in a closed container.

*If you have any questions, consult your doctor, pharmacist, or health care provider.*

| Generic Name Brand Name Example | Supplied As | Generic Available |
|---|---|---|
| Rx **Flumazenil** | | |
| *Romazicon* | **Injection:** 0.1 mg/mL[1] | No |

[1] Contains EDTA and parabens.

## Type of Drug:

Antidote for benzodiazepine (eg, diazepam)-induced sedation.

## How the Drug Works:

Flumazenil reverses the effects of benzodiazepines by inhibiting their activity. It counteracts sedation, memory loss and impaired movement.

## Uses:

To reverse the sedative effects of benzodiazepines in cases of general anesthesia, diagnostic or therapeutic sedation, and overdose.

## Precautions:

*Do not use in the following situations:*

allergy to benzodiazepines
allergy to flumazenil
benzodiazepine use to control a potentially life-threatening condition
cyclic antidepressant (eg, amitriptyline) overdose, serious

*Use with caution in the following situations:*

alcoholism
drug dependency
head injury
intensive care unit use
liver disease
mixed drug overdose
panic disorder, history
neuromuscular blocker use

*Seizures:* The reversal of benzodiazepine effects may be associated with seizures in certain individuals. Risk factors include: withdrawal from sedative-hypnotics (eg, triazolam); recent therapy with repeated doses of injectable benzodiazepines, jerking or seizure activity prior to flumazenil use in overdose; cyclic antidepressant poisoning.

*Amnesia:* Flumazenil does not consistently reverse amnesia. Patients cannot be expected to remember information told to them following administration. Therefore, instructions should be written down or given to a responsible family member.

*Hypoventilation:* Monitor patients who have received flumazenil for reversal of benzodiazepine effects (after conscious sedation or general anesthesia) for resedation, respiratory depression or other residual benzodiazepine effects for up to 120 minutes.

*Pregnancy:* Adequate studies have not been done in pregnant women. Use only if clearly needed and potential benefits outweigh the possibie hazards to the fetus.

*Breastfeeding:* It is not known if flumazenil appears in breast milk. Consult your doctor before you begin breastfeeding.

*Children:* Safety and effectiveness in children have not been established. Use is not recommended.

## Drug Interactions:

Tell your doctor or pharmacist if you are taking or if you are planning to take any over-the-counter or prescription medications or dietary supplements with flumazenil. Doses of one or both drugs may need to be modified or a different drug may need to be prescribed.

## Side Effects:

Every drug is capable of producing side effects. Many flumazenil users experience no, or minor, side effects. The frequency and severity of side effects depend on many factors including dose, duration of therapy and individual susceptibility. Possible side effects include:

*Digestive Tract:* Nausea; vomiting.

*Nervous System:* Seizures; dizziness; headache, fatigue; weakness; agitation; anxiety; nervousness; tremor; sleeplessness; vertigo (feeling of whirling motion); incoordination; emotional changes (eg, depression); abnormal sensations.

*Other:* Pain at injection site; reaction at injection site (eg, rash); sweating; abnormal or blurred vision; general body discomfort; flushing; hot flushes; dry mouth; palpitations (pounding in the chest); difficulty breathing.

---

### Guidelines for Use:

- The reversal of benzodiazepine effects may be associated with seizures in certain individuals. Consult your doctor regarding sedative-hypnotic drug withdrawal, recent therapy with repeated doses of injectable benzodiazepines, jerking or seizures prior to flumazenil use, and cyclic antidepressant poisoning.
- Inform your doctor of any benzodiazepine, alcohol or sedative use prior to flumazenil therapy.
- Benzodiazepine effects may recur despite alertness at the time of discharge. Memory and judgment may be impaired.
- *Do not* drive or perform other tasks requiring alertness until at least 18 to 24 hours after discharge.
- *Do not* take any alcohol or nonprescription drugs for 18 to 24 hours after flumazenil use or if sedation persists.

---

*If you have any questions, consult your doctor, pharmacist, or health care provider.*

| Generic Name | Supplied As | Generic Available |
|---|---|---|
| otc/ **Ipecac**[1] Rx | **Syrup** | Yes |

[1] Contains alcohol.

## Type of Drug:

Emetic; an agent that induces vomiting.

## How the Drug Works:

Ipecac irritates the stomach lining and stimulates the vomiting center (chemoreceptor trigger zone, CTZ) in the brain.

## Uses:

To treat drug overdoses and certain poisonings caused by swallowing.

## Precautions:

*Do not use in the following situations:*
> breastfeeding
> corrosives (eg, alkalies, strong acids)
> poisoning by petroleum distillates
> pregnancy
> semiconscious or unconscious patients
> strychnine poisoning

*Ipecac syrup abuse:* Ipecac syrup may be abused by bulimic and anorexic patients. It has been implicated as the cause of severe heart problems and even death in several persons with eating disorders who used it regularly to cause vomiting.

*Pregnancy:* Not recommended for use during pregnancy. Adequate studies have not been done in pregnant women. Use only if clearly needed and potential benefits outweigh the possible hazards to the fetus.

*Breastfeeding:* It is not known if ipecac appears in breast milk. Use is not recommended. Contact your doctor.

## Drug Interactions:

Tell your doctor or pharmacist if you are taking or if you are planning to take any over-the-counter or prescription medications or dietary supplements with ipecac. Doses of one or both drugs may need to be modified or a different drug may need to be prescribed. The following drugs and drug classes interact with ipecac.

> carbonated beverages
> charcoal, activated
> milk

## Side Effects:

Every drug is capable of producing side effects. Many ipecac syrup users experience no, or minor, side effects. The frequency and severity of side effects depend on many factors including dose, duration of therapy and individual susceptibility. Possible side effects include diarrhea, drowsiness, stomach ache and vomiting.

When ipecac syrup does not cause vomiting, absorption may occur and may cause heart conduction disturbances, or even fatal inflammations of the heart muscle (see Precautions).

---

### Guidelines for Use:

- Do not give to semiconscious or unconscious individuals. Have patient sit upright with head forward before administering dose.
- Always consult your doctor or poison control center in cases of accidental ingestion of toxic substances.
- Ipecac syrup may not work on an empty stomach. Give with plenty of water. Do not exceed recommended dosage.
- Do not take with milk or carbonated drinks (eg, soda).
- Do not confuse ipecac syrup with ipecac fluid extract, which is 14 times stronger and has caused some deaths.
- *Children (6 months to 1 year)* — 5 to 10 mL (1 to 2 tsp) followed by one-half to one glass of water. Syrup of ipecac should probably be given only with a doctor's advice or supervision. It is not recommended that ipecac be given to children less than 6 months of age.
- *Children (1 to 12 years)* — 15 mL (1 tbsp) followed by 1 to 2 glasses of water.
- *Adults* — 15 to 30 mL (1 to 2 tbsp) followed by 3 to 4 glasses of water.
- Repeat the dosage once if vomiting does not occur within 30 minutes.
- If vomiting does not occur within 30 minutes after the second dose, contact your doctor or poison control center.
- If vomiting does not occur after taking ipecac syrup, or if excessive doses are used, it may be absorbed into the body and cause problems with the heart. Contact your doctor.

---

*If you have any questions, consult your doctor, pharmacist, or health care provider.*

| Generic Name<br>*Brand Name Example* | Supplied As | Generic<br>Available |
|---|---|---|
| *Rx* **Dexrazoxane**<br>*Zinecard* | **Injection:** 10 mg/mL | No |

## Type of Drug:
Cardioprotective (heart protective) agent.

## How the Drug Works:
Dexrazoxane heaps protect women from heart problems caused by doxorubicin (chemotherapy) treatment of breast cancer.

## Uses:
To reduce the chances and severity of heart problems caused by doxorubicin(chemotherapy) treatment of breast cancer. This medicine should not be used at the beginning of doxorubicin therapy. It is added after a certain amount of doxorubicin has been given.

## Precautions:
*Do not use in the following situations:*
> allergy to dexrazoxanle or to any of its components
> chemotherapy that does not contain an anthracyclinle drug

*Use with caution in the following situations:*
> FAC therapy (fluorouracil, doxorubicin, cyclophosphamide), initiation
> myelosuppression (bone marrow suppression)

*Pregnancy:* Adequate studies have not been done in pregnant women, or animal studies may have shown a risk to the fetus. Use only if clearly needed and potential benefits outweigh the possible hazards to the fetus.

*Breastfeeding:* It is not known if dexrazoxane appears in breast milk. Consult your doctor before you begin breastfeeding.

*Children:* Safety and effectiveness for use have not been established.

*Lab tests* will be required durinlg treatment with dexrazoxane. Tests will include frequent blood counts.

## Side Effects:
Every drug is capable of producing side effects. Many patients experience no, or minor, side effects. The frequency or severity of side effects depend on many factors including dose, duration of therapy and individual susceptibility. Possible side effects include:

*Digestive Tract:* Nausea, vomiting; diarrhea; appetite loss; difficulty swallowing; stomach ache; inflammation of mouth and throat.

*Skin:* Pain on injection; pain at injection site; redess/streaking; flushing; bruising; hives; rash; numbness.

*Other:* Fatigue; general body discomfort; fever; infection; blood clots; hair loss; bleeding.

**Guidelines for Use:**

- This medicine will be prepared and administered by a healthcare provider.
- *Infections* — This medicine, along with chemotherapy medicines, may lower your body's ability to fight infection. Notify your doctor of any signs of infection, including: fever, sore throat, rashes or chills.
- Lab tests and exams will be required to monitor therapy. Be sure to keep appointments.

*If you have any questions, consult your doctor, pharmacist, or health care provider.*

| Generic Name<br>*Brand Name Example* | Supplied As | Generic<br>Available |
|---|---|---|
| *Rx* **Nalmefene HCl** | | |
| *Revex* | **Injection:** 1 mg/mL | No |

## Type of Drug:

Anti-opioid; antinarcotic; narcotic antagonist.

## How the Drug Works:

Nalmefene prevents or reverses the effects of narcotics (opioids), including respiratory depression, sedation and hypotension (low blood pressure). Nalmefene can cause acute withdrawal symptoms in individuals who are narcotic addicts/abusers. Nalmefene does not produce tolerance, nor cause physical or psychological dependence.

## Uses:

To completely or partially reverse narcotic effects, including respiratory depression. To manage known or suspected narcotic overdose.

## Precautions:

*Do not use in the following situations:*
allergy to nalmefene

*Use with caution in the following situations:*
heart disease, preexisting
kidney disease
liver disease
patients who have received potentially cardiotoxic drugs
physical dependence on narcotics
surgery involving high use of narcotics

*Pregnancy:* Studies in pregnant women or in animals have been judged not to show a risk to the fetus. However, no drug should be used during pregnancy unless clearly needed.

*Breastfeeding:* Nalmefene appears in breast milk. Consult your doctor before you begin breastfeeding.

*Children:* Safety and effectiveness for use have not been established.

## Drug Interactions:

Tell your doctor or pharmacist if you are taking or if you are planning to take any over-the-counter or prescription medications or dietary supplements while taking this medicine. Doses of one or both drugs may need to be modified or a different drug may need to be prescribed. Nalmefene may interact with flumazenil (*Romazicon*).

## Side Effects:

Every drug is capable of producing side effects. Many patients experience no, or minor, side effects. The frequency or severity of side effects depend on many factors including dose, duration of therapy and individual susceptibility. Possible side effects include:

*Digestive Tract:* Nausea; vomiting.

*Circulatory System:* Rapid heartbeat; changes in blood pressure.

*Other:* Fever; dizziness; headache; chills; flushing; pain.

---

## Guidelines for Use:

- This medicine will be administered by a healthcare provider.
- Difficulty breathing may occur even after using this medicine. Contact your doctor if you are experiencing difficulties.
- Patients using this medicine require careful monitoring by their healthcare providers.
- This medicine should be used with caution in patients with previous heart problems or who are taking drugs which affect the heart.
- This medicine can cause severe withdrawal symptoms and should be used with extreme caution in patients with a known physical dependence on or tolerance to narcotics, or following surgery involving high doses of narcotics.
- This medicine has no demonstrated abuse potential, is not addictive and is not a controlled substance, nor will it relieve pain.
- This medicine is not effective in cases where narcotics were not responsible for sedation and shortness of breath.
- Dosage adjustments may be necessary in patients with kidney failure.

---

*If you have any questions, consult your doctor, pharmacist, or health care provider.*

| Generic Name<br>*Brand Name Example* | Supplied As | Generic<br>Available |
|---|---|---|
| *Rx* **Naloxone HCl**<br>    *Narcan*[1] | **Injection:** 0.02 mg/mL,<br>0.4 mg/mL,[2] 1 mg/mL[2] | Yes |

[1] Contains sodium chloride.
[2] Available with or without methyl and propylparabens.

## Type of Drug:

Anti-opioid; antinarcotic; narcotic antagonist.

## How the Drug Works:

Naloxone prevents or reverses the effects of narcotics (opioids) and certain narcotic analgesics (eg, codeine). The exact mechanism of action is not fully understood. Evidence suggests that narcotic effects are blocked by competition for the same receptor sites.

Naloxone does not produce tolerance, nor cause dependence. Naloxone will produce withdrawal symptoms in individuals who are narcotic addicts/abusers.

## Uses:

To completely or partially reverse narcotic effects, including respiratory depression induced by narcotics (opioids). To diagnose suspected acute narcotic overdosage.

*Unlabeled Use(s):* Occasionally doctors may prescribe naloxone for improved circulation in refractory shock, reversal of alcoholic coma, dementia of the Alzheimer type and schizophrenia.

## Precautions:

*Do not use in the following situations:*
    allergy to naloxone

*Use with caution in the following situations:*
    heart disease, preexisting
    patients who have received potentially cardiotoxic drugs
    physical dependence on narcotics, known or suspected (including newborns of dependent mothers)

*Pregnancy:* Studies in pregnant women or in animals have been judged not to show a risk to the fetus. However, no drug should be used during pregnancy unless clearly needed.

*Breastfeeding:* It is not known if naloxone appears in breast milk. Consult your doctor before you begin breastfeeding.

## Side Effects:

Every drug is capable of producing side effects. Many patients experience no, or minor, side effects. The frequency and severity of side effects depend on many factors including dose, duration of therapy and individual susceptibility. Possible side effects include:

*Digestive Tract:* Nausea; vomiting.

*Circulatory System:* Increased heart rate; changes in blood pressure; heart attack.

*Other:* Sweating; seizures; excitement; tremors; fluid in the lungs.

---

### Guidelines for Use:

- Naloxone does not produce tolerance or cause physical or psychological dependence.
- In the presence of physical dependence on narcotics, naloxone will produce withdrawal symptoms.
- Since the duration of action of some narcotics may exceed that of naloxone, patients should be kept under continued supervision and given repeated doses of naloxone if necessary.

---

*If you have any questions, consult your doctor, pharmacist, or health care provider.*

| Generic Name<br>*Brand Name Example* | Supplied As | Generic<br>Available |
|---|---|---|
| *Rx* **Succimer** | | |
| *Chemet* | **Capsules:** 100 mg | No |

## Type of Drug:
Chelating agent.

## How the Drug Works:
Succimer binds to lead in the body and then is excreted in the urine. This results in a reduction in the total amount of lead (which is poisonous) in the body.

## Uses:
To treat lead poisoning in children with blood lead levels greater than 45 µg/dL. When using this drug, the source of the lead poisoning should always be identified and removed.

## Precautions:
*Do not use in the following situations:* Allergy to succimer or any of its ingredients.

*Use with caution in the following situations:*
    kidney disease
    liver disease, history of

*Pregnancy:* Adequate studies have not been done in pregnant women. Use only when clearly needed and potential benefits to the mother outweigh the possible hazards to the fetus.

*Breastfeeding:* It is not known if succimer appears in breast milk. Consult your doctor before you begin breastfeeding.

*Children:* Safety and effectiveness for use in children under 1 year of age have not been established.

*Lab tests* will be required during treatment with succimer. Tests may include bloodcounts, blood lead levels, and liver function tests.

## Side Effects:
Every drug is capable of producing side effects. Many succimer users experience no, or minor, side effects. The frequency and severity of side effects depend on many factors including dose, duration of therapy, and individual susceptibility. Possible side effects include:

*Digestive Tract:* Nausea; vomiting; diarrhea; appetite loss; stomach ache or cramps; loose stools.

*Nervous System:* Headache; dizziness; drowsiness.

*Circulatory System:* Irregular heartbeat.

*Respiratory System:* Cough; runny nose; nasal congestion.

*Skin:* Rash; itching; eruptions of skin and mucous membranes; abnormal skin sensations (burning, prickling, tingling).

*Other:* Fever; chills; head or body aches or pain; heavy head feeling; cloudy film in eyes; watery eyes; ear infection; plugged ears; cold or flu-like symptoms; sore throat; metallic taste in mouth; hemorrhoidal symptoms; fungal infections; decreased or difficult urination; protein in urine; abnormal blood counts; abnormal blood tests.

## Guidelines for Use:

- Dosage is individualized.
- Do not stop taking or change the dose of the drug unless advised to do so by your doctor.
- Drink plenty of fluids.
- If dose is missed, take it as soon as possible. If several hours have passed or if it is nearing time for the next dose, do not double the dose to catch up, unless advised to do so by your doctor. If more than one dose is missed, contact your doctor or pharmacist.
- Identification of the source of the lead poisoning and its removal are critical to successful therapy. Succimer should not be used prophylactically to prevent further exposure to lead.
- In young children who are unable to swallow capsules, the contents of the capsule may be sprinkled on a small amount of food or on a spoon and followed with fruit drink.
- Contact your doctor immediately if you experience a rash.
- Uninterrupted therapy for greater than 3 weeks is generally not recommended.
- Patients should promptly report any indication of infection (eg, sore throat, fever), which may be a sign of low white blood cell count.
- Experience with this drug is limited; therefore, close observation by a doctor is required.
- Lab tests will be required to monitor therapy. Be sure to keep appointments.
- Store between 59° and 77°F and avoid excessive heat.

*If you have any questions, consult your doctor, pharmacist, or health care provider.*

| Generic Name<br>*Brand Name Examples* | Supplied As | Generic<br>Available |
|---|---|---|
| *Rx* **Ambenonium Chloride** | | |
| *Mytelase Caplets* | **Tablets:** 10 mg | No |
| *Rx* **Edrophonium Chloride** | | |
| *Enlon,[1] Reversol,[1] Tensilon[1]* | **Injection:** 10 mg/mL | No |
| *Rx* **Edrophonium Chloride and Atropine Sulfate** | | |
| *Enlon-Plus[1]* | **Injection:** 10 mg edrophonium chloride and 0.14 mg atropine sulfate/mL | No |
| *Rx* **Neostigmine Bromide** | | |
| *Prostigmin* | **Tablets:** 15 mg | No |
| *Rx* **Neostigmine Methylsulfate** | | |
| *Prostigmin* | **Injection:** 0.25 mg/mL, 0.5 mg/mL, 1 mg/mL | Yes |
| *Rx* **Pyridostigmine Bromide** | | |
| *Mestinon* | **Tablets:** 60 mg | No |
| *Mestinon Timespan* | **Tablets, sustained-release:** 180 mg | No |
| *Mestinon* | **Syrup:** 60 mg/5 mL | No |
| *Regonol* | **Injection:** 5 mg/mL | No |

[1] Contains sodium sulfite.

## Type of Drug:

Muscle stimulants; anticholinesterase; cholinesterase inhibitor.

## How the Drug Works:

Anticholinesterase muscle stimulants improve the transmission of nerve impulses in muscles so that the muscles are better able to work.

## Uses:

To diagnose and treat myasthenia gravis (a disease which causes muscle weakness).

Used as an antidote for certain muscle relaxant drugs used during surgery.

To prevent and treat distention and urinary retention following surgery (neostigmine methylsulfate only).

## Precautions:

*Do not use in the following situations:*

allergy to anticholinesterase muscle stimulants or any of their ingredients

allergy to bromides (neostigmine bromide and pyridostigmine only)

intestinal obstruction

peritonitis (inflammation of the lining of abdomen) (neostigmine methylsulfate only)

urinary obstruction

*Use with caution in the following situations:*

abnormal heart rhythm

asthma

epilepsy

kidney disease (pyridostigmine only)

obstruction of coronary artery, recent

overactive thyroid

peptic ulcer

slow heartbeat

*Overdosage:* Overdosage may result in cholinergic crisis which causes increased muscle weakness. Muscle weakness involving the respiratory muscles may lead to death.

*Pregnancy:* Safety for use during pregnancy has not been established. Although cholinesterase inhibitors are apparently safe for the fetus, they may ultimately affect the condition of the infant. Temporary muscular weakness has occurred in infants whose mothers used these drugs during pregnancy. Use only if clearly needed and the potential benefits outweigh the possible hazards to the fetus.

*Breastfeeding:* It is not known if anticholinesterase muscle stimulants appear in breast milk. Consult your doctor before you begin breastfeeding.

*Children:* Safety and effectiveness for use in children have not been established.

*Sulfites:* Some of these products may contain sulfite preservatives, which can cause allergic reactions in some individuals (eg, patients with asthma). Check package label when available or consult your doctor or pharmacist.

## Drug Interactions:

Tell your doctor or pharmacist if you are taking or if you are planning to take any over-the-counter or prescription medications or dietary supplements with anticholinesterase muscle stimulants. Doses of one or both drugs may need to be modified or a different drug may need to be prescribed. The following drugs and drug classes interact with anticholinesterase muscle stimulants:

aminoglycosides (eg, gentamicin)

atropine

corticosteroids (eg, prednisone)

mecamylamine (eg, *Inversine*)

succinylcholine (eg, *Anectine*)

## Side Effects:

Every drug is capable of producing side effects. Many anticholinesterase muscle stimulant users experience no, or minor, side effects. The frequency and severity of side effects depend on many factors including dose, duration of therapy, and individual susceptibility. Possible side effects include:

*Muscular System:* Muscle cramps or spasms; muscle twitching; joint pain; weakness.

*Eyes or Ocular:* Increased tearing; blurred vision; double vision; redness; visual changes; decreased pupil size.

*Digestive Tract:* Nausea; vomiting; diarrhea; stomach pain or cramping; gas.

*Nervous System:* Convulsions; loss of consciousness; dizziness; drowsiness; headache.

*Circulatory System:* Changes in heart rate; abnormal heart rhythm; decreased blood pressure.

*Skin:* Rash; itching; sweating; flushing; hives.

*Other:* Vocal problems or difficulty speaking; difficulty swallowing; uncontrolled urination; increased urination; increased salivation; difficult or painful breathing; fainting.

---

### Guidelines for Use:

- Dosage is individualized.
- Close supervision by your doctor is required during treatment to avoid overdosage.
- Do not crush or chew sustained-release tablets.
- Do not change the dose or stop taking unless advised to do so by your doctor. Frequently, therapy is required day and night (except ambenonium).
- *Oral products* — If a dose is missed, take it as soon as possible. If several hours have passed or if it is nearing time for the next dose, do not double the dose to catch up, unless advised to do so by your doctor. If more than one dose is missed or it is necessary to establish a new dosage schedule, contact your doctor or pharmacist.
- *Pyridostigmine* — Sustained-release tablets may develop some patchy discoloration over time. This does not change the effectiveness of the medicine and is no cause for concern.
- Keep a daily record of doses and note times of greatest fatigue or weakness.
- Contact your doctor immediately if you experience periods of extreme muscle weakness, diarrhea, vomiting, stomach cramps, increased salivation, decreased pupil size, or difficulty speaking or swallowing.
- Store at controlled room temperature (59° to 86°F).

---

*If you have any questions, consult your doctor, pharmacist, or health care provider.*

| Generic Name<br>*Brand Name Example* | Supplied As | Generic<br>Available |
|---|---|---|
| *Rx* **Acetohydroxamic Acid** | | |
| *Lithostat* | **Tablets:** 250 mg | No |

## Type of Drug:
Urinary enzyme inhibitor.

## How the Drug Works:
Acetohydroxamic acid (AHA) inhibits the bacterial enzyme urease, thereby inhibiting ammonia production and urea decomposition in the urine. These two effects enable antibiotics to be more effective in treating chronic urinary tract infections.

## Uses:
To aid antibiotic treatment of chronic urinary tract infections due to urea-splitting bacteria.

## Precautions:
*Do not use in the following situations:*
   allergy to acetohydroxamic acid or any of its ingredients
   female patients who do not use adequate contraception
   infection treatable with antibiotics alone
   kidney disease, moderate to severe infection treatable with surgery and antibiotics
   pregnancy
   urinary infection with nonurease-producing bacteria

*Use with caution in the following situations:*
   hemolytic anemia (Coombs negative)
   kidney disease, mild

*Pregnancy:* Do not use during pregnancy. May cause fetal harm when given to a pregnant woman. The risk of use in a pregnant woman clearly outweighs any possible benefit. If you become pregnant while taking this medicine or plan to become pregnant, consult your doctor.

*Breastfeeding:* It is not known if acetohydroxamic acid appears in breast milk. Consult your doctor before you begin breastfeeding.

*Children:* Children with chronic recalcitrant urinary tract infections caused by urea-splitting bacteria may benefit from this drug. However, detailed studies involving dosage and dose intervals in children have not been established. If used in children, close monitoring will be required.

*Lab tests* may be required during treatment with acetohydroxamic acid. Tests may include complete blood counts, kidney function tests, urine cultures, and liver function tests.

## Drug Interactions:

Tell your doctor or pharmacist if you are taking or planning to take any over-the-counter or prescription medications or dietary supplements with acetohydroxamic acid. Doses of one or both drugs may need to be modified or a different drug may need to be prescribed. The following drugs and drug classes interact with acetohydroxamic acid:

alcohol
heavy metals (eg, iron)

## Side Effects:

Every drug is capable of producing side effects. Many acetohydroxamic acid users experience no, or minor, side effects. The frequency and severity of side effects depend on many factors including dose, duration of therapy, and individual susceptibility. Possible side effects include:

*Digestive Tract:* Nausea; vomiting; appetite loss.

*Nervous System:* Mild headache; shakiness; depression; anxiety; nervousness; fatigue.

*Skin:* Rash (especially after ingesting alcohol); hair loss.

*Other:* Vein inflammation of the lower extremities; palpitations (pounding in the chest); leg pain; abnormal blood counts; abnormal lab tests; general body discomfort.

---

## Guidelines for Use:

- Read the patient package insert before using.
- Dosage is individualized.
- Do not stop taking or change the dose unless advised to do so by your doctor.
- Take on an empty stomach at least 1 hour before or 2 hours after a meal or snack.
- If dose is missed, take it as soon as possible. If several hours have passed or if it is nearing time for the next dose, do not double the dose to catch up, unless advised to do so by your doctor. If more than one dose is missed, contact your doctor or pharmacist.
- Do not take iron tablets or multivitamins with minerals at the same time. Take between dose of *Lithostat*.
- Avoid alcoholic beverages. A rash commonly appears 30 to 45 minutes after drinking alcohol. It is associated with a general feeling of warmth and spontaneously disappears within 30 to 60 minutes.
- Contact your doctor if you experience tiredness, nausea, vomiting, rash, lower extremity pain, appetite loss, or fatigue.
- Lab tests may be required to monitor therapy. Be sure to keep appointments.
- Store at room temperature (59° to 86°F) in a dry place.

---

*If you have any questions, consult your doctor, pharmacist, or health care provider.*

| Generic Name<br>*Brand Name Examples* | Supplied As | Generic<br>Available |
|---|---|---|
| Rx **Potassium Acid Phosphate** | | |
| *K-Phos Original* | **Tablets:** 500 mg | No |
| Rx **Potassium Acid Phosphate and Sodium Acid Phosphate** | | |
| *K-Phos M.F.* | **Tablets:** 155 mg potassium acid bphosphate and 350 mg sodium acid phosphate | No |
| *K-Phos No. 2* | **Tablets:** 305 mg potassium acid phosphate and 700 mg sodium acid phosphate | No |

Although controversy exists regarding the effectiveness of ascorbic acid as a urinary acidifier, it is often used for this purpose. For more information on ascorbic acid, see the Vitamin C (Ascorbic Acid) monograph in the Nutritionals chapter.

## Type of Drug:
Urinary tract acidifiers.

## How the Drug Works:
Urinary tract acidifiers increase the amount of acid in the urine. This lowers the pH of the urine.

## Uses:
Makes the urine more acid and therefore less likely to support the growth of some bacteria. Also helps calcium dissolve in the urine, thereby reducing the risk of calcium stone formation. Increases the effect of the urinary tract anti-infective methenamine. Reduces odor and skin irritation caused by urine with high ammonia concentrations.

## Precautions:
*Do not use in the following situations:*

increased blood phosphate levels

increased blood potassium levels

infected phosphate stones

kidney disease, severe

*Use with caution in the following situations:*

Addison disease

dehydration

edema (fluid retention), body or lungs (sodium acid phosphate only)

heart disease (eg, heart failure)

high blood pressure (sodium acid phosphate only)

hypoparathyroidism (decreased function)

kidney disease, mild-to-moderate

liver disease (eg, cirrhosis)

pancreas, inflamed

rickets (vitamin D deficiency)

sodium in the blood, increased (sodium acid phosphate only)

sodium-restricted diet (sodium acid phosphate only)

tissue breakdown, extensive (eg, burns)

toxemia of pregnancy (sodium acid phosphate only)

*Kidney stones:* Patients with kidney stones may pass old stones when therapy is started.

*Antacids:* Avoid antacids which contain aluminum, calcium, or magnesium. These ingredients may prevent phosphate absorption.

*Potassium supplements:* Consider the potassium content of urinary acidifiers if potassium supplements, salt substitutes, or potassium sparing diuretics are being used. Potassium levels should be monitored in these situations.

*Pregnancy:* Adequate studies have not been done in pregnant women. Use only if clearly needed and potential benefits outweigh the possible hazards to the fetus.

*Breastfeeding:* It is not known if urinary acidifiers appear in breast milk. Consult your doctor before you begin breastfeeding.

*Lab tests* may be required during treatment with urinary acidifiers. Tests may include: Liver and kidney function tests; blood electrolyte (sodium, potassium, phosphorus, calcium) levels.

## Drug Interactions:

Tell your doctor or pharmacist if you are taking or if you are planning to take any over-the-counter or prescription medications or dietary supplements with urinary acidifiers. Doses of one or both drugs may need to be modified or a different drug may need to be prescribed. The following drugs and drug classes interact with urinary acidifiers:

aluminum-, calcium-, or magnesium-containing antacids (eg, *Maalox*)

amiloride *(Midamor)*

corticosteroids (eg, prednisone)

corticotropin (eg, *Acthar*)

diazoxide (eg, *Proglycem*)

guanethidine (eg, *Ismelin*)

hydralazine (eg, *Apresoline*)

methyldopa (eg, *Aldomet*)

potassium supplements

reserpine (eg, *Serpasil*)

salicylates (eg, aspirin)

salt substitutes (eg, *Morton Salt Substitute*)

spironolactone (eg, *Aldactone*)

triamterene (*Dyrenium*)

## Side Effects:

Every drug is capable of producing side effects. Many urinary acidifier users experience no, or minor, side effects. The frequency and severity of side effects depend on many factors including dose, duration of therapy, and individual susceptibility. Possible side effects include:

*Digestive Tract:* Stomach pain; nausea; vomiting; diarrhea.

*Nervous System:* Confusion; seizures; unusual tiredness; dizziness; headache.

*Circulatory System:* Fast or irregular heartbeat.

*Respiratory System:* Shortness of breath; difficulty breathing.

*Other:* Weakness or heaviness of legs; muscle cramps; numbness, tingling, pain or weakness in hands or feet; numbness or tingling around lips; swelling of feet or legs; low urine output; unusual thirst; bone or joint pain; weight gain; edema (fluid retention).

---

### Guidelines for Use:

- Do not change the dose or stop taking this medicine unless advised to do so by your doctor.
- If a dose is missed, take it as soon as possible. If several hours have passed or if it is nearing time for the next dose, do not double the dose in order to catch up, unless advised to do so by your doctor. If more than one dose is missed or it is necessary to establish a new dosage schedule, contact your doctor or pharmacist.
- *Potassium Acid Phosphate and Sodium Acid Phosphate Tablets* — Take each dose with a full glass of water.
- *Potassium Acid Phosphate Tablets* — Dissolve prescribed number of tablets in a full glass of water before taking. Let tablets soak for 2 to 5 minutes. You may crush and stir the tablets to speed the dissolving time.
- Notify your doctor if stomach pain, nausea or vomiting, heart irregularities, or edema (fluid retention) occurs.
- Avoid antacids containing aluminum, calcium, or magnesium.
- Some patients experience a mild laxative effect. If this effect persists, contact your doctor.
- Inform your doctor if you are pregnant, become pregnant, are planning to become pregnant, or are breastfeeding.
- Lab tests may be required during therapy. Be sure to keep appointments.
- Store at controlled room temperature (59° to 86°F).

---

*If you have any questions, consult your doctor, pharmacist, or health care provider.*

| Generic Name<br>*Brand Name Examples* | Supplied As | Generic<br>Available |
|---|---|---|
| Rx **Potassium Citrate** | | |
| *Urocit-K* | **Tablets:** 5 mEq, 10 mEq | No |
| Rx **Potassium Citrate Combinations** | | |
| *Polycitra-LC* | **Solution:** 550 mg potassium citrate, 500 mg sodium citrate and 334 mg citric acid/5 mL | No |
| *Polycitra-K* | **Solution:** 1100 mg potassium citrate and 334 mg citric acid/ 5 mL | No |
| otc **Sodium Bicarbonate** | **Tablets:** 650 mg | Yes |
| | **Powder** | Yes |
| Rx **Sodium Citrate and Citric Acid (Shohl's Solution, Modified)** | | |
| *Bicitra* | **Solution:** 500 mg sodium citrate and 334 mg citric acid/ 5 mL | No |
| *Oracit* | **Solution**: 490 mg sodium citrate and 640 mg citric acid/ 5 mL | No |

## Type of Drug:

Urinary alkalinizer.

## How the Drug Works:

Urinary alkalinizers make the urine less acidic (alkaline). This may help dissolve certain types of kidney stones and enhance the elimination of certain acidic drugs and other substances in the urine.

## Uses:

To correct acid urine and systemic acidosis (excessive acid in the blood) due to disorders of the kidney tubules (renal tubular acidosis).

To limit the formation of uric acid crystals in the urine during the treatment of gout.

To help dissolve some types of kidney stones.

To alter the kidneys' elimination of certain medications.

## Precautions:

*Do not use in the following situations:*

Addison disease, untreated
adrenal insufficiency
allergy to urinary alkalinizers or
any of their ingredients
anticholinergic drug therapy,
concurrent
dehydration, acute
delayed stomach emptying
(potassium citrate tablets only)
diabetes mellitus, uncontrolled
diuretic therapy, concurrent
esophageal compression (potassium citrate tablets only)
heart damage, severe
heat cramps
hyperkalemia (high blood potassium levels)
intestinal obstruction or stricture
(potassium citrate tablets only)
kidney disease, severe
kidney failure, chronic (potassium products only)
peptic ulcer (potassium citrate
tablets only)
strenuous physical exercise in
unconditioned patients
tissue breakdown, extensive
(eg, severe trauma)
urinary tract infection

*Use with caution in the following situations:*

congestive heart failure (sodium
products only)
disorders which cause swelling
(sodium products only)
high blood pressure (sodium
products only)
kidney disease
low urine output
sodium-restricted diet (sodium
products only)
toxemia of pregnancy (sodium
products only)

*Pregnancy:* There are no adequate and well-controlled studies in pregnant women. Use only if clearly needed and the potential benefits to
the mother outweigh the possible risks to the fetus.

*Breastfeeding:* It is not known if urinary alkalinizers appear in breast milk.
Consult your doctor before you begin breastfeeding.

*Children:* Safety and effectiveness of potassium citrate tablets in children
have not been established.

*Lab tests* may be required to monitor therapy. Tests may include serum
potassium determinations and acid-base determinations.

## Drug Interactions:

Tell your doctor or pharmacist if you are taking or if you are planning to
take any over-the-counter or prescription medications or dietary
supplements with urinary alkalinizers. Doses of one or both drugs may
need to be modified or a different drug may need to be prescribed. The
following drugs and drug classes interact with urinary alkalinizers:

ACE inhibitors (eg, captopril)
aluminum-based antacids
(eg, *Amphojel*)
anorexiants (eg, amphetamine)
anticholinergic drugs
(eg, atropine) (potassium citrate tablets only)
chlorpropamide (eg, diabenese)
lithium (eg, *Eskalith*)
potassium-sparing diuretics
(eg, amiloride, triamterene)
salicylates (eg, aspirin)
sympathomimetics (eg, pseudoephedrine)
tetracyclines (eg, doxycycline)

## Side Effects:

Every drug is capable of producing side effects. Many urinary alkalinizer users experience no, or minor, side effects. The frequency and severity of side effects depend on many factors including dose, duration of therapy, and individual susceptibility. Possible side effects include:

*Digestive Tract:* Stomach discomfort; vomiting; diarrhea; loose stools; nausea.

*Other:* Edema (fluid retention) (sodium products); gas; sour taste (citrate products); high blood pressure (sodium products).

---

### Guidelines for Use:

- Dosage will be individualized.
- Do not change the dose or stop taking unless advised to do so by your doctor.
- Take with or after meals or a snack to avoid stomach discomfort.
- If a dose is missed, take it as soon as possible. If several hours have passed or if it is nearing time for the next dose, do not double the dose in order to catch up, unless advised to do so by your doctor. If several doses are missed, or it is necessary to establish a new dosage schedule, contact your doctor or pharmacist.
- *Potassium citrate tablets* — Stop taking and notify your doctor if you experience severe vomiting, severe stomach pain, vomiting of blood, or dark, tarry stools.
  Do not crush, chew, or suck on the tablet. Swallow whole.
  Following the release of the potassium citrate, the wax matrix of the tablet, which is not absorbable, is excreted in the stool. This is normal and no cause for concern.
- *Solutions* — Dilute with water; follow with more water, if desired. Refrigerate to mask taste.
- *Tablets* — Talk to you doctor if you have trouble swallowing the tablets or they seem to stick in your throat.
- *Sodium bicarbonate* — Dissolve each dose in a glass of water. Do not take until completely dissolved in water. Do not take if you are overly full from food or drink.
- Lab tests may be required to monitor therapy. Be sure to keep appointments.
- Store at controlled room temperature (59° to 86°F).

---

*If you have any questions, consult your doctor, pharmacist, or health care provider.*

| Generic Name<br>*Brand Name Examples* | Supplied As | Generic<br>Available |
|---|---|---|
| *Rx* **Bethanechol Chloride** | | |
| *Urecholine* | **Tablets:** 5 mg, 10 mg, 25 mg, 50 mg | Yes |
| *Urecholine* | **Injection:** 5 mg/mL | No |

## Type of Drug:

Cholinergic stimulant; bladder stimulant.

## How the Drug Works:

Bethanechol chloride stimulates the muscles in the bladder to contract, which causes urination. It also stimlates digestive tract movement.

## Uses:

To treat urinary retention (incomplete emptying of the bladder) after surgery or childbirth or due to neurogenic atony (nerve damage).

*Unlabeled Use(s):* Occasionally doctors may prescribe bethanechol for reflux esophagitis in adults and for gastroesophageal reflux in infants and children.

## Precautions:

*Do not use in the following situations:*

allergy to bethanechol chloride
  or any of its ingredients
bladder obstruction
bladder surgery, recent
bronchial asthma, latent or
  active
coronary artery disease
digestive tract obstruction
digestive tract lesions, acute
epilepsy

intestinal surgery, recent
low blood pressure
overactive thyroid
Parkinson's disease
peptic ulcer
peritonitis
slow heart rate
spastic digestive tract disorders
vagotonia, marked
vasomotor instability

*Use with caution in the following situations:* Bladder infection.

*Pregnancy:* There are no adequate and well-controlled studies in pregnant women. Use only if clearly needed and potential benefits to the mother outweigh the possible hazards to the fetus.

*Breastfeeding:* It is not known if bethanechol appears in breast milk. Consult your doctor before you begin breastfeeding.

*Children:* Safety and effectiveness in children have not been established.

## Drug Interactions:

Tell your doctor or pharmacist if you are taking or if you are planning to take any over-the-counter or prescription medications or dietary supplements with bethanechol. Doses of one or both drugs may need to be modified or a different drug may need to be prescribed. The following drugs and drug classes interact with bethanechol:

> cholinergic drugs (eg, ambenonium)
> ganglion-blocking compounds
> procainamide (eg, *Pronestyl*)
> quinidine (eg, *Cin-Quin*)

## Side Effects:

Every drug is capable of producing side effects. Many bethanechol users experience no, or minor, side effects. The frequency and severity of side effects depend on many factors including dose, duration of therapy, and individual susceptibility. Possible side effects include:

*Digestive Tract:* Belching; diarrhea; stomach pain, cramps, or discomfort; rumbling stomach; nausea; abnormal salivation.

*Respiratory System:* Asthma attack; difficulty breathing.

*Other:* General body discomfort; urinary urgency; headache; fall in blood pressure with fast heart rate; sweating; flushing producing a feeling of warmth; facial warmth; visual disturbances; tearing of eyes; change in pupil size.

---

### Guidelines for Use:

- Dosage is individualized.
- Do not stop taking or change the dose unless advised to do so by your doctor.
- Take tablets on an empty stomach at least 1 hour before or 2 hours after meals to avoid nausea or vomiting.
- If a dose is missed, take it as soon as possible. If several hours have passed or if it is nearing time for the next dose, do not double the dose in order to catch up, unless advised to do so by your doctor. If several doses are missed, or it is necessary to establish a new dosage schedule, contact your doctor or pharmacist.
- Injection is for subcutaneous (SC) (beneath the skin) administration only. It will be prepared and administered by your health care provider in a medical setting.
- May cause increased salivation, sweating, flushing, or stomach ache. Notify your doctor if these symptoms persist or become severe.
- May cause dizziness, lightheadedness, or fainting, especially when rising from a seated or lying position.
- Store tablets at controlled room temperature (59° to 86°F).

---

*If you have any questions, consult your doctor, pharmacist, or health care provider.*

| Generic Name<br>*Brand Name Example* | Supplied As | Generic<br>Available |
|---|---|---|
| Rx **Cellulose Sodium Phosphate** | | |
| *Calcibind* | **Powder** | No |

## Type of Drug:
Urinary tract product.

## How the Drug Works:
Cellulose sodium phosphate alters the levels of calcium, magnesium, phosphate, and oxalate in the urine. Urine phosphate and oxalate levels increase. Urine calcium and magnesium levels decrease. Lowering of calcium in the urine leads to decreased formation of calcium-containing kidney stones.

## Uses:
To reduce the formation of calcium containing kidney stones in absorptive hypercalciuria Type I (excess calcium levels in the urine).

## Precautions:
*Do not use in the following situations:*
   allergy to cellulose sodium phosphate or any of its ingredients
   calcium levels in blood or urine, decreased
   hyperparathyroidism (overactive parathyroid)
   increased urine calcium levels other than absorptive hyper calciuria Type I
   magnesium levels, decreased in blood
   osteomalacia (softening of bone)
   osteitis (inflammation of bone)
   osteoporosis (brittle bones)
   oxalic acid or oxalates, increased in urine
   phosphate levels, decreased in blood

*Use with caution in the following situations:*
   ascites (fluid in the abdominal cavity)
   congestive heart failure

*Pregnancy:* Adequate studies have not been done in pregnant women. Because of the increased dietary calcium requirement in pregnant women, use only when clearly needed and potential benefits to the mother outweigh possible hazards to the fetus.

*Breastfeeding:* It is not known if cellulose sodium appears in breast milk. Consult your doctor before you begin breastfeeding.

*Children:* Because of the increased requirement for dietary calcium in growing children, use in children under 16 years of age is not recommended.

*Lab tests* will be required to monitor therapy. Tests may include blood levels of calcium, magnesium, copper, zinc, iron and parathyroid hormone, and complete blood counts.

## Side Effects:

Every drug is capable of producing side effects. Many cellulose sodium phosphate users experience no, or minor, side effects. The frequency and severity of side effects depend on many factors including dose, duration of therapy, and individual susceptibility.

*Digestive Tract:* Diarrhea; indigestion; loose bowel movements; poor taste of the drug.

*Circulatory System:* Calcium and magnesium depletion; depletion of trace metals (ie, copper, zinc, iron).

## Guidelines for Use:

- Dosage is individualized and may be adjusted over time.
- Do not stop taking or change the dose of the drug unless advised to do so by your doctor.
- Dietary changes are recommended, including:
  Avoid dairy products and reduce intake of calcium from other sources.
  Restrict oxalate in the diet by avoiding spinach and other dark greens, rhubarb, chocolate, and brewed tea.
  Avoid vitamin C supplements.
  Reduce your sodium intake.
  Drink plenty of fluids.
- Dissolve prescribed amount of the powder for each dose in water, soft drinks, or fruit juices. Take within 30 minutes of a meal, but do not take at the same time as magnesium supplements (eg, magnesium gluconate).
- Lab tests will be required to monitor therapy. Be sure to keep appointments.
- Store in a dry place at room temperature (59° to 86°F).

*If you have any questions, consult your doctor, pharmacist, or health care provider.*

| Generic Name Brand Name Example | Supplied As | Generic Available |
|---|---|---|
| Rx **Cysteamine Bitartrate** | | |
| *Cystagon* | **Capsules:** 50 mg, 150 mg | No |

## Type of Drug:

Urinary tract product.

## How the Drug Works:

Cysteamine lowers the cystine content of cells in patients with cystinosis.

## Uses:

To manage nephropathic cystinosis (a rare, serious kidney disease) in children and adults. This disease may cause kidney failure, other organ damage or growth reduction in children.

## Precautions:

*Do not use in the following situations:*
allergy to cysteamine or penicillamine (eg, *Cuprimine*)

*Use with caution in the following situations:*

| | |
|---|---|
| depression | neurologic problems |
| drowsiness | rash |
| lethargy | seizures |
| liver, digestive or blood disorders | |

*Rash:* Do not begin or continue use if a skin rash is present.

*Pregnancy:* Adequate studies have not been done in pregnant women. Use only if clearly needed and potential benefits outweigh the possible hazards to the fetus.

*Breastfeeding:* It is not known if cysteamine appears in breast milk. Consult your doctor before you begin breastfeeding.

*Children:* Cysteamine is a safe and effective drug for use in children once nephropathic cystinosis is diagnosed.

*Lab tests:* Cysteamine may cause abnormal blood counts (low white blood cells) and abnormal liver function tests. Lab tests will be required to monitor therapy.

## Side Effects:

Every drug is capable of producing side effects. Many cysteamine users experience no, or minor, side effects. The frequency and severity of side effects depend on many factors including dose, duration of therapy and individual susceptibility. Possible side effects include:

*Digestive Tract:* Vomiting; diarrhea; constipation; appetite loss; nausea; bad breath; stomach ache; indigestion.

*Nervous System:* Fever; tiredness; weakness; drowsiness; headache; convulsions; seizures; incoordination; confusion; tremor; impaired hearing; dizziness; jitteriness; abnormal dreams; lightheadedness; nervousness; abnormal thinking; depression; emotional instability; hallucinations.

*Skin:* Rash; hives.

*Other:* Dehydration; flushing; abnormal blood counts; abnormal liver function tests.

---

### Guidelines for Use:

- Take in 4 divided doses about 6 hours apart, or as directed by your doctor.
- Young children may not be able to swallow the capsules. Contents of the capsules should be sprinkled over food or mixed in formula for children under 6 years of age. Other patients should follow their doctor's instructions with regard to food.
- Do not increase or decrease this medication without your doctor's approval.
- Upset stomach and indigestion are common side effects. If these are severe or become a nuisance, contact your doctor.
- If a dose is missed, take it as soon as possible. If several hours have passed or if it is nearing time for the next dose, do not double the dose to catch up (unless advised to do so by your doctor). If more than one dose is missed or if it is necessary to establish a new dosage schedule, contact your doctor or pharmacist. Use exactly as prescribed.
- If a skin rash develops, discontinue use of this medicine and contact your doctor immediately.
- Notify your doctor if any of the following occurs: fever; seizures; weakness; tiredness; drowsiness; incoordination; difficulty breathing; strange behavior; unusual thinking or emotions, depression; nausea; diarrhea; vomiting; appetite loss; abdominal pain.
- May cause drowsiness, dizziness or confusion. Avoid driving or performing other tasks requiring alertness or coordination until effects are known, then use caution.
- Lab tests will be required every 3 months. Tests will include: liver function tests and complete blood counts. Be sure to keep appointments.
- Store in a dry, safe place away from light and the reach of children.

---

*If you have any questions, consult your doctor, pharmacist, or health care provider.*

| Generic Name<br>*Brand Name Example* | **Supplied As** | Generic<br>Available |
|---|---|---|
| *Rx* **Dimethyl Sulfoxide<br>(DMSO)** | | |
| *Rimso-50* | **Solution, aqueous:** 50% | No |

Dimethyl sulfoxide (DMSO) is available in a variety of forms not intended for human use (eg, veterinary and industrial solvents). Human use of such products should be discouraged because of their unknown purity. Because of its skin transport characteristics, impurities and contaminants may be systemically absorbed from topical use.

## Type of Drug:
Local anti-inflammatory agent.

## How the Drug Works:
DMSO has a broad range of pharmacological properties that include: Anti-inflammatory action, nerve blockade, diuresis, cholinesterase inhibition, vasodilation and muscle relaxation.

## Uses:
For symptomatic relief of bladder inflammation.

There is no clinical evidence of effectiveness for treatment of bacterial urinary tract infections.

*Unlabeled Use(s):* DMSO has been used in the topical treatment of a wide variety of musculoskeletal disorders and collagen diseases and to enhance the absorption of other drugs through the skin. Such unlabeled uses, as well as many others, have not been approved by the FDA.

## Precautions:
*Allergic reaction:* DMSO can cause an allergic reaction. Consult your doctor.

*Pregnancy:* Adequate studies have not been done in pregnant women. Use only if clearly needed and potential benefits outweigh the possible hazards to the fetus.

*Breastfeeding:* It is not known if DMSO appears in breast milk, but presence is likely. Consult your doctor before you begin breastfeeding.

*Children:* Safety and effectiveness have not been established.

*Lab tests* will be required at least every 6 months during treatment with DMSO. Tests may include: Liver and kidney function tests, full eye exams and complete blood counts.

## Drug Interactions:
Tell your doctor or pharmacist if you are taking or if you are planning to take any over-the-counter or prescription medications or dietary supplements with DMSO. Doses of one or both drugs may need to be modified or a different drug may need to be prescribed.

Sulindac *(Clinoril)* interacts with DMSO.

## Side Effects:

Every drug is capable of producing side effects. Many DMSO users experience no, or minor, side effects. The frequency and severity of side effects depend on many factors including dose, duration of therapy and individual susceptibility. Possible side effects include:

*Topical Use:* Garlic-like taste and odor on breath and skin; dermatitis; sedation; nausea; vomiting; headache; burning or aching eyes.

*Other:* Inflamed bladder.

---

### Guidelines for Use:

- Caution — Use of veterinary and industrial forms of this drug is not recommended because of unknown purity.
- A garlic-like taste, breath and odor on skin may develop within a few minutes of use. The taste may linger for several hours. Odor on the breath and skin may be present for up to 72 hours.
- Obtain a complete eye exam before and during treatment with this drug.
- Lab tests will be required every 6 months. Tests will include: Liver and kidney function tests and complete blood counts.

---

*If you have any questions, consult your doctor, pharmacist, or health care provider.*

| Generic Name<br>*Brand Name Example* | Supplied As | Generic<br>Available |
|---|---|---|
| *Rx* **Flavoxate HCl** | | |
| *Urispas* | **Tablets:** 100 mg | No |

## Type of Drug:
Urinary tract antispasmodic.

## How the Drug Works:
Flavoxate relieves smooth muscle spasm of the urinary tract. It aids in the retention of urine and has local anesthetic and pain-relieving properties.

## Uses:
For relief of painful urination, frequency, urgency, nighttime urination, incontinence and pain associated with urinary tract disorders. It is not a definitive treatment, but is compatible with other urinary tract drugs.

## Precautions:
*Do not use in the following situations:*

achalasia (failure of certain sphincter muscles to relax)
bleeding of digestive tract
intestinal obstruction
stomach obstruction
urinary tract obstruction

*Use with caution in the following situations:* glaucoma

*Pregnancy:* Adequate studies have not been done in pregnant women. Use only if clearly needed and potential benefits outweigh the possible hazards to the fetus.

*Breastfeeding:* It is not known if flavoxate appears in breast milk. Consult your doctor before you begin breastfeeding.

*Children:* Safety and effectiveness in children under 12 have not been established.

## Side Effects:
Every drug is capable of producing side effects. Many flavoxate users experience no, or minor, side effects. The frequency and severity of side effects depend on many factors including dose, duration of therapy and individual susceptibility. Possible side effects include:

*Digestive Tract:* Nausea; vomiting.

*Nervous System:* Nervousness; vertigo (feeling of whirling motion); headache; drowsiness; confusion.

*Other:* Dry mouth; high fever; painful or difficult urination; increased heart rate; palpitations (pounding in the chest); vision problems (eg, blurred vision); hives; skin disorders; abnormal blood counts.

## Guidelines for Use:

- May cause drowsiness or blurred vision. Use caution while driving or performing other tasks requiring alertness, coordination or physical dexterity.
- May cause dry mouth, hives and rash. If these or other side effects persist or worsen, contact your doctor.

*If you have any questions, consult your doctor, pharmacist, or health care provider.*

| Generic Name<br>*Brand Name Examples* | Supplied As | Generic Available |
|---|---|---|
| Rx **Oxybutynin Chloride** | | |
| *Ditropan* | **Tablets:** 5 mg | Yes |
| *Ditropan* | **Syrup:** 5 mg/5 mL | Yes |

## Type of Drug:

Urinary tract antispasmodic.

## How the Drug Works:

Oxybutynin chloride reduces muscle spasms of the bladder by exerting direct relaxing effects on the muscle around the bladder and inhibiting the effect of chemicals which can cause bladder spasm.

## Uses:

For symptomatic relief of certain bladder conditions, such as frequent or painful urination, urge, incontinence, and urinary leakage.

## Precautions:

*Do not use in the following situations:*

glaucoma, angle-closure
intestinal weakness, elderly or debilitated
intestinal tract problems, paralyzed, obstructed, or inflammed
megacolon (dilated or enlarged colon)
myasthenia gravis
urinary tract obstruction
unstable blood pressure from blood loss

*Use with caution in the following situations:*

autonomic nervous system disorders
congestive heart failure
coronary artery disease
diarrhea
elderly
hiatal hernia
high blood pressure
hot weather
hyperthyroidism
ileostomy or colostomy
increased heart rate
irregular heartbeat
kidney disease
liver disease
prostate, enlarged
sweating, decreased
ulcerative colitis

*Hot weather:* Oxbutynin can cause heat prostration (fever and heatstroke) due to decreased sweating.

*Diarrhea:* Diarrhea may be a sign of partial intestinal obstruction especially in ileostomy or colostomy patients. If diarrhea is severe, discontinue use and contact your doctor.

*Pregnancy:* Adequate studies have not been done in pregnant women. Use only if clearly needed and potential benefits outweigh the possible hazards to the fetus.

*Breastfeeding:* It is not known if oxybutynin appears in breast milk. Consult your doctor before you begin breastfeeding.

*Children:* Safety and effectiveness in children under 5 years old have not been established.

## Drug Interactions:

Tell your doctor or pharmacist if you are taking or if you are planning to take any over-the-counter or prescription medications or dietary supplements with oxybutynin. Doses of one or both drugs may need to be modified or a different drug may need to be prescribed. The following drugs and drug classes interact with oxybutynin.

digoxin (eg, *Lanoxin)*
haloperidol (eg, *Haldol)*
phenothiazines (eg, promethazine)
atenolol (eg, *Tenormin)*
acetaminophen (eg, *Tylenol)*
levodopa (eg, *Larodopa)*
nitrofurantoin (eg, *Macrodantin)*
amantadine (eg, *Symmetrel)*

## Side Effects:

Every drug is capable of producing side effects. Many oxybutynin users experience no, or minor, side effects. The frequency and severity of side effects depend on many factors including dose, duration of therapy and individual susceptibility. Possible side effects include:

*Digestive Tract:* Nausea; vomiting; constipation.

*Nervous System:* Dizziness; sleeplessness; weakness; restlessness; drowsiness; hallucinations.

*Circulatory System:* Palpitations (pounding in the chest); rapid heart rate; flushing.

*Other:* Difficulty or inability to urinate; impotence; decreased tearing of eyes; vision problems; suppression of breast milk production; decreased sweating; dry mouth; rash; dilated pupils; fever; vision problems.

---

### Guidelines for Use:

- Usual adult dose is 1 tablet 2 or 3 times per day. Adjust dosage to control symptoms.
- If a dose is missed, take it as soon as possible. If several hours have passed or if it is nearing time for the next dose, do not double the dose to catch up (unless advised by your doctor). If more than 1 dose is missed, contact your doctor or pharmacist.
- May cause drowsiness or blurred vision. Alcohol or sedatives may enhance these effects. Use caution when driving or performing other tasks requiring alertness, coordination, or physical dexterity until tolerance is determined.
- May cause dry mouth. If this or other side effects, especially diarrhea, persist or worsen, contact your doctor.
- Use caution in hot weather.
- Store at room temperature.

---

*If you have any questions, consult your doctor, pharmacist, or health care provider.*

| Generic Name<br>*Brand Name Example* | Supplied As | Generic<br>Available |
|---|---|---|
| *Rx* **Tolterodine Tartrate** | | |
| *Detrol* | **Tablets:** 1 mg, 2 mg | No |

## Type of Drug:
Bladder muscle relaxant.

## How the Drug Works:
Tolterodine acts on the muscles of the bladder, decreasing the pressures and urge to empty the bladder.

## Uses:
For the treatment of patients with an overactive bladder with the symptoms of urinary frequency, urgency, and urinary incontinence.

## Precautions:
*Do not use in the following situations:*

allergy to tolterodine
digestive tract obstruction
narrow-angle glaucoma, uncontrolled
urinary retention

*Use with caution in the following situations:*

bladder outflow obstruction
gastrointestinal obstructive disorders (pyloric stenosis)
kidney function, reduced
liver function, reduced
narrow-angle glaucoma, controlled

*Pregnancy:* There are no studies of tolterodine in pregnant women. Use only if the potential benefit justifies the potential risk to the fetus.

*Breastfeeding:* It is not known if tolterodine appears in breast milk. Therefore, tolterodine should be discontinued during breastfeeding.

*Children:* Safety and effectiveness in children have not been established.

## Drug Interactions:
Tell your doctor or pharmacist if you are taking or if you are planning to take any over-the-counter or prescription medications or dietary supplements with tolterodine. Doses of one or both drugs may need to be modified or a different drug may need to be prescribed. The following drugs and drug classes interact with tolterodine.

azole antifungal agents (eg, ketoconazole, itraconazole, miconazole)
fluoxetine
macrolide antibiotics (eg, erythromycin, clarithromycin)

## Side Effects:

*Nervous System:* Abnormal skin sensations; dizziness; drowsiness; feeling of whirling motion; nervousness; headache.

*Digestive Tract:* Abdominal pain; constipation; diarrhea; gas; indigestion; nausea; vomiting.

*Respiratory System:* Bronchitis; coughing; sore throat; upper respiratory tract infection; runny nose.

*Urinary and Reproductive Tract:* Painful, difficult, or frequent urination; urine retention; urination disorders; urinary tract infection.

*Other:* Dry mouth; dry skin; back, chest, and joint pain; fatigue; flu-like symptoms; falling; itching; rash; skin flushing or redness; abnormal vision; dry eyes; night blindness; weight gain; high blood pressure; infection; blurred vision.

---

### Guidelines for Use:

- The recommended dose is 2 mg twice daily but it can be lowered to 1 mg twice daily based on individual need.
- For patients with reduced liver function or for those taking macrolide antibiotics or azole antifungal agents, the recommended dose is 1 mg twice daily.
- May cause dry mouth. If this or other side effects persist or worsen, contact your doctor.
- May cause drowsiness or blurred vision. Use caution while driving or performing other tasks that require alertness until tolerance is determined.
- Store at controlled room temperature (68° to 77°F).

---

*If you have any questions, consult your doctor, pharmacist, or health care provider.*

| Generic Name<br>*Brand Name Examples* | Supplied As | Generic<br>Available |
|---|---|---|
| **Phenazopyridine HCl** | | |
| *otc Azo-Standard, Azo-<br>Gesic, Uristat* | **Tablets:** 95 mg | No |
| *otc Baridium, ReAzo* | **Tablets:** 97 mg | No |
| *Rx Pyridium, Urogesic* | **Tablets:** 100 mg, 200 mg | Yes |

For more information on urinary tract combinations containing phenazo-pyridine, see Urinary Anti-Infective Combinations in the Anti-Infectives chapter.

## Type of Drug:

Urinary tract pain reliever.

## How the Drug Works:

Phenazopyridine exerts a local analgesic (pain-relieving) action on the inner lining of the urinary tract. It relieves symptoms of pain, burning, urgency, and frequency only. It does not treat the cause of the pain (eg, infection).

## Uses:

For symptomatic relief of pain, burning, urgency, frequent urination, and other discomforts due to irritation of the lower urinary tract.

## Precautions:

*Do not use in the following situations:*
> allergy to phenazopyridine
> kidney function, reduced
> liver disease

*Urinary tract infection:* Treatment of the discomforting symptoms of a lower urinary tract infection with phenazopyridine should not exceed 2 days.

*Kidney/liver dysfunction:* Yellowing of skin or eyes may indicate accumulation of the drug due to impaired kidney or liver function. The drug may need to be discontinued. Consult your doctor.

*Pregnancy:* Adequate studies have not been done in pregnant women. Use only if clearly needed and potential benefits outweigh the possible hazards to the fetus.

*Breastfeeding:* It is not known if phenazopyridine appears in breast milk. Consult your doctor before you begin breastfeeding.

*Children:* Phenazopyridine should not be given to children under 12 years of age unless prescribed by your doctor.

*Lab tests:* Phenazopyridine may interfere with some urine tests for sugar and ketones.

## Side Effects:

Every drug is capable of producing side effects. Many phenazopyridine users experience no, or minor, side effects. The frequency and severity of side effects depend on many factors including dose, duration of therapy, and individual susceptibility. Possible side effects include: Stomach upset; headache; rash; itching; blue lips and fingertips; anemia; liver and kidney damage; fever; staining of contact lenses.

## Guidelines for Use:

- Take exactly as prescribed or as the package labeling directs (OTC products).
- May cause stomach upset. Take with or after meals to decrease irritation.
- May cause urine to turn reddish orange. This is not harmful but may stain bedding or undergarments. Staining of contact lenses may occur.
- Treatment of urinary tract pain associated with a urinary tract infection should not exceed 2 days.
- Notify your doctor if any of the following occurs: Symptoms persist for more than 2 days or get worse; fever; chills; back pain; bloody urine.
- This medicine can interfere with lab tests including urine tests for sugar and ketones.
- Provides symptom (eg, pain, burning, urgency, frequency) relief only; it does not treat the cause of the symptoms (eg, infection).
- Store at room temperature.

*OTC drugs —*
- If symptoms persist for more than 5 days, contact your doctor.
- Do not give OTC drugs to children under 12 years of age unless instructed by your doctor.
- Do not use if you have liver or kidney problems unless instructed by your doctor.

*If you have any questions, consult your doctor, pharmacist, or health care provider.*

| Generic Name<br>*Brand Name Example* | Supplied As | Generic<br>Available |
|---|---|---|
| *Rx* **Azathioprine**[1] | | |
| *Imuran* | **Tablets:** 50 mg | No |

[1] This product is also available as an injection.

## Type of Drug:

Drug used to suppress the immune system.

## How the Drug Works:

The exact mechanism is not known. Azathioprine alters the immune response in the body, alters the production of antibodies and, in some instances, reduces inflammation.

## Uses:

To prevent rejection of kidney transplants.

To treat severe rheumatoid arthritis that does not respond to other therapies.

*Unlabeled Use(s):* Occasionally doctors may prescribe azathioprine for treatment of chronic ulcerative colitis and generalized myasthenia gravis. However, serious side effects may offset any benefits the drug may offer. It also may be prescribed for controlling Behcet syndrome, especially eye disease. It may be effective in treating Crohn disease.

## Precautions:

*Do not use in the following situations:*
    allergy to azathioprine
    pregnant rheumatoid arthritis patients

*Serious infections* are a constant hazard for patients on chronic immuno-suppression, especially transplant recipients. Fungal, viral, bacterial and protozoal infections may be fatal and should be treated vigorously. Infection may occur as a result of bone marrow suppression or decreased white-cell counts. Azathioprine dose may have to be reduced or other drugs used.

*Chronic use:* Long-term use of azathioprine may increase the risk of developing tumors. Consult your doctor.

*Pregnancy:* Studies have shown a potential effect to the fetus. Use only if clearly needed and potential benefits outweigh the possible risks. Do not give to pregnant rheumatoid arthritis patients.

*Breastfeeding:* Azathioprine or its metabolites appear in breast milk. Use of azathioprine in nursing mothers is not recommended. Consult your doctor before you begin breastfeeding.

*Children:* Safety and efficacy in children have not been established. However, it has been used in children.

*Lab tests* will be required during treatment with azathioprine. Tests may include: Complete blood and platelet counts to monitor for blood disorders; liver function tests; and cultures to check for infections.

## Drug Interactions:

Tell your doctor or pharmacist if you are taking or if you are planning to take any over-the-counter or prescription medications or dietary supplements while taking this medicine. Doses of one or both drugs may need to be modified or a different drug may need to be prescribed. The following drugs and drug classes interact with azathioprine.

ACE inhibitors (eg, captopril)
allopurinol (eg, *Zyloprim)*
anticoagulants (eg, warfarin)
sulfamethoxazole/trimethoprim (eg, *Bactrim)*

cyclosporine (eg, *Sandimmune)*
nondepolarizing neuromuscular blockers (eg, rocuronium bromide)
methotrexate (eg, *Folex PFS)*

## Side Effects:

Every drug is capable of producing side effects. Most patients experience side effects. The frequency and severity of side effects depend on many factors including dose, duration of therapy and individual susceptibility. Possible side effects include:

*Digestive Tract:* Nausea; vomiting; diarrhea.

*Other:* Rash; fever; general body discomfort; muscle pain; infection; tumors; abnormal blood counts.

---

## Guidelines for Use:

- Take exactly as prescribed.
- If stomach upset occurs, take in divided doses or with food.
- If a dose is missed, take it as soon as possible. If several hours have passed or if it is nearing time for the next dose, do not double the dose in order to catch up (unless advised to do so by your doctor). If more than one dose is missed or it is necessary to establish a new dosage schedule, contact your doctor or pharmacist.
- Notify your doctor if any of the following occurs: Unusual bleeding or bruising, fever, sore throat, mouth sores, signs of infection, stomach pain, pale stools or darkened urine.
- May cause nausea, vomiting, rash, fever, muscle pain and diarrhea. Notify your doctor if these persist or become bothersome.
- Contraceptive measures (birth control) are recommended during treatment to avoid birth defects. Inform your doctor if you are pregnant, become pregnant, are planning to become pregnant or if you are breast-feeding.
- Lab tests will be required to monitor therapy. Be sure to keep appointments.
- Visually inspect injection solution for particles or discoloration before use.
- Store at room temperature (59° to 77°F), away from moisture and light.

---

*If you have any questions, consult your doctor, pharmacist, or health care provider.*

| Generic Name<br>*Brand Name Examples* | Supplied As | Generic<br>Available |
|---|---|---|
| Rx **Cyclosporine**<br>*Sandimmune* | **Capsules, soft gelatin:** 25 mg,<br>50 mg, 100 mg | No |
| *Neoral* | **Capsules, soft gelatin for<br>microemulsion:** 25 mg,<br>100 mg | No |
| *Sandimmune*[1] | **Oral solution:** 100 mg/mL | No |
| *Neoral* | **Oral solution for<br>microemulsion:** 100 mg/mL | No |
| *Sandimmune* | **IV solution:** 50 mg/mL | No |

[1] Contains alcohol.

## Type of Drug:

Immunosuppressive; drug used to suppress the immune system in organ transplants.

## How the Drug Works:

Cyclosporine is a potent immunosuppressive agent which increases the survival of transplants involving skin, kidney, liver, heart, pancreas, bone marrow, small intestine and lung. It is not known how cyclosporine suppresses the immune system.

## Uses:

To prevent rejection of organ (eg, kidney, liver, heart) transplants. May be used with corticosteroids.

To treat chronic rejection in patients previously treated with other immunosuppressive agents (*Sandimmune* only).

*Unlabeled Use(s):* Occasionally doctors may prescribe cyclosporine for Crohn disease, Graves ophthalmopathy, severe psoriasis, aplastic anemia, multiple sclerosis, alopecia areata, pemphigus and pemphigoid, dermatomyositis, polymyositis, lichen planus, Behcet's disease, uveitis, pulmonary sarcoidosis, biliary cirrhosis, myasthenia gravis, atopic dermatitis, insulin-dependent diabetes mellitus, lupus nephritis, nephrotic syndrome, psoriatic arthritis, pyoderma gangrenosum, rheumatoid arthritis, ulcerative colitis and corneal transplantation or other diseases of the eye which have an autoimmune component; pancreas, bone marrow and heart/lung transplants.

## Precautions:

*Do not use in the following situations:* An allergy to cyclosporine or polyoxyethylated castor oil or coadministration of potassium-sparing diuretics.

*Use with caution in the following situations:*

high blood levels of aluminum, potassium and uric acid (eg, gout)
high blood pressure
high dose methylprednisolone therapy
kidney disease (other than transplant)
liver disease (other than transplant)
low blood levels of cholesterol or magnesium
malabsorption problems
seizures

*Nervous system toxicity:* Symptoms including headache, flushing, confusion, seizures, incoordination, hallucinations, mania, depression, sleep problems and blurred vision have been observed. Various studies have associated the symptoms with low cholesterol and magnesium levels, high levels of aluminum, kidney problems, high dose methylprednisolone and high blood pressure.

*Diabetes:* Kidney transplant patients have developed insulin-dependent diabetes meltitus after treatment with cyclosporine and prednisolone.

*Immunosuppression:* Increases susceptibility to infection and the possible development of lymphoma and other tumors may result from the degree of immunosuppression.

*Pregnancy:* Adequate studies have not been done in pregnant women, or studies in animals may have shown a risk to the fetus. Use only if clearly needed and potential benefits outweigh the possible hazards to the fetus.

*Breastfeeding:* Cyclosporine appears in breast milk. Avoid breastfeeding while taking this drug.

*Children:* Safety and effectiveness have not been established. Patients as young as 6 months have received the drug with no unusual side effects.

*Lab tests* may be required to monitor therapy. Be sure to keep appointments. Liver and kidney problems have occurred during therapy; therefore, close monitoring is needed.

## Drug Interactions:

Tell your doctor or pharmacist if you are taking or if you are planning to take any over-the-counter or prescription medications or dietary supplements while taking this medicine. Doses of one or both drugs may need to be modified or a different drug may need to be prescribed. The following drugs and drug classes interact with this medicine.

allopurinol (eg, *Zyloprim*)
aminoglycosides (eg, gentamicin)
amiodarone (eg, *Cordarone*)
amphotericin B
azathioprine (eg, *Imuran*)
azole antifungals (eg, fluconazole)
bromocriptine (*Parlodel*)
calcium channel blockers (eg, nifedipine)
carbamazepine (eg, *Tegretol*)
clarithromycin (eg, *Biaxin*)
colchicine
contraceptives, oral (eg, *Ortho-Novum*)
corticosteroids (eg, prednisolone)
cyclophosphamide (eg, *Cytoxan*)
danazol (*Danocrine*)
digoxin (eg, *Lanoxin*)
erythromycin (eg, *EES*)
histamine H$_2$ antagonists (eg, cimetidine)

imipenem-cilastatin (*Primaxin*)
lovastatin (eg, *Mevacor*)
melphalan (*Alkeran*)
methyltestosterone (eg, *Testred*)
metoclopramide (eg, *Reglan*)
nafcillin (eg, *Nafcil*)
nondepolarizing muscle relaxants (eg, rocuronium bromide)
NSAIDs (eg, indomethacin)
octreotide (*Sandostatin*)
phenobarbital
phenytoin (eg, *Dilantin*)
potassium-sparing diuretics (eg, spironolactone)
quinolones (eg, ciprofloxacin)
rifabutin (*Mycobutin*)
rifampin (eg, *Rifadin*)
sulfamethoxazole/trimethoprim (eg, *Septra*)
tacrolimus (*Prograf*)
ticlopidine (eg, *Ticlid*)
vaccines
vancomycin (eg, *Vancocin*)

## Side Effects:

Every drug is capable of producing side effects. Many patients experience no, or minor, side effects. The frequency and severity of side effects depend on many factors including dose, duration of therapy and individual susceptibility. Possible side effects include:

*Digestive Tract:* Nausea; vomiting; stomach pain or discomfort; appetite loss; diarrhea; hiccups; peptic ulcer.

*Nervous System:* Confusion; seizures; tremors; headache; abnormal skin sensations.

*Skin:* Acne; unusual hair growth; brittle fingernails; flushing.

*Other:* Unusual growth of the gums; swelling of the breast (male or female); swelling; fever; hearing loss; ringing in the ears; signs of infection; muscle pain; sinus inflammation; weight loss; anemia; high blood sugar; cramps; blood clots; high blood pressure.

## Guidelines for Use:

- Take exactly as directed by your doctor.
- Do not take with food or grapefruit juice.
- To improve the flavor of the oral solution, dilute with milk, chocolate milk, apple juice or orange juice (preferably at room temperature). Try to be consistent with the mixture you use. The combination of milk and *Neoral* may be unpalatable.
- If a dose is missed, take it as soon as possible. If several hours have passed or if it is nearing time for the next dose, do not double the dose in order to catch up (unless advised to do so by your doctor). If more than one dose is missed or it is necessary to establish a new dosage schedule, contact your doctor or pharmacist.
- Do not change from one brand of this drug to another without consulting your doctor or pharmacist. These products are not equivalent to each other.
- Do not stop taking this medication unless advised to do so by your doctor.
- See your doctor regularly to assure that the drug is working properly and that no serious side effects are developing.
- Use a glass container when mixing this medication. Stir well and drink at once. Rinse glass and drink again to assure that the entire dose was taken. Do not allow it to stand before drinking.
- *Oral solution* — Do not rinse the syringe used for measuring dosages before or after use. Getting water or chemicals in the medicine can cause variation in the dose. After use, replace the syringe in its protective cover.
- Injection should only be used in patients who cannot take the capsules or oral suspension.
- Contact your doctor if fever, sore throat, tiredness, urinary problems or unusual bleeding or bruising occurs.
- Discontinue use at first first appearance of signs of allergic reaction. Symptoms may include: Flushing of the face or upper chest, difficulty breathing, wheezing, changes in blood pressure and rapid heartbeat.
- Use mechanical contraceptive measures (eg, diaphragm, condom) during cyclosporine treatment. Do not use oral contraceptives. Contact your doctor if pregnancy is suspected.
- Diabetic patients may experience loss of glucose control. Be prepared to monitor blood sugar more often.
- Lab tests will be required to monitor therapy. Be sure to keep appointments.
- Visually inspect solutions for particles or discoloration.
- Store at room temperature (below 86°F). Protect from light.
- *Oral solution* — Store at room temperature (68° to 77°F). Do not refrigerate. If Neoral solution gets too cold, it may gel. If this happens, allow to warm to room temperature (77°F) before use. Once opened, contents must be used within 2 months.

*If you have any questions, consult your doctor, pharmacist, or health care provider.*

| Generic Name<br>*Brand Name Examples* | Supplied As | Generic<br>Available |
|---|---|---|
| Rx **Mycophenolate Mofetil** | | |
| *CellCept* | **Capsules:** 250 mg | No |
| *CellCept* | **Tablets:** 500 mg | No |
| **Mycophenolate Mofetil HCl** | | |
| *CellCept Intravenous* | **Powder for injection:** 500 mg | No |

## Type of Drug:

Immunosuppressant used to prevent rejection of transplanted organs.

## How the Drug Works:

Inhibits an enzyme needed by T-cells and B-cells to produce an immune response to foreign proteins in the body.

## Uses:

To prevent organ rejection in patients receiving allogenic kidney or heart transplants. Mycophenolate is used in combination with cyclosporine and corticosteroids.

## Precautions:

*Do not use in the following situations:*

allergy to mycophenolate, mycophenolic acid (active metabolite), or any ingredient of this medicine

*Use with caution in the following situations:*

digestive system disease, active, serious
kidney disease, severe, chronic
women of childbearing potential

*Pregnancy:* Adequate studies have not been done in pregnant women. Use only if clearly needed and potential benefits outweigh the possible hazards to the fetus.

*Breastfeeding:* It is not known if mycophenolate or mycophenolic acid appears in breast milk. Because of the potential for serious adverse reactions in nursing infants, a decision should be made whether to discontinue nursing or discontinue the drug, taking into account the importance of the drug to the mother. Consult your doctor before you begin breastfeeding.

*Children:* Safety and effectiveness for use in children have not been established.

*Lab tests* will be required to monitor therapy. Tests will include complete blood counts and pregnancy tests.

## Drug Interactions:

Tell your doctor or pharmacist if you are taking or if you are planning to take any over-the-counter or prescription medications or dietary supplements while taking mycophenolate mofetil. Doses of one or both drugs may need to be modified or a different drug may need to be prescribed. The following drugs and drug classes interact with mycophenolate mofetil:

acyclovir (eg, *Zovirax*)
antacids with magnesium and aluminum (eg, *Maalox*)
azathioprine (eg, *Imuran*)
cholestyramine (eg, *Questran*)
contraceptives, oral (eg, *Ortho-Novum*)
cyclosporine (eg, *Sandimmune*)

ganciclovir (*Cytovene*)
phenytoin (eg, *Dilantin*)
probenecid (eg, *Benemid*)
salicylates (eg, aspirin)
theophylline (eg, *Theo-Dur*)
trimethoprim/sulfamethoxazole (eg, *Bactrim*)

## Side Effects:

Every drug is capable of producing side effects. Many mycophenolate mofetil users experience no, or minor, side effects. The frequency and severity of side effects depend on many factors including dose, duration of therapy, and individual susceptibility. Possible side effects include:

*Digestive Tract:* Diarrhea; constipation; nausea; indigestion; stomach pain; vomiting; mouth sores; inflammation of the gums; appetite loss; gas; enlarged abdomen; inflammation of the esophagus.

*Urinary and Reproductive Tract:* Urinary tract infection; blood in urine; painful or difficult urination; infrequent urination; impotence.

*Pulmonary:* Difficulty breathing; cough; sore throat; bronchitis; pneumonia; asthma; sinus infection; sinus congestion.

*Circulatory System:* Chest pain; irregular heartbeat; rapid or slow heartbeat; pounding in the chest (palpitations); changes in blood pressure; blood clots; heart problems; heart failure.

*Nervous System:* Tremors; dizziness; headache; weakness; sleeplessness; anxiety; depression; drowsiness; abnormal skin sensations; agitation; confusion; nervousness.

*Skin:* Acne; rash; hair loss; excessive hairiness; itching; sweating; skin ulcers; skin infection; skin growth; bruising; skin disorder.

*Muscular System:* Pelvic, back, joint, and muscle pain; muscle weakness; leg cramps; muscle tightness.

*Eyes or Ocular:* Changes in vision; infection.

*Other:* Pain; chills; fever; infection; edema (fluid retention); swelling of the arms and legs; high blood sugar levels; general body discomfort; bleeding; weight gain; change in potassium levels; elevated cholesterol; low blood phosphorus levels; anemia; decreased blood platelets; change in white blood counts.

## Guidelines for Use:

- Use exactly as prescribed.
- Injectable form is only used when patients cannot take medicines by mouth. The injectable form will be prepared and administered by your health care provider.
- Usual dosage for kidney transplant is 1 g taken orally twice daily on an empty stomach in combination with corticosteroids and cyclosporine. Usual dosage for heart transplant is 1.5 g taken orally twice daily.
- Take each dose 1 hour before or 2 hours after meals.
- Do not open or crush capsules. Do not crush tablets. Avoid inhalation or direct contact of the powder contained in the tablets or capsules with skin or mucous membranes. If contact occurs, wash skin thoroughly with soap and water; rinse eyes with plain water.
- Stagger doses of antacids and mycophenolate by at least 1 hour.
- This medicine is used in conjunction with corticosteroids (eg, predni-sone) and cyclosporine.
- Use caution when rising from a sitting or lying position. Sit or lie down if you feel lightheaded. If dizziness or lightheadedness become bother-some, notify your doctor.
- If a dose is missed, take it as soon as possible. If several hours have passed or if it is nearing time for the next dose, do not double the dose in order to catch up (unless advised to do so by your doctor). If more than one dose is missed or it is necessary to establish a new dosage schedule, contact your doctor or pharmacist.
- Increased susceptibility to infection and the possible development of lymphoma may result from immunosuppression. Contact your doctor if you develop fever, fatigue, unusual bruising or bleeding, swollen lymph nodes, or skin growths.
- This medicine increases the chances of infections, lymphomas, and other malignancies, particularly of the skin. Tell your doctor is any of the following occur: Fever; chills; tiredness; bruising or bleeding; sore throat; mouth sores.
- For patients at increased risk of skin cancer, limit exposure to sunlight and UV light (eg, tanning beds) by wearing protective clothing and using a sunscreen with a high protection factor.
- Inform your doctor if you are pregnant, become pregnant, are planning to become pregnant, or if you are breastfeeding. Effective contracep-tion must be used before beginning therapy, during therapy, and for 6 weeks following discontinuation of therapy. Use 2 reliable forms of con-traception. Women of childbearing potential must have a negative pregnancy test result 1 week before beginning mycophenolate therapy.
- Lab tests will be required. Be sure to keep appointments.
- Store at room temperature (59° to 86°F).

*If you have any questions, consult your doctor, pharmacist, or health care provider.*

| Generic Name Brand Name Example | Supplied As | Generic Available |
|---|---|---|
| Rx **Muromonab-CD3** | | |
| *Orthoclone OKT3* | **Injection:** 5 mg/5 mL | No |

## Type of Drug:

Drug used to suppress the immune system; immunosuppressant.

## How the Drug Works:

Muromonab-CD3 blocks the function of blood cells (T-cells) which play a major role in heart, kidney and liver transplant (organ) rejection.

## Uses:

To treat heart, kidney or liver transplant rejection.

## Precautions:

*Do not use in the following situations:*

allergy to this medicine or any
 of its relatives
breastfeeding
fluid retention problems

heart failure
pregnancy
seizures, history of

*Use with caution in the following situations:*

angina, unstable
calcium levels, low
cardiac or respiratory arrest
cardiovascular collapse
cerebrovascular disease
chronic obstructive pulmonary
 disease (COPD)
 (eg, breathing difficulties)
coma
dehydration, severe
electrolyte imbalances, history
 of fever
fluid in the lungs

head trauma, history of
heart attack, recent
heart disease
high blood pressure
infection
low blood sugar
medications affecting the
 central nervous system
septic shock
shock
uremia (eg, kidney disease)
vascular disease

*Immunosuppression:* As a result of immunosuppression, organ transplant patients have an increased risk of developing serious infections and various types of cancer.

*First Dose Effect:* Fever (up to 107° F), chills, rigidity, headache, tremors, nausea, vomiting, diarrhea, stomach pain, general body discomfort, muscle/joint aches and pains, generalized weakness, fluid in the lungs or difficulty breathing can occur within 30 to 60 minutes of the first few doses.

*Pregnancy:* Adequate studies have not been done in pregnant women, or animal studies may have shown a risk to the fetus. Use only if clearly needed and potential benefits outweigh the possible hazards to the fetus.

*Breastfeeding:* It is not known if muromonab-CD3 appears in breast milk. Consult your doctor before you begin breastfeeding.

*Children:* Safety and effectiveness have not been established. Careful and frequent monitoring is required for children more than for adults. It is not known whether there may be significant long-term effects from the high fever, seizures, infections or meningitis from this treatment, especially in children under 1 year of age.

*Lab tests* and chest x-rays will be required before and during treatment with this medicine. Be sure to keep appointments.

## Drug Interactions:
Tell your doctor or pharmacist if you are taking or if you are planning to take any over-the-counter or prescription medications or dietary supplements while taking this medicine. Doses of one of both drugs may need to be modified or a different drug may need to be prescribed. The following drug and drug classes interact with this medicine.

azathioprine (eg, *Imuran*)
corticosteroids (eg, predniso-lone)

cyclosporine (eg, *Sandimmune*)
indomethacin (eg, *Indocin*)

## Side Effects:
Every drug is capable of producing side effects. Many patients experience no, or minor, side effects. The frequency and severity of side effects depend on many factors including dose, duration of therapy and individual susceptibility. Possible side effects include:

*Digestive Tract:* Nausea; vomiting; diarrhea; appetite loss; stomach pain; stomach bleeding.

*Circulatory System:* Chest pain or tightness; changes in heart rhythm; blood pressure changes; shock; heart attack.

*Respiratory System:* Shortness of breath; wheezing; difficult or painful breathing; hyperventilation; pneumonia; bronchospasm.

*Skin:* Rash; hives; itching; redness; flushing; excessive sweating.

*Senses:* Blindness; blurred vision; double vision; eye irritation; light sensitivity; hearing loss; ringing in the ears; ear infection.

*Other:* Infections (some severe); tremors; headache; fever; rigidity; chills; general body discomfort; flu-like syndrome; tiredness; weakness; muscle and joint pain/stiffness; vertigo (feeling of whirling motion); nasal/ear stuffiness; neck stiffness; meningitis; seizures.

## Guidelines for Use:

- Use exactly as prescribed.
- If a dose is missed, inject it as soon as possible. If several hours have passed or it is nearing time for the next dose, do not double the dose in order to "catch up," unless advised by your doctor. If more than one dose is missed, contact your doctor or pharmacist.
- *First Dose Effect:* Fever, chills, rigidity, headache, tremors, nausea, vomiting, diarrhea, stomach or muscle/joint aches/pains, general body discomfort, weakness or difficulty breathing can occur within 30 to 60 minutes of the first few doses. Contact your doctor immediately if any of these occur.
- Notify your doctor immediately if any of the following occurs: Rash, hives, rapid heartbeat, chest pain, difficulty breathing or swallowing.
- Patients should know how they might react before driving or performing other tasks requiring alertness, coordination or physical dexterity.
- Lab tests will be required to monitor treatment. Be sure to keep appointments.
- Visually inspect solution for particles or discoloration before use.
- Store in the refrigerator between 36° and 46°F. Do not freeze or shake. After use, discard any unused solution.

*If you have any questions, consult your doctor, pharmacist, or health care provider.*

| Generic Name Brand Name Example | Supplied As | Generic Available |
|---|---|---|
| Rx **Tacrolimus** | | |
| *Prograf*[1] | **Capsules:** 1 mg, 5 mg | No |

[1] Some of these products are also available as an injection.

## Type of Drug:

Drug used to suppress the immune system after organ (liver) transplants.

## How the Drug Works:

Although the exact mechanism of action is not known, it appears tacrolimus suppresses organ graft rejection by inhibiting the activation of T-lymphocyte cells.

## Uses:

To prevent organ (liver) transplant rejection. It is recommended that tacrolimus be used in conjunction with adrenal corticosteroids.

*Unlabeled Use(s):* Tacrolimus is being investigated for the treatment of kidney, bone marrow, heart, pancreas, pancreatic island cell and small bowel transplantation. It has also been used for the treatment of autoimmune disease and severe recalcitrant psoriasis.

## Precautions:

*Do not use in the following situations:*
>      allergy to tacrolimus
>      allergy to HCO-60 polyoxyl 60 hydrogenated castor oil
>           (injection only)
>      cyclosporine use within 24 hours
>      potassium-sparing diuretic use
>      other immunosuppressive use (except adrenal corticosteroids)

*Use with caution in the following situations:*

| | |
|---|---|
| diabetes | liver disease |
| Epstein-Barr virus | long-term immunosuppressive |
| high blood pressure |  use |
| high potassium levels | lymphomas or skin cancer |
| kidney disease | |

*Liver and kidney function:* Due to the possibility of kidney damage, patients with kidney or liver disease should receive the lowest recommended dose. Further reductions in dosage may be required.

*Diabetes:* Transplant patients have developed insulin-dependent diabetes mellitus after treatment with tacrolimus.

*Infection:* Patients using immunosuppressants are at a higher risk of developing lymphomas and other malignancies (tumors), especially of the skin.

*Nerve damage:* Over half of liver transplant recipients experience nerve damage including tremors, headaches, changes in muscle coordination, mental status and sensory function. Seizures, coma and delirium have also been observed.

*Pregnancy:* Adequate studies have not been done in pregnant women. Use only if clearly needed and potential benefits outweigh the possible hazards to the fetus.

*Breastfeeding:* Tacrolimus appears in breast milk. Avoid breastfeeding while taking this drug. Consult your doctor before you begin breast-feeding.

*Children:* Tacrolimus has been used successfully in liver transplants in children less than 12 years of age. Younger patients usually require higher doses than adults.

*Lab tests* will be required during treatment with tacrolimus. Tests may include routine monitoring of kidney, blood and metabolic systems.

## Drug Interactions:

Tell your doctor or pharmacist if you are taking or if you are planning to take any over-the-counter or prescription medications or dietary supplements while taking tacrolimus. Doses of one or both drugs may need to be modified or a different drug may need to be prescribed. The following drugs and drug classes interact with tacrolimus.

aminoglycosides (eg, kanamycin sulfate)
antifungals (eg, amphotericin B)
bromocriptine (eg, *Parlodel*)
calcium channel blockers (eg, nifedipine)
carbamazepine (eg, *Tegretol*)
cimetidine (eg, *Tagamet*)
cisplatin (eg, *Platinol*)
clarithromycin (*Biaxin*)
clotrimazole (eg, *Lotrimin*)
cyclosporine (eg, *Sandimmune*)
danazol (eg, *Danocrine*)
diltiazem (eg, *Cardizem*)
erythromycin (eg, *E-Mycin*)

fluconazole (*Diflucan*)
immunosuppressive agents (except adrenal corticosteroids)
itraconazole (*Sporanox*)
ketoconazole (eg, *Nizoral*)
methylprednisolone (eg, *Medrol*)
metoclopramide (eg, *Reglan*)
phenobarbital (eg, *Solfoton*)
phenytoin (eg, *Dilantin Infatab*)
potassium-sparing diuretics (eg, amiloride HCl)
rifabutin (*Mycobutin*)
rifampin (eg, *Rifadin*)
vaccines

## Side Effects:

Every drug is capable of producing side effects. Many tacrolimus users experience no, or minor, side effects. The frequency and severity of side effects depend on many factors including dose, duration of therapy and individual susceptibility. Possible side effects include:

*Digestive Tract:* Diarrhea; enlarged abdomen; nausea; constipation; appetite changes; vomiting; stomach pain; bloating; indigestion; gas; liver damage or disease; hepatitis; intestinal bleeding or other problems.

*Nervous System:* Mood swings; stiffness; tremor; headache; sleeplessness; abnormal skin sensations; abnormal dreams; anxiety; confusion; depression; dizziness; hallucinations; incoordination; drowsiness; seizures; coma.

*Circulatory System:* High blood pressure; abnormal blood counts; chest pain; low blood pressure; fast heartbeat; abnormal heart rhythms; abnormal blood clotting; bleeding.

*Respiratory System:* Difficulty breathing; cough; asthma; sore throat; pneumonia; bronchitis; voice alteration; sinus infection.

*Skin:* Skin cancer; itching; hives; rash; bruising; hair loss; abnormal hair growth; sweating.

*Urinary and Reproductive Tract:* Urinary tract infection; infrequent urination; blood in the urine.

*Other:* Yellowing of the skin and eyes; weight loss; non-Hodgkin's lymphoma; infections related to Epstein-Barr virus; elevated blood sugar levels; fever; weakness; back pain; mouth infections; swelling of the arms and legs; vision changes; ringing in the ears; speech impairment; kidney failure; abnormal healing; abscesses; chills; hernia; sensitivity to sunlight; joint, muscle, back and general body pain; leg cramps; herpes; tumors; oral thrush; abnormal sensations.

---

## Guidelines for Use:

- Take exactly as prescribed.
- The possibility of serious infection, nerve or kidney damage, diabetes and some cancers is increased with the use of this medicine.
- *Capsules* — Take in two divided doses every 12 hours on an empty stomach, or as directed by your doctor.
- Administer injectable form only in facilities that can handle emergency situations.
- If a dose is missed, take it as soon as possible. If several hours have passed or if it is nearing time for the next dose, do not double the dose in order to "catch up" (unless advised to do so by your doctor). If more than one dose is missed or it is necessary to establish a new dosage schedule, contact your doctor or pharmacist.
- Lab tests will be required to monitor therapy. Be sure to keep appointments.
- Notify your doctor immediately if you have any of the following: tremors, headache, dizziness, incoordination, abnormal sensations, suspected infections, changes in mental status, or decreased urination.
- *Injection patients* — Notify your doctor immediately if any of the following signs of an allergic reaction occurs: hives, itching, fluid retention or difficulty breathing.
- May cause drowsiness, dizziness or visual problems. Use caution while driving or performing other tasks requiring alertness, coordination or physical dexterity.
- Store at room temperature.

*If you have any questions, consult your doctor, pharmacist, or health care provider.*

| Generic Name<br>*Brand Name Example* | Supplied As | Generic<br>Available |
|---|---|---|
| Rx **Isotretinoin** | | |
| *Accutane*[1] | **Capsules**: 10 mg, 20 mg,<br>40 mg | No |

[1] Contains edetate disodium, methyl- and propylparabens.

## Type of Drug:

Agent for severe, disfiguring nodular acne resistant to standard therapies.

## How the Drug Works:

The exact mechanism by which isotretinoin exerts its beneficial effect is not known. The drug reduces sebum (oil) secreted by specialized glands in the skin (sebaceous glands), changes some of the characteristics of the sebum, and may prevent abnormal hardening of skin cells (keratinization).

## Uses:

To treat severe disfiguring nodular (red, swollen, tender lumps in the skin) acne unresponsive to conventional therapy including antibiotics.

*Unlabeled Use(s):* Occasionally doctors may prescribe isotretinoin for Darier-White disease, pityriasis rubra pilaris, lamellar ichthyosis, congenital ichthyosiform erythroderma, hyperkeratosis palmaris and plantaris, cutaneous T-cell lymphoma and leukoplakia, rosacea, lichen planus, psoriasis, or for prevention of second primary tumors in skin cancer of the head and neck.

## Precautions:

*Do not use in the following situations:*

allergy to isotretinoin or any of its ingredients (eg, parabens)
breastfeeding
depression
pregnancy or likelihood of becoming pregnant
psychosis
sexually active women of childbearing age not using 1 or more methods of effective contraception
suicidal thoughts
tetracycline therapy, concurrent
vitamin A use, concurrent

*Use with caution in the following situations:*

alcohol use
blood donors
diabetes
high cholesterol or triglyceride levels
liver disease

*Depression:* Depression and mood swings, including suicidal ideation, suicide attempts and suicide have been associated with isotretinoin use. Discontinuation of the drug may be insufficient; further testing may be necessary.

*Pseudotumor cerebri:* Pseudotumor cerebri (benign intracranial hypertension) has occurred with isotretinoin. Early signs and symptoms include headache, swelling of optic disk, nausea, vomiting, and visual disturbances. If present, discontinue drug immediately and consult your doctor or a neurologist.

*Inflammatory bowel disease:* Inflammatory bowel disease (including regional ileitis) has been temporally associated with isotretinoin in patients with no history of intestinal disorders. Discontinue treatment immediately if abdominal pain, rectal bleeding or severe diarrhea occur.

*Visual disturbances:* Visual disturbances such as decreased night vision and clouding in the eye have occurred during therapy with isotretinoin. Because the onset may be sudden, use caution when driving or operating any vehicle, especially at night. Stop using the drug and see your eye doctor if any visual problems occur.

*Hearing impairment:* Hearing impairment has been reported in patients taking isotretinoin and, in some cases, has persisted after discontinuing treatment. Discontinue drug immediately and consult your doctor if ringing in the ears or impared hearing occurs.

*Pregnancy:* Women who are pregnant or who may become pregnant must not use isotretinoin. There is an extremely high risk that serious birth defects will result if pregnancy occurs while taking this drug in any amount, even for short periods. Potentially, all exposed fetuses can be adversely affected.

*Breastfeeding:* It is not known if isotretinoin appears in breast milk. Because of the potential for side effects, do not take while breast-feeding.

*Children:* Safety and effectiveness in children have not been established.

*Lab tests* and eye exams may be required before and during treatment with isotretinoin. Tests may include: liver function tests, blood lipid tests (cholesterol, triglycerides, and lipoproteins), glucose tests, CPK tests, and pregnancy tests.

## Drug Interactions:

Tell your doctor or pharmacist if you are taking or planning to take any over-the-counter or prescription medications or dietary supplements with isotretinoin. Doses of one or both drugs may need to be modified or a different drug may need to be prescribed. The following drugs and drug classes interact with isotretinoin:

> vitamin A
> tetracyclines (eg, minocycline)

## Side Effects:

Every drug is capable of producing side effects. Many isotretinoin users experience side effects. The frequency and severity of side effects depend on many factors including dose, duration of therapy, and individual susceptibility. Possible side effects include:

*Nervous System:* Headache; depression; mood swings, suicidal thoughts; psychosis; pseudotumor cerebri; fatigue; dizziness; drowsiness; sleeplessness; lethargy; nervousness; seizures; suicidal thoughts.

*Skin:* Dry skin; rash; sloughing of skin; thinning of hair; sensitivity to sunlight; hives; crusty or oily skin; redness; fragile skin; itching; brittle nails; cracking around corners of mouth; bruising; chapped or swollen lips; drying of mucous membranes; peeling of palms and soles; nosebleed, bleeding gums.

*Senses:* Visual disturbances; corneal clouding; cataracts; eye infection; dry eyes; decreased night vision; sensitivity to light.

*Other:* Dry nose or mouth; inflammatory bowel disease (see Precautions); blood or protein in urine; abnormal menstrual flow; bone, joint, or muscle pain or stiffness; chest pain; nausea; vomiting; stomachache; appetite loss; change in blood lipids; increase in liver enzymes; hepatitis; changes in blood counts; delayed wound healing; pus-filled swollen sores; increased blood sugar; swelling; rapid heart rate; weight loss; nausea; anemia; low platelet counts.

## Guidelines for Use:

- Dosage is individualized. Take exactly as prescribed.
- Usually taken in 2 divided daily doses with meals for 15 to 20 weeks.
- Read the patient information leaflet available with the product and complete patient consent form prior to use.
- Do not crush or chew the capsules. Swallow whole.
- Take with food.
- If a dose is missed, take it as soon as possible. If several hours have passed or it is nearing time for the next dose, do not double the dose to catch up unless advised to do so by your doctor. If more than one dose is missed or it is necessary to establish a new dosage schedule, contact your doctor or pharmacist.
- Avoid drinking alcohol.
- Do not take vitamin supplements containing vitamin A while taking isotretinoin.
- A prescription will not be issued until a report of a negative pregnancy test has been received by your doctor and pregnancy testing will be repeated on a monthly basis. For your health and well-being, be sure to keep appointments.
- Sexually active women of childbearing potential should practice contraception 1 month before starting therapy, during therapy, and for 1 month after therapy is stopped.
- Two separate, reliable forms of contraception should be used at the same time unless abstinence is the chosen method.
- Contact the doctor immediately if pregnancy is suspected during therapy. Major birth defects have been associated with isotretinoin use. Discuss continuation of the pregnancy with your doctor.
- Worsening of acne may occur during the initial period of therapy. This does not suggest a therapeutic failure or a need to stop therapy.
- Isotretinoin may cause photosensitivity (sensitivity to sunlight). Avoid prolonged exposure to the sun or other forms of ultraviolet (UV) light (eg, tanning beds). Use sunscreens and wear protective clothing until tolerance is determined.
- Discontinue the drug and contact your doctor immediately if depression, visual disturbances, abdominal pain, rectal bleeding, severe diarrhea, or difficulty in controlling blood sugar occur.
- Do not donate blood for transfusion during therapy and for 30 days after stopping therapy.
- Patients may experience decreased tolerance to contact lenses during and after therapy.
- Avoid skin smoothing procedures, including waxing, dermabrasion, or laser procedures, during therapy and for 6 months after stopping therapy. There is an increased possibility of scarring.
- If the total nodule count has been reduced by 70% or more before completing 15 to 20 weeks of treatment, therapy may be stopped. After 2 months or more of therapy and if the acne returns, a second course of therapy may be started. Contraceptive measures must be followed for any following course of therapy.
- Lab tests will be required before and during therapy. Be sure to keep appointments.
- Store at 59° to 86°F. Protect from light.

*If you have any questions, consult your doctor, pharmacist, or health care provider.*

| Generic Name<br>*Brand Name Example* | Supplied As | Generic<br>Available |
|---|---|---|
| *Rx* **Leflunomide** | | |
| *Arava* | **Tablets:** 10 mg, 20 mg, 100 mg | No |

## Type of Drug:

Agent for treating active rheumatoid arthritis.

## How the Drug Works:

Leflunomide appears to inhibit enzymes responsible for abnormal tissue development or growth. It may also have anti-inflammatory activity (ie, reduces swelling, pain).

## Uses:

For the treatment of active rheumatoid arthritis (RA) in adults to reduce signs and symptoms and to slow damage to the joints. May be used in combination with aspirin, nonsteroidal anti-inflammatory agents (NSAIDs) (eg, ibuprofen), or low-dose corticosteroids (eg, prednisone).

## Precautions:

*Do not use in the following situations:*
>   allergy to the drug or any of its ingredients
>   pregnancy or the possibility of pregnancy

*Use with caution in the following situations:*

| | |
|---|---|
| bone marrow dysplasia | positive hepatitis B or C |
| immunodeficiency, severe | serologies |
| kidney disease | uncontrolled infections, severe |
| liver disease | vaccination with live vaccine |

*Pregnancy:* Do not use during pregnancy or in women of childbearing potential who are not using reliable contraception. The risk of use in a pregnant woman clearly outweighs any possible benefit. Pregnancy must be excluded before the start of treatment, and patients must be fully counseled on the potential for serious risks to the fetus, such as birth defects. Pregnancy must be avoided during treatment and prior to the completion of the drug elimination procedure after treatment. If there is any delay in the onset of menses or any other reason to suspect pregnancy, the physician must be notified immediately. In addition, to minimize any possible risk, men taking leflunomide who are considering fathering a child should discuss discontinuing use of leflunomide and completing the drug elimination procedure with their doctor.

*Breastfeeding:* It is not known if leflunomide is excreted in breast milk. Because of the potential for serious adverse reactions in nursing infants from leflunomide, decide whether to discontinue breastfeeding or the drug, taking into account the importance of the drug to the mother.

*Children:* Safety and effectiveness have not been established. Use of leflunomide in patients younger than 18 years of age is not recommended.

*Lab tests* will be required before, during, and after therapy. Tests include liver enzymes and kidney function tests, and blood cell counts.

## Drug Interactions:

Tell your doctor or pharmacist if you are taking or planning to take any over-the-counter or prescription medications or dietary supplements while taking this drug. Drug doses may need to be modified or a different drug prescribed. The following drugs and drug classes interact with this drug:

charcoal
cholestyramine (eg, *Questran*)
hepatotoxic drugs (eg, methotrexate, isoniazid)
immunosuppression medica-
  tions (eg, azathioprine, cyclosporine)

NSAIDs (eg, ibuprofen,
  naproxen)
rifampin (eg, *Rifadin*)

## Side Effects:

Every drug is capable or producing side effects. Many patients experience no, or minor, side effects. The frequency and severity of side effects depend on many factors including dose, duration of therapy, and individual susceptibility. Possible side effects include:

*Digestive Tract:* Stomach pain; appetite loss; diarrhea; indigestion; stomach or intestinal irritation; nausea; mouth ulcer; vomiting; gallstones; colitis; constipation; heartburn; gas; gum inflammation; dark, bloody stools; mouth fungal infection; enlarged salivary gland; dry mouth; mouth inflammation; tooth disorder; taste changes.

*Nervous System:* Weakness; dizziness; headache; abnormal skin sensations; migraine; anxiety; depression; sleeplessness; nerve pain; sleep disorder; sweating; feeling of whirling motion.

*Circulatory System:* High blood pressure; chest pain; pounding in the chest (palpitations); fast heartbeat; blood vessel inflammation; varicose veins; anemia; flushing.

*Respiratory System:* Bronchitis; increased cough; respiratory tract infection; sore throat; pneumonia; runny nose; sinus infection; asthma; difficulty breathing; lung disorder.

*Urinary and Reproductive Tract:* Protein in urine; bladder inflammation; painful or difficult urination; blood in the urine; menstrual disorder; vaginal fungal infection; prostate disorder; urinary frequency; urinary tract infection.

*Skin:* Hair loss; rash; inflamed and itching skin; dry skin; acne; contact dermatitis; fungal skin infection; hair discoloration; skin nodule; skin disorder; skin discoloration; skin ulcer; nail disorder; herpes simplex; herpes zoster; increased sweating; unusual bruising.

*Eyes or Ocular:* Blurred vision; cataract; eye inflammation; eye disorder.

*Other:* Abnormal liver enzymes; allergic reaction; flu-like syndrome; infection; accidental injury; muscle, back, neck, joint, pelvic, or bone pain; low blood potassium levels; weight loss; leg cramps; joint disorder; abscess; cyst; hernia; general body discomfort; swelling of arms and legs; hyperlipidemia; bursitis; muscle cramps; bone necrosis; tendon rupture; fever; high blood sugar levels; nosebleed; overactive thyroid.

## Guidelines for Use:

- Dosage is individualized. Take exactly as prescribed.
- Do not stop taking or change the dose, unless instructed by your doctor.
- Aspirin, nonsteroidal anti-inflammatory agents (eg, ibuprofen), or low-dose corticosteroids (eg, prednisone) may be continued during therapy with leflunomide.
- Take without regard to meals. Take with food if stomach upset occurs.
- Stop taking and notify your doctor immediately if you experience skin rash, mouth sores, unusual bruising, paleness, unexplained tiredness, or increased incidence of infections.
- Do not use if you are pregnant or may become pregnant. Pregnancy must be excluded before the start of treatment. Pregnancy must also be avoided prior to the completion of the drug elimination procedure after treatment. If there is any reason to suspect pregnancy (eg, delayed menstrual period), the physician must be notified immediately.
- To minimize any possible risk to the fetus, men taking leflunomide who are considering fathering a child should discuss discontinuing use of leflunomide with their doctor.
- There is a potential for immunosuppression with leflunomide.
- Vaccination with live vaccines during leflunomide therapy is not recommended.
- Beneficial effects should be noted within 1 month of starting therapy, but further improvement in symptoms may progress during the first 6 months of therapy.
- Leflunomide is converted in the body to a very long-acting by-product (metabolite) that may remain in the body for up to 2 years following discontinuation of therapy. In situations in which the metabolite needs to be eliminated more rapidly (eg, planned pregnancy or toxicity), a drug elimination procedure using cholestyramine will need to be used.
- Lab tests will be required before, during, and after therapy. Be sure to keep appointments.
- Store at controlled room temperature (59° to 86°F).

*If you have any questions, consult your doctor, pharmacist, or health care provider.*

| Generic Name Brand Name Examples | Supplied As | Generic Available |
|---|---|---|
| Rx **Bromocriptine Mesylate** | | |
| Parlodel | **Capsules:** 5 mg | No |
| Parlodel | **Tablets:** 2.5 mg | No |

## Type of Drug:

Ergot alkaloid derivative; antiparkinson drug; fertility drug.

## How the Drug Works:

Bromocriptine suppresses prolactin secretion from the pituitary gland in the brain. Excessive prolactin activity can be responsible for galactorrhea (excessive milk flow), amenorrhea (absence of menstruation) and infertility. By inhibiting prolactin release, bromocriptine can suppress galactorrhea and reinstate normal menstrual cycles.

Bromocriptine also reduces the secretion of growth hormones from the pituitary gland. This can help in the treatment of acromegaly (abnormal enlargement of the bones of the hands, feet or face).

It also acts on the chemicals in the brain to relieve some of the symptoms of Parkinson disease.

## Uses:

To treat female infertility and other disorders (eg, menstrual irregularities, reduced sex gland activities) caused by the secretion of too much prolactin, acromegaly and Parkinson's disease; also to reduce the size of some pituitary gland tumors before surgery.

Unlabeled Use(s): Occasionally doctors may prescribe bromocriptine mesylate to treat neuroleptic malignant syndrome, hyperprolactinemia associated with pituitary gland tumors, cocaine addiction and cyclical mastalgia. Bromocriptine mesylate was previously used to reduce or prevent breast milk production in mothers who do not want to breastfeed following delivery. It is not used for this condition anymore.

## Precautions:

Do not use in the following situations:
allergy to ergot alkaloids
high blood pressure, uncontrolled
heart or vascular disease, severe
pregnancy in patients with hyperprolactinemia

Use with caution in the following situations:
kidney disease
liver disease
peptic ulcers

Pregnancy: Studies in pregnant women or in animals have been judged not to show a risk to the fetus. However, no drug should be used during pregnancy unless clearly needed.

*Breastfeeding:* Since bromocriptine prevents lactation, mothers who wish to breastfeed should not use this drug.

*Children:* Safety and effectiveness in children under 15 years of age have not been established.

*Lab tests or exams* may be required to monitor treatment. Be sure to keep appointments.

## Drug Interactions:

Tell your doctor or pharmacist if you are taking or if you are planning to take any over-the-counter or prescription medications or dietary supplements while taking this medicine. Doses of one or both drugs may need to be modified or a different drug may need to be prescribed. The following drugs and drug classes interact with this medicine.

> erythromycin (eg, *E-Mycin*)
> blood-pressure-lowering agents (eg, clonidine)
> phenothiazines (eg, chlorpromazine)
> sympathomimetics (eg, phenylpropanolamine)

## Side Effects:

Every drug is capable of producing side effects. Many patients experience no, or minor, side effects. The frequency and severity of side effects depend on many factors including dose, duration of therapy and individual susceptibility. Possible side effects include:

*Digestive Tract:* Nausea; vomiting; diarrhea; constipation; stomach cramps; indigestion; appetite loss; dry mouth.

*Nervous System:* Psychological disturbances; headache; dizziness; tiredness; lightheadedness; fainting; drowsiness.

*Other:* Low blood pressure; orthostatic hypotension (dizziness or lightheadedness when rising from a seated or lying position); coldness or numbness in hands or feet; nasal congestion.

## Guidelines for Use:

- Take with meals or food.
- Take the first dose while lying down. May cause drowsiness, dizziness or fainting, especially following the first dose. Avoid sudden changes in posture, such as rising from a sitting or lying position. Use caution when driving or performing other tasks requiring alertness, coordination or physical dexterity.
- Do not stop taking or change the dose unless advised to do so by your doctor.
- If a dose is missed, take it as soon as possible. If several hours have passed or it is nearing time for the next dose, do not double the dose in order to "catch up" (unless advised to do so by your doctor). If more than one dose is missed or it is necessary to establish a new dosage schedule, contact your doctor or pharmacist. Use exactly as prescribed.
- Contact your doctor immediately if you experience a persistent runny nose.
- Use mechanical contraceptive measures (eg, diaphragm, condom) during treatment. Do not use oral contraceptives. Perform a pregnancy test every 4 weeks during the amenorrheal (non-menstrual) period or if menstruation does not occur within 3 days of the expected date.
- Inform your doctor if you are pregnant, become pregnant, are planning to become pregnant or if you are breastfeeding.
- *Medical exams* may be required to monitor treatment. Be sure to keep appointments.
- Store below 77°F. Protect from light.

*If you have any questions, consult your doctor, pharmacist, or health care provider.*

| Generic Name<br>*Brand Name Example* | Supplied As | Generic<br>Available |
|---|---|---|
| *Rx* **Cabergoline** | | |
| *Dostinex* | **Tablets:** 0.5 mg | No |

## Type of Drug:

Dopamine receptor agonist.

## How the Drug Works:

Inhibits secretion of prolactin from the pituitary gland; reduces prolactin levels in blood.

## Uses:

For hyperprolactinemic disorders, either from an unknown cause or caused by pituitary adenomas (tumors).

*Unlabeled Use(s):* To shrink pituitary tumors; to treat Parkinson's disease; normalize androgen levels and improve menstrual cyclicity in polycystic ovary syndrome.

## Precautions:

*Do not use in the following situations:*
uncontrolled high blood pressure

allergy to ergot derivatives

*Use with caution in the following situations:*
pregnancy-induced high blood pressure
liver impairment
use in conjuction with other medicines used to lower blood pressure
suppression of physiologic lactation

*Pregnancy:* Studies in pregnanct women or in animals have been judged not to show a risk to the fetus. However, no drug should be used during pregnancy unless clearly needed.

*Breastfeeding:* It is not known if cabergoline appears in breast milk. Consult your doctor before you begin breastfeeding.

*Children:* Safety and effectiveness have not been established.

*Lab tests* are required to monitor treatment. Be sure to keep appointments.

## Drug Interactions:

Tell your doctor or pharmacist if you are taking or planning to take any over-the-counter or prescription medications or dietary supplements while taking this medicine. Doses of one or both drugs may need to be modified or a different drug may need to be prescribed. The following drugs and drug classes interact with cabergoline: Dopamine ($D_2$)-antagonists (eg, phenothiazines); antihypertensive drugs (eg, methyldopa).

## Side Effects:

*Digestive Tract:* Nausea; constipation; abdominal pain; indigestion; vomiting; diarrhea; gas.

*Nervous System:* Headache; dizziness; drowsiness; depression; nervousness; feeling of whirling motion; abnormal skin sensations; abnormal movements; confusion; hallucinations.

*Circulatory System:* Low blood pressure.

*Urinary and Reproductive Tract:* Breast pain; painful menstruation.

*Other:* Weakness; fatigue; dry mouth; pain; hot flashes; abnormal vision; itching; swelling of feet or ankles.

### Guidelines for Use:

- May take with or without food. Take with food if GI upset occurs.
- Take this medicine twice a week as directed by your doctor. Increases in dosage of medication should occur no less often than every 4 weeks after physician assessment of response.
- If response is not noted after increase in dose, the lowest dose that achieves benefit should be used and other therapies considered.
- After normal serum prolactin levels are maintained for 6 months, therapy may be discontinued.
- This medicine may cause drowsiness or dizziness. Use caution while driving or performing other tasks requiring mental alertness, coordination or dexterity.
- Inform your doctor if you are pregnant, become pregnant or are planning to become pregnant.
- Lab tests or exams will be required to monitor treatment. Be sure to keep appointments. Tests will include serum prolactin levels.
- Store at controlled room temperature (68° to 77°F).

*If you have any questions, consult your doctor, pharmacist, or health care provider.*

| Generic Name<br>*Brand Name Example* | Supplied As | Generic<br>Available |
|---|---|---|
| Rx **Chymopapain**<br>*Chymodiactin*[1] | **Powder for injection,<br>lyophilized:** 4000 pKat units<br>chymopapain | No |

[1] Preservative free.

## Type of Drug:
Enzyme that breaks down proteins.

## How the Drug Works:
When injected into the cushioning disc between the bones in the lower spine (lumbar), chymopapain breaks down the proteins in the disc. This reduces pressure in the disc and relieves symptoms of disc compression.

## Uses:
To treat documented herniated (protruding) intervertebral discs in the lumbar (lower) spine which have not responded to conservative therapy.

## Precautions:
*Do not use in the following situations:*
- allergy to chymopapain, papaya, or papaya derivatives
- circulating chymopapain-specific IgE antibodies
- displaced vertebrae
- injection of chymopapain, history
- lesions producing spinal motor or sensory dysfunction (eg, cauda equina lesion)
- paralysis, severe and progressing as indicated by rapidly progressing neurological dysfunction
- spinal cord tumor
- spinal stenosis, significant
- use in any other region of the spinal cord other than the lumbar area

*Use with caution in the following situations:*
- beta blocker therapy, current use
- cerebrovascular disorders (eg, stroke), history or family history
- females (particularly black females)
- general anesthesia use
- high blood pressure, history
- injections at 2 or more disc sites
- iodine allergy
- surgery of lumbar spine, history

*Allergic reactions* (mild to severe) have occurred rarely with chymopapain use. The reactions have occurred more frequently in females (particularly black females) and patients receiving general anesthesia.

Symptoms can be immediate or delayed up to 2 hours. They can last for a few minutes to several hours or longer. Symptoms may include decreased blood pressure, dizziness, difficulty breathing, and irregular heartbeat. A delayed reaction (rash, hives, itching) may occur for up to 15 days after injection.

*Pregnancy:* Adequate studies have not been done in pregnant women. Use only if clearly needed and potential benefits outweigh the possible hazards to the fetus.

*Children:* Safety and effectiveness have not been established; do not use chymopapain in children.

*Lab tests and exams* may be required before therapy. Tests include preoperative screening test for chymopapain-specific IgE antibody.

## Side Effects:

Every drug is capable of producing side effects. Chymopapain may cause no, or minor, side effects. The frequency and severity of side effects depend on many factors including dose, duration of therapy, and individual susceptibility. Possible side effects include:

*Symptoms of Anaphylaxis:* Difficulty breathing; palpitations (pounding in the chest); redness; flushing; rash; goosebumps; itching; stomach problems; skin inflammation; low blood pressure; bronchospasm; irregular heartbeat; cardiac arrest; hives; redness or discharge around the eye; runny nose; coma.

*Other:* Back pain, stiffness, or soreness; tingling, weakness, or pain in the legs; foot drop; cramping in calves; paraplegia or paraparesis (eg, cauda equina syndrome); back spasm; subarachnoid or cerebral hemorrhage; seizures; burning sensation in the lower back; decreased sensitivity to pain; abnormal skin sensations; numbness in the legs or toes; disc inflammation.

---

### Guidelines for Use:

- This medication will be prepared and administered by your health care provider.
- Chymopapain is *only* used in a hospital setting by doctors experienced and trained in the diagnosis of lumbar disc disease and all standard treatment methods, including surgery. Doctors and their support personnel are to be competent in the diagnosis and management of all potential complications from chymopapain use.
- *Postinjection pain* — You may experience pain or involuntary muscle spasm in the lower back for several days. A lingering stiffness or soreness may persist for several months. This is not uncommon.
- Notify your doctor immediately if you experience a rash of any type, hives, or itching as late as 15 days after the procedure. These symptoms may be signs of an allergic reaction.
- Lab tests may be required to monitor therapy. Be sure to keep appointments.

---

*If you have any questions, consult your doctor, pharmacist, or health care provider.*

| Generic Name *Brand Name Example* | Supplied As | Generic Available |
|---|---|---|
| Rx **Cromolyn Sodium** | | |
| *Gastrocrom* | **Oral concentrate:** 100 mg/5 mL | No |

Cromolyn sodium is also available as a respiratory inhalant and antiallergy agent for the eyes. See the corresponding monographs.

## Type of Drug:
Mast cell stabilizer; antiallergy.

## How the Drug Works:
Cromolyn sodium is a mast cell stabilizer. Mast cells, which are distributed throughout the body, contain storage granules containing potent inflammatory materials (eg, histamine) that are released by a variety of stimuli. Patients with mastocytosis have a greater than normal accumulation of mast cells. Oral cromolyn sodium reduces histamine release from these cells and decreases symptoms caused by histamine.

## Uses:
To prevent attacks and relieve the symptoms of mastocytosis. These symptoms include diarrhea, flushing, headaches, vomiting, hives, stomach pain, nausea, and itching.

## Precautions:
*Do not use in the following situations:* Allergy to cromolyn sodium or any of its ingredients.

*Use with caution in the following situations:*
    kidney disease
    liver disease

*Pregnancy:* There are no adequate and well-controlled studies in pregnant women. Use only if clearly needed and the potential benefits to the mother outweigh the possible risks to the fetus.

*Breastfeeding:* It is not known if cromolyn sodium appears in breast milk. Consult your doctor before you begin breastfeeding.

*Children:* Use in children under 2 years of age is not recommended and should be used only in those patients with severe diseases where the benefits clearly outweigh the risks.

## Drug Interactions:
Tell your doctor or pharmacist if you are taking or if you are planning to take any over-the-counter or prescription medications or dietary supplements with cromolyn sodium. Doses of one or both drugs may need to be modified or a different drug may need to be prescribed.

## Side Effects:

Every drug is capable of producing side effects. Many oral cromolyn sodium users experience no, or minor, side effects. The frequency and severity of side effects depend on many factors including dose, duration of therapy, and individual susceptibility. Possible side effects include:

*Digestive Tract:* Diarrhea; nausea; stomach pain.

*Nervous System:* Headache; irritability; anxiety.

*Other:* Rash; itching; general body discomfort; muscle or joint pain; sensitivity to light; pounding in the chest; rapid heart rate; fluid retention.

---

### Guidelines for Use:

- Dosage will be individualized. Your doctor may increase or decrease your dose depending on your response to the medication.
- For maximum effectiveness, take at regular intervals as directed by your doctor. To prevent relapses, maintain the dosage regimen prescribed by your doctor.
- Break open ampule(s) and squeeze liquid contents into a glass of water. Stir solution and drink all of the liquid. Discard the empty ampule.
- Mix with water only. Do not mix with milk, fruit juice, or foods.
- Take at least one-half hour before meals and at bedtime.
- Do not use if ampule contains particles or becomes discolored.
- Store between 59° and 86°F. Protect from light. Leave ampules in foil pouch until ready for use.

---

*If you have any questions, consult your doctor, pharmacist, or health care provider.*

| Generic Name<br>*Brand Name Example* | Supplied As | Generic<br>Available |
|---|---|---|
| *Rx* **Disulfiram** | | |
| *Antabuse* | **Tablets:** 250 mg, 500 mg | Yes |

## Type of Drug:

Anti-alcoholic.

## How the Drug Works:

Disulfiram blocks the normal breakdown of alcohol and allows an unpleasant by-product (acetaldehyde) to accumulate. This by-product produces numerous side effects, including flushing, throbbing in the head and neck, throbbing headache, nausea, vomiting, painful and difficult breathing, sweating, thirst, chest pain, heart pounding, increased heart rate, low blood pressure, feeling of whirling motion, weakness, blurred vision, marked uneasiness, fainting, hyperventilation, and confusion.

## Uses:

To aid in the management of selected chronic alcoholic patients who wish to remain in a state of enforced sobriety so that supportive and psychotherapeutic treatment may be applied to best advantage.

Disulfiram is not a cure for alcoholism. When used alone, without proper motivation and support therapy, it is unlikely that it will have any substantive effect on the drinking pattern of the chronic alcoholic patient.

## Precautions:

*Do not use in the following situations:*

alcohol or alcohol-containing products (eg, some cough syrups, sauces, aftershave lotions), use of
allergy to disulfiram or any of its ingredients
allergy to rubber
allergy to thiuram derivatives used in pesticides
heart disease, severe
metronidazole use, current or recent
paraldehyde use, current or recent
psychosis

*Use with caution in the following situations:*

brain damage
diabetes mellitus
epilepsy
kidney disease
liver disease
rubber contact dermatitis
underactive thyroid

*Disulfiram-alcohol reaction:* Disulfiram plus alcohol, even small amounts, produces flushing, throbbing in the head and neck, throbbing headaches, fainting, nausea, vomiting, sweating, thirst, chest pain, heart pounding, painful and difficult breathing, increased heart rate, weakness, feeling of whirling motion, blurred vision, low blood pressure, hyperventilation, marked uneasiness, and confusion. In severe reactions, there may be collapse, irregular heart rhythm, heart attack, acute congestive heart failure, unconsciousness, convulsions, and death. The intensity of the reaction is generally proportional to the amounts of disulfiram and alcohol ingested. Mild reactions may occur in the sensitive individual when the blood-alcohol level is low. The reaction may last from 30 to 60 minutes to several hours, or as long as there is alcohol in the blood.

*Ethylene dibromide* (a fumigant also found in antiknock gasolines) and its vapors may be harmful to patients receiving disulfiram. Avoid exposure.

*Pregnancy:* Safety for use during pregnancy has not been established. Use only if clearly needed and the potential benefits to the mother outweigh the potential risks to the fetus.

*Breastfeeding:* It is not known if disulfiram appears in breast milk. Consult your doctor before you begin breastfeeding.

*Lab tests* will be required during treatment with disulfiram. Tests may include: Liver function tests and complete blood counts. Patients with a history of rubber contact dermatitis should be tested for allergy to disulfiram before administration.

## Drug Interactions:
Tell your doctor or pharmacist if you are taking or if you are planning to take any over-the-counter or prescription medications or dietary supplements with disulfiram. Doses of one or both drugs may need to be modified or a different drug may need to be prescribed. The following drugs and drug classes interact with disulfiram.

| | |
|---|---|
| alcohol | hydantoins (eg, phenytoin) |
| anticoagulants, oral (eg, warfarin) | isoniazid (eg, *Laniazid*) |
| | metronidazole (eg, *Flagyl*) |
| benzodiazepines (eg, diazepam) | theophyllines (eg, amino- |
| chlorzoxazone (eg, *Paraflex*) | phylline) |

## Side Effects:
Every drug is capable of producing side effects. Many disulfiram users experience no, or minor, side effects. The frequency and severity of side effects depend on many factors including dose, duration of therapy, and individual susceptibility. Possible side effects include:

*Nervous System:* Drowsiness; fatigue; headache; psychotic reaction.

*Other:* Rash; acne; metallic or garlic-like aftertaste; impotence; abnormal liver function; optic neuritis; peripheral neuritis; polyneuritis; peripheral neuropathy.

## Guidelines for Use:

- Dosage will be individualized. Use exactly as prescribed.
- Tablets may be crushed and mixed with liquid to insure ingestion.
- Depending on the individual patient, maintenance dosage may be required for months or even years.
- Never use in intoxicated individuals or without an individual's knowledge. Patient's relatives should be instructed accordingly.
- Do not take for at least 12 hours after drinking alcohol. A reaction may occur for up to 2 weeks after disulfiram has been stopped.
- If a dose is missed, take it as soon as possible. If several hours have passed or if it is nearing time for the next dose, do not double the dose to catch up, unless advised to do so by your doctor. If more than one dose is missed, or it is necessary to establish a new dosage schedule, contact your doctor or pharmacist.
- Avoid alcohol in all forms. This includes: Alcoholic beverages including beer and wine, vinegars, many liquid medications (including prescription and nonprescription products), some sauces, aftershave lotions, colognes, liniments, backrubs, etc.
- Always read product labels or ask your pharmacist about alcohol content of all liquid medications before choosing one.
- May cause drowsiness. Use caution while driving or performing other tasks requiring alertness, coordination, or physical dexterity.
- The alcohol-disulfiram reaction can have serious adverse effects on the heart and respiratory systems.
- When taking disulfiram, always carry identification that describes the symptoms most likely to occur as a result of the disulfiram-alcohol reaction. Include the phone numbers of your doctor or the medical facility that should be contacted in case of an emergency.
- Lab tests will be required during therapy. Be sure to keep appointments.
- Store at room temperature.

*If you have any questions, consult your doctor, pharmacist, or health care provider.*

| Generic Name<br>*Brand Name Example* | Supplied As | Generic<br>Available |
|---|---|---|
| Rx **Naltrexone HCl** | | |
| *ReVia* | **Tablets:** 50 mg | No |

## Type of Drug:

Pure opioid antagonist; anti-opioid; antinarcotic.

## How the Drug Works:

Naltrexone blocks the effects of alcohol and intravenous (IV) opioids (eg, narcotic pain relievers, heroin). The exact mechanism of action is unknown. It is believed that naltrexone blocks the effects of opioids by competitive binding at opioid receptors. Therefore, if patients self-administer alcohol, heroin or any other opiate they will not feel the effects ("high") of the drug.

## Uses:

To aid in the treatment of alcohol dependence and narcotic addiction by blocking the drug's effects. It has not been shown to provide any benefit except as part of a full plan of management for the addictions.

*Unlabeled Use(s):* Occasionally doctors may prescribe naltrexone for the treatment of postconcussional syndrome unresponsive to other treatments. It has also been used in eating disorders.

## Precautions:

*Do not use in the following situations:*

acute opioid withdrawal
allergy to naltrexone
failure of NARCAN challenge test
hepatitis, acute

liver failure
opioid dependency
opioid use (within 7 to 10 days)
opioid analgesic use

*Use with caution in the following situations:*

liver disease, active or history of

*Drug-free* condition should be maintained for at least 7 to 10 days before starting naltrexone.

*Severe opioid withdrawal syndromes* have been reported in addicts currently using narcotics who have ingested naltrexone. Symptoms usually appear within 5 minutes and last up to 48 hours. Symptoms may include confusion, severe drowsiness and hallucinations. Fluid loss due to vomiting and diarrhea may require IV fluid replacement.

*Self-administering* large amounts of opioids in an attempt to overcome the blockade is very dangerous and may lead to a fatal overdose.

*Pregnancy:* Adequate studies have not been done in pregnant women. Use only if clearly needed and potential benefits outweigh the possible hazards to the fetus.

*Breastfeeding:* It is not known if naltrexone appears in breast milk. Consult your doctor before you begin breastfeeding.

*Children:* Safety and effectiveness have not been established in children under 18.

## Drug Interactions:

Tell your doctor or pharmacist if you are taking or if you are planning to take any over-the-counter or prescription medications or dietary supplements while taking naltrexone. Doses of one or both drugs may need to be modified or a different drug may need to be prescribed. The following drugs and drug classes may interact with naltrexone:

> disulfiram (eg, *Antabuse*)
> opioid containing medicines (eg, opioid analgesics, narcotic pain relievers)
> thioridazine (eg, *Mellaril*)

## Side Effects:

Every drug is capable of producing side effects. Many naltrexone users experience no, or minor, side effects. The frequency and severity of side effects depend on many factors including dose, duration of therapy and individual susceptibility. Possible side effects include:

*Digestive Tract:* Nausea; vomiting; stomach cramps/pain; appetite loss; diarrhea; constipation.

*Nervous System:* Sleeplessness; anxiety; headache; changes in energy level; irritability; dizziness; fatigue; depression; drowsiness; suicidal thoughts.

*Other:* Bone, joint or muscle pain; skin rash; chills; increased thirst; delayed ejaculation; impotence; abnormal blood counts and liver function tests; liver problems; tearfulness; nasal symptoms; yawning.

## Guidelines for Use:

- Always carry identification indicating that you are taking naltrexone.
- Take without regard to food.
- If a dose is missed, take it as soon as possible. If several hours have passed or if it is nearing time for the next dose, do not double the dose in order to "catch up" (unless advised to do so by your doctor). If more than one dose is missed or it is necessary to establish a new dosage schedule, contact your doctor or pharmacist.
- Do not share your medication with anyone else.
- Do not take this medicine until you are opioid-free for at least 7 to 10 days, and after successful completion of the NARCAN challenge test.
- Take only as directed by your doctor. Attempts to self-administer heroin or any other opiate in small doses will result in no perceived effect. However, self-administration of large doses may result in serious injury, coma or death.
- Patients taking naltrexone may not benefit from opioid-containing medicines, such as cough and cold preparations, antidiarrheals and some pain relievers. Use a nonopioid-containing alternative, if available.
- Naltrexone may cause liver injury when taken in large doses, or in people who develop liver disease from other causes. If you develop abdominal pain lasting more than a few days, white bowel movements, dark urine or yellowing of the eyes, stop taking naltrexone and contact your doctor immediately.
- Lab tests will need to be done often to detect early liver damage. Be sure to keep appointments.
- Naltrexone should be used only as part of a comprehensive alcohol or drug treatment program.
- Store in a dry, dark place at room temperature.

*If you have any questions, consult your doctor, pharmacist, or health care provider.*

| Generic Name<br>*Brand Name Example* | Supplied As | Generic<br>Available |
|---|---|---|
| *C-II* **Levomethadyl Acetate<br>Hydrochloride (LAAM)** | | |
| *ORLAAM* | **Oral Solution:** 10 mg | No |

## Type of Drug:

Synthetic opioid analgesic used as an anti-opioid/antinarcotic.

## How the Drug Works:

LAAM suppresses the symptoms of withdrawal in opiate-dependent individuals by acting as a substitute for morphine-like opiates. Chronic administration also can produce enough tolerance to block the "high" associated with injectable opiates.

## Uses:

For the management of opiate (eg, heroin, morphine) dependence. LAAM is intended for use as part of a comprehensive treatment plan.

## Precautions:

*Do not use in the following situations:* allergy to LAAM

*Use with caution in the following situations:*

Addison disease
asthma and other respiratory
 conditions
elderly or debilitated
head injury
heart conduction abnormality,
 existing or potential
hypothyroidism (underactive
 thyroid)

increased intracranial pressure
kidney disease
liver disease
prostatic hypertrophy
stomach conditions, acute
urethral stricture

*Pregnancy:* Adequate studies have not been done in pregnant women. LAAM use is not recommended during pregnancy.

*Breastfeeding:* It is not known if LAAM appears in breast milk. Consult your doctor before you begin breastfeeding.

*Children:* LAAM is not recommended in children under 18 years of age.

## Drug Interactions:

Tell your doctor or pharmacist if you are taking or if you are planning to take any over-the-counter or prescription medications or dietary supplements with levomethadyl acetate hydrochloride. Doses of one or both drugs may need to be modified or a different drug may need to be prescribed. The following drugs and drug classes interact with levomethadyl acetate hydrochloride.

alcohol
antidepressants
antifungals (eg, ketoconazole)
antihistamines
benzodiazepines (eg, diazepam)
carbamazepine (eg, *Tegretol)*
cimetidine (eg, *Tagamet)*
erythromycin (eg, *E-Mycin)*
meperidine (eg, *Demerol)*
methadone (eg, *Dolophine)*

narcotic antagonists/agonists
opioids
phenobarbital (eg, *Barbita)*
phenytoin (eg, *Dilantin- 125)*
propoxyphene (eg, *Darvon)*
rifampin
sedatives (eg, benzodiazepines)
tranquilizers (eg, phenothiazines)

## Side Effects:

Every drug is capable of producing side effects. Many LAAM users experience no, or minor, side effects. The frequency and severity of side effects depend on many factors including dose, duration of therapy and individual susceptibility. Possible side effects include:

*Digestive Tract:* Abdominal pain; constipation; diarrhea; dry mouth; nausea; vomiting.

*Nervous System:* Abnormal dreams; anxiety; decreased sex drive; depression; euphoria (exaggerated sense of well being); headache; decreased sensitivity to stimulation; sleeplessness; nervousness; sleepiness.

*Circulatory System:* Slow heart beat; light-headedness upon rising.

*Respiratory System:* Nasal congestion; cough; yawning.

*Skin:* Rash; sweating.

*Other:* Weakness; back pain; chilis; edema (fluid retention); hot flashes; flu-like symptoms;general body discomfort; blurred vision; tearing; difficult ejaculation; impotence; muscle and joint pain.

## Guidelines for Use:

- Do not take more frequently than prescribed. These drugs can be addicting.
- Do not take daily. Daily use of the usual doses will lead to serious overdose.
- The full effects of LAAM will not be felt for several days.
- Use or abuse of other psychoactive drugs or alcohol may result in fatal overdose.
- If transferring from LAAM to methadone, wait 48 hours after the last dose of LAAM before taking the first dose of methadone or other narcotics.
- May impair mental and/or physical abilities. Use caution while driving or performing other tasks requiring alertness, coordination and/or physical dexterity.
- Current regulations mandate monthly pregnancy tests in female patients of childbearing potential.
- Patients should inform their adult family members that, in the event of overdose, the treating physician or emergency room staff should be told that the patient physically dependent on narcotics, is being treated with LAAM, a long-acting opioid that is likely to outlast naloxone-induced reversal and which requires prolonged observation and careful monitoring.

*If you have any questions, consult your doctor, pharmacist, or health care provider.*

| Generic Name Brand Name Examples | Supplied As | Generic Available |
|---|---|---|
| *Rx* **Penicillamine** | | |
| *Cuprimine* | **Capsules:** 125 mg, 250 mg | No |
| *Depen* | **Tablets:** 250 mg | No |

## Type of Drug:

Arthritis agent, chelating agent; antidote. Drug to decrease cystine kidney stone formation.

## How the Drug Works:

The exact manner by which penicillamine works in arthritis is unknown. It may have anti-inflammatory activity or it may interfere with immune mechanisms which are responsible for arthritis-type problems.

Penicillamine is a chelating agent. Chelating agents combine with metal. Penicillamine removes excess copper from the systems of people with Wilson's disease. It may also be used in poisoning by binding with metals (iron, mercury, lead, arsenic).

Penicillamine reduces excessive excretion of amino acids in the urine, which leads to kidney stone formation, by chemically reacting with the stones, making them more soluble.

## Uses:

To treat rheumatoid arthritis.

To treat Wilson disease (disease characterized by copper deposits in the body due to faulty copper metabolism).

To treat kidney stone formation due to cystinuria.

*Unlabeled Use(s):* Occasionally doctors may prescribe penicillamine for treatment of primary biliary cirrhosis and scleroderma (thickening and hardening of the skin).

## Precautions:

*Do not use in the following situations:*
>   breastfeeding
>   kidney disease
>   penicillamine-related aplastic anemia, history
>   penicillamine-related decrease in white blood cells
>   pregnancy

*Use with caution in the following situations:* myasthenic syndrome. Progression to myasthenia gravis has occurred. Symptoms usually disappear when the drug is stopped.

*Pregnancy:* Use only when clearly needed and when the potential benefits outweigh the possible hazards to the fetus. There are possible hazards of penicillamine to the developing fetus. Report promptly any missed menstrual periods or other indications of possible pregnancy to your doctor.

*Breastfeeding:* Safety of penicillamine use while breastfeeding is not established. Do not breastfeed while taking this drug.

*Children:* The safety and effectiveness of penicillamine in juvenile rheumatoid arthritis have not been established.

*Lab tests* will be required during treatment with penicillamine. Tests may include: Urine tests, liver function tests, x-rays, complete blood count and platelet count and an antinuclear antibody (ANA) test.

## Drug Interactions:

Tell your doctor or pharmacist if you are taking or if you are planning to take any over-the-counter or prescription medications or dietary supplements with penicillamine. Doses of one or both durgs may need to be modified or a different drug may need to be prescribed. The following drugs and drug classes interact with penicillamine.

antacids
anticancer drugs (eg, methotrexate)
antimalarial drugs (eg, quinine sulfate)
digoxin (eg, *Lanoxin)*

gold therapy (eg, auranofin)
iron salts (eg, ferrous sulfate)
oxyphenbutazone
phenylbutazone
 (eg, *Butazolidin)*

## Side Effects:

Every drug is capable of producing side effects. Many penicillamine users experience side effects. The frequency and severity of side effects depend on many factors including dose, duration of therapy and individual susceptibility. Possible side effects include:

*Digestive Tract:* Nausea; vomiting; stomach pain; appetite loss; diarrhea; reactivated peptic ulcer; colitis.

*Respiratory System:* Breathing difficulty; coughing or wheezing; shortness of breath.

*Skin:* Rash; itching; unusual bruising or bleeding; yellowing of skin or eyes; hot flashes.

*Other:* Fever; chills; joint pain; mouth sores; ringing in the ears; hair loss; muscle weakness; sore throat; breast enlargement; altered taste perception; abnormal liver function tests; protein and blood in urine; abnormal blood counts.

**Guidelines for Use:**

- Take on an empty stomach (1 hour before meals or 2 hours after meals). Take at least 1 hour apart from any other drugs, food or milk.
- Drink ample water while taking this drug.
- Notify your doctor promptly if fever, sore throat, chills, bruising or bleeding occurs.
- Periodically see your doctor to make certain that the drug is working properly and to insure that no serious side effects are developing.
- Do not stop taking this medication without first consulting your doctor. If therapy is interrupted, do not start taking the medication again without first consulting your doctor.
- May increase the dietary need for pyridoxine and iron. Daily supplements may be required.

*If you have any questions, consult your doctor, pharmacist, or health care provider.*

| Generic Name<br>*Brand Name Example* | **Supplied As** | **Generic<br>Available** |
|---|---|---|
| *Rx* **Anakinra** | | |
| *Kineret* | **Injection**: 100 mg/mL | No |

## Type of Drug:

Agent for treating active rheumatoid arthritis; human interleukin-1 receptor antagonist; immune system modulator.

## How the Drug Works:

Interleukin-1 (IL-1) is one of the chemicals produced by the body that can cause pain, inflammation, and bone and joint loss in rheumatoid arthritis. Anakinra relieves signs and symptoms of rheumatoid arthritis by blocking these destructive actions of IL-1.

## Uses:

For the reduction in signs and symptoms of moderately to severely active rheumatoid arthritis in patients 18 years of age and older who have failed one or more disease modifying antirheumatic drugs (DMARDs). The drug can be used alone or in combination with DMARDs other than tumor necrosis factor (TNF) blocking agents (eg, etanercept).

## Precautions:

*Do not use in the following situations:*
allergy to the drug, any of its ingredients, or *Escherichia coli*-derived proteins
infections, active

*Use with caution in the following situations:*
immunosuppression
kidney disease
live vaccines, concurrent administration

*Pregnancy:* There are no adequate and well-controlled studies in pregnant women. Use only if clearly needed and the potential benefits outweigh the possible risks to the fetus.

*Breastfeeding:* It is not known if anakinra appears in breast milk. Consult your doctor before you begin breastfeeding.

*Children:* Safety and effectiveness have not been established.

*Elderly:* No overall differences in safety or effectiveness were observed in elderly patients compared with younger patients. Because there is a higher incidence of infection in the elderly population, caution should be used in treating the elderly.

*Lab tests* will be required during treatment. Tests include blood cell counts.

## Drug Interactions:

Tell your doctor or pharmacist if you are taking or planning to take any over-the-counter or prescription medications or dietary supplements with this drug. Drug doses may need to be modified or a different drug prescribed. Etanercept (*Enbrel*) interacts with this drug.

## Side Effects:

Every drug is capable of producing side effects. Many patients experience no, or minor, side effects. The frequency and severity of side effects depend on many factors, including dose, duration of therapy, and individual susceptibility. Possible side effects include injection-site reaction, sinus infection, flu-like symptoms, headache, nausea, diarrhea, stomach pain, and upper respiratory infection.

## Guidelines for Use:

- Review the patient information leaflet before starting therapy and when you receive each refill.
- Dosage is individualized. Take exactly as prescribed.
- Do not stop taking or change the dose, unless instructed by your doctor.
- Anakinra is intended for use under the guidance and supervision of your doctor. Patients may self-inject only if their doctor determines that it is appropriate and with medical follow-up as necessary after proper training in injection technique.
- Carefully follow the storage, preparation, administration, and disposal techniques taught to you by your health care provider.
- This drug is injected subcutaneously (SC; beneath the skin).
- Doses should be administered at the same time every day. New injections should be given at least 1 inch from an old site and never into areas where the skin is tender, bruised, red, or hard.
- Visually inspect the solution for particles or discoloration before use. Do not use if the solution is discolored, cloudy, or has particles.
- Contact your doctor immediately if you experience persistent fever, sore throat, or other signs of infection.
- Stop taking anakinra and contact your doctor immediately if an anaphylactic reaction or other serious allergic reaction occurs.
- Inform your doctor if you are pregnant, become pregnant, plan to become pregnant, or are breastfeeding.
- Live vaccines should not be given concurrently with anakinra.
- Injection-site reactions generally occur in the first month of use and subsequently decrease in frequency. The duration of reactions is typically 14 to 28 days. Notify your doctor if this becomes intolerable.
- Lab tests will be required to monitor therapy. Be sure to keep appointments.
- Store in refrigerator at 36° to 46°F. Do not freeze or shake. Protect from light. Do not use beyond the date stamped on the carton.

*If you have any questions, consult your doctor, pharmacist, or health care provider.*

| Generic Name Brand Name Example | Supplied As | Generic Available |
|---|---|---|
| Rx **Etanercept** | | |
| *Enbrel* | **Powder for injection:** 25 mg[1] | No |

[1] Contains 0.9% benzyl alcohol.

## Type of Drug:

Agent for rheumatoid arthritis and psoriatic arthritis.

## How the Drug Works:

Etanercept binds to and inhibits one of the chemical mediators (tumor necrosis factor) that is responsible for the inflammation and joint destruction of rheumatoid arthritis and psoriatic arthritis.

## Uses:

For reducing the signs and symptoms and delaying structural damage in patients with moderately to severely active rheumatoid arthritis. Etanercept can be used in combination with methotrexate in patients who do not respond adequately to methotrexate alone.

For reducing the signs and symptoms of moderately to severely active polyarticular-course juvenile rheumatoid arthritis (JRA) in patients who have had an inadequate response to one or more disease-modifying antirheumatic drugs (DMARDs).

For reducing the signs and symptoms of active arthritis in patients with psoriatic arthritis. Etanercept can be used in combination with methotrexate in patients who do not respond adequately to methotrexate alone.

## Precautions:

*Do not use in the following situations:*

allergy to the drug or any of its ingredients
diabetes, poorly controlled
infection, active
sepsis (blood infection)
vaccines, live

*Use with caution in the following situations:*

blood abnormalities, history of
demylelinating disorders of the central nervous system (eg, multiple sclerosis)
heart failure
immunosuppression
infections, chronic or history of recurring

*Immunosuppression:* There is a possibility that etanercept may reduce the body's defense mechanism against infections and cancers. The safety and efficacy of etanercept in patients with immunosuppression or chronic infections have not been evaluated.

*Pregnancy:* There are no adequate and well-controlled studies in pregnant women. Use only if clearly needed and potential benefits outweigh the possible risks to the fetus.

*Breastfeeding:* It is not known if etanercept appears in breast milk. Consult your doctor before you begin breastfeeding.

*Children:* Safety and effectiveness have not been established in children younger than 4 years of age. Childhood immunizations should be up-to-date before starting etanercept therapy. Pediatric patients who receive etanercept and have a significant exposure to varicella virus (chickenpox) should temporarily stop etanercept therapy and be evaluated for treatment with varicella-zoster immune globulin.

*Elderly:* No overall differences in safety or effectiveness were observed in elderly patients compared with younger patients. Because there is a higher incidence of infections in the elderly population, caution should be used in treating the elderly.

## Drug Interactions:

Tell your doctor or pharmacist if you are taking or planning to take any over-the-counter or prescription medications or dietary supplements while taking this drug. Drug doses may need to be modified or a different drug prescribed.

## Side Effects:

Every drug is capable of producing side effects. Many patients experience no, or minor, side effects. The frequency and severity of side effects depend on many factors including dose, duration of therapy, and individual susceptibility. Possible side effects include:

*Injection Site Reaction:* Mild to moderate redness; itching; pain; swelling.

*Digestive Tract:* Stomach pain; indigestion; vomiting; nausea.

*Nervous System:* Headache; dizziness.

*Respiratory System:* Upper respiratory tract infection; sinus infection; pneumonia; difficulty breathing; runny nose; cough; sore throat.

*Other:* Kidney, joint, skin, bone, blood, or wound infection; rash; skin or mouth ulcer; hair loss; weakness; swelling of the feet or ankles.

## Guidelines for Use:

- Dosage is individualized. Take exactly as prescribed.
- Etanercept is intended for use under the guidance and supervision of your doctor. Patients may self-inject only if their doctor determines that it is appropriate, and with medical follow-up as necessary after proper training in injection technique.
- Carefully follow the storage, preparation, administration, and disposal techniques taught to you by your health care provider.
- The usual dosage is administered subcutaneously (SC; beneath the skin) twice weekly.
- Doses should be separated by 72 to 96 hours and injection sites should be rotated. New injections should be given at least 1 inch from an old site and never into areas where the skin is tender, bruised, red, or hard.
- Visually inspect the solution for particles or discoloration before use. Do not use if the solution is discolored, cloudy, or has particles.
- Contact your doctor immediately if you experience persistent fever, bruising, bleeding, or pale skin while taking this medicine.
- Stop taking and contact your doctor immediately if an anaphylactic or other serious allergic reaction occurs.
- If you are sensitive to latex, do not handle the needle cover of the syringe containing the diluent.
- Live vaccines should not be given concurrently with etanercept.
- JRA patients should be up-to-date with all immunizations prior to initiating therapy with etanercept.
- Methotrexate, corticosteroids (eg, prednisone), salicylates, nonsteroidal anti-inflammatory drugs (NSAIDs), or analgesics may be continued during treatment with etanercept. Methotrexate should not be continued in JRA patients receiving high doses of etanercept.
- Injection-site reactions generally occur in the first month of use and subsequently decrease in frequency. The duration of reactions is typically 3 to 5 days.
- Improvement in symptoms may be noted within 1 to 2 weeks of starting therapy, but may take up to 3 months in some cases.
- Arthritis symptoms will recur, usually within 1 month, following discontinuation of etanercept.
- Dose tray must be refrigerated at 36° to 46°F. Do not freeze. Do not use a dose tray beyond the date stamped on the carton.

*If you have any questions, consult your doctor, pharmacist, or health care provider.*

| Generic Name Brand Name Example | Supplied As | Generic Available |
|---|---|---|
| Rx **Peginterferon alfa-2a** | | |
| Pegasys | Injection 180 mcg/mL | No |

## Type of Drug:

Immunomodulator; alpha interferon; viral replication inhibitor.

## How the Drug Works:

The exact mechanism of action is not known. Peginterferon may inhibit viral replication in infected cells, inhibit viral cell growth, or modify viral cell activity (immunomodulation).

## Uses:

For use alone or in combination with ribavirin for the treatment of adults with chronic hepatitis C virus infection who have compensated liver disease and have not been previously treated with interferon alfa. Patients in whom efficacy was demonstrated included patients with compensated liver disease and histological evidence of cirrhosis (Child-Pugh class A).

*Unlabeled Use(s):* Has been used to treat renal cell carcinoma.

## Precautions:

*Do not use in the following situations:*

allergy to the drug or any of its ingredients
autoimmune liver disease
blood disease (eg, sickle cell anemia, thalassemia)
liver decompensation
men whose female partners are pregnant
newborns and infants
pregnant women

*Use with caution in the following situations:*

autoimmune disorders (eg, psoriasis, rheumatoid arthritis, hepatitis)
bone marrow disease
colon disease
depression
heart disease
infection, severe
kidney disease
lung disease
overactive or underactive thyroid
pancreatic disease
suicidal ideation
viral infections
vision disorders (eg, retinopathy)

*Pregnancy:* There are no adequate and well-controlled studies in pregnant women. Use only if clearly needed and the potential benefits outweigh the possible risks to the fetus. When used in combination with ribavirin, do not use during pregnancy. The risk of use in a pregnant woman clearly outweighs any possible benefit.

*Breastfeeding:* It is not known if peginterferon alfa-2a appears in breast milk. Consult your doctor before you begin breastfeeding.

*Children:* Safety and effectiveness in children younger than 18 years of age have not been established.

*Elderly:* Safety and effectiveness in patients 65 years of age and older have not been established.

*Lab tests* are required during treatment. Tests include blood cell counts and liver and kidney function tests.

## Drug Interactions:

Tell your doctor or pharmacist if you are taking or planning to take any over-the-counter or prescription medications or dietary supplements with this drug. Drug doses may need to be modified or a different drug prescribed. Theophylline (eg, *Theolair*) interacts with this drug.

## Side Effects:

Every drug is capable of producing side effects. Many patients experience no, or minor, side effects. The frequency and severity of side effects depend on many factors, including dose, duration of therapy, and individual susceptibility. Possible side effects include:

*Digestive Tract:* Nausea; vomiting; diarrhea; stomach pain; colitis; dry mouth; upset stomach; appetite loss.

*Nervous System:* Headache; dizziness; memory impairment; irritability; anxiety; nervousness; sleeplessness; depression; concentration impairment.

*Skin:* Hair loss; increased sweating; rash; skin inflammation; itching; hives; injection-site reaction; dry skin.

*Other:* Blurred vision; difficulty breathing; cough; back, muscle, or joint pain; fatigue; weakness; stiffness; pain; fever; flu-like symptoms; high blood pressure; thyroid disorder; anemia; rigors; weight loss.

## Guidelines for Use:

- Dosage is individualized. Take exactly as prescribed.
- Peginterferon alfa-2a is intended for use under the guidance and supervision of a doctor. Patients may self-inject only if their doctor determines that it is appropriate, and with medical follow-up as necessary after proper training in injection technique.
- Carefully follow the storage, preparation, administration, and disposal techniques taught to you by your health care provider.
- New injections should be given at least 1 inch from an old site and never into areas where the skin is tender, bruised, red, or hard.
- Visually inspect the solution for particles or discoloration before use. Do not use if the solution is discolored, cloudy, or has particles.
- Report any changes in vision to your doctor.
- Report signs or symptoms of depression or suicidal thoughts to your doctor.
- Stop taking peginterferon alfa-2a and contact your doctor immediately if you experience weakness, severe diarrhea, rash, hives, difficulty breathing, fever, or a serious allergic reaction.
- Inform your doctor if you are pregnant, become pregnant, plan to become pregnant, or are breastfeeding.
- Lab tests will be required during treatment. Be sure to keep appointments.
- Store in the refrigerator (36° to 46°F). Do not freeze or shake. Protect from light. Vials are for single use only. Discard any unused portion.

*If you have any questions, consult your doctor, pharmacist, or health care provider.*

| Generic Name<br>*Brand Name Example* | Supplied As | Generic<br>Available |
|---|---|---|
| *Rx* **Peginterferon alfa-2b** | | |
| *PEG-Intron* | **Powder for Injection**: 50 mcg/<br>0.5 mL, 80 mcg/0.5 mL,<br>120 mcg/0.5 mL, 150 mcg/<br>0.5 mL | No |

## Type of Drug:

Immunomodulator; alpha interferon; viral replication inhibitor.

## How the Drug Works:

The exact mechanism of action is not known. Peginterferon may inhibit viral replication in infected cells, inhibit viral cell growth, or modify viral cell activity (immunomodulation).

## Uses:

For use alone or in combination with ribavirin for the treatment of chronic hepatitis C in patients with compensated liver disease who have not been previously treated with interferon alfa and are at least 18 years of age.

*Unlabeled Use(s):* Has been used to treat renal carcinoma.

## Precautions:

*Do not use in the following situations:*

allergy to the drug or any of its ingredients
autoimmune liver disease
blood disease
liver disease, decompensated
men whose female partners are pregnant
pregnant women

*Use with caution in the following situations:*

autoimmune disorders (eg, psoriasis, rheumatoid arthritis, hepatitis)
bone marrow disease
colon disease
depression
heart disease
infection, severe
kidney disease
lung disease
overactive or underactive thyroid
pancreatic disease
suicidal ideation
vision disorders (eg, retinopathy)

*Pregnancy:* There are no adequate and well-controlled studies in pregnant women. Use only if clearly needed and potential benefits outweigh the possible risks to the fetus. When used in combination with ribavirin, do not use during pregnancy. The risk of use in a pregnant woman clearly outweighs any possible benefit.

*Breastfeeding:* It is not known if peginterferon alfa-2b appears in breast milk. Consult your doctor before begin breastfeeding.

*Children:* Safety and effectiveness in children younger than 18 years of age have not been established.

*Elderly:* Safety and effectiveness in patients 65 years of age and older have not been established.

*Lab tests* may be required during treatment. Tests include blood cell counts and liver and kidney function tests.

## Drug Interactions:

Tell your doctor or pharmacist if you are taking or planning to take any over-the-counter or prescription medications or dietary supplements with this drug. Drug doses may need to be modified or a different drug prescribed.

## Side Effects:

Every drug is capable of producing side effects. Many patients experience no, or minor, side effects. The frequency and severity of side effects depend on many factors, including dose, duration of therapy, and individual susceptibility. Possible side effects include:

*Digestive Tract:* Nausea; appetite loss; diarrhea; vomiting; stomach pain; upset stomach; constipation; dry mouth.

*Nervous System:* Dizziness; sleeplessness; depression; anxiety; irritability; impaired concentration; agitation; nervousness.

*Respiratory System:* Difficulty breathing; cough; sore throat; runny nose; sinus infection.

*Skin:* Hair loss; itching; rash; dry skin; increased sweating; injection-site reaction.

*Other:* Flushing; fatigue; headache; fever; weight loss; chest, muscle, or joint pain; weakness; menstrual pain; fungal infection; viral infection; taste changes; blurred vision; stiffness; blood disorders; rigors.

## Guidelines for Use:

- Dosage is individualized. Take exactly as prescribed.
- Peginterferon alfa-2b is intended for use under the guidance and supervision of a physician. Patients may self-inject only if their physician determines that it is appropriate, and with medical follow-up as necessary after proper training in injection technique.
- Carefully follow the storage, preparation, administration, and disposal techniques taught to you by your health care provider.
- New injections should be given at least 1 inch from an old site and never into areas where the skin is tender, bruised, red, or hard.
- Visually inspect the solution for particles or discoloration before use. Do not use if the solution is discolored, cloudy, or has particles.
- Notify your doctor if you experience severe or bloody diarrhea, rash, hives, difficulty breathing, fever, depression, suicidal thoughts, change in vision, severe chest pain, unusual bruising or bleeding, severe stomach pain, or lower back pain.
- Stop taking peginterferon alfa-2b and contact your doctor immediately if a serious allergic reaction occurs.
- Inform your doctor if you are pregnant, become pregnant, plan to become pregnant, or are breastfeeding.
- Lab tests will be required to monitor treatment. Be sure to keep appointments.
- Store at 77°F. After reconstitution with supplied diluent, the solution should be used immediately, but may be stored up to 24 hours at 36° to 46°F.

*If you have any questions, consult your doctor, pharmacist, or health care provider.*

| Generic Name<br>*Brand Name Example* | Supplied As | Generic<br>Available |
|---|---|---|
| *Rx* **Bupropion HCl** | | |
| *Zyban* | **Tablets, sustained release**:<br>150 mg | No |

## Type of Drug:

Nonnicotine smoking deterrent; antidepressant.

## How the Drug Works:

The exact mechanism by which bupropion helps patients stop smoking is unknown. It may alter chemicals in the brain (neurotransmitters) that suppress the urge to smoke.

## Uses:

An aid to smoking cessation treatment.

Bupropion is also used as an antidepressant. See the Antidepressants-Bupropion monograph in the Central Nervous System Drugs chapter.

*Unlabeled Use(s):* Occasionally, doctors may prescribe bupropion for the treatment of attention deficit hyperactivity disorder and sustained-release bupropion for the treatment of neuropathic pain or to enhance weight loss.

## Precautions:

*Do not use in the following situations:*

abrupt discontinuation of alcohol or sedatives (benzodiazepines)
allergy to the drug or any of its ingredients
anorexia nervosa, active or history of
bulimia, active or history of
bupropion (eg, *Wellbutrin*), current use for depression
monoamine oxidase inhibitor (MAOI) use, current or within 14 days
seizure disorders

*Use with caution in the following situations:*

alcohol use, excessive
attempted suicide, history of
bipolar manic depression
brain tumor
diabetes treated with oral hypoglycemics or insulin
drug abuse
head injury, history of
heart attack, recent
heart disease
kidney disease
liver disease
sedative (benzodiazepine) use, current
seizure, history or risk of
therapy that lowers seizure threshold (eg, antipsychotics, antidepressants, theophyllines, systemic steroids)

*Pregnancy:* There are no adequate and well-controlled studies in pregnant women. Use only if clearly needed and the potential benefits outweigh the possible risks to the fetus.

*Breastfeeding:* Bupropion is excreted in breast milk. Serious side effects could potentially occur in the nursing infant. Decide whether to discontinue the drug or discontinue breastfeeding, taking into account the importance of the drug to the mother. Consult your doctor before you begin breastfeeding.

*Children:* Safety and effectiveness have not been established in children younger than 18 years of age.

*Elderly:* Older patients are known to metabolize drugs more slowly and to be more sensitive to antidepressant drugs. Use the lowest effective dose.

## Drug Interactions:

Tell your doctor or pharmacist if you are taking or planning to take any over-the-counter or prescription medications or dietary supplements with this drug. Drug doses may need to be modified or a different drug prescribed. The following drugs and drug classes interact with this drug:

amantadine (eg, *Symmetrel*)
antidepressants (eg, fluoxetine, amitriptyline)
antipsychotics (eg, phenothiazines)
beta blockers (eg, metoprolol)
carbamazepine (eg, *Tegretol*)
cimetidine (eg, *Tagamet*)
corticosteroids, systemic (eg, prednisone)
levodopa (eg, *Sinemet*)

MAOIs (eg, phenelzine)
nicotine transdermal system (eg, *Nicoderm*)
phenobarbital (eg, *Solfoton*)
phenytoin (eg, *Dilantin*)
ritonavir (eg, *Norvir*)
theophylline (eg, *Slo-Phyllin*)
type 1C antiarrythmics (eg, propafenone, flecainide)
warfarin (eg, *Coumadin*)

## Side Effects:

Every drug is capable of producing side effects. Many patients experience no, or minor, side effects. The frequency and severity of side effects depend on many factors including dose, duration of therapy, and individual susceptibility. Possible side effects include:

*Parkinson Disease-Like Symptoms:* Stumbling walk; movement disorders.

*Digestive Tract:* Nausea; vomiting; constipation; indigestion; appetite changes; stomach pain; dry mouth; mouth sores; diarrhea; difficulty swallowing; increased salivation.

*Nervous System:* Seizures; tremor; dizziness; agitation; anxiety; headache; activation of psychosis or mania; sleeplessness; depression; nervousness; irritability; disturbed concentration; delusions; hallucinations; confusion; decreased memory; sleep disturbances; drowsiness; restlessness; exaggerated sense of well-being; hostility; paranoia; sedation; fatigue; CNS stimulation; sensory disturbance; migraine headache.

*Circulatory System:* Changes in blood pressure; pounding in chest (palpitations); chest pain; changes in heart rate or rhythm; fainting.

*Skin:* Rash; itching; excessive sweating; flushing; hives; feeling of hot or cold skin.

*Other:* Taste sensation changes; blurred vision; ringing in the ears; frequent urination; fever; joint or muscle pain; weakness; hot flashes; sore throat; weight changes; abnormal skin sensations; facial swelling; increased cough; sinus infection; hearing problems; impotence; menstrual problems; chills; changes in sex drive; urinary retention; muscle spasms; urinary tract infection; twitch; vaginal bleeding; sore throat; upper respiratory complaints; vision problems; ringing in ears; infection.

## Guidelines for Use:

- Dosage is individualized. Take exactly as prescribed.
- Do not exceed 300 mg of bupropion sustained-release tablets daily for smoking cessation. Single doses should not exceed 150 mg because of the risk of seizures.
- Do not crush, chew, or divide tablets. Tablets are designed to gradually release medication.
- Do not change the dose or stop taking, unless advised to do so by your doctor.
- May be taken without regard to meals. Take with food if stomach upset occurs.
- If a dose is missed, take it as soon as possible. If several hours have passed or it is less than 8 hours before your next dose, do not double the dose to catch up, unless instructed by your doctor. Never take more than 150 mg at one time. If several doses are missed or it is necessary to establish a new dosage schedule, contact your doctor or pharmacist.
- Usual duration of therapy is 7 to 12 weeks. Longer periods of therapy are acceptable under your doctor's guidance.
- To maximize your chance of quitting smoking, you should not stop smoking until you have been taking bupropion for 1 week. You should set a date to stop smoking during the second week you are taking bupropion.
- This medicine should not be used in combination with *Wellbutrin* or any other medication containing bupropion.
- It is not physically dangerous to smoke and use this medicine at the same time. However, continuing to smoke after the date you set to stop smoking will seriously reduce your chance of breaking your smoking habit.
- Using bupropion and nicotine patches (eg, *Nicoderm CQ*) at the same time can raise your blood pressure. Use both only under your doctor's supervision.
- Do not smoke if you are using bupropion and nicotine patches at the same time.
- Avoid or minimize alcohol consumption to reduce the risk of seizures caused by bupropion.
- Do not take in combination with MAOIs or within 14 days of discontinuing treatment with an MAOI.
- May cause drowsiness. Use caution while driving or performing other tasks requiring alertness, coordination, or physical dexterity until tolerance is determined.

## Guidelines for Use (cont.):

- Sustained-release bupropion has a characteristic odor; this is normal and no cause for concern.
- Counseling and support are an important component of smoking cessation.
- Store at 68° to 77°F.

*If you have any questions, consult your doctor, pharmacist, or health care provider.*

| Generic Name<br>*Brand Name Examples* | Supplied As | Generic<br>Available |
|---|---|---|
| **Nicotine** | | |
| *Rx Nicotrol* | **Inhaler:** 10 mg/cartridge | No |
| *Rx Nicotrol NS* | **Nasal Spray:** 10 mg/mL | No |
| *otc Nicotrol* | **Transdermal System:** 5 mg/day, 10 mg/day, 15 mg/day | No |
| *otc Nicoderm CQ* | **Transdermal System:** 7 mg/day, 14 mg/day, 21 mg/day | Yes |
| *otc Commit* | **Lozenge:** 2 mg/lozenge, 4 mg/lozenge | No |
| *otc Nicorette* | **Chewing Gum:** 2 mg/square, 4 mg/square | Yes |

## Type of Drug:

Smoking deterrents. Aids to stop smoking and for the relief of nicotine-withdrawal symptoms. Smoking deterrents should be used as part of a comprehensive behavioral smoking-cessation program.

## How the Drug Works:

Nicotine has a variety of effects on the body. It is possible to become dependent on and abuse nicotine. Smoking deterrents containing nicotine provide low levels of nicotine in the body but without the tars and carbon monoxide found in cigarette smoke. This low level of nicotine may help prevent physical signs of nicotine withdrawal after stopping smoking to help reduce the urge to smoke nicotine.

## Uses:

To temporarily aid a cigarette smoker who is trying to quit smoking.

*Unlabeled Use(s):* Occasionally doctors may prescribe nicotine gum with haloperidol to improve symptoms of Tourette syndrome.

## Precautions:

*Do not use in the following situations:* Allergy to the drug or any of its ingredients (eg, menthol).

*Use with caution in the following situations:*

allergy to adhesive tape (transdermal system only)
angina, severe
asthma (nasal spray, inhaler only)
cardiovascular disease
diabetes
heart attack, history of or recent
high blood pressure, accelerated (inhaler, transdermal system only)
high blood pressure, uncontrolled
irregular heart rhythm
kidney disease, severe
liver disease
mouth, teeth, or jaw problems (gum only)
nasal disorders, chronic (eg, allergy, congestion, polyps, sinus problems) (nasal spray only)
nonnicotine smoking deterrents (eg, bupropion)
overactive thyroid
peptic ulcer
peripheral vascular disease
pheochromocytoma (tumor of the adrenal gland)
pregnancy
skin disorders (transdermal system only)
temporomandibular disease (TMJ), active (gum only)

*Pregnancy:* Smoking and smoking deterrents are not recommended during pregnancy. Studies have shown a potential adverse effect on the fetus. Use only if clearly needed and potential benefits outweigh the possible risks to the fetus.

*Breastfeeding:* Nicotine is excreted in breast milk. Do not use during breastfeeding. Consult your doctor before breastfeeding.

*Children:* Safety and effectiveness have not been established. These products are not intended for use by children or adolescents. The amounts of nicotine in nicotine-containing smoking deterrents that are tolerated by adult smokers can produce symptoms of poisoning and could prove fatal if applied or ingested by children. Therefore, keep these products out of the reach of children. Contact your doctor if a child chews or swallows a piece of nicotine gum.

## Drug Interactions:

Tell your doctor or pharmacist if you are taking or planning to take any over-the-counter or prescription medications or dietary supplements while taking this medicine. Drug doses may need to be modified or a different drug prescribed. Stopping smoking, with or without nicotine substitutes, may change the response to the following drugs and drug classes:

acetaminophen (eg, *Tylenol)*
adrenergic antagonists
  (eg, prazosin, labetalol)
alcohol
benzodiazepines (eg, diazepam,
  chlordiazepoxide)
beta adrenergic blockers
  (eg, atenolol)
caffeine
catecholamines
  (eg, isoproterenol)
clorazepate (eg, *Tranxene*)
clozapine (eg, *Clozaril*)
cortisol (eg, hydrocortisone)

estradiol (eg, *Estrace*)
flecainide (eg, *Tambocor*)
fluvoxamine (eg, *Luvox*)
heparin
insulin
mexiletine (*Mexitil*)
olanzapine (*Zyprexa*)
opioids (eg, dextropropoxy-
  phene)
tacrine (*Cognex*)
theophylline (eg, *Theolair*)
tricyclic antidepressants
  (eg, imipramine)

## Side Effects:

Every drug is capable of producing side effects. Many patients experience no, or minor, side effects. The frequency and severity of side effects depend on many factors including dose, duration of therapy, and individual susceptibility. Possible side effects include:

*Chewing gum* – Mouth or tongue sores; injury to teeth or lining of the mouth; jaw ache; sore throat or mouth; belching; increased salivation.

*Inhaler* – Mouth or throat irritation; coughing; runny nose; indigestion; headache; taste complaints; jaw, back, or neck pain; tooth disorder; sinus infection; flu-like symptoms; abnormal skin sensations; fever; gas; chest discomfort; bronchitis; high blood pressure; nausea; diarrhea; hiccups.

*Lozenge* – Nausea; heartburn; indigestion; hiccups; sleeplessness; headache; gas; coughing.

*Nasal spray* – Nasal irritation, ulcers, or blisters; congestion; runny nose; sore throat; hoarseness; watery eyes; sneezing; cough; smell or taste sensation changes; numbness or burning of nose or mouth; earache; flushing; sinus problems; eye irritation or burning; chest tightness; indigestion; abnormal skin, mouth, nose, or head sensations; constipation; mouth inflammation; nosebleed; sore throat; headache; back, muscle, stomach, or joint pain; difficulty breathing; nausea; menstrual disorder; pounding in the chest (palpitations); gas; tooth or gum disorder; acne; itching; painful menstruation.

*Transdermal system* – Burning; itching; redness; rash; swelling; diarrhea; indigestion; muscle pain; abnormal dreams; drowsiness; joint pain; rapid heartbeat; pounding in the chest (palpitations).

## Guidelines for Use:

- Use exactly as prescribed. Read patient information sheet carefully before starting therapy and with each refill.
- Stop smoking completely when starting this medicine. People who smoke while taking this medicine may experience side effects more profound than those experienced from smoking alone.
- Keep these products, including both used and unused patches, nasal spray, lozenges, and gum, out of the reach of children and pets.
- Stop using and notify your doctor if you experience paleness, cold sweat, persistent nausea, dizziness, weakness, tremor, or mental confusion.
- Do not use different nicotine-containing smoking deterrents at the same time.
- *Chewing gum* — Most patients require approximately 9 to 12 pieces of gum per day during the first month of treatment. Do not exceed 24 pieces of 4 mg gum per day.
  Avoid eating and drinking for 15 minutes before and during chewing nicotine gum.
  It may take a few days for you to adjust to the unpleasant taste of the gum.
  Slowly chew one piece of gum whenever you have an urge to smoke. Chew each piece slowly until it tingles, then leave it between your cheek and gum until the tingle is gone. Begin chewing again until the tingle returns. Repeat until most of the tingle is gone (about 30 minutes). Chewing quickly can release the nicotine too quickly, leading to effects similar to oversmoking (eg, nausea, hiccups, throat irritation).
  If you experience strong or frequent cravings, you may use a second piece of gum within the hour. Do not use one piece continuously after another.
  Stop using the gum at the end of 12 weeks, unless instructed by your doctor.
  Place used gum in a wrapper and dispose in a safe place.
  Stop using this gum if the gum sticks to dental work or you experience jaw pain.
  Store below 77°F, away from heat and light.
- *Inhaler* — Use at least 6 cartridges/day for the first 3 to 6 weeks of treatment. Additional doses may be needed to control the urge to smoke; however, do not exceed 16 cartridges/day.
  Best effect is achieved by frequent, continuous puffing over 20 minutes.
  Gradual reduction of dose may begin after 12 weeks of initial treatment and may last up to 12 weeks. If you are unable to stop smoking within 4 weeks, discontinue therapy. Do not continue for longer than 6 months because of the harmful and addictive nature of nicotine.
  After using inhaler, separate mouthpiece, remove used cartridge, and throw it away. Store mouthpiece in the plastic storage case for further use. The mouthpiece is reusable and should be cleaned regularly with soap and water.
  Store at room temperature below 77°F. Protect cartridges from light.
- *Lozenge* — Place lozenge in mouth and allow it to dissolve slowly. Do not chew or swallow it whole. Occasionally shift lozenge from one side of mouth to the other. It will take about 20 to 30 minutes to dissolve. You may feel a warm or tingling sensation in mouth. This is normal.

## Guidelines for Use (cont.):

- *Lozenge* (cont.):
  Do not eat or drink 15 minutes before or during lozenge use.
  Do not use more than one lozenge at a time or continuously use one lozenge after another. Do not use more than 5 lozenges in 6 hours, or more than 20 lozenges/day.
  Stop using and consult your doctor if you experience heartburn, nausea, indigestion, or sore throat.
- *Nasal Spray* — Administer the spray with head tilted back slightly.
  Usual starting dose is 1 to 2 doses (2 to 4 sprays) per hour. The recommended minimum dose is 8 doses (16 sprays) per day. Dose may be increased as tolerated and needed to a maximum of 5 doses (10 sprays) per hour or 40 doses (80 sprays) per day.
  Do not sniff, swallow, or inhale through the nose as spray is administered. Avoid contact with eyes, mouth, or ears. If solution comes into contact with skin, lips, mouth, eyes, or ears, rinse immediately with water only. Contact your doctor if this occurs and tissue irritation is still present, even after flushing with water.
  If solution is spilled, clean up immediately with an absorbent cloth or paper towel. Avoid contact with skin. Wash area of spill several times.
  This medicine may cause nasal irritation.
  Do not continue for longer than 6 months because of the harmful and addictive effects of nicotine.
  Discard bottle with the child-resistant cap in place.
  Store at room temperature below 86°F.
- *Transdermal system* — Dosage may vary. Refer to patient package insert or consult your doctor for recommended dosing schedules. Once the appropriate dosage has been selected, continue therapy at that dosage for the prescribed time.
  Apply patch promptly upon removal from the protective pouch. Use only if pouch is intact. Apply patch once a day to nonhairy, clean, dry skin on the upper body or upper outer arm or hip. After 24 hours (16 hours for *Nicotrol*), remove the used patch and apply a new patch to an alternate skin site. Skin sites should not be reused for at least a week. (Note: Remove *Nicotrol* at bedtime. It is for waking use only.) Do not use the same patch for more than 24 hours.
  Do not wear more than one patch at a time. Do not cut the patch into smaller pieces to reduce the dose.
  If the patch falls off, discard and apply a new patch. Remove and replace the new patch at the regular time to keep your schedule the same.
  If you are unable to stop smoking within 4 weeks, therapy should be discontinued. Therapy should not continue for longer than 6 weeks for *Nicotrol*, or 8 weeks for *Nicoderm*, in patients who have stopped smoking because of the harmful and addictive effects of nicotine.
  Following application or removal, wash hands with water only. Do not use soap. Avoid contact with eyes.
  Discontinue use and consult your doctor if you experience severe or persistent skin reactions.
  After use, fold patch over itself, place in pouch and discard.
  Store *Nicotrol* below 86°F. Store *Nicoderm* and *Habitrol* below 77°F. A slight discoloration of the patch is not significant. Do not store out of the pouch. Once out of the protective pouch, apply promptly since nicotine evaporates and the patch may lose its strength.

*If you have any questions, consult your doctor, pharmacist, or health care provider.*

| Generic Name<br>*Brand Name Examples* | Supplied As | Generic<br>Available |
|---|---|---|
| *Rx* **Alprostadil** | | |
| *Caverject* | **Injection:** 6.15 mcg, 11.9 mcg, 23.2 mcg, 46.4 mcg/vial | No |
| *Edex* | **Injection:** 6.225 mcg, 12.45 mcg, 24.90 mcg, 49.80 mcg | No |
| *Muse* | **Pellets:** 125 mcg, 250 mcg, 500 mcg, 1000 mcg | No |

## Type of Drug:
Agent for impotence.

## How the Drug Works:
Alprostadil induces penile erection by relaxing certain muscles of the penis and increasing arterial blood flow to the penis. When the effect of alprostadil wears off, blood flow to the penis returns to normal and the erection disappears.

## Uses:
To treat erectile dysfunction (impotence) in adult males. The injection may also be used with other tests to diagnose erectile dysfunction.

## Precautions:
*Do not use in the following situations:*

allergy to the drug or any of its
 ingredients
bone marrow tumors
children
leukemia
men who are advised not to
 engage in sexual activity
newborns
penile deformity
penile implants
sickle cell anemia or trait
women

*Use with caution in the following situations:*

anticoagulant (eg, warfarin) use, current
fainting, history of (pellets only)

## Drug Interactions:
Tell your doctor or pharmacist if you are taking or planning to take any over-the-counter or prescription medications or dietary supplements with this drug. Drug doses may need to be modified or a different drug prescribed. Anticoagulants (eg, warfarin) interact with this medicine (causing an increased risk of bleeding after injection).

## Side Effects:

Every drug is capable of producing side effects. Many patients experience no, or minor, side effects. The frequency or severity of side effects depend on many factors including dose, duration of therapy, and individual susceptibility. Possible side effects include:

*Nervous System:* Headache; dizziness; light-headedness.

*Respiratory System:* Upper respiratory infection; flu syndrome; sinus infection; nasal congestion; cough.

*Urinary and Reproductive Tract:* Injection-site bruising or bleeding; prolonged erection; prostate disorder or pain (possibly difficult urination); penile pain; itching, redness, rash, swelling, hardening (lumps) or discoloration of the skin; curving of the penis; testicular pain; burning sensation in urethra; pelvic pain.

*Other:* High blood pressure; back pain; heart disease; abnormal vision; swelling of leg veins; leg pain; rapid pulse; fainting.

## Guidelines for Use:

- Review patient instruction leaflet before beginning therapy and with each refill.
- Erections usually occur within 5 to 20 minutes after injection and last about 1 hour. If erection lasts longer than 4 hours, contact your doctor immediately, or, if unavailable, seek immediate medical assistance.
- This medicine does not protect against HIV (the virus that causes AIDS) or any other sexually transmitted diseases. A small amount of bleeding at the injection or insertion site can increase the risk of transmitting serious blood-borne diseases between partners.
- This medicine may cause dizziness or fainting. Use caution while driving or performing other tasks requiring alertness, coordination, or physical dexterity until tolerance is determined.
- Regular medical checkups are necessary to monitor treatment. Be sure to keep appointments.
- *Injection* — Follow the administration, reconstitution (mixing), storage, and disposal techniques taught to you by your health care provider. Many side effects can be reduced if the proper administration technique is used.
  Dosage is individualized. The proper dose is usually determined by injections being given in your doctor's office.
  Visually inspect solution for particles or discoloration before use. Discard such vials. Do not shake the contents of reconstituted vials.
  The reconstituted vial is designed for one use only. Use it immediately or within 24 hours of mixing. Discard any solution that remains after the proper dose has been withdrawn from the vial or if stored for more than 24 hours after mixing.
  Discard needle properly after each use. Do not reuse or share needles or syringes. Do not allow anyone to access or use your medicine.
  Do not use this medicine more than 3 times per week. Wait at least 24 hours between each use.
  Contact your doctor immediately if you experience penile redness, swelling, tenderness, pain, lumps, hardening of the skin, or curving of the erect penis.
  A small amount of bleeding at the injection site may occur. This is normal.
  Store *Caverject* at or below 77°F. Store *Edex* at controlled room temperature (59° to 86°F).
- *Pellets* — Carefully follow the insertion technique taught to you by your health care provider.
  Allow the delivery system to warm to room temperature before using.
  Wash hands before and after handling delivery system.
  Urinate immediately before inserting the pellet.
  If you experience dizziness or feel faint, lie down immediately and raise your legs. Contact your doctor if symptoms persist or worsen.
  Mild vaginal itching or burning in female partner may occur. Contact your doctor if this becomes bothersome.
  Do not use more than twice in 24 hours.
  Use a condom barrier during intercourse with a pregnant woman.
  Store in refrigerator (36° to 46°F). May be stored at room temperature (less than 86°F) for up to 14 days. Avoid exposure to temperatures greater than 86°F or exposure to direct sunlight. Do not freeze, store in checked luggage during air travel, or leave in a closed automobile.

*If you have any questions, consult your doctor, pharmacist, or health care provider.*

| Generic Name *Brand Name Example* | Supplied As | Generic Available |
|---|---|---|
| Rx **Sildenafil Citrate** | | |
| *Viagra* | **Tablets:** 25 mg, 50 mg, 100 mg | No |

## Type of Drug:

Agent for impotence (erectile dysfunction).

## How the Drug Works:

Sildenafil citrate produces smooth muscle relaxation in the penis, allowing blood to flow in and cause an erection.

Sildenafil citrate has no effect in the absence of sexual stimulation or arousal.

## Uses:

To treat erectile dysfunction (eg, impotence) due to a variety of causes.

## Precautions:

*Do not use in the following situations:*

allergy to sildenafil or any of its ingredients
children
women
organic nitrates, regular or intermittent use in any dose form (eg, nitroglycerin, isosorbide dinitrate as sublingual tablets, tablets, capsules, transdermal patches, ointments, nasal sprays)

*Use with caution in the following situations:*

abnormal heart rhythm, life-threatening (within the last 6 months)
bleeding disorders (eg, hemophilia)
cardiovascular disease, preexisting
elderly (65 years of age or older)
heart failure or coronary artery disease causing unstable angina
high blood pressure (BP greater than 170/110)
kidney function impairment, severe
leukemia
liver disease
low blood pressure, resting (BP less than 90/50)
multiple myeloma
myocardial infarction (within the last 6 months)
penile deformity (eg, Peyronie disease)
penile implants or other erectile dysfunction treatments
priapism (eg, prolonged or painful erections)
retinitis pigmentosa
sickle cell anemia
stroke (within the last 6 months)
ulcers, active peptic

*Pregnancy:* There are no adequate and well-controlled studies in pregnant women. Sildenafil citrate is not indicated for use in women, children, or newborns.

*Elderly:* The elimination of sildenafil citrate is reduced in healthy patients over 65 years of age. The starting dose should not be over 25 mg.

*Lab tests* may be required before beginning treatment with sildenafil. A thorough medical history and physical exam must be done to determine erectile dysfunction, underlying causes, and appropriate treatment.

## Drug Interactions:

Tell your doctor or pharmacist if you are taking or if you are planning to take any over-the-counter or prescription medications or dietary supplements with sildenafil. Doses of one or both drugs may need to be modified or a different drug may need to be prescribed. The following drugs interact with sildenafil.

> amlodipine (eg, *Norvasc*)
> beta blockers, non-specific (eg, atenolol, propranolol)
> cytochrome P450 3A4 inducers (eg, rifampin)
> cytochrome P450 3A4 inhibitors (eg, cimetidine, erythromycin, itraconazole)
> high-fat meals may slow absorption with concurrent drug administration
> loop diuretics (eg, furosemide)
> organic nitrates (eg, nitroglycerin, all dose forms)
> potassium-sparing diuretics (eg, spironolactone)

## Side Effects:

Every drug is capable of producing side effects. Many sildenafil users experience no, or minor, side effects. The frequency and severity of side effects depend on many factors including dose, duration of therapy, and individual susceptibility. Possible side effects include:

*Circulatory System:* Chest pain; heart block; heart muscle damage; flushing; fast heartbeat; low blood pressure; heart failure; blood clots in brain; palpitations (pounding in chest); dizziness; fainting; low blood pressure when rising from a seated or lying position; abnormal heart rhythm; angina; cardiac arrest.

*Digestive Tract:* Vomiting; colon inflammation; difficulty swallowing; stomach pain; dry mouth; gum, stomach, tongue, or mouth inflammation; rectal bleeding; indigestion; diarrhea.

*Nervous System:* Dizziness; vertigo (feeling of a whirling motion); headache; migraine; tremors; depression; sleeplessness; drowsiness; decreased reflexes; abnormal dreams; abnormal skin sensations; nerve pain; nerve disease; incoordination; muscle stiffness or weakness; decreased sensitivity to touch.

*Respiratory System:* Asthma; difficulty breathing; laryngitis; increased cough; increased sputum; sinus inflammation; sore throat; nasal congestion; bronchitis; respiratory tract infections.

*Skin:* Sweating; skin ulcers; herpes simplex; hives; itching; skin inflammation; flushing; rash.

*Senses:* Eye pain; cataract; dry eyes; ear pain; ringing in ears; sensitivity to light; eye inflammation; pupil dilation; abnormal vision; color tinge to vision; blurred vision; double vision; deafness; eye bleeding.

*Urinary and Reproductive Tract:* Frequent urination; urinary tract infection; breast enlargement; inability to control bladder; abnormal ejaculation; genital swelling; bladder inflammation; excessive nighttime urination; inability to achieve orgasm; prolonged erection; priapism (painful erection longer than 6 hours in duration); blood in the urine.

*Other:* Back, muscle, joint, or bone pain; gout; thirst; high blood sugar; low blood sugar; shock; weakness; pain; chills; accidental injuries or falling; allergic reactions; facial swelling; flu-like syndrome; swelling; unstable diabetes; tendon rupture or inflammation; swelling of hands or feet; abnormal liver function tests; joint pain or inflammation; anemia; high blood uric acid levels; high blood sodium levels; decreased white blood cell counts.

## Guidelines for Use:

- Sildenafil is not indicated for use in women, children, or newborns.
- A thorough physical exam and medical history assessing cardiovascular and general health status and confirming erectile dysfunction, including a determination of potential underlying causes, is necessary prior to beginning treatment.
- Recommended dosage is 50 mg taken approximately 1 hour before sexual activity. It may be taken 30 minutes to 4 hours before sexual activity. Dose may be increased to a maximum recommended dose of 100 mg or decreased to 25 mg based on effectiveness and patient tolerance. Maximum dosage frequency is once daily.
- Sildenafil has no effect in the absence of sexual stimulation or arousal.
- Do not use sildenafil citrate in combination with any nitrate medications (eg, nitroglycerin, isosorbide in any dose form) as it may cause a severe, possibly fatal drop in blood pressure.
- After therapy with sildenafil, it is not known when nitrates, if needed, can be safely administered.
- Patients who experience symptoms (eg, chest pain, dizziness, nausea) upon initiation of sexual activity should be advised to refrain from further activity and notify their doctor of the episode.
- Contact your doctor if you experience any unusual side effects.
- There is a potential for cardiac risk associated with sexual activity in patients with preexisting cardiovascular disease. Therefore, treatments for erectile dysfunction should not be generally used in men for whom sexual activity is inadvisable because of their underlying cardiovascular status.
- Prior to prescribing sildenafil, physicians should carefully consider whether their patients with underlying cardiovascular disease could be affected adversely by vasodilatory effects (transient decreases in supine blood pressure), especially in combination with sexual activity.
- Taking sildenafil citrate with a high-fat meal reduces the absorption rate which can result in a delay in onset of effect.
- Do not use sildenafil in combination with any other erectile dysfunction treatment.
- This medicine offers no protection from sexually transmitted diseases such as HIV (the virus that causes AIDS).
- Seek immediate medical assistance in the event of an erection that persists longer than 4 hours. If priapism (painful erection longer than 6 hours in duration) is not treated immediately, penile tissue damage and permanent loss of potency could result.
- Store at controlled room temperature (59° to 86°F).

*If you have any questions, consult your doctor, pharmacist, or health care provider.*

| Generic Name<br>*Brand Name Examples* | Supplied As | Generic<br>Available |
|---|---|---|
| *Rx* **Yohimbine** | | |
| *Aphrodyne, Yocon,*<br>*Yohimex* | **Tablets:** 5.4 mg | No |

## Type of Drug:

Alpha adrenergic blocker. Drug for impotence (unlabeled).

## How the Drug Works:

Yohimbine causes the release of the nervous system chemical norepinephrine. Norepinephrine affects the body in a variety of ways including: Increased blood flow to the penis, stimulation of mood, local
anesthesia, mild decrease in urine output, and changes in blood pressure.

## Uses:

Yohimbine has no FDA approved uses.

*Unlabeled Use(s):* Occasionally doctors may prescribe yohimbine for orthostatic hypotension and to dilate the pupil. Yohimbine may also be used
as an aphrodisiac.

## Precautions:

*Do not use in the following situations:*
 allergy to yohimbine
 kidney disease

*Use with caution in the following situations:*
 duodenal ulcers
 heart disease
 psychiatric patients
 stomach ulcers

*Pregnancy:* Do not use during pregnancy.

*Children:* Not intended for use in children.

*Elderly:* Not intended for use in elderly patients.

## Drug Interactions:

Tell your doctor or pharmacist if you are taking or if you are planning to
take any over-the-counter or prescription medications or dietary
supplements with yohimbine. Doses of one or both drugs may need to
be modified or a different drug may need to be prescribed. Antidepressants and other mood-modifying drugs interact with yohimbine.

## Side Effects:

Every drug is capable of producing side effects. Many yohimbine users experience no, or minor, side effects. The frequency and severity of side effects depend on many factors including dose, duration of therapy and individual susceptibility. Possible side effects include:

*Nervous System:* Nervousness; irritability; tremors; dizziness; headache; increased motor activity; incoordination.

*Circulatory System:* Increased heart rate; heart pounding (palpitations); increased blood pressure.

*Other:* Runny nose; "goosebumps"; flushing; decreased urination.

### Guidelines for Use:

- Yohimbine has no FDA approved use.
- If the inability to urinate, elevated blood pressure and heart rate, increased motor activity, nervousness, irritability or tremor occurs, reduce the dosage by half, followed by gradual increases to the original dose. Consult your doctor.
- Results of therapy for longer than 10 weeks are unknown.

*If you have any questions, consult your doctor, pharmacist, or health care provider.*

| Generic Name<br>*Brand Name Examples* | Supplied As | Generic<br>Available |
|---|---|---|
| *Rx* **Interferon Beta-1a** | | |
| *Avonex* | **Powder for Injection**<br>**(lyophilized):** 0.33 mg<br>(6.6 mIU) | No |
| *Rx* **Interferon Beta-1b** | | |
| *Betaseron* | **Powder for Injection**<br>**(lyophilized):** 0.3 mg (9.6 mIU) | No |

## Type of Drug:
An antiviral and immunoregulatory.

## How the Drug Works:
The mechanisms by which interferon beta works on multiple sclerosis are not clearly understood.

## Uses:
For use in ambulatory patients with relapsing-remitting multiple sclerosis (MS) to slow the accumulation of physical disability or reduce the frequency and severity of attacks. Relapsing-remitting MS is characterized by recurrent attacks of neurologic dysfunction followed by complete or incomplete recovery.

*Unlabeled Use(s):* Occasionally, doctors may prescribe interferon beta to treat AIDS, AIDS-related Kaposi's sarcoma, herpes of the lips or genitals, certain cancers and acute non-A/non-B hepatitis.

## Precautions:
*Do not use in the following situations:* Do not use if you are allergic to interferon beta, albumin human or any other component of the formulation.

*Use with caution in the following situations:*

| | |
|---|---|
| depression | seizure disorder |
| heart disease | suicidal thoughts |

*Mental disorders/suicidal thoughts:* Depression and thoughts of suicide can be a side effect of interferon beta. These symptoms should be reported immediately to your doctor.

*Pregnancy:* Adequate studies have not been done in pregnant women, or animal studies may have shown a risk to the fetus. Use only if clearly needed and potential benefits outweigh the possible hazards to the fetus. Spontaneous abortions have occurred during this therapy.

*Breastfeeding:* It is not known if interferon beta appears in breast milk. Consult your doctor before you begin breastfeeding.

*Children:* Safety and efficacy in children under 18 years of age have not been established.

*Lab tests* may be required before starting and during treatment with interferon beta. Be sure to keep appointments.

## Drug Interactions:

Tell your doctor or pharmacist if you are taking or if you are planning to take any over-the-counter or prescription medications or dietary supplements while taking this medicine. Doses of one or both drugs may need to be modified or a different drug may need to be prescribed. Antidepressants and other mood-modifying drugs interact with this medicine.

## Side Effects:

Every drug is capable of producing side effects. Many patients experience no, or minor, side effects. The frequency and severity of side effects depend on many factors including dose, duration of therapy and individual susceptibility. Possible side effects include:

*Digestive Tract:* Diarrhea; constipation; vomiting; nausea; appetite loss; indigestion; stomach pain; dry mouth.

*Nervous System:* Sleeplessness; depression; confusion; weakness; slurred speech; convulsions; dizziness; drowsiness; migraines; headache.

*Circulatory System:* Palpitations (pounding in the chest); rapid heartbeat; chest pain; flushing; fainting; high blood pressure; unusual bleeding/bruising; cold hands and feet.

*Respiratory System:* Sinus infection; difficulty breathing; laryngitis.

*Skin:* Sweating; hair loss; sunlight sensitivity; hives; herpes; shingles; splotchiness.

*Urinary and Reproductive Tract:* Painful menstruation; heavy menstrual bleeding; breast pain; fibrous cysts in the breast or ovaries; pelvic pain; frequent urination; vaginal infection; lumps in the breast.

*Other:* Pain and tenderness at the injection site; fever; flu-like symptoms; pain; chills; general body discomfort; joint and muscle pains or spasms; weight changes; eye irritation; vision problems; inner ear infections; hearing loss; infections; goiter; swelling; suicidal thoughts; abnormal lab values.

## Guidelines for Use:

- Use exactly as prescribed.
- *Beta-1a* — usual dose is 1 vial once a week.
- *Beta-1b* — usual dose is 1 vial every other day.
- Follow the mixing process and injection procedure taught to you by your healthcare provider. Your first self-administered injection should be given under the supervision of a health care professional. A patient informa- tion sheet is provided.
- If a dose is missed, inject it as soon as possible. If it is nearing the next dose, do not double the dose in order to catch up (unless advised to do so by your doctor). If more than one dose is missed or it is neces- sary to establish a new dosage schedule, contact your doctor or pharmacist.
- If you become pregnant or plan to become pregnant, discontinue using the medicine and talk to your doctor. Spontaneous abortions have occurred during use of interferon beta.
- May cause sunlight sensitivity. Avoid long exposure to the sun. Use sun- screens and protective clothing until tolerance is known.
- Flu-like symptoms are not uncommon following the beginning of therapy. Acetaminophen may be used to relieve fever and muscle pain.
- Contact your doctor immediately if depression or suicidal thoughts occur.
- Lab tests may be required to monitor therapy. Be sure to keep appointments.
- Store in the refrigerator (36°-46°F). If refrigerator is unavailable, inter- feron beta-1a may be stored at room temperature for up to 30 days. Use reconstituted solution within 3 hours (6 hours for Beta-1a). Discard any unused solution.

*If you have any questions, consult your doctor, pharmacist, or health care provider.*

| Generic Name<br>*Brand Name Example* | Supplied As | Generic<br>Available |
|---|---|---|
| *Rx* **Riluzole** | | |
| *Rilutek* | **Tablets:** 50 mg | No |

## Type of Drug:
Neuroprotective agent.

## How the Drug Works:
Riluzole may prevent damage to certain brain cells (motor neurons) responsible for controlling muscle functions.

## Uses:
To prolong survival in patients with amyotrophic lateral sclerosis (ALS, Lou Gehrig disease).

## Precautions:
*Do not use in the following situations:*
allergy to this medicine or its ingredients

*Use with caution in the following situations:*
kidney disease
liver disease

*Pregnancy:* Adequate studies have not been done in pregnant women, or animal studies may have shown a risk to the fetus. Use only if clearly needed and potential benefits outweigh the possible hazards to the fetus.

*Breastfeeding:* It is not known if riluzole appears in breast milk. Breastfeeding is not recommended. Contact your doctor before you begin breastfeeding.

*Children:* Safety and efficacy in children have not been established.

*Elderly:* Dosage may need to be adjusted due to reduced kidney or liver function in the elderly.

*Lab tests* will be required to monitor therapy. Be sure to keep appointments.

## Drug Interactions:
Tell your doctor or pharmacist if you are taking or if you are planning to take any over-the-counter or prescription medications or dietary supplements with this medicine. Doses of one or both drugs may need to be modified or a different drug may need to be prescribed. The following drugs or drug classes interact with this medicine.

amitriptyline (eg, *Elavil)*
caffeine
cigarette smoke
food, charcoal broiled
omeprazole (eg, *Prilosec)*

quinolones (eg, ciprofloxacin)
rifampin (eg, *Rifadin)*
tacrine (*Cognex)*
theophylline (eg, *Theo-Dur)*

## Side Effects:

Every drug is capable of producing side effects. Many patients experience no, or minor, side effects. The frequency and severity of side effects depend on many factors including dose, duration of therapy and individual susceptibility. Possible side effects include:

*Digestive Tract:* Nausea; vomiting; diarrhea; appetite loss; indigestion; weight loss; stomach pain; gas; dry mouth; inflamed or sore mouth; teeth problems.

*Skin:* Rash; itching; eczema; hair loss.

*Nervous System:* Dizziness; vertigo (feeling of whirling motion); headache; weakness; drowsiness; abnormal skin sensations; depression; sleeplessness.

*Other:* General body discomfort; joint or back pain; difficulty breathing; pneumonia; nasal congestion; cough; swelling of hands and feet; high blood pressure; fast heartbeat; vein inflammation; postural hypotension (dizziness or lightheadedness when rising quickly from a sitting or lying position); difficult or painful urination; tight muscles; soreness; stiffness; inflexibility.

## Guidelines for Use:

- Use exactly as prescribed.
- Usual dose is one tablet every 12 hours. Take at the same time of day (eg, in the morning and evening) each day.
- Take on an empty stomach, at least 1 hour before or 2 hours after a meal.
- Women and Japanese patients may require a lower dose.
- If a dose is missed, take the next tablet as originally planned. Do not try to catch up (unless advised to do so by your doctor).
- This medicine may cause drowsiness or dizziness, especially when rising or standing. If these symptoms should occur, sit or lie down and contact your doctor. Use caution while driving or performing other tasks requiring alertness, coordination or dexterity.
- To reduce the risk of liver damage, avoid drinking excessive alcohol while taking this medicine.
- Tell your doctor if you smoke. It may reduce the effectiveness of this medicine.
- Contact your doctor immediately if fever or any illness occurs.
- Lab tests will be required to monitor therapy. Be sure to keep appointments.
- Store at room temperature (68°-77°F), away from bright light.

*If you have any questions, consult your doctor, pharmacist, or health care provider.*

| Generic Name<br>*Brand Name Example* | Supplied As | Generic<br>Available |
|---|---|---|
| *Rx* **Glatiramer Acetate** | | |
| *Copaxone* | **Powder for Injection,**<br>**lyophilized:** 20 mg glatiramer<br>acetate and 40 mg mannitol/<br>2 mL vial | No |

## Type of Drug:

Agent to reduce frequency of relapses in relapsing-remitting multiple sclerosis (MS).

## How the Drug Works:

The mechanism of action by which glatiramer acetate works on MS is unknown. Glatiramer is thought to possibly modify the immune process that may cause MS.

## Uses:

Indicated in the reduction or frequency or relapses in patients with relapsing-remitting MS.

## Precautions:

*Do not use in the following situations:*
    allergy to glatiramer acetate or mannitol

*Use with caution in the following situations:*
    immune disorders

*Pregnancy:* There are no adequate or well controlled studies in pregnant women. However, no drug should be used during pregnancy unless clearly needed.

*Breastfeeding:* It is not known if glatiramer acetate appears in breast milk. Consult your doctor before you begin breastfeeding.

*Children:* The safety and effectiveness of glatiramer acetate have not been established in individuals less than 18 years of age.

## Side Effects:

Every drug is capable of producing side effects. Many patients experience side effects. The frequency and severity of side effects depend on many factors including dose, duration of therapy and individual susceptibility. Possible side effects include:

*Digestive Tract:* Nausea; appetite loss; diarrhea; stomach irritation; stomach disorder; vomiting; stomach pain; indigestion; gum disease; mouth sores.

*Nervous System:* Anxiety; depression; dizziness; tremor; agitation; confusion; foot drop; nervousness; rapid eye movement; speech disorder; feeling of whirling motion; migraine.

*Circulatory System:* Fast heartbeat; pounding in the chest; fainting; unusual bruising; lymph node disorder; high blood pressure

*Respiratory System:* Difficulty breathing; bronchitis; difficulty swallowing; nasal congestion; laryngitis; rapid breathing.

*Urinary and Reproductive Tract:* Urinary urgency; painful menstruation; impotence; vaginal and yeast infections; menstrual disorder; blood in urine.

*Skin:* Hives; rash; flushing; itching; skin nodule; sweating; redness.

*Senses:* Ear pain; eye disorder.

*Body as a Whole:* Injection site reactions; chest pain; weakness; infection; pain; joint pain; muscle soreness or tightness; chills; cyst; facial swelling; fever; flu syndrome; neck pain or rigidity; general swelling; swelling of arms and legs; accidental injury; general body discomfort.

---

### Guidelines for Use:

- The usual dose is 20 mg/day.
- Deliver by subcutaneous route only.
- Follow the injection procedure taught to you by your healthcare provider. Patient instructions for use are enclosed in each package; follow the instructions provided with the medicine exactly. Perform your first self-administered injection under the supervision of a healthcare professional.
- Do not stop taking this medicine or change the dose without checking with your doctor.
- Inform your physician if you are pregnant, if you are planning to become pregnant or if you become pregnant while taking this medication.
- Inform your physician if you are nursing.
- The reconstituted product contains no preservative; it should be used immediately. Before reconstitution with diluent, store in freezer at -4° to 14°F. Store diluent at room temperature.

---

*If you have any questions, consult your doctor, pharmacist, or health care provider.*

| Generic Name<br>*Brand Name Example* | Supplied As | Generic<br>Available |
|---|---|---|
| Rx **Thalidomide** | | |
| *Thalomid* | **Capsules:** 50 mg | No |

## Type of Drug:
Immune system modulator.

## How the Drug Works:
The exact mechanism of action is unknown. It appears that thalidomide modifies some immune system effects which are responsible for the skin changes seen in erythema nodosum leprosum (ENL).

## Uses:
For the acute treatment of the cutaneous (skin) manifestations of moderate to severe erythema nodosum leprosum (ENL).

Also for maintenance therapy for prevention and suppression of the cutaneous (skin) manifestations of ENL recurrence.

This drug is not indicated as monotherapy for ENL treatment in the presence of moderate to severe neuritis (nerve inflammation).

Thalidomide is approved for marketing only under a special restricted distribution program called "System for Thalidomide Education and Prescribing Safety (S.T.E.P.S.)." Only prescribers and pharmacists registered under the program are allowed to prescribe and dispense the product. Patients must be advised of, agree to, and comply with the requirements of the S.T.E.P.S. program to receive the product.

## Precautions:
*Do not use in the following situations:*
allergy to thalidomide or any of its ingredients
neuritis, moderate to severe
pregnancy or the possibility of pregnancy

*Use with caution in the following situations:*
HIV infection
low blood pressure
neuritis, preexisting

*Pregnancy:* Do not use during pregnancy. The risk of use in a pregnant woman clearly outweighs any possible benefit. If thalidomide is taken during pregnancy, it can cause severe birth defects or death to an unborn baby. Even a single dose (50 mg) taken by a pregnant woman can cause severe birth defects. When there is no alternative treatment, women of childbearing potential may be treated with thalidomide, provided adequate precautions are taken to avoid pregnancy. Women must commit either to abstain continuously from sexual intercourse or use 2 methods of reliable birth control, including at least 1 highly effective method (eg, IUD, hormonal contraception) and 1 additional effective method (eg, latex condom, diaphragm, cervical cap), beginning 4 weeks prior to initiating treatment with thalidomide, during therapy, and for

4 weeks following discontinuation of therapy. This should be done even when there has been a history of infertility, unless due to a hysterectomy or because the patient has been postmenopausal for at least 24 months.

Women of childbearing potential must have pregnancy testing (sensitivity of at least 50 mIU/mL). A written report of a negative pregnancy test must be obtained before the prescription is written. The test should be performed within the 24 hours before beginning thalidomide therapy and then weekly during the first month of therapy, then monthly thereafter in women with regular menstrual cycles or every 2 weeks in women with irregular menstrual cycles. Perform pregnancy testing and counseling if a patient misses her period or if there is any abnormality in menstrual bleeding. If pregnancy occurs during treatment, thalidomide must be discontinued immediately. Under these conditions, the patient should be referred to an OB/GYN experienced in reproductive toxicity for further evaluation and counseling.

Because it is not known whether thalidomide is present in the ejaculate of males receiving the drug, males receiving thalidomide must always use a latex condom when engaging in sexual activity with women of childbearing potential.

*Breastfeeding:* It is not known whether thalidomide appears in breast milk. A decision should be made whether to discontinue nursing or discontinue the drug, taking into account the importance of the drug to the mother. Consult your doctor before you begin breastfeeding.

*Children:* Safety and efficacy in children under 12 years of age have not been established.

*Lab tests* will be required before, during, and after treatment. Tests may include: Pregnancy tests, peripheral neuropathy detection, blood counts, and viral load in HIV patients.

## Drug Interactions:

Tell your doctor or pharmacist if you are taking or planning to take any over-the-counter or prescription medications or dietary supplements with thalidomide. Doses of one or both drugs may need to be modified or a different drug may need to be prescribed. The following drugs may interact with thalidomide:

> alcohol
> barbiturates (eg, phenobarbital)
> chlorpromazine (eg, *Thorazine*)
> drugs associated with neuropathy (eg, isoniazid, amiodarone, clofibrate)
> reserpine

A variety of drugs (eg, protease inhibitors, phenytoin, carbamazepine, rifampin, rifabutin, griseofulvin, broad-spectrum antibiotics) may interact with oral contraceptives and render them less effective. This increases the risk of pregnancy.

## Side Effects:

Every drug is capable of producing side effects. Many thalidomide users experience no, or minor, side effects. The frequency and severity of side effects depend on many factors including dose, duration of therapy, and individual susceptibility. Possible side effects include:

*Nervous System:* Agitation; dizziness; sleeplessness; nervousness; abnormal skin sensations; drowsiness; tremor; feeling of whirling motion; headache; dizziness when rising; numbness, tingling, or pain in hands or feet.

*Skin:* Acne; fungal skin inflammation; nail disorder; itching; rash; sweating.

*Digestive Tract:* Loss of appetite; stomach pain; constipation; diarrhea; dry mouth; gas; nausea; fungal infection (mouth); tooth pain.

*Urinary and Reproductive Tract:* Protein in urine; blood in urine; impotence.

*Respiratory System:* Sore throat; sinus infection; congested or runny nose.

*Other:* Anemia; swelling of feet or ankles; decreased white blood cell count; increased viral load (in HIV patients); low blood pressure; slow heart hate; accidental injury; weakness; back pain; infection; neck pain; neck stiffness; pain; liver function test abnormalities; chills; fever; general body discomfort; swollen glands.

## Guidelines for Use:

- Thalidomide must only be administered in strict compliance with all of the terms outlined in the S.T.E.P.S. (System for Thalidomide Education and Prescribing Safety) program. Thalidomide may only be prescribed by prescribers registered with the S.T.E.P.S. program and only dispensed by pharmacists registered with the S.T.E.P.S. program.
- For an episode of cutaneous ENL, the recommended dose is 100 to 300 mg once daily with water, preferably at bedtime and at least 1 hour after the evening meal. Patients weighing less than 110 lbs. should be started at the low end of the dose range.
- In patients with a severe cutaneous ENL reaction, or in those who have previously required higher doses to control the reaction, thalidomide dosing may be initiated at higher doses, up to 400 mg once daily at bedtime or in divided doses with water, at least 1 hour after meals.
- Dosing with thalidomide should usually continue until signs and symptoms of active reaction have subsided, usually a period of at least 2 weeks. Patients may then be tapered off medication in 50 mg decrements every 2 to 4 weeks.
- Patients who have a documented history of requiring prolonged maintenance treatment to prevent the recurrence of cutaneous ENL or who flare during tapering off medication, should be maintained on the minimum dose necessary to control the reaction. Tapering off medication should be attempted every 3 to 6 months, in decrements of 50 mg every 2 to 4 weeks.

## Guidelines for Use (cont.):

- Thalidomide should never be used by women who are pregnant or who could become pregnant while taking the drug.
- Women of childbearing potential must have pregnancy testing before and during therapy.
- Women must commit either to abstain continuously from sexual intercourse or use 2 methods of reliable birth control, including at least 1 highly effective method (eg, IUD, hormonal contraception) and 1 additional effective method (eg, latex condom, diaphragm, cervical cap), beginning 4 weeks prior to initiating treatment with thalidomide, during therapy, and continuing 4 weeks following discontinuation of therapy.
- Discontinue thalidomide immediately if pregnancy is suspected or identified.
- Males receiving thalidomide must always use a latex condom when engaging in sexual activity with women of childbearing potential.
- Women using oral contraceptives to prevent pregnancy should be aware that HIV-protease inhibitors, griseofulvin, rifampin, phenytoin, carbamazepine, and broad-spectrum antibiotic therapy can reduce the effectiveness of oral contraceptives.
- Thalidomide is known to cause nerve damage that may be permanent. Peripheral neuropathy is a common, potentially severe and irreversible, side effect of treatment. Symptoms (eg, numbness, tingling, or pain in the hands and feet) may occur after thalidomide treatment has been stopped and may resolve slowly or not at all. If symptoms develop, notify your physician immediately. If appropriate, your physician will discontinue thalidomide immediately to limit further damage. Testing at monthly intervals will be required for the first 3 months of therapy and periodically thereafter during treatment.
- Contact your doctor immediately if you experience a skin rash, fever, fast heartbeat, or low blood pressure. These may be signs of an allergic reaction and may necessitate therapy discontinuation.
- May cause drowsiness, dizziness, or blurred vision. Use caution while driving or performing other tasks requiring alertness, coordination, or physical dexterity until tolerance is determined. Patients should sit upright for a few minutes prior to standing up.
- May cause photosensitivity (sensitivity to sunlight). Avoid prolonged exposure to the sun or other forms of ultraviolet (UV) light (eg, tanning beds). Use sunscreens and wear protective clothing until tolerance is determined.
- In patients with moderate to severe neuritis associated with a severe ENL reaction, corticosteroids may be started along with thalidomide. Steroid usage may be tapered or discontinued when the neuritis has improved.
- Do NOT share this medication with anyone else.
- Patients taking thalidomide cannot donate blood. Male patients should not donate sperm.
- Lab tests will be required during therapy. Be sure to keep appointments.
- Store between 59° and 86°F. Protect from light.

*If you have any questions, consult your doctor, pharmacist, or health care provider.*

**Glucose (Blood) Tests,** 1751

**Glucose (Urine) Tests,** 1754

**Ketone Tests,** 1758

**Occult Blood Tests,** 1761

**Ovulation Tests,** 1764

**Pregnancy Tests,** 1766

**Protein Tests,** 1768

**Urinary Tract Infection
  Tests,** 1770

**Miscellaneous Tests (Urine),** 1772

| | Brand Name Examples | Supplied As | Test For |
|---|---|---|---|
| *otc* | *Accu-Chek Advantage* | **Test Strips:** For blood | Glucose meter (*Accu-Chek*) |
| *otc* | *Chemstrip bG* | **Test Strips:** For blood | Visual glucose and glucose meter (*Accu-Chek*) |
| *otc* | *Dextrostix, Glucostix* | **Test Strips:** For blood | Visual glucose and glucose meter (*Glucometer*) |
| *otc* | *Diascan* | **Test Strips:** For blood | Visual glucose and glucose meter (*Diascan*) |
| *otc* | *Glucofilm, Glucometer Elite, Glucometer Encore* | **Test Strips:** For blood | Glucose meter (*Glucometer*) |
| *otc* | *One Touch* | **Test Strips:** For blood | Glucose meter (*One Touch*) |
| *otc* | *First Choice* | **Test Strips:** For blood | Glucose meter (*Diascan, Glucometer, One Touch*) |
| *otc* | *Tracer bG* | **Test Strips:** For blood | Glucose meter (*Tracer*) |

Diagnostic or therapeutic decisions should not be based on a single test result. If you have any questions regarding your test results, contact your doctor. For information on diabetes and diabetes medications, see the insulin and sulfonylureas monographs in the Hormones chapter.

## Type of Drug:

For detection of glucose (sugar) in blood.

## How the Drug Works:

Specially treated test strips indicate the blood glucose concentration. Regular monitoring of glucose aids in the control of diabetes. It will help determine medication, dietary and exercise needs and help decrease the complications (eg, neuropathies, retinopathies) and problems during pregnancy.

## Uses:

To monitor blood glucose levels in diabetics. To aid in control of the condition.

To aid in determining medication regimes, diet, and exercise programs for diabetics.

To help prevent development of complications during pregnancy.

## Precautions:

*Do not use in the following situations:*

| | |
|---|---|
| dehydration, severe | internal use |
| illness, severe | shock |

*Normal blood glucose levels — Approximate ranges:*

*Nondiabetic fasting adults –* 60 to 110 mg/dL.

*Nondiabetic adults (1 to 2 hours after eating) –* 110 to 180 mg/dL.

*Diabetics –* Results will vary depending on diet, medication dose, exercise, etc. Consult your doctor to determine your target blood glucose level.

*Newborns –* Not all tests strips or glucose meters are intended for testing newborn blood samples. Read manufacturers' instructions carefully.

*Specimen collection and handling:* All blood glucose test strips require a finger or earlobe stick. An automatic lancet device punctures the skin to obtain a single drop of blood. A manual lancet is more painful and laceration size and puncture depth cannot be predicted. These are important because they control the volume of the drop of blood. The size of the test pad varies among manufacturers. It must be completely covered with blood.

A single drop of blood is placed on the test strip. Begin timing when the test pad is covered completely. In some tests, the blood drop is wiped from the test strip at the end of the timed period. Timing is critical. The wiping or blotting technique and the recommended tissue paper or cotton for blotting may vary by manufacturer. The test strip is placed in the glucose meter. The results are read from the meter display. The visual test is read against the color key.

*Storage and handling:* A bottle of test strips can be used for 4 months after being opened. Always write the date the bottle is first opened on the bottle label. Never use the test strips past the expiration date indicated on the bottle label or foil packet. Use of strips beyond the expiration date may yield inaccurate results.

Keep unused test strips in the original bottle with cap tightly closed. Always replace the cap immediately and tightly. Never transfer test strips to another bottle.

Leave the drying agent in the bottle. The drying agent absorbs moisture and keeps the strips dry. Never put cotton or other material in the bottle. Do not use discolored strips. Keep your fingers or other objects from touching the test pads before testing. Touching the pads could cause inaccurate test results.

Keep strip vial away from small children. A child could choke on the cap or drying agent, which could be harmful if swallowed.

Store at room temperature (59° to 86°F). Do not store bottle in direct sunlight. Do not freeze. Do not store in cabinets with bleach or products containing bleach.

## Drug Interactions:

Tell your doctor or pharmacist if you are taking or planning to take any over-the-counter or prescription medications or dietary supplements while testing for blood glucose. The following drugs and drug classes may interact with the test to cause questionable results:

acetaminophen (eg, *Tylenol*)
aspirin (large amounts)
dopamine (large amounts)

fluoride
methyldopa (large amounts)
vitamin C

## Guidelines for Use:

- Follow instructions on the label exactly.
- Monitor blood for glucose as prescribed. Monitor urine ketones if your blood glucose level has been greater than 300 mg/dL for 2 consecutive blood glucose determinations.
- Blood glucose monitoring is recommended to achieve normal blood sugar levels. Keep track of your blood glucose results so that adjustments in your treatment program can be made more easily.
- Participate in a thorough diabetes education program so that you understand diabetes and all aspects of its treatment, including diet, exercise, personal hygiene and how to self-monitor blood glucose.
- Apply the blood drop, time the reaction, blot the test pads and read the test results the same way each time you do the test.
- *Diabetics — Monitor glucose:*
  When you have a cold, the flu or any other kind of illness.
  When you "feel" the signs of low or high blood sugar (greater than 240 mg/dL) or when your blood sugar is well over the range your doctor has set for you (if you do blood glucose monitoring).
  When you are under unusual physical or emotional stress.
  During pregnancy or after a testing pattern has been established with your doctor or educator.
- Have all the materials you need before beginning the test: Test strips, timer (stop-watch or watch with a second hand), sterile lancet, cotton or rayon balls, alcohol wipes, and glucose meter.
- Color vision is needed to properly read visual, but not meter, test results. Have someone else confirm the visual test results if in doubt.
- Quality control and sample tests may be required before testing.
- If test results seem questionable, check expiration date on the label, repeat the test using a new test strip, run controls, check glucose meter and check procedure (timing).
- If you are unable to identify the cause of a low or high test result, contact your doctor or diabetes educator. Know the symptoms of hyperglycemia (high blood sugar), which include thirst, hunger and frequent and excessive urination and those of hypoglycemia (low blood sugar), which include trembling, sweating, blurred vision, rapid heartbeat, and tingling or numbness around mouth or fingertips.
- If you experience stomach pain, vomiting or difficulty breathing, contact your doctor immediately.
- Individuals with high uric acid, bilirubin cholesterol, triglyceride or hematocrit levels may have lowered glucose levels.
- Diabetes education may be obtained through your local chapter of the American Diabetes Association.

*If you have any questions, consult your doctor, pharmacist, or health care provider.*

| | Brand Name Examples | Supplied As | Test For |
|---|---|---|---|
| otc | Chemstrip uGK, Keto-Diastix | **Test strips:** for urine | Glucose and ketones (acetoacetic acid) |
| otc | Chemstrip 2GP | **Test strips:** for urine | Glucose and protein |
| otc | Chemstrip bG, Clinistix, Diastix | **Test strips:** for urine | Glucose |
| otc | Clinitest | **Tablets:** for urine | Glucose, lactose, fructose, galactose and pentose |

Diagnostic or therapeutic decisions should not be based on a single test result. If you have any questions regarding your test results, contact your doctor. For information on diabetes and diabetes medications see the insulin and sulfonylureas monographs in the Hormones chapter.

## Type of Drug:

For detection of glucose (sugar) in urine.

## How the Drug Works:

Glucose does not normally appear in the urine, but when too much glucose builds up in the blood, the excess spills over from the kidney into the urine where it can be detected by specially designed plastic test strips and reagent tablets containing chemicals which detect glucose in urine. Color changes occur according to the amount of sugar present.

Regular monitoring of glucose levels aids in the control of diabetes. It will help determine medication, exercise and dietary needs and help decrease complications (eg, kidney and eye problems) and problems during pregnancy.

Ketones appear in the urine when the body breaks down body fats to use as a source of energy or food. This can occur in fasting individuals, out-of-control diabetics and individuals on starvation diets.

Proteins in the urine may be an early sign of kidney disease.

## Uses:

To detect glucose in urine.

To aid diabetics in monitoring medication regimens, diet and exercise programs.

To help prevent the development of complications and problems during pregnancy.

## Precautions:

*Not for internal use.*

*Avoid contact with skin, mucous membranes or clothing.* If contact occurs, flush the affected area with large amounts of water. If test strips, tape, or tablets are eaten or rubbed in the eyes, contact your doctor or local poison control center immediately. If eaten, do not induce vomiting; instead, drink large amounts of water or milk. If contact with the eyes occurs, flush with water for 15 minutes. Get prompt medical attention.

*Specimen collection and handling:* Collect fresh urine in a clean, dry container and test as soon as possible. (An alternate method is to pass the test strips directly through the urine stream). If testing cannot be done within an hour after collection, refrigerate. Let it return to room temperature before testing. Prolonged exposure of unpreserved urine to room temperature (59° to 86°F) may result in bacterial contamination and bacterial consumption of the glucose. Urine preservatives may also affect the accuracy of test results.

*Storage and handling:*

*For bottled strips –* Store at room temperature (59° to 86 F). Do not store the bottle in direct sunlight. Protect from light, heat, and moisture.
Keep unused test strips in the original bottle with the cap tightly closed. Always replace the cap immediately and tightly. A new bottle of test strips can be used for 6 months after first being opened. Always write the date you first opened the bottle on the bottle label. Do not use the product after the expiration date. Use of strips beyond the expiration date may yield inaccurate test results. Never transfer strips to another bottle. Do not remove drying agent from the bottle. The agent absorbs moisture and keeps the strips dry. Never put cotton or other materials in the bottle. If test areas are discolored or darkened, throw the strip away and use a strip from a new bottle.

*For tablets –* Tablets have prolonged stability in the unopened container if stored at room temperature between 59° and 86°F. Do not refrigerate. Do not store in direct sunlight. Once the bottle is opened, protect from moisture. Excessive moisture may cause a chemical reaction and a bottle explosion may occur. Use tablets on a regular basis and do not store for extended periods of time after the bottle is opened. Recap the bottle tightly immediately after removing a tablet. Tablets in foil must be used immediately upon opening. Protect tablets from light, heat and moisture. Do not open the bottle in a steamy bathroom. Moisture causes tablets to turn a deeper shade of blue. If tablets darken or if test results seem questionable or inconsistent with expected findings:
Confirm that product is within expiration date shown on label or foil. Check performance with a positive control. If proper result is not obtained, discard and retest with a fresh tablet.

*Tablets:* Sugars other than glucose will cause a positive test result. These sugars include: Lactose, fructose, galactose, and pentose.

*Ketones:* High levels of ketones may cause false positive test results for urine containing small amounts of glucose.

## Drug Interactions:

Tell your doctor or pharmacist if you are taking or planning to take any over-the-counter or prescription medication or dietary supplements while testing for urine glucose. The following drugs and drug classes may interact with the test to cause questionable results:

aspirin (large amounts)
nalidixic acid *(NegGram)*
nitrofurantoin (eg, *Furadantin)*
phenazopyridine (eg, *Pyridium)*

riboflavin
sulfa drugs (eg, sulfonamides)
vitamin C (ascorbic acid)

*Clinitest only —*

cephalosporins (eg, cephalexin)
penicillin

probenecid (eg, *Benemid)*
x-ray contrast media (IV)

Consider all drug interactions reported for protein test strips and ketone test strips when appropriate.

## Guidelines for Use:

- Follow instructions on the label exactly.
- Glucose is not normally detected in urine.
- Monitor urine for glucose and ketones as prescribed. Monitor urine ketones if your blood glucose level has been greater than 300 mg/dL for 2 consecutive blood glucose determinations. Blood glucose monitoring is recommended to achieve normal blood sugar levels. Keep track of your blood glucose results so that adjustments in your treatment program can be made more easily.
- Participate in a thorough diabetes education program so that you understand diabetes and all aspects of its treatment, including diet, exercise, personal hygiene, and how to self-monitor blood or urine glucose.
- *Diabetics — Monitor glucose:*
    When you have a cold, the flu or any other kind of illness.
    When you "feel" the signs of high blood sugar (more than 240 mg/dL) or when your blood sugar is well over the range your doctor has set for you (if you do blood glucose monitoring).
    When you are under unusual physical or emotional stress.
    During pregnancy after a testing pattern has been established with your doctor or educator.
- Have all the materials you need before beginning the test: Test strips, timer (stopwatch or watch with a second hand), and a clean dry container.
- Color vision is needed to properly read test results. Have someone else confirm the test results if in doubt.
- If test results seem questionable, check expiration date on the label, repeat the test using a new test strip or tablet and a fresh urine specimen.
- If your are unable to identify the cause of a low or high test result, contact your doctor or diabetes educator. Know the symptoms of hyperglycemia (high blood sugar), which include thirst, hunger and frequent and excessive urination and those of hypoglycemia (low blood sugar), which include trembling, sweating, blurred vision, rapid heartbeat, and tingling or numbness around mouth or fingertips.
- Individuals with high uric acid, bilirubin cholesterol, triglyceride, or hematocrit levels may have lowered glucose levels.
- Diabetes education may be obtained through your local chapter of the American Diabetes Association.
- Some of these items can cause burns. Avoid contact with skin, eyes, mucous membranes, and clothing. Keep away from children.

*If you have any questions, consult your doctor, pharmacist, or health care provider.*

| | Brand Name Examples | Supplied As | Test For |
|---|---|---|---|
| otc | Acetest | **Tablets:** For blood, serum, plasma, or urine | Acetoacetic acid and acetone |
| otc | Chemstrip K | **Test strips:** For urine | Acetoacetic acid and acetone |
| otc | Ketostix | **Test strips:** For urine | Acetoacetic acid |

Diagnostic or therapeutic decisions should not be based on a single test result. If you have any questions regarding your test results, contact your doctor.

## Type of Drug:

For detection of ketones (acetone, acetoacetate, or acetoacetic acid, also known as "ketone bodies" or "ketones").

## How the Drug Works:

Specially treated tablets *(Acetest)* or plastic test strips *(Chemstrip K, Ketostix)* detect the presence of ketones in the urine and blood (*Acetest* only). Ketones are substances that are formed when the body breaks down fats and carbohydrates for energy or food. When there are too many ketones in the body, they spill over into the urine. Ketones may be found in the urine of people who are fasting, on starvation diets, or in diabetics who have a very high blood sugar level because of lack of insulin. Ketones are not present in normal urine.

## Uses:

To detect ketones in urine.

To monitor for diabetic ketoacidosis, a complication of diabetes that may lead to diabetic coma. Ketoacidosis occurs in uncontrolled diabetes.

*Acetest only* — To detect ketones in urine and in blood.

## Precautions:

*Not for internal use.* Do not chew or swallow.

*Do not touch the testing patch of test strips with skin or mucous membranes.* If contact occurs, flush the affected area with large amounts of water. If test pads are eaten or rubbed in the eyes, contact your doctor immediately.

*Liver and kidney function tests* requiring the administration of phthalein compounds such as bromsulfophthalein, phenolsulfonphthalein (PSP), or phenylketones (large quantities) may interfere with the ketone tests.

*Specimen collection and preparations:* Collect fresh urine in clean dry container and test as soon as possible. If testing cannot be done within an hour, refrigerate immediately. Let urine return to room temperature (59° to 86°F) before testing. Mix urine thoroughly before testing. Urine that is not tested right away or use of urine preservatives may affect test results.

*Storage and handling:*

*For Acetest tablets* – These tablets are stable in the unopened container if stored at temperatures between 59° and 86°F. Protect from heat, moisture, and light. Once opened, stability is decreased with exposure to moisture, heat, and light. The bottle must be recapped promptly after removing a tablet. Tablets should be used on a regular basis and not stored for an extended period of time after the bottle is opened. Tan-to-brown discoloration or darkening of the tablet is an indication of deterioration.

*For ChemStrip K* – Avoid contact with skin and mucous membranes. Keep unused test strips in the original bottle with the cap tightly closed. *ChemStrip K* will remain stable in the original capped vial until the listed expiration date. To avoid moisture, replace the original stopper, which contains a drying agent, immediately after use. Store at room temperature (59° to 86°F). Protect from heat, moisure, and light. Do not freeze.

*For Ketostix* – Keep fingers or other objects from touching the reagent area before testing. Store at room temperatures between 59° and 86°F. Protect from heat, moisture, and light. Keep unused test strips in the original bottle with the cap tightly closed. Always replace the cap immediately and tightly. A new bottle can be used for 6 months. Always write the date you first opened the bottle on the bottle label. Do not use the strips after the expiration date has passed. Never transfer strips to another bottle. Do not remove the drying agent from bottle. It absorbs moisture and keeps the strips dry. Never put cotton or other materials in the bottle. If the reagent area becomes discolored or darkened, throw the strip away and use a strip from a new bottle. If using the individual foil-wrapped strips, do not remove strips until just prior to use.

## Drug Interactions:

Tell your doctor or pharmacist if you are taking or if you are planning to take any over-the-counter or prescription medications or dietary supplements while testing for ketones. The following drugs and drug classes interact with the tests to cause questionable results.

8-hydroxyquinolone
levodopa (eg, *Larodopa)*
mesna (eg, *Mesnex)*
nitrofurantoin (*Furadantin)*
phenazopyridine (eg, *Pyridium)*
phenylketone (see Precautions)

phthalein compounds (eg, brom-sulfophthalein) (see Precautions)
sulfhydryls
sulfisoxazole and phenazo-pyridine (eg, *Azo-Sulfisoxazole)*
vitamin $B_2$ (riboflavin)

## Guidelines for Use:

- Follow the instructions on the label EXACTLY.
- Monitor urine for glucose and ketones as prescribed. Monitor urine ketones especially if your blood glucose level has been more than 250 mg/dL for 2 consecutive blood glucose determinations. Blood glucose monitoring is essential to achieve normal blood sugar levels. Keep track of your blood glucose results so that adjustments in your treatment program can be made more easily.
- Ketones are not present in normal urine. Ketones in urine could be a sign of illness, stress, or poor diabetes control. Immediately report any positive test result to your doctor.
- Have all of the materials you need before beginning the test: Test strips or tablets, timer (stopwatch or watch with second hand), and a clean dry container. For *Acetest* you will need a dropper and a clean, white piece of paper.
- Color vision is needed to properly read test results. Have someone else confirm results if in doubt.
- If test results seem questionable, confirm that product is within the expiration date on the bottle. Repeat the test using a new test strip or tablet and fresh urine specimen.
- *Acetest* — When a drop of urine is put onto a tablet, the drop should be absorbed within 30 seconds. If absorption takes more than 30 seconds, the tablets have been exposed to moisture and may not give good results.
- As with all laboratory tests, definitive diagnostic or therapeutic decisions should not be based on any single result or method.
- Patients with diabetes should test for ketones:
  When you have a cold, the flu, or any other kind of illness.
  When your urine sugar test results show you are spilling large amounts of sugar (at least 2% for at least 2 tests in a row or several days).
  When you feel the signs of high blood sugar (more than 240 mg/dL) or when your blood sugar is well over the range your doctor or educator has set for you.
  When you are under unusual physical or emotional stress.
  Regularly during pregnancy.
- Participate in a diabetes education program so that you understand diabetes and all aspects of its treatment, including diet, exercise, personal hygiene, and how to self-monitor blood glucose.
- Diabetes education materials may be obtained through your local chapter of the American Diabetes Association.
- Do not use opened or unopened product after expiration date.
- For storage and stability see Precautions.

*If you have any questions, consult your doctor, pharmacist, or health care provider.*

| Brand Name Examples | Supplied As | Test For |
|---|---|---|
| otc  ColoCare[1] | **Pads:** For toilet bowl | Occult blood |
| otc  ColoScreen[2], ColoScreen-ES[2] | **Slides:** For stool | |
| otc  EZ Detect[1] | **Tissue:** For toilet bowl | |
| otc  Heme-Chek [2] | **Slides:** For stool | |
| otc  Hemoccult [2] | **Slides:** For stool | |
| otc  Hemoccult SENSA[2] | **Slides:** For stool | |

[1] Flushable.
[2] Return test results to doctor's office.

Diagnostic or therapeutic decisions should not be based on a single test result. If you have any questions regarding your test results, contact your doctor.

## Type of Drug:

For detection of occult blood ("hidden" blood or blood that is difficult to see) in the stool (feces).

## How the Drug Works:

Tests for occult blood screen for unseen blood cells in the stool itself or in the toilet water around the stool. Specially treated pads turn a different color in the presence of blood.

Occult blood in the stool (feces) may be an indication of a disease in the digestive or gastrointestinal tract such as hemorrhoids, diverticulitis, fissures, ulcers, polyps, colitis, or colorectal cancer (cancer in colon or rectal area).

## Uses:

To screen for early signs of digestive tract diseases, including ulcers, colitis, polyps, fissures, diverticulitis, hemorrhoids, and colorectal cancer.

Recommended for people older than 40 years of age and for those who have a personal or family history of lower intestinal disorders or colorectal cancers.

These tests *do not* replace regular physical and rectal examinations by your doctor. However, they may show the need for further examinations.

## Precautions:

*Not for internal use.*

*Diet:* Eat a normal, well-balanced diet for 2 days before and throughout the testing period (eg, well-cooked poultry, raw beef, lamb), tuna fish, peanuts, high fiber foods such as bran cereal and popcorn, and plenty of raw or cooked lettuce, spinach, corn, prunes, grapes, plums, and apples.). Such a diet reduces the number of false positive results and at the same time the roughage helps to uncover "silent" lesions which may bleed only intermittently. Do not eat red or rare meat, horserad-ish, turnips, radishes, broccoli, cauliflower, cantaloupe, melons, or large amounts of citrus fruits. Consult your doctor before altering or discon-tinuing a special diet.

*Do not use* until 3 days after menstrual bleeding has ceased, or while you have bleeding hemorrhoids or constipation. Do not use any rectal oint-ments, suppositories, or certain medications (see Drug Interactions) for 2 days prior to or during the test period. Contact your doctor before stopping any drug therapy.

*Kits containing a positive control package:* Avoid contact with eyes, skin, clothing, heat, or open flame. In case of an accidental spill or direct con-tact, wash the affected area with large amounts of water. If ingested, administer large amounts of water. Do not induce vomiting. Call the poison control center.

*Toilet cleaners, disinfectants, and deodorizers* in the toilet bowl and tank can interfere with test results. Remove these items and flush repeat-edly until water is clear.

*Perform the test on* 3 consecutive bowel movements. If the sequence is broken, continue the test until 3 bowel movements have been tested. Some digestive tract bleeding occurs intermittently. Checking 3 consecu-tive bowel movements will offer a better chance of finding lower intesti-nal bleeding.

*Quality control tests or tests for toilet water quality* may be required. Read individual test directions carefully.

*Specimen collection and preparation of slides, collection papers, and filter papers returned to doctor's office:*
1. Provide all information requested on outside of packet: Name, address, date, doctor, etc.
2. Collect sample from the toilet bowl.
3. Using the applicator provided, apply a thin smear to the slide or paper.
4. Close the cover. Place slide away from heat and light.
5. Mail or deliver to doctor's office.

*Specimen collection and preparation of flushable tissue and pads:* Care-fully drop tissue or pad into toilet bowl. Wait the required length of time, then read the results as directed.

## Drug Interactions:

Tell your doctor or pharmacist if you are taking or planning to take any over-the-counter or prescription medications or dietary supplements while testing for occult blood. The following drugs and drug classes may inter-act with the test, leading to questionable results.

anticoagulants (eg, warfarin)
antimetabolites (eg, methotrexate)
aspirin

cancer chemotherapeutic drugs
corticosteroids (eg, hydrocortisone)
dipyridamole (eg, *Persantine*)

iron
mineral oil
nonsteroidal anti-inflammatory
 drugs (eg, indomethacin)
phenylbutazone
 (eg, *Butazolidin)*

reserpine (eg, *Serpasil)*
vitamin C (ascorbic acid), large
 amounts

## Guidelines for Use:
- Read the product instructions carefully prior to testing. Follow the directions on the package label EXACTLY.
- A positive test indicates the presence of blood but does not necessarily mean that a serious condition exists. Discuss all positive test results with your doctor.
- *False negative results* (a false reading even though blood is actually present) can be caused by an improper sampling technique, ingestion of more than 250 mg a day of vitamin C (ascorbic acid), large amounts of citrus fruits, use of expired reagents or kits that have been improperly stored, or lesions not bleeding at the time of the test.
- *False positive results* (a positive reading even though no blood is actually present) can be caused by drugs causing gastrointestinal bleeding (see Drug Interactions), red or rare meat, foods such as horseradish, turnips, broccoli, cauliflower, or melons (eg, cantaloupe), toilet bowl cleaners, and sources of nongastrointestinal bleeding such as nosebleeds, menstruation, and hematuria (blood in the urine).
- The best results are achieved when 3 consecutive stool specimens are tested.
- Follow special diet for 2 days prior to testing (see Precautions). Do not change diet or prescription medications without first discussing it with your doctor.
- Have all the materials you need on hand before beginning the test: Testing package, pencil or pen, timer (stopwatch or watch with a second hand), and a clean, dry container.
- For some tests, color vision may be needed to properly read the test results. Have someone else confirm results if in doubt.
- Hema-Chek *slide test* — Use a clean container or toilet paper to collect sample. Do not collect from the toilet bowl.
- Store slide tests at room temperature in a dry place. Protect from heat and light. Keep bottle tightly closed.
- *Pad and tissue tests* —
Remove all toilet cleaners and disinfectants from the toilet bowl and tank. Flush several times.
Flush the toilet after urinating. Then have bowel movement.
Do not throw toilet paper in toilet following bowel movement.
Protect from heat, sunlight, or fluorescent light. Store at room temperature (59° to 86°F). Do not store in the bathroom or in an area where there is a high humidity or moisture level. Do not store in the refrigerator or in an area where the temperature will exceed 86°F. Keep out of the reach of children. Do not use after expiration date on pouch.

*If you have any questions, consult your doctor, pharmacist, or health care provider.*

|  | Brand Name Examples | Supplied As | Test For |
|---|---|---|---|
| otc | Answer Quick & Simple | **Test kit:** For urine (5 days) | Luteinizing hormone |
| otc | Clearplan Easy | **Test kit:** For urine (5 days) | |
| otc | First Response Ovulation Predictor | **Test kit:** For urine (5 days) | |
| otc | Healthcheck Ovulation Detector | **Test kit:** For urine (6 days) | |
| otc | OvuKIT Self-Test | **Test kit:** For urine (9 days) | |
| otc | OvuQUICK Self-Test | **Test kit:** For urine (6 days) | |
| otc | OvuSign | **Test kit:** For urine (7 days) | |
| otc | SureStep | **Test kit:** For urine (5 days) | |

Diagnostic or therapeutic decisions should not be based on a single test result. If you have any questions regarding your test results, contact your doctor.

## Type of Drug:

Tests to predict time of ovulation and fertility.

## How the Drug Works:

Ovulation predictor kits test for the presence of luteinizing hormone (LH) in the urine. The pituitary gland increases LH production 12 to 16 days before menstruation begins. This "LH surge" causes an ovarian follicle to rupture and releases a mature egg in 1 to 1.5 days (24 to 40 hours). The onset of the LH surge (and therefore ovulation) can be estimated by using the ovulation predictor tests for several days.

An egg survives for 12 to 24 hours after ovulation. If the egg and sperm are not united shortly after ovulation, conception will not occur.

It is possible the LH surge and ovulation will not occur during every menstrual cycle. Onset of menstrual bleeding does not always mean ovulation has occurred.

## Uses:

To aid in planning pregnancy; to determine fertile time of menstrual cycle.

## Precautions:

*Not for internal use.*

*Menopause:* Women entering menopause may have high LH levels during their entire menstrual cycle.

*Day for beginning testing* is determined by the approximate length of the menstrual cycle, the first day being the onset of bleeding (even spotting), the last being the day before bleeding onset. Test kits vary regarding the date to begin testing. Follow manufacturers' instructions carefully.

*Specimen collection and handling:* Collect urine in the urine cup from the kit or in a clean, dry container. If testing cannot be done in 3 to 4 hours after collecting the urine specimen, cover and refrigerate immediately. Let it return to room temperature before testing. Do not freeze specimen. For best results, do the test the same day as the urine was collected.

*Time:* Allow enough time to complete the test.

## Drug Interactions:

Tell your doctor or pharmacist if you are taking or if you are planning to take any over-the-counter or prescription medications or dietary supplements while testing for LH surge (ovulation). The following drugs and drug classes may interact with the test to cause questionable results:

> thyroid stimulating hormone (eg, *Thyrogen)*
> hCG injection (eg, *A.P.L., Profasi HP)*
> menopropins (eg, *Pergonal)*
> steroids (eg, prednisone)

---

### Guidelines for Use:

- *Do not use as a contraceptive aid.* Results cannot guarantee that pregnancy will not occur.
- Follow the directions on the label EXACTLY.
- Results may not be accurate during menopause, pregnancy, in the presence of ovarian cysts, or after an abortion.
- Not all women ovulate during every menstrual cycle.
- Drinking large quantities of water before the test may dilute the urine and interfere with the results.
- Have all the materials you need on hand before beginning the test: Test kit, timer (second hand and 30-minute timer), clean dry container, and pen or pencil for dating test. Be near a cold water faucet.
- Do test at the same time in the same room with the same lighting each day, if possible. It is best to test in the mid-morning (10 a.m.).
- Color vision is needed to properly read the test results. Have someone else confirm results if in doubt.
- Look for the FIRST noticeable change in color, not the darkest.

---

*If you have any questions, consult your doctor, pharmacist, or health care provider.*

|       | Brand Name Examples                                                                           | Supplied As     | Test For                               |
| ----- | --------------------------------------------------------------------------------------------- | --------------- | -------------------------------------- |
| otc   | Answer Plus, Answer Quick & Simple, Conceive Pregnancy, Fact Plus, Fortel Plus, RapidVue       | **Test Kit**    | Human chorionic gonadotropin           |
| otc   | Advance, Clearblue Easy, e.p.t. Quick Stick, First Response, One Step Midstream, QTest          | **Test Stick**  | Human chorionic gonadotropin           |
| otc   | Nimbus Quick Strip                                                                             | **Test Strips** | Human chorionic gonadotropin           |
| otc   | Pregnosis                                                                                      | **Slide Tests** | Human chorionic gonadotropin           |

## Type of Drug:

For detection of pregnancy.

## How the Drug Works:

Pregnancy home tests detect the presence of human chorionic gonadotropin (HCG) in the urine. HCG is a hormone produced by the placenta during pregnancy. HCG will cause menstruation to stop. HCG slowly builds up in the body and appears in measurable levels in the urine 1 to 3 days after the first missed period.

## Uses:

To detect pregnancy.

## Precautions:

*Not for internal use.*

*Use only once and discard.*

*False results:* False positive results (test result is positive when no pregnancy actually exists) and false negative results (pregnancy is present, but test result is negative) may occur: during menopause; when protein, blood or excessive thyroid hormone are present in the urine; with cold urine; in the presence of an ovarian cyst or ectopic pregnancy (outside the uterus); with certain drugs (see Drug Interactions); performing the test too early; or when the test directions are not followed exactly.

*Specimen collection and preparation:* Collect fresh urine in a clean dry container or container provided. Do not use a wax cup. (Some products, however, may not require urine collection in a container.) For the best results, the sample should be the first morning urine. If testing cannot be done immediately, cover and refrigerate. Do not freeze. Let urine return to room temperature before testing. Do not mix or shake urine. Use the urine at the top of the container. Be sure to test the urine the same day.

*Time:* Depending on the test kit chosen, the time required for the test is often less than 5 minutes. Most test kits require 3 minutes or less to complete. Allow enough time to complete the test.

## Drug Interactions:

Tell your doctor or pharmacist if you are taking or if you are planning to take any over-the-counter or prescription medications or dietary supplements while testing for pregnancy. The following drugs and drug classes may interact with the test to cause questionable results.

anticonvulsants (eg, carbamaze-pine)

antiparkinson agents (eg, biperiden)

HCG (eg, *A.P.L., Profasi HP*)

methadone (eg, *Dolophine*)

oral contraceptives (eg, *Ortho-Novum)*

phenothiazines (eg, chlorproma-zine)

steroids (eg, prednisone)

### Guidelines for Use:

- Follow the instructions EXACTLY.
- For best results, use the first urine of the day.
- Consult your doctor or pharmacist if you are taking any medication (eg, birth control pills) which could cause questionable tests results.
- If urine is cloudy, pink or red or has a strong odor, do not do the test. Wait 1 to 2 days and try the test then.
- Read instructions before beginning the test. Have all of the materials you need on hand: test kit, clean dry container, timer, and sink with cold running water.
- If test results seem questionable, check the expiration date on the test kit and repeat the test. Follow directions exactly.
- *Negative results* — Recount the number of days since your last period. Retest in 3 to 7 days. It is possible that not enough HCG has accumulated to cause a positive result. If you still do not have your period, contact your doctor. A health condition other than pregnancy may be causing your missed periods.
- *Positive results* — Contact your doctor to confirm the test results.
- Regardless of test results, contact your doctor if there are any signs of pregnancy (eg, delayed menstrual cycle, morning sickness).
- For some tests, color vision may be needed to properly read test results. Have someone else confirm results if in doubt.

*If you have any questions, consult your doctor, pharmacist, or health care provider.*

| Brand Name Examples | Supplied As | Test For |
|---|---|---|
| otc Albustix, Chemstrip Micral | **Test strips:** For urine | Protein |

## Type of Drug:

For detection of protein in urine.

## How the Drug Works:

Specially treated plastic test strips can detect protein in urine (protein-uria), which can be an early sign of kidney disease. Protein is not usually detected in urine. However, occasionally people with normal kidney function may have "trace" urine protein results. Contact your doctor if test results are positive.

## Uses:

To detect protein in the urine. To screen for early signs of kidney disease, eclampsia (toxemia) in pregnant women.

## Precautions:

*Not for internal use.*

*Specimen collection and preparation:* Collect urine in a clean container according to product instructions and test it as soon as possible. If testing cannot be done within an hour, refrigerate immediately. Let it return to room temperature before testing.

*Storage/handling:* Keep all unused strips in original bottle. Transfer to any other container may cause deterioration. Do not remove drying agent from bottle. Replace cap immediately and tightly after removing strip. Do not touch test area of the strip. Keep work area and containers free of detergents and other contaminants. Discoloration of the test area on the strip indicates deterioration.

## Drug Interactions:

Tell your doctor or pharmacist if you are taking or if you are planning to take any over-the-counter or prescription medications or dietary supplements while testing for protein in the urine. The following drugs and drug classes may interact with the test results.

antiseptics
detergents
nitrofurantoin (*Furadantin*)
phenazopyridine (eg, *Pyridium*)
skin cleansers (eg, chlorhexidine)

sulfa drugs and phenazopyridine (eg, *Azo Gantanol*)
urinary alkalinizers (eg, antacids, sodium bicarbonate)
vitamin $B_2$ (riboflavin)

## Guidelines for Use:

- Follow the directions on the label EXACTLY.
- Proteins are not usually detected in urine. Contact your doctor to confirm test results.
- Have all of the materials you need on hand before beginning the test: test strips, timer (stopwatch or watch with a second hand), and clean dry container.
- If test results seem questionable, check the expiration date on the bottle and repeat the test using a new test strip and fresh urine specimen.
- Color vision is needed to properly read test results. Have someone else confirm results if in doubt.

*If you have any questions, consult your doctor, pharmacist, or health care provider.*

| | Brand Name Examples | Supplied As | Test For |
|---|---|---|---|
| otc | Chemstrip 2 LN | **Test strips:** For urine | Leukocytes (white blood cells) and nitrites |
| otc | Microstix-3 | **Test strips:** For urine | Nitrites and bacteria |
| otc | UTI | **Test strips:** For urine | Nitrites |

Diagnostic or therapeutic decisions should not be based on a single test result. If you have any questions regarding your test results, contact your doctor.

## Type of Drug:
Aid in the detection of urinary tract infections (UTIs).

## How the Drug Works:
Nitrites can be detected in the first morning urine specimen in up to 90% of all people with UTIs (infections in kidneys or bladder). Urinary nitrate is often associated with UTIs. Specially treated plastic test strips are used to test for nitrites that are converted from nitrates by bacteria in the urine. Normally no nitrites are detectable in urine.

Leukocytes (white blood cells [WBCs]) are present in the urine of people with UTIs. Specially treated plastic strips detect enzymes from certain WBCs (neutrophils) in the urine. Red blood cells and cells from the urinary tract do not usually interfere with the test.

Bacteria may be detected in the urine specimens of people with UTIs. Specially treated plastic strips containing nutrients to support bacterial growth detect total bacterial and Gram-negative bacterial counts in the urine.

## Uses:
To detect WBCs, bacteria, and nitrites. To aid in the detection of UTIs.

## Precautions:
*Not for internal use.*

*Caution:* Nitrites are produced by some *(not all)* UTI causing bacteria. Therefore, a negative test result does not necessarily mean no infection exists.

*White blood cell test strips:* Avoid contact with skin and mucous membranes. If contact occurs, flush affected areas with large amounts of water. If test pads are eaten or rubbed in the eyes, contact your doctor or a poison control center immediately.

*High urine protein (albumin) and vitamin C (ascorbic acid) levels* will interfere with the test results for WBCs.

## Drug Interactions:

Tell your doctor or pharmacist if you are taking or if you are planning to take any over-the-counter or prescription medications or dietary supplements while testing for UTIs. The following drugs and drug classes may interact with the tests to cause questionable results.

antibiotics (eg, cephalexin, gentamicin, nitrofurantoin)
phenazopyridine (eg, *Pyridium)*
vitamin C (ascorbic acid), large amounts

## Guidelines for Use:

- A negative result with a test kit *does not* rule out the possibility that you may have a urinary tract infection (UTI).
- Consult your doctor if you experience symptoms of a UTI: Frequent urination, painful or burning urination, lower backache.
- Read the test instructions carefully before use. Follow the instructions on the label EXACTLY.
- Have all of the materials you need before beginning the test: Test strips, timer (stopwatch or watch with a second hand), and clean dry container.
- Do not open the vial in humid conditions, such as a steamy bathroom.
- Handle strips with clean, dry hands. Do not touch the test area of the strips.
- Do not use test strips if they are discolored or damaged.
- *Chemstrip 2 LN* — May be used on any fresh urine specimen or on urine collected under special conditions, such as first-morning specimens. Collect urine in a clean container and test as soon as possible after collection. If testing cannot be performed within one hour, refrigerate immediately. Return to room temperature before testing. Mix thoroughly before use. Do not use preservatives.
- Color vision is needed to properly read test results. Have someone else confirm results if in doubt.
- If test results seem questionable, check the expiration date on the bottle and repeat the test using a new test strip and a fresh urine specimen.
- Contact your doctor if the test results are positive or if you are unsure what your test results mean.
- Some medications may cause abnormal urine color and affect the readability of the test strip. Consult your doctor.
- *Vitamin C* (ascorbic acid) — Large doses of vitamin C (25 mg/dL or more) will give incorrect test results for nitrites.
- Store at room temperature (59° to 86°F) in a cool, dry place. Do not refrigerate. Keep out of direct sunlight. Close vial immediately after removing the test strip because prolonged exposure to air will cause the test strips to deteriorate.

*If you have any questions, consult your doctor, pharmacist, or health care provider.*

| | Brand Name Examples | Glucose | Protein | pH | Blood | Ketones | Bilirubin | Urobilinogen | Nitrites | Leukocytes |
|---|---|---|---|---|---|---|---|---|---|---|
| otc | Chemstrip uG | x | | | | | | | | |
| otc | Nitrazine | | | x | | | | | | |
| otc | Hemastix | | | | x | | | | | |
| otc | Chemstrip K | | | | | x | | | | |
| otc | Chemstrip 2 GP, Uristix | x | x | | | | | | | |
| otc | Chemstrip uGK | x | | | | x | | | | |
| otc | Combistix | x | x | x | | | | | | |
| otc | Hema-Combistix | x | x | x | x | | | | | |
| otc | Uristix 4 | x | x | | | | | | x | x |
| otc | Chemstrip 4 the OB | x | x | | x | | | | | x |
| otc | Chemstrip 6 | x | x | x | x | x | | | | x |
| otc | Labstix | x | x | x | x | x | | | | |
| otc | Bili-Labstix, Bili-Labstix SG¹ | x | x | x | x | x | x | | | |
| otc | Chemstrip 7 | x | x | x | x | x | x | | | x |
| otc | Multistix, Multistix SG¹ | x | x | x | x | x | x | x | | |
| otc | Multistix 7, Multistix 8 SG¹ | x | x | x | x | x | | | x | x |
| otc | N-Multistix, N-Multistix SG¹ | x | x | x | x | x | x | x | x | |
| otc | Multistix 8, Multistix 9 SG¹ | x | x | x | x | x | x | | x | x |
| otc | Chemstrip 9, Chemstrip 10 SG¹, Multistix 9, Multistix 10 SG¹ | x | x | x | x | x | x | x | x | x |

¹ Also tests specific gravity.

Do not base diagnostic or therapeutic decisions on a single test result. If you have any questions regarding your test results, contact your doctor.

## Type of Drug:

Miscellaneous urine tests.

## Uses:

Specialized test strips and test tapes detect:

*Glucose* — To detect glucose in urine. To aid diabetics in monitoring medication regimens and diet and exercise needs. To help reduce complications and problems during pregnancy.

*Protein* — To detect protein in the urine. To screen for early signs of kidney disease.

*pH* — To determine if urine is too acidic or too alkaline (basic). Normal pH range 4 to 8 (average pH is 6). Urine pH is influenced by diet and some disease states that affect the kidneys.

*Blood* — To detect occult (hidden/unseen) blood in urine. Blood may appear when there is disease or trauma in the urinary tract (kidney, bladder, etc.), with some drug therapy (eg, cyclophosphamide), or after extreme exertion (eg, running a marathon).

*Ketones* — To detect ketones in urine and blood. To monitor for diabetic ketoacidosis, a complication of diabetes, which may lead to diabetic coma.

*Bilirubin* — To detect bilirubin (a product of hemoglobin metabolism) in the urine. Used to diagnose and follow conditions such as hepatitis or gallbladder disease.

*Urobilinogen* — To detect urobilinogen (a product of bilirubin metabolism) in the urine. It is normally found in the urine. Increased levels of urobilinogen may occur when there is liver damage.

*Nitrite* — To detect nitrites in the urine. To aid in the detection of urinary tract infections (UTIs).

*Leukocytes (white blood cells)* — To detect white blood cells in the urine. To aid in the detection of UTIs.

*Specific gravity* — To detect the kidney's ability to concentrate urine. (Most accurate if patient is fluid-restricted).

## Drug Interactions:

Tell your doctor or pharmacist if you are taking or if you are planning to take any over-the-counter or prescription medications or dietary supplements while using these tests. The following drugs and drug classes may interact with the tests to cause questionable results.

| | |
|---|---|
| nitrofurantoin (eg, *Furadantin)* | vitamin B$_2$ (riboflavin) |
| phenazopyridine (eg, *Pyridium)* | vitamin C (ascorbic acid), large |
| sulfa drugs and phenazo-pyridine (eg, *Azo-Sulfisoxazole)* | amounts |

Consider all drug interactions reported for the individual test kits when using urine tests.

## Guidelines for Use:

- Have all the materials you need before beginning the test: Testing packet, pencil or pen, timer (stopwatch or watch with a second hand), and clean, dry container.
- Follow instructions EXACTLY as provided.
- If test results seem questionable, check the expiration date on the packet and repeat the test.
- Color vision is needed to properly read test results. Have someone else confirm results if in doubt.

*If you have any questions, consult your doctor, pharmacist, or health care provider.*

# APPENDIX

**The Home Medicine Cabinet**, A-3

**Oral Dosage Forms that Should Not Be Crushed or Chewed**, A-7

**International System of Units**, A-21

**Normal Laboratory Values**, A-23

**FDA Pregnancy Categories**, A-31

**Poison Center Hotline**, A-33

**Drug Names that Look Alike and Sound Alike**, A-35

The cost associated with office visits to doctors for diagnosis and treatment of minor conditions due to accidental injury or illness amounts to hundreds of millions of dollars annually. In many instances, the time and money spent visiting the doctor can be avoided if you have a properly stocked home medicine cabinet and a basic knowledge of first aid and self care.

A properly stocked home medicine cabinet must include, but not be limited to, typical first-aid items. Having key drugs and devices available and knowing how to use them may prevent delays in treating discomforting symptoms. However, if significant relief is not achieved or the condition worsens during the first 24 hours after the accident or onset of symptoms, do not hesitate to contact a pharmacist or doctor.

When we refer to the home medicine cabinet, the tendency is to think of a bathroom cabinet or drawer. However, the humidity and temperature fluctuations of the bathroom may accelerate the deterioration of certain drugs. The bathroom is a less than ideal place to store these health care items. Also, some items are bulky (eg, cool mist vaporizer, heating pad, ice pack) and it may not be practical to store them with other items. Think primarily of storing the items for the home medicine cabinet in a cool, dry area out of the reach of children. The upper portion of a hall or bedroom closet are good storage areas. Consolidation of many of the items in a locked fishing tackle box or plastic tub is a good idea.

## Basic Inventory

The ideal inventory for a home medicine cabinet varies widely. Contents should reflect the nature, size, lifestyle, location, age, and health status of the individual or family. The basic inventory for a household that includes one or more children is included in the following table. These items may prevent costly and unnecessary trips to the emergency room or doctor's office, but must not be used as substitutes for appropriate medical attention.

*First-aid Items:* First-aid items are most frequently employed to manage cuts, scrapes, bites, stings, sprains, and strains. Thoroughly clean all wounds involving broken skin. Mild soap and warm water are very effective. Hydrogen peroxide (3%) may be used if the wound is dirty and very sensitive. The bubbling action of the peroxide helps to physically remove debris. The antiseptic/antibacterial action of hydrogen peroxide is limited, however, and should not be overestimated. If the wound is painful, a local anesthetic spray may be applied. If no allergies to the drug exist, a thin layer of multiple antibiotic ointment or cream may be applied to a superficial wound each time the dressing is changed. Cover all wounds involving broken skin with a loose protective dressing for a few days and change the dressing at least once daily.

Hydrocortisone ointment or cream (0.5% or 1%) is useful in treating local pain, irritation, itching, and inflammation associated with bites, stings, sunburn, and contact dermatitis associated with poison ivy, oak, or sumac. If the allergic reaction is severe, oral diphenhydramine (eg, *Benadryl*) capsules or tablets may be required to provide relief. Oatmeal baths and calamine lotion may be useful if local inflammation is widespread, such as chickenpox. Isopropyl alcohol is included as an agent to rub on sprains and strains. If used as an antiseptic on a fresh wound, it will burn for several seconds.

An ice pack is recommended to control inflammation, pain, and swelling of bites, stings, sprains, and strains. Apply it as soon after the injury as possible. Heat should not generally be applied to a sprain or strain for 24 to 48 hours after the acute injury.

| Home Medicine Cabinet — Basic Inventory |
|---|

**First Aid Items**
- Assorted adhesive bandages (eg, *Band-Aids*) — 1 box
- Sterile gauze pads (2" × 2") — 1 box
- Waterproof adhesive tape (½" to 5 yards) — 1 roll
- Blunt scissors
- Elastic bandage (2" to 3" wide)
- Ice pack (6" to 9" diameter)
- Heating pad (dry or moist heat)
- Hydrogen peroxide (3%) — 8 oz
- Triple antibiotic ointment (eg, *Neosporin*, *Mycitracin*)
- Local anesthetic spray (eg, *Bactine*, *Medi-Quick*) — 1 aerosol can
- Isopropyl ("rubbing") alcohol (70%) — 16 oz
- Hydrocortisone ointment or cream (0.5% or 1%) — ½ oz tube

**Cold and Allergy Items**
- Diphenhydramine (eg, *Benadryl*) 25 mg capsule or tablet — 24 count
- Chlorpheniramine maleate (eg, *Chlor-Trimeton*) 4 mg tablet — 24 count
- Pseudoephedrine (30 or 60 mg) tablet — 24 count

**Gastrointestinal items**
- Antacid (eg, *Maalox*, *Mylanta*) — 12 oz
- $H_2$ antagonist (eg, *Pepcid AC*)
- Antidiarrheal (eg, *Kaopectate*, *Donnagel*, *Imodium A-D*) — 8 oz

**Analgesic items**
- Aspirin (325 mg) tablet — 50 count
- Nonsteroidal anti-inflammatory drug (eg, *Advil*, *Motrin*, *Aleve*)
- Acetaminophen (325 mg) tablet, capsule, or gelcap — 50 count

**Sunscreen**
- Waterproof or water-resistant sunscreen with an SPF rating of at least 15

**Miscellaneous Items**
- Oral fever thermometer
- Rectal fever thermometer (for small children)
- Tweezers
- Cool mist humidifier
- Syrup of ipecac — 1 oz
- Phone number of nearest poison control center

*Cold and Allergy Items:* Antihistamines, decongestants or both will provide symptomatic relief of seasonal allergic rhinitis and the common cold. Antihistamines work best in relieving allergic symptoms and are sometimes overvalued in treating the common cold.

*Gastrointestinal Products:* Stomach upset, heartburn, and acid indigestion may be relieved with gastrointestinal products. Simple uncomplicated diarrhea should respond to *Kaopectate, Donnagel,* or *Imodium A-D.*

*Analgesic Items:* Fever-reducing drugs and pain relievers are essential components of the home medicine cabinet. Standard fever-reducing drugs are aspirin and acetaminophen. Pain is the most common medical symptom. Over 30 million Americans suffer from headaches each week. Because of the suspected link between aspirin use and Reye syndrome, do not give aspirin to children experiencing pain or fever. Acetaminophen is as effective as aspirin as an analgesic and fever-reducing drug. Therefore, treat children with symptoms of neuralgia, arthralgia, myalgia, headache, fever, or general discomfort associated with viral conditions such as chickenpox or influenza with acetaminophen. Liquid or chewable acetaminophen may be preferable for children. Nonsteroidal anti-inflammatory drugs (eg, ibuprofen, naproxen) are alternatives to aspirin or acetaminophen as analgesics and fever-reducing agents in a variety of clinical situations.

*Sunscreens:* The association of excessive exposure to ultraviolet (UV) light and skin cancers of various types is real. Sunscreens are strongly recommended, regardless of skin type, if exposure to sunlight is to be lengthy.

*Miscellaneous Items:* Tweezers are useful for removing splinters and other foreign objects embedded in the skin.

A cool mist humidifier, properly maintained and cleaned after use, helps to provide symptomatic relief from dry mucous membranes of the nasal passages and throat associated with colds and flu.

Finally, one ounce of ipecac syrup is an emergency drug that should be in every home in the event of childhood poisoning. Doses for children are smaller than adult doses. Call the nearest poison control center before administering ipecac to determine the proper dose or whether it should be used at all. Ipecac must not be used to treat some types of poisoning.

## Conclusion

A host of other items may be appropriate additions to the home medicine cabinet. These often include foot powder; antifungal ointments, solutions, creams, or sprays; laxatives; vitamins; minerals; eye drops; lotions; and so forth. The core items recommended should serve most families well. Other items may be added as need.

Do not neglect your home medicine cabinet. At times, medicine cabinets need first aid themselves. Remove and discard old, outdated, and deteriorate items periodically. Throw away any product that has changed its color, consistency, or odor, as it has probably "gone bad." Keep remaining items orderly so they may be found when needed. If symptoms do not respond to treatment or worsen rapidly after being treated with appropriate items in the home, do not hesitate to contact a pharmacist or doctor.

The purpose of this feature is to alert health care professionals about medications that should not be crushed because of their special pharmaceutical formulations or characteristics, such as oral dosage forms that are sustained-release in nature. Crushing or chewing such products may substantially alter their intended pharmacokinetics. Other reasons for not chewing or crushing drugs include poor taste, irritant properties, or carcinogenic potential. Alternative liquid forms of these products are listed if available. Refer to the end of the table for a complete explanation of references.

Anyone who visits any acute- or long-term care facility can observe personnel meticulously grinding tablets or the contents of capsules in a mortar and pestle. Their rationale is well-intentioned: they have an order to administer medication to a patient with an nasogastric tube or who cannot swallow solids and have to incorporate the drug into a liquid vehicle. However, they do so at the risk of changing the pharmacokinetics of the solid dosage formulation. Examples of special formulations include sublingual or buccal, enteric-coated, and extended-release tablets or capsules. Products containing extended-release dosage forms frequently have an abbreviation affixed to their brand name that serves as a clue that crushing may affect the formulation (Table 1). In addition, some medications are inherently corrosive to the oral mucosa and/or upper gastrointestinal tract, remarkably bitter to the taste, or capable of staining the oral mucosa and teeth.

Finally, several medications are potentially carcinogenic and require limited handling by medical personnel. Crushing or breaking of products that have carcinogenic/teratogenic potential (ie, antineoplastics) may not alter the dosage form or delivery mechanisms but may cause aerosolization of particles, exposing health care workers handling these products. The reader is encouraged to review the American Society of Health-System Pharmacists' (previously the American Society of Hospital Pharmacists) bulletin on handling cytotoxic and hazardous drugs.

A more detailed description of the dosage forms mentioned above has been published in previous versions of this article and is summarized in Table 2.

*Alternatives to Crushing:* For patients who cannot swallow whole tablets or capsules, the most logical approach is to use liquid suspension forms of the same medication. Table 3 identifies examples of medications that have a liquid form commercially available. In some cases, there must be a dosage adjustment when the liquid is substituted. This is especially true if the tablet or capsule is an extended-release medication. If a liquid or suspension is not commercially available, the pharmacist should be consulted to determine if a liquid formulation could be extemporaneously prepared.

Occasionally, it is possible to substitute the injectable form of the medication by placing the appropriate amount of injection in some suitable fluid, such as juice. This should be done, however, only after consultation with a pharmacist to ensure that there are no problems regarding compatibility or changes in absorption of the drug. Another alternative is to use a chemically different but clinically similar medication that is available in a liquid form. Some medications that cannot be crushed may be administered in other ways, such as administering the contents of a capsule in soft food. This type of information is provided in Table 3 and indexed in the footnote.

*Updates to List:* Inherent with a listing of this type is the difficulty in keeping such lists current. The author encourages manufacturers, pharmacist, nurses, and other health professionals to notify us of any changes or updates.

*References:*

1. American Society of Hospital Pharmacists. ASHP technical assistance bulletin on handling cytotoxic and hazardous drugs. *Am J Hosp Pharm.* 1990;47:1033-1049.

2. Mitchell JF. Oral dosage forms that should not be crushed: 2000 update. *Hosp Pharm.* 2000;35:553-567.

| Table 1: Common Abbreviations for Extended-Release Products | |
|---|---|
| CR | controlled release |
| CRT | controlled release tablet |
| LA | long acting |
| SR | sustained release |
| TR | time release |
| TD | time delay |
| SA | sustained action |
| XL | extended release |
| XR | extended release |

| Table 2: Summary of Drug Formulations that Preclude Crushing | |
|---|---|
| **Type** | **Reason(s) for the formulation** |
| Enteric coated | Designed to pass through the stomach intact with drug being released in the intestines to:<br>(1) prevent destruction of drug by stomach acids<br>(2) prevent stomach irritation<br>(3) delay onset of action |

### Table 2: Summary of Drug Formulations that Preclude Crushing

| Type | Reason(s) for the formulation |
|---|---|
| Extended release | Designed to release drug over an extended period of time. Such products include: |
| | (1) multiple-layered tablets releasing drug as each layer is dissolved |
| | (2) mixed release pellets that dissolve at different time intervals |
| | (3) special matrixes that are themselves inert, but slowly release drug from the matrix |
| Sublingual | Designed to dissolve quickly in oral fluids for rapid absorption by the abundant blood supply of the mouth. |
| Miscellaneous | Drugs that: |
| | (1) produce oral mucosa irritation |
| | (2) are extremely bitter |
| | (3) contain dyes or inherently could stain teeth and mucosal tissue |
| | (4) drugs that, if handled without adequate protection, are potenially carcinogenic |

### Table 3: Medications That Should Not Be Crushed or Chewed

| Drug Product | Dosage Form | Reason/Comments |
|---|---|---|
| Aciphex | Tablet | Slow Release |
| Accutane | Capsule | Mucous membrane irritant |
| Actifed 12 Hour | Capsule | Slow release[1] |
| Acutrim (Various) | Tablet | Slow release |
| Adalat CC | Tablet | Slow release |
| Aerolate SR, JR, III | Capsule | Slow release[1,2] |
| Allegra D | Tablet | Slow release |
| Allerest 12 Hour | Capsule | Slow release |
| Artane Sequels | Capsule | Slow release[1,2] |
| Arthritis Bayer Time Release | Capsule | Slow release |
| Arthrotec | Tablet | Enteric coated |
| ASA Enseals | Tablet | Enteric coated |

## Table 3: Medications That Should Not Be Crushed or Chewed

| Drug Product | Dosage Form | Reason/Comments |
|---|---|---|
| Asacol | Tablet | Slow release |
| Ascriptin A/D | Tablet | Enteric coated |
| Ascriptin Extra Strength | Tablet | Enteric coated |
| Atrohist LA | Tablet | Slow release[1] |
| Atrohist Pediatric | Capsule | Slow release[1,2] |
| Atrohist Plus | Tablet | Slow release[1] |
| Azulfidine EN-tabs | Tablet | Enteric coated |
| Baros | Tablet | Effervescent tablet[3] |
| Bayer Enteric-Coated | Caplet | Enteric coated |
| Bayer Low Adult 81 mg | Tablet | Enteric coated |
| Bayer Regular Strength 325 mg Caplet | Caplet | Enteric coated |
| Betachron | Capsule | Slow release |
| Betapen-VK | Tablet | Taste[4] |
| Biaxin-XL | Tablet | Slow release |
| Bisacodyl | Tablet | Enteric coated[5] |
| Bontril-SR | Capsule | Slow release |
| Breonesin | Capsule | Slow release[1] |
| Brexin L.A. | Capsule | Slow release |
| Calan SR | Tablet | Slow release[6] |
| Cama Arthritis Pain Reliever | Tablet | Multiple compressed tablet |
| Carbatrol | Capsule | Slow release[2] |
| Carbiset-TR | Tablet | Slow release |
| Cardene SR | Capsule | Slow release |
| Cardizem | Tablet | Slow release |
| Cardizem CD | Capsule | Slow release[2] |
| Cardizem SR | Capsule | Slow release[2] |
| Carter's Little Pills | Tablet | Enteric coated |
| CartiaXT | Capsule | Slow release |
| Ceclor CD | Tablet | Slow release |
| Ceftin | Tablet | Taste[1] Note: Use suspension for children |
| CellCept | Capsule, Tablet | Teratogenic potential[7] |
| Charcoal Plus | Tablet | Enteric coated |
| Chloral Hydrate | Capsule | Note: Product is in liquid form within a special capsule[1] |

### Table 3: Medications That Should Not Be Crushed or Chewed

| Drug Product | Dosage Form | Reason/Comments |
|---|---|---|
| Chlor-Trimeton 12-Hour | Tablet | Slow release[1] |
| Choledyl SA | Tablet | Slow release[1] |
| Cipro | Tablet | Taste[4] |
| Claritin-D | Tablet | Slow release |
| Claritin-D 24 Hour | Tablet | Slow release |
| Codimal-LA | Capsule | Slow release |
| Codimal-LA Half | Capsule | Slow release |
| Colace | Capsule | Taste[4] |
| Colestid | Tablet | Slow release |
| Comhist LA | Capsule | Slow release[2] |
| Compazine Spansule | Capsule | Slow release[1] |
| Condrin-LA | Tablet | Slow release |
| Congress SR, JR | Capsule | Slow release |
| Contac 12-Hour | Capsule | Slow release[1,2] |
| Contac Maximum Strength | Capsule | Slow release[1,2] |
| Cotazym-S | Capsule | Enteric coated[2] |
| Covera-HS | Tablet | Slow release |
| Creon 10, 20, 25 | Capsule | Enteric coated[2] |
| Cystospaz-M | Capsule | Slow release |
| Cytovene | Capsule | Skin irritant |
| Cytoxan | Tablet | Note: Drug may be crushed, but manufacturer recommends injection |
| D.A. II | Tablet | Slow release[6] |
| Dallergy | Capsule | Slow release |
| Dallergy-D | Capsule | Slow release |
| Dallergy-JR | Capsule | Slow release |
| Deconamine SR | Capsule | Slow release[1] |
| Defen-LA | Tablet | Slow release[6] |
| Depakene | Capsule | Slow release, mucous membrane irritant[1] |
| Depakote | Capsule | Enteric coated |
| Desoxyn Gradumets | Tablet | Slow release |
| Desyrel | Tablet | Taste[4] |
| Dexatrim, Extended Duration | Tablet | Slow release |
| Dexedrine Spansule | Capsule | Slow release |
| Diamox Sequels | Capsule | Slow release |
| Dilacor XR | Capsule | Slow release |

## Table 3: Medications That Should Not Be Crushed or Chewed

| Drug Product | Dosage Form | Reason/Comments |
|---|---|---|
| Dilatrate-SR | Capsule | Slow release |
| Disobrom | Tablet | Slow release |
| Disophrol Chronotab | Tablet | Slow release |
| Dital | Capsule | Slow release |
| Ditropan XL | Tablet | Slow release |
| Dolobid | Tablet | Irritant |
| Donnatal Extentab | Tablet | Slow release[1] |
| Donnazyme | Tablet | Enteric coated |
| Drisdol | Capsule | Liquid filled[8] |
| Drixoral | Tablet | Slow release[1] |
| Drixoral Plus | Tablet | Slow release |
| Drixoral, Various | Tablet | Slow release |
| Dulcolax | Tablet | Enteric coated[5] |
| Duratuss-GP | Tablet | Slow release[6] |
| Dura-Vent/A | Tablet | Slow release[6] |
| Dura-Vent/DA | Tablet | Slow release[6] |
| Dynabac | Tablet | Enteric coated |
| DynaCirc CR | Tablet | Slow release |
| Easprin | Tablet | Enteric coated |
| EC-Naprosyn | Tablet | Enteric coated |
| Ecotrin Adult Low Strength | Tablet | Enteric coated |
| Ecotrin Maximum Strength | Tablet | Enteric coated |
| Ecotrin Regular Strength | Tablet | Enteric coated |
| E.E.S. 400 | Tablet | Enteric coated[1] |
| Effexor XR | Capsule | Slow release |
| Efidac/24 | Tablet | Slow release |
| Efidac/24 Chlorphenir-amine | Tablet | Slow release |
| E-Mycin | Tablet | Enteric coated |
| Endafed | Capsule | Slow release |
| Entex LA | Tablet | Slow release[1] |
| Entex PSE | Tablet | Slow release |
| Equanil | Tablet | Taste[4] |
| Ergomar | Tablet | Sublingual form[9] |
| Eryc | Capsule | Enteric coated[2] |
| Ery-Tab | Tablet | Enteric coated |
| Erythrocrin Stearate | Tablet | Enteric coated |
| Erythromycin Base | Tablet | Enteric coated |
| Eskalith CR | Tablet | Slow release |

### Table 3: Medications That Should Not Be Crushed or Chewed

| Drug Product | Dosage Form | Reason/Comments |
|---|---|---|
| *Exgest LA* | Tablet | Slow release |
| *Extendryl JR* | Capsule | Slow release |
| *Extendryl S-R* | Capsule | Slow release[1] |
| *Fe 50* | Tablet | Slow release |
| *Fedahist Gyrocaps* | Capsule | Slow release[1] |
| *Fedahist Timecaps* | Capsule | Slow release[1] |
| *Feldene* | Capsule | Mucous membrane irritant |
| *Feocyte* | Tablet | Slow release |
| *Feosol* | Tablet | Enteric coated[1] |
| *Feosol* | Capsule | Slow release[1,2] |
| *Feratab* | Tablet | Enteric coated[1] |
| *Fergon* | Capsule | Slow release[2] |
| *Fero-Grad 500 mg* | Tablet | Slow release |
| *Ferro-Sequels* | Tablet | Slow release |
| *Feverall Sprinkle* | Capsule | Taste[2] Note: Capsule contents intended to be placed in a teaspoon of water or soft food |
| *Flomax* | Capsule | Slow release |
| *Fumatinic* | Capsule | Slow release |
| *Gastrocrom* | Capsule | Note: Contents may be dissolved in water for administration |
| *Geocillin* | Tablet | Taste |
| *Glucotrol XL* | Tablet | Slow release |
| *Gris-PEG* | Tablet | Note: Crushing may result in precipitation as larger particles |
| *Guaimax-D* | Tablet | Slow release |
| *Guiafed* | Capsule | Slow release |
| *Guiafed-PD* | Capsule | Slow release |
| *Guiafenex LA* | Tablet | Slow release[6] |
| *Guaifenex PPA* | Tablet | Slow release |
| *Guaifenex PSE* | Tablet | Slow release[6] |
| *Humibid DM* | Tablet | Slow release |
| *Humibid DM Sprinkle* | Capsule | Slow release[2] |
| *Humibid LA* | Tablet | Slow release |
| *Humibid Sprinkle* | Capsule | Slow release[2] |

**Table 3: Medications That Should Not Be Crushed or Chewed**

| Drug Product | Dosage Form | Reason/Comments |
|---|---|---|
| Hydergine LC | Capsule | Note: Product is in liquid form within a special capsule[1] |
| Iberet | Tablet | Slow release[1] |
| Iberet 500 | Tablet | Slow release[1] |
| ICaps Plus | Tablet | Slow release |
| ICaps Time Release | Tablet | Slow release |
| Ilotycin | Tablet | Enteric coated |
| Imdur | Tablet | Slow release[6] |
| Inderal LA | Capsule | Slow release |
| Inderide LA | Capsule | Slow release |
| Indocin SR | Capsule | Slow release[1,2] |
| Ionamin | Capsule | Slow release |
| Isoptin SR | Tablet | Slow release |
| Isordil Sublingual | Tablet | Sublingual form[9] |
| Isordil Tembid | Tablet | Slow release |
| Isosorbide Dinitrate Sublingual | Tablet | Sublingual form[9] |
| Isosorbide SR | Tablet | Slow release |
| K + 8 | Tablet | Slow release[1] |
| K + 10 | Tablet | Slow release[1] |
| Kadian | Capsule | Slow release[2] |
| Kaon Cl | Tablet | Slow release[1] |
| K-Dur | Tablet | Slow release |
| K-Lease | Capsule | Slow release[1,2] |
| Klor-Con | Tablet | Slow release[1] |
| Klotrix | Tablet | Slow release[1] |
| K-Lyte | Tablet | Effervescent tablet[3] |
| K-Lyte CL | Tablet | Effervescent tablet[3] |
| K-Lyte DS | Tablet | Effervescent tablet[3] |
| K-Norm | Capsule | Slow release |
| K-Tab | Tablet | Slow release[1] |
| Levbid | Tablet | Slow release[6] |
| Levsinex Timecaps | Capsule | Slow release |
| Lexxel | Tablet | Slow release |
| Lithobid | Tablet | Slow release |
| Lodine XL | Tablet | Slow release |
| Lodrane LD | Capsule | Slow release[2] |
| Mag-Tab SR | Tablet | Slow release |

## Table 3: Medications That Should Not Be Crushed or Chewed

| Drug Product | Dosage Form | Reason/Comments |
| --- | --- | --- |
| Mestinon Timespan | Tablet | Slow release[1] |
| Mi-Cebrin | Tablet | Enteric coated |
| Mi-Cebrin T | Tablet | Enteric coated |
| Micro K | Capsule | Slow release[1,2] |
| Monafed | Tablet | Slow release |
| Monafed DM | Tablet | Slow release |
| Motrin | Tablet | Taste[4] |
| MS Contrin | Tablet | Slow release[1] |
| Muco-Fen-DM | Tablet | Slow release[6] |
| Muco-Fen-LA | Tablet | Slow release[6] |
| Naldecon | Tablet | Slow release[1] |
| Naprelan | Tablet | Slow release |
| Nasatab LA | Tablet | Slow release[6] |
| Nexium | Capsule | Slow release[2] |
| Nicotinic Acid | Capsule, Tablet | Slow release |
| Nitroglyn | Capsule | Slow release[2] |
| Nitromed | Tablet | Slow release |
| Nitrong | Tablet | Sublingual form[9] |
| Nitrostat | Tablet | Sublingual form[9] |
| Nitro-Time | Capsule | Slow release |
| Nolamine | Tablet | Slow release |
| Nolex LA | Tablet | Slow release |
| Norflex | Tablet | Slow release |
| Norpace CR | Capsule | Slow release form within a special capsule |
| Ondrox | Tablet | Slow release |
| Optilets 500 | Tablet | Enteric coated |
| Optilets-M 500 | Tablet | Enteric coated |
| Oragrafin | Capsule | Note: product is in liquid form within a special capsule |
| Oramorph SR | Tablet | Slow release[1] |
| Ornade Spansule | Capsule | Slow release |
| OxyContin | Tablet | Slow release |
| Pabalate | Tablet | Enteric coated |
| Pabalate SF | Tablet | Enteric coated |
| Pancrease | Capsule | Enteric coated[2] |
| Pancrease MT | Capsule | Enteric coated[2] |

**Table 3: Medications That Should Not Be Crushed or Chewed**

| Drug Product | Dosage Form | Reason/Comments |
|---|---|---|
| PanMist Jr, LA | Tablet | Slow release[6] |
| Panmycin | Capsule | Taste |
| Pannaz | Tablet | Slow release[6] |
| Papaverine Sustained Action | Capsule | Slow release |
| Pathilon Sequels | Capsule | Slow release[2] |
| Pavabid Plateau | Capsule | Slow release[2] |
| PBZ-SR | Tablet | Slow release[1] |
| Pentasa | Tablet | Slow release |
| Perdiem Fiber Therapy | Granules | Wax coated |
| Peritrate SA | Tablet | Slow release[6] |
| Permitil Chronotab | Tablet | Slow release[1] |
| Phazyme | Tablet | Slow release |
| Phazyme 95, 125 | Tablet | Slow release |
| Phenergan | Tablet | Taste[5] |
| Phyllocontin | Tablet | Slow release |
| Plendil | Tablet | Slow release |
| Pneumomist | Tablet | Slow release[6] |
| Polaramine Repetabs | Tablet | Slow release[1] |
| Prelu-2 | Capsule | Slow release |
| Prevacid | Capsule | Slow release |
| Prilosec | Capsule | Slow release |
| Pro-Banthine | Tablet | Taste |
| Procainamide HCl SR | Tablet | Slow release |
| Procanbid | Tablet | Slow release |
| Procardia | Capsule | Delays absorption[1,4] |
| Procardia XL | Tablet | Slow release Note: AUC is unaffected |
| Profen II | Tablet | Slow release[6] |
| Profen-LA | Tablet | Slow release[6] |
| Pronestyl SR | Tablet | Slow release |
| Propecia | Tablet | Note: Women who are or may become pregnant should not handle crushed or broken tablets |
| Proscar | Tablet | Note: Women who are or may become pregnant should not handle crushed or broken tablets |
| Protonix | Tablet | Slow release |

## Table 3: Medications That Should Not Be Crushed or Chewed

| Drug Product | Dosage Form | Reason/Comments |
|---|---|---|
| Proventil Repetabs | Tablet | Slow release[1] |
| Prozac | Capsule | Slow release[2] |
| Quibron-T SR | Tablet | Slow release[1] |
| Quinaglute Dura-Tabs | Tablet | Slow release |
| Quinidex Extentabs | Tablet | Slow release |
| Quin-Release | Tablet | Slow release |
| Respa-1st | Tablet | Slow release[6] |
| Respa-DM | Tablet | Slow release[6] |
| Respa-GF | Tablet | Slow release[6] |
| Respahist | Capsule | Slow release[2] |
| Respaire SR | Capsule | Slow release |
| Respbid | Tablet | Slow release |
| Ritalin SR | Tablet | Slow release |
| Robimycin | Tablet | Enteric coated |
| Rondec TR | Tablet | Slow release[1] |
| Ru-Tuss DE | Tablet | Slow release |
| Sinemet CR | Tablet | Slow release |
| Singlet for Adults | Tablet | Slow release |
| Slo-Bid Gyrocaps | Capsule | Slow release[2] |
| Slo-Niacin | Tablet | Slow release[6] |
| Slo-Phyllin GG | Tablet | Slow release[1] |
| Slo-Phyllin Gyrocaps | Capsule | Slow release[1,2] |
| Slow-FE | Tablet | Slow release[1] |
| Slow-FE Folic Acid | Tablet | Slow release |
| Slow-K | Tablet | Slow release[1] |
| Slow-Mag | Tablet | Slow release |
| Sorbitrate SA | Tablet | Slow release |
| Sorbitrate Sublingual | Tablet | Sublingual form |
| S-P-T | Capsule | Note: Liquid gelatin thyroid suspension |
| Sudafed 12 hour | Capsule | Slow release[1] |
| Sudal 60/500 | Tablet | Slow release |
| Sudal 120/600 | Tablet | Slow release |
| Sudex | Tablet | Slow release[6] |
| Sular | Tablet | Slow release |
| Sustaire | Tablet | Slow release[1] |
| Syn-RX | Tablet | Slow release |
| Syn-RX DM | Tablet | Slow release |

## Table 3: Medications That Should Not Be Crushed or Chewed

| Drug Product | Dosage Form | Reason/Comments |
|---|---|---|
| Tavist-D | Tablet | Multiple compressed tablet |
| Teczam | Tablet | Slow release |
| Tedral SA | Tablet | Slow release[1] |
| Tegretol-XR | Tablet | Slow release |
| Teldrin Maximum Strength | Capsule | Slow release[2] |
| Tepanil Ten-Tab | Tablet | Slow release |
| Tessalon Perles | Capsule | Slow release |
| Theo-24 | Tablet | Slow release[1] |
| Theobid Duracaps | Capsule | Slow release[1,2] |
| Theochron | Tablet | Slow release |
| Theoclear L.A. | Capsule | Slow release[1] |
| Theo-Dur | Tablet | Slow release[1] |
| Theo-Dur Sprinkle | Capsule | Slow release[1,2] |
| Theolair SR | Tablet | Slow release[1] |
| Theo-Sav | Tablet | Slow release[6] |
| Theo-Span-SR | Capsule | Slow release |
| Theo-Time SR | Tablet | Slow release |
| Theovent | Capsule | Slow release[1] |
| Theo-X | Tablet | Slow release |
| Thorazine Spansule | Capsule | Slow release |
| Tiamate | Tablet | Slow release |
| Tiazac | Capsule | Slow release |
| Toprol XL | Tablet | Slow release[6] |
| Touro A&D | Capsule | Slow release |
| Touro EX | Tablet | Slow release |
| Touro LA | Tablet | Slow release |
| T-Phyl | Tablet | Slow release |
| Trental | Tablet | Slow release |
| Triaminic | Tablet | Enteric coated[1] |
| Triaminic 12 | Tablet | Slow release[1] |
| Triaminic TR | Tablet | Multiple compressed tablet[1] |
| Tri-Phen-Chlor Time Released | Tablet | Slow release |
| Tri-Phen-Mine SR | Tablet | Slow release |
| Triptone | Tablet | Slow release |
| Tuss LA | Tablet | Slow release |
| Tuss Ornade Spansule | Capsule | Slow release |

## Table 3: Medications That Should Not Be Crushed or Chewed

| Drug Product | Dosage Form | Reason/Comments |
|---|---|---|
| *Tylenol Extended Relief* | Capsule | Slow release |
| *ULR-LA* | Tablet | Slow release |
| *Ultrace* | Capsule | Enteric coated[2] |
| *Ultrace MT* | Capsule | Enteric coated[2] |
| *Uni-Dur* | Tablet | Slow release |
| *Uniphyl* | Tablet | Slow release |
| *Urocit-K* | Tablet | Wax coated |
| *Verelan* | Capsule | Slow release[2] |
| *Volmax* | Tablet | Slow release |
| *Wellbutrin SR* | Tablet | Anesthetize mucous membrane |
| *Wyamycin S* | Tablet | Slow release |
| *Wygesic* | Tablet | Taste |
| *ZORprin* | Tablet | Slow release |
| *Zyban* | Tablet | Slow release |
| *Zymase* | Capsule | Enteric coated[2] |

[1] Liquid dosage forms of the product are available; however, dose, frequency of administration, and manufacturers may differ from that of the solid dosage form.

[2] Capsule may be opened and the contents taken without crushing or chewing; soft food such as applesauce or pudding may facilitate administration; contents may generally be administered via nasogastric tube using an appropriate fluid, provided entire contents are washed down the tube.

[3] Effervescent tablets must be dissolved in the amount of diluent recommended by the manufacturer.

[4] The taste of this product in a liquid form would likely be unacceptable to the patient; administration via nasogastric tube should be acceptable.

[5] Antacids and/or milk may prematurely dissolve the coating of the tablet.

[6] Tablet is scored and may be broken in half without affecting release characteristics.

[7] Skin contact may enhance tumor production; avoid direct contact.

[8] Capsule may be opened and the liquid contents removed for administration.

[9] Tablets are made to disintegrate under the tongue.

Revised by John F. Mitchell, PharmD, FASHP, from an article that originally appeared in *Hosp Pharm*. 1996.;1:27–37.

The *Système international d 'unités* (International System of Units) or *SI* is a modernized version of the metric system. The primary goal of the conversion to SI units is to revise the present confused measurement system and to improve test-result communications.

The SI has 7 basic units from which other units are derived:

| Base Units of SI | | |
|---|---|---|
| Physical quantity | Base unit | SI symbol |
| length | meter | m |
| mass | kilogram | kg |
| time | second | s |
| amount of substance | mole | mol |
| thermodynamic temperature | kelvin | K |
| electric current | ampere | A |
| luminous intensity | candela | cd |

Combinations of these base units can express any property, although, for simplicity, special names are given to some of these derived units.

| Representative Derived Units | | |
|---|---|---|
| Derived unit | Name and symbol | Derivation from base units |
| area | square meter | $m^2$ |
| volume | cubic meter | $m^3$ |
| force | newton (N) | $kg{\cdot}m{\cdot}s^{-2}$ |
| pressure | pascal (Pa) | $kg{\cdot}m^{-1}{\cdot}s^{-2}(N/m^2)$ |
| work, energy | joule (J) | $kg{\cdot}m^2{\cdot}s^{-2}$ (N${\cdot}$m) |
| mass density | kilogram per cubic meter | $kg/m^3$ |
| frequency | hertz (Hz) | 1 cycles/s$^{-1}$ |
| temperature degree | Celsius (°C) | °C = °K −273.15 |
| concentration | | |
|   mass | kilogram/liter | kg/L |
|   substance | mole/liter | mol/L |
| molality | mole/kilogram | mol/kg |
| density | kilogram/liter | kg/L |

Prefixes to the base unit are used in this system to form decimal multiples and submultiples. The preferred multiples and submultiples listed below change the quantity by increments of $10^3$ or $10^{-3}$. The exceptions to these recommended factors are within the middle rectangle.

| Prefixes and Symbols for Decimal Multiples and Submultiples | | |
|---|---|---|
| Factor | Prefix | Symbol |
| $10^{18}$ | exa | E |
| $10^{15}$ | peta | P |
| $10^{12}$ | tera | T |
| $10^{9}$ | giga | G |
| $10^{6}$ | mega | M |
| $10^{3}$ | kilo | k |
| $10^{2}$ | hecto | h |
| $10^{1}$ | deka | da |
| $10^{-1}$ | deci | d |
| $10^{-2}$ | centi | c |
| $10^{-3}$ | milli | m |
| $10^{-6}$ | micro | $\mu$ |
| $10^{-9}$ | nano | n |
| $10^{-12}$ | pico | p |
| $10^{-15}$ | femto | f |
| $10^{-18}$ | atto | a |

To convert drug concentrations to or from SI units:

Conversion factor (CF) = 1000/mol wt
Conversion *to* SI units: $\mu g/mL \times CF = \mu mol/L$
Conversion *from* SI units: $\mu mol/L \div CF = \mu g/mL$

In the following tables, normal reference values for commonly requested laboratory tests are listed in traditional units and in SI units. The tables are a guideline only. Values are method dependent and "normal values" may vary between laboratories.

| BLOOD, PLASMA OR SERUM | | |
|---|---|---|
| | Reference Value | |
| Determination | Conventional units | SI units |
| Alpha-fetoprotein | *Adult:* < 15 ng/mL *Pregnant (16-18 weeks):* 38-45 ng/mL | *Adult:* < 15 mcg/L *Pregnant (16-18 weeks):* 38-45 mcg/L |
| Ammonia ($NH_3$) - diffusion | 20-120 mcg/dL | 12-70 mcmol/L |
| Ammonia Nitrogen | 15-45 µg/dL | 11-32 µmol/L |
| Amylase | 35-118 IU/L | 0.58-1.97 mckat/L |
| Anion gap ($Na^+$-[$Cl^-$ + $HCO_3^-$]) (P) | 7-16 mEq/L | 7-16 mmol/L |
| Antithrombin III (AT III) | 80-120 U/dL | 800-1200 U/L |
| Bicarbonate: Arterial | 21-28 mEq/L | 21-28 mmol/L |
| Venous | 22-29 mEq/L | 22-29 mmol/L |
| Bilirubin: Conjugated (direct) | ≤ 0.2 mg/dL | ≤ 4 mcmol/L |
| Total | 0.1-1 mg/dL | 2-18 mcmol/L |
| Calcitonin | < 100 pg/mL | < 100 ng/L |
| Calcium: Total | 8.6-10.3 mg/dL | 2.2-2.74 mmol/L |
| Ionized | 4.4-5.1 mg/dL | 1-1.3 mmol/L |
| Carbon dioxide content (plasma) | 21-32 mmol/L | 21-32 mmol/L |
| Carcinoembryonic antigen | < 3 ng/mL | < 3 mcg/L |
| Chloride | 95-110 mEq/L | 95-110 mmol/L |
| *Coagulation screen:* Bleeding time | 3-9.5 min | 180-570 sec |
| Prothrombin time | 10-13 sec | 10-13 sec |
| Partial thromboplastin time (activated) | 22-37 sec | 22-37 sec |
| Protein C | 0.7-1.4 µ/mL | 700-1400 U/mL |
| Protein S | 0.7-1.4 µ/mL | 700-1400 U/mL |
| Copper, total | 70-160 mcg/dL | 11-25 mcmol/L |
| Corticotropin (ACTH adrenocorticotropic hormone) - 0800 hr | < 60 pg/mL | < 13.2 pmol/L |
| Cortisol: 0800 hr | 5-30 mcg/dL | 138-810 nmol/L |
| 1800 hr | 2-15 mcg/dL | 50-410 nmol/L |
| 2000 hr | ≤ 50% of 0800 hr | ≤ 50% of 0800 hr |
| Creatine kinase: Female | 20-170 IU/L | 0.33-2.83 mckat/L |
| Male | 30-220 IU/L | 0.5-3.67 mckat/L |

| BLOOD, PLASMA OR SERUM | | |
|---|---|---|
| | Reference Value | |
| Determination | Conventional units | SI units |
| Creatinine kinase isoen-zymes, MB fraction | 0-12 IU/L | 0-0.2 mckat/L |
| Creatinine | 0.5-1.7 mg/dL | 44-150 mcmol/L |
| Fibrinogen (coagulation factor I) | 150-360 mg/dL | 1.5-3.6 g/L |
| Follicle-stimulating hor-mone (FSH): Female<br>Midcycle<br>Male | 2-13 mLU/mL<br>5-22 mLU/mL<br>1-8 mLU/mL | 2-13 IU/L<br>5-22 IU/L<br>1-8 IU/L |
| Glucose, fasting | 65-115 mg/dL | 3.6-6.3 mmol/L |
| Glucose Tolerance Test (Oral)<br>Fasting<br>60 min<br>90 min<br>120 min | mg/dL<br>*Normal   Diabetic*<br>70-105      140<br>120-170    ≥ 200<br>100-140    ≥ 200<br>70-120      ≥ 140 | mmol/L<br>*Normal   Diabetic*<br>3.9-5.8      7.8<br>6.7-9.4    ≥ 11.1<br>5.6-7.8    ≥ 11.1<br>3.9-6.7    ≥ 7.8 |
| (γ) -Glutamyltransferase (GGT): Male<br>Female | 9-50 units/L<br>8-40 units/L | 9-50 units/L<br>8-40 units/L |
| Haptoglobin | 44-303 mg/dL | 0.44-3.03 g/L |
| *Hematologic tests:*<br>Fibrinogen<br>Hematocrit (Hct): Female<br><br>Male<br><br>Hemoglobin A$_{1C}$<br><br>Hemoglobin (Hb):<br>Female<br>Male<br>Leukocyte count (WBC)<br>Erythrocyte count (RBC):<br>Female<br>Male<br>Mean corpuscular volume (MCV)<br>Mean corpuscular hemo-globin (MCH)<br>Mean corpuscular hemo-globin concentrate (MCHC)<br>Erythrocyte sedimenta-tion rate (sedrate, ESR) | 200-400 mg/dL<br>36%-44.6%<br><br>40.7%-50.3%<br><br>5.3%-7.5% of total Hgb<br><br><br>12.1-15.3 g/dL<br>13.8-17.5 g/dL<br>3800-9800/mcL<br><br>3.5-5 × 10$^6$/mcL<br>4.3-5.9 × 10$^6$/mcL<br>80-97.6 mcm$^3$<br><br>27-33 pg/cell<br><br>33-36 g/dL<br><br><br>≤ 30 mm/hr | 2-4 g/L<br>0.36-0.446 fraction of 1<br>0.4-0.503 fraction of 1<br>0.053-0.075<br><br><br>121-153 g/L<br>138-175 g/L<br>3.8-9.8 × 10$^9$/L<br><br>3.5-5 × 10$^{12}$/L<br>4.3-5.9 × 10$^{12}$/L<br>80-97.6 fl<br><br>1.66-2.09 fmol/cell<br><br>20.3-22 mmol/L<br><br><br>≤ 30 mm/hr |

| BLOOD, PLASMA OR SERUM | | |
|---|---|---|
| | Reference Value | |
| Determination | Conventional units | SI units |
| Erythrocyte enzymes: Glucose-6-phosphate dehydrognase (G-6-PD) | 250-5000 units/ $10^6$ cells | 250-5000 mcunits/ cell |
| Ferritin | 10-383 ng/mL | 23-862 pmol/L |
| Folic acid: normal | > 3.1-12.4 ng/mL | 7-28.1 nmol/L |
| Platelet count | 150-450 × $10^3$/ mcL | 150-450 × $10^9$/L |
| Reticulocytes | 0.5%-1.5% of erythrocytes | 0.005-0.015 |
| Vitamin $B_{12}$ | 223-1132 pg/mL | 165-835 pmol/L |
| Iron: Female | 30-160 mcg/dL | 5.4-31.3 mcmol/L |
| Male | 45-160 mcg/dL | 8.1-31.3 mcmol/L |
| Iron binding capacity | 220-420 mcg/dL | 39.4-75.2 mcmol/L |
| Isocitrate dehydrogenase | 1.2-7 units/L | 1.2-7 units/L |
| Isoenzymes Fraction 1 | 14%-26% of total | 0.14-0.26 fraction of total |
| Fraction 2 | 29%-39% of total | 0.29-0.39 fraction of total |
| Fraction 3 | 20%-26% of total | 0.20-0.26 fraction of total |
| Fraction 4 | 8%-16% of total | 0.08-0.16 fraction of total |
| Fraction 5 | 6%-16% of total | 0.06-0.16 fraction of total |
| Lactate dehydrogenase | 100-250 IU/L | 1.67-4.17 mckat/L |
| Lactic acid (lactate) | 6-19 mg/dL | 0.7-2.1 mmol/L |
| Lead | ≤ 50 mcg/dL | ≤ 2.41 mcmol/L |
| Lipase | 10-150 units/L | 10-150 units/L |
| *Lipids:* Total Cholesterol | | |
| Desirable | < 200 mg/dL | < 5.2 mmol/L |
| Borderline-high | 200-239 mg/dL | < 5.2-6.2 mmol/L |
| High | > 239 mg/dL | > 6.2 mmol/L |
| LDL | | |
| Desirable | < 130 mg/dL | < 3.36 mmol/L |
| Borderline-high | 130-159 mg/dL | 3.36-4.11 mmol/L |
| High | > 159 mg/dL | > 4.11 mmol/L |
| HDL (low) | < 35 mg/dL | < 0.91 mmol/L |
| Triglycerides | | |
| Desirable | < 200 mg/dL | < 2.26 mmol/L |
| Borderline-high | 200-400 mg/dL | 2.26-4.52 mmol/L |
| High | 400-1000 mg/dL | 4.52-11.3 mmol/L |
| Very high | > 1000 mg/dL | > 11.3 mmol/L |
| Magnesium | 1.3-2.2 mEq/L | 0.65-1.1 mmol/L |

| BLOOD, PLASMA OR SERUM | | |
|---|---|---|
| | Reference Value | |
| **Determination** | **Conventional units** | **SI units** |
| Osmolality | 280-300 mOsm/kg | 280-300 mmol/kg |
| Oxygen saturation (arterial) | 94%-100% | 0.94 - fraction of 1 |
| $PCO_2$, arterial | 35-45 mmHg | 4.7-6 kPa |
| pH, arterial | 7.35-7.45 | 7.35-7.45 |
| $PO_2$, arterial: Breathing room air[1]<br>On 100% $O_2$ | 80-105 mmHg<br>> 500 mmHg | 10.6-14 kPa |
| Phosphatase (acid), total at 37°C | 0.13-0.63 IU/L | 2.2-10.5 IU/L or 2.2-10.5 mckat/L |
| Phosphatase alkaline[2] | 20-130 IU/L | 20-130 IU/L or 0.33-2.17 mckat/L |
| Phosphorus, inorganic,[3] (phosphate) | 2.5-5 mg/dL | 0.8-1.6 mmol/L |
| Potassium | 3.5-5 mEq/L | 3.5-5 mmol/L |
| *Progesterone*<br>Female<br>   Follicular phase<br>   Luteal phase<br>Male | 0.1-1.5 ng/mL<br>0.1-1.5 ng/mL<br>2.5-28 ng/mL<br>< 0.5 ng/mL | 0.32-4.8 nmol/L<br>0.32-4.8 nmol/L<br>8-89 nmol/L<br>< 1.6 nmol/L |
| Prolactin | 1.4-24.2 ng/mL | 1.4-24.2 mcg/L |
| Prostate specific antigen<br>Protein: Total<br>   Albumin<br>   Globulin | 0-4 ng/mL<br>6-8 g/dL<br>3.6-5 g/dL<br>2.3-3.5 g/dL | 0-4 ng/mL<br>60-80 g/L<br>36-50 g/L<br>23-35 g/L |
| Rheumatoid factor | < 60 IU/mL | < 60 kIU/L |
| Sodium | 135-147 mEq/L | 135-147 mmol/L |
| Testosterone: Female<br>Male | 6-86 ng/dL<br>270-1070 ng/dL | 0.21-3 nmol/L<br>9.3-37 nmol/L |
| *Thyroid Hormone Function Tests:*<br>Thyroid-stimulating hormone (TSH) | <br>0.35-6.2 mcU/mL | <br>0.35-6.2 mU/L |
| Thyroxine-binding globulin capacity | 10-26 mcg/dL | 100-260 mcg/L |
| Total triiodothyronine ($T_3$) | 75-220 ng/dL | 1.2-3.4 nmol/L |
| Total thyroxine by RIA ($T_4$) | 4-11 mcg/dL | 51-142 nmol/L |
| $T_3$ resin uptake | 25%-38% | 0.25-0.38 fraction of 1 |
| Transaminase, AST (aspartate aminotransferase, SGOT) | 11-47 IU/L | 0.18-0.78 mckat/L |

| BLOOD, PLASMA OR SERUM | | |
|---|---|---|
| | Reference Value | |
| Determination | Conventional units | SI units |
| Transaminase, ALT (alanine aminotransferase, SGPT) | 7-53 IU/L | 0.12-0.88 mckat/L |
| Transferrin | 220-400 mg/dL | 2.20-4.00 g/L |
| Urea nitrogen (BUN) | 8-25 mg/dL | 2.9-8.9 mmol/L |
| Uric acid | 3-8 mg/dL | 179-476 mcmol/L |
| Vitamin A (retinol) | 15-60 mcg/dL | 0.52-2.09 mcmol/L |
| Zinc | 50-150 mcg/dL | 7.7-23 mcmol/L |

[1] Age dependent.
[2] Infants and adolescents up to 104 U/L.
[3] Infants in the first year up to 6 mg/dL.

| URINE | | |
|---|---|---|
| | Reference value | |
| Determination | Conventional units | SI units |
| Calcium[1] | 50-250 mcg/day | 1.25-6.25 mmol/day |
| Catecholamines: | | |
| Epinephrine | < 20 mcg/day | < 109 nmol/day |
| Norepinephrine | < 100 mcg/day | < 590 nmol/day |
| Catecholamines, 24-hr | < 110 µg | < 650 nmol |
| Copper[1] | 15-60 mcg/day | 0.24-0.95 mcmol/day |
| Creatinine: Child | 8-22 mg/kg | 71-195 µmol/kg |
| Adolescent | 8-30 mg/kg | 71-265 µmol/kg |
| Female | 0.6-1.5 g/day | 5.3-13.3 mmol/day |
| Male | 0.8-1.8 g/day | 7.1-15.9 mmol/day |
| pH | 4.5-8 | 4.5-8 |
| Phosphate[1] | 0.9-1.3 g/day | 29-42 mmol/day |
| Potassium[1] | 25-100 mEq/day | 25-100 mmol/day |
| Protein | | |
| Total | 1-14 mg/dL | 10-140 mg/L |
| At rest | 50-80 mg/day | 50-80 mg/day |
| Protein, quantitative | < 150 mg/day | < 0.15 g/day |
| Sodium[1] | 100-250 mEq/day | 100-250 mmol/day |
| Specific gravity, random | 1.002-1.030 | 1.002-1.030 |
| Uric acid, 24-hr | 250-750 mg | 1.48-4.43 mmol |

[1] Diet Dependent

| DRUG LEVELS* | | |
|---|---|---|
| | Reference value | |
| Drug determination | Conventional units | SI units |
| **Aminoglycosides** | | |
| Amikacin | | |
| (trough) | 1-8 mcg/mL | 1.7-13.7 mcmol/L |
| (peak) | 20-30 mcg/mL | 34-51 mcmol/L |
| Gentamicin | | |
| (trough) | 0.5-2 mcg/mL | 1-4.2 mcmol/L |
| (peak) | 6-10 mcg/mL | 12.5-20.9 mcmol/L |
| Kanamycin | | |
| (trough) | 5-10 mcg/mL | nd[1] |
| (peak) | 20-25 mcg/mL | nd |
| Netilimicin | | |
| (trough) | 0.5-2 mcg/mL | nd |
| (peak) | 6-10 mcg/mL | nd |
| Streptomycin | | |
| (trough) | < 5 mcg/mL | nd |
| (peak) | 5-20 mcg/mL | nd |
| Tobramycin | | |
| (trough) | 0.5-2 mcg/mL | 1.1-4.3 mcmol/L |
| (peak) | 5-20 mcg/mL | 12.8-21.8 mcmol/L |
| **Antiarrhythmics** | | |
| Amiodarone | 0.5-2.5 mcg/mL | 1.5-4 mcmol/L |
| Bretylium | 0.5-1.5 mcg/mL | nd |
| Digitoxin | 9-25 mcg/L | 11.8-32.8 nmol/L |
| Digoxin | 0.8-2 ng/mL | 0.9-2.5 nmol/L |
| Disopyramide | 2-8 mcg/mL | 6-18 mcmol/L |
| Flecainide | 0.2-1 mcg/mL | nd |
| Lidocaine | 1.5-6 mcg/mL | 4.5-21.5 mcmol/L |
| Mexiletine | 0.5-2 mcg/mL | nd |
| Procainamide | 4-8 mcg/mL | 17-34 mcmol/mL |
| Propranolol | 50-200 ng/mL | 190-770 nmol/L |
| Quinidine | 2-6 mcg/mL | 4.6-9.2 mcmol/L |
| Tocainide | 4-10 mcg/mL | nd |
| Verapamil | 0.08-0.3 mcg/mL | nd |
| **Anticonvulsants** | | |
| Carbamazepine | 4-12 mcg/mL | 17-51 mcmol/L |
| Phenobarbital | 10-40 mcg/mL | 43-172 mcmol/L |
| Phenytoin | 10-20 mcg/mL | 40-80 mcmol/L |
| Primidone | 4-12 mcg/mL | 18-55 mcmol/L |
| Valproic Acid | 40-100 mcg/mL | 280-700 mcmol/L |

| DRUG LEVELS* | | |
| --- | --- | --- |
| | Reference value | |
| Drug determination | Conventional units | SI units |
| **Antidepressants** | | |
| Amitriptyline | 110-250 ng/mL[2] | 500-900 nmol/L |
| Amoxapine | 200-500 ng/mL | nd |
| Bupropion | 25-100 ng/mL | nd |
| Clomipramine | 80-100 ng/mL | nd |
| Desipramine | 115-300 ng/mL | nd |
| Doxepin | 110-250 ng/mL[2] | nd |
| Imipramine | 225-350 ng/mL[2] | nd |
| Maprotiline | 200-300 ng/mL | nd |
| Nortriptyline | 50-150 ng/mL | nd |
| Protriptyline | 70-250 ng/mL | nd |
| Trazodone | 800-1600 ng/mL | nd |
| **Antipsychotics** | | |
| Chlorpromazine | 50-300 ng/mL | 150-950 nmol/L |
| Fluphenazine | 0.13-2.8 ng/mL | nd |
| Haloperidol | 5-20 ng/mL | nd |
| Perphenazine | 0.8-1.2 ng/mL | nd |
| Thiothixene | 2-57 ng/mL | nd |
| **Miscellaneous** | | |
| Amantadine | 300 ng/mL | nd |
| Amrinone | 3.7 mcg/mL | nd |
| Chloramphenicol | 10-20 mcg/mL | 31-62 mcmol/L |
| Cyclosporine[3] | 250-800 ng/mL (whole blood, RIA) 50-300 ng/mL (plasma, RIA) | nd nd |
| Ethanol[4] | 0 mg/dL | 0 mmol/L |
| Hydralazine | 100 ng/mL | nd |
| Lithium | 0.6-1.2 mEq/L | 0.6-1.2 mmol/L |
| Salicylate | 100-300 mg/L | 724-2172 mcmol/L |
| Sulfonamide | 5-15 mg/dL | nd |
| Terbutaline | 0.5-4.1 ng/mL | nd |
| Theophylline | 10-20 mcg/mL | 55-110 mcmol/L |
| Vancomycin (trough) | 5-15 ng/mL | nd |
| (peak) | 20-40 mcg/mL | nd |

* The values given are generally accepted as desirable for treatment without toxicity for most patients. However, exceptions are not uncommon.
[1] nd = No data available.
[2] Parent drug plus N-desmethyl metabolite.
[3] 24-hour trough values.
[4] Toxic: 50-100 mg/dL (10.9-21.7 mmol/L).

The following table is adopted from the Sixth Report of the Joint National Committee on Prevention, Detection, Evaluation, and Treatment of High Blood Pressure, National Institutes of Health.

| CLASSIFICATION OF BLOOD PRESSURE* | | | |
|---|---|---|---|
| | Reference value | | |
| Category | Systolic (mmHg) | | Diastolic (mmHg) |
| Optimal[1] | < 120 | and | < 80 |
| Normal | < 130 | and | < 85 |
| High-normal | 130-139 | or | 85-89 |
| Hypertension[2] | | | |
| Stage 1 | 140-159 | or | 90-99 |
| Stage 2 | 160-179 | or | 100-109 |
| Stage 3 | $\geq$ 180 | or | $\geq$ 110 |

* For adults age 18 and older who are not taking antihypertensive drugs and not acutely ill. When systolic and diastolic blood pressures fall into different categories, the higher category should be selected to classify the individual's blood pressure status. In addition to classifying stages of hypertension on the basis of average blood pressure levels, clinicians should specify presence or absence of target organ disease and additional risk factors.

[1] Optimal blood pressure with respect to cardiovascular risk is below 120/88 mmHg. However, unusually low readings should be evaluated for clinical significance.

[2] Based on the average of two or more readings taken at each of two or more visits after an initial screening.

The rational use of any medication requires a risk vs benefit assessment. Among the myriad of risk factors which complicate this assessment, pregnancy is one of the most perplexing.

The FDA has established 5 categories to indicate the potential of a systemically absorbed drug for causing birth defects. The key differentiation among the categories rests upon the degree (reliability) of documentation and the risk vs benefit ratio. Pregnancy Category X is particularly notable in that if any data exists that may implicate a drug as a teratogen and the risk vs benefit ratio does not support use of the drug, the drug is contraindicated during pregnancy. These categories are summarized below:

| FDA Pregnancy Categories | |
|---|---|
| Pregnancy Category | Definition |
| A | Controlled studies show no risk. Adequate, well-controlled studies in pregnant women have failed to demonstrate risk to the fetus. |
| B | No evidence of risk in humans. Either animal findings show risk, but human findings do not; or if no adequate human studies have been done, animal findings are negative. |
| C | Risk cannot be ruled out. Human studies are lacking, and animal studies are either positive for fetal risk or lacking. However, potential benefits may justify the potential risks. |
| D | Positive evidence of risk. Investigational or postmarketing data show risk to the fetus. Nevertheless, potential benefits may outweigh the potential risks. If needed in a life-threatening situation or a serious disease, the drug may be acceptable if safer drugs cannot be used or are ineffective. |
| X | Contraindicated in pregnancy. Studies in animals or human, or investigational or post-marketing reports have shown fetal risk which clearly outweighs any possible benefit to the patients. |

*Regardless of the designated pregnancy category or presumed safety, no drug should be administered during pregnancy unless it is clearly needed and potential benefits outweigh potential hazards to the fetus.*

The American Association of Poison Control Centers (AAPCC) has established a national toll-free poison center hotline. Now everyone in the United States can call 1-800-222-1222 to reach the local poison center. Poison Center services are available 24 hours a day, 7 days a week.

The phone number can be used for a poison emergency, or questions about poisons and poison prevention.

Regardless of where the call is placed, the hotline automatically connects callers to the closest poison control center. Existing local poison center numbers will still connect callers to their poison centers.

Callers who use a TTY/TDD and non-English speaking callers can also use this hotline.

This list has been prepared to sensitize health professionals and their support personnel for the need to properly communicate when writing, speaking, reading, and hearing drug names.

No drug name is without problems. Any name can be written or spoken poorly enough so that it can be mistaken for another.

Listed in the accompanying table are drug names that can look and/or sound alike. Some are dangerously close, whereas others require incomplete prescribing information, poor communications skills, poor listening, and/or lack of knowledge about the drugs for an error to result.

To reduce errors, practitioners must share the common goal of drug name safety with pharmaceutical manufacturers, the Food and Drug Administration (FDA), the World Health Organization (WHO), the United States Adopted Name Council (USANC), and the United States Pharmacopeia (USP).

The potential errors can be reduced by:
- Pretesting proposed names for error potential
- Careful selection of brand names and generic names by manufacturers, FDA, WHO, and USANC
- Legible handwriting
- Clear oral communications
- Writing complete drug orders
- Specifying the dosage form (eg, tablet)
- Specifying the drug strength (eg, 100 mg)
- Specifying directions (eg, take one daily with breakfast)
- Specifying the purpose/indication (eg, take one daily with breakfast to control blood pressure)
- Printing orders for new or rarely prescribed drugs
- Using computer-generated orders
- For those involved in drug dispensing and administration, being aware of the drugs that are available and paying careful attention tot he work at hand
- Knowing the patient's condition/problems, to ascertain if the drug name which has been read or heard is indicated
- Double-checking completed prescriptions in the pharmacy
- Educating patients about their drug regimens (this serves as another final check that the prescription was properly read and dispensed)

Proprietary names are capitalized; other names are in lower case letters.

| | | |
|---|---|---|
| Accolate.............Accupril | Aciphex.............Accupril | Afrin..................aspirin |
| Accolate.............Aclovate | Aciphex.............Aricept | Aggrastat............Aggrenox |
| Accupril.............Accolate | Aclovate.............Accolate | Aggrenox............Aggrastat |
| Accupril.............Accutane | Acthar.................Acthrel | Albutein.............albuterol |
| Accupril.............Aciphex | Acthar.................Acular | albuterol.............Albutein |
| Accurbron...........Accutane | Acthrel.............Acthar | albuterol.............atenolol |
| Accutane.............Accupril | Acular.................Acthar | Alcaine..............Alcare |
| Accutane.............Accurbron | adapalene...........Adapin | Alcare................Alcaine |
| acetazolamide......acetohexamide | Adapin...............adapalene | Aldactazide.........Aldactone |
| acetohexamide.....acetazolamide | Adderall.............Inderal | Aldactone...........Aldactazide |
| acetylocholine......acetylcysteine | Adeflor M............Aldoclor | Aldoclor..............Adeflor M |
| acetylcysteine......acetaylcholine | Adriamycin..........Idamycin | Aldoclor..............Aldoril |

| | |
|---|---|
| Aldomet | Aldoril |
| Aldomet | Anzemet |
| Aldoril | Aldoclor |
| Aldoril | Aldomet |
| Alesse | Aleve |
| Aleve | Alesse |
| Alfenta | Sufenta |
| alfentanil | Anafranil |
| alfentanil | fentanyl |
| alfentanil | sufentanil |
| Alkeran | Leukeran |
| Alor 5/500 | Alora |
| Alora | Alor 5/500 |
| alprazolam | lorazepam |
| alprazolam | alprostadil |
| alprostadil | alprazolam |
| Altace | alteplase |
| Altace | Artane |
| alteplase | Altace |
| alteplase | anistreplase |
| Alupent | Atrovent |
| Amaryl | Amerge |
| Ambenyl | Aventyl |
| Ambien | Amen |
| Amen | Ambien |
| Amerge | Amaryl |
| Amicar | amikacin |
| Amicar | Amikin |
| amikacin | Amicar |
| Amikin | Amicar |
| amiloride | amiodarone |
| amiloride | amlodipine |
| aminophylline | amitriptyline |
| aminophylline | ampicillin |
| amiodarone | amiloride |
| amitriptyline | aminophylline |
| amitriptyline | nortriptyline |
| amlodipine | amiloride |
| amoxapine | amoxicillin |
| amoxicillin | amoxapine |
| ampicillin | aminophylline |
| Anafranil | alfentanil |
| Anafranil | enalapril |
| Anafranil | nafarelin |
| Anaprox | Anaspaz |
| Anaspaz | Anaprox |
| Ancobon | Oncovin |
| anisindione | anisotropine |
| anisotropine | anisindione |
| anistreplase | alteplase |
| Antabuse | Anturane |
| Anturane | Antabuse |
| Anturane | Artane |
| Anusol | Aplisol |
| Anusol | Aquasol |

| | |
|---|---|
| Anzemet | Aldomet |
| Aplisol | Anusol |
| Aplisol | Aplitest |
| Aplisol | Atropisol |
| Aplitest | Aplisol |
| Apresazide | Apresoline |
| Apresoline | Apresazide |
| Aquasol | Anusol |
| Aricept | Aciphex |
| Aricept | Ascriptin |
| Artane | Altace |
| Artane | Anturane |
| Asacol | Os-Cal |
| Ascriptin | Aricept |
| Asendin | aspirin |
| aspirin | Afrin |
| aspirin | Asendin |
| Atarax | Ativan |
| Atarax | Marax |
| atenolol | albuterol |
| atenolol | timolol |
| Atgam | Ativan |
| Ativan | Atarax |
| Ativan | Atgam |
| Ativan | Avitene |
| Atropisol | Aplisol |
| Atrovent | Alupent |
| Avelox | Avonex |
| Aventyl | Ambenyl |
| Aventyl | Bentyl |
| Avitene | Ativan |
| Avonex | Avelox |
| azatadine | azathioprine |
| azathioprine | azatadine |
| azathioprine | azidothymidine |
| azathioprine | Azulfidine |
| azidothymidine | azathioprine |
| azithromycin | erythromycin |
| Azulfidine | azathioprine |
| bacitracin | Bactrim |
| bacitracin | Bactroban |
| baclofen | Bactroban |
| baclofen | Becolvent |
| Bactrim | bacitracin |
| Bactroban | bacitracin |
| Bactroban | baclofen |
| Banthine | Brethine |
| Becolvent | baclofen |
| Beminal | Benemid |
| Benadryl | benazepril |
| Benadryl | Bentyl |
| Benadryl | Benylin |
| benazepril | Benadryl |
| Benemid | Beminal |
| Benoxyl | Brevoxyl |

| | |
|---|---|
| Benoxyl | Peroxyl |
| Bentyl | Aventyl |
| Bentyl | Benadryl |
| Benylin | Benadryl |
| Benylin | Ventolin |
| benztropine | bromocriptine |
| bepridil | Prepidil |
| Betadine | betaine |
| Betagan | Betagen |
| Betagen | Betagan |
| betaine | Betadine |
| betaxolol | bethanechol |
| bethanechol | betaxolol |
| Betoptic | Betoptic S |
| Betoptic S | Betoptic |
| Bicillin | Wycillin |
| Brethaire | Brethine |
| Brethine | Banthine |
| Brethine | Brethaire |
| Brevoxyl | Benoxyl |
| bromocriptine | benztropine |
| Bronkodyl | Bronkosol |
| Bronkosol | Bronkodyl |
| bupivacaine | mepivacaine |
| bupropion | buspirone |
| buspirone | bupropion |
| butabarbital | Butalbital |
| Butalbital | butabarbital |
| Cafergot | Carafate |
| Caladryl | calamine |
| calamine | Caladryl |
| calcifediol | calcitriol |
| calciferol | calcitriol |
| calcitonin | calcitriol |
| calcitriol | calcifediol |
| calcitriol | calcitonin |
| calcium glubio-nate | calcium gluco-nate |
| calcium gluco-nate | calcium glubio-nate |
| Capastat | Cepastat |
| Capitrol | Captopril |
| Captopril | Capitrol |
| Carafate | Cafergot |
| Carbatrol | Cartrol |
| Carbex | Surbex |
| Carboplatin | Cisplatin |
| Cardene | Cardura |
| Cardene | codeine |
| Cardene SR | Cardizem SR |
| Cardizem SR | Cardene SR |
| Cardura | Cardene |
| Cardura | Cordarone |
| Cardura | Coumadin |
| Cardura | K-Dur |
| carteolol | carvedilol |

Cartrol ...............Carbatrol
carvedilol ...........carteolol
Catapres ............Cetapred
Catapres ............Combipres
cefamandole........cefmetazole
cefazolin.............cefprozil
cefmetazole.........cefamandole
Cefobid ..............cefonicid
cefonicid.............Cefobid
Cefotan ..............Ceftin
cefotaxime ..........cefoxitin
cefotaxime ..........ceftizoxime
cefotaxime ..........cefuroxime
cefotetan ............cefoxitin
cefoxitin .............cefotaxime
cefoxitin .............cefotetan
cefoxitin .............Cytoxan
cefprozil .............cefazolin
ceftazidime..........ceftizoxime
Ceftin ................Cefotan
Ceftin ................Cefzil
ceftizoxime..........cefotaxime
ceftizoxime..........ceftazidime
cefuroxime ..........cefotaxime
cefuroxime ..........deferoxamine
Cefzil.................Ceftin
Cefzil.................Kefzol
Celebrex.............Cerebyx
Cepastat.............Capastat
cephapirin...........cephradine
cephradine..........cephapirin
Cerebyx .............Celebrex
Cerebyx .............Cerezyme
Ceredase............Cerezyme
Cerezyme ...........Cerebyx
Cerezyme ...........Ceredase
Cetaphil .............Cetapred
Cetapred ............Catapres
Cetapred ............Cetaphil
Chenix...............Cystex
chlorambucil ........Chloromycetin
Chloromycetin......chlorambucil
chlorpromazine.....chlorpropamide
chlorpromazine.....clomipramine
chlorpromazine.....prochlorperazine
chlorpropamide ....chlorpromazine
Chorex...............Chymex
Chymex .............Chorex
Cidex.................Lidex
Ciloxan ..............cinoxacin
Ciloxan ..............Cytoxan
cimetidine ...........simethicone
cinoxacin ............Ciloxan
Cisplatin .............Carboplatin
Citracal ..............Citrucel

Citrucel ..............Citracal
Clinoril ...............Clozaril
clofazimine..........clozapine
clofibrate ............clorazepate
clomiphene .........clomipramine
clomiphene .........clonidine
clomipramine .......chlorpromazine
clomipramine .......clomiphene
clonazepam.........lorazepam
clonidine.............clomiphene
clonidine.............quinidine
clorazepate .........clofibrate
clotrimazole.........co-trimoxazole
Cloxapen............clozapine
clozapine ............clofazimine
clozapine ............Cloxapen
Clozaril ..............Clinoril
Clozaril ..............Colazal
co-trimoxazole......clotrimazole
codeine ..............Cardene
codeine ..............Lodine
Colazal ..............Clozaril
Combipres ..........Catapres
Combivent ..........Combivir
Combivir.............Combivent
Compazine..........Copaxone
Comvax .............Recombivax
Copaxone ...........Compazine
Cordarone...........Cordran
Cordarone...........Cardura
Cordran..............Cordarone
Cort-Dome ..........Cortone
Cortone..............Cort-Dome
Cortrosyn............Cotazym
Cotazym.............Cortrosyn
Coumadin ...........Cardura
Coumadin ...........Kemadrin
Cozaar...............Zocor
cyclobenzaprine....cycloserine
cyclobenzaprine....cyproheptadine
cyclophosphamide.cyclosporine
cycloserine..........cyclobenzaprine
cycloserine..........cyclosporine
cyclosporine .......cyclophospha-mide
cyclosporine ........cycloserine
cyclosporine ........Cyklokapron
Cyklokapron ........cyclosporine
cyproheptadine.....cyclobenzaprine
Cystex ...............Chenix
Cytadren ............cytarabine
cytarabine...........Cytadren
cytarabine...........vidarabine
CytoGam............Cytoxan
Cytosar U ..........Cytovene

Cytosar U ..........Cytoxan
Cytotec ..............Cytoxan
Cytovene............Cytosar U
Cytoxan .............cefoxitin
Cytoxan .............Ciloxan
Cytoxan .............CytoGam
Cytoxan .............Cytosar U
Cytoxan .............Cytotec
dacarbazine ........Dicarbosil
dacarbazine ........procarbazine
Dacriose.............Danocrine
dactinomycin .......daunorubicin
dactinomycin .......doxorubicin
Dalmane.............Demulen
Dalmane.............Dialume
Danocrine...........Dacriose
Dantrium ............Daraprim
dapsone .............Diprosone
Daranide ............Daraprim
Daraprim ............Dantrium
Daraprim ............Daranide
Darvocet-N..........Darvon-N
Darvon-N............Darvocet-N
daunorubicin........dactinomycin
daunorubicin........doxorubicin
deferoxamine.......cefuroxime
Delsym ..............Desyrel
Demerol .............Demulen
Demerol .............Dymelor
Demulen.............Dalmane
Demulen.............Demerol
Depen ...............Endep
Depo-Estradiol .....Depo-Testadiol
Depo-Medrol........Solu-Medrol
Depo-Testadiol .....Depo-Estradiol
Dermatop ...........Dimetapp
Desferal .............Disophrol
desipramine ........disopyramide
desipramine ........imipramine
desoximetasone ...dexamethasone
Desoxyn.............digoxin
Desyrel ..............Delsym
Desyrel ..............Zestril
dexamethasone ....desoximetasone
Dexedrine...........Dextran
Dexedrine...........Excedrin
Dextran..............Dexedrine
DiaBeta..............Zebeta
Dialume .............Dalmane
Diamox ..............Trimox
diazepam............diazoxide
diazepam............Ditropan
diazoxide ...........diazepam
diazoxide ...........Dyazide
Dicarbosil ..........dacarbazine

| | | |
|---|---|---|
| dichloroacetic acid................trichloracetic acid | doxorubicin .........doxacurium | Ethmozine..........Erythrocin |
| diclofenac ...........Diflucan | doxorubicin .........doxapram | Ethmozine..........erythromycin |
| diclofenac ...........Duphalac | doxorubicin .........doxazosin | ethosuximide .......methsuximide |
| dicyclomine .........doxycycline | doxorubicin .........idarubicin | Ethyol...............ethanol |
| dicyclomine .........dyclonine | Doxy ................Doxil | etidocaine ..........etidronate |
| Diflucan.............diclofenac | doxycycline .........dicyclomine | etidronate ..........etidocaine |
| Diflucan.............disulfiram | doxycycline .........doxylamine | etidronate ..........etomidate |
| digoxin ..............Desoxyn | doxylamine.........doxycycline | etomidate ..........etidronate |
| digoxin ..............doxepin | dronabinol..........droperidol | Eurax ................Evoxac |
| Dilantin .............Dilaudid | droperidol ..........dronabinol | Eurax ................Serax |
| Dilaudid.............Dilantin | Duphalac...........diclofenac | Eurax ................Urex |
| dimenhydrinate.....diphenhydra-mine | Dyazide.............diazoxide | Evoxac.............Eurax |
| Dimetane...........Dimetapp | dyclonine ...........dicyclomine | Excedrin............Dexedrine |
| Dimetapp...........Dermatop | Dymelor ............Demerol | Factrel ..............Sectral |
| Dimetapp...........Dimetane | Dynabac............Dynacin | fentanyl ............alfentanil |
| diphenhydramine ..dimenhydrinate | Dynabac............DynaCirc | Feosol ..............Fer-in-Sol |
| Diprosone...........dapsone | Dynacin.............Dynabac | Fer-in-Sol ..........Feosol |
| dipyridamole .......disopyramide | Dynacin.............DynaCirc | Feridex .............Fertinex |
| Disophrol...........Desferal | DynaCirc ...........Dynabac | Fertinex.............Feridex |
| disopyramide ......desipramine | DynaCirc ...........Dynacin | Fioricet.............Fiorinal |
| disopyramide ......dipyridamole | Ecotrin .............Edecrin | Fiorinal.............Fioricet |
| disulfiram...........Diflucan | Edecrin .............Ecotrin | Fiorinal.............Florinef |
| dithranol ...........Ditropan | Efidac...............Efudex | flecainide ..........fluconazole |
| Ditropan ...........diazepam | Efudex ..............Efidac | Flexeril..............Floxin |
| Ditropan ...........dithranol | Elavil ...............Equanil | Flexon ..............Floxin |
| dobutamine ........dopamine | Elavil ...............Mellaril | Flomax.............Fosamax |
| Dolobid .............Slo-bid | Eldepryl.............enalapril | Flomax.............Volmax |
| Donnagel...........Donnatal | Eldopaque Forte...Eldoquin Forte | Florinef .............Fiorinal |
| Donnatal...........Donnagel | Eldoquin Forte .....Eldopaque Forte | Florvite.............Flovite |
| dopamine ..........dobutamine | Elmiron .............Imuran | Floxin ..............Flexeril |
| dopamine ..........Dopram | Emcyt...............Eryc | Floxin ..............Flexon |
| Dopar ...............Dopram | enalapril ............Anafranil | fluconazole.........flecainide |
| Dopram.............dopamine | enalapril ............Eldepryl | Fludara .............FUDR |
| Dopram.............Dopar | Endep................Depen | Flumadine..........flunisolide |
| doxacurium ........doxapram | Enduronyl Forte....Inderal 40 mg | Flumadine..........flutamide |
| doxacurium ........doxorubicin | enflurane ...........isoflurane | flunisolide ..........Flumadine |
| doxapram ..........doxacurium | Entex................Tenex | flunisolide ..........fluocinonide |
| doxapram ..........doxazosin | ephedrine ..........epinephrine | fluocinolone........fluocinonide |
| doxapram ..........doxepin | epinephrine ........ephedrine | fluocinonide........flunisolide |
| doxapram ..........Doxinate | Epogen .............Neupogen | fluocinonide........fluocinolone |
| doxapram ..........doxorubicin | Equagesic...........EquiGesic (veterinary) | fluoxetine ..........fluvastatin |
| doxazosin ..........doxapram | Equanil .............Elavil | flutamide ...........Flumadine |
| doxazosin ..........doxepin | EquiGesic (veterinary).........Equagesic | fluvastatin ..........fluoxetine |
| doxazosin ..........doxorubicin | | folic acid............folinic acid |
| doxepin .............digoxin | Eryc ................Emcyt | folinic acid..........folic acid |
| doxepin .............doxapram | Erythrocin ..........Ethmozine | Folvite ..............Florvite |
| doxepin .............doxazosin | erythromycin........azithromcyin | Fosamax ...........Flomax |
| doxepin .............Doxidan | erythromycin........Ethmozine | fosinopril............lisinopril |
| Doxidan ............doxepin | Esimil ...............Estinyl | FUDR...............Fludara |
| Doxil.................Doxy | Esimil ...............Ismelin | Fulvicin .............Furacin |
| Doxil.................Paxil | Estinyl ..............Esimil | Furacin .............Fulvicin |
| Doxinate............doxapram | Estraderm..........Testoderm | furosemide .........Torsemide |
| doxorubicin .........dactinomycin | Ethamolin ..........ethanol | Gantanol ...........Gantrisin |
| doxorubicin .........daunorubicin | ethanol..............Ethamolin | Gantrisin............Gantanol |
| | ethanol..............Ethyol | Genpril..............Genprin |

| | | |
|---|---|---|
| Genprin............Genpril | hydroxyurea .......hydroxyzine | K-Phos Neutral.....Neutra-Phos-K |
| Glaucon............glucagon | hydroxyzine.........hydralazine | Kaochlor............K-Lor |
| glimepiride.........glipizide | hydroxyzine.........hydroxyurea | Kefzol................Cefzil |
| glipizide.............glimepiride | Hygroton............Regroton | Kemadrin............Coumadin |
| glipizide.............glyburide | Hyperstat............Nitrostat | Klaron................Klor-Con |
| glucagon............Glaucon | Hytone...............Vytone | Klor-Con.............Klaron |
| Glucotrol............glyburide | Idamycin..............Adriamycin | lactose..............lactulose |
| glutethimide........guanethidine | idarubicin............doxorubicin | lactulose............lactose |
| glyburide...........glipizide | Iletin..................Lente | Lamictal.............Lamisil |
| glyburide...........Glucotrol | imipenem............Omnipen | Lamictal.............Lomotil |
| GoLYTELY.........NuLytely | imipramine..........desipramine | Lamisil...............Lamictal |
| gonadorelin.........gonadotropin | Imodium..............Indocin | lamivudine.........lamotrigine |
| gonadorelin.........guanadrel | Imodium..............Ionamin | lamotrigine.........lamivudine |
| gonadotropin.......gonadorelin | Imuran...............Elmiron | Lanoxin.............Levsinex |
| guaifenesin........guanfacine | Imuran...............Inderal | Lanoxin.............Lonox |
| guanabenz.........guanadrel | indapamide.........iodamide | Lantus...............Lente |
| guanabenz.........guanfacine | indapamide.........iopamidol | Lasix.................Lidex |
| guanadrel..........gonadorelin | indapamide.........Iopidine | Lasix.................Luvox |
| guanadrel..........guanabenz | Inderal...............Adderall | Lasix.................Luxiq |
| guanethidine.......glutethimide | Inderal...............Imuran | Lente.................Iletin |
| guanethidine.......guanidine | Inderal...............Inderide | Lente.................Lantus |
| guanfacine.........guaifenesin | Inderal...............Isordil | Leukeran............Alkeran |
| guanfacine.........guanabenz | Inderal 40 mg......Enduronyl Forte | Leukeran............Leukine |
| guanfacine.........guanidine | Inderide.............Inderal | Leukine..............Leukeran |
| guanidine...........guanethidine | Indocin..............Imodium | Leustatin...........lovastatin |
| guanidine...........guanfacine | Indocin..............Vicodin | Levatol..............Lipitor |
| halcinonide.........Halcion | interferon 2.........interleukin 2 | Levbid..............Lithobid |
| Halcion.............halcinonide | interferon alfa-2a..interferon alfa-2b | levothyroxine.......liothyronine |
| Halcion.............Haldol | interferon alfa-2b..interferon alfa-2a | Levsinex............Lanoxin |
| Halcion.............Healon | interleukin 2.......interferon 2 | Librax...............Librium |
| Haldol...............Halcion | interleukin 2.......interleukin 11 | Librium..............Librax |
| Haldol...............Halog | interleukin 11......interleukin 2 | Lidex................Cidex |
| Halog...............Haldol | Intropin.............Isoptin | Lidex................Lasix |
| Halotestin..........Halotex | iodamide...........indapamide | Lioresal.............lisinopril |
| Halotestin..........halothane | iodapamide........Iopidine | liothyronine.........levothyroxine |
| Halotex.............Halotestin | iodine...............Iopidine | Lipitor...............Levatol |
| halothane..........Halotestin | iodine...............Lodine | lisinopril.............fosinopril |
| Healon..............Halcion | Ionamin.............Imodium | lisinopril.............Lioresal |
| heparin.............Hespan | iopamidol...........indapamide | Lithobid..............Levbid |
| Hespan.............heparin | Iopidine.............indapamide | Lithobid..............Lithostat |
| Humalog............Humulin | Iopidine.............iodapamide | Lithobid..............Lithotabs |
| Humulin.............Humalog | Iopidine.............iodine | Lithonate...........Lithostat |
| Hycodan............Hycomine | Iopidine.............Lodine | Lithostat............Lithobid |
| Hycodan............Vicodin | Ismelin..............Esimil | Lithostat............Lithonate |
| Hycomine..........Hycodan | Ismelin..............Isuprel | Lithostat............Lithotabs |
| hydralazine........hydroxyzine | isoflurane...........enflurane | Lithotabs...........Lithobid |
| hydrochlorothia-zide...hydroflumethia-zide | Isoptin..............Intropin | Lithotabs...........Lithostat |
| hydrocortisone.....hydroxychloro-quine | Isopto Carbachol..Isopto Carpine | Livostin.............lovastatin |
| | Isopto Carpine.....Isopto Carbachol | Lodine..............codeine |
| hydroflumethia-zide...hydrochlorothia-zide | Isordil...............Inderal | Lodine..............iodine |
| | Isordil...............Isuprel | Lodine..............Iopidine |
| hydromorphone....morphine | Isuprel..............Ismelin | Lomotil..............Lamictal |
| hydroxychloro-quine...hydrocortisone | Isuprel..............Isordil | Loniten..............Lotensin |
| | K-Dur...............Cardura | Lonox...............Lanoxin |
| hydroxyproges-terone...medroxypro-gesterone | K-Lor................Kaochlor | Lonox...............Loprox |

| | | |
|---|---|---|
| Lopressor ...........Lopurin | metaproterenol .....metipranolol | Mylanta .............Milontin |
| Loprox ...............Lonox | metaproterenol .....metoprolol | Mylanta .............Mynatal |
| Lopurin ..............Lopressor | Metatensin ..........Mestinon | Myleran ..............Mylicon |
| Lopurin ..............Lupron | methazolamide.....metolazone | Mylicon ..............Myleran |
| Lorabid ..............Lortab | methenamine.......methionine | Mynatal ..............Mylanta |
| lorazepam...........alprazolam | methicillin ...........mezlocillin | Myoflex ..............Mycelex |
| lorazepam...........clonazepam | methionine ..........methenamine | nafarelin .............Anafranil |
| Lortab................Lorabid | methocarbamol ....mephobarbital | Naldecon............Nalfon |
| Lotensin .............Loniten | methsuximide ......ethosuximide | Nalfon...............Naldecon |
| Lotensin .............lovastatin | methylpredniso-   medroxypro- | naloxone ............naltrexone |
| Lotronex.............Lovenox | lone .................gesterone | naltrexone...........naloxone |
| Lotronex.............Protonix | methyltestos-   medroxypro- | Narcan...............Norcuron |
| lovastatin ...........Leustatin | terone...............gesterone | Nasarel .............Nizoral |
| lovastatin ...........Livostin | metipranolol .......metaproterenol | Navane .............Norvasc |
| lovastatin ...........Lotensin | metolazone .........methiazolamine | Navane .............Nubain |
| Lovenox .............Lotronex | metolazone .........metoprolol | Nembutal............Myambutol |
| Luminal..............Tuinal | metoprolol...........metaproterenol | Nephro-Calci .......Nephrocaps |
| Lupron ...............Lopurin | metoprolol...........metolazone | Nephrocaps.........Nephro-Calci |
| Lupron ...............Nuprin | metyrapone ........metyrosine | Neumega............Neupogen |
| Luvox ................Lasix | metryrosine ........metyrapone | Neupogen...........Epogen |
| Luxiq ................Lasix | Mevacor.............Mivacron | Neupogen...........Neumega |
| Maalox...............Maolate | mezlocillin ..........methicillin | Neupogen...........Nutramigen |
| Maalox...............Marax | miconazole.........Micronase | Neurontin............Noroxin |
| magnesium sul-   manganese | miconazole.........Micronor | Neutra-Phos-K .....K-Phos Neutral |
| fate ...................sulfate | Micro-K .............Micronase | niacin ................Minocin |
| manganese sul-   magnesium | Micronase..........miconazole | nicardipine .........nifedipine |
| fate ...................sulfate | Micronase..........Micro-K | Nicobid .............Nitro-Bid |
| Maolate.............Maalox | Micronase..........Micronor | Nicoderm...........Nitroderm |
| Maranox.............Marax | Micronor............miconazole | Nicorette............Nordette |
| Marax................Atarax | Micronor............Micronase | nifedipine...........nicardipine |
| Marax................Maalox | Midrin ...............Mydfrin | nifedipine...........nimodipine |
| Marax................Maranox | Mifeprex ............Mirapex | Nilstat................Nitrostat |
| Maxidex ............Maxzide | Milontin .............Miltown | Nilstat................Nystatin |
| Maxzide ............Maxidex | Milontin .............Mylanta | nimodipine ..........nifedipine |
| Mebaral.............Medrol | Miltown .............Milontin | Nitro-Bid............Nicobid |
| Mebaral.............Mellaril | Minocin .............Mithracin | Nitroderm ..........Nicoderm |
| mecamylamine .....mesalamine | Minocin .............niacin | nitroglycerin.........nitroprusside |
| Medrol ..............Mebaral | MiraLax.............Mirapex | Nitrol ................Nizoral |
| medroxypro-   hydroxyproges- | Mirapex.............Mifeprex | nitroprusside........nitrogylcerin |
| gesterone ...........terone | Mirapex.............MiraLax | Nitrostat .............Hyperstat |
| medroxypro-   methylpredniso- | Mithracin ...........Minocin | Nitrostat .............Nilstat |
| gesterone ...........lone | mithramycin.........mitomycin | Nitrostat .............Nystatin |
| medroxypro-   methyltestos- | mitomycin ..........mithramycin | Nizoral ..............Nasarel |
| gesterone ...........terone | Mivacron ...........Mevacor | Nizoral ..............Nitrol |
| Mellaril...............Elavil | Moban ..............Mobidin | Norcuron ............Narcan |
| Mellaril...............Mebaral | Mobidin.............Moban | Nordette.............Nicorette |
| melphalan...........Mephyton | Modane.............Mudrane | Norgesic #40 .......Norgesic Forte |
| mephenytoin........Mephyton | Monopril............Monurol | Norgesic Forte .....Norgesic #40 |
| mephenytoin........phenytoin | Monurol.............Monopril | Noroxin ..............Neurontin |
| mephobarbital ......methocarbamol | morphine ...........hydromorphone | nortriptyline ........amitriptyline |
| Mephyton ..........melphalan | Mudrane............Modane | Norvasc .............Navane |
| Mephyton ..........mephenytoin | Myambutol..........Nembutal | Norvasc .............Vascor |
| mepivacaine .......bupivacaine | Mycelex .............Myoflex | Nubain...............Navane |
| mesalamine.........mecamylamine | Myciguent ..........Mycitracin | NuLytely.............GoLYTELY |
| Mesantoin...........Mestinon | Mycitracin ..........Myciguent | Nuprin ...............Lupron |
| Mestinon ............Mesantoin | Mydfrin..............Midrin | |
| Mestinon ............Metatensin | | |

| | |
|---|---|
| Nutramigen | Neupogen |
| Nystatin | Nilstat |
| Nystatin | Nitrostat |
| OctreoScan | octreotide |
| OctreoScan | OncoScint |
| octreotide | OctreoScan |
| Ocufen | Ocuflox |
| Ocuflox | Ocufen |
| olanzapine | olsalazine |
| olsalazine | olanzapine |
| Omnipen | imipenem |
| Omnipen | Unipen |
| OncoScint | OctreoScan |
| Oncovin | Ancobon |
| Ophthaine | Ophthetic |
| Ophthetic | Ophthaine |
| Optiray | Optival |
| Optivar | Optiray |
| Oretic | Oreton |
| Oreton | Oretic |
| Orinase | Ornade |
| Orinase | Ornex |
| Ornade | Orinase |
| Os-Cal | Asacol |
| oxaprozin | oxazepam |
| oxazepam | oxaprozin |
| oxybutynin | OxyContin |
| OxyContin | oxybutynin |
| oxymetazoline | oxymetholone |
| oxymetholone | oxymetazoline |
| oxymetholone | oxymorphone |
| oxymorphone | oxymetholone |
| paclitaxel | paroxetine |
| paclitaxel | Paxil |
| Panadol | pindolol |
| pancuronium | pipecuronium |
| Paraplatin | Platinol |
| paregoric | Percogesic |
| Parlodel | pindolol |
| paroxetine | paclitaxel |
| paroxetine | pyridoxine |
| Patanol | Platinol |
| Pathilon | Pathocil |
| Pathocil | Pathilon |
| Pathocil | Placidyl |
| Paxil | Doxil |
| Paxil | paclitaxel |
| Paxil | Plavix |
| Paxil | Taxol |
| Pediapred | Pediazole |
| Pediazole | Pediapred |
| Penetrex | Pentrax |
| penicillamine | penicillin |
| penicillin | penicillamine |

| | |
|---|---|
| penicillin G potassium | penicillin G procaine |
| penicillin G procaine | penicillin G potassium |
| pentobarbital | phenobarbital |
| pentosan | pentostatin |
| pentostatin | pentosan |
| Pentrax | Penetrex |
| Pentrax | Permax |
| Perative | Periactin |
| Percocet | Percodan |
| Percodan | Percocet |
| Percodan | Percogesic |
| Percodan | Periactin |
| Percogesic | paregoric |
| Percogesic | Percodan |
| Periactin | Perative |
| Periactin | Percodan |
| Periactin | Persantine |
| Peridex | Precedex |
| Permax | Pentrax |
| Permax | Pernox |
| Pernox | Permax |
| Peroxyl | Benoxyl |
| Persantine | Periactin |
| phenobarbital | pentobarbital |
| phentermine | phentolamine |
| phentolamine | phentermine |
| phenytoin | mephenytoin |
| pHisoDerm | pHisoHex |
| pHisoHex | pHisoDerm |
| pHisoHex | Phos-Ex |
| Phos-Ex | pHisoHex |
| Phos-Flur | PhosLo |
| PhosChol | PhosLo |
| PhosChol | Phosphocol P32 |
| PhosLo | Phos-Flur |
| PhosLo | PhosChol |
| Phosphocol P32 | PhosChol |
| physostigmine | Prostigmin |
| physostigmine | pyridostigmine |
| pindolol | Panadol |
| pindolol | Parlodel |
| pindolol | Plendil |
| pipecuronium | pancuronium |
| Pitocin | Pitressin |
| Pitressin | Pitocin |
| Placidyl | Pathocil |
| Platinol | Paraplatin |
| Platinol | Patanol |
| Plavix | Paxil |
| Plendil | pindolol |
| Plendil | Pletal |
| Pletal | Plendil |
| Polocaine | prilocaine |
| Ponstel | Pronestyl |

| | |
|---|---|
| Posicor | Proscar |
| Posicor | Psorcon |
| pralidoxime | Pramoxine |
| pralidoxime | pyridoxine |
| Pramoxine | pralidoxime |
| Pravachol | Prevacid |
| Pravachol | propranolol |
| PreCare | Precose |
| Precedex | Peridex |
| Precose | PreCare |
| prednisolone | prednisone |
| prednisone | prednisolone |
| prednisone | primidone |
| Premarin | Primaxin |
| Premarin | Remeron |
| Premphase | Prempro |
| Prempro | Premphase |
| Prepidil | bepridil |
| Prevacid | Pravachol |
| Prevacid | Prevpac |
| Preven | Prevnar |
| Prevnar | Preven |
| Prevpac | Prevacid |
| prilocaine | Polocaine |
| prilocaine | Prilosec |
| Prilosec | prilocaine |
| Prilosec | Prinivil |
| Prilosec | Prozac |
| Primaxin | Premarin |
| primidone | prednisone |
| Prinivil | Prilosec |
| Prinivil | Proventil |
| ProAmatine | protamine |
| probenecid | Procanbid |
| procaine | Prokine |
| Procanbid | probenecid |
| procarbazine | dacarbazine |
| prochlorperazine | chlorpromazine |
| Prokine | procaine |
| Proloprim | Protropin |
| promazine | promethazine |
| promethazine | promazine |
| Pronestyl | Ponstel |
| propranolol | Pravachol |
| Proscar | Posicor |
| Proscar | ProSom |
| Proscar | Prozac |
| Proscar | Psorcon |
| ProSom | Proscar |
| ProSom | Prozac |
| ProSom | Psorcon |
| Prostigmin | physostigmine |
| protamine | ProAmatine |
| protamine | Protopam |
| protamine | Protropin |

Protonix .............Lotronex
Protopam............protamine
Protopam............Protropin
Protropin ............Proloprim
Protropin ............protamine
Protropin ............Protopam
Proventil..............Prinivil
Prozac...............Prilosec
Prozac...............Proscar
Prozac...............ProSom
Psorcon .............Posicor
Psorcon .............Proscar
Psorcon .............ProSom
Pyridium.............pyridoxine
pyridostigmine......physostigmine
pyridoxine ..........paroxetine
pyridoxine ..........pralidoxime
pyridoxine ..........Pyridium
Quarzan..............quazepam
Quarzan..............Questran
quazepam...........Quarzan
Questran ............Quarzan
quinidine.............clonidine
quinidine.............quinine
quinidine.............Quinora
quinine...............quinidine
Quinora...............quinidine
ranitidine ...........rimantadine
ranitidine ...........ritodrine
Recombivax ........Comvax
Reglan...............Regonol
Reglan...............Renagel
Regonol .............Reglan
Regonol .............Regroton
Regonol .............Renagel
Regranex............Repronex
Regroton ............Hygroton
Regroton ............Regonol
Remeron ............Premarin
Remicade ..........Renacidin
Renacidin ..........Remicade
Renagel .............Reglan
Renagel .............Regonol
Repronex............Regranex
reserpine ............risperidone
Restasis .............Retavase
Restoril ..............Vistaril
Restoril ..............Zestril
Retavase............Restasis
Retrovir..............ritonavir
Revex................ReVia
ReVia ...............Revex
Ribavirin..............riboflavin
riboflavin.............Ribavirin
rifabutin..............rifampin

Rifadin...............Ritalin
Rifamate.............rifampin
rifampin..............rifabutin
rifampin..............Rifamate
rifampin..............rifapentine
rifapentine...........rifampin
rimanatadine........ranitidine
risperidone ..........reserpine
Ritalin................Rifadin
ritodrine..............ranitidine
ritonavir..............Retrovir
Roxanol .............Roxicet
Roxicet ..............Roxanol
Sandimmune .......Sandoglobulin
Sandimmune .......Sandostatin
Sandoglobulin ......Sandimmune
Sandoglobulin ......Sandostatin
Sandostatin.........Sandimmune
Sandostatin.........Sandoglobulin
saquinavir ...........Sinequan
Sarafem .............Serophene
Sectral...............Factrel
Sectral...............Septra
selegiline ............Stelazine
Septa ................Septra
Septra ...............Sectral
Septra ...............Septa
Serax ................Eurax
Serax ................Xerac
Serentil ..............Serevent
Serentil ..............sertraline
Serevent.............Serentil
Serophene ..........Sarafem
sertraline ............Serentil
simethicone.........cimetidine
Sinequan............saquinavir
Slo-bid ...............Dolobid
Slow FE ..............Slow-K
Slow-K...............Slow FE
Solu-Medrol.........Depo-Medrol
somatrem ...........somatropin
somatropin..........somatrem
somatropin..........sumatriptan
sotalol................Stadol
Sporanox............Suprax
Stadol................sotalol
Stelazine ............selegiline
Sufenta ..............Alfenta
Sufenta ..............Survanta
sufentanil............alfentanil
sulfadiazine.........sulfasalazine
sulfamethizole......sulfamethoxazole
sulfamethoxazole ..sulfamethizole
sulfasalazine........sulfadiazine
sulfasalazine........sulfisoxazole

sulfisoxazole........sulfasalazine
sumatriptan .........somatropin
Suprax...............Sporanox
Surbex...............Carbex
Surbex...............Surfak
Surfak................Surbex
Survanta.............Sufenta
Synagis..............Synalgos-DC
Synalgos-DC .......Synagis
Taxol .................Paxil
Taxol .................Taxotere
Taxotere.............Taxol
Tazicef...............Tazidime
Tazidime.............Tazicef
Tegretol..............Toradol
Tegretol..............Trental
Ten-K ................Tenex
Tenex ................Entex
Tenex ................Ten-K
Tenex ................Xanax
terbinafine...........terbutaline
terbutaline...........terbinafine
terbutaline...........tolbutamide
terconazole .........tioconazole
Testoderm...........Estraderm
testolactone........testosterone
testosterone ........testolactone
Theolair..............Thyrolar
Thera-Flur...........TheraFlu
TheraFlu.............Thera-Flur
thiamine .............Thorazine
thioridazine .........thiothixene
thioridazine .........Thorazine
thiothixene ..........thioridazine
Thorazine ...........thiamine
Thorazine ...........thioridazine
Thyrogen............Thyrolar
Thyrolar .............Theolair
Thyrolar .............Thyrogen
timolol................atenolol
Timoptic .............Viroptic
tioconazole..........terconazole
TobraDex............Tobrex
tobramycin ..........Trobicin
Tobrex ...............TobraDex
tolazamide ..........tolbutamide
tolbutamide .........terbutaline
tolbutamide .........tolazamide
tolnafate .............Tornalate
Toradol ..............Tegretol
Toradol ..............Torecan
Toradol ..............tramadol
Torecan..............Toradol
Tornalate ............tolnaftate
Torsemide...........furosemide

tramadol.............*Toradol*
tramadol.............*Trandate*
*Trandate*.............tramadol
*Trandate*.............*Trental*
*Travatan*.............*Xalatan*
*Trental*.............*Tegretol*
*Trental*.............*Trandate*
tretinoin.............trientine
triamcinolone.......*Triaminicin*
triamcinolone.......*Triaminicol*
*Triaminic*.............*Triaminicin*
*Triaminic*.............*TriHemic*
*Triaminicin*.........triamcinolone
*Triaminicin*.........*Triaminic*
*Triaminicol*.........triamcinolone
triamterene.........trimipramine
trichloracetic      dichlotoacetic
acid.................acid
trientine.............tretinoin
trifluoperazine......triflupromazine
triflupromazine.....trifluoperazine
*TriHemic*.............*Triaminic*
trimeprazine........trimipramine
trimipramine........triamterene
trimipramine........trimeprazine
*Trimox* .............*Diamox*
*Trimox* .............*Tylox*
*Trobicin*.............tobramycin
*Tronolane* ..........*Tronothane*
*Tronothane*..........*Tronolane*
*Tuinal* ...............*Luminal*
*Tuinal* ...............*Tylenol*
*Tylenol*..............*Tuinal*
*Tylenol*..............*Tylox*
*Tylox* ................*Trimox*
*Tylox* ................*Tylenol*
*Ultane*...............*Ultram*
*Ultram* ...............*Ultane*
*Unicap*..............*Unipen*
*Unipen*..............*Omnipen*
*Unipen*..............*Unicap*
*Urex*.................*Eurax*

*Urised*...............*Urispas*
*Urispas* .............*Urised*
*Valcyte*..............*Valium*
*Valium* ..............*Valcyte*
valsartan ............*Valstar*
*Valstar*...............valsartan
*Vancenase*..........*Vanceril*
*Vanceril*..............*Vancenase*
*Vanceril*..............*Vansil*
*Vaniqa* ...............*Viagra*
*Vansil* ................*Vanceril*
*Vantin*................*Ventolin*
*Vascor* ..............*Norvasc*
*Vasocidin*...........*Vasodilan*
*Vasodilan*...........*Vasocidin*
*Vasosulf* .............*Velosef*
*Velosef* .............*Vasosulf*
*Ventolin*.............*Benylin*
*Ventolin*.............*Vantin*
*VePesid* .............*Versed*
*Verelan* ..............*Virilon*
*Verelan* ..............*Vivarin*
*Verelan* ..............*Voltaren*
*Versed*...............*VePesid*
*Vexol*................*VoSol*
*Viagra*................*Vaniqa*
*Vicodin*..............*Hycodan*
*Vicodin*..............*Indocin*
vidarabine...........cytarabine
vinblastine..........vincristine
vinblastine..........vinorelbine
vincristine ..........vinblastine
vinorelbine ..........vinblastine
*Vioxx*.................*Zyvox*
*Virilon*................*Verelan*
*Viroptic* .............*Timoptic*
*Visine* ................*Visken*
*Visken* ..............*Visine*
*Vistaril* ...............*Restoril*
*Vivarin* ..............*Verelan*
*Volmax* ..............*Flomax*
*Voltaren* ............*Verelan*

*VoSol* ...............*Vexol*
*Vytone* ..............*Hytone*
*Wellbutrin* ..........*Wellcovorin*
*Wellbutrin* ..........*Wellferon*
*Wellcovorin* .........*Wellbutrin*
*Wellcovorin* .........*Wellferon*
*Wellferon*............*Wellbutrin*
*Wellferon*............*Wellcovorin*
*Wycillin* ..............*Bicillin*
*Xalatan* ..............*Travatan*
*Xanax*................*Tenex*
*Xanax*................*Xopenex*
*Xanax*................*Zantac*
*Xerac* ................*Serax*
*Xopenex*.............*Xanax*
*Zagam* ...............*Zyban*
*Zantac* ...............*Xanax*
*Zantac* ...............*Zofran*
*Zarontin* .............*Zaroxolyn*
*Zaroxolyn* ...........*Zarontin*
*Zebeta* ...............*DiaBeta*
*Zestril* ................*Desyrel*
*Zestril* ................*Restoril*
*Zestril* ................*Zostrix*
*Zocor*.................*Cozaar*
*Zofran*................*Zantac*
*Zofran*................*Zosyn*
*ZORprin* .............*Zyloprim*
*Zostrix* ..............*Zestril*
*Zostrix* ..............*Zovirax*
*Zosyn* ................*Zofran*
*Zosyn* ................*Zyvox*
*Zovirax*...............*Zostrix*
*Zyban*................*Zagam*
*Zyloprim* .............*ZORprin*
*Zyprexa*..............*Zyrtec*
*Zytrec*................*Zyprexa*
*Zyvox* ................*Vioxx*
*Zyvox* ................*Zosyn*

This list was compiled by Neil M. Davis MS, PharmD, FASHP, President, Safe Medication Practices Consulting, Inc., 1143 Wright Drive, Huntingdon Valley, PA, 19006.

# Patient
# Drug Facts

The *Patient Drug Facts* Annual Index lists all generic names (in bold), brand names, and drug group names included in *Patient Drug Facts.* Index entries may refer to more than one doseform of a product (ie, tablets, capsules, elixir, cream) when all forms are included on a single page. Separate index entries are included when multiple forms of a product appear on different pages or when products are listed in more than one therapeutic group.

## GENERAL INDEX

.44 Magnum, 583
**2-Ethylhexyl p-methoxy-cinnamate, 1506**
**2-Ethylhexyl salicylate, 1508**
4-Way 12 Hour Nasal Spray, 500
4-Way Fast Acting Nasal Spray, 500
5-Aminosalicylic acid agents, 1001
5-HT$_3$ receptor antagonists, 684
**6-MP. see Mercaptopurine**
8-Hour Bayer Caplets, 605
**8-Methoxypsoralen, 1447**
357 HR Magnum, 583
666 Cold Preparation, Maximum Strength Liquid, 547

**A**-200, 1229
A and D, 1483
A•E•R, 1519
A/G Pro, 54
A/T/S, 1041
**Abacavir, 1176**
**Abacavir sulfate/lamivudine/zidovudine, 1176**
Abilify, 780
Absorbine Jr., 1114, 1504
Abuval Sport, 1509, 1510
**Acacia, 983**
**Acarbose, 264**
Accolate, 467
Accu-Chek, 1751

Accupril, 385
Accuretic Tablets, 429
Accutane, 1681
**Acebutolol HCl, 376**
Aceon, 385
Acephen, 602
Aceta, 601
Aceta-Gesic Tablets, 530, 613
**Acetaminophen, 601**
in analgesic combinations, 635
in antacid combinations, 914
buffered, 602
in migraine combinations, 670
in narcotic pain relievers, 626-631
in nonnarcotic pain relievers, 612, 613
in nonprescription sleep aids, 810
in skeletal muscle relaxants, 875
in upper respiratory combinations, 521-523, 530, 538-542, 547, 548, 550-555, 559-564, 566-568
Acetaminophen Uniserts, 602
Acetaminophen w/Codeine Elixir, 626
Acetaminophen w/Codeine Tablets, 626, 627

Acetasol, 1382
Acetasol-HC, 1382
**Acetazolamide**
as anticonvulsant, 813
as diuretic, 305
Acetest, 1758
**Acetic acid**
in anorectal preparations, 1412
in antifungal combinations, 1119
in douche products, 1407
in otic preparations, 1382
**Acetohexamide, 270**
**Acetohydroxamic acid, 1642**
**Acetone**
in acne products, 1430
in antifungal combinations, 1118
**Acetylcholine chloride, intraocular, 1303**
**Acetylcysteine, 484**
**N-Acetylcysteine, 54**
Achromycin, 1077
Acidifiers, urinary tract, 1644
**Acidulated phosphate fluoride, 34**
Aciphex, 953
**Acitretin, 1441**
Aclovate, 238
Acne products
adapalene, 1422

**I-2 Acn/Alc**

Acne products *(cont.)*
  alitretinoin, 1425
  azelaic acid, 1419
  benzoyl peroxide, 1416
  combinations, 1430
  sulfur, 1421
  tazarotene, 1451
  tretinoin, 1427
Acno Cleanser, 1433
Acno Lotion, 1430
Acnomel Cream, 1430
Acnotex Lotion, 1430
**Acrivastine, 532**
ACT, 34
ACT for Kids, 34
ActHIB, 1254
Acticin, 1229
Actidose-Aqua, 1625
Actidose with Sorbitol, 1625
Actifed Cold & Allergy Tablets, 534
Actifed Cold & Sinus Maximum Strength Tablets, 539
Actigall, 957
Actimmune, 1227
Actinex, 1519
Actiq, 618
Actisite, 1394
Activase, 109
**Activated charcoal, 1625**
Active immunization agents, 1243
Activella, 150
Actonel, 297
Actos, 267
ACU-dyne, 1494
Acular, 1338
Adalat, 364
Adalat CC, 364
**Adapalene, 1422**
Adderall, 579
Adderall XR, 579
**Adefovir, 1149**
**Adefovir dipivoxil, 1149**
**Adenine arabinoside. see Vidarabine**
Adipex-P, 587
Adprin-B, 605
Adprin-B Coated Caplets, 610
Adprin-B, Extra Strength, 605
Adrenal cortical steroids
  corticosteroid combinations, 245

Adrenal cortical steroids *(cont.)*
  corticosteroids, topical, 238
  corticotropin, 226
  glucocorticoids, 230
  mineralocorticoid, 249
Adrenal steroid inhibitors, aminoglutethimide, 253
Adrenalin Chloride, 455, 500
Adriamycin PFS, 1553
Adriamycin RDF, 1553
Adsorbocarpine, 1303
Advair Diskus, 470
Advance, 1766
Advanced Formula Di-Gel, 907
Advantage, 1751
Advicor, 450
Advil, Children's, 640
Advil Cold & Sinus Tablets, 523
Advil Flu & Body Ache Tablets, 523
Advil Gelcaps and Liqui-Gels, 640
Advil, Infants', 640
Advil, Junior Strength, 640
Advil Migraine, 640
Advil Tablets and Caplets, 640
AeroBid, 470
AeroBid-M, 470
Aerocaine, 1472
Aerotherm, 1472
Aerozoin, 1487
Afrin Children's Nasal Decongestant Spray, 500
Afrin Extra Moisturizing Nasal Spray, 500
Afrin Original 12 Hour Decongestant Nasal Spray, 500
Afrin Saline Nasal Spray, 502
Afrin Severe Congestion Nasal Spray with Menthol, 500
Afrin Sinus 12 Hour Nasal Spray, 500
Aftate for Athlete's Foot, 1114
Aftate for Jock Itch, 1114
**Agar, 983**
Agenerase, 1169
Aggregation inhibitors, 84

Aggregation inhibitors/vasodilators, 88
Aggrenox, 94
Agoral, 983
Agrylin, 90
AH-chew D, 500
AH-chew Tablets, 542
Airet, 455
AK-Cide, 1354
AK-Cide Suspension, 1354
AK-Con, 1322
AK-Dex, 1331
AK-Dilate, 1322
AK-Homatropine, 1328
AK-Nefrin, 1322
AK-Neo-Dex Solution, 1352
AK-Pentolate, 1328
AK-Pred, 1331
AK-Spore H.C., 1353
AK-Spore H.C. Ophthalmic Suspension, 1352
AK-Spore H.C. Otic, 1379
AK-Sulf, 1348
AK-Tob, 1348
AK-Tracin, 1348
AK-Trol, 1354
AK-Trol Suspension, 1353
Akarpine, 1303
Akineton, 877
Akne-mycin, 1081
AKPro, 1309
Akwa Tears, 1365, 1368
Ala-Cort, 240
Ala-Quin Cream, 245
Ala-Scalp, 240
Alacol DM Syrup, 549
Alamag Plus Suspension, 910
Alamag Suspension, 910
Alamast, 1336
Alasulf, 1093
Albalon, 1322
**Albendazole, 1185**
Albenza, 1185
Albustix, 1768
**Albuterol sulfate, 455**
**Alclometasone dipropionate, 238**
**Alcohol**
  in acne products, 1421, 1430
  in anorectal preparations, 1411
  in antifungal combinations, 1118

# INDEX

**Alcohol** *(cont.)*
  in poison ivy treatment products, 1502
  in topical antihistamines, 1491
Aldactazide, 319
Aldactone, 312
Aldomet, 418
Aldoril 15 Tablets, 428
Aldoril 25 Tablets, 428
Aldoril D30 Tablets, 428
Aldoril D50 Tablets, 428
**Alemtuzumab, 1613**
**Alendronate sodium, 297**
Alesse, 170
Aleve Caplets, 641
Aleve Cold & Sinus Tablets, 523
Aleve Sinus & Headache Tablets, 523
Alferon N, 1222
**Alginic acid, 907**
**Alitretinoin, 1425**
Alka-Mints, 29, 903
Alka-Seltzer, 914
Alka-Seltzer, Extra Strength, 914
Alka-Seltzer Extra Strength Antacid and Pain Relief Effervescent Tablets, 610
Alka-Seltzer Flavored Antacid and Pain Relief Effervescent Tablets, 610
Alka-Seltzer, Original, 914
Alka-Seltzer Original Antacid and Pain Relief Effervescent Tablets, 610
Alka-Seltzer Plus Cold & Cough Liqui-Gels, 551
Alka-Seltzer Plus Cold & Cough Medicine Effervescent Tablets, 550
Alka-Seltzer Plus Cold & Flu Liqui-Gels, 547
Alka-Seltzer Plus Cold & Sinus Liqui-Gels, 521
Alka-Seltzer Plus Cold & Sinus Tablets, 521
Alka-Seltzer Plus Cold Medicine Effervescent Tablets, 538
Alka-Seltzer Plus Cold Medicine Liqui-Gels, 538
Alka-Seltzer Plus Flu Medicine Effervescent Tablets, 550

Alka-Seltzer Plus Liqui-Gels Flu Medicine, 547
Alka-Seltzer Plus Night-Time Cold Medicine Effervescent Tablets, 554
Alka-Seltzer Plus Night-Time Cold LiquiGels, 554
Alkalinizers, urinary tract, 1647
Alkeran, 1590
Alkets, 903, 908
Alkets, Extra Strength, 903
Alkylating agents
  carmustine, 1581
  estrogen/nitrogen mustard, 1588
  lomustine, 1584
  nitrogen mustards, 1590
  streptozocin, 1586
All-Nite Children's Cold/Cough Relief Liquid, 562
All-Nite Liquid, 554
**Allantoin**
  in mouth and throat products, 1402
  in topical agents, 1520
  in upper respiratory combinations, 576
Allegra, 494
Allegra-D Tablets, 534
Aller-Chlor, 493
Allercreme Skin, 1486
Allercreme Ultra, 1486
Allerest Eye Drops, 1322
Allerest Maximum Strength Tablets, 533
Allerfrim Syrup, 534
Allerfrim Tablets, 534
Allergan Enzymatic, 1375
Allergen Ear Drops, 1382
Allergy, 493
Allergy Drops, 1322
Allergy Drops, Maximum Strength, 1322
AllerMax, 494, 676, 877
AlleRx-D Tablets, 543
AlleRx Dose Pack Tablets, 544
Allfen-DM Tablets, 574
**Allopurinol**
  as antineoplastic agent, 1536
  as gout agent, 657
Almacone, 907, 910

Almacone II Double Strength Suspension, 910
Almora, 38
**Almotriptan malate, 673**
Alocril, 1336
**Aloe vera**
  in acne products, 1430
  in anorectal preparations, 1412
  in diaper rash products, 1497
Alomide, 1336
Alophen Pills, 973
Alora, 144
Alpha-1-adrenergic blockers, 382
Alpha-2 adrenergic agonist, 1295
Alpha-adrenergic blocking agents, 1320
Alpha-glucosidase inhibitors, 264
Alpha Keri, 1488
Alpha Keri Shower and Bath, 1516
Alpha Keri Therapeutic, 1487
Alphagan, 1295
Alphatrex, 238
**Alprazolam, 698**
**Alprostadil, 1729**
Alramucil, 962
Alrex, 1334
Altace, 385
**Alteplase, recombinant, 109**
ALternaGEL, 903
Altinac, 1427
**Altretamine, 1601**
Alu-Cap, 903
Alu-Tab, 903
Aludrox Suspension, 910
**Alumina-magnesia, 610**
Alumina, Magnesia, and Simethicone Suspension, 910
**Aluminum acetate**
  in astringents, 1517
  in otic preparations, 1382
**Aluminum carbonate gel, basic, 903**
**Aluminum chloride hexahydrate, 1435, 1518**
**Aluminum hydroxide**
  in analgesics, 610

**Aluminum hydroxide**
*(cont.)*
  in antacid combinations,
  907, 910
  in nonnarcotic analge-
  sics, 613
**Aluminum hydroxide gel,
903**
**Aluminum magnesium
hydroxide sulfate, 903**
**Aluminum oxide, 1433**
Aluminum Paste, 1520
**Aluminum sulfate, 1521**
Alupent, 456
Amacodone Tablets, 627
**Amantadine, 1154**
**Amantadine HCl**
  as antiparkinson agent,
  881
  as antiviral agent, 1154
Amaphen w/Codeine No. 3
  Capsules, 627
Amaryl, 270
**Ambenonium chloride,
1639**
Ambien, 805
**Amcinonide, 238**
Amerge, 673
Americaine First Aid, 1472
Americaine Otic, 1382
Amigesic, 606
**Amiloride and hydro-
chlorothiazide, 319**
**Amiloride HCl, 312**
Amino acid combinations,
  54
Amino acids, 53
**Aminoglutethimide, 253**
Aminoglycosides, oral,
  1013
**Aminophylline, 461**
Aminoquinolines, 1124
Aminoxin, 17
**Amiodarone, 338**
Amitone, 29, 903
**Amitriptyline HCl, 749**
**Amitriptyline HCl and
chlordiazepoxide, 795**
**Amitriptyline HCl and
perphenazine, 795**
Amlexanox, 1396
**Amlodipine, 363, 430**
**Ammonium alum, 1407**
**Ammonium Cl, 321**
**Amobarbital sodium, 800**
Amosan, 1402
**Amoxapine, 749**

**Amoxicillin**
  for Helicobacter pylori
  infections, 932
  as oral antibiotic, 1067
**Amoxicillin and potas-
sium clavulanate, 1067**
Amoxil, 1067
Amoxil Pediatric Drops,
  1067
**Amphetamine mixtures,
579**
Amphetamines, 579
Amphojel, 903
**Amphotericin B, 1113**
**Ampicillin, 1067**
**Amprenavir, 1169**
Amylase, 946
Amytal Sodium, 800
Anabolic steroids, 130
Anacin Caplets and Tab-
  lets, 614
Anacin Maximum Strength,
  Aspirin Free, 601
Anacin P.M. Caplets, 612
Anacin Tablets, Maxi-
  mum Strength, 614
Anadrol-50, 130
Anafranil, 749
**Anagrelide HCl, 90**
AnaGuard, 455
**Anakinra, 1709**
Analeptics, 583
Analgesic Balm, 1504
Analgesics
  acetaminophen, 601
  aspirin and salicylates,
  605
  buffered aspirin, 610
  butorphanol tartrate,
  633
  and decongestant and
  antihistamine combi-
  nations, 538
  pediatric, 542
  and decongestants, 521
  pediatric, 523
  diflunisal, 616
  narcotic pain reliever
  combinations, 626
  narcotic pain relievers,
  618
  nonnarcotic combina-
  tions, 612
  pentazocine, 635
  topical, capsaicin, 1489
  tramadol, 638
Analpram-HC Cream, 245

Analpram-HC Cream 2.5,
  245
Anaplex-DM Liquid, 549
Anaplex HD Liquid, 556
Anaprox, 641
Anaprox DS, 641
Anaspaz, 916
**Anastrozole, 1574**
Anbesol, 1402, 1468
Anbesol Cool Mint, 1402
Anbesol, Maximum
  Strength, 1402, 1468
Ancef, 1019
Andehist DM Oral Drops,
  561
Andehist-DM Syrup, 549
Andehist Drops, 536
Andehist Syrup, 532
Androderm, 137
Androgen inhibitors, 141
Androgens
  as antineoplastic
  agents, 1562
  in estrogen combina-
  tions, 150
  as sex hormones, 137
Android, 137
Anestacon, 1468
Anesthetics
  local, in anorectal
  preparations, 1411
  topical for mucous
  membranes, 1468
  for skin disorders, 1472
Anexsia 5/500 Tablets, 627
Anexsia 7.5/650 Tablets,
  628
Angiotensin converting
  enzyme inhibitors
  as antihypertensive
  agents, 385
  in antihypertensive
  combinations, 428
Angiotensin II receptor
  antagonists
  as antihypertensive
  agents, 390
  in antihypertensive
  combinations, 429
**Anisindione, 104**
**Anistreplase, 109**
Anodynos DHC Tablets,
  627
Anorectal preparations,
  1411
Anorexiants, 587
Ansaid, 640

# INDEX

Answer Plus, 1766
Answer Quick & Simple, 1764, 1766
Antabuse, 1697
Antacid Suspension, 910
Antacid Tablets, 903
Antacid Tablets, Extra Strength, 903
Antacids, 903
  combinations capsules and tablets, 907
  liquids, 910
  powders and effervescent tablets, 914
**Antazoline phosphate, 1326**
Anthra-Derm, 1437
Anthracyclines
  daunorubicin, 1551
  doxorubicin, 1553
  epirubicin, 1556
  idarubicin, 1558
  valrubicin, 1560
**Anthralin, 1437**
Anti-infectives.
  see also Antibiotics; Antifungals; Antimalarials; Antiviral agents
  antiparasitics
    albendazole, 1185
    ivermectin, 1193
    mebendazole, 1187
    pyrantel, 1189
    thiabendazole, 1191
  antiretroviral agents
    non-nucleoside reverse transcriptase inhibitors, 1181
    nucleoside reverse transcriptase inhibitors, 1176
    nucleotide analog reverse transcriptase inhibitors, 1173
    protease inhibitors, 1169
  antituberculosis drugs, 1207
  atovaquone, 1217
  interferon alfa-N3, 1222
  interferon alfacon-1, 1224
  interferon gamma-1B, 1227
  pediculicides, 1229
  pentamidine isethionate, 1219

Anti-infectives. *(cont.)*
  scabicides, 1229
  sulfonamides, 1084
  erythromycin ethylsuccinate and sulfisoxazole, 1087
  trimethoprim and sulfamethoxazole, 1090
  urinary, 1195
  combinations, 1204
  fosfomycin tromethamine, 1197
  methenamine, 1195
  nalidixic acid, 1199
  nitrofurantoin, 1201
  vaginal, 1093
  combinations, 1093
Anti-inflammatory agents, nonsteroidal
  ophthalmic, 1338
  systemic, 640
Anti-obesity agents, orlistat, 1006
Anti-Tuss, 513
Anti-ulcer agents
  misoprostol, 940
  sucralfate, 942
Antiandrogens, 1564
Antianginals, nitrates, 330
Antianxiety agents
  benzodiazepines, 698
  buspirone, 703
  hydroxyzine, 706
  meprobamate, 708
Antiarrhythmics
  amiodarone, 338
  disopyramide, 341
  dofetilide, 344
  flecainide, 347
  mexiletine, 349
  moricizine, 351
  procainamide, 354
  propafenone, 356
  quinidine, 358
  tocainide, 361
Antibiotic and steroid combinations, 1352
Antibiotic combinations, 1087
Antibiotics
  aminoglycosides, 1013
  aztreonam, 1016
  carbapenem, 1055
  cephalosporins, 1019
  chloramphenicol, 1027
  ertapenem, 1057
  erythromycin, 1041

Antibiotics *(cont.)*
  fluoroquinolones, 1049
  imipenem-cilastatin, 1059
  lincosamides, 1030
  macrolides, 1034
  meropenem, 1057
  metronidazole, 1062
  multiple, 1081
  mupirocin, 1065
  ophthalmic, 1348
  otic, 1379
  oxalodinones, 1046
  penicillins, 1067
  spectinomycin hydrochloride, 1039
  tetracyclines, 1072
  topical, 1077
  topical, 1081
  trimethoprim, 1079
  triple, 1082
  vancomycin, 1043
Anticholinergic and decongestant and antihistamine combinations, 542
  pediatric, 545
Anticholinergic combinations, 921
Anticholinergics, 916
  as antiemetic/antivertigo agents, 676
  as antiparkinson agents, 877
Anticholinesterase muscle stimulants, 1639
Anticoagulants
  coumarin derivatives, 104
  heparin, 97
  low molecular weight, 100
Anticonvulsants
  acetazolamide, 813
  carbamazepine, 816
  clonazepam, 820
  felbamate, 824
  gabapentin, 827
  hydantoins, 829
  lamotrigine, 849
  levetiracetam, 855
  oxazolidinediones, 834
  oxcarbazepine, 836
  primidone, 841
  succinimides, 846
  tiagabine, 852
  topiramate, 843

Anticonvulsants *(cont.)*
  valproic acid and
    derivatives, 857
  zonisamide, 839
Antidepressants
  bupropion, 711
  citalopram hydrobro-
    mide, 726
  escitalopram, 717
  fluoxetine, 719
  fluvoxamine, 723
  monoamine oxidase
    inhibitors, 732
  nefazodone, 714
  paroxetine, 738
  sertraline, 741
  tetracyclic compounds,
    729
  trazodone, 743
  tricyclic, 749
  venlafaxine, 746
Antidiabetic agents
  alpha-glucosidase
    inhibitors, 264
  glyburide/metformin,
    281
  insulin, 255
  meglitinides, 275
  metformin, 278
  sulfonylureas, 270
  thiazolidinediones, 267
Antidiarrheals
  bismuth subsalicylate,
    989
  combination products,
    998
  difenoxin, 992
  diphenoxylate, 992
  lactobacillus, 995
  loperamide, 996
Antidotes
  charcoal, activated,
    1625
  dexrazoxane, 1631
  flumazenil, 1627
  ipecac, 1629
  nalmefene HCl, 1633
  naloxone, 1635
Antiemetic/antivertigo
  agents
  5-HT$_3$ receptor antago-
    nists, 684
  anticholinergics, 676
  cannabinoids, 681
  phenothiazines, 687
  phosphorated carbohy-
    drate, 693

Antiestrogens, 1571
Antiflatulents, 944
Antifungal combinations,
  topical, 1118
Antifungals
  clotrimazole, 1096
  fluconazole, 1098
  griseofulvin, 1100
  itraconazole, 1102
  ketoconazole, 1105
  nystatin, 1109
  topical preparations,
    1113
  vaginal preparations,
    1121
  voriconazole, 1111
Antiherpes virus agents,
  1151
Antihist-1, 493
Antihistamine and analge-
  sic combinations, 530
Antihistamine and decon-
  gestant and analgesic
  combinations, 538
  pediatric, 542
Antihistamine and decon-
  gestant and anticholin-
  ergic combinations, 542
  pediatric, 545
Antihistamine and decon-
  gestant combinations,
  532
  pediatric, 536
Antihistamine and expectorant and decongestant
  combinations, 531
  pediatric, 531
Antihistamines, 493
  azelastine, 1342
  ketotifen fumarate, 1346
  levocabastine, 1340
  olopatadine, 1344
  topical, 1491
Antihyperlipidemic combi-
  nations, niacin/lova-
  statin, 450
Antihyperlipidemics
  bile acid sequestrants,
    434
  ezetimibe, 438
  fenofibrate, 440
  gemfibrozil, 443
  HMG-CoA reductase
    inhibitors, 446
Antihypertensive combina-
  tions, 427

Antihypertensives
  alpha-1-adrenergic
    blockers, 382
  angiotensin converting
    enzyme inhibitors,
    385
  angiotensin II receptor
    antagonists, 390
  carvedilol, 410
  clonidine, 394
  guanabenz acetate, 398
  guanadrel sulfate, 400
  guanethidine mono-
    sulfate, 402
  guanfacine, 405
  hydralazine, 407
  labetalol, 413
  mecamylamine, 416
  methyldopa, 418
  minoxidil, 421
  miscellaneous, 430
  reserpine, 424
  selective aldosterone
    receptor antago-
    nists, 432
Antihypotensive agents.
  see Vasopressor/anti-
  hypotensive agents
Antimalarials
  aminoquinolines, 1124
  atovaquone and pro-
    guanil HCl, 1136
  halofantrine HCl, 1134
  mefloquine, 1127
  pyrimethamine, 1129
  quinine sulfate, 1138
  sulfadoxine and pyri-
    methamine, 1131
Antimetabolites
  folic acid analogs, 1533
  purine analogs, 1536
  pyrimidine analogs,
    1539
Antiminth, 1189
Antineoplastic agents,
  1529. see also Alkylat-
  ing agents; Anthracy-
  clines; Hormones;
  Monoclonal antibodies
  antimetabolites folic
    acid analogs, 1533
  purine analogs, 1536
  pyrimidine analogs,
    1539
  busulfan, 1545
  camptothecins, 1542
  enzymes, 1607

# INDEX

Antineoplastic agents, (cont.)
etoposide, 1547
immunologic agents, interferons, 1594
miscellaneous, 1601
mitotic inhibitors, vinorelbine tartrate, 1549
porfimer sodium, 1610
retinoids, tretinoin, 1598
Antiparasitics
albendazole, 1185
ivermectin, 1193
mebendazole, 1187
pyrantel, 1189
thiabendazole, 1191
Antiparkinson agents
anticholinergics, 877
dopaminergics, 881
entacapone, 898
pergolide mesylate, 892
pramipexole, 886
ropinirole, 889
selegiline, 895
Antiplatelet agents
aggregation inhibitors, 84
aggregation inhibitors/ vasodilators, 88
anagrelide, 90
dipyridamole, 92
dipyridamole and aspirin, 94
Antipsychotic agents
benzisoxazole derivatives, 758
dibenzapine derivatives, 761
dihydroindolone derivatives, 765
phenothiazine derivatives, 768
phenylbutylpiperadine derivatives, 776
quinolone derivatives, 780
thioxanthene derivatives, 782
**Antipyrine, 1382**
Antiretroviral agents
nonnucleoside reverse transcriptase inhibitors, 1181
nucleoside reverse transcriptase inhibitors, 1176

Antiretroviral agents (cont.)
nucleotide analog reverse transcriptase inhibitors, 1173
protease inhibitors, 1169
Antirheumatic agents
gold compounds, 648
hydroxychloroquine, 651
leflunomide, 1685
methotrexate, 653
Antiseborrheic products
combinations, 1466
miscellaneous, 1462
selenium sulfide, 1460
Antiseptics, topical, 1494
Antispasmodics, 916
**Antithymocyte globulin (equine), 1236**
**Antithymocyte globulin (rabbit), 1235**
Antithyroid agents, 286
Antituberculosis drugs, 1207
Antitussive and expectorant combinations, 565
pediatric, 571
Antitussive combinations, 545
pediatric, 559
Antitussives
narcotic, 506
nonnarcotic, 509
Antitussives with expectorants, 571
pediatric, 576
Antivert, 676
Antivert/25, 676
Antivert/50, 676
Antivertigo agents. see Antiemetic/antivertigo agents
Antiviral agents
adefovir, 1149
amantadine, 1154
antiherpes virus agents, 1151
cidofovir, 1157
foscarnet, 1140
ganciclovir, 1143
ophthalmic, 1358
oseltamivir phosphate, 1167
ribavirin, 1160
rimantadine, 1163
valganciclovir, 1146

Antiviral agents (cont.)
zanamivir, 1165
Anturane, 668
Anucort-HC, 1411
Anumed-HC, 1411
Anusol, 1411, 1412
Anusol HC-1, 240, 1411
Anzemet, 684
AOSEPT, 1376
AOSEPT Disinfecting, 1376
Apacet, 601
**APAP. see Acetaminophen**
Apatate Liquid, 46
Apatate Tablets, 46
Aphrodyne, 1736
Aphthasol, 1396
Aplisol, 1289
Aplitest, 1289
**Apple blossom oil, 1522**
**Apraclonidine HCl, 1312**
Apresoline, 407
Apri, 170
Aprodine Syrup, 534
Aprodine Tablets, 534
Aqua-Ban, 321
Aqua-Ban Plus, 321
Aquacare, 1483
Aquachloral Supprettes, 805
Aquafresh Sensitive Teeth, 1400
AquaMEPHYTON, 114
Aquanil, 1516
AquaSite, 1365
Aquatab C Tablets, 569
Aquatab DM Tablets, 574
AquatabD Dose Pack Tablets, 526
Aquatab D Tablets, 526
Aquatensen, 315
Aquavit-E, 26
AR Eye Drops - Astringent Redness Reliever, 1322
**Ara-A. see Vidarabine**
Aralen HCl, 1124
Aranesp, 118
Arava, 1685
Arcobee with C Caplets, 47
Aredia, 297
Argesic Cream, 1505
Argesic-SA, 606
**L-Arginine pyroglutamate, 54**
Aricept, 791

Arimidex, 1574
**Aripiprazole, 780**
Aristocort, 232
Aristocort A, 241
Aristocort Forte, 232
Aristocort Intralesional, 232
Aristospan Intra-articular, 232
Aristospan Intralesional, 232
Armour Thyroid, 291
**Arnica, 1518**
Aromasin, 1574
Aromatase inhibitors, 1574
Artane, 878
Artane Sequels, 878
Arth-Rx Lotion, 1505
Artha-G, 606
ArthriCare Lotion, 1505
ArthriCare Rub, 1504
ArthriCare Ultra Rub, 1505
Arthritis Foundation Pain Reliever, 605
Arthritis Foundation Pain Reliever Aspirin Free, 601
Arthritis Pain Ascriptin Coated Caplets, 610
Arthritis Pain Formula Aspirin Free, 601
Arthropan, 605
Arthrotec Tablets, 614
ArthroTherapy Gel, 1505
Artificial Tears, 1365, 1368
Artificial tears, 1365
Artificial Tears Plus, 1365
Asacol, 1001
**Ascorbic acid, 6, 19**
**Ascorbic acid with iron, 73**
Ascriptin Coated Caplets, Arthritis Pain, 610
Ascriptin Coated Caplets, Maximum Strength, 610
Ascriptin Regular Strength Coated Tablets, 610
Asendin, 749
**Asparaginase, 1607**
Aspercreme, 1504
Aspercreme Rub, 1504
Aspergum, 605
**Aspirin, 605**
    in analgesic combinations, 635
    in antacid combinations, 914
    buffered, 610

**Aspirin,** *(cont.)*
    children's, 605
    in migraine combinations, 670
    in narcotic pain relievers, 626-631
    in nonnarcotic pain relievers, 613, 614
    and salicylates, 605
    in skeletal muscle relaxants, 875
    in upper respiratory combinations, 550
**Aspirin and dipyridamole, 94**
Aspirin Free Anacin Maximum Strength, 601
Aspirin Free Excedrin Caplets, 612
Aspirin Free Pain Relief, 601
Aspirin Regimen Bayer Adult Low Strength with Calcium Caplets, 610
Aspirin w/Codeine Tablets No. 2, 626
Aspirin w/Codeine Tablets No. 3, 626
Aspirin w/Codeine Tablets No. 4, 627
Asprimox Extra Protection for Arthritis Pain, 605
Astelin, 493
AsthmaHaler Mist, 455
Astramorph PF, 619
Astringents, aluminum acetate, 1517
Atacand, 390
Atacand HCT 16/12.5 Tablets, 429
Atacand HCT 32/12.5 Tablets, 429
Atarax, 494, 706
Atarax 100, 494, 706
**Atenolol, 376, 427**
**ATG. see Antithymocyte globulin (equine)**
**ATG rabbit. see Antithymocyte globulin (rabbit)**
Atgam, 1236
Ativan, 698
**Atorvastatin calcium, 446**
**Atovaquone, 1217**
**Atovaquone and proguanil HCl, 1136**
Atropine-1, 1328

Atropine Care, 1328
**Atropine sulfate**
    in anticholinergic combinations, 921
    in antidiarrheal combination products, 992
    in cycloplegic mydriatics, 1328
    in upper respiratory combinations, 543
    in urinary anti-infective combinations, 1204
**Atropine sulfate and edrophonium chloride, 1639**
Atropisol, 1328
Atrosept, 1205
Atrovent, 477
**Attapulgite**
    in acne products, 1431
    in antidiarrheal combination products, 998
Attenuvax, 1265
Atuss EX Syrup, 575
Atuss-G Syrup, 569
Atuss HD Liquid, 557
Atuss MS Liquid, 557
Augmentin, 1067
**Auranofin, 648**
Auro-Dri, 1382
Auro Ear Drops, 1382
Aurocaine 2, 1382
Aurolate, 648
**Aurothioglucose, 648**
Auroto Otic, 1382
Avalide Tablets, 429
Avandia, 267
Avapro, 390
AVC, 1093
Aveeno, 1486, 1502
Aveeno Acne Treatment, 1516
Aveeno Cleansing for Acne-Prone Skin, 1432
Aveeno Combination Skin, 1516
Aveeno Dry Skin, 1516
Aveeno Oilated Bath, 1487
Aveeno Regular, 1487
Avelox, 1049
Aventyl, 749
Aventyl Pulvules, 749
Avita, 1427
**Avobenzone, 1507**
Avodart, 141
Avonex, 1738
Axert, for migraine, 673

# INDEX

Axid AR, 935
Axid Pulvules, 935
Axocet Capsules, 612
Aygestin, 156
Ayr Saline, 502
Ayr Saline Nasal Drops and Spray, 502
Azactam, 1016
**Azatadine maleate, 493, 534**
**Azathioprine, 1666**
Azdone Tablets, 628
**Azelaic acid, 1419**
**Azelastine**
in antihistamines, 493
ophthalmic, 1342
Azelex, 1419
**Azithromycin, 1034**
Azmacort, 470
Azo-Gesic, 1664
Azo-Standard, 1664
Azo-Sulfisoxazole, 1204
Azopt, 1314
**Aztreonam, 1016**
Azulfidine, 1084
Azulfidine EN-tabs, 1084

**B**& O Supprettes No. 15A Suppositories, 629
B-50 Caps Capsules, 49
B-50 Super B Complex Tablets, 49
B-100 Ultra B Complex Timed-Release Tablets, 49
B C w/Folic Acid Plus Tablets, 47
B-Complex and B-12 Tablets, 46
B-Complex plus C High Potency Timed-Release Tablets, 47
B Complex Tablets, 46
B-Complex with Vitamin B-12 Tablets, 49
B-Plex Tablets, 47
Babee Teething, 1402
Baby Ayr Saline Nasal Drops and Spray, 502
Baby Numz•it, 1402
Baby Orajel, 1402
**Bacampicillin HCl, 1067**
Bacid, 995
Baciguent, 1081
**Bacitracin**
ophthalmic, 1348

**Bacitracin** *(cont.)*
topical, 1081
Backache Maximum Strength Relief, 606
**Baclofen, 862**
Bactine Antiseptic Anesthetic, 1472
Bactrim, 1090, 1204
Bactrim DS, 1090, 1204
Bactrim Pediatric, 1204
Bactroban, 1065
Bactroban Nasal, 1065
Bain de Soleil All Day Extended Protection, 1507, 1510
Bain de Soleil GentleBlock, 1507
Bain de Soleil Kids, 1507
Bain de Soleil Mademoiselle, 1510
Bain de Soleil Mega Tan, 1511
Bain de Soleil Orange Gelee, 1509, 1510, 1511
Bain de Soleil Tanning Mist, 1511
Bain de Soleil Tropical Deluxe, 1511
Balamine DM Oral Drops, 562
Balamine DM Syrup, 549, 562
Balanced B-50 Capsules, 49
Balanced B-100 Capsules, 49
Balmex, 1484, 1486
Balmex Diaper Rash, 1497
Balneol Perianal Cleansing, 1412
Balnetar, 1462
**Balsalazide disodium, 1001**
**Balsam peru**
in anorectal preparations, 1411
in diaper rash products, 1497
in topical agents, 1520
Banalg Hospital Strength Lotion, 1504
Banalg Muscle Pain Reliever, 1504
Banana Boat Action Sport, 1509
Banana Boat Baby, 1506

Banana Boat Dark Tanning, 1511
Banana Boat Faces Plus, 1509
Banana Boat Kids, 1507
Banana Boat Maximum, 1506
Banana Boat Sport, 1506, 1510
Banana Boat Ultra, 1507
Bancap HC Capsules, 627
Banophen, 494, 676, 877
Banophen Softgels, 494
Barbidonna, 921
Barbidonna No. 2, 921
Barbiturate combinations, 800
Barbiturates, 800
Baridium, 1664
**Barley malt extract, 961**
Basaljel, 903
**Basic fuchsin, 1118**
Basis All Clear, 1516
Basis Cleaner Clean Face Wash, 1516
Basis Comfortably Clean Face Wash, 1516
Basis Sensitive Skin, 1516
Bath products, 1462
Bayer Adult Low Strength with Calcium Caplets, Aspirin Regimen, 610
Bayer Aspirin Tablets and Caplets, Genuine, 605
Bayer Aspirin Tablets and Caplets, Maximum, 605
Bayer Buffered, 605
Bayer Children's, 605
Bayer Enteric 500, Extra Strength, 605
Bayer Enteric Coated Caplets, Regular Strength, 605
Bayer Low Adult Strength, 605
Bayer Plus, Extra Strength, 605
Bayer PM Aspirin Plus Sleep Aid Caplets, Extra Strength, 614
Bayer Select Maximum Strength Backache, 606
BayGam, 1235
BayHep B, 1235
BayRab, 1237
BayRho-D Full Dose, 1237
BayRho-D Mini Dose, 1237

BayTet, 1237
BC Powder Original Formula, 613
**Becaplermin, 1454**
**Beclomethasone dipropionate, 470, 489**
Beconase, 489
Beconase AQ, 489
Beepen-VK, 1068
**Beeswax**
in anorectal preparations, 1411
in topical agents, 1521
Beldin, 509
Belix, 676, 877
Bell/ans, 904
**Belladonna**
in anticholinergic combinations, 921
in antidiarrheal combination products, 998
in narcotic pain relievers, 629
**Belladonna alkaloids**
in migraine combinations, 670
in upper respiratory combinations, 543
Bellergal-S, 922
Ben Gay, 1504
Ben Gay Ultra Strength Cream, 1504
Benadryl, 494, 676, 877, 1491
Benadryl, 2, Maximum Strength, 1491
Benadryl 25, 877
Benadryl Allergy, 494, 676, 877
Benadryl Allergy & Cold Tablets, 540
Benadryl Allergy & Sinus Fastmelt Dissolving Tablets, 534
Benadryl Allergy & Sinus Headache Tablets and Gelcaps, 540
Benadryl Allergy & Sinus Liquid, 534
Benadryl Allergy & Sinus Tablets, 534
Benadryl Allergy Chewables, 676
Benadryl Allergy Kapseals, 676, 877
Benadryl Allergy Ultratab, 494, 676

Benadryl Children's Allergy & Cold Fastmelt Tablets, 537
Benadryl Children's Allergy & Sinus Liquid, 537
Benadryl Dye-Free, 877
Benadryl Dye-Free Allergy, 494
Benadryl Dye-Free Allergy Liqui Gels, 494, 877
Benadryl Kapseals, 877
Benadryl Maximum Strength Severe Allergy & Sinus Headache Tablets, 541
**Benazepril, 428, 430**
**Benazepril HCl, 385**
**Bendroflumethiazide, 315, 427**
Benegyn, 1093
Benicar, 390
Benoquin, 1519
Benoxyl 5, 1416
Benoxyl 10, 1416
Bensulfoid, 1421
Bensulfoid Cream, 1430
**Bentonite, 1421, 1521**
**Bentonite magma, 1502**
Bentyl, 916
Benylin, 509
Benylin Cough, 877
Benylin Expectorant Liquid, 572
Benylin Pediatric, 509
Benz-all, 1495
Benza, 1495
Benzac 5 and 10, 1416
Benzac W 2.5, 5 and 10, 1416
Benzac W Wash 5 and 10, 1416
Benzagel, 1416
**Benzalkonium chloride**
in acne products, 1433
in antiseptics/germicides, 1495
in douche products, 1407
in mouth and throat products, 1404
in poison ivy treatment products, 1502
in topical agents, 1521
in topical antihistamines, 1491
Benzamycin, 1416
Benzedrex, 502

**Benzethonium chloride**
in acne products, 1434
in diaper rash products, 1497
in topical antihistamines, 1491
Benzisoxazole derivatives, 758
**Benzocaine**
in anorectal preparations, 1411
in antifungal combinations, 1118
in antitussives, 509
in lozenges, 1399
in mouth and throat products, 1402
for mucous membranes, 1468
in otic preparations, 1382
in poison ivy treatment products, 1502
for skin disorders, 1472
in topical agents, 1520
in topical antihistamines, 1491
Benzodent, 1402
Benzodiazepines, 698
**Benzoic acid**
in antifungal combinations, 1118
in urinary anti-infective combinations, 1204
Benzoin, 1487
**Benzonatate, 509**
**Benzophenone-3, 1506**
**Benzoyl peroxide**
in acne products, 1416
cleansers, 1416
combinations, 1416
creams, 1416
gels, 1416
lotions, 1416
in topical corticosteroids, 245
**Benzphetamine HCl, 587**
**Benzthiazide, 315**
**Benztropine mesylate, 877**
**Benzyl acetate, 1119**
**Benzyl alcohol**
in acne products, 1431
in anorectal preparations, 1411
in antifungal combinations, 1118

# INDEX

Benzyl alcohol *(cont.)*
in mouth and throat
products, 1398
in topical agents, 1522
**Benzyl alcohol tincture
compound, 1403**
**Benzyl benzoate, 1411**
**Bepridil HCl, 363**
Berocca Tablets, 47
Beta-adrenergic blocking
agents, 376
Beta-blockers
in antihypertensive
combinations, 427
as glaucoma agents,
1297
Beta-Val, 238
Betadine, 1494
Betadine Medicated Dis-
posable Douche, 1407
Betagan Liquifilm, 1297
Betalin S, 10
**Betamethasone, 230**
**Betamethasone dipropio-
nate, 238**
**Betamethasone sodium
phosphate, 230**
**Betamethasone sodium
phosphate and beta-
methasone acetate, 230**
**Betamethasone valer-
ate, 238**
Betapace, 376
Betapace AF, 376
Betaseron, 1738
Betatrex, 238
**Betaxolol HCl**
ophthalmic, 1297
systemic, 376
Betaxon, 1297
**Bethanechol chloride,
1650**
Bethaprim, 1090
Bethaprim DS, 1090
Bethaprim SS, 1090
Betoptic S, 1297
Bextra, 642
Biavax II, 1265
Biaxin, 1034
Biaxin XL, 1034
**Bicalutamide, 1564**
Bicitra, 1647
BiCNU, 1581
Bicozene, 1472
Bile acid sequestrants, 434
Bili-Labstix, 1772
Bili-Labstix SG, 1772

**Bimatoprost, 1306**
Bioflavonoids, 56
Biohist-LA Tablets, 534
Biosun Faces, 1509
Biosun Professional Sun
Protection, 1506
Biotin, 49
**Biperiden, 877**
**Biphasic oral contracep-
tives, 171**
**Bisacodyl**
in bowel evacuation
kits, 987
in laxatives, 973
BiscoLax, 973
**Bismuth subcarbonate,
998**
**Bismuth subgallate**
in anorectal prepara-
tions, 1412
in antidiarrheal combi-
nation products, 998
**Bismuth subnitrate, 1520**
**Bismuth subsalicylate**
in antidiarrheal prod-
ucts, 989
for Helicobacter pylori
infections, 929
**Bisoprolol fumarate**
in antihypertensive
combinations, 427
as beta-adrenergic
blocking agent, 376
Bisphosphonates, 297
**Bitolterol mesylate, 455**
Black-Draught, 974, 983
Blairex Sterile Saline, 1375
Bleph-10, 1348
Blephamide, 1354
Blephamide Suspension,
1354
Blis-To-Sol, 1118
BlisterGard, 1487
Blistex, 1512
Blistex DCT, 1511
Blistex Lip, 1402
Blistex Lip Medex, 1403
Blocadren, 376
Blood tests
glucose, 1751
ketone, 1758
Bluboro Powder, 1517
B&O Suprettes, 998
Boil-Ease, 1472, 1520
Bonine, 676
Bontril PDM, 587
Bontril Slow-Release, 587

**Boric acid**
in antifungal combina-
tions, 1118
in otic preparations,
1382
in topical agents, 1518
Borofair Otic, 1382
Borofax, 1518
Boropak, 1517
**Bosentan, 336**
Boston Advance Cleaner,
1372
Boston Advance Comfort,
1372
Boston Advance Comfort
Formula Convenience
Pack, 1372
Boston Cleaner (original
formula), 1372
Boston Conditioning, 1372
Boston One Step Liquid,
1372
Boston Reconditioning
Drops, 1372
Boston Rewetting Drops,
1369, 1372
Boston Simplicity Multi-
Action, 1372
Bowel evacuants
kits for, 987
polyethylene glycol, 985
Brasivol, 1432
Bravelle, 200
Breathe Free Nasal Spray,
502
Breathe Right Children's
Colds Nasal Strips, 576
Breathe Right Colds Nasal
Strips, 576
Breathe Right Saline Nasal
Spray, 502
Breezee Mist, 1114
Breonesin, 513
Brethine, 456
Brevicon, 170
Brewers Yeast 500 Tab-
lets, 46
Brexin-L.A. Capsules, 533
**Brimonidine tartrate,
1295**
**Brinzolamide, 1314**
Brite-Life Children's Ibu-
profen, 640
Brofed Liquid, 532
Bromanate DM Cold &
Cough Elixir, 561
Bromanate Elixir, 536

Bromatane DX Syrup, 549
Bromfed Capsules, 533
Bromfed DM Cough Syrup, 549
Bromfed-PD Capsules, 536
Bromfed Syrup, 532
Bromfed Tablets, 532
Bromfenex Capsules, 533
Bromfenex PD Capsules, 536
Bromo Seltzer, 602, 914
**Bromocriptine mesylate, 881, 1688**
**Brompheniramine maleate, 532, 533, 536, 538, 549, 556, 561**
Brompheniramine Maleate/Pseudoephedrine HCl Syrup, 532, 536
Bronchodilators
  sympathomimetics, 455
  xanthine derivatives, 461
Broncholate Syrup, 524
Brondelate Elixir, 520
Bronkaid Dual Action Tablets, 524
**Budesonide, 470, 489**
Buf-Puf Acne Cleansing, 1432
**Buffered acetaminophen, 602**
**Buffered aspirin, 610**
Buffered Aspirin Enteric Coated Tablets, 610
Bufferin Arthritis Strength Pain Reliever Caplets, 610
Bufferin Coated Tablets, 610
Bufferin Extra Strength Coated Caplets, 610
Bulk-reducing laxatives, 961
Bullfrog Body Gel, 1507
Bullfrog Body Lotion, 1507
Bullfrog for Babies, 1506
Bullfrog for Kids, 1507
Bullfrog Magic Block, 1507
Bullfrog Quik Gel, 1509
Bullfrog Quik Stick, 1507
Bullfrog Sport Lotion, 1507
Bullfrog SuperBlock, 1506
**Bumetanide, 309**
Bumex, 309
Bupap Tablets, 612
Buphenyl, 116

**Bupropion HCl**
  as antidepressant, 711
  as smoking deterrent, 1720
Burn preparations
  mafenide, 1456
  silver sulfadiazine, 1458
Buro-Sol, 1517
Burow's Solution, 1517
Burow's Solution, Modified, 1382, 1517
BuSpar, 703
**Buspirone HCl, 703**
**Busulfan, 1545**
**Butabarbital sodium**
  in anticholinergic combinations, 922
  as sedative, 800
**Butalbital**
  in narcotic analgesics, 627
  in nonnarcotic analgesics, 612, 613
Butalbital, Acetaminophen and Caffeine Tablets, 613
Butalbital Compound Capsules and Tablets, 614
**Butamben picrate, 1472**
Butesin Picrate, 1472
Butibel, 922
Butisol, 800
**Butoconazole nitrate, 1121**
**Butorphanol tartrate, 633**
**Butylene glycol, 1434**
Bydramine Cough, 509

**C** Factors "1000" Plus, 56
C-PHED Tannate Suspension, 535
**Cabergoline, 1691**
Cafatine-PB, 670
Cafergot, 670
Caffedrine, 583
**Caffeine**
  as CNS stimulant, 583
  in diuretics, 321
  in migraine combinations, 670
  in narcotic analgesics, 627, 629, 631
  in nonnarcotic analgesics, 612, 613, 614
  in skeletal muscle relaxants, 875
**Caffeine citrate, 538, 565**

Cal-Carb Forte, 28, 29
Cal-Citrate, 28
Cal-Mint, 29
Cala-gen, 1491, 1502
Calaclear, 1502
Calagesic, 1502
**Calamine**
  in poison ivy treatment products, 1502
  in topical agents, 1520
  in topical antihistamines, 1491
Calamycin, 1491
Calan, 364
Calan SR, 364
Calcarb 600 with Vitamin D Tablets, 51
Calcet Tablets, 51
Calcibind, 1652
Calcichew, 29, 903
**Calcifediol, 22**
Calciferol, 22
Calciferol Drops, 22
Calcijex, 22
Calcimar, 294
Calcionate, 28
**Calcipotriene, 1439**
Calciquid, 28
**Calcitonin, 294**
**Calcitonin-Salmon, 294**
**Calcitriol, 22**
Calcium 500 mg with D Tablets, 51
Calcium 600-D Tablets, 51
Calcium 600 mg with D Tablets, 51
Calcium 600 with Vitamin D Tablets, 51
**Calcium and vitamin D, 51**
**Calcium ascorbate, 19**
**Calcium carbonate**
  in analgesics, 610
  in antacid combinations, 907, 910
  in antacids, 903
  in histamine $H_2$ antagonists, 935
  in laxatives, 962
  nutritional, 28
Calcium channel blocking agents, 363
**Calcium citrate, 28**
**Calcium glubionate, 28**
**Calcium gluconate, 28**
**Calcium hydroxide, 1502**
**Calcium lactate, 28**

# INDEX

**Calcium, 5, 28**
**Calcium pantothenate, 16**
Calcium Rich Rolaids, 907
**Calcium salts of senno-sides A & B, 973**
Caldecort, 240
Calderol, 22
Calglycine, 908
Calicylic Creme, 1480
Calm-X, 676
Calmol 4, 1412
Caltrate 600, 28
Caltrate 600 Plus, 28, 29
Caltrate 600+D, 28
Caltrate 600+D Tablets, 51
Caltrate 600+Soy, 28
Cameo, 1487
Campath, 1613
Campho-Phenique, 1520
**Camphor**
    in anorectal prepara-tions, 1412
    in antifungal combina-tions, 1118
    in mouth and throat products, 1402
    in poison ivy treatment products, 1502
    in rubs and liniments, 1504
    in topical agents, 1520
    in topical antihista-mines, 1491
    in upper respiratory combinations, 576
Camptosar, 1542
Camptothecins, 1542
Cancer drugs. see Antineo-plastic agents
**Candesartan cilexetil, 390, 429**
Cankaid, 1387
Cannabinoids, 681
Cantil, 916
Cantri, 1093
Capastat Sulfate, 1207
**Capecitabine, 1539**
Capital w/Codeine Suspen-sion, 626
Capitrol, 1462
Capoten, 385
Capozide 25/15 Tablets, 428
Capozide 25/25 Tablets, 428

Capozide 50/15 Tablets, 428
Capozide 50/25 Tablets, 428
**Capreomycin, 1207**
**Capsaicin, 1489**
Capsin Lotion, 1505
**Captopril**
    in antihypertensive combinations, 428
    in antihypertensives, 385
Carafate, 942
**Carbachol**
    intraocular, 1303
    topical, 1303
**Carbamazepine, 816**
**Carbamide peroxide**
    in mouth and throat products, 1387
    in otic preparations, 1382
Carbapenem antibiotics
    ertapenem, 1057
    imipenem-cilastatin, 1059
    meropenem, 1055
Carbastat, 1303
**Carbenicillin indanyl sodium, 1067**
**Carbetapentane citrate, 565**
**Carbetapentane tannate, 545, 559**
Carbex, 895
**Carbidopa, 881**
**Carbidopa/levodopa, 881**
Carbinoxamine Com-pound Drops, 562
Carbinoxamine Compound Syrup, 550
**Carbinoxamine maleate, 533, 536, 537, 543, 549, 550, 558, 561, 562**
Carbinoxamine Oral Drops, 537
Carbinoxamine Syrup, 537
Carbodex DM Drops, 561
Carbodex DM Syrup, 549
Carbofed DM Oral Drops, 561
Carbofed DM Syrup, 549
Carbohydrate, 961
**Carbomer 940, 1521**
Carbonic anhydrase inhibi-tors
    as diuretic, 305

Carbonic anhydrase inhibi-tors *(cont.)*
    as glaucoma agent, 1314
Carboptic, 1303
Cardec DM Syrup, 550
Cardec-S Liquid, 533
Cardene, 363
Cardene SR, 363
Cardiac glycosides, 322
Cardioquin, 358
Cardizem, 363
Cardizem CD, 363
Cardizem SR, 363
Cardura, 382
Carimune, 1236
**Carisoprodol, 871, 875**
**Carisoprodol compound, 875**
Carmol 10, 1483
Carmol 20, 1483
Carmol 40, 1483
Carmol HC, 1411
Carmol HC Cream, 245
**Carmustine, 1581**
**L-Carnitine, 54, 60**
Carnitor, 60
**Carteolol HCl**
    as beta-adrenergic blocking agent, 376
    for glaucoma, 1297
Cartia XT, 363
Cartrol, 376
**Carvedilol, 410**
**Casanthranol, 980, 983**
**Cascara sagrada**
    as laxative, 973
    in laxative combina-tions, 980
Cascara Sagrada Aromatic Fluid Extract, 973
Casodex, 1564
Castaderm, 1118
Castel Minus, 1118
Castel Plus, 1118
Castellani Paint, 1118
**Castor oil**
    in acne products, 1433
    in topical agents, 1520
Cataflam, 640
Catapres, 394
Catapres-TTS-1, 394
Catapres-TTS-2, 394
Catapres-TTS-3, 394
Catrix, 1486
Caverject, 1729
**CCNU. see Lomustine**

Ceclor, 1019
Ceclor CD, 1019
Cecon, 19
Cedax, 1020
CeeNu, 1584
**Cefaclor, 1019**
**Cefadroxil, 1019**
Cefadyl, 1021
**Cefazolin sodium, 1019**
**Cefdinir, 1019**
**Cefepime hydrochloride, 1019**
**Cefixime, 1019**
Cefizox, 1020
**Cefmetazole sodium, 1019**
Cefobid, 1020
**Cefonicid sodium, 1019**
**Cefoperazone sodium, 1020**
Cefotan, 1020
**Cefotaxime sodium, 1020**
**Cefotetan disodium, 1020**
**Cefoxitin sodium, 1020**
**Cefprozil, 1020**
**Ceftazidime, 1020**
**Ceftibuten, 1020**
Ceftin, 1021
**Ceftizoxime sodium, 1020**
**Ceftriaxone sodium, 1021**
**Cefuroxime, 1021**
Cefzil, 1020
Celebrex, 640
**Celecoxib, 640**
Celestone, 230
Celestone Phosphate, 230
Celestone Soluspan, 230
Celexa, 726
CellCept, 1672
CellCept Intravenous, 1672
**Cellulose sodium phosphate, 1652**
Celluvisc, 1365
Celontin Kapseals, 846
Cenafed Plus Tablets, 534
Cenestin, 144
Cenolate, 19
Centrax, 698
Cpacol (lozenges), 1399
Cpacol (mouthwash), 1400
Cpacol ColdCare, 1399
Cpacol Maximum Strength (lozenges), 1399

Cpacol Maximum Strength (throat spray), 1400
Cpacol Sore Throat Liquid, 521
Cpacol Sugar Free, Maximum Strength, 1399
Cpastat Cherry, 1399
Cpastat Extra Strength, 1399
Cpastat Fast-Acting, 1399
**Cephalexin HCl monohydrate, 1021**
**Cephalexin monohydrate, 1021**
Cephalosporins, 1019
**Cephapirin sodium, 1021**
**Cephradine, 1021**
Cephulac, 967
Ceptaz, 1020
Cerebyx, 829
**Ceresin wax, 1520**
Cerezyme, 301
Cerumenex Drops, 1382
Cervical cap, 160
Ceta Cleanser, 1516
Cetacaine, 1473
Cetacort, 240
**Cetalkonium chloride, 1402**
Cetaphil, 1516
Cetaphil Oily Skin, 1516
Cetapred, 1354
**Cetethyl morpholinium ethosulfate, 1412**
**Cetirizine HCl**
    as antihistamine, 493
    in upper respiratory combinations, 533
**Cetyl alcohol**
    in acne products, 1431
    in topical agents, 1524
**Cetylpyridinium chloride**
    in douche products, 1407
    in lozenges, 1399
    in mouth and throat products, 1403
    in mouthwash, 1400
Cevi-Bid, 19
Chapstick Flava-Craze, 1512
Chapstick Ultra, 1511
CharcoAid, 1625
**Charcoal, 944**
**Charcoal, activated, 1625**

CharcoCaps, 944
Chardonna-2, 922
Chelated magnesium, 38
Chelating agents, succimer, 1637
Chemet, 1637
Chemical disinfection systems, for soft (hydrogel) contact lenses, 1376
Chemotherapy. see Antineoplastic agents
Chemstrip 2 GP, 1754, 1772
Chemstrip 2 LN, 1770
Chemstrip 4 the OB, 1772
Chemstrip 6, 1772
Chemstrip 7, 1772
Chemstrip 9, 1772
Chemstrip 10 SG, 1772
Chemstrip bG, 1751, 1754
Chemstrip K, 1758, 1772
Chemstrip Micral, 1768
Chemstrip uG, 1772
Chemstrip uGK, 1754, 1772
Cheracol Cough Syrup, 571
Cheracol D Cough Formula Syrup, 572
Cheracol Plus Liquid, 572
Chigger-Tox, 1472
Chiggerex, 1472
Children's Advil, 640
Children's Decofed, 501
Children's Dramamine, 676
Children's Elixir DM Cough & Cold Elixir, 561
Children's Feverall, 602
Children's Genapap, 601
Children's Halenol, 602
Children's Kaopectate, 998
Children's Mapap, 601
Children's Motrin, 640
Children's Nasalcrom, 474
Children's Panadol, 601, 602
Children's Silapap, 601
Children's Silfedrine, 501
Children's Sudafed, 501
Children's Tylenol, 601, 602
Chlo-Amine, 493
Chlor-Trimeton, 493
Chlor-Trimeton Allergy 8-Hour, 493
Chlor-Trimeton Allergy 12-Hour, 493

# INDEX

Chlor-Trimeton Allergy-D 4 Hour Tablets, 534
Chlor-Trimeton Allergy-D 12 Hour Tablets, 535
**Chloral hydrate, 805**
**Chlorambucil, 1590**
**Chloramphenicol**
in ophthalmic anti-infectives, 1348, 1352
in otic antibiotics, 1379
systemic, 1027
topical, 1081
**Chlorbutanol, 1521**
**Chlorcyclizine HCl, 245**
**Chlordiazepoxide**
as antianxiety agent, 698
in anticholinergic combinations, 922
**Chlordiazepoxide and amitriptyline HCl, 795**
Chloresiom, 1518
Chloresium, 1518
**Chlorhexidine, 1389**
**Chlorhexidine gluconate**
as antiseptic, 1494
as mouth and throat product, 1389
**Chloride, 32**
Chloromycetin, 1081, 1348
Chloromycetin/Hydro-cortisone for Suspension, 1352
Chloromycetin Otic, 1379
Chloromycetin Sodium Succinate, 1027
**Chlorophyll derivatives, 1118, 1518**
**Chlorophyllin, 1118**
Chloroptic, 1348
**Chloroquine hydrochloride, 1124**
**Chloroquine phosphate, 1124**
Chlorostat, 1494
**Chlorothiazide, 315**
**Chloroxine, 1462**
**Chloroxylenol**
in antifungal combinations, 1118
in otic preparations, 1382
in topical antihistamines, 1491
**Chlorphenesin carbamate, 871**

**Chlorpheniramine maleate, 537**
systemic, 493
topical, 1491
in upper respiratory combinations, 530-535, 538-545, 550-553, 556, 557, 562-564, 566, 570
Chlorpheniramine maleate/ pseudoephedrine HCl ER capsules, 533
**Chlorpheniramine tannate, 532, 535, 536, 537, 545, 559**
Chlorpheniramine Tannate/ Pseudoephedrine Tannate Suspension, 537
**Chlorpromazine, 687**
**Chlorpromazine HCl, 768**
**Chlorpropamide, 270**
**Chlorthalidone, 315, 427, 429**
**Chlorzoxazone, 871, 875**
**Chlorzoxazone with APAP, 875**
Cholac, 967
**Cholecalciferol, 22**
Choledyl SA, 461
**Cholestyramine, 434**
**Choline, 49, 62**
**Choline bitartrate, 62**
**Choline salicylate, 605, 606**
**Choline theophyllinate, 461**
Cholinesterase inhibitors
for dementia, 791
ophthalmic, 1300
Chooz, 29, 903
**Choriogonadotropin alfa, 195**
**Chorionic gonadotropin, 197**
Chromelin Complexion Blender, 1518
Chronulac, 967
Chymodiactin, 1693
**Chymopapain, 1693**
Ciba Vision Daily Cleaner, 1375
Ciba Vision Saline, 1375
**Ciclopirox olamine, 1113**
Cidex, 1495
Cidex Formula-7, 1495
Cidex PA, 1495
Cidex Plus, 1495

**Cidofovir, 1157**
**Cilostazol, 84**
Ciloxan, 1348
**Cimetidine, 935**
**Cinoxate, 1509**
Cipro, 1049
**Ciprofloxacin, 1049**
**Ciprofloxacin HCl, 1348**
**Citalopram hydrobromide, 726**
Citra pH, 904
Citracal, 28
Citracal Caplets + D, 28
Citracal Liquitab, 28
**Citrate, 32**
Citrate of Magnesia, 971
**Citric acid**
in acne products, 1434
in analgesics, 602, 610
in anorectal preparations, 1412
in antacid combinations, 914
in laxatives, 962
**Citric acid and sodium citrate, 1647**
Citrocarbonate, 914
Citrucel, 961
Citrucel Sugar Free, 961
Citrus Calcium+D Tablets, 51
Claforan, 1020
**Clarithromycin**
for Helicobacter pylori infections, 932
as macrolide, 1034
Claritin, 495
Claritin-D 12 Hour Tablets, 535
Claritin-D 24 Hour Tablets, 535
Claritin Reditabs, 495
Clean-N-Soak, 1370
Cleaning and soaking solutions
for hard contact lenses, 1370
for rigid gas permeable contact lenses, 1372
Cleaning, soaking, and wetting solutions, for hard contact lenses, 1369
Cleaning solutions and gels, for hard contact lenses, 1369
Cleaning solutions, for rigid gas permeable contact lenses, 1372

Clear Eyes, 1322
Clear Eyes ACR, 1322, 1326
Clear Total Lice Elimination System, 1229
Clearasil 10, 1416
Clearasil Adult Care Cream, 1430
Clearasil Antibacterial Soap, 1432
Clearasil Clearstick Maximum Strength, 1430
Clearasil Clearstick Regular Strength, 1430
Clearasil Double Clear Maximum Strength Pads, 1430
Clearasil Double Clear Regular Strength Pads, 1430
Clearasil Double Textured Pads Maximum Strength, 1433
Clearasil Double Textured Pads Regular Strength, 1433
Clearasil Maximum Strength, 1416
Clearasil Medicated Deep Cleaner, 1433
Clearblue Easy, 1766
Clearly Cala-gel, 1491
Clearplan Easy, 1764
**Clemastine fumarate**
    as antihistamine, 493
    in upper respiratory combinations, 540
Cleocin, 1093
Cleocin HCl, 1030
Cleocin Pediatric, 1030
Cleocin Phosphate, 1030
Cleocin T, 1030
Clerz 2, 1369
Clerz 2 Lubricating and Rewetting Drops, 1376
**Clidinium bromide, 922**
Climara, 144
Clinacort, 232
Clinalog, 232
Clinda-Derm, 1030
**Clindamycin HCl, 1030**
Clinistix, 1754
Clinitest, 1754
Clinoril, 642
**Clobetasol propionate, 238**

**Clocortolone pivalate, 238**
Cloderm, 238
Clomid, 206
**Clomiphene citrate, 206**
**Clomipramine HCl, 749**
**Clonazepam**
    as antianxiety agent, 698
    as anticonvulsant, 820
**Clonidine HCl**
    in antihypertensive combinations, 429
    in antihypertensives, 394
**Clopidogrel bisulfate, 84**
Clopra, 950
**Clorazepate dipotassium, 698**
Clorpactin WCS-90, 1496
Clorpres 0.1 Tablets, 429
Clorpres 0.2 Tablets, 429
Clorpres 0.3 Tablets, 429
**Clotrimazole**
    in topical antifungals, 1096, 1113
    in vaginal preparations, 1121
**Clove, 1402**
**Cloxacillin sodium, 1068**
**Clozapine, 761**
Clozaril, 761
**CMV-IGIV. see Cytomegalovirus immune globulin intravenous (human)**
CNS stimulants
    amphetamines, 579
    analeptics, 583
    anorexiants, 587
    dexmethylphenidate, 592
    methylphenidate, 594
    pemoline, 598
**Coal tar, in antifungal combinations, 1118**
**Cocaine HCl, 1468**
**Cocamidopropyl betaine, 1434**
**Cocoa butter**
    in anorectal preparations, 1411
    in mouth and throat products, 1403
**Cod liver oil, 1497**
Cod Liver Oil USP, 45
Codal-DH Syrup, 558

Codal-DM Syrup, 555
**Codeine, 618**
**Codeine phosphate**
    in antitussives, 506
    in narcotic pain relievers, 618, 626, 627
    in skeletal muscle relaxant combinations, 875
    in upper respiratory combinations, 545, 546, 565, 571
Codeine Phosphate and Guaifenesin Tablets, 571
**Codeine sulfate**
    in antitussives, 506
    in narcotic pain relievers, 618
Codiclear DH Syrup, 575
Codimal DH Syrup, 558
Codimal DM Syrup, 555
Codimal PH Syrup, 546
Cogentin, 877
Cognex, 791
Col-Probenecid, 660, 664
Colace, 977
Colace-T, 977
Colax Tablets, 980
Colazal, 1001
**Colchicine, 660**
**Colchicine and probenecid, 660, 664**
Cold & Cough Tussin Softgels, 567
Cold Symptoms Relief Maximum Strength Tablets, 552
Coldec D Tablets, 533
Coldec DM Syrup, 549
Coldmist JR Tablets, 525
Coldmist LA Tablets, 526
**Colesevelam HCl, 434**
Colestid, 434
Colestid, Flavored, 434
**Colestipol HCl, 434**
Colfed-A Capsules, 533
**Colistin, 1379**
**Colloidal alumina, 1119**
**Colloidal bentonite, 1421**
**Colloidal oatmeal**
    in acne products, 1432
    in poison ivy treatment products, 1502
Collyrium Fresh, 1322
ColoCare, 1761
Colony-stimulating factor, 121
ColoScreen, 1761

# INDEX

ColoScreen-ES, 1761
Coly-Mycin S Otic, 1379
Colyte, 985
Colyte Flavored, 985
Combination diuretics, 319
Combination oral contra-
ceptives, 160
CombiPatch, 151
Combistix, 1772
Combivent, 480
Combivir, 1176
Comfort Eye Drops, 1322
Commit, 1724
Compazine, 687, 768
Compazine Spansules,
687
Complete Allergy Relief,
494
Complex 15, 1486
Compound W, 1480
Compound W Wart
Remover for Kids, 1480
Compoz Nighttime Sleep
Aid, Maximum Strength,
810
Compro, 768
Comtan, 898
Comtrex Acute Head Cold
& Sinus Pressure Relief,
Multi-Symptom Maxi-
mum Strength Tablets,
538
Comtrex Allergy-Sinus
Treatment, Maximum
Strength Tablets, 539
Comtrex Cough and Cold
Relief, Multi-Symptom
Maximum Strength Tab-
lets, 552
Comtrex Day & Night Cold
& Cough Relief, Multi-
Symptom Maximum
Strength Tablets, 552
Comtrex Flu Therapy &
Fever Relief Day & Night,
Multi-Symptom Maxi-
mum Strength Tablets,
539
Comtrex Multi-Symptom
Deep Chest Cold & Con-
gestion Relief Softgels,
566
Comtrex Multi-Symptom
Maximum Strength
Non-Drowsy Cold &
Cough Relief Tablets, 548
Comtussin HC Syrup, 556

Comvax, 1257
Conceive Pregnancy, 1766
Concentrated Phillips' Milk
of Magnesia, 904
Conceptrol, 1409
Conceptrol Contraceptive
Inserts, 1409
Concerta, 594
Condoms
female, 160
male, 160
Condylox, 1478
Congestac Tablets, 526
**Conjugated estrogens,
144, 150**
Constilac, 967
Constulose, 967
Contac Day & Night
Allergy/Sinus Relief Tab-
lets, 541
Contac Day & Night Cold
& Flu Tablets, 553
Contac Severe Cold & Flu
Maximum Strength Tab-
lets, 552
Contact lenses
hard, products for, 1369
rigid gas permeable,
products for, 1372
soft (hydrogel), prod-
ucts for, 1375
Contraceptive(s), 161
emergency, 179
oral, 170
Contraceptive methods,
160
Contraceptive systems
intrauterine proges-
terone, 182
levonorgestrel implant,
185
levonorgestrel-releasing
intrauterine system,
188
Contraceptive transdermal
system, norelgestromin/
ethinyl estradiol, 192
Contrin Capsules, 75
ConvaTec Aloe Vesta Peri-
neal, 1412
Cool Hot Gel, 1504
Cool'n'Hot Gel, 1504
Copaxone, 1743
Cope Analgesic Tablets,
614
Copper, 49

Coppertone All Day, 1506,
1507, 1510
Coppertone Aloe and Vita-
min E, 1512
Coppertone Bug & Sun,
1507, 1510
Coppertone Gold Dark
Tanning, 1511
Coppertone Gold Dark
Tanning Dry Oil, 1511
Coppertone Gold Tan Mag-
nifier, 1511
Coppertone Kids, 1507,
1508
Coppertone Kids Color-
block, 1507
Coppertone Kids Spray 'n
Splash, 1508
Coppertone Kids Wacky
Foam, 1507
Coppertone Moisturizing
Suntan, 1511
Coppertone Natural Fruit
Flavor, 1512
Coppertone Oil-Free, 1506,
1507, 1510
Coppertone Shade, 1506,
1507, 1508
Coppertone Shade UVA
Guard, 1508
Coppertone Sport, 1506,
1508, 1510
Coppertone to Go, 1508,
1510
Coppertone Water Babies
(lip balm), 1511
Coppertone Water Babies
(sunscreen), 1506, 1508
Coppertone Water Babies
Lotion, 1506
Cordarone, 338
Cordran, 239
Cordran SP, 239
Coreg, 410
Corgard, 376
Coricidin 'D' Cold, Flu, &
Sinus Tablets, 541
Coricidin HBP Cold & Flu
Tablets, 530
Coricidin HBP Cough &
Cold Tablets, 550
Coricidin HBP Maximum
Strength Flu Tablets,
550
Corn Huskers, 1486
**Corn starch, 1497**
**Cornmint oil, 1434**

Correctol, 977
Correctol Extra Gentle, 977
Correctol Tablets, 980
CortaGel, 240
Cortaid Intensive Therapy, 240
Cortaid Maximum Strength, 240
Cortaid Sensitive Skin with Aloe, 240
Cortastat, 230
Cortastat 10, 230
Cortastat LA, 230
Cortef, 230, 231
Cortenema, 230
Cortic Ear Drops, 1382
Corticaine, 1411
CortiCool, 240
Corticosteroid combinations, 245
Corticosteroids
    inhalants, 470
    as ophthalmic anti-inflammatory agents, 1331
    topical, 238
Corticotropin, 226
Cortifoam, 230
Cortisol. see Hydrocortisone
Cortisone acetate, 230
Cortisporin, 1353
Cortisporin Otic, 1379
Cortisporin Suspension, 1352
Cortisporin-TC, 1379
Cortizone-5, 240
Cortizone-10, 240
Cortizone-10 External Anal Itch Relief, 240
Cortizone-10 Plus, 240
Cortizone-10 Quick Shot, 240
Cortizone for Kids, 240
Corzide 40/5 Tablets, 427
Corzide 80/5 Tablets, 427
Cosopt, 1316
Cosyntropin, 226
Cotrim, 1090, 1204
Cotrim DS, 1090, 1204
Cotrim Pediatric, 1090, 1204
Cottonseed oil, 1522
Coumadin, 104
Coumarin derivatives, 104
Covera-HS, 364
Covicone, 1487

Cozaar, 390
C.P.-DM Drops, 561
CP-TANNIC Suspension, 535
CPM 8/PSE 90/MSC 2.5 Tablets, 543
Creon 5 Delayed-Release Capsules, 946
Creon 10 Delayed-Release Capsules, 946
Creon 20 Delayed-Release Capsules, 947
Crest Sensitivity Protection, 1400
m-cresyl acetate, 1382
Cresylate, 1382
Crinone, 156
Crixivan, 1169
Crolom, 1336
Cromolyn sodium
    inhalant, 474
    ophthalmic, 1336
    oral, 1695
Crotamiton, 1229
Cruex, 1096, 1113
Cuprimine, 1706
Curel, 1486
Curel Moisturizing, 1486
Cutar Bath Oil, 1462
Cutemol, 1486
Cuticura Medicated Antibacterial, 1516
Cuticura Ointment, 1430
Cutivate, 239
Cyanocobalamin, 6
Cyclizine HCl, 676
Cyclobenzaprine, 871
Cyclocort, 238
Cyclogyl, 1328
Cyclomydril, 1328
Cyclopentolate HCl, 1328
Cyclophosphamide, 1590
Cycloplegic mydriatics, 1328
Cycloserine, 1207
Cyclosporine, 1668
Cycofed Syrup, 545
Cydec-DM Drops, 562
Cydec-DM Syrup, 550, 562
Cydec Oral Drops, 537
Cylert, 598
Cyproheptadine HCl, 493
Cystagon, 1654
Cysteamine bitartrate, 1654
L-Cysteine, 54
Cystex, 1205

Cystospaz, 916
Cystospaz-M, 916
Cytadren, 253
CytoGam, 1235
Cytomegalovirus immune globulin intravenous (human), 1235
Cytomel, 291
Cytotec, 940
Cytovene, 1143
Cytoxan, 1590
Cytuss HC Liquid, 556

D-S-S, 977
Daily Cleaner, 1375
Dakin's Solution Full Strength, 1495
Dakin's Solution Half Strength, 1495
Dalalone, 230
Dalalone D.P., 230
Dalalone L.A., 230
Dallergy Extended Release Tablets, 543
DALLERGY-JR Capsules, 536
Dallergy Syrup, 542
Dallergy Tablets, 542
Dalmane, 805
d'ALPHA E 400, 26
d'ALPHA E 1000, 26
Dalteparin sodium, 100
Damason-P Tablets, 628
Danazol, 215
Danocrine, 215
Dantrium, 865
Dantrium Intravenous, 865
Dantrolene sodium, 865
Dapa, 601
Dapa Extra Strength, 601
Dapiprazole HCl, 1320
Daptacel, 1250
Daranide, 305
Daraprim, 1129
Darbepoetin alfa, 118
Darvocet-N 50 Tablets, 630
Darvocet-N 100 Tablets, 631
Darvon Compound-65 Pulvules, 631
Darvon-N, 619
Darvon Pulvules, 619
Daunorubicin, 1551
Daunorubicin citrate liposome, 1551
DaunoXome, 1551

# INDEX

Dayhist-1, 493
Daypro Caplets, 642
Dayto Sulf, 1093
DC Softgels, 977
DDAVP, 218
**ddI. see Didanosine**
De-Sensitize Plus, 1400
Debrox Drops, 1382
Deca-Durabolin, 130
Decadron, 230
Decadron Phosphate, 230, 1331
Decaject, 230
Decaject-L.A., 230
Declomycin, 1072
Decodult Tablets, 538
Decofed, Children's, 501
Decohistine DH Liquid, 545
Decolate Tablets, 531
Deconamine SR Capsules, 533
Deconamine Syrup, 533
Deconamine Tablets, 533
Decongestant(s)
  nasal, 500
  ophthalmic, 1322
  combinations, 1326
Decongestant and analgesic combinations, 521
  pediatric, 523
Decongestant and antihistamine combinations, 532
  pediatric, 536
Decongestant and expectorant combinations, 524
  pediatric, 529
Decongestant, antihistamine, and analgesic combinations, 538
  pediatric, 542
Decongestant, antihistamine, and anticholinergic combinations, 542
  pediatric, 545
Decongestant, antihistamine, and expectorant combinations, 531
  pediatric, 531
Decongestant combinations, 502
Decongestant inhalers, 502
Deconomed SR Capsules, 533
Deconsal II Tablets, 526
Deep-Down Rub, 1504
Defen-LA Tablets, 526
Degest 2, 1322

Dehistine Syrup, 542
Del Aqua-5, 1416
Del Aqua-10, 1416
Del-Mycin, 1041
Delatestryl, 137
**Delavirdine mesylate, 1181**
Delestrogen, 144
Delfen Contraceptive, 1409
Delsym, 509
Delta-D2, 22
Delta D3, 22
Deltasone, 231
Deltavac, 1093
Demadex, 309
**Demecarium bromide, 1300**
**Demeclocycline HCl, 1072**
Demerol, 618
Demulen 1/35, 170
Demulen 1/50, 170
Denorex Extra Strength, 1462
Denorex Medicated, 1462
Depakene, 857
Depakote, 857
Depakote ER, 857
Depen, 1706
depMedalone 40, 231
depMedalone 80, 231
Depo-Estradiol, 144
Depo-Medrol, 231
Depo-Provera, 161
Depo-Testadiol, 150
Depo-Testosterone, 137
Depogen, 144
Depoject-40, 231
Depoject-80, 231
Deponit, 331
Depopred, 231
Depotest 100, 137
Depotest 200, 137
Depotestogen, 150
Dequasine, 54
Derma-Pax, 1491
Derma Viva, 1486
Dermacoat, 1472
Dermacort, 240
DermaFlex, 1472
Dermamycin, 1491
Dermarest, 1491
Dermarest Plus, 1491
Dermasept Antifungal, 1118
Dermoplast, 1472
Desenex, 1113

**Desipramine HCl, 749**
Desitin, 1484, 1497
Desitin Creamy, 1497
Desitin with Zinc Oxide, 1497
**Desmopressin acetate, 218**
Desogen, 170
**Desogestrel, 170, 171**
Desogestrel and Ethinyl Estradiol, 170
**Desonide, 238**
DesOwen, 238
**Desoximetasone, 239**
Desoxyn, 579
Desquam-E, 1416
Desquam-X 5 and 10, 1416
Desquam-X Wash, 1416
Desyrel, 743
Desyrel Dividose, 743
Detane, 1472
Detrol, 1662
**Detropropoxyphene, 619**
Detussin Liquid, 555
Devrom, 998
Dex GG TR Tablets, 574
Dexacidin, 1354
Dexacine Suspension, 1353
Dexameth, 230
**Dexamethasone**
  ophthalmic, 1331, 1353
  systemic, 230
**Dexamethasone acetate, 230**
Dexamethasone Intensol, 230
**Dexamethasone phosphate, 1352**
**Dexamethasone sodium phosphate**
  ophthalmic, 1331
  systemic, 230
Dexasporin, 1354
**Dexbrompheniramine maleate, 535, 541**
**Dexchlorpheniramine maleate**
  as antihistamine, 493
  in upper respiratory combinations, 531
Dexedrine, 579
Dexedrine Spansules, 579
**Dexmethylphenidate, 592**
**Dexpanthenol, 1483**
**Dexrazoxane, 1631**

Dextroamphetamine sulfate, 579
Dextromethorphan HBr, as antitussive, 509, 546-555, 559-564, 566-569, 571-574, 576
Dextromethorphan HCl, 1399
Dextrose, 693
DextroStat, 579
Dextrostix, 1751
DHS Tar, 1462
DHS Zinc, 1462
DHT, 22
DHT. see Dihydrotachysterol
DHT Intensol, 22
Di-Delamine, 1491
Di-Gel, 910
Di-Gel, Advanced Formula, 907
DiaBeta, 270
Diabetic Tussin DM Liquid, 572
Diabetic Tussin Maximum Strength DM Liquid, 573
Diabetic ulcer agent, becaplermin, 1454
Diabinese, 270
Dialose, 977
Dialose Plus Capsules, 980
Dialose Plus Capsules and Tablets, 980
Diamox, 305, 813
Diamox Sequels, 305, 813
Diaparene, 1497
Diaparene Medicated, 1497
Diaparene Peri-Anal Medicated, 1497
Diaper rash products, 1497
Diaphragm, 160
Diascan, 1751
Diasorb, 998
Diastix, 1754
Diazepam
  as antianxiety agent, 698
  as muscle relaxant, 871
Diazepam Intensol, 698, 871
Diazolidinyl urea
  in acne products, 1434
  in douche products, 1407

Dibasic calcium phosphate dihydrate, 28
Dibasic sodium phosphate, 987
Dibenzazepine derivatives, 761
Dibucaine
  in anorectal preparations, 1411
  for skin disorders, 1472
Dical-D Tablets, 51
Dicarbosil, 29
Dichloralphenazone, 670
Dichlorphenamide, 305
Diclofenac potassium, 640
Diclofenac sodium
  in nonnarcotic analgesics, 614
  as nonsteroidal anti-inflammatory agent, 640
  ophthalmic, 1338
  topical, 1476
Dicloxacillin sodium, 1068
Dicomal-DH Syrup, 558
Dicomal-DM Syrup, 555
Dicumarol, 104
Dicyclomine, 916
Didanosine, 1176
Didrex, 587
Didronel, 297
Dienestrol, 144
n,n-diethyl m-toluamide, 1507
Diethylpropion HCl, 587
Diethylstilbestrol diphosphate, 1569
Difenoxin, 992
Difenoxin with atropine sulfate, 992
Differin, 1422
Diflorasone diacetate, 239
Diflucan, 1098
Diflunisal, 616
Digestive aids
  digestive enzymes, 946
  metoclopramide, 950
Digestive enzymes, 946
Digitek, 322
Digoxin, 322
Dihistine DH Elixir, 545
Dihistine Expectorant Liquid, 565
Dihydrocodeine bitartrate, 629

Dihydroindolone derivatives, 765
Dihydrotachysterol, 22
Dihydroxyacetone, 1518
Dihydroxypropyl theophylline, 461
Dilacor XR, 363
Dilantin-125, 829
Dilantin Infatab, 829
Dilantin Kapseals, 829
Dilantin with Phenobarbital Kapseals, 829
Dilatrate-SR, 330
Dilaudid, 618
Dilaudid Cough Syrup, 575
Dilor, 461
Dilor-400, 461
Dilor-G Liquid, 520
Dilor-G Tablets, 520
Diltia XT, 363
Diltiazem HCl, 363
Dimaphen DM Cold & Cough Elixir, 561
Dimaphen Elixir, 536
Dimenhydrinate, 676
Dimetane-DX Cough Syrup, 549
Dimetapp 12 Hour Non-Drowsy Extentabs, 501
Dimetapp Children's Nighttime Flu Syrup, 561
Dimetapp Children's Non-Drowsy Flu Syrup, 560
Dimetapp Cold & Allergy Elixir, 536
Dimetapp Decongestant Infant Drops, 501
Dimetapp Decongestant Liqui-Gels, 501
Dimetapp Decongestant Plus Cough Infant Drops, 559
Dimetapp DM Cold & Cough Elixir, 561
Dimethicone, 1468
Dimethyl sulfoxide, 1656
Diocto, 977
Diocto C, 983
Diocto-K, 977
Diocto-K Plus Capsules, 980
Dioctolose Plus Capsules, 980
Dioeze, 977
Diovan, 390
Diovan HCT Tablets, 429
Dipentum, 1001

# INDEX

Diphen, 494

Diphen AF, 494, 509

Diphen Cough, 494, 509, 676, 877

Diphenhist, 494, 877

Diphenhist Captabs, 494, 877

**Diphenhydramine**
as antiparkinson agent, 877
in nonnarcotic analgesics, 614

**Diphenhydramine citrate, 534, 537**

**Diphenhydramine HCl**
as antiemetic/antivertigo agent, 676
as antihistamine, 494
as antiparkinson agent, 877
as antitussive, 509
in nonnarcotic analgesics, 612
in nonprescription sleep aids, 810
as topical antihistamine, 1491
in topical corticosteroids, 245
in upper respiratory combinations, 530, 534, 537, 540, 541, 553

**Diphenoxylate, 992**

**Diphenoxylate with atropine sulfate, 992**

**Diphtheria and tetanus toxoids, adsorbed, 1250**

**Diphtheria and tetanus toxoids and acellular pertussis vaccine adsorbed, 1250**

**Diphtheria, tetanus, pertussis, haemophilus b vaccine, 1259**

**Diphtheria, tetanus, pertussis vaccine, 1250**

**Dipivefrin, 1309**

Diprolene, 238

Diprolene AF, 238

Diprosone, 238

**Dipyridamole, 92**

**Dipyridamole and aspirin, 94**

Direct-acting miotics, 1303

**Dirithromycin, 1034**

Disalcid, 606

Disalcid Amigesic, 606

Disanthrol Capsules, 980

Disinfecting Solution, 1376

Disinfecting/wetting/ soaking solutions, for rigid gas permeable contact lenses, 1372

**Disodium, 1430**

**Disodium cocoamphodiacetate, 1412**

**Disodium lauryl sulfosuccinate, 1434**

Disolan Capsules, 980

Disolan Forte Capsules, 980

Disonate, 977

Disoplex Capsules, 980

**Disopyramide phosphate, 341**

**Disulfiram, 1697**

D.I.T.1-2, 1093

Ditropan, 1660

Diucardin, 315

Diurese, 315

Diuretics
carbonic anhydrase inhibitors, 305
combinations, 319
loop diuretics, 309
nonprescription, 321
potassium-sparing diuretics, 312
thiazides and related diuretics, 315

Diurigen, 315

Diuril, 315

**Divalproex sodium, 857**

**DMDM hydantoin**
in anorectal preparations, 1412
in topical agents, 1521

DML, 1486

**DMSO. see Dimethyl sulfoxide**

Doan's, Original, 606

Doan's PM, Extra Strength, 606

Docucal-P Softgels, 980

**Docusate calcium, 977**

**Docusate potassium, 977**

**Docusate sodium**
in laxative combinations, 980, 983
in laxatives, 977

**Dofetilide, 344**

DOK, 977

Dolacet Capsules, 627

Dolanex, 601

**Dolasetron mesylate, 684**

Dolobid, 616

Dolophine HCl, 618

Dolsed, 1205

Dome-Paste, 1520

Domeboro Powder Packets, 1517

Domeboro Tablets, 1517

Domol Bath and Shower, 1487

Donatussin DC Syrup, 569

Donatussin Drops, 531

Donatussin Syrup, 566

**Donepezil HCl, 791**

Donnagel, 998

Donnamar, 916

Donnatal, 921

Donnatal Extentabs, 921

Dopaminergics, 881

Doral, 805

Dormarex 2, 877

**Dornase Alfa, 484**

Doryx, 1072

**Dorzolamide HCl, 1314**

**Dorzolamide HCl/timolol maleate, 1316**

DOS Softgel, 977

Dosalax, 974

Dostinex, 1691

Double Strength Gaviscon-2, 907

Douche products, 1407

Dovonex, 1439

**Doxazosin mesylate, 382**

**Doxepin HCl**
in topical antihistamines, 1491
in tricyclic antidepressants, 749

Doxidan Capsules, 980

Doxidan LiquiGels, 980

Doxil, 1553

Doxinate, 977

**Doxorubicin, 1553**
conventional, 1553
liposome, 1553

**Doxycycline**
as antibiotic, 1072
as mouth and throat product, 924

**Doxylamine succinate**
in nonprescription sleep aids, 810

**Doxylamine succinate**
  *(cont.)*
    in upper respiratory
      combinations, 541,
      553, 554
**DPT. see Diphtheria, teta-
  nus, pertussis vaccine**
Dr. Caldwell Senna, 974
Dr. Dermi-Heal, 1520
Dr. Scholl's Cracked Heel
  Relief, 1472
Dr. Scholl's Fungi Solution,
  1114
Dramamine, 676
Dramamine, Children's,
  676
Dri/Ear, 1382
Drisdol, 22
Dristan 12-hr Nasal Spray,
  500
Dristan Cold Multi-
  Symptom Formula Tab-
  lets, 538
Dristan Cold Non-Drowsy
  Maximum Strength Tab-
  lets, 522
Dristan Fast Acting For-
  mula Nasal Spray, 502
Dristan Sinus Tablets, 523
Dritho-Scalp, 1437
Drithocreme, 1437
Drithocreme HP 1, 1437
Drixomed Tablets, 535
Drixoral Allergy Sinus Tab-
  lets, 541
Drixoral Cold & Allergy Tab-
  lets, 535
Drixoral Non-Drowsy 12
  Hour Relief, 501
**Dronabinol, 681**
Drug Names that Look
  Alike and Sound Alike,
  A-35
Dry E 400, 26
Dry Eye Therapy, 1365
Dry Eyes, 1365, 1368
Dryphen Multi-Symptom
  Formula Tablets, 538
Drysol, 1518
Drytex Lotion, 1433
DSMC Plus Capsules, 980
**DTaP. see Diphtheria and
  tetanus toxoids and
  acellular pertussis vac-
  cine adsorbed**
**DTP. see Diphtheria, teta-
  nus, pertussis vaccine**

Dulcagen, 973
Dulcolax, 973
Dull-C, 19
Duofilm, 1480
Duonate-12 Suspension,
  536
DuoNeb, 480
Duoplant Gel, 1480
Duphalac, 967
Duplex T, 1462
Duraclon, 394
Duradrin, 670
Duradryl JR Capsules, 545
Duradryl Syrup, 542
Duragesic, 618
Duramist Plus Nasal Spray,
  500
Duramorph, 619
DuraScreen, 1508, 1510
Duratears Naturale, 1365,
  1368
Duration 12 Hour Nasal
  Spray, 500
Duratuss DM Elixir, 573
Duratuss GP Tablets, 528
Duratuss HD Elixir, 570
Duratuss Tablets, 527
Durex, 1409
Duricef, 1019
**Dutasteride, 141**
Dy-G Liquid, 520
Dyazide, 319
Dycill, 1068
Dyclone, 1468
**Dyclonine HCl**
  in lozenges, 1399
  in mouth and throat
    products, 1400
  for mucous membranes,
    1468
Dyflex-G Tablets, 520
Dynabac, 1034
Dynacin, 1072
DynaCirc, 363
DynaCirc CR, 363
Dynafed Asthma Relief
  Tablets, 524
Dynapen, 1068
Dynex Tablets, 527
**Dyphylline**
  as bronchodilator, 461
  in upper respiratory
    combinations, 521
Dyphylline-GG Elixir, 520
Dyrenium, 312

**E**-400, 26
E-LOR Tablets, 631
E-Mycin, 1034
E-Pherol, 26
E•R•O Ear Drops, 1382
Ear-Dry, 1382
EarSol-HC, 1382
Eastprin, 605
EC-Naprosyn, 641
**Echothiophate iodide,
  1300**
**Econazole nitrate, 1113**
Econopred, 1331
Econopred Plus, 1331
Ed A-Hist Liquid, 532
Ed A-Hist Tablets, 532
Ed-DOXY Caps, 1072
Ed-Flex Capsules, 530
ED-TLC Liquid, 556
ED Tuss HC Syrup, 557
Edecrin, 309
Edex, 1729
**Edrophonium chloride,
  1639**
**Edrophonium chloride
  and atropine sulfate,
  1639**
**EDTA**
  in acne products, 1430
  in anorectal prepara-
    tions, 1411
  in antacid combinations,
    911
  in antifungal combina-
    tions, 1119
E.E.S. 200, 1034
E.E.S. 400, 1034
E.E.S. Granules, 1034
**Efavirenz, 1181**
Effer-K, 40
Effer-syllium, 962
Effexor, 746
Effexor XR, 746
Efidac 24, 493
Efidac 24 Pseudoephed-
  rine, 501
**Eflornithine HCl, 1525**
**Egg albumin, 983**
Elavil, 749
Eldepryl, 895
Electrolyte mixtures, oral,
  32
Eligard, 1577
Elimite, 1229
Elixophyllin, 461
Elixophyllin-GG Liquid, 520

# INDEX

Elixophyllin-KI Elixir, 520
Ellence, 1556
Elocon, 241
Elspar, 1607
Elta Block, 1507
Eltroxin, 291
Emcyt, 1588
Emergency contraceptives, 179
Emetrol, 693
Emgel, 1041
Eminase, 109
EMLA, 1473
Emollients, 1463, 1483
Empirin, 605
Empirin w/Codeine No. 3 Tablets, 626
Empirin w/Codeine No. 4 Tablets, 627
Emulsoil, 973
**Enalapril, 385**
**Enalapril maleate, 428, 430**
Enbrel, 1711
Encare, 1409
Endagen-HD Liquid, 556
Endal Tablets, 524
Enduron, 315
Engerix-B, 1278
Enlon, 1639
Enlon-Plus, 1639
**Enoxaparin sodium, 100**
**Entacapone, 898**
Entertainer's Secret, 1391
Entex HC Liquid, 569
Entex LA Tablets, 524
Entex Liquid, 524
Entex PSE Tablets, 527
Enulose, 967
Enviro-Stress Tablets, 47
Enzymatic cleaners
    for hard contact lenses, 1370
    for rigid gas permeable contact lenses, 1372
    for soft (hydrogel) contact lenses, 1375
Enzymes, 1607
    asparaginase, 1607
    pegaspargase, 1607
EPA Capsules, 58
EPA Capsules, Max, 58
**Ephedrine HCl, 521, 524**
**Ephedrine sulfate**
    in anorectal preparations, 1412
    as bronchodilator, 455

**Ephedrine sulfate** (cont.)
    as decongestant, 500
    in upper respiratory combinations, 524
**Ephedrine tannate, 545, 559**
Epifoam Aerosol Foam, 245
Epifrin, 1309
Epilyt, 1486
Epinal, 1309
**Epinephrine, 455**
**Epinephrine bitartrate and pilocarpine HCl, 1319**
**Epinephrine borate, 1309**
**Epinephrine HCl**
    as decongestant, 500
    ophthalmic, 1309
**Epirubicin HCl, 1556**
Epitol, 816
Epivir, 1176
Epivir-HBV, 1176
**Eplerenone, 432**
**Epoetin alfa, 118**
Epogen, 118
**Epoprostenol sodium, 370**
**Eprosartan mesylate, 390**
Epsom Salt, 971
e.p.t. Quick Stick, 1766
Equagesic Tablets, 614
Equalactin, 961
Equanil, 708
**Ergocalciferol, 22**
**Ergoloid mesylates, 785**
**Ergotamine tartrate, 670**
**Ertapenem, 1057**
Ery-Tab, 1034
Eryc, 1034
Erycette, 1041
Eryderm 2, 1041
Erygel, 1041
Erymax, 1041
EryPed, 1034
EryPed Drops, 1034
Erythra-Derm, 1041
**Erythromycin**
    in acne products, 1416
    ophthalmic, 1348
    topical, 1041, 1081
**Erythromycin base, 1034**
**Erythromycin estolate, 1034**
**Erythromycin ethylsuccinate, 1034**

**Erythromycin ethylsuccinate and sulfisoxazole, 1087**
**Erythromycin stearate, 1035**
Eryzole, 1087
Escitalopram, 717
**Escitalopram oxalate, 717**
Esclim, 144
Eserine Sulfate, 1300
Esgic-Plus Tablets, 612
Esgic Tablets, 613
Esidrix, 315
Eskalith, 787
Eskalith CR, 787
**Esomeprazole magnesium, 953**
Esoterica, 1486
Espotabs, 973
Estar, 1463
**Estazolam, 805**
Ester-C Plus 500 mg Vegicaps, 56
Ester-C Plus Multi-Mineral Formula Vegicaps, 56
**Esterified estrogens, 144, 150**
Estinyl, 144
Estrace, 144
Estraderm, 144
**Estradiol, 144, 150, 151**
**Estradiol cypionate, 144, 150**
**Estradiol hemihydrate, 144**
**Estradiol valerate in oil, 144**
**Estramustine phosphate sodium, 1588**
Estratab, 144
Estratest, 150
Estratest H.S., 150
Estring, 144
Estrogen(s)
    as antineoplastic agents, 1569
    as sex hormones, 144
Estrogen and nitrogen mustard, 1588
Estrogen combinations, 150
**Estrone aqueous, 144**
**Estropipate, 144**
Estrostep, 172
Estrostep Fe, 172
**Etanercept, 1711**

Ethacrynic acid, 309
Ethambutol hydrochloride, 1207
Ethanol, 1118
Ethchlorvynol, 805
Ethinyl estradiol, 144, 150, 170, 171, 172, 179
Ethinyl estradiol/levonorgestrel, 179
Ethionamide, 1207
Ethmozine, 351
Ethopropazine, 877
Ethosuximide, 846
Ethotoin, 829
Ethyl alcohol, 1435
Ethylhexyl p-methoxycinnamate, 1506
Ethynodiol diacetate, 170
Etidronate disodium, 297
Etodolac, 640
Etonogestrel/ethinyl estradiol, 166
Etoposide, 1547
Etrafon, 795
Etrafon 2-10, 795
Etrafon Forte, 795
Eucalyptamint, 1504
Eucalyptamint 2000 Gel, 1505
Eucalyptol
  in douche products, 1407
  in mouth and throat products, 1402
  in mouthwash, 1400
  in topical agents, 1521
  in topical antihistamines, 1491
Eucalyptol acetate, 1119
Eucalyptus oil
  in acne products, 1434
  in douche products, 1407
  in lozenges, 1399
  in topical agents, 1520
  in upper respiratory combinations, 576
Eucerin, 1486
Eulexin, 1564
Eurax, 1229
Evac-Q-Kwik, 987
Evac-U-Gen, 973
Evac-U-Lax Tablets, 973
Everone 200, 137
Evista, 153
Ex-Histine Syrup, 542
Ex-Lax Chocolated, 973

Ex-Lax Extra Gentle Pills, 980
Ex-Lax Gentle Nature, 973
Ex-Lax Maximum Relief, 973
Ex-Lax Unflavored, 973
Exact, 1433
Excedrin Caplets, Aspirin Free, 612
Excedrin Extra Strength Caplets, Geltabs, and Tablets, 613
Excedrin Migraine, 670
Excedrin PM Tablets, 612
Exelderm, 1114
Exelon, 791
Exemestane, 1574
Exna, 315
Exocaine Odor Free Creme, 1504
Exocaine Plus Rub, 1504
Expectorants, 513
  and antitussives, 565, 571
  pediatric, 571, 576
  and decongestants, 524
  pediatric, 529
  and decongestants and antihistamines, 531
Extendryl Chewable Tablets, 542
Extendryl JR Capsules, 545
Extendryl SR Capsules, 543
Extendryl Syrup, 542
Extra Action Cough Syrup, 572
Extra Potency Ester-C Plus, 56
Extra Strength Adprin-B, 605
Extra Strength Alka-Seltzer, 914
Extra Strength Alkets, 903
Extra Strength Antacid Tablets, 903
Extra Strength Bayer Enteric 500, 605
Extra Strength Bayer Plus, 605
Extra Strength Bayer PM Aspirin Plus Sleep Aid Caplets, 614
Extra Strength Doan's PM, 606
Extra Strength Gas-X, 944

Extra Strength Genaton, 908
Extra Strength Goody's Tablets, 613
Extra Strength Maalox, 907
Extra Strength Maalox Plus, 907
Extra Strength Maalox Plus Suspension, 911
Extra Strength Maalox Suspension, 911
Extra Strength Mintox Plus, 911
Extra Strength Tylenol PM Geltabs, 810
Eye Drops, 1322
Eye Drops Extra, 1322
Eyesine, 1322
EZ Detect, 1761
Ezetimibe, 438
Ezide, 315

Fact Plus, 1766
Famotidine, 935
Famvir, 1151
Fansidar, 1131
Fareston, 1571
Fat, 962
Father John's Medicine Plus Liquid, 550
FDA Pregnancy Categories, A-31
Fe-O.D. Tablets, 73
Fe-Tinic 150 Forte Capsules, 74
Feen-a-mint, 973
Feen-a-mint Chocolated, 973
Feen-a-mint Pills, 980
Felbamate, 824
Felbatol, 824
Feldene, 642
Felodipine, 363, 430
Fem-1 Tablets, 612
Female condoms, 160
Femara, 1574
Femcare, 1121
femhrt, 150
Femilax Tablets, 980
Femiron, 69
FemPatch, 144
Femstat, 1121
Fen-gen-sol, 69
Fenesin, 513
Fenofibrate, 440
Fenoprofen calcium, 640

# INDEX

**Fentanyl, 618**
Feosol, 69
Feostat, 69
Fer-In-Sol, 69
Fer-Iron, 69
Ferancee Tablets, 73
Feratab, 69
Fergon, 69
Fermalox, 70
Fero-Folic-500 Filmtabs, 74
Fero-Grad-500 Filmtabs, 73
Fero-Gradumet Filmtab, 69
Ferocyl, 70
Ferospace, 69
Ferra-TD, 69
Ferralet, 69
Ferralet Slow Release, 69
Ferralyn Lanacaps, 69
Ferretts, 69
Ferro-Docusate T.R., 70
Ferro-Dok TR, 70
Ferro-DSS S.R., 70
Ferro-Sequels, 70
Ferromar Caplets, 73
**Ferrous fumarate, 69**
**Ferrous gluconate, 69**
**Ferrous sulfate, 69**
**Ferrous sulfate exsiccated, 69**
Fertility agents
  choriogonadotropin alfa, 195
  chorionic gonadotropin, 197
  clomiphene, 206
  follitropin alfa, 202
  follitropin beta, 204
  menotropins, 209
  urofollitropin, 200
Fertinex, 200
Feverall, Children's, 602
Feverall, Infants', 602
Feverall Sprinkle Caps, 601
**Fexofenadine HCl, 494, 534**
Fiber-Lax, 961
Fiberall, 961, 962
Fiberall Natural Flavor, 961
Fiberall Orange Flavor, 961
FiberCon, 961
FiberNorm, 961
**Filgrastim, 121**

Finac Lotion, 1430
**Finasteride, 141**
Finevin, 1419
Fioricet Tablets, 613
Fioricet w/Codeine Capsules, 627
Fiorinal Capsules, 614
Fiorinal w/Codeine No. 3 Capsules, 627
Fiortal Capsules, 613
First Choice, 1751
First Response, 1766
First Response Ovulation Predictor, 1764
Fish oils, 58
Fisher-Price Sensitive Skin Sunblock for Kids, 1509
Fisher-Price Spray Mist Sunscreen for Kids, 1509
Fisher-Price Sunscreen for Kids, 1507
Flagyl, 1062
Flagyl 375, 1062
Flagyl ER, 1062
Flanders Buttocks, 1497
Flarex, 1331
Flatulex, 944
Flavons, 56
Flavored Colestid, 434
**Flavoxate HCl, 1658**
**Flecainide acetate, 347**
Fleet, 973
Fleet Babylax, 965
Fleet Bisacodyl Uniserts, 973
Fleet Flavored Castor Oil, 973
Fleet Phospho-soda, 971
Fleet Prep Kit #1, 987
Fleet Prep Kit #2, 987
Fleet Prep Kit #3, 987
Fletcher's Castoria, 974
Flexaphen, 875
Flexeril, 871
Flextra-DS Tablets, 612
Flolan, 370
Flomax, 382
Flonase, 489
Florical, 28, 29
Florinef Acetate, 249
Florone, 239
Florone E, 239
Flovent, 470
Flovent Rotadisk, 470
Floxin, 1049
**Fluconazole, 1098**

**Fludrocortisone acetate, 249**
Flumadine, 1163
**Flumazenil, 1627**
**Flunisolide**
  inhalant, 470
  intranasal, 489
**Fluocinolone acetonide, 239**
**Fluocinonide, 239**
Fluogen, 1270
Fluonid, 239
Fluor-Op, 1331
**Fluoride**
  oral, 34
  topical, 34
Fluorigard, 34
Fluorinse, 34
Fluoritab, 34
**Fluorometholone**
  in ophthalmic anti-infectives, 1354
  in ophthalmic anti-inflammatory agents, 1331
Fluoroquinolones, 1049
**Fluoxetine HCl, 719**
**Fluoxymesterone, 137**
**Fluphenazine HCl, 768**
**Flurandrenolide, 239**
**Flurazepam HCl, 805**
**Flurbiprofen, 640**
**Flurbiprofen sodium, 1338**
FluShield, 1270
**Flutamide, 1564**
**Fluticasone propionate**
  inhalant, 470
  intranasal, 489
  topical, 239
**Fluticasone propionate/salmeterol, 470**
**Fluvastatin sodium, 446**
Fluvirin, 1270
**Fluvoxamine maleate, 723**
Fluzone, 1270
FML, 1331
FML Forte, 1331
FML-S Suspension, 1354
FML S.O.P., 1331
Foamicon, 907
Focalin, 592
Foille Medicated FirstAid, 1472
Foille Plus, 1472
**Folate. see Folic acid**

**Folic acid, 6, 77**
with iron, 74, 75
vitamin B with, 49
Folic acid analogs, 1533
Follistim, 204
**Follitropin alfa, 202**
**Follitropin beta, 204**
Foltrin Capsules, 75
Folvite, 77
**Fomivirsen sodium, 1360**
**Formic acid, 1524**
Formula 405 AHA, 1516
Formula 405 Moisturizing, 1516
Formula E-400, 26
Fortaz, 1020
Fortel Plus, 1766
Fortovase, 1169
Fosamax, 297
**Foscarnet, 1140**
**Foscarnet sodium, 1140**
Foscavir, 1140
**Fosfomycin tromethamine, 1197**
**Fosinopril sodium, 385, 428**
**Fosphenytoin, 829**
Fostex, 1416
Fostex 10 Wash, 1416
Fostex Acne Cleansing Bar, 1432
Fostex Acne Cleansing Cream, 1430
Fostex Medicated Cover-Up, 1421
Fostril Lotion, 1430
Fototar, 1463
Fragmin, 100
Frova, 673
**Frovatriptan succinate, 673**
**Fructose, 693**
Fulvicin P/G, 1100
Fumasorb, 69
Fumatinic Capsules, 74
Fumerin, 69
Fungi•Nail, 1118
FungiCure, 1114
Fungizone, 1113
Fungoid, 1096, 1113
Fungoid Tincture, 1113
Furadantin, 1201
**Furosemide, 309**

**G**/P 1200/60 Tablets, 526
**Gabapentin, 827**

Gabitril Filmtab, 852
**Galantamine HBr, 791**
Gallstone dissolving agents
infusion, 959
oral, 957
Gamimune N, 1236
**Gamma benzene hexachloride. see Lindane**
**Gamma globulin. see Immune globulin (human)**
Gammagard S/D, 1236
Gammar-P I.V., 1236
**Ganciclovir, 1143**
**Ganciclovir sodium, 1143**
Gani-Tuss-DM NR Liquid, 572
Gani-Tuss NR Liquid, 571
Gantanol, 1084
Gantanol DS, 1084
Gantrisin, 1084
Garamycin, 1348
Gas-Ban, 908
Gas-Ban DS, 910
Gas-X, 944
Gas-X, Extra Strength, 944
Gastro-Relief, 903
Gastrocrom, 1695
**Gatifloxacin, 1049**
Gaviscon, 907, 911
Gaviscon-2, Double Strength, 907
Gaviscon Extra Strength Relief Formula, 908, 911
Gee-Gee, 513
Gel-Kam, 34
Gel-Tin, 34
**Gelatin, 1520**
Gelusil, 907, 910
**Gemfibrozil, 443**
**Gemtuzumab, 1615**
Gen-Xene, 698
Genac Tablets, 534
Genacol Maximum Strength Cold & Flu Relief Tablets, 552
Genafed, 501
Genagesic Tablets, 631
Genahist
as antiemetic/antivertigo agent, 676
as antihistamine, 494
as antiparkinson agent, 877
Genapap, Children's, 601
Genapap Extra Strength, 601

Genapap Infants' Drops, 602
Genapax, 1121
Genasal Nasal Spray, 500
Genasoft Plus Softgels, 980
Genaton, 907, 911
Genaton, Extra Strength, 908
Genatuss, 513
Genatuss DM Syrup, 572
Genebs, 601
Genebs Extra Strength, 601
Generet-500 Tablets, 74
Geneye, 1322
Geneye AC Allergy Formula, 1326
Geneye Extra, 1322
Genoptic, 1348
Genotropin, 223
Genpril, 640
Genprin, 605
Gentacidin, 1348
Gentak, 1348
**Gentamicin**
ophthalmic, 1348
topical, 1081
**Gentamicin sulfate, 1352**
GenTeal Multidose, 1365
**Gentian violet**
topical, 1113
vaginal, 1121
Gentlax, 974
Gentlax S Tablets, 980
Genuine Bayer Aspirin Tablets and Caplets, 605
Geocillin, 1067
Geodon, 758
Gerber Pediatric Electrolyte Solution, 32
Germicides, topical, 1494
Gets-It, 1480
Gevrabon Liquid, 46
GFN 600/Phenylephrine 20 Tablets, 524
GFN 1000/DM 60 Tablets, 574
GFN 1200/DM 60/PSE 120 Tablets, 569
GFN 1200/DM 60 Tablets, 574
GFN/PSE Tablets, 528
**Glatiramer acetate, 1743**
Glaucoma agents
alpha-2 adrenergic agonist, 1295

# INDEX

Glaucoma agents *(cont.)*
apraclonidine, 1312
beta-blockers, 1297
carbonic anhydrase
inhibitors, 1314
combinations, 1319
dorzolamide and timo-
lol, 1316
miotics cholinesterase
inhibitor, 1300
direct-acting, 1303
prostaglandin agonists,
1306
sympathomimetics,
1309
Glaucon, 1309
Gliadel, 1581
**Glibenclamide, 270**
**Glimepiride, 270**
**Glipizide, 270**
**Glucagon, 284**
Glucagon Diagnostic Kit,
284
Glucagon Emergency Kit,
284
Glucocorticoids, 230
Glucofilm, 1751
Glucometer Elite, 1751
Glucometer Encore, 1751
Glucophage, 278
Glucophage XR, 278
Glucose elevating agents,
glucagon, 284
Glucose tests
blood, 1751
urine, 1754
Glucostix, 1751
Glucotrol, 270
Glucotrol XL, 270
Glucovance, 281
**L-Glutamine, 54**
**Glutaraldehyde, 1495**
Glutofac Caplets, 47
Gly-Oxide Liquid, 1387
**Glyburide, 270**
**Glyburide/metformin, 281**
**Glycerin**
in acne products, 1432
in anorectal prepara-
tions, 1411
in diaper rash products,
1497
in laxative combina-
tions, 983
in laxatives, 965
in otic preparations,
1382

**Glycerin** *(cont.)*
in poison ivy treatment
products, 1502
in topical agents, 1521
**Glycerin rectal liquid, 965**
**Glycerin, USP, 965**
**Glyceryl cocoate, 1435**
**Glyceryl guaiacolate, 513**
**Glyceryl stearate**
in anorectal prepara-
tions, 1412
in topical agents, 1521
**Glycine, 908**
**Glycopyrrolate, 916**
Glynase PresTab, 270
Glyset, 264
Glytuss, 513
Gold Alka-Seltzer, 914
Gold compounds, 648
**Gold sodium thiomalate,
648**
GoLYTELY, 985
Gonadotropin-releasing
hormone analogs, 1577
Gonadotropin-releasing
hormones, nafarelin, 212
Gonal-F, 202
Good Sense Maximum
Strength Dose Sinus Tab-
lets, 539
Good Sense Maximum
Strength Pain Relief
Allergy Sinus Gelcaps,
539
Goody's Body Pain Pow-
der, 613
Goody's Extra Strength
Headache Powder, 613
Goody's Tablets, Extra
Strength, 613
Gordochom, 1118
Gordofilm, 1480
Gordogesic Cream, 1504
**Goserelin acetate, 1577**
Gout agents
allopurinol, 657
colchicine, 660
probenecid, 664
sulfinpyrazone, 668
GP-500 Tablets, 527
**Gramicidin, 1081**
**Granisetron HCl, 684**
Gris-PEG, 1100
Grisactin Ultra, 1100
**Griseofulvin, 1100**
**Griseofulvin ultramicro-
size, 1100**

Growth hormones
somatrem, 221
somatropin, 223
Guai-Vent/PSE Tablets,
527
Guaifed Capsules, 527
Guaifed-PD Capsules, 525
Guaifed Syrup, 525
**Guaifenesin, 521, 531**
as expectorant, 513
in upper respiratory
combinations, 520,
524-529, 565-576
Guaifenesin 1000 mg and
Dextromethorphan HBr
60 mg LA Tablets, 574
Guaifenesin-DM NR Liq-
uid, 572
Guaifenesin DM Syrup,
572
Guaifenesin/Pseudo-
ephedrine HCl Tablets,
526
Guaifenex DM Tablets, 574
Guaifenex GP Tablets, 528
Guaifenex PSE 60 Tab-
lets, 526
Guaifenex PSE 120 Tab-
lets, 527
Guaifenex-Rx DM Tablets,
568
Guaifenex-Rx Tablets, 526
GuaiMAX-D Tablets, 527
Guaipax PSE Tablets, 527
**Guanabenz acetate, 398**
**Guanadrel sulfate, 400**
**Guanethidine mono-
sulfate, 402**
**Guanfacine HCl, 405**
Guiadrine DM Tablets, 574
Guiatuss, 513
Guiatuss AC Syrup, 571
Guiatuss CF Syrup, 566
Guiatuss DAC Liquid, 565
Guiatuss-DM Syrup, 572
Guiatuss PE Liquid, 524
**Gum benzoin, 1404**
Gyne-Lotrimin, 1121
Gyne-Lotrimin Combina-
tion Pack, 1121
Gyne-Sulf, 1093
Gynecort 5, 240
Gynecort 10, 240
Gynodiol, 144
Gynol II Extra Strength,
1409

Gynol II Original Formula, 1409

**H**9600 SR Tablets, 526
H. pylori agents. see Helicobacter pylori agents
**Haemophilus b conjugate and hepatitis B vaccine, 1257**
**Haemophilus b conjugate vaccine, 1254**
Hair dressings, 1466
**Halazepam, 698**
**Halcinonide, 239**
Halcion, 805
Haldol, 776
Halenol, Children's, 602
Haley's M-O, 983
Halfan, 1134
Halfprin, 605
Halfprin 81, 605
Hall's Mentho-Lyptus, 1399
**Halobetasol propionate, 239**
**Halofantrine HCl, 1134**
Halog, 239
Halog-E, 239
**Haloperidol, 776**
Halotestin, 137
Halotussin AC Liquid, 571
Halotussin DAC Syrup, 565
Haltran, 640
**Hamamelis water. see Witch hazel**
Hard contact lens products, 1369
**Hard fat, 1412**
Havrix, 1275
Hawaiian Tropic 15 Plus, 1510
Hawaiian Tropic 30 Plus, 1508
Hawaiian Tropic 45 Plus, 1506
Hawaiian Tropic Baby Faces, 1506
Hawaiian Tropic Dark Tanning, 1511
Hawaiian Tropic Super Waterproof, 1508, 1510
**HBIG. see Hepatitis B immune globulin (human)**
HC Derma-Pax Liquid, 245
**HCTZ. see Hydrochlorothiazide**

Head and Shoulders Dandruff, 1462
Head and Shoulders Intensive Treatment, 1460
Healthcheck Ovulation Detector, 1764
Heet Spray, 1505
Helicobacter pylori agents
   bismuth subsalicylate, metronidazole and tetracycline HCl, 929
   lansoprazole/amoxicillin/clarithromycin, 932
   ranitidine bismuth citrate, 927
Helidac, 929
Hem-Prep, 1412
Hema-Combistix, 1772
Hemaspan Tablets, 73
Hemastix, 1772
Heme-Chek, 1761
Hemoccult, 1761
Hemoccult SENSA, 1761
Hemocyte, 69
Hemocyte-F Tablets, 74
Hemocyte Plus Tablets, 74
Hemorrhoidal HC, 1411
**Heparin, 97**
   low molecular weight, 100
Heparin Sodium, Multiple Dose Vials, 97
Heparin Sodium, Single Dose Ampules and Vials, 97
Heparin Sodium, Unit Dose, 97
**Hepatitis A, inactivated and hepatitis B, recombinant vaccine, 1282**
**Hepatitis A vaccine, 1275**
**Hepatitis A vaccine, inactivated, 1275**
**Hepatitis B immune globulin (human), 1235**
**Hepatitis B vaccine, 1278**
Hepsera, 1149
Herbal Laxative Tablets, 980
Herceptin, 1621
**Hexachlorophene, 1494**
Hexalen, 1601
Hi-Vegi-Lip Tablets, 946
Hibiclens, 1494

Hibiclens Antiseptic/Antimicrobial Skin, 1494
Hibistat Germicidal Hand, 1494
HibTITER, 1254
Hiprex, 1195
Hista-Vent DA Tablets, 543
Histade Capsules, 534
Histamine $H_2$ antagonists, 935
Histatab Plus Tablets, 532
Histex Liquid, 533
Histex SR Capsules, 533
Histinex HC Syrup, 556
Histinex PV Syrup, 557
Histussin D Liquid, 555
Histussin HC Syrup, 556
Hivid, 1176
HMG-CoA reductase inhibitors, 446
HMS, 1331
Hold DM, 509
**Homatropine HBr, 1328**
**Homatropine MBr, 555**
Home Medicine Cabinet, A-3
Home tests
   glucose tests blood, 1751
   urine, 1754
   ketone tests, 1758
   occult blood tests, 1761
   ovulation tests, 1764
   pregnancy tests, 1766
   protein tests, 1768
   urinary tract infection tests, 1770
**Homosalate, 1506**
Hormones. see also Sex hormones
   androgens, 1562
   antiandrogens, 1564
   antiestrogens, 1571
   aromatase inhibitors, 1574
   estrogens, 1569
   gonadotropin-releasing hormone analogs, 1577
   progestins, 1567
H.P. Acthar Gel, 226
Humalog, 256
Humalog Mix 50/50, 256
Humalog Mix 75/25, 256
Human Erythropoietin, Recombinant, 118
Humatin, 1013

# INDEX

Humatrope, 223
Humibid DM Tablets, 574
Humibid L.A., 513
Humibid Sprinkle, 513
HuMist Moisturizing Nasal
  Mist, 502
Humorsol, 1300
Humulin 50/50, 256
Humulin 70/30, 256
Humulin L, 255
Humulin N, 255
Humulin R, 255
Humulin R Regular U-500
  (Concentrated), 255
Humulin U Ultralente, 255
Hurricaine, 1468
Hy-Phen Tablets, 628
Hycamtin, 1542
Hycodan Syrup, 555
Hycodan Tablets, 555
Hycosin Expectorant
  Syrup, 575
Hycotuss Expectorant
  Syrup, 575
Hydantoins, 829
Hydergine, 785
Hydergine LC, 785
Hydra-Zide Capsules, 427
**Hydralazine, 427**
**Hydralazine HCl**
  in antihypertensive
    combinations, 427
  in antihypertensives,
    407
Hydramine, 676
Hydramine Cough, 494,
  509
Hydramyn, 877
Hydrate, 676
Hydrea, 1601
Hydrisalic, 1480
Hydrisinol, 1486
Hydro-Par, 315
Hydro-PC II Liquid, 556
Hydro-PC Liquid, 556
Hydro-Tussin DM Liquid,
  573
Hydro-Tussin HC Syrup,
  557
Hydro-Tussin HD Liquid,
  570
Hydrocet Capsules, 628
**Hydrochlorothiazide**
  in antihypertensive
    combinations, 427,
    428, 429, 430
  as diuretic, 315

Hydrocil Instant, 961
**Hydrocodone bitartrate**
  in narcotic pain reliev-
    ers, 627
  in upper respiratory
    combinations,
    555-558, 570, 574,
    575
Hydrocodone Bitartrate
  5 mg/Pseudoephedrine
  HCl 30 mg/Carbinox-
  amine Maleate 2 mg
  Liquid, 558
Hydrocodone Bitartrate
  and Acetaminophen Cap-
  sules and Tablets, 628
Hydrocodone Bitartrate
  and Guaifenesin Liquid,
  575
Hydrocodone CP Syrup,
  556
Hydrocodone GF Syrup,
  575
Hydrocodone HD Liquid,
  556
**Hydrocortisone**
  in acne products, 1416
  as adrenal cortical
    steroid, 230, 240, 245
  in anorectal prepara-
    tions, 1411
  in ophthalmic anti-
    infectives, 1352
  in otic preparations,
    1379, 1382
**Hydrocortisone acetate**
  as adrenal cortical ste-
    roid, 230, 240
  in anorectal prepara-
    tions, 1411
  in ophthalmic anti-
    infectives, 1352
**Hydrocortisone cypio-
  nate, 231**
**Hydrocortisone probu-
  tate, 240**
**Hydrocortisone sodium
  phosphate, 231**
**Hydrocortisone sodium
  succinate, 231**
**Hydrocortisone valerate,
  240**
Hydrocortone, 230
Hydrocortone Phosphate,
  231
HydroDIURIL, 315

**Hydroflumethiazide, as
  diuretic, 315**
Hydrogel contact lenses.
  see Soft (hydrogel)
  contact lens products
**Hydrogen peroxide, 1404**
Hydromet Syrup, 555
Hydromide Syrup, 555
**Hydromorphone, 618**
**Hydromorphone HCl, in
  upper respiratory
  combinations, 575**
Hydromox, 315
Hydron KGS Liquid, 575
Hydropane Syrup, 555
Hydropel, 1487
**Hydroxyamphetamine
  HBr, 1328**
**Hydroxychloroquine, 651**
**Hydroxychloroquine
  sulfate, 1124**
**Hydroxyethylcellulose,
  1118**
**Hydroxypropyl cellulose,
  1365**
**Hydroxyurea, 1601**
**Hydroxyzine, 494**
**Hydroxyzine HCl, 706**
**Hydroxyzine pamoate,
  706**
Hygroton, 315
Hylorel, 400
**Hyoscine HBr. see
  Scopolamine HBr**
**Hyoscyamine**
  in upper respiratory
    combinations, 543
  in urinary anti-infective
    combinations, 1204
**L-Hyoscyamine, 922**
**Hyoscyamine HBr, 921**
**Hyoscyamine sulfate**
  as anticholinergic/
    antispasmodic agent,
    916
  in anticholinergic combi-
    nations, 922
  in upper respiratory
    combinations, 543
  in urinary anti-infective
    combinations, 1204
Hyosophen, 921
Hyphed Liquid, 557
Hypnotics, 805
HypoTears, 1365, 1368
HypoTears PF, 1365
Hyrexin-50, 494, 676

Hytakerol, 22
Hytinic, 70
Hytone, 240
Hytrin, 382
Hytuss, 513
Hytuss 2X, 513
Hyzaar Tablets, 429
Hyzine 50, 706

**I**beret-500 Filmtabs, 74
Iberet Filmtabs, 74
Iberet-Folic-500 Filmtabs, 74
**Ibritumomab tiuxetan, 1617**
**Ibuprofen**
  as nonsteroidal anti-inflammatory agent, 640
  in upper respiratory combinations, 523
**Ichthammol, 1520**
Icy Hot, 1504
Idamycin, 1558
Idamycin PFS, 1558
**Idarubicin HCl, 1558**
Ifex, 1590
**Ifosfamide, 1590**
IG. see Immune globulin (human)
IgG. see Immune globulin (human)
IGIM. see Immune globulin (human)
IGIV. see Immune globulin intravenous (human)
Imdur, 330
**Imiglucerase, 301**
**Imipenem-cilastatin, 1059**
**Imipramine HCl, 749**
**Imipramine pamoate, 749**
Imitrex, 673
**Immune globulin (human), 1235**
**Immune globulin intravenous (human), 1236**
Immune globulins, 1235
Immunologic agents, interferons, 1594
Immunomodulators
  anakinra, 1709
  etanercept, 1711
  peginterferon alfa-2a, 1714
  peginterferon alfa-2b, 1717

Immunosuppressives
  azathioprine, 1666
  cyclosporine, 1668
  muromonab-CD3, 1675
  mycophenolate mofetil, 1672
  tacrolimus, 1678
Imodium, 996
Imodium A-D, 996
Imodium A-D Caplets, 996
Imogam Rabies-HT, 1237
Impotence agents
  alprostadil, 1729
  sildenafil citrate, 1732
Imuran, 1666
**Inamrinone lactate, 326**
**Indapamide, 315**
Inderal, 376
Inderal LA, 376
Inderide LA Capsules, 427
Inderide Tablets, 427
**Indinavir sulfate, 1169**
Indocin, 641
**Indomethacin, 641**
Infalyte Oral Solution, 32
Infanrix, 1250
Infants' Advil, 640
Infants' Feverall, 602
Infants' Motrin, 640
Infergen, 1224
Inflamase Forte, 1331
Inflamase Mild, 1331
**Infliximab, 1004**
**Influenza virus vaccine, 1270**
Infumorph, 619
**INH. see Isoniazid**
Inhalants
  corticosteroids, 470
  cromolyn sodium, 474
  ipratropium bromide, 477
  ipratropium bromide/albuterol sulfate, 480
  mucolytics, 484
  nedocromil sodium, 487
Inhalers, nasal decongestant, 502
Innohep, 100
**Inositol, 49, 62**
Inspra, 432
**Insulin, 255**
**Insulin analog injection, 256**
**Insulin glargine injection, 256**

**Insulin injection**
  concentrated, 255
  regular insulin, 255
**Insulin zinc suspension, 255**
**Insulin zinc suspension, extended, 255**
Intal Inhaler, 474
Intal Nebulizer Solution, 474
Interferon(s), 1594
**Interferon alfa-2a, 1594**
**Interferon alfa-2b, 1594**
**Interferon alfa-n3, 1222**
**Interferon alfacon-1, 1224**
**Interferon beta, 1738**
**Interferon beta-1a, 1738**
**Interferon beta-1b, 1738**
**Interferon gamma-1b, 1227**
International System of Units, A-21
Intranasal steroids, 489
Intrauterine progesterone, 182
Intrinsic factor with iron, 75
Intron A, 1594
Invanz, 1057
Inversine, 416
Invirase, 1169
Iobid DM Tablets, 574
Iodex, 1494
Iodex w/Menthyl Salicylate Ointment, 1505
**Iodine**
  as antiseptic, 1494
  nutritional, 5
**Iodine products**
  as expectorants, 513
  as thyroid drugs, 289
**Iodochlorhydroxyquin, 245**
**Iodoquinol, 245**
Iodotope, 286
Ionamin, 587
Ionax, 1432
Ionax Astringent Cleanser, 1433
Ionax Foam, 1433
Ionil, 1466
Ionil T, 1466
Iopidine, 1312
Iosal II Tablets, 526
Iosopan, 903
**Ipecac, 1629**
IPOL, 1261
**Ipratropium bromide, 477**

# INDEX

**Ipratropium bromide/ albuterol sulfate, 480**
Iprin, 640
**Irbesartan, 390, 429**
Ircon, 69
Ircon-FA Tablets, 74
**Irinotecan, 1542**
**Irish moss, 983**
Iron, 5
in diuretics, 321
with vitamin B$_{12}$ and intrinsic factor, 75
with vitamin C, 73
with vitamins, 49, 74
Iron-containing products, 69
Iron-Folic 500 Tablets, 74
**Iron oxides, 1521**
Irospan Capsules, 73
Irospan Tablets, 73
Ismelin, 402
Ismo, 330
**Isobutane, 1502**
**Isocarboxazid, 732**
**Isoetharine HCl, 455**
**Isometheptene mucate, 670**
**Isoniazid, 1207**
**Isoniazid with rifampin, 1207**
**Isoniazid with rifampin and pyrazinamide, 1207**
**Isophane insulin suspension, 255**
**Isophane insulin suspension (NPH) and regular insulin injection combined, 256**
**Isopropanol, 1435**
**Isopropyl alcohol**
in acne products, 1421, 1430
in antifungal combinations, 1118
in otic preparations, 1382
in topical agents, 1521
**Isopropyl myristate, 1502**
**Isoproterenol, 455**
Isoptin SR, 364
Isopto Atropine, 1328
Isopto Carbachol, 1303
Isopto Carpine, 1303
Isopto Cetapred Suspension, 1354
Isopto Homatropine, 1328
Isopto Hyoscine, 1328

Isopto P-ES, 1319
Isopto Plain, 1365
Isopto Tears, 1365
Isordil, 330
Isordil Titradose, 330
**Isosorbide dinitrate, 330**
**Isosorbide mononitrate, 330**
**Isotretinoin, 1681**
**Isoxsuprine HCl, 372**
**Isradipine, 363**
Isuprel, 455
Itch-X, 1472
**Itraconazole, 1102**
IUD, 160
Iveegam, 1236
**Ivermectin, 1193**
Ivy-Rid, 1502

**J**enest, 171
Jets, 54
Junior Strength Advil, 640
Junior Strength Motrin, 640
Junior Strength Motrin Caplets, 640
**Juniper tar, 1520**
Just for Kids, 34
Just Tears, 1365

**K**+ 8, 40
K+ 10, 40
K-99, 40
K-C, 998
K-Dur 10, 40
K-Dur 20, 40
K-Lor, 40
K-Lyte/Cl, 40
K-Lyte/Cl 50, 40
K-Lyte DS, 40
K-Pek, 998
K-Phos M.F., 1644
K-Phos No. 2, 1644
K-Phos Original, 1644
K-Tab, 40
Kadian, 619
Kaletra, 1169
**Kanamycin sulfate, 1013**
Kanka, 1403
Kantrex, 1013
Kao-Spen, 998
Kao-Tin, 998
Kaochlor, 40
Kaochlor-SF, 40
Kaodene Non-Narcotic, 998

**Kaolin**
in antidiarrheal combination products, 998
in diaper rash products, 1497
Kaolin with Pectin, 998
Kaon-Cl, 40
Kaon-Cl 10, 40
Kaon Elixir, 40
Kaopectate, 998
Kaopectate, Children's, 998
Kaopectate II Caplets, 996
Kapectolin, 998
Karigel, 34
Karigel Maintenance Neutral, 34
Kasof, 977
Kay Ciel, 40
Keep Alert, 583
Keflex, 1021
Keftab, 1021
Kefurox, 1021
Kefzol, 1019
Kemadrin, 877
Kenaject, 232
Kenalog, 241
Kenalog-10, 232
Kenalog-40, 232
Kenalog in Orabase, 1403
Keppra, 855
Keratolytics
diclofenac, 1476
podofilox, 1478
salicylic acid, 1480
Keri, 1486
Keri Creme, 1486
Keri-Light, 1486
KeriCort-10, 240
Kerlone, 376
Kerodex, 1487
Kestrone 5, 144
Keto-Diastix, 1754
**Ketoconazole, 1105**
Ketone tests, 1758
**Ketoprofen, 641**
**Ketorolac tromethamine**
as nonsteroidal anti-inflammatory agent, 641
ophthalmic, 1338
Ketostix, 1758
**Ketotifen fumarate, 1346**
Key-Pred, 231
Kid Kare Children's Cough/ Cold Liquid, 563
KIE Syrup, 524

Kineret, 1709
Kiss My Face, 1507, 1508, 1509
Klonopin, 698, 820
Klor-Con, 40
Klor-Con 8, 40
Klor-Con 10, 40
Klor-Con/25, 40
Klor-Con/EF, 40
Klotrix, 40
Kobee Tablets, 49
Kolephrin/DM Tablets, 551
Kolephrin GG/DM Liquid, 573
Kolephrin Tablets, 538
Kondremul Plain, 969
Kondremul with Phenolphthalein, 983
Konsyl, 961
Konsyl Fiber, 961
Konsyl-Orange, 961
Koromex, 1409
Koromex Clear, 1409
**KPAB. see Potassium para-amino-benzoate**
Kronofed-A Capsules, 533
Kronofed-A Jr. Capsules, 533
Ku-Zyme Capsules, 946
Ku-Zyme HP Capsules, 946
Kudrox Double Strength Suspension, 911
Kutrase Capsules, 946
Kwelcof Liquid, 575
Kytril, 684

**L**AAM. see Levomethadyl acetate HCl
**Labetalol HCl, 413**
Labstix, 1772
Lac-Hydrin, 1486
Lac-Hydrin Five, 1486
Lacri-Lube S.O.P., 1368
Lacrisert, 1365
**Lactic acid, 1407**
LactiCare, 1486
Lactinex, 995
**Lactobacillus, 995**
**Lactulose, 967**
Lamictal, 849
Lamisil AT, 1114
**Lamivudine, 1176**
**Lamivudine/abacavir sulfate/zidovudine, 1176**
**Lamivudine/zidovudine, 1176**

**Lamotrigine, 849**
Lanabiotic, 1082
Lanacane, 1472
Lanacort 5, 240
Lanacort 10, 240
Lanacort Cool, 240
**Lanolin**
  in acne products, 1416, 1431
  in anorectal preparations, 1412
  in diaper rash products, 1497
  in mouth and throat products, 1403
  in topical agents, 1520
**Lanolin and petrolatum, 1483**
**Lanolin calcium caseinate, 1497**
Lanoxicaps, 322
Lanoxin, 322
Lanoxin Pediatric, 322
**Lansoprazole**
  for Helicobacter pylori infections, 932
  as proton pump inhibitor, 953
Lantus, 256
Lariam, 1127
Larodopa, 881
Lasix, 309
**Latanoprost, 1306**
**Laureth-4, 1421**
Lax Pills, 973
Laxative Pills, 973
Laxatives
  bulk-reducing, 961
  combinations capsules and tablets, 980
  liquids, 983
  glycerin, 965
  lactulose, 967
  mineral oil, 969
  saline, 971
  stimulant, 973
  stool softeners, 977
LC-65, 1369, 1375
LC-65 Daily Cleaner, 1372
Lecithin, 49, 62
**Leflunomide, 1685**
Lens Drops, 1369, 1372, 1376
Lens Plus, 1375
Lens Plus Daily Cleaner, 1375

Lens Plus Rewetting Drops, 1376
Lente Iletin I, 255
Lente Iletin II, 255
**Lente insulin, 255, 258**
Lescol, 446
Lescol XL, 446
**Letrozole, 1574**
**Leucovorin, 79**
**Leucovorin calcium, 79**
Leukeran, 1590
Leukine, 121
Leukotriene receptor antagonists/formation inhibitors, 467
**Leuprolide acetate, 1577**
**Levalbuterol HCl, 455**
Levall 5.0 Liquid, 569
Levall Liquid, 565
Levaquin, 1049
Levatol, 376
**Levetiracetam, 855**
Levlen, 170
Levlite, 170
**Levmetamfetamine, 430**
Levo-Dromoran, 618
Levo-T, 291
**Levobetaxolol HCl, 1297**
**Levobunolol HCl, 1297**
**Levocabastine HCl, 1340**
**Levocarnitine, 60**
**Levodopa, 881**
**Levodopa/carbidopa, 881**
**Levofloxacin**
  ophthalmic, 1348
  systemic, 1049
**Levomethadyl acetate HCl, 618, 1703**
**Levonorgestrel, 170, 171, 179, 185, 188**
Levonorgestrel implants, 160, 185
Levonorgestrel-releasing intrauterine system, 188
Levora, 170
**Levorphanol tartrate, 618**
Levothroid, 291
**Levothyroxine sodium, 291**
Levoxine, 291
Levoxyl, 291
Levsin, 916
Levsin Drops, 916
Levsin-PB Drops, 922
Levsin with Phenobarbital, 922
Levsinex Timecaps, 916

# INDEX

Lexapro, 717
Lexxel Extended-Release Tablets, 430
Librax, 922
Libritabs, 698
Librium, 698
Lidex, 239
Lidex-E, 239
**Lidocaine**
    for skin disorders, 1472
    in topical agents, 1521
    in topical antibiotics, 1082
**Lidocaine HCl, for mucous membranes, 1468**
LIG. see Lymphocyte immune globulin
Limbitrol, 795
Limbitrol DS, 795
**Lime water, 1522**
Lincocin, 1030
**Lincomycin, 1030**
Lincorex, 1030
Lincosamides, 1030
**Lindane, 1229**
**Linezolid, 1046**
Liniments, 1504
Lioresal, 862
Lioresal Intrathecal, 862
**Liothyronine sodium, 291**
**Liotrix, 291**
**Lipase, 946**
Lipitor, 446
Lipotropic combinations, 62
Lipotropic products, 62
Lipram 4500 Delayed-Release Capsules, 946
Lipram-CR5 Delayed-Release Capsules, 946
Lipram-CR10 Delayed-Release Capsules, 946
Lipram-CR20 Delayed-Release Capsules, 947
Lipram-PN10 Delayed-Release Capsules, 946
Lipram-PN16 Delayed-Release Capsules, 946
Lipram-PN20 Delayed-Release Capsules, 947
Lipram-UL12 Delayed-Release Capsules, 946
Lipram-UL18 Delayed-Release Capsules, 947
Lipram-UL20 Delayed-Release Capsules, 947

Liqui-Char, 1625
Liqui-Doss, 983
Liquibid-D Tablets, 524
Liquid PedvaxHIB, 1254
Liquifilm Tears, 1365
Liquifilm Wetting, 1369
Liquimat, 1421
Liquiprin, 601
Liquiprin Infants' Drops, 602
**Lisinopril, 385, 428**
Listerex Scrub, 1432
Listerine, 1400
Lithium, 787
**Lithium carbonate, 787**
**Lithium citrate, 787**
Lithobid, 787
Lithostat, 1642
Little Licks, 1511
Little Noses Moisturizing Saline, 502
Little Noses Saline Nasal Drops and Spray, 502
Live yeast cell derivative, 1412
Livostin, 1340
Lo/Ovral, 170
Lobana Body, 1486
Lobana Derm-Ade, 1484
Lobana Peri-Garde, 1484
Local anesthetics, in anorectal preparations, 1411
Local vasoconstrictors, in anorectal preparations, 1412
LoCHOLEST, 434
LoCHOLEST Light, 434
Lodine, 640
Lodine XL, 640
Lodosyn, 881
**Lodoxamide trometh-amine, 1336**
Lodrane LD Capsules, 532
Lodrane Liquid, 532
Loestrin 1/20, 170
Loestrin 1.5/30, 170
Loestrin Fe 1/20, 170
Loestrin Fe 1.5/30, 170
**Lomefloxacin HCl, 1049**
Lomotil, 992
**Lomustine, 1584**
Long-Acting Nasal Relief Spray, 500
Loniten, 421
Lonox, 992
Loop diuretics, 309

**Loperamide, 996**
Lopid, 443
**Lopinavir/ritonavir, 1169**
Lopressor, 376
Lopressor HCT 50/25 Tablets, 427
Lopressor HCT 100/25 Tablets, 427
Lopressor HCT 100/50 Tablets, 427
Loprox, 1113
Lorabid, 1021
**Loracarbef, 1021**
**Loratadine**
    as antihistamine, 495
    in upper respiratory combinations, 535
**Lorazepam, 698**
Lorazepam Intensol, 698
Lorcet 10/650 Tablets, 629
Lorcet-HD Capsules, 628
Lorcet Plus Tablets, 628
Lorcet Tablets, 628
Loroxide, 1416
Lortab 5/500 Tablets, 628
Lortab 7.5/500 Tablets, 628
Lortab ASA Tablets, 628
Lortab Liquid, 627
Lortab Tablets, 627
**Losartan potassium, 390, 429**
Lotemax, 1334
Lotensin, 385
Lotensin HCT Tablets, 428
**Loteprednol etabonate, 1334**
Lotrel Capsules, 430
Lotrimin, 1096
Lotrimin AF, 1096, 1113
**Lovastatin, 446**
**Lovastatin and niacin, 450**
Lovenox, 100
Low molecular weight heparins, 100
Low-Ogestrel, 170
Lowila Cake, 1516
Lowsium, 903
Lowsium Plus Suspension, 912
**Loxapine succinate, 761**
Loxitane, 761
Lozenges, 1399
Lozol, 315
LubraSol, 1487
Lubricants, ocular, 1368
Lubriderm (lotion), 1486

Lubriderm (oil), 1487
Lubriderm (soap), 1516
Lufyllin, 461
Lufyllin-400, 461
Lufyllin-EPG Tablets, 521
Lufyllin-GG Elixir, 520
Lufyllin-GG Tablets, 520
Lugol's Solution, 289
Lumigan, 1306
Lunelle, 163
Lupron, 1577
Lupron Depot, 1577
Lupron Depot-3 Month, 1577
Lupron Depot-4 Month, 1577
Lupron Depot-Ped, 1577
Lupron for Pediatric Use, 1577
Luride, 34
Luride Lozi-Tabs, 34
Luvox, 723
**Lymphocyte immune globulin, 1236**
**L-Lysine, 53, 54**
Lysodren, 1601

**M**-M-R II, 1265
M-R-Vax II, 1265
Maalox, 907
Maalox Anti-Diarrheal Caplets, 996
Maalox Daily Fiber Therapy, 961
Maalox, Extra Strength, 907
Maalox Heartburn Relief, 912
Maalox Plus, 907
Maalox Plus, Extra Strength, 907
Maalox Plus Suspension, Extra Strength, 911
Maalox Suspension, 910
Maalox Suspension, Extra Strength, 911
Maalox Therapeutic Concentrate Suspension, 911
Macrobid, 1201
Macrodantin, 1201
Macrolides, 1034
**Mafenide, 1456**
Mag-Carb, 38
Mag-Ox 400, 38, 904
Mag-SR, 38

Mag-Tab SR, 38
**Magaldrate, 903, 908, 912**
Magaldrate Plus Suspension, 912
Magalox Plus, 907
Magan, 606
Magnalox, 910
Magnaprin Film Coated Tablets, 610
**Magnesia, 904**
**Magnesium, 5, 38**
Magnesium AA, 38
**Magnesium amino acid chelate, 38**
**Magnesium carbonate**
  in analgesics, 610
  in antacid combinations, 908, 911
  nutritional, 38
**Magnesium chloride hexahydrate, 38**
**Magnesium citrate**
  in bowel evacuation kits, 987
  in laxatives, 971
  nutritional, 38
**Magnesium gluconate dihydrate, 38**
**Magnesium hydroxide**
  in analgesics, 610
  in antacid combinations, 907, 910
  in antacids, 904
  in histamine H$_2$ antagonists, 935
  in laxative combinations, 983
  in laxatives, 971
  in nonnarcotic analgesics, 613
**Magnesium lactate, 38**
**Magnesium oxide**
  in analgesics, 610
  in antacids, 904
  nutritional, 38
**Magnesium salicylate**
  in analgesics, 606
  in nonnarcotic analgesics, 613
**Magnesium salicylate tetrahydrate, 614**
**Magnesium sulfate, in bowel evacuation kits, 987**
**Magnesium trisilicate, 907**
Magnox Suspension, 910

Magonate, 38
Magonate Natal, 38
Magsal Tablets, 614
Magtrate, 38
Major-gesic Tablets, 530
Malarone, 1136
Malarone Pediatric, 1136
**Malathion, 1229**
Male condoms, 160
Mallamint, 29, 903
Mallazine Eye Drops, 1322
Maltsupex, 961
Mammol, 1520
Mandelamine, 1195
Manganese, 49
Mantadil Cream, 245
Maolate, 871
Mapap, Children's, 601
Mapap Cold Formula Tablets, 551
Mapap Extra Strength, 601
Mapap Infants' Drops, 602
Mapap Regular Strength, 601
Mapap Sinus Maximum Strength Geltabs, 522
**Maprotiline HCl, 729**
Maranox, 601
Marblen, 908, 912
Marcof Expectorant Syrup, 575
Marezine, 676
Margesic Capsules, 613
Margesic H Capsules, 628
Margesic No. 3 Tablets, 626
Marine Lipid Concentrate Capsules, 58
Marinol, 681
Marplan, 732
Marthritic, 606
**Masoprocol, 1519**
Masse Breast, 1486
Massengill Disposable Douche, 1407
Massengill Douche, 1407
Massengill Extra Cleansing Disposable Douche, 1407
Massengill Extra Mild Disposable Douche, 1407
Massengill Medicated Disposable Douche, 1407
Massengill "Scented" Disposable Douche, 1407
Mast cell stabilizers, 1336
Matulane, 1601
Mavik, 385

# INDEX

Max EPA Capsules, 58
Maxair Autohaler, 456
Maxalt, 673
Maxalt-MLT, 673
Maxaquin, 1049
Maxi-Tuss DM Liquid, 573
Maxi-Tuss HC Liquid, 557
Maxidex, 1331
Maxifed DM Tablets, 568
Maxifed-G Tablets, 526
Maxifed Tablets, 526
Maxiflor, 239
Maximum Bayer Aspirin Tablets and Caplets, 605
Maximum Cramp Relief Pamprin Caplets, 613
Maximum Strength Allergy Drops, 1322
Maximum Strength Anacin Tablets, 614
Maximum Strength Anbesol, 1402, 1468
Maximum Strength Ascriptin Coated Caplets, 610
Maximum Strength Benadryl, 2, 1491
Maximum Strength Compoz Nighttime Sleep Aid, 810
Maximum Strength Midol Cramp, 640
Maximum Strength Midol Menstrual Caplets and Gelcaps, 612
Maximum Strength Midol PMS Caplets and Gelcaps, 612
Maximum Strength Midol Teen Caplets, 612
Maximum Strength Multi-Symptom Pamprin Caplets and Tablets, 612
Maximum Strength NoDoz, 583
Maximum Strength Nytol QuickGels, 810
Maximum Strength Sleepinal Softgels, 810
Maximum Strength Sominex, 810
Maximum Strength Unisom SleepGels, 810
Maxipime, 1019
Maxitrol, 1354
Maxitrol Suspension, 1353
Maxivate, 238
Maxolon, 950

Maxzide, 319
Maxzide-25MG, 319
**Measles (rubeola) and rubella virus vaccine, live, 1265**
**Measles, mumps, and rubella virus vaccine, 1265**
**Measles, mumps, and rubella virus vaccine, live, 1265**
**Measles (rubeola) virus vaccine, live, attenuated, 1265**
Mebaral, 800
**Mebendazole, 1187**
**Mecamylamine HCl, 416**
**Mechlorethamine HCl, 1590**
Meclan, 1077
**Meclizine HCl, 676**
**Meclocycline sulfosalicylate, 1077**
**Meclofenamate sodium, 641**
MED-Rx DM Tablets, 569
Meda Cap, 601
Meda Tab, 601
Medent-DM Tablets, 569
Medi-First Sinus Decongestant, 501
Medi-Quik, 1472
Medicated Acne Cleanser, 1430
Medicated hair dressings, 1466
Medicone, 1411, 1412
Medigesic Capsules, 613
Medilax, 973
Mediplast, 1480
Medotar, 1463
Medrol, 231
**Medroxyprogesterone acetate, 150, 156, 161**
**Medroxyprogesterone acetate/estradiol cypionate, 163**
Medroxyprogesterone injection, 160
**Medrysone, 1331**
**Mefenamic acid, 641**
**Mefloquine, 1127**
Mefoxin, 1020
Mega-B Tablets, 49
Mega-MaxEPA Capsules, 58
Megace, 156, 1567

**Megestrol acetate**
  as antineoplastic agents, 1567
  as sex hormone, 156
Meglitinides, **275**
Melfiat-105 Unicelles, 587
Mellaril, 768
Mellaril-S, 768
**Meloxicam, 641**
**Melphalan, 1590**
Menadol Captabs, 640
Menest, 144
Meni-D, 676
**Menotropins, 209**
**Menthol**
  in acne products, 1430
  in antifungal combinations, 1118
  in douche products, 1407
  in laxative combinations, 983
  in lozenges, 1399
  in mouth and throat products, 1402
  in mouthwash, 1400
  in poison ivy treatment products, 1502
  in rubs and liniments, 1504
  in topical agents, 1520
  in topical antihistamines, 1491
  in upper respiratory combinations, 576
Mentholatum Cherry Chest Rub for Kids, 576
Mentholatum ointment, 576
**Menthyl anthranilate, 1506**
**Mepenzolate bromide, 916**
Mepergan Fortis Capsules, 630
**Meperidine, 630**
**Meperidine HCl, 618, 630**
**Mephenytoin, 829**
**Mephobarbital, 800**
Mephyton, 114
**Meprobamate**
  as antianxiety agent, 708
  in nonnarcotic analgesics, 614
Mepron, 1217
**Mercaptopurine, 1536**

Meropenem, 1055
Merrem I.V., 1055
Meruvax II, 1265
Mesalamine, 1001
Mesantoin, 829
Mescolor Tablets, 544
Mesoridazine, 768
Mestinon, 1639
Mestinon Timespan, 1639
Mestranol, 170
Metadate CD, 594
Metadate ER, 594
Metahydrin, 315
Metallic aluminum, 1520
Metamucil, 961, 962
Metamucil Lemon-Lime
   Flavor, 962
Metamucil Orange Flavor,
   961, 962
Metamucil Sugar Free, 961
Metaproterenol sulfate,
   456
Metaxalone, 871
Meted, Maximum Strength,
   1466
Metformin, 278
Methacort 40, 231
Methacort 80, 231
Methadone HCl, 618
Methadone HCl Diskets,
   618
Methadone HCl Intensol,
   618
Methadose, 618
Methagual, 1505
Methamphetamine HCl,
   579
Methazolamide, 305
Methenamine, 1195, 1204
Methenamine combina-
   tions, 1204
Methenamine hippurate,
   1195
Methenamine mandelate,
   1195, 1204
Methenamine salts, 1195
Methimazole, 286
Methionine, 1497
L-Methionine, 54
Methocarbamol, 871, 875
Methocarbamol with
   ASA, 875
Methotrexate
   as antineoplastic agent,
      1533
   as antipsoriatic, 1444

Methotrexate (cont.)
   as antirheumatic agent,
      653
Methotrexate LPF Sodium,
   1444
Methotrexate Sodium For
   Injection, 1444
Methotrexate Sodium
   Injection, 1444
Methoxsalen, 1447
Methscopolamine bro-
   mide, 916
Methscopolamine nitrate,
   542, 543, 544, 545
Methsuximide, 846
Methyclothiazide, 315
Methyl nicotinate, 1504
Methyl salicylate
   in douche products,
      1407
   in laxative combina-
      tions, 983
   in mouthwash, 1400
   in rubs and liniments,
      1504
Methylbenzethonium
   chloride, 1497
Methylbenzethonium
   HCl, 1118
Methylcellulose, 961
Methyldopa
   in antihypertensive
      combinations, 428
   in antihypertensives,
      418
Methylene blue, 1204
Methylene chloride, 1502
Methylin, 594
Methylin ER, 594
Methylparaben
   in acne products, 1432
   in anorectal prepara-
      tions, 1411
Methylphenidate HCl, 594
Methylprednisolone, 231
Methylprednisolone
   acetate, 231
Methylprednisolone
   sodium succinate, 231
Methyltestosterone, 137,
   150
Meticorten, 231
Metimyd Suspension, 1354
Metipranolol HCl, 1297
Metoclopramide, 950
Metoclopramide Intensol,
   950

Metolazone, 315
Metoprolol, 376
Metoprolol tartrate, 427
MetroCream, 1062
MetroGel, 1062, 1093
MetroGel Vaginal, 1062
MetroLotion, 1062
Metronidazole
   as antibiotic, 1062
   for Helicobacter pylori
      infections, 929
Mevacor, 446
Mexiletine, 349
Mexitil, 349
Mexsana Medicated, 1497
MG217, 1462
MG217 Medicated Inten-
   sive Strength, 1463
Mi-Acid, 910
Miacalcin, 294
Micardis, 390
Micardis HCT Tablets, 429
Micatin, 1113
Miconazole nitrate
   topical, 1113
   vaginal, 1121
Micrainin Tablets, 614
MICRhoGAM, 1237
Micro-K 10 Extencaps, 40
Micro-K Extencaps, 40
Microcrystalline sulfur,
   1421
Micronase, 270
microNefrin, 455
Micronor, 172
Microstix-3, 1770
Midamor, 312
Midodrine HCl, 695
Midol Cramp, Maximum
   Strength, 640
Midol Menstrual Caplets
   and Gelcaps, Maxi-
   mum Strength, 612
Midol PMS Caplets and
   Gelcaps, Maximum
   Strength, 612
Midol Teen Caplets, Maxi-
   mum Strength, 612
Midrin, 670
Mifeprex, 134
Mifepristone, 134
Miglitol, 264
Migraine agents
   combinations, 670
   serotonin 5-HT$_1$ recep-
      tor agonists, 673
Migratine, 670

# INDEX

Milex Shur-Seal, 1409
Milk of Magnesia, 904, 971
Milk of Magnesia, Con-
centrated, 971
Milkinol, 969
**Milrinone lactate, 328**
Miltown, 708
**Mineral oil**
in acne products, 1416
in anorectal prepara-
tions, 1411
in antacid combinations,
911
as laxative, 969
in laxative combina-
tions, 983
in mouth and throat
products, 1403
in topical agents, 1520
Mineralocorticoid, 249
Minerals, 5
Minerals and electrolytes
calcium, 28
fluoride, 34
magnesium, 38
oral electrolyte mix-
tures, 32
potassium, 40
zinc, 43
Mini Two-Way Action Tab-
lets, 524
Minipress, 382
Minitran, 331
Minocin, 1072
**Minocycline HCl, 1072**
**Minoxidil**
systemic, 421
topical, 1499
Mintezol, 1191
Mintox, 907
Mintox Plus, 907
Mintox Plus, Extra
Strength, 911
Miochol-E, 1303
Miostat, 1303
Miotics
cholinesterase inhibitor,
1300
direct-acting, 1303
Miradon, 104
MiraFlow Extra Strength,
1369, 1375
Mirapex, 886
Miraphen PSE Tablets, 527
Mircette, 171
Mirena, 188
**Mirtazapine, 729**

**Misoprostol**
as anti-ulcer agent, 940
in nonnarcotic analge-
sics, 614
**Mitotane, 1601**
Mitotic inhibitors, vinorel-
bine tartrate, 1549
Mitran, 698
Mitrolan, 961
Mixed E 400, 26
Mixed E 1000, 26
Moban, 765
Mobic, 641
Mobidin, 606
Mobigesic Backache Pain
Reliever Tablets, 614
Mobisyl Creme, 1504
Moctanin, 959
**Modafinil, 583**
Modane, 973
Modane Plus Tablets, 980
Modane Soft, 977
Modicon, 170
Modified bar soaps, 1432,
1516
Modified Burow's Solution,
1382, 1517
**Modified iron products,
70**
Modified Shohl's Solution,
1647
Moduretic, 319
**Moexipril HCl, 385, 429**
Moi-Stir, 1391
Moi-Stir 10, 1391
Moi-Stir Swabsticks, 1391
Moisture Eyes, 1365
Moisture Eyes PM, 1368
Moisturel, 1486
Moisturizing Nasal Spray,
502
Mol-Iron, 69
Mol-Iron w/Vitamin C Tab-
lets, 73
Molie, 583
**Molindone HCl, 765**
Mollifene Ear Wax
Removal Aid, 1382
Momentum Muscular Back-
ache Formula, 606
**Mometasone furoate, 241**
**Mometasone furoate
monohydrate, 489**
Monistat 3, 1121
Monistat 7, 1121
Monistat 7 Combination
Pack, 1121

Monistat-Derm, 1113, 1121
Monistat Dual-Pak, 1121
Mono-Gesic, 606
Mono-Vacc Test (O.T.),
1289
Monoamine oxidase inhibi-
tors, 732
**Monobasic sodium phos-
phate, 987**
**Monobenzone, 1519**
Monocid, 1019
Monoclonal antibodies
alemtuzumab, 1613
gemtuzumab, 1615
ibritumomab tiuxetan,
1617
palivizumab, 1241
rituximab, 1619
trastuzumab, 1621
**Monoctanoin, 959**
Monodox, 1072
Monoket, 330
**Monophasic oral contra-
ceptives, 170**
Monopril, 385
Monopril-HCT 10/12.5 Tab-
lets, 428
Monopril-HCT 20/12.5 Tab-
lets, 428
**Montelukast sodium, 467**
Monurol, 1197
More-Dophilus, 995
**Moricizine, 351**
**Morphine, 998**
**Morphine sulfate, 619**
Motion Sickness, 676
Motofen, 992
Motrin, 640
Motrin Caplets, Junior
Strength, 640
Motrin, Children's, 640
Motrin Children's Cold Sus-
pension, 523
Motrin IB, 640
Motrin IB Gelcaps, 640
Motrin, Infants', 640
Motrin, Junior Strength,
640
Motrin Migraine Pain
Caplets, 640
Motrin Sinus Headache
Tablets, 523
Mouth and throat products
amlexanox, 1396
benzyl alcohol, 1398
carbamide peroxide,
1387

Mouth and throat products
   (cont.)
   chlorhexidine, 1389
   doxycycline, 924
   lozenges, 1399
   miscellaneous, 1402
   mouthwashes and
      sprays, 1400
   preparations for sensi-
      tive teeth, 1400
   saliva substitutes, 1391
   tetracycline, 1394
MouthKote, 1391
Mouthwashes, 1400
**Moxifloxacin HCl, 1049**
MS Contin, 619
MSIR, 619
**MTX. see Methotrexate**
Muco-Fen-DM Tablets, 574
Mucolytics, 484
Mucomyst, 484
Mucosil-10, 484
Mucosil-20, 484
Mucous membranes, topi-
   cal anesthetics for, 1468
Multiparous cervical cap,
   160
Multiple antibiotics, 1081
Multiple sulfonamides,
   1084
Multistix, 1772
Multistix 7, 1772
Multistix 8, 1772
Multistix 8 SG, 1772
Multistix 9, 1772
Multistix 9 SG, 1772
Multistix 10 SG, 1772
Multistix SG, 1772
**Mumps virus vaccine,
   live, 1265**
Mumpsvax, 1265
**Mupirocin, 1065**
Murine Ear Drops, 1382
Murine Ear Wax Removal
   System, 1382
Murine Plus, 1322
Muro 128 2, 1365
Muro 128 5, 1365
Murocel, 1365
Murocoll-2, 1328
**Muromonab-CD3, 1675**
Muscle relaxants
   baclofen, 862
   dantrolene sodium, 865
   skeletal, 871
   combinations, 875
   tizanidine, 868

Muse, 1729
Mustargen, 1590
Myambutol, 1207
Myapap Drops, 602
Mycelex, 1096
Mycelex-7, 1121
Mycelex-G, 1121
Mycelex Twin Pack, 1121
Myciguent, 1081
Mycinettes, 1399
Mycitracin Triple Antibiotic,
   1082
Mycobutin, 1207
Mycolog-II, 1118
**Mycophenolate mofetil,
   1672**
Mycostatin, 1109, 1121
Mycostatin Pastilles, 1109
Mydfrin 2.5, 1322
Mydriacyl, 1328
Mydriatic combinations,
   1328
Mygel II Suspension, 910
Mygel Suspension, 910
Mykrox, 315
Mylagen, 910
Mylagen Gelcaps, 908
Mylagen II, 910
Mylanta, 907, 910
Mylanta Double Strength,
   907, 911
Mylanta Gelcaps, 908
Mylanta Natural Fiber
   Supplement, 961
Myleran, 1545
Mylicon, 944
Mylicon-125, 944
Mylotarg, 1615
Myoflex Creme, 1505
Mysoline, 841
Mytelase Caplets, 1639
Mytussin, 513
Mytussin AC Cough Syrup,
   571
Mytussin DAC Liquid, 565
Mytussin DM Syrup, 572

**N**D Clear Capsules, 533
N-Multistix, 1772
N-Multistix SG, 1772
Nabi-HB, 1235
**Nabumetone, 641**
**Nadolol**
   in antihypertensive
      combinations, 427
   as beta-adrenergic
      blocking agent, 376

**Nafarelin acetate, 212**
Nafazair, 1322
**Naftifine HCl, 1113**
Naftin, 1113
Naldecon Senior DX Liq-
   uid, 573
Naldecon Senior EX, 513
Nalfon, 640
**Nalidixic acid, 1199**
**Nalmefene HCl, 1633**
**Naloxone, 1635**
**Naloxone HCl, 635**
**Naltrexone HCl, 1700**
Nandrolone decanoate,
   130
**Naphazoline HCl**
   in nasal decongestants,
      500
   in ophthalmic decon-
      gestant combina-
      tions, 1326
   in ophthalmic decon-
      gestants, 1322
Naphazoline Plus, 1326
Naphcon, 1322
Naphcon-A, 1326
Naphcon Forte, 1322
Naprelan, 641
Naprosyn, 641
**Naproxen, 641**
**Naproxen sodium**
   as nonsteroidal anti-
      inflammatory agent,
      641
   in upper respiratory
      combinations, 523
Naqua, 315
**Naratriptan HCl, 673**
Narcan, 1635
Narcotic antitussives, 506
Narcotic pain reliever
   combinations, 626
Narcotic pain relievers, 618
Nardil, 732
Nasacort, 489
Nasacort AQ, 489
Nasal decongestant combi-
   nations, 502
Nasal decongestant inhal-
   ers, 502
Nasal Decongestant Sinus
   Non-Drowsy Tablets, 522
Nasal decongestants, 500
Nasal Moist, 502
Nasal Moist Nasal Spray,
   502

# INDEX

NaSal Nasal Drops and Spray, 502
Nasal products, 502
Nasal Relief Spray, 500
Nasalcrom, 474
Nasalcrom, Children's, 474
Nasalide, 489
Nasarel, 489
Nasatab LA Tablets, 527
Nasonex, 489
Natacyn, 1356
**Natamycin, 1356**
**Nateglinide, 275**
Natru-vent Nasal Spray, 501
Natru-vent Saline Nasal Spray, 502
Natural Brewers Yeast 71/2 grs Tablets, 46
Nature's Remedy Tablets, 981
Naturetin, 315
Nausetrol, 693
Navane, 782
Navelbine, 1549
N.B.P., 1082
NebuPent, 1219
Necon 0.5/35, 170
Necon 1/35, 170
Necon 1/50, 170
Necon 10/11, 171
**Nedocromil sodium**
  as inhalant, 487
  ophthalmic, 1336
**Nefazodone HCl, 714**
NegGram, 1199
**Nelfinavir mesylate, 1169**
Nelova 0.5/35E, 170
Nelova 1/35E, 170
Nelova 1/50M, 170
Nelova 7/14, 171
Nelova 10/11, 171
Nembutal, 800
Nembutal Sodium, 800
Neo-Castaderm, 1118
Neo-Cultol, 969
Neo-Dexameth, 1352
Neo-fradin, 1013
Neo-Synephrine, 1322
Neo-Synephrine 12-Hour Extra Moisturizing Nasal Spray, 500
Neo-Synephrine 12-Hour Nasal Spray, 500
Neo-Synephrine Extra Strength Nasal Drops and Spray, 500

Neo-Synephrine Mild Strength Nasal Spray, 500
Neo-Synephrine Regular Strength Nasal Drops and Spray, 500
Neo-Synephrine Viscous, 1322
Neodecadron, 1353
Neodecadron Solution, 1352
Neoloid, 973
Neomac, 1082
Neomixin, 1082
**Neomycin sulfate**
  in ophthalmic anti-infectives, 1352
  in otic antibiotics, 1379
  systemic, 1013
  topical, 1081
Neopap, 602
Neoral, 1668
Neosporin, 1081, 1082
**Neostigmine bromide, 1639**
**Neostigmine methyl-sulfate, 1639**
Neotricin HC, 1353
Nephro-Calci, 28
Nephro-Fer, 69
Nephro-Vite OTC Tablets, 47
Nephro-Vite Rx Tablets, 47
Nephrocaps Capsules, 47
Nephron FA Tablets, 74
Nephron S-2, 455
Nephrox, 911
Neptazane, 305
Nervine, 810
Nestrex, 17
Neulasta, 121
Neupogen, 121
NeuRecover-DA, 54
NeuRecover-SA, 54
Neurodep-Caps Capsules, 46
Neurontin, 827
NeuroSlim, 54
NeutraCare, 34
**Neutral sodium fluoride, 34**
Neutrogena, 1516
Neutrogena Acne-Prone Skin, 1516
Neutrogena Antiseptic Cleanser for Acne-Prone Skin, 1433, 1516

Neutrogena Body, 1486
Neutrogena Dry Skin, 1516
Neutrogena Drying Gel, 1430
Neutrogena Kids, 1508
Neutrogena Moisture, 1510
Neutrogena Non-Drying, 1516
Neutrogena Norwegian Formula, 1486
Neutrogena Oil-Free, 1508, 1509
Neutrogena Oil-Free Acne Wash, 1434, 1516
Neutrogena Oily Skin, 1516
Neutrogena Sensitive Skin, 1509
Neutrogena Sunblock, 1506, 1508, 1510
Neutrogena T/Gel, 1462
Neutrogena T/Gel Extra Strength, 1462
**Nevirapine, 1181**
New-Skin, 1487
New-Skin Antiseptic, 1487
Nexium, 953
Niacin, 6
**Niacin and lovastatin, 450**
Niacor, 13
**Nicardipine HCl, 363**
N'ice, 1399
N'ice Vitamin C Drops, 19
Nicoderm CQ, 1724
Nicorette, 1724
**Nicotinamide/niacin-amide, 13**
**Nicotine, 1724**
Nicotinex, 13
**Nicotinic acid/niacin, 13**
Nicotrol, 1724
Nicotrol NS, 1724
Nidryl, 877
Nifedical XL, 364
**Nifedipine, 364**
Niferex, 70
Niferex-150, 70
Niferex-150 Forte Cap-sules, 74
Niferex w/Vitamin C Tab-lets, 73
Nil, 1093
Nilandron, 1564
Nilstat, 1109
**Nilutamide, 1564**
Nimbus Quick Strip, 1766

**Nimodipine, 364**
Nimotop, 364
Nipent, 1601
**Nisoldipine, 364**
Nite Time Children's Liquid, 562
Nite Time Cold Formula for Adults Liquid, 554
Nitrates, 330
Nitrazine, 1772
Nitrek, 331
Nitro-Bid, 330
Nitro-Dur, 331
Nitro-Time, 330
Nitrodisc, 331
**Nitrofurantoin, 1201**
**Nitrofurantoin macrocrystals, 1201**
Nitrogard, 330
Nitrogen mustards, 1590
Nitrogen mustards and estrogen, 1588
**Nitroglycerin, 330**
Nitroglycerin Transdermal, 331
Nitrolingual, 330
NitroQuick, 330
Nitrostat, 330
NitroTab, 330
Nivea Creme, 1516
Nivea Moisturizing, 1486
Nivea Skin, 1486
Nivea Visage, 1516
Nix, 1229
**Nizatidine, 935**
Nizoral, 1105
NoDoz, Maximum Strength, 583
Nolahist, 495
Nolvadex, 1571
Non-nucleoside reverse transcriptase inhibitors, 1181
Nonbarbiturate sedatives, hypnotics, 805
Nonnarcotic analgesic combinations, 612
Nonnarcotic antitussive combinations, 509
Nonnarcotic antitussives, 509
**Nonoxynol-9, 1409**
Nonprescription diuretics, 321
Nonprescription sleep aids, 810

Nonsteroidal anti-inflammatory agents
ophthalmic, 1338
systemic, 640
Nor-QD, 172
Nordette, 170
Norditropin, 223
**Norelgestromin/ethinyl estradiol, 192**
**Norethindrone, 170, 171, 172**
**Norethindrone acetate, 150, 151, 156, 170, 172**
Norethindrone and Ethinyl Estradiol, 170
Norethindrone and Ethinyl Estradiol (7/14), 171
Norethindrone and Ethinyl Estradiol (10/11), 171
Norflex, 871
**Norfloxacin, 1049**
Norgesic, 875
Norgesic Forte, 875
**Norgestimate, 150, 171**
**Norgestrel, 170, 172**
Norinyl 1+35, 170
Norinyl 1+50, 170
Noritate, 1062
Normal Laboratory Values, A-23
Normodyne, 413
Noroxin, 1049
Norpace, 341
Norpace CR, 341
Norplant System, 185
Norpramin, 749
**Nortriptyline HCl, 749**
Norvasc, 363
Norvir, 1169
Norwegian Cod Liver Oil, 45
Norwegian Cod Liver Oil Capsules, 45
Nose Better Gel, 576
Nostrilla 12 Hour Nasal Spray, 500
Novacet Lotion, 1431
Novagest Expectorant with Codeine Liquid, 565
Novolin 70/30, 256
Novolin 70/30 PenFill, 256
Novolin 70/30 Prefilled, 256
Novolin L, 255
Novolin N, 255
Novolin N PenFill, 256
Novolin N Prefilled, 256

Novolin R, 255
Novolin R PenFill, 255
Novolin R Prefilled, 255
NovoLog, 256
NP•27, 1114
NPH Iletin I, 255
NPH Iletin II, 255
**NPH insulin, 258**
Nu-Iron 150, 70
Nucleoside reverse transcriptase inhibitors, 1176
Nucleotide analog reverse transcriptase inhibitors, 1173
Nucofed Capsules, 545
Nucofed Expectorant Syrup, 565
Nucofed Pediatric Expectorant Syrup, 571
Nucofed Syrup, 545
Nucotuss Expectorant Syrup, 565
Nucotuss Pediatric Expectorant Syrup, 571
Nulliparous cervical cap, 160
Numorphan, 619
Numz•it, Baby, 1402
Nupercainal
as adrenal cortical steroid, 240
as anorectal preparation, 1411, 1412
as topical anesthetic, 1472
Nutra-Soothe, 1487
Nutracort, 240
Nutraderm (lotion), 1486
Nutraderm (oil), 1487
Nutraplus, 1483
Nutritional supplements
amino acid combinations, 54
amino acids, 53
bioflavonoids, 56
fish oils, 58
levocarnitine, 60
lipotropic products, 62
para-aminobenzoic acid, 64
Nutropin, 223
Nutropin AQ, 223
NuvaRing, 166
Nydrazid, 1207
**Nystatin, 1109**
in antifungal combinations, 1118

# INDEX

**Nystatin, 1109** *(cont.)*
  in topical antifungals, 1113
  in vaginal antifungals, 1121
Nystex, 1109
Nytol QuickCaps, 810
Nytol QuickGels, Maximum Strength, 810

**O**cclusal-HP, 1480
Occult blood tests, 1761
Ocean Nasal Drops and Spray, 502
OCL, 985
Octamide, 950
**Octocrylene, 1506**
**Octoxynol-9**
  in douche products, 1407
  in spermicides, 1409
**Octreotide acetate, 127**
**Octyl dimethyl PABA, 1510**
**Octyl methoxycinnamate, 1506**
**Octyl salicylate, 1506**
OcuClear, 1322
Ocufen, 1338
Ocuflox, 1348
Ocular lubricants, 1368
Ocupress, 1297
Ocusert Pilo, 1303
Ocusulf-10, 1348
Odor-Eaters, 1114
Off-Ezy Wart Remover, 1480
**Ofloxacin**
  ophthalmic, 1348
  systemic, 1049
Ogen, 144
Oil of Olay Foaming Face Wash Liquid, 1434
Oilatum, 1516
Oilatum-AD, 1516
**Olanzapine, 761**
Old, 1289
**Old tuberculin, multiple puncture devices, 1289**
**Oleostearine, 1523**
**Olive oil, 1522**
**Olmesartan medoxomil, 390**
**Olopatadine, 1344**
**Olsalazine sodium, 1001**
Omega-3 700 Capsules, 58

Omega-3 fatty acids, 58
**Omeprazole, 953**
OMNI, 34
Omnicef, 1019
OMNIhist L.A. Tablets, 543
OMS Concentrate, 619
Oncaspar, 1607
**Ondansetron HCl, 684**
One Step Midstream, 1766
One Touch, 1751
Opcon-A, 1326
Operand, 1494
Ophthalmic anti-infectives
  antibiotics, 1348
  antiviral agents, 1358
  natamycin, 1356
  steroid and antibiotic combinations, 1352
Ophthalmic anti-inflammatory agents, corticosteroids, 1331
Ophthalmic drug therapy, 1293
Ophthalmic phototherapy, 1362
Ophthalmic vasoconstrictors, decongestants, 1322
  combinations, 1326
Ophthocort, 1353
Opiates, in antidiarrheal combination products, 998
**Opium**
  in antidiarrheal combination products, 998
  in narcotic pain relievers, 629
Opium and Belladonna Suppositories, 629
Opium Tincture, 998
Opti-Clean II, 1369, 1372, 1375
Opti-Clean Daily Cleaner, 1369, 1372, 1375
Opti-Free, 1376
Opti-Free Daily Cleaner, 1369, 1372, 1375
Opti-Free Enzymatic Cleaner, 1375
Opti-Free Enzymatic Cleaner Especially for Sensitive Eyes, 1370
Opti-Free Express, 1376
Opti-Free Rewetting Drops, 1376

Opti-Free Supra Clens Daily Protein Remover, 1372, 1375
Opti-Soft, 1375
Opti-Soft Disinfecting, 1376
Opti-Tears Soothing Drops, 1369, 1372, 1376
Opti-Zyme Enzymatic Cleaner, 1372
Opti-Zyme Enzymatic Cleaner Especially for Sensitive Eyes, 1375
Opti-Zyme Especially for Sensitive Eyes, 1372
Opticyl, 1328
Optigene 3, 1322
Optimal Omega Capsules, 58
Optimine, 493
Optimoist, 1391
Optimum Stress Formula Capsules, 47
OptiPranolol, 1297
Optivar, 1342
**OPV. see Poliovirus vaccine, live, oral, trivalent**
Orabase-B, 1403
Orabase-B Gel, 1468
Orabase Gel, 1403
Orabase-Plain, 1403
Oracit, 1647
Orajel, 1403
Orajel, Baby, 1402
Orajel Denture, 1403
Orajel, Maximum Strength, 1403
Orajel Mouth-Aid, 1404, 1468
Orajel Perioseptic, 1387
Oral-B Sensitive with Fluoride, 1400
Oral contraceptives, 160, 170
Oral Dosage Forms that Should Not Be Crushed or Chewed, A-7
Oramorph SR, 619
Orap, 776
Oraphen-PD, 601
Orazinc 110, 43
Orazinc 220, 43
Oretic, 315
Orexin Chewable Tablets, 46
Original Alka-Seltzer, 914
Original Doan's, 606

Orimune, 1261
Orinase, 270
ORLAAM, 618, 1703
**Orlistat, 1006**
Ornex No Drowsiness Maximum Strength Tablets, 522
Ornex No Drowsiness Tablets, 521
**Ornithine aspartate, 54**
**Orphenadrine citrate, 871, 875**
**Orphenadrine citrate with ASA, 875**
Ortho-Cept, 170
Ortho-Cyclen, 170
Ortho Dienestrol, 144
Ortho-Est, 144
Ortho Evra, 192
Ortho-Gynol Contraceptive, 1409
Ortho-Novum 1/35, 170
Ortho-Novum 1/50, 170
Ortho-Novum 7/7/7, 171
Ortho-Novum 10/11, 171
Ortho-Prefest, 150
Ortho Tri-Cyclen, 171
Orthoclone OKT3, 1675
Orudis, 641
Orudis KT, 641
Oruvail, 641
Os-Cal, 29
Os-Cal 250+D, 28
Os-Cal 250+D Tablets, 51
Os-Cal 500, 28
Os-Cal 500+D, 28
Os-Cal 500+D Tablets, 51
**Oseltamivir phosphate, 1167**
Osteocalcin, 294
Ostiderm, 1521
Otic antibiotics, 1379
Otic preparations, miscellaneous, 1382
Otocain, 1382
Otrivin Nasal Drops and Spray, 501
Otrivin Pediatric Nasal Drops, 501
Outgro, 1521
Ovcon 35, 170
Ovcon 50, 170
Ovide, 1229
Ovidrel, 195
Ovral, 170
Ovrette, 172
OvuKIT Self-Test, 1764

Ovulation tests, 1764
OvuQUICK Self-Test, 1764
OvuSign, 1764
**Oxacillin sodium, 1068**
Oxalodinones, 1046
Oxandrin, 130
**Oxandrolone, 130**
**Oxaprozin, 642**
**Oxazepam, 698**
Oxazolidinediones, 834
**Oxcarbazepine, 836**
**Oxiconazole nitrate, 1113**
Oxipor VHC, 1463
Oxistat, 1113
Oxsoralen, 1447
Oxsoralen-Ultra, 1447
**Oxtriphylline, 461**
Oxy 10 Balance, 1416
Oxy Balance, 1416
Oxy Medicated Cleanser & Pads Regular Strength, 1434
Oxy Medicated Pads Maximum Strength, 1434
Oxy Medicated Pads Sensitive Skin, 1434
Oxy Medicated Soap, 1432
Oxy Night Watch Maximum Strength Lotion, 1431
Oxy Night Watch Sensitive Skin Lotion, 1431
Oxy ResiDON'T Medicated Face Wash, 1434
**Oxybenzone, 1506**
**Oxybutynin chloride, 1660**
Oxycet Tablets, 629
**Oxychlorosene sodium, 1496**
Oxycodone 2 Aspirin Tablets, 630
**Oxycodone HCl, 619, 629, 630**
Oxycodone HCl and Acetaminophen Tablets, 629
**Oxycodone, in narcotic pain relievers, 629**
**Oxycodone terephthalate, 629**
Oxycodone with Acetaminophen Capsules, 630
OxyContin, 619
OxyFast, 619
OxyIR, 619
**Oxymetazoline HCl, 1322**
**Oxymetholone, 130**

**Oxymorphone HCl, 619**
**Oxyquinoline, 1430**
**Oxyquinolone sulfate, 1521**
Oxysept Disinfection System, 1376
**Oxytetracycline**
in ophthalmic anti-infectives, 1352
in topical antibiotics, 1081
in urinary anti-infective combinations, 1204
**Oxytetracycline HCl, 1072**
Oxyzal Wet Dressing, 1521
Oysco 500, 28
Oysco 500+D Tablets, 51
Oysco D Tablets, 51
Oyst-Cal 500, 28
Oyst-Cal-D, 28
Oyst-Cal-D 500, 28
Oyst-Cal-D 500 Tablets, 51
Oyst-Cal-D Tablets, 51
Oystercal 500, 28
Oystercal-D 250, 28
Oystercal-D 250 Tablets, 51
Oystercal-D 500 Tablets, 51

**P** & S (hair dressing), 1466
P & S (shampoo), 1466
P-1000, 56
P-A-C Analgesic Tablets, 614
P-V-Tussin Syrup, 557
P-V-Tussin Tablets, 555
$P_1E_1$, 1319
$P_2E_1$, 1319
$P_3E_1$, 1319
$P_4E_1$, 1319
$P_6E_1$, 1319
**PABA. see Para-aminobenzoic acid**
Pacerone, 338
**Paclitaxel, 1601**
**Padimate O, 1511**
Pain Bust-R II Cream, 1504
Pain Relief Cream, 1505
Pain relievers, narcotic, 618
Palgic-D Tablets, 533
Palgic DS Syrup, 536
**Palivizumab, 1241**

# INDEX

Palmitate-A 5000, 7
**Pamabrom, 612, 613**
Pamelor, 749
**Pamidronate disodium, 297**
Pamine, 916
Pamprin Caplets and Tablets, Maximum Strength Multi-Symptom, 612
Pamprin Caplets, Maximum Cramp Relief, 613
Pan-C 500, 56
Panadol, 601
Panadol, Children's, 601, 602
Panadol Infants' Drops, 602
Panadol Junior Strength, 601
Panalgesic Gold Cream, 1504
Panama Jack, 1511
Panama Jack Dark Tanning, 1511
Pancof-HC Liquid, 557
Pancof-XP Liquid, 570
Pancrease Capsules, 946
Pancrease MT 4 Capsules, 946
Pancrease MT 10 Capsules, 946
Pancrease MT 16 Capsules, 946
Pancrease MT 20 Capsules, 947
Pancrecarb MS-4 Delayed-Release Capsules, 946
Pancrecarb MS-8 Delayed-Release Capsules, 946
Pandel, 240
Panex, 601
Panfil-G Capsules, 520
Pangestyme CN-10 Delayed-Release Capsules, 946
Pangestyme CN-20 Delayed-Release Capsules, 947
Pangestyme EC Capsules, 946
Pangestyme MT16 Capsules, 946
Pangestyme UL12 Capsules, 946
Pangestyme UL18 Capsules, 947

Pangestyme UL20 Capsules, 947
Panglobulin, 1236
PanMist-DM Syrup, 567, 568
PanMist JR Tablets, 525
PanMist LA Tablets, 526
PanMist-S Syrup, 525
Pannaz S Syrup, 543
Pannaz Tablets, 543
Panokase 16 Tablets, 947
PanOxyl, 1416
PanOxyl 5 and 10, 1416
PanOxyl AQ 2.5, 5 and 10, 1416
Panretin, 1425
Panthoderm, 1483
**Pantoprazole sodium, 953**
**Pantothenic acid, 16**
**Papaverine HCl, 374**
**Para-aminobenzoic acid (PABA), 49, 64**
**Parabens**
  in acne products, 1416, 1430
  in anorectal preparations, 1411
  in topical agents, 1522
**Paraffin, 1520**
Paraflex Caplets, 871
Parafon Forte DSC Caplets, 871
Paregoric, 998
Paremyd, 1328
**Paricalcitol, 22**
Parlodel, 881, 1688
Parlodel SnapTabs, 881
Parnate, 732
**Paromomycin sulfate, 1013**
**Paroxetine HCl, 738**
Parsidol, 877
Parva-Cal 250 Tablets, 51
Parva-Cal 500 Tablets, 51
Parvlex Tablets, 49, 74
Patanol, 1344
Pavabid Plateau Caps, 374
Paxil, 738
Paxil CR, 738
Paxipam, 698
Pazo Hemorrhoid, 1412
PCE Dispertab, 1034
PDP Liquid Protein, 54
**Peanut oil, 1522**
**Pectin, 998**

Pedameth, 1497
Pedi-Bath Salts, 1488
Pedi-Boro Soak Packs, 1517
Pedi-Dri, 1109, 1113
Pedi-Vit A, 1486
Pedia Care Children's Long-Lasting Cough Plus Cold Liquid, 560
Pedia Care Cough-Cold Liquid, 563
Pedia Care Infants' Decongestant & Cough Drops, 559
Pedia Care Multi-Symptom Cold Liquid, 563
Pedia Care NightRest Cough & Cold Liquid, 564
Pedia Relief Decongestant Plus Cough Infants' Drops, 559
PediaCare Children's Cold & Allergy Liquid, 537
PediaCare Infants' Drops, 501
Pediaflor, 34
Pedialyte Freezer Pops, 32
Pedialyte Solution, 32
Pediamist Nasal Spray, 502
Pediapred, 231
Pediatex-D Liquid, 536
Pediatex-DM Liquid, 561
Pediatric Electrolyte Solution, 32
Pediatrics
  antitussive and expectorant combinations, 571, 576
  antitussive combinations, 559
  decongestant and analgesic combinations, 523
  decongestant and antihistamine combinations, 536
  decongestant and expectorant combinations, 529
  decongestant, antihistamine, and analgesic combinations, 542
  decongestant, antihistamine, and anticholinergic combinations, 545

Pediculicides, 1229
PedvaxHIB, 1254
**PEG-8 stearate, 1521**
**PEG-100 stearate, 1521**
PEG-Intron, 1717
Peganone, 829
**Pegaspargase, 1607**
Pegasys, 1714
**Pegfilgrastim, 121**
**Peginterferon alfa-2a, 1714**
**Peginterferon alfa-2b, 1717**
PemADD, 598
PemADD CT, 598
**Pemirolast potassium, 1336**
**Pemoline, 598**
Pen-Kera, 1486
**Penbutolol sulfate, 376**
Penecort, 240
**Penicillamine, 1706**
**Penicillin V potassium, 1068**
Penicillins, oral, 1067
Penlac Nail Lacquer, 1113
**Pentamidine isethio-nate, 1219**
**Pentazocine, 635**
**Pentazocine combina-tions, 635**
**Pentobarbital, 800**
**Pentobarbital sodium**
   in migraine combina-tions, 670
   in sedatives, 800
Pentolair, 1328
**Pentostatin, 1601**
**Pentoxifylline, 112**
Pentrax, 1462
Pentrax Gold, 1462
Pepcid, 935
Pepcid AC, 935
Pepcid Complete, 935
Pepcid RPD, 935
**Peppermint oil**
   in acne products, 1434
   in mouth and throat products, 1402
Pepto-Bismol, 989
Pepto-Bismol, Maximum Strength, 989
Pepto Diarrhea Control, 996
**Peracetic acid, 1495**
Percocet Tablets, 629

Percodan-Demi Tablets, 630
Percodan Tablets, 630
Percogesic Extra Strength Tablets, 530
Percogesic Tablets, 530
Percolone, 619
Perdiem Fiber, 962
**Pergolide mesylate, 892**
Pergonal, 209
Peri-Colace, 983
Peri-Colace Capsules, 980
Peri-Dos Softgels, 980
Periactin, 493
Perianal hygiene products, 1412
Peridex, 1389
Peridin-C, 56
**Perindopril erbumine, 385**
PerioMed, 34
Periostat, 924, 1072
Peripheral vasodilators
   epoprostenol, 370
   isoxsuprine, 372
   papaverine, 374
Permax, 892
**Permethrin, 1229**
Pernox Lathering Abradant Scrub Lotion, 1433
Pernox Scrub for Oily Skin, 1433
Peroxyl, 1404
**Perphenazine, 687, 768**
**Perphenazine and ami-triptyline HCl, 795**
Persa-Gel W, 1416
Persantine, 92
Pertussin CS, 509
Pertussin DM, 509
**Peruvian balsam. see Balsam peru**
**Petrolatum**
   in anorectal prepara-tions, 1411
   in diaper rash products, 1497
   in mouth and throat products, 1402
   in sunscreens, 1509
   in topical agents, 1520
**Petrolatum and lanolin, 1483**
**PFA. see Foscarnet sodium**
Pfeiffer's Cold Sore, 1404

Phanatuss DM Cough Syrup, 572
Pharmadine, 1494
Pharmaflur, 34
Pharmaflur 1.1, 34
Phazyme, 944
Phazyme 95, 944
Phazyme 125, 944
Phenapap Tablets, 521
Phenaphen-650 w/Codeine Tablets, 626
Phenaphen w/Codeine No. 3 Capsules, 626
Phenaphen w/Codeine No. 4 Capsules, 627
**Phenazopyridine HCl**
   in urinary anti-infective combina-tions, 1204
   in urinary tract prod-ucts, 1664
**Phendimetrazine tartrate, 587**
Phendry, 877
**Phenelzine, 732**
Phenergan, 495, 687
Phenergan Fortis, 495, 687
Phenergan Plain, 495, 687
Phenergan VC Syrup, 532
**Phenindamine tartrate, 495**
**Pheniramine maleate**
   in nasal products, 502
   in ophthalmic decon-gestant combina-tions, 1326
   in topical antihista-mines, 1491
   in upper respiratory combinations, 534, 537, 538, 565
**Phenobarbital**
   in anticholinergic combi-nations, 921
   in sedatives, 800
   in upper respiratory combinations, 521
**Phenobarbital with phenytoin sodium, 829**
**Phenol**
   in acne products, 1430
   in antifungal combi-nations, 1118
   in douche products, 1407
   in lozenges, 1399

# INDEX

**Phenol** *(cont.)*
in mouth and throat
products, 1402
in poison ivy treatment
products, 1502
in topical agents, 1520
Phenolated Calamine,
1502
**Phenolphthalein**
as laxative, 973
in laxative combina-
tions, 980, 983
Phenoptic, 1322
Phenothiazine derivatives,
768
Phenothiazines, 687
**Phentermine HCl, 587**
**Phenyl, 1118**
**Phenyl salicylate, 1204**
**Phenylalanine**
in antacid combinations,
914
in laxatives, 961
**L-Phenylalanine, 54**
**Phenylbenzimidazole**
**sulfonic acid, 1508**
Phenylbutylpiperadine
derivatives, 776
**Phenylcarbinol, 1502**
**Phenylephrine HCl**
in anorectal prepara-
tions, 1412
in cycloplegic mydriat-
ics, 1328
in decongestants, 500
in lozenges, 1399
in nasal products, 502
in ophthalmic decon-
gestant combina-
tions, 1326
in ophthalmic decon-
gestants, 1322
in otic preparations,
1382
in upper respiratory
combinations, 521,
524, 531, 532, 538,
542, 543, 545, 546,
549, 550, 554, 555,
557, 558, 565, 566,
569
**Phenylephrine tannate,**
**536, 545, 559**
Phenylephrine Tannate/
Chlorpheniramine
Tannate/Pyrilamine Tan-
nate Pediatric Suspen-
sion, 536

Phenylgesic Tablets, 530
**Phenylpropanolamine**
**HCl, 1399**
**Phenyltoloxamine citrate**
in nonnarcotic analge-
sics, 612, 613, 614
in upper respiratory
combinations, 530,
534, 537
**Phenyltoloxamine dihy-**
**drogen citrate, 614**
**Phenytoin, 829**
Phenytoin Sodium, 829
**Phenytoin sodium,**
**extended, 829**
**Phenytoin sodium,**
**prompt, 829**
**Phenytoin sodium with**
**phenobarbital, 829**
Phillips' Laxative Gelcaps,
980
Phillips' LaxCaps, 980
Phillips' Milk of Magnesia,
904, 971
Phillips' Milk of Magnesia,
Concentrated, 904, 971
pHisoDerm Acne, 1516
pHisoDerm Baby, 1516
pHisoDerm Normal to Dry,
1516
pHisoDerm Normal to Oily,
1516
pHisoDerm Sensitive Skin,
1516
pHisoHex, 1494
Phos-Flur, 34
PhosChol, 62
**Phospho-soda, 987**
Phospholine Iodide, 1300
**Phosphonoformic acid.**
**see Foscarnet sodium**
**Phosphorated carbohy-**
**drate, 693**
**Phosphoric acid, 693**
Phosphorus, 5
Photofrin, 1610
Phototherapy, ophthalmic,
1362
Phrenilin Forte Capsules,
612
Phrenilin Tablets, 613
**Physostigmine, for glau-**
**coma, 1300**
**Physostigmine salicylate**
**and Pilocarpine HCl,**
**1319**
**Phytonadione, 114**

Pilagan, 1303
Pilocar, 1303
**Pilocarpine HCl**
as glaucoma agent,
1303
as saliva substitute,
1392
**Pilocarpine HCl and epi-**
**nephrine bitartrate,**
**1319**
**Pilocarpine HCl and**
**physostigmine salicy-**
**late, 1319**
**Pilocarpine nitrate, 1303**
Pilopine HS, 1303
Piloptic, 1303
Pilopto-Carpine, 1303
Pilostat, 1303
Pima, 513
**Pimozide, 776**
Pin-Rid, 1189
Pin-X, 1189
**Pindolol, 376**
**Pioglitazone HCl, 267**
**Piperazine estrone sul-**
**fate. see Estropipate**
**Pirbuterol acetate, 456**
**Piroxicam, 642**
**PIV. see Poliovirus vac-**
**cine, inactivated**
Placidyl, 805
Plan B, 179
Plaquenil, 1124
Plaquenil Sulfate, 651
Plaretase 8000 Tablets,
946
Plavix, 84
Plendil, 363
Pletal, 84
**Pneumococcal 7-valent**
**conjugate vaccine, 1287**
**Pneumococcal vac-**
**cine, 1285**
Pneumotussin 2.5 Cough
Syrup, 574
Pneumotussin Tablets, 574
Pneumovax 23, 1285
Pnu-Imune 23, 1285
Podiacin Soak'n Massage
Gel, 1504
**Podofilox, 1478**
Poison Center Hotline,
A-33
Poison ivy treatment prod-
ucts, 1502
Polaramine, 493

Polaramine Expectorant Liquid, 531
Polaramine Repetabs, 493
**Polio vaccine, 1261**
**Polio vaccine, inactivated, 1261**
Poliovax, 1261
**Poliovirus vaccine, inactivated, 1261**
**Poliovirus vaccine, live, oral, trivalent, 1261**
Poly-Pred Suspension, 1352
**Polycarbophil, 961**
Polycitra-K, 1647
Polycitra-LC, 1647
Polydine, 1494
**Polyethylene glycol, 985**
Polygam S/D, 1236
**Polymyxin B sulfate**
   in ophthalmic anti-infectives, 1348, 1352
   in otic antibiotics, 1379
   in topical antibiotics, 1081
**Polyquaternium-10, 1524**
**Polysaccharide-iron complex, 70**
**Polysorbate 80, 1435**
Polysporin, 1081, 1082
Polytar (shampoo), 1462
Polytar (soap), 1462
**Polythiazide, 315**
**Polyvinyl alcohol, 1433**
Ponstel, 641
Pontocaine, 1473
Pontocaine HCl, 1468
**Porfimer sodium, 1610**
Posterior pituitary hormones, desmopressin acetate, 218
Posture, 28
Posture-D, 28
Posture D-Chewable Tablets, 51
Posture D-Tablets, 51
Potassium 99, 40
**Potassium acid phosphate, 1644**
**Potassium acid phosphate and sodium acid phosphate, 1644**
**Potassium bicarbonate**
   in antacid combinations, 914
   in laxatives, 962
**Potassium chloride, 40**

**Potassium citrate, 1647**
**Potassium citrate combinations, 1647**
**Potassium gluconate, 40**
**Potassium guaiacolsulfonate, 570, 575**
**Potassium iodide**
   in expectorants, 513
   as thyroid drug, 289
   in upper respiratory combinations, 520, 524
**Potassium**
   in combinations, 40
   in electrolyte mixtures, 32
   in laxatives, 961
   nutritional, 40
**Potassium nitrate, 1400**
**Potassium para-aminobenzoate (KPAB), 64**
Potassium-sparing diuretics, 312
**Povidone-iodine**
   in antiseptics, 1494
   in douche products, 1407
   in topical agents, 1521
PrameGel, 1472
Pramipexole, 886
**Pramipexole dihydrochloride, 886**
Pramosone Cream, 245
Pramosone Cream 2.5, 245
**Pramoxine HCl**
   in anorectal preparations, 1411
   in otic preparations, 1382
   in poison ivy treatment products, 1502
   for skin disorders, 1472
   in topical corticosteroids, 245
Prandin, 275
Pravachol, 446
**Pravastatin sodium, 446**
Prax, 1472
**Prazepam, 698**
**Prazosin HCl, 382**
Pre-Hist-D Tablets, 543
Precose, 264
Pred Forte, 1331
Pred-G S.O.P., 1353
Pred-G Suspension, 1352
Pred Mild, 1331

Predalone 50, 231
**Prednisolone, 231**
**Prednisolone acetate**
   as adrenal cortical steroids, 231
   in ophthalmic anti-infectives, 1352
   in ophthalmic anti-inflammatory agents, 1331
**Prednisolone sodium phosphate**
   as adrenal cortical steroids, 231
   in ophthalmic anti-inflammatory agents, 1331
**Prednisone, 231**
Prednisone Intensol Concentrate, 231
Prefrin Liquifilm, 1322
Pregnancy tests, 1766
Pregnosis, 1766
Pregnyl, 197
Prelone, 231
Prelu-2, 587
Premarin, 144
Premarin Intravenous, 144
Premphase, 150
Prempro, 150
Premsyn PMS Caplets, 612
Preparation H, 1412
Preparation H Anti-Itch, 240
Preservative Free Moisture Eyes, 1365
Preservative free saline solutions, for soft (hydrogel) contact lenses, 1375
Preserved saline solution, for soft (hydrogel) contact lenses, 1375
PreSun Ultra, 1507, 1509
Pretz-D Nasal Spray, 500
Pretz Irrigation, 502
Pretz Nasal Spray, 502
Prevacid, 953
Prevacid SoluTab, 953
Prevalite, 434
Preven, 179
PreviDent, 34
PreviDent 5000 Plus, 34
Prevnar, 1287
Prevpac, 932
Priftin, 1207
Prilosec, 953

# INDEX

Primacor, 328
**Primaquine phosphate, 1124**
Primatene Mist, 455
Primatene Tablets, 524
Primaxin I.M., 1059
Primaxin I.V., 1059
**Primidone, 841**
Principen, 1067
Prinivil, 385
Prinzide Tablets, 428
Privine Nasal Drops and Spray, 500
Pro-Banthine, 916
Pro-Cal-Sof, 977
Pro-Cute, 1486
Pro-Sof Capsules, 977
Pro-Sof Plus Capsules, 980
ProAmatine, 695
**Probenecid, 664**
**Probenecid and colchicine, 660, 664**
**Procainamide, 354**
Procan SR, 354
**Procarbazine, 1601**
Procardia, 364
Procardia XL, 364
**Prochlorperazine, 687, 768**
Procrit, 118
Proctocort, 1411
ProctoCream-HC 2.5, 240
ProctoFoam, 1411
ProctoFoam-HC, 1411
ProctoFoam-HC Aerosol Foam, 245
**Procyclidine, 877**
Proderm Topical, 1521
Profasi, 197
Profen Forte DM Tablets, 569
Profen Forte Tablets, 527
Profen II DM Liquid, 566
Profen II DM Tablets, 569
Profen II Tablets, 525
Profenal, 1338
ProFree/GP Weekly Enzymatic Cleaner Tablets, 1372
Progestasert, 182
**Progesterone, 156**
  intrauterine, 182
Progesterone in oil, 156
Progestin-only oral contraceptives, 160, 172

Progestins
  as antineoplastic agents, 1567
  as sex hormones, 150, 156
Prograf, 1678
**Proguanil HCl and atovaquone, 1136**
Prolex DH Liquid, 575
Proloprim, 1079
Prometh VC Plain Syrup, 532
Prometh VC w/Codeine Cough Syrup, 546
Prometh w/Codeine Cough Syrup, 546
Prometh w/Dextromethorphan Syrup, 555
**Promethazine**
  as antiemetic/antivertigo agent, 687
  in upper respiratory combinations, 555
**Promethazine HCl**
  as antihistamine, 495
  in narcotic pain reliever combinations, 630
  in upper respiratory combinations, 532, 546
Promethazine HCl and Phenylephrine HCl Syrup, 532
Promethazine HCl w/Codeine Syrup, 546
Promethazine VC w/Codeine Cough Syrup, 546
Promethazine w/Dextromethorphan Cough Syrup, 555
Prometrium, 156
Promise Sensitive, 1400
Pronestyl, 354
Pronestyl-SR, 354
Pronto, 1229
Propacet 100 Tablets, 631
**Propafenone HCl, 356**
**Propantheline bromide, 916**
PROPApH Acne Maximum Strength Cream, 1431
PROPApH Cleansing for Oily Skin Lotion, 1431
PROPApH Cleansing for Sensitive Skin Pads, 1434

PROPApH Cleansing Lotion for Normal/Combination Skin, 1431
PROPApH Cleansing Maximum Strength Pads, 1434
PROPApH Cleansing Pads, 1431
PROPApH Foaming Face Wash, 1434
PROPApH Peel-Off Acne Mask, 1433
Propecia, 141
Prophyllin, 1118
Propine, 1309
**Propoxyphene, 619**
**Propoxyphene HCl, 631**
Propoxyphene HCl Compound Capsules, 631
Propoxyphene HCl w/Acetaminophen Tablets, 631
**Propoxyphene napsylate, 630**
Propoxyphene Napsylate and Acetaminophen Tablets, 630, 631
**Propranolol HCl**
  in antihypertensive combinations, 427
  as beta-adrenergic blocking agent, 376
Propranolol Intensol, 376
**Propylene glycol**
  in acne products, 1416, 1430
  in anorectal preparations, 1411
  in antifungal combinations, 1119
  in douche products, 1407
  in topical agents, 1521
**Propylene glycol alginate, 1521**
**Propylhexedrine, 502**
**Propylthiouracil, 286**
Proscar, 141
Prosed/DS, 1204
ProSom, 805
Prostaglandin agonists, 1306
Prostigmin, 1639
**Protease, 946**
Protease inhibitors, 1169
ProTech First-Aid Stik, 1472, 1521

Protein, 5, 54
Protein hydrolysate, 54
Protein tests, 1768
Proton pump inhibitors, 953
Protonix, 953
Protriptyline HCl, 749
Protropin, 221
Protuss-D Liquid, 570
Protuss DM Tablets, 568
Protuss Liquid, 575
Proventil, 455
Proventil HFA, 455
Proventil Repetabs, 455
Provera, 156
Provigil, 583
Proxigel, 1387
Prozac, 719
Prozac Weekly, 719
Prulet, 973
PSE 120/MSC 2.5 Tablets, 543
Pseudoephedrine HCl
    as decongestant, 501
    in upper respiratory combinations, 521-529, 532-534, 536-571
Pseudoephedrine sulfate
    as decongestant, 501
    in upper respiratory combinations, 531, 534, 535, 541
Pseudoephedrine tannate, 535, 536, 537
Pseudovent Capsules, 527
Pseudovent-PED Capsules, 529
Psoralens, 1447
Psorcon, 239
Psorcon E, 239
Psoriasis agents
    acitretin, 1441
    anthralin, 1437
    calcipotriene, 1439
    methotrexate, 1444
    psoralens, 1447
    tazarotene, 1451
PsoriGel, 1463
Psychotherapeutic agents
    ergoloid mesylates, 785
    lithium, 787
Psychotherapeutic combinations, 795
Psyllium, 961
PTU. see Propylthiouracil
Pulmicort Respules, 470

Pulmicort Turbuhaler, 470
Pulmozyme, 484
Puralube, 1365
Pure Eyes Cleaner/Rinse, 1375
Pure Eyes Disinfecting/ Soaking, 1375
Purge, 973
Purified water, 1407
Purine analogs, 1536
Purinethol, 1536
Purpose, 1516
Purpose DrySkin, 1486
Pyrantel, 1189
Pyrazinamide, 1207
Pyrazinamide with rifampin and isoniazid, 1207
Pyrethrins, 1229
Pyridium, 1664
Pyridostigmine bromide, 1639
Pyridoxine, 6, 17
Pyridoxine HCl
    in analgesics, 612
    nutritional, 17
Pyrilamine maleate
    in nonnarcotic analgesics, 612
    in topical agents, 1522
    in topical antihistamines, 1491
    in upper respiratory combinations, 534, 537, 546, 555, 557, 558
Pyrilamine tannate, 536
Pyrimethamine, 1129
Pyrimethamine and sulfadoxine, 1131
Pyrimidine analogs, 1539
Pyrinyl Plus, 1229
Pyrithione zinc, 1462

QTest, 1766
Quad Tann Tablets, 545
Quadra-Hist D Capsules, 534
Quadra-Hist D PED Capsules, 537
Quazepam, 805
Quercetin, 56
Questran, 434
Questran Light, 434
Quetiapine fumarate, 761
Quibron Capsules, 520
Quibron-300 Capsules, 520

Quibron-T Accudose, 461
Quibron-T/SR Accudose, 461
Quick Care Starting Solution, 1376
Quin B Strong B-25 Tablets, 49
Quinalan, 358
Quinapril, 429
Quinapril HCl, 385
Quinethazone, 315
Quinidex Extentabs, 358
Quinidine, 358
Quinidine gluconate, 358
Quinidine polygalacturonate, 358
Quinidine sulfate, 358
Quinine sulfate, 1138
Quinolone derivatives, 780
Quinora, 358
Quinsana Plus, 1114
Quixin, 1348
QVAR, 470

R/S Lotion, 1431
R-Tanna 12 Suspension, 536
R-Tannic-S A/D Suspension, 536
RA Lotion, 1431
RabAvert, 1248
Rabeprazole sodium, 953
Rabies immune globulin (human), 1237
Rabies vaccine, 1248
Raloxifene HCl, 153
Ramipril, 385
Ranitidine, 935
Ranitidine bismuth citrate, 927
RapidVue, 1766
Ray Block, 1510
R&C, 1229
Rea-Lo, 1483
ReAzo, 1664
Rebetol, 1160
Reclomide, 950
Recombinant Human Erythropoietin, 118
Recombivax HB, 1278
Rectagene Medicated Rectal Balm, 1412
Red petrolatum. see Petrolatum
Redutemp, 601
Reese's Pinworm, 1189

# INDEX

Refenesen Plus Severe Strength Cough & Cold Medicine Tablets, 526
Refresh, 1365
Refresh Plus, 1365
Refresh PM, 1368
Refresh Tears, 1365
Reglan, 950
Regonol, 1639
Regranex, 1454
Regulace Capsules, 980
Regular Iletin II, 255
**Regular Insulin, 258**
Regular Strength Bayer Enteric Coated Caplets, 605
Regulax SS, 977
Rehydrate Solution, 32
Relafen, 641
Relenza, 1165
Relief, 1322
Remeron, 729
Remeron SolTab, 729
Remicade, 1004
Reminyl, 791
Remodulin, 88
Remular-S, 871
Renese, 315
Renova, 1427
ReNu 1 Step, 1375
ReNu Effervescent, 1375
ReNu Lubricating and Rewetting Drops, 1376
ReNu Multi-Purpose, 1376
ReNu MultiPlus, 1376
**Repaglinide, 275**
Repan CF Tablets, 612
Repan Tablets, 613
Reposans, 698
**Repository corticotropin, 226**
Repronex, 209
Requip, 889
Rescon 12 Hour Capsules, 534
Rescon-DM Liquid, 551
Rescon-GG Liquid, 524
Rescon-Jr. Capsules, 537
Rescon-MX Tablets, 544
Rescriptor, 1181
Rescula, 1306
**Reserpine, 424**
**Resorcinol**
  in acne products, 1430
  in antifungal combinations, 1118

**Resorcinol** *(cont.)*
  in topical antihistamines, 1491
Respa-1st Tablets, 525
Respa A.R. Tablets, 543
Respa-DM Tablets, 573
Respahist Capsules, 532
Respaire-60 SR Capsules, 525
Respaire-120 SR Capsules, 527
Respbid, 461
RespiGam, 1237
**Respiratory syncytial virus immune globulin intravenous (human), 1237**
Restore, 961
Restoril, 805
Retavase, 109
**Reteplase, recombinant, 109**
Retin-A, 1427
Retin-A Micro, 1427
Retinoids
  adapalene, 1422
  alitretinoin, 1425
  isotretinoin, 1681
  tretinoin, 1427, 1598
Retrovir, 1176
Rv-Eyes, 1320
Reversol, 1639
Revex, 1633
ReVia, 1700
Rewetting solutions
  for hard contact lenses, 1369
  for rigid gas permeable contact lenses, 1372
  for soft (hydrogel) contact lenses, 1376
Rezamid Lotion, 1431
Rheaban, 998
Rheumatrex Dose Pack, 653, 1444, 1533
Rhinall Nose Drops and Spray, 500
Rhinatate-NF Pediatric Suspension, 536
Rhinatate Pediatric Suspension, 536
Rhinocort, 489
Rhinocort Aqua, 489
RhoGAM, 1237
**Rh$_o$(D) immune globulin (human), 1237**

**Rh$_o$(D) immune globulin IV (human), 1237**
**Rh$_o$(D) immune globulin micro-dose, 1237**
Rhuli Aerosol, 1502
Rhuli Gel, 1502
Rhuli Spray, 1502
**Ribavirin, 1160**
**Riboflavin, 6, 12**
RID, 1229
Rid-A-Pain Cream, 1505
Rid-A-Pain Dental, 1404
Rid-A-Pain HP Cream, 1505
Ridafed, 501
Ridaura, 648
Ridenol, 601
**Rifabutin, 1207**
Rifadin, 1207
Rifamate, 1207
**Rifampin, 1207**
**Rifampin with isoniazid, 1207**
**Rifampin with isoniazid and pyrazinamide, 1207**
**Rifapentine, 1207**
Rifater, 1207
**RIG. see Rabies immune globulin (human)**
Rigid gas permeable contact lens products, 1372
Rilutek, 1741
**Riluzole, 1741**
Rimactane, 1207
**Rimantadine, 1163**
**Rimantadine HCl, 1163**
**Rimexolone, 1331**
Rimso-50, 1656
Rinade B.I.D. Capsules, 533
Riopan Plus, 908
Riopan Plus Double Strength, 908
Riopan Plus Double Strength Suspension, 912
Riopan Plus Suspension, 912
**Risedronate, 297**
Risperdal, 758
**Risperidone, 758**
Ritalin, 594
Ritalin-SR, 594
**Ritonavir, 1169**
**Ritonavir/lopinavir, 1169**
Rituxan, 1619
**Rituximab, 1619**

**Rivastigmine tartrate, 791**
**Rizatriptan benzoate, 673**
RMS, 619
Robafen CF Syrup, 566
Robafen PE Liquid, 524
Robaxin, 871
Robaxin-750, 871
Robaxisal, 875
Robinul, 916
Robinul Forte, 916
Robitussin, 513
Robitussin Allergy & Cough Liquid, 549
Robitussin CF Syrup, 566
Robitussin Cold, Cold & Congestion Softgels and Tablets, 567
Robitussin Cold, Cold & Cough Softgels, 567
Robitussin Cold, Multi-Symptom Cold & Flu Softgels, 566
Robitussin Cold Sinus & Congestion Tablets, 525
Robitussin Cough & Cold Infant Drops, 571
Robitussin Cough & Congestion Formula Liquid, 573
Robitussin DM Infant Drops, 576
Robitussin-DM Liquid, 572
Robitussin Flu Liquid, 551
Robitussin Honey Cough & Cold Liquid, 546
Robitussin Honey Flu Multi-Symptom Liquid, 547
Robitussin Honey Flu Nighttime Syrup, 552
Robitussin Honey Flu Non-Drowsy Syrup, 548
Robitussin Maximum Strength Cough & Cold Syrup, 546
Robitussin Night Relief Liquid, 555
Robitussin PE Liquid, 524
Robitussin Pediatric Cough & Cold Formula Liquid, 560
Robitussin Pediatric Night Relief Cough & Cold Liquid, 564
Robitussin Severe Congestion Liqui-Gels, 525

Robitussin Sugar Free Cough Liquid, 572
Rocaltrol, 22
Rocephin, 1021
**Rofecoxib, 642**
Roferon-A, 1594
Rogaine Extra Strength for Men, 1499
Rogaine for Men, 1499
Rogaine for Women, 1499
Rolaids, 29
Rolaids, Calcium Rich, 907
Romazicon, 1627
Romilar AC Liquid, 571
Rondamine DM Syrup, 549
Rondec-DM Oral Drops, 561
Rondec-DM Syrup, 549
Rondec Oral Drops, 536
Rondec Syrup, 532
Rondec Tablets, 533
Rondec-TR Tablets, 533
**Ropinirole HCl, 889**
**Rosiglitazone maleate, 267**
**Rosin, 1520**
Rowasa, 1001
Roxanol, 619
Roxanol 100, 619
Roxanol T, 619
Roxicet 5/500 Caplets, 630
Roxicet Tablets and Solution, 629
Roxicodone, 619
Roxicodone Intensol, 619
Roxilox Capsules, 630
Roxiprin Tablets, 630
**RSV-IGIV. see Respiratory syncytial virus immune globulin intravenous (human)**
**Rubella and mumps virus vaccine, live, 1265**
**Rubella virus vaccine, live, 1265**
Rubex, 1553
Rubs, 1504
RuLox, 907
Rulox #1, 907
Rulox #2, 907
Rulox Plus Suspension, 911
Rulox Suspension, 910
Rum-K, 40
Rutin, 56
RVPaque, 1509

Ryna-12 S Suspension, 536
Ryna-C Liquid, 545
Ryna Liquid, 533
Rynatan Pediatric Suspension, 536
Rynatan Tablets, 532
Rynatuss Pediatric Suspension, 559
Rynatuss Tablets, 545
Rythmol, 356

**S**-P-T, 291
S-T Forte 2 Liquid, 556
**Sabin vaccine. see Poliovirus vaccine, live, oral, trivalent**
**Saccharin, 961**
Safe Tussin Liquid, 573
Sal-Clens Acne Cleanser Gel, 1431
SalAc Cleanser, 1434
Salactic Film, 1480
Salagen, 1392
Saleto Tablets, 613
Salflex, 606
**Salicylamide**
   in nonnarcotic analgesics, 613
   in upper respiratory combinations, 530
Salicylate combinations, 606
Salicylates and aspirin, 605
**Salicylic acid**
   in antifungal combinations, 1118
   in mouth and throat products, 1403
   topical, 1480
Salicylic Acid and Sulfur Soap, 1432
Salicylic Acid Cleansing Bar, 1432
Saline laxatives, 971
Saline Solution, 1375
SalineX Nasal Drops and Spray, 502
Saliva Substitute, 1391
Saliva substitutes, 1391
Salivart, 1391
Salix, 1391
**Salk vaccine. see Poliovirus vaccine, inactivated**
**Salmeterol/fluticasone propionate, 470**

# INDEX

**Salmeterol xinafoate, 456**
**Salsalate, 606**
Salsitab, 606
Saluron, 315
Sam-EPA Capsules, 58
Sandimmune, 1668
Sandostatin, 127
Sani-Supp, 965
**Sanitized water, 1407**
**Saquinavir, 1169**
Sarafem, 719
Saratoga, 1521
**Sargramostim, 121**
Sarna Anti-Itch, 1521
SAStid Soap, 1432
Scabicides, 1229
**Scarlet red, 1522**
Scarlet Red Ointment
 Dressings, 1522
Schamberg, 1522
Schamberg's, 1522
Scopace, 676
Scope, 1400
**Scopolamine HBr**
 in anticholinergic combi-
 nations, 921
 as antiemetic/antiver-
 tigo agent, 676
 as cycloplegic mydri-
 atic, 1328
 in upper respiratory
 combinations, 543
**Scopolamine, in upper**
**respiratory combina-**
**tions, 543**
Scot-tussin, 513
Scot-Tussin Allergy, 494,
 877
Scot-Tussin DM Cough
 Chasers, 509
Scot-Tussin DM Liquid,
 550
Scot-Tussin Hayfebrol Liq-
 uid, 533
Scot-Tussin Original 5-
 Action Cold and Allergy
 Formula Syrup, 538
Scot-Tussin Original Clear
 5-Action Cold and Allergy
 Formula Liquid, 538
Scot-Tussin Senior Clear
 Liquid, 573
Scott's Emulsion, 45
**SD alcohol**
 in acne products, 1432
 in poison ivy treat-
 ment products, 1502

**SD alcohol 40**
 in acne products, 1431
 in douche products,
 1407
Sea-Omega 30 Capsules,
 58
Sea-Omega 50 Capsules,
 58
Seale's Lotion Modified,
 1431
Seba-Nil Cleansing Mask,
 1433
Seba-Nil Oily Skin
 Cleanser, 1434
Sebasorb Lotion, 1431
Sebex, 1466
Sebizon, 1462
Sebucare, 1466
Sebulex, 1466
Sebulex with Conditioners,
 1466
Sebulon, 1462
**Secobarbital sodium, 800**
Seconal Sodium, 800
Sectral, 376
Sedapap Tablets, 612
Sedatives
 barbiturates, 800
 hypnotics, 805
Selective aldosterone
 receptor antagonists, 432
Selective estrogen receptor
 modulator, 153
**Selegiline HCl, 895**
**Selenium, 5**
**Selenium sulfide, 1460**
Selsun, 1460
Selsun Blue, 1460
Semicid, 1409
**Semilente Insulin, 258**
Semprex-D Capsules, 532
Senexon, 973, 974
**Senna**
 in bowel evacuation
 kits, 987
 as laxative, 974
 in laxative combina-
 tions, 980, 983
Senna-Gen, 974
**Sennosides, 987**
Senokot, 974
Senokot-S Tablets, 980
SenokotXTRA, 974
Senolax, 974
Sensitive Eyes Daily
 Cleaner, 1375

Sensitive Eyes Drops,
 1376
Sensitive Eyes Enzymatic
 Cleaner, 1375
Sensitive Eyes Plus Saline,
 1375
Sensitive Eyes Saline,
 1375
Sensitive Eyes Saline/
 Cleaning Solution, 1375
Sensitive Eyes Sterile
 Saline Spray, 1375
Sensitive teeth prepara-
 tions, 1400
Sensodyne Cool Gel for
 Sensitive Teeth and Cav-
 ity Prevention, 1400
Sensodyne Extra Whiten-
 ing for Sensitive Teeth,
 1400
Sensodyne-SC Original
 Formula for Sensitive
 Teeth, 1400
Sensodyne w/Baking Soda
 for Sensitive Teeth and
 Cavity Prevention, 1400
Septa, 1082
Septi-Soft, 1494
Septra, 1090, 1204
Septra DS, 1090, 1204
Serax, 698
Sereine, 1369
Serentil, 768
Serevent, 456
Serevent Diskus, 456
Seromycin Pulvules, 1207
Serophene, 206
Seroquel, 761
Serostim, 223
Serotonin 5-HT$_1$ receptor
 agonists, 673
**Sertraline HCl, 741**
Serutan, 962
Serzone, 714
Severe Congestion Tussin
 Softgels, 525
Sex hormones
 anabolic steroids, 130
 androgens, 137
 emergency contracep-
 tives, 179
 estrogen combinations,
 150
 estrogens, 144
 etonogestrel/ethinyl
 estradiol, 166

Sex hormones *(cont.)*
  medroxyprogesterone
    acetate, 161
  medroxyprogesterone
    acetate/estradiol
    cypionate, 163
  mifepristone, 134
  oral contraceptives, 170
  progestins, 156
  selective estrogen
    receptor modulator,
    153
**Sexadecyl alcohol, 1520**
SF 1.1, 34
SF 5000 Plus, 34
SFC, 1516
Shampoos, 1460, 1462,
  1466
**Shark liver oil, 1412**
Shepard's Skin, 1486
Shohl's Solution, Modified,
  1647
Siblin, 962
Silace, 977
Silace-C, 983
Siladryl, 877
Silafed Syrup, 534
Silapap, Children's, 601
Silapap Infants' Drops, 602
Sildec-DM Oral Drops, 561
Sildec-DM Syrup, 549
**Sildenafil citrate, 1732**
Silfedrine, Children's, 501
**Silica**
  in douche products,
    1407
  in topical agents, 1521
Silicone No. 2, 1487
Silphen-DM, 509
Siltussin DM Cough Syrup,
  573
Silvadene, 1458
**Silver sulfadiazine, 1458**
**Simethicone**
  in antacid combinations,
    907, 910
  as antiflatulent, 944
  in topical agents, 1522
Simplet Tablets, 539
Simply Saline Nasal Spray,
  502
Simron, 69
**Simvastatin, 446**
Sine-Off Night Time For-
  mula Sinus, Cold, & Flu
  Medicine Geltabs, 541

Sine-Off No-Drowsiness
  Formula Tablets, 522
Sine-Off Sinus Medicine
  Tablets, 539
Sinemet 10-100, 881
Sinemet 25-100, 881
Sinemet 25-250, 881
Sinemet CR, 881
Sinequan, 749
Singlet for Adults Tablets,
  539
Singular, 467
Sinumist-SR, 513
Sinus-Relief Maximum
  Strength Tablets, 522
Sinustop, 501
Sinutab Non-Drying Liquid
  Caps, 525
Sinutab Sinus Without
  Drowsiness Maximum
  Strength Tablets, 522
Sinutab Sinus Without
  Drowsiness Regular
  Strength Tablets, 521
Skeeter Stik, 1472
Skelaxin, 871
Skeletal muscle relaxants,
  871
  combinations, 875
Skelid, 297
Skin cleansers, 1516
Skin disorders, topical
  anesthetics for, 1472
Sleep aids, nonprescrip-
  tion, 810
Sleepinal Softgels, Maxi-
  mum Strength, 810
Slo-Niacin, 13
Slo-Phyllin, 461
Slo-Phyllin GG Syrup, 520
Sloan's Liniment, 1505
Slow FE, 69
Slow-K, 40
Slow-Mag, 38
SLT Lotion, 1466
Smoking deterrents
  bupropion HCl, 1720
  nicotine, 1724
Snaplets-FR, 601
Soac-Lens, 1369
Soap-free cleansers, 1516
Soaps, modified bar, 1432,
  1516
**Sodium**
  in antacid combinations,
    907, 914

**Sodium** *(cont.)*
  in electrolyte mixtures,
    32
  in laxatives, 961
**Sodium acetate, 1412**
**Sodium acid phosphate
  and potassium acid
  phosphate, 1644**
**Sodium acid phosphate
  monohydrate, 1204**
**Sodium alginate, 911**
**Sodium ascorbate, 73**
**Sodium bicarbonate**
  in analgesics, 602, 610
  in antacid combina-
    tions, 907, 914
  in antacids, 904
  in douche products,
    1407
  in laxatives, 962
  in urinary tract prod-
    ucts, 1647
**Sodium biphosphate**
  in laxatives, 971
  in urinary anti-infective
    combinations, 1204
**Sodium bisulfite**
  in anorectal prepara-
    tions, 1411
  in antifungal combina-
    tions, 1118
**Sodium C$_{12-14}$olefin
  sulfonate, 1412**
**Sodium carboxymethyl-
  cellulose**
  as antidiarrheal agent,
    995
  in laxative combina-
    tions, 980
**Sodium chloride**
  in douche products,
    1407
  in nasal products, 430
**Sodium citrate**
  in antacid combinations,
    914
  in antacids, 904
  in upper respiratory
    combinations, 538,
    565
**Sodium citrate and citric
  acid, 1647**
**Sodium cocoyl isethio-
  nate, 1434**
**Sodium fluoride**
  nutritional, 28, 29, 34
  in toothpaste, 1400

# INDEX

Sodium hypochlorite, **1495**
Sodium iodide I 131, **286**
Sodium lactate, **1407**
Sodium laureth sulfate, **1434**
Sodium lauryl sulfate, **1407**
Sodium perborate mono-hydrate, **1407**
Sodium peroxyborate monohydrate, **1402**
Sodium phenylbutyrate, **116**
Sodium phosphate
  in bowel evacuation kits, 987
  in laxatives, 971
Sodium propionate, **1118**
Sodium salicylate
  in analgesics, 606
  in upper respiratory combinations, 538, 565
Sodium stearate, **1119**
Sodium sulfacetamide
  in acne products, 1431
  in ophthalmic anti-infectives, 1354
Sodium thiosulfate
  in acne products, 1431
  in antifungal combinations, 1119
Sodol Compound, 875
Soft (hydrogel) contact lens products, 1375
Solaraze, 1476
Solarcaine, 1472
Solarcaine Aloe Extra Burn Relief, 1472
SolBar PF, 1506, 1507
Solganal, 648
Soltice Quick-Rub, 1505
Solu-Cortef, 231
Solu-Medrol, 231
Solurex, 230
Solurex-LA, 230
Soma, 871
Soma Compound, 875
Soma Compound w/ Codeine, 875
Somatrem, **221**
Somatropin, **223**
Sominex, 810
Sominex, Maximum Strength, 810
Sominex Pain Relief, 810

Somnote, 805
Sonata, 805
Soothaderm, 1522
Sorbitol, **1412**
Sorbitrate, 330
Soriatane, 1441
Sorine, 376
Sotalol HCl, **376**
Span C, 56
Span-FF, 69
Sparfloxacin, **1049**
Spec-T, 1399
Spec-T Cough Suppressant, 509
Spectazole, 1113
Spectinomycin HCl, **1039**
Spectro-Jel, 1516
Spectrobid, 1067
Spectrocin, 1081
Spermicides, 160, 1409
Spironolactone, **312**
Spironolactone and hydrochlorothiazide, **319**
Spirozide, 319
Sporanox, 1102
Sportscreme, 1504
SSD, 1458
SSD AF, 1458
SSKI, 513
St. Joseph Adult Chewable Aspirin, 605
St. Joseph Aspirin-Free Fever Reducer for Children, 602
St. Joseph Aspirin-Free for Children, 601
St. Joseph Aspirin-Free Infants' Drops, 602
Stadol NS, 633
Stahist Tablets, 543
Stamoist E Tablets, 527
Stannous fluoride, **34**
Stanozolol, **130**
Star-Otic, 1382
Starlix, 275
Staticin, 1041
Statuss Green Liquid, 557
Stavudine, **1176**
Stay Awake, 583
Stearyl alcohol, **1430, 1431**
Stelazine, 768
Step 2, 1524
Sterapred, 231
SteriNail, 1119

Steroids. see also Adrenal cortical steroids; Anabolic steroids
  in anorectal preparations, 1411
  and ophthalmic antibiotic combinations, 1352
Stilphostrol, 1569
Stimate, 218
Stimulant laxatives, 973
Sting-Eze, 1491
Sting-Kill, 1472
Stool softeners, 977
Storzine 2, 1303
Streptase, 109
Streptokinase, **109**
Streptozocin, **1586**
Stri-Dex Cleansing Bar, 1432
Stri-Dex Pads Maximum Strength, 1434
Stri-Dex Pads Oil Fighting Formula, 1434
Stri-Dex Pads Regular Strength, 1435
Stri-Dex Pads Sensitive Skin, 1435
Stridex Clear Gel, 1431
Stromectol, 1193
Strong Iodine Solution, 289
Strovite Tablets, 47
Stypto-Caine, 1522
SU-TUSS DM Liquid, 573
Su-Tuss HD Elixir, 570
Succimer, **1637**
Succinimides, 846
Sucralfate, **942**
Sucrets, 1399
Sucrets 4-Hour Cough Suppressant, 509
Sucrets, Children's, 1399
Sucrets Maximum Strength, 1400
Sucrose, **961**
Sudafed, 501
Sudafed 12 Hour Caplets, 501
Sudafed 24 Hour, 501
Sudafed, Children's, 501
Sudafed Children's Non-Drowsy Cold & Cough Liquid, 559
Sudafed Cold & Allergy Maximum Strength Tablets, 533
Sudafed Cold & Sinus Non-Drowsy Liqui-Caps, 521

Sudafed Maximum Strength Sinus Nighttime Plus Pain Relief Tablets, 541
Sudafed Multi-Symptom Cold & Cough Liquid Caps, 566
Sudafed Non-Drowsy Non-Drying Sinus Liquid Caps, 525
Sudafed Non-Drowsy Severe Cold Formula Maximum Strength Tablets, 548
Sudafed Sinus Headache Non-Drowsy Tablets, 522
Sudafed Sinus Nighttime Maximum Strength Tablets, 534
Sudal 60/500 Tablets, 526
Sudal-DM Tablets, 573
Sudodrin, 501
SudoGest, 501
SudoGest Sinus Maximum Strength Tablets, 522
Sular, 364
**Sulconazole nitrate, 1114**
Sulf-10, 1348
Sulfa-Trip, 1093
Sulfacet-R Lotion, 1431
**Sulfacetamide sodium**
  ophthalmic, 1348
  topical, 1462
**Sulfadiazine, 1084**
**Sulfadoxine and pyrimethamine, 1131**
Sulfalax Calcium, 977
**Sulfamethizole**
  as sulfonamide, 1084
  in urinary anti-infective combinations, 1204
**Sulfamethoxazole and trimethoprim, 1090**
Sulfamylon, 1456
**Sulfanilamide, 1093**
**Sulfasalazine, 1084**
Sulfatrim, 1090, 1204
Sulfatrim DS, 1090
**Sulfinpyrazone, 668**
**Sulfisoxazole, 1204**
**Sulfisoxazole and erythromycin ethylsuccinate, 1087**
Sulfoil, 1516
Sulfonamides, 1084
  combinations, 1204

Sulfonamides, 1084 *(cont.)*
  erythromycin ethylsuccinate and sulfisoxazole, 1087
  multiple, 1084
  trimethoprim and sulfamethoxazole, 1090
Sulfonylureas, 270
Sulforcin Lotion, 1432
Sulfoxyl Regular, 1416
Sulfoxyl Strong, 1416
**Sulfur**
  in acne products, 1416, 1421
  in topical agents, 1520
Sulfur Soap, 1432
**Sulindac, 642**
Sulmeprim, 1090
Sulpho-Lac, 1421
Sulster Solution, 1354
Sultrin Triple Sulfa, 1093
**Sumatriptan succinate, 673**
Summer's Eve, 240
Summer's Eve Disposable Douche, 1407
Summer's Eve Douche, 1407
Summer's Eve Medicated Disposable Douche, 1407
Summer's Eve Post-Menstrual Disposable Douche, 1407
Summit Extra Strength Coated Tablets, 613
Sumycin 250, 1072
Sumycin 500, 1072
Sumycin Syrup, 1072
Sun Splash, 1508
Sunscreens, 1506
Super B Complex Capsules, 46
Super Calcium 1200, 29
Super DEC B-100 Tablets, 49
Super Quints B-50 Tablets, 49
Superchar, 1625
Suphedrine 12 Hour, 501
Suppap, 602
Suprax, 1019
**Suprofen, 1338**
Surbex-T Filmtabs, 47
Surbex with C Filmtabs, 47
SureStep, 1764

Surfactant cleaning solutions, for soft (hydrogel) contact lenses, 1375
Surfak Liquigels, 977
Surmontil, 749
Sustiva, 1181
Sweet'n fresh clotrimazole-7, 1121
Swim Ear, 1382
Symmetrel, 881, 1154
Sympathomimetics
  as bronchodilators, 455
  as glaucoma agents, 1309
Synagis, 1241
Synalar, 239
Synalgos-DC Capsules, 629
Synarel, 212
Synemol, 239
**Synthetic Conjugated Estrogens, A, 144**
Synthroid, 291

**T**/Derm, 1463
T-Phyl, 461
T-Stat, 1041
T-Vites Tablets, 47
**T$_3$, 291**
**T$_4$, 291**
Tabloid, 1536
**Tacrine HCl, 791**
**Tacrolimus, 1678**
Tagamet, 935
Tagamet HB 200, 935
Talacen Caplets, 635
**Talc, 1497**
Talwin Compound Caplets, 635
Talwin Nx, 635
Tambocor, 347
Tamiflu, 1167
**Tamoxifen citrate, 1571**
**Tamsulosin HCl, 382**
Tanac, 1404
Tanafed Suspension, 535
Tannic-12 Suspension, 559
Tannic-12 Tablets, 545
**Tannic acid**
  in antifungal combinations, 1118
  in mouth and throat products, 1403
  in topical agents, 1521
Tapanol Extra Strength, 601

# INDEX

Tapazole, 286
**Tar derivatives**
 in bath products, 1462
 in emollients, 1462
 in shampoos, 1462
Tarka Extended-Release
 Tablets, 430
Tarsum, 1466
**Tartrazine, 1430**
Tavist Allergy, 493
Tavist Allergy/Sinus/Head-
 ache Tablets, 540
Tavist Sinus Maximum
 Strength Tablets, 522
Taxol, 1601
**Tazarotene, 1451**
Tazicef, 1020
Tazidime, 1020
Tazorac, 1451
Teargen, 1365
Teargen II, 1365
Tearisol, 1365
Tears Naturale, 1365
Tears Naturale II, 1365,
 1368
Tears Naturale Free, 1365
Tears Plus, 1365
Tears Renewed, 1365
Tebamide, 676
**Tegaserod maleate, 1009**
Tegretol, 816
Tegretol-XR, 816
Tegrin, 1463
Tegrin Medicated
 Advanced Formula, 1462
**Telmisartan, 390, 429**
**Temazepam, 805**
Temovate, 238
Temovate E, 238
Tempo, 907
Tempra Drops, 602
**Tenecteplase, 109**
Tenex, 405
**Tenofovir disoproxil
 fumarate, 1173**
Tenoretic 50 Tablets, 427
Tenoretic 100 Tablets, 427
Tenormin, 376
Tensilon, 1639
Tenuate, 587
Tenuate Dospan, 587
Tequin, 1049
Teraseptic, 1516
Terazol 3, 1121
Terazol 7, 1121
**Terazosin HCl, 382**
**Terbinafine HCl, 1114**

**Terbutaline sulfate, 456**
**Terconazole, 1121**
Terra-Cortril Suspension,
 1352
Terramycin, 1072
Terramycin with Polymyxin
 B Sulfate, 1081, 1093
Teslac, 1562
Tessalon Perles, 509
Testoderm, 137
Testoderm TTS, 137
**Testolactone, 1562**
Testopel, 137
**Testosterone aqueous,
 137**
**Testosterone cypionate,
 137, 150**
**Testosterone enanthate,
 137**
**Testosterone pellets, 137**
**Testosterone propio-
 nate, 137**
**Testosterone trans-
 dermal, 137**
Testred, 137
**Tetanus immune glob-
 ulin (human), 1237**
**Tetanus toxoid adsorbed,
 1250**
**Tetracaine HCl**
 for mucous membranes,
  1468
 for skin disorders, 1473
 in topical agents, 1522
Tetracyclic compounds,
 729
**Tetracycline HCl**
 as antibiotic, 1072
 for Helicobacter pylori
  infections, 929
 topical, 1077, 1394
Tetracyclines
 systemic, 1072
 topical, 1077
**Tetrahydrozoline HCl**
 in nasal decongestants,
  501
 in ophthalmic decon-
  gestant combina-
  tions, 1326
 in ophthalmic decon-
  gestants, 1322
Tetrasine, 1322
Tetrasine Extra, 1322
Teveten, 390
**Thalidomide, 1745**
Thalitone, 315

Thalomid, 1745
Theo-24, 461
Theo-Dur, 461
Theo-X, 461
Theochron, 461
Theolair, 461
Theolair-SR, 461
Theolate Liquid, 520
**Theophylline, 461**
**Theophylline ethylene-
 diamine, 261**
Thera-Flur-N, 34
Thera-gesic, 1504
Thera-Hist Cold & Allergy
 Syrup, 537
Thera-Hist Cold & Cough
 Syrup, 563
Thera-Hist Expectorant
 Chest Congestion Liquid,
 529
Therac Lotion, 1432
TheraFlu Cold & Cough
 Night Time Powder, 552
TheraFlu Flu & Cold Medi-
 cine for Sore Throat,
 Maximum Strength Pow-
 der, 540
TheraFlu Flu & Cough
 Night Time, Maximum
 Strength Powder, 553
TheraFlu Flu & Sore
 Throat, Maximum
 Strength Powder, 540
TheraFlu Flu & Sore Throat
 Night Time, Maximum
 Strength Powder, 540
TheraFlu Flu and Cold
 Medicine Original For-
 mula Powder, 539
TheraFlu Flu, Cold &
 Cough and Sore Throat,
 Maximum Strength
 Powder, 553
TheraFlu Flu, Cold &
 Cough Night Time, Maxi-
 mum Strength Powder,
 553
TheraFlu Flu, Cold &
 Cough Powder, 552
TheraFlu Maximum
 Strength Flu & Conges-
 tion Non-Drowsy Powder,
 568
TheraFlu Maximum
 Strength Flu, Cold &
 Cough Powder, 568

TheraFlu Maximum Strength NightTime Formula Flu, Cold & Cough Medicine Tablets, 552
TheraFlu Non-Drowsy Flu, Cold & Cough Maximum Strength Powder, 548
TheraFlu Non-Drowsy Formula Maximum Strength Tablets, 548
Theraflu Severe Cold & Congestion Night Time Maximum Strength Powder, 553
Theraflu Severe Cold & Congestion Non-Drowsy, Maximum Strength Powder, 548
Theramycin Z, 1041
TheraPatch Vapor Patch for Kids Cough Suppressant, 576
Therapeutic B Complex with C Capsules, 47
Therapeutic Bath, 1487
ThexForte Caplets, 47
**Thiabendazole, 1191**
Thiamilate, 10
Thiamin HCl, 10
**Thiamine, 6, 10**
**Thiazide diuretic and beta-blockers, 427**
**Thiazide diuretic and hydralazine, 427**
Thiazide diuretics, 315
**Thiazide diuretics and angiotensin converting enzyme inhibitors, 428**
**Thiazide diuretics and angiotensin II receptor antagonists, 429**
**Thiazide diuretics and clonidine, 429**
**Thiazide diuretics and methyldopa, 428**
Thiazolidinediones, 267
**Thiethylperazine, 687**
**Thimerosal, 1494**
**Thioguanine, 1536**
**Thioridazine HCl, 768**
Thiosulfil Forte, 1084
**Thioxanthene, 782**
Thioxanthene derivatives, 782
**Thonzonium bromide, 1379**

Thorazine
as antiemetic/antivertigo agent, 687
as antipsychotic, 768
Thorazine Spansules, 687
Throat and mouth products. see Mouth and throat products
Throat sprays, 1400
Thrombolytic agents, 109
**Thyme oil, 1523**
Thymoglobulin, 1235
**Thymol**
in douche products, 1407
in mouth and throat products, 1402
in mouthwash, 1400
in topical agents, 1520
Thyrar, 291
Thyro-Block, 289
**Thyroid desiccated, 291**
Thyroid drugs
antithyroid agents, 286
iodine products, 289
Thyroid hormones, 291
Thyroid Strong, 291
Thyrolar, 291
**L-Thyroxine, 291**
Ti•Baby Natural, 1509
Ti•Screen (lip balm), 1512
Ti•Screen (sunscreen), 1508, 1509, 1510
Ti•Screen Natural, 1509
Ti•Screen Sports Gel, 1509
**Tiagabine HCl, 852**
Tiamate, 363
Tiazac, 363
Ticlid, 84
**Ticlopidine HCl, 84**
**TIG. see Tetanus immune globulin (human)**
Tigan, 676
Tikosyn, 344
Tilade, 487
**Tiludronate disodium, 297**
Time-Hist Capsules, 533
Timolide Tablets, 427
**Timolol maleate**
in antihypertensive combinations, 427
as beta-adrenergic blocking agent, 376
ophthalmic, 1297

**Timolol maleate and dorzolamide HCl, 1316**
Timoptic, 1297
Timoptic in Ocudose, 1297
Timoptic-XE, 1297
Tinactin, 1114
Tinactin for Jock Itch, 1114
TinBen, 1487
TinCoBen, 1487
Tine Test, 1289
Tine Test PPD, 1289
Ting, 1113, 1114, 1119
Tinver, 1119
**Tinzaparin sodium, 100**
**Tioconazole, 1121**
Tisit, 1229
**Titanium dioxide**
in acne products, 1432
in antifungal combinations, 1119
in sunscreens, 1506
Titralac, 908
Titralac Extra Strength, 908
Titralac Plus, 908, 911
**Tizanidine HCl, 868**
**TMP. see Trimethoprim**
**TMP-SMZ. see Trimethoprim and sulfamethoxazole**
TNKase, 109
TobraDex, 1353
TobraDex Suspension, 1352
**Tobramycin, 1348, 1352**
Tobrex, 1348
**Tocainide, 361**
Tofranil, 749
Tofranil-PM, 749
**Tolazamide, 270**
**Tolbutamide, 270**
Tolectin 600, 642
Tolectin DS, 642
Tolfrinic Tablets, 74
Tolinase, 270
**Tolmetin sodium, 642**
**Tolnaftate**
in antifungal combinations, 1118
in topical antifungal preparations, 1114
**Tolterodine tartrate, 1662**
Tolu-Sed DM Liquid, 573
Tom's of Maine Natural Cough & Cold Rub Cough Suppressant, 576
Tonocard, 361

# INDEX

Toothpaste, for sensitive teeth, 1400
Top Care LiquiCaps Nite Time Multi-Symptom Cold/Flu Relief Capsules, 554
Top Care Maximum Strength Flu, Cold & Cough Medicine Night Time Powder, 553
Top Care Maximum Strength Soothing Cough & Head Congestion Relief D Liquid, 546
Top Care Multi-Symptom Pain Relief Cold Tablets, 547, 551
Topamax, 843
Topic, 1522
Topical analgesics, capsaicin, 1489
Topical anesthetics
 for mucous membranes, 1468
 for skin disorders, 1472
Topical antibiotics, 1081
Topical antifungal combinations, 1118
Topical antifungal preparations, 1113
Topical antihistamines, 1491
Topical antiseptics, 1494
Topical combinations, 576
Topical germicides, 1494
**Topical starch, 1412**
Topicort, 239
Topicort LP, 239
Topicycline, 1077
**Topiramate, 843**
**Topotecan, 1542**
Toprol XL, 376
**TOPV. see Poliovirus vaccine, live, oral, trivalent**
Toradol, 641
Torecan, 687
**Toremifene citrate, 1571**
Tornalate, 455
**Torsemide, 309**
Totacillin, 1067
Total, 1369
Touro Allergy Capsules, 532
Touro CC Tablets, 568
Touro DM Tablets, 573
Touro LA Tablets, 527
Trac Tabs 2X, 1204

Tracer bG, 1751
Tracleer, 336
**Tragacanth, 983**
**Tramadol HCl, 638**
Trandate, 413
**Trandolapril, 385, 430**
Trans-Ver-Sal, 1480
Transact, 1421
Transderm-Nitro, 331
Transderm Scop, 676
Tranxene, 698
Tranxene-SD, 698
Tranxene-SD Half-Strength, 698
**Tranylcypromine sulfate, 732**
**Trastuzumab, 1621**
Travatan, 1306
**Travoprost, 1306**
**Trazodone HCl, 743**
Trecator-SC, 1207
Trental, 112
**Treprostinil sodium, 88**
**Tretinoin**
 as acne product, 1427
 as antineoplastic agent, 1598
Tri-Acting Cold & Allergy Syrup, 537
Tri-Acting Cold & Cough Syrup, 563
Tri-K, 40
Tri Levlen, 171
Tri-Norinyl, 171
Tri Super Flavons, 56
Tri-Vi-Sol Drops, 45
Triacin-C Cough Syrup, 546
Triacting Cold & Allergy Liquid, 537
Triacting Liquid, 529
Triad Capsules, 613
Triam-A, 232
Triam Forte, 232
Triamcin, 232
**Triamcinolone, 232**
**Triamcinolone acetonide**
 in antifungal combinations, 1118
 in glucocorticoids, 232
 in inhaled corticosteroids, 470
 in intranasal steroids, 489
 in mouth and throat products, 1403

**Triamcinolone acetonide** *(cont.)*
 in topical corticosteroids, 241
**Triamcinolone diacetate, 232**
**Triamcinolone hexacetonide, 232**
Triaminic Allergy Congestion Softchews, 501
Triaminic AM, 501
Triaminic AM Non-Drowsy Cough & Decongestant Liquid, 560
Triaminic Chest Congestion Liquid, 529
Triaminic Cold & Allergy Liquid, 537
Triaminic Cold & Cough Liquid, 563
Triaminic Cold & Cough Softchews Tablets, 563
Triaminic Cold & Night Time Cough Liquid, 564
Triaminic Cold, Cough & Fever Liquid, 564
Triaminic Cough & Congestion Liquid, 560
Triaminic Cough & Sore Throat Liquid, 560
Triaminic Cough Softchews Tablets, 563
Triaminic Softchews Allergy Sinus & Headache Tablets, 523
Triaminic Softchews Tablets, 537
Triaminic Throat Pain & Cough Softchews Tablets, 560
Triaminic Vapor Patch for Cough, 576
Triaminicin Cold, Allergy, Sinus Medicine Tablets, 539
Triamonide 40, 232
**Triamterene, 312**
**Triamterene and hydrochlorothiazide, 319**
**Triazolam, 805**
**Tribasic calcium phosphate, 28**
**Trichlormethiazide, as diuretic, 315**
Trichotine Douche, 1407
Trichotine Liquid Douche Concentrate, 1407

**Triclosan, 1432**
Tricodene Cough & Cold Liquid, 546
Tricodene Sugar Free Liquid, 550
Tricor, 440
Tricyclic antidepressants, 749
Triderm, 241
Tridesilon, 238
Tridione, 834
Tridrate Dry Bowel Cleansing System, 987
**Triethanolamine polypeptide oleate-condensate, 1382**
**Triethanolamine salicylate**
in rubs and liniments, 1504
in sunscreens, 1511
**Trifluoperazine HCl, 768**
**Trifluorothymidine. see Trifluridine**
**Triflupromazine HCl, 687**
**Trifluridine, 1358**
TriHemic 600 Tablets, 75
Trihexy-2, 878
Trihexy-4, 878
**Trihexyphenidyl HCl, 878**
TriHIBit, 1259
Trilafon, 687, 768
Trileptal, 836
Trilisate, 606
Trimazide, 676
**Trimethadione, 834**
**Trimethobenzamide HCl, 676**
**Trimethoprim**
systemic, 1079
in urinary anti-infective combinations, 1204
**Trimethoprim and sulfamethoxazole, 1090**
**Trimipramine maleate, 749**
Trimox, 1067
Trimox Pediatric Drops, 1067
Trinalin Repetabs Tablets, 534
Trinsicon Capsules, 75
Trionate Tablets, 545
Triostat, 291
Triotann Pediatric Suspension, 536

Triotann-S Pediatric Suspension, 536
**Trioxsalen, 1447**
Tripedia, 1250
**Tripelennamine HCl, 1491**
Triphasic oral contraceptives, 171
Triphasil, 171
Triple antibiotics, 1082
Triple Sulfa, 1084
**Triple sulfa, 1093**
Triple Sulfa No. 2, 1084
**Triprolidine HCl, 534, 546**
Triprolidine HCl w/Pseudoephedrine HCl Syrup, 534
Triptone, 676
**Trisodium EDTA, 1434**
Trisoralen, 1447
Tristoject, 232
Tritec, 927
Trivora, 171
Trizivir, 1176
Trobicin, 1039
Trocaine, 1400
Tronolane, 1411, 1412
Tronothane HCl, 1472
Tropicacyl, 1328
**Tropicamide, 1328**
**Trovafloxacin mesylate, 1049**
Trovan, 1049
Trusopt, 1314
Trysul, 1093
Tuberculin, 1289
**Tuberculin PPD multiple puncture device, 1289**
**Tuberculin purified protein derivative, 1289**
Tuberculin tests, 1289
Tubersol, 1289
Tucks, 1412
Tucks Hemorrhoidal, 1519
Tucks Take-Alongs, 1412
Tuinal 100 mg Pulvules, 800
Tuinal 200 mg Pulvules, 800
Tums, 29, 903
Tums 500, 29
Tums E-X, 29, 903
Tums E-X Sugar Free, 29
Tums Ultra, 29, 903
Tur-Bi-Kal Nasal Drops, 500
Tuss-DM Tablets, 573
Tussafed Ex Syrup, 566

Tussafed HC Syrup, 569
Tussafed-LA Tablets, 568
Tussafed Syrup, 550
Tussend Syrup, 557
Tussend Tablets, 557
Tussex Cough Syrup, 566
Tussi-12 S Suspension, 559
Tussi-12 Tablets, 545
TUSSI-bid Tablets, 574
Tussi-Organidin-DM NR Liquid, 573
Tussi-Organidin NR Liquid, 571
Tussi-Organidin-S NR Liquid, 571
Tussigon Tablets, 555
Tussionex Pennkinetic Suspension, 557
Tussirex Sugar Free Liquid, 565
Tussirex Syrup, 565
Tusstat, 509, 877
Tusstat Cough, 676
Twice-A-Day 12 Hour Nasal Spray, 500
Twilite, 810
Twinrix, 1282
Tylenol Allergy Sinus, Maximum Strength Tablets, Gelcaps, and Geltabs, 539
Tylenol Allergy Sinus Night-Time, Maximum Strength Tablets, 541
Tylenol Caplets, 601
Tylenol, Children's, 601, 602
Tylenol Children's Cold Chewable Tablets, 542
Tylenol Children's Cold Liquid, 542
Tylenol Children's Cold Plus Cough Chewable Tablets, 562
Tylenol Children's Cold Plus Cough Suspension, 563
Tylenol Children's Flu Suspension, 564
Tylenol Children's Sinus Suspension, 523
Tylenol Cold Complete Formula Tablets, 551
Tylenol Cold Non-Drowsy Formula Gelcaps and Tablets, 547

# INDEX

Tylenol Extended Relief, 601

Tylenol Extra Strength, 601, 602

Tylenol Flu Maximum Strength Non-Drowsy Gelcaps, 548

Tylenol Flu NightTime, Maximum Strength Gelcaps, 541

Tylenol Flu NightTime, Maximum Strength Liquid, 554

Tylenol Infant's Cold Concentrated Drops, 523

Tylenol Infants' Cold Decongestant & Fever Reducer Plus Cough Concentrated Drops, 559

Tylenol Infants' Drops, 602

Tylenol Junior Strength, 601

Tylenol Multi-Symptom Cold Severe Congestion Tablets, 567

Tylenol Multi-Symptom Menstrual Relief Caplets, Women's, 612

Tylenol PM Extra Strength Tablets, Gelcaps, and Geltabs, 530

Tylenol PM Geltabs, Extra Strength, 810

Tylenol Regular Strength, 601

Tylenol Severe Allergy Tablets, 530

Tylenol Sinus NightTime, Maximum Strength Tablets, 541

Tylenol Sinus Non-Drowsy Maximum Strength Geltabs, Tablets, and Gelcaps, 522

Tylenol w/Codeine Elixir, 626

Tylenol w/Codeine No. 2 Tablets, 626

Tylenol w/Codeine No. 3 Capsules and Tablets, 626

Tylenol w/Codeine No. 4 Tablets, 627

Tylox Capsules, 630

Tympagesic, 1382

**L-Tyrosine, 54**

Tyrosum Cleanser Liquid and Packets, 1435

Tyzine Nasal Drops and Spray, 501

Tyzine Pediatric Nasal Drops, 501

**U**AA, 1205

Ultra Derm (lotion), 1486

Ultra Derm (oil), 1487

Ultra Mide 25, 1483

Ultra Tears, 1365

ULTRAbrom Capsules, 533

ULTRAbrom PD Capsules, 536

**Ultralente Insulin, 258**

Ultram, 638

Ultrase Capsules, 946

Ultrase MT12 Capsules, 946

Ultrase MT18 Capsules, 947

Ultrase MT20 Capsules, 947

Ultravate, 239

Ultrazyme, 1375

**Undecylenic acid, 1118**

**Undecylenic acid and derivatives, 1114**

Unguentine, 1523

Unguentine Plus, 1472

Uni-Ace, 602

Unifiber, 961

Unilax Capsules, 980

Uniphyl, 461

Uniretic Tablets, 429

Unisol, 1375

Unisol 4, 1375

Unisom Nighttime Sleep Aid, 810

Unisom SleepGels, Maximum Strength, 810

Unisom with Pain Relief, 810

Univasc, 385

**Unoprostone isopropyl, 1306**

Upper respiratory combinations, 517

Uracid, 1497

**Urea**
   in anorectal preparations, 1411
   in emollients, 1483
   in mouth and throat products, 1402

**Urea** (cont.)
   in topical corticosteroids, 245

Ureacin-10, 1483

Ureacin-20, 1483

Urecholine, 1650

Urex, 1195

Uridon Modified, 1205

Urimar-T, 1204

Urinary anti-infectives combinations, 1204
   fosfomycin tromethamine, 1197
   methenamine, 1195
   methenamine salts, 1195
   nalidixic acid, 1199
   nitrofurantoin, 1201

Urinary Antiseptic No. 2, 1205

Urinary tract infection tests, 1770

Urinary tract products
   acetohydroxamic acid, 1642
   acidifiers, 1644
   alkalinizers, 1647
   bethanechol chloride, 1650
   cellulose sodium phosphate, 1652
   cysteamine bitartrate, 1654
   dimethyl sulfoxide, 1656
   flavoxate, 1658
   oxybutynin chloride, 1660
   phenazopyridine HCl, 1664
   tolterodine tartrate, 1662

Urine tests
   glucose, 1754
   ketone, 1758
   miscellaneous, 1772
   ovulation, 1764
   pregnancy, 1766
   protein, 1768
   urinary tract infection, 1770

Urised, 1205

Urisedamine, 1204

Urispas, 1658

Uristat, 1664

Uristix, 1772

Uristix 4, 1772

Uritin, 1205

## I-60   Uro/Vic

Uro-Mag, 38, 904
Uro-Phosphate, 1204
Urobak, 1084
Urobiotic-250, 1204
Urocit-K, 1647
**Urofollitropin, 200**
Urogesic, 1664
Urogesic Blue, 1204
Uroplus DS, 1090
Uroplus SS, 1090
Uroquid-Acid No.2, 1204
**Ursodiol, 957**
UTI, 1770

**V**-Dec-M Tablets, 527
V.V.S., 1093
Vaccines
　diphtheria, tetanus, per-
　　tussis, 1250
　diphtheria, tetanus, per-
　　tussis, haemophilus b,
　　1259
　haemophilus b, 1254
　haemophilus b/hepatitis
　　B, 1257
　hepatitis A, 1275
　hepatitis A/hepatitis B,
　　1282
　hepatitis B, 1278
　influenza, 1270
　measles, mumps and
　　rubella virus, 1265
　pneumococcal, 1285
　pneumococcal 7-valent
　　conjugate, 1287
　polio, 1261
　rabies, 1248
　varicella, 1268
Vagifem, 144
Vaginal anti-infectives,
　1093
　combinations, 1093
Vaginal antifungals, 1121
Vaginal preparations,
　douche products, 1407
Vagisec Plus, 1093
Vagisil, Maximum Strength,
　1468
Vagisil, New Improved,
　1468
Vagistat-1, 1121
Valcyte, 1146
**Valdecoxib, 642**
Valergen 20, 144
Valergen 40, 144
**Valganciclovir, 1146**

**Valganciclovir HCl, 1146**
Valium
　as antianxiety agent,
　　698
　as muscle relaxant, 871
**Valproic acid, 857**
Valproic acid derivatives,
　857
Valrelease, 698
**Valrubicin, 1560**
**Valsartan, 390, 429-430**
Valstar, 1560
Valtrex, 1151
Vancenase AQ, 489
Vanceril, 470
Vanceril Double Strength,
　470
Vancocin, 1043
Vancoled, 1043
**Vancomycin, 1043**
Vanex HD Liquid, 556
Vaniqa, 1525
Vanoxide-HC, 1416
Vanoxide-HC Lotion, 245
Vanquish Caplets, 613
Vantin, 1020
VAQTA, 1275
**Varicella vaccine, 1268**
**Varicella virus vaccine,
　live, 1268**
**Varicella-zoster immune
　globulin (human), 1238**
Varivax, 1268
Vascor, 363
Vaseretic Tablets, 428
Vasocidin, 1354
Vasocidin Solution, 1354
VasoClear, 1322
VasoClear A, 1326
Vasocon-A, 1326
Vasoconstrictors, local, in
　anorectal preparations,
　1412
Vasodilan, 372
Vasodilators
　bosentan, 336
　peripheral epopros-
　　tenol, 370
　isoxsuprine, 372
　papaverine, 374
Vasodilators/aggregation
　inhibitors, 88
Vasopressor/antihypoten-
　sive agents, midodrine,
　695
Vasotec, 385
Vectrin, 1072

Veetids, 1068
Velosef, 1021
Velosulin BR, 255
**Venlafaxine HCl, 746**
Venoglobulin-S, 1236
Ventolin, 455
Ventolin Nebules, 455
Ventolin Rotocaps, 455
VePesid, 1547
Veracolate Tablets, 981
**Verapamil, 430**
**Verapamil HCl, 364**
Verelan, 364
Verelan PM, 364
Vermox, 1187
Versacaps Capsules, 525
**Verteporfin, 1362**
Vesanoid, 1598
Vesprin, 687
Vexol, 1331
Vfend, 1111
Vi-Daylin ADC Oral Solu-
　tion, 45
Viadur, 1577
Viagra, 1732
Vibra-Tabs, 1072
Vibramycin, 1072
Vicks 44D Cough & Head
　Congestion Relief Liq-
　uid, 546
Vicks 44E Cough & Chest
　Congestion Relief Liq-
　uid, 572
Vicks 44M Cough, Cold, &
　Flu Relief Liquid, 551
Vicks Children's NyQuil
　Cold/Cough Relief Liquid,
　562
Vicks Chloraseptic, 1399
Vicks DayQuil LiquiCaps
　Multi-Symptom Cold/
　Flu Relief Capsules, 547
Vicks DayQuil Multi-
　Symptom Cold/Flu Relief
　Liquid, 547
Vicks NyQuil Cough Syrup,
　553
Vicks NyQuil Multi-
　Symptom Cold & Flu
　Relief LiquiCaps Cap-
　sules, 554
Vicks NyQuil Multi-
　Symptom Cold/Flu Relief
　Liquid, 554
Vicks Pediatric 44E Cough
　& Chest Congestion
　Relief Liquid, 576

# INDEX

Vicks Pediatric 44M Cough & Cold Relief Liquid, 562
Vicks Sinex 12 Hour Nasal Spray and Ultra Fine Mist, 500
Vicks Sinex Nasal Spray and Ultra Fine Mist, 500
Vicks Vapo Rub, 1505
Vicks Vapor Inhaler, 502
Vicks VapoRub Cream, 576
Vicodin ES Tablets, 628
Vicodin Tablets, 628
Vicon-C Capsules, 47
**Vidarabine, 1358**
Videx, 1176
Videx EC, 1176
**Vinegar, 1407**
**Vinorelbine tartrate, 1549**
Viogen-C Capsules, 47
Viokase 8 Tablets, 946
Viokase 16 Tablets, 947
Viokase Powder, 947
Vioxx, 642
Vira-A, 1358
Viracept, 1169
Viramune, 1181
Virazole, 1160
Viread, 1173
Virilon, 137
Viroptic, 1358
Visine, 1322
Visine Allergy Relief, 1326
Visine L.R., 1322
Visine Moisturizing, 1322
Visken, 376
Vistaril, 494, 706
Vistide, 1157
Visudyne, 1362
Vita-Bee w/C Captabs, 47
Vita-C, 19
Vita-Plus E, 26
Vitamin(s)
    combinations calcium and vitamin D, 51
    vitamin B, 46
    vitamin B with C, 47
    vitamin B with folic acid, 49
    vitamins A and D, 45
    fat-soluble, 6
    iron with, 74
    water-soluble, 6
**Vitamin A**
    in emollients, 1484
    nutritional, 6, 7, 45
Vitamin A & D Tablets, 45

Vitamin A and Beta Carotene, 7
Vitamin A Palmitate, 7
**Vitamin B**
    with folic acid, 49
    nutritional, 46
Vitamin B-100 Complex Tablets, 49
**Vitamin B$_1$, 6, 10, 46, 47, 49**
**Vitamin B$_2$, 6, 12, 46, 47, 49**
**Vitamin B$_3$, 6, 13, 46, 47, 49**
**Vitamin B$_5$, 16, 46, 47, 49**
**Vitamin B$_6$, 6, 17, 46, 47, 49**
**Vitamin B$_{12}$, 46, 47, 49, 81**
    with iron, 74, 75
    nutritional, 6
Vitamin B$_{12}$ with Folic Acid Tablets, 49
**Vitamin C**
    with iron, 73, 74, 75
    nutritional, 6, 19, 45, 47
**Vitamin D**
    calcium and, 51
    in emollients, 1484
    nutritional, 6, 22, 45
**Vitamin D$_2$, 22**
**Vitamin D$_3$, 22**
**Vitamin E**
    in emollients, 1484
    nutritional, 6, 26
Vitamin E 400 I.U., 26
Vitamin E 1000 I.U., 26
**Vitamin E acetate, 1432**
**Vitamin K**
    as antihemorrhagic, 114
    nutritional, 6
Vite E, 1484
Vitec, 1484
Vitelle Lurline PMS Tablets, 612
Vitravene, 1360
Vitron-C Tablets, 73
Vitron-C-Plus Tablets, 73
Vitussin Syrup, 575
Vivactil, 749
Vivarin, 583
Vivelle, 144
Vivelle-Dot, 144
Volmax, 455
Voltaren, 640, 1338
Voltaren-XR, 640
**Voriconazole, 1111**

VōSol HC Otic, 1382
VōSol Otic, 1382
Vytone Cream, 245
**VZIG. see Varicellazoster immune globulin (human)**

**W**arfarin sodium, 104
Wart-Off Maximum Strength, 1480
Welchol, 434
Wellbutrin, 711
Wellbutrin SR, 711
Wellcovorin, 79
Westcort, 240
Wet-N-Soak, 1372
Wet-N-Soak Plus, 1369, 1372
Wetting & Soaking, 1369
Wetting/soaking solutions, for hard contact lenses, 1369
Wetting solutions, for hard contact lenses, 1369
**Wheat bran, 961**
White Cloverine Salve, 1487
**White petrolatum. see Petrolatum**
Whitfield's, 1119
Wigraine, 670
WinRho SDF, 1237
Winstrol, 130
**Wisteria oil, 1522**
**Witch hazel, 1519**
    in acne products, 1430
    in anorectal preparations, 1412
Women's Tylenol Multi-Symptom Menstrual Relief Caplets, 612
Wondra, 1486
Wygesic Tablets, 631
Wytensin, 398

**X**-Prep Bowel Evacuant Kit-1, 987
X-Prep Bowel Evacuant Kit-2, 987
X-Prep Senna Liquid Bowel Evacuant, 987
X-Seb T Pearl, 1466
X-Seb T Plus, 1466
Xalatan, 1306
Xanax, 698
Xanthine combinations, 520

Xanthine derivatives, 461
Xanthine-sympathomimetic
  combinations, 521
Xeloda, 1539
Xenical, 1006
Xerac, 1421
Xerac AC, 1435
Xiral Tablets, 544
Xopenex, 455
Xylocaine, 1468, 1472
Xylocaine 10
Oral, 1468
Xylocaine-MPF, 1468
Xylocaine Viscous, 1468
**Xylometazoline HCl, 501**

**Y**ellow wax, 1520
Yocon, 1736
**Yohimbine, 1736**
Yohimex, 1736

**Z**-Cof DM Syrup, 567
Zaditor, 1346
**Zafirlukast, 467**
Zagam, 1049
**Zalcitabine, 1176**
**Zaleplon, 805**
Zanaflex, 868
**Zanamivir, 1165**
Zanosar, 1586
Zantac, 935
Zantac 75, 935
Zantac 150, 935
Zantac 150 EFFERdose,
  935
Zantac 300, 935
Zarontin, 846
Zaroxolyn, 315
Zeasorb-AF, 1113
Zebeta, 376
Zefazone, 1019
Zelnorm, 1009
Zemplar, 22
Zephiran, 1495
Zerit, 1176
Zestoretic Tablets, 428
Zestril, 385

Zetar (emulsion), 1462
Zetar (shampoo), 1462
Zetia, 438
Zevalin, 1617
Ziac Tablets, 427
Ziagen, 1176
**Zidovudine, 1176**
**Zidovudine/lamivudine,
  1176**
**Zidovudine/lamivudine/
  abacavir sulfate, 1176**
Zilactin, 1398
Zilactin-L, 1472
**Zileuton, 467**
Zinacef, 1021
**Zinc**
  in lozenges, 1399
  nutritional, 5, 43
Zinc 15, 43
Zinc-220, 43
**Zinc acetate**
  in poison ivy treatment
    products, 1502
  in topical antihista-
    mines, 1491
**Zinc bacitracin**
  in ophthalmic anti-
    infectives, 1353
  topical, 1081
**Zinc chloride**
  in antifungal combina-
    tions, 1118
  in mouth and throat
    products, 1404
**Zinc gluconate, 43**
**Zinc oxide, 1519**
  in acne products, 1430
  in anorectal prepara-
    tions, 1411
  in antifungal combina-
    tions, 1119
  in diaper rash products,
    1497
  in emollients, 1484
  in poison ivy treatment
    products, 1502
  in sunscreens, 1507

**Zinc oxide, 1519** *(cont.)*
  in topical antihista-
    mines, 1491
**Zinc stearate, 1119**
**Zinc sulfate**
  nutritional, 43
  in ophthalmic decon-
    gestant combina-
    tions, 1326
Zincate, 43
Zincfrin, 1326
Zincon, 1462
Zinecard, 1631
**Ziprasidone HCl, 758**
Ziradryl, 1491
**Zirconium oxide, 1491**
Zithromax, 1034
Zocor, 446
Zofran, 684
Zofran ODT, 684
Zoladex, 1577
**Zoledronic acid, 297**
**Zolmitriptan, 673**
Zoloft, 741
**Zolpidem tartrate, 805**
Zometa, 297
Zomig, 673
Zomig-ZMT, 673
Zonalon, 1491
Zone-A Forte Lotion, 245
Zonegran, 839
**Zonisamide, 839**
Zonite Douche, 1407
ZORprin, 605
Zostrix, 1489
Zostrix-HP, 1489
Zōtō-HC Ear Drops, 1382
Zovia 1/35E, 170
Zovia 1/50E, 170
Zovirax, 1151
ZTuss Expectorant Liquid,
  570
Zyban, 1720
Zydone Capsules, 628
Zyflo Filmtabs, 467
Zyloprim, 657, 1536
Zyprexa, 761
Zyrtec, 493
Zyrtec-D 12 Hour Tablets,
  533
Zyvox, 1046